MOSBY'S COMPREHENSIVE REVIEW OF NURSING

Editor

DOLORES F. SAXTON, R.N., B.S. in Ed., M.A., M.P.S., Ed.D.

Associate Editors

PATRICIA M. NUGENT, R.N., A.A.S., B.S., M.S., Ed.M.

PHYLLIS K. PELIKAN, R.N., A.A.S., B.S., M.A.

THIRTEENTH EDITION

Illustrated

THE C. V. MOSBY COMPANY

St. Louis • Baltimore • Philadelphia • Toronto   1990

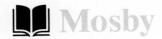

Editor: Nancy L. Coon
Sr. developmental editor: Susan R. Epstein
Project manager: Kathleen L. Teal
Designer: Susan E. Lane
Production editor: Teresa Breckwoldt

THIRTEENTH EDITION

Previous editions copyrighted 1949, 1951, 1955, 1958, 1961, 1965, 1969, 1973, 1977, 1981, 1984, 1987

Printed in the United States of America

Library of Congress Cataloging in Publication Data

Mosby's comprehensive review of nursing/editor, Dolores F. Saxton;
　　associate editors, Patricia M. Nugent, Phyllis K. Pelikan.—13th ed.
　　　p.　　cm.
　　Bibliography: p.
　　Includes index.
　　ISBN 0-8016-3573-X
　　1. Nursing—Examinations, questions, etc.　2. Nursing—Outlines,
syllabi, etc.　I. Saxton, Dolores F.　II. Nugent, Patricia Mary.
III. Pelikan, Phyllis K.　IV. Title: Comprehensive review
of nursing.
　　[DNLM:　1. Nursing—examination question.　2. Nursing—
outlines.
WY 18 M8944]
RT55.M64　1990
610.73'076—dc20
DNLM/DLC
for Library of Congress　　　　　　　　　　　　　　89-9469
　　　　　　　　　　　　　　　　　　　　　　　　　　CIP

C/VH/VH　9　8　7　6　5　4　3　2　1

Contributors

JOANN FESTA, R.N., A.A.S., B.S., M.S., Ph.D.
Associate Professor, Department of Nursing, Nassau Community College
Garden City, New York

MARY ANN HELLMER, R.N., A.A.S., B.S., M.S., Ph.D.
Associate Professor, Department of Nursing, Nassau Community College
Garden City, New York

CHRISTINA ALGIERE KASPRISIN, R.N., M.S.
Assistant Clinical Professor, College of Nursing, University of Oklahoma, Tulsa, Oklahoma
Quality Attainment Coordinator-Nursing, St. Francis Hospital, Tulsa, Oklahoma

MILDRED L. MONTAG, R.N., B.A., B.S., M.A., Ed.D., LL.D., L.H.D., D.Sc.
Professor Emeritus, Teachers College, Columbia University
New York, New York

THERESA A. MORAN, R.N., A.A.S., B.S., Ed.M.
Assistant Professor, Department of Nursing, Nassau Community College
Garden City, New York

SELMA NEEDLEMAN, R.N., B.A., M.A.
Professor Emeritus, Nassau Community College
Garden City, New York

PATRICIA A. NUTZ, R.N., B.S., B.S.N., M.Ed.
Instructor, School of Nursing, St. Francis Hospital
New Castle, Pennsylvania

TERRY F. O'DWYER, B.S., Ph.D.
Professor, Department of Engineering Science/Physics/Technology, Nassau Community College
Garden City, New York

JOSEPH E. PELLICCIA, B.A., M.A.
Professor, Department of Biology, Nassau Community College
Garden City, New York

MARY SIROTNIK, Reg. N., B.Sc.N.
Mack Centre of Nursing Education, Niagara College of Applied Arts and Technology
St. Catharines, Ontario, Canada

Preface

The material in *Mosby's Comprehensive Review of Nursing* has been revised and updated for this thirteenth edition. The progression of subject matter in each area reflects the consistent approach that has been used throughout the book. Selected information incorporates the latest knowledge, newest trends, and current practices in the profession of nursing.

The medical-surgical, maternity, pediatric, and psychiatric chapters incorporate material from the basic sciences, nutrition, pharmacology, and rehabilitation. Chapter 1 gives directions on how to study and use the review to prepare for the licensing examination.

The chapter, "Components of Nursing Practice," includes a conceptual introduction covering the health-illness continuum and health resources; nursing practice and the law in the United States and Canada; and the nurse's role. Highlighted in the section on the nurse's role are those topics the student of today needs to know to function as tomorrow's practitioner: communication; the nursing process; the teaching-learning environment, leadership, and the administration of medications. A list of nursing diagnoses as developed by the North American Nursing Diagnosis Association at the National Conference, held in 1988 has also been included.

We have continued to present the material in the traditional clinical groupings, for we still believe that, even in preparing for the comprehensive examination, the average student will study all the distinct parts before attempting to put them together. However, recognizing the universal acceptance of the nursing process we have, in this edition, highlighted this material to include nursing diagnoses based on assessment and the essential nursing care based on the nursing diagnoses. To avoid needless repitition, and recognizing the abilities of our readers, we have not divided the nursing process into its distinct steps since we believe that in practice the process is an evolving one rather than a clearly defined step by step procedure.

This edition contains, for every question following the individual chapters as well as for every question in the two comprehensive tests, the reasons why the incorrect answers are incorrect as well as why the correct answer is correct. In the two 375-question comprehensive tests we have also analyzed each question as to the step in the nursing process required, the level of cognitive ability required, the clinical area involved, the area of human needs involved, and the category of concern.

The comprehensive tests at the end of the text give the reader an opportunity to apply material from the specific clinical areas to any nursing situation. Since Canada and the United States use comprehensive examinations, these tests will help students from both countries prepare for this experience. The movement from specific learning to general application is educationally sound, and the reader should follow this approach in studying.

All the questions used in this book have been submitted by outstanding educators and practitioners of nursing. Initially the editorial panel reviewed all questions selecting the most pertinent for inclusion in a mass field-testing project. Students graduating from baccalaureate, associate degree, and diploma nursing programs in various locations in the United States and Canada provided a diverse testing group. The results were statistically analyzed. This analysis was used to select questions for inclusion in the book and to provide the reader with a general idea of each question's level of difficulty.

We would like to take this opportunity to express our sincere appreciation to our many colleagues for their contributions and support: to Edith Augustson for her careful processing of the manuscript; to our editors Nancy Coon and Susan Epstein for their help and support; and last, but not least, to our families for their love and encouragement.

Dolores F. Saxton
Patricia M. Nugent
Phyllis K. Pelikan

Contents

MOSBY'S
COMPREHENSIVE
REVIEW OF NURSING

CHAPTER 1

Introduction for Students Preparing for the Licensing Examination

Licensing examinations in the United States and Canada have been integrated and comprehensive for many years. Nursing candidates in both countries are required to answer questions that necessitate a recognition and understanding of the physiologic, biologic, and social sciences, as well as the specific nursing skills and abilities involved in a given client situation.

Both tests contain objective multiple-choice questions. To answer the questions appropriately, a candidate needs to understand and correlate certain aspects of anatomy and physiology, the behavioral sciences, basic nursing, the effects of medications administered, the client's attitude toward illness, and other pertinent factors (e.g., legal responsibilities). Most questions are based on nursing situations similar to those with which candidates have had experience, since both the United States and Canada emphasize the nursing care of clients with representative common national health problems. Some questions, however, require candidates to apply basic principles and techniques to clinical situations with which they have had little, if any, actual experience.

To prepare adequately for an integrated comprehensive examination, it is necessary to understand the discrete parts that compose the universe under consideration. This is one of the major principles of learning on which *Mosby's Comprehensive Review of Nursing* has been developed.

Using this principle, the text first presents a review of each major clinical area. Each review is followed by questions that test the student's knowledge of principles and theories underlying nursing care in a variety of situations (acute, critical, and long term), in a variety of settings (acute care hospitals, nursing homes, and the community), and with a variety of nursing goals (preventive, curative, palliative, and restorative).

Answers to the questions as well as rationales supporting the answers are provided on tear sheets (pp. 532-704) following the comprehensive tests. Explanations are also presented to document why the other answers are inappropriate. By reviewing the rationales the student is able to verify information and reinforce knowledge.

The text concludes with two integrated comprehensive tests reflecting the licensing examinations. In other words, the questions require the student to cross clinical disciplines and respond to individual and specific needs associated with given health problems. Rationales are also provided for answers to these questions.

Similar to those in the comprehensive licensing examinations, questions in the comprehensive tests have been classified by phases of the nursing process and area of client needs. To provide a more inclusive study guide for the student, we have three additional categories of classifica-

tion: (1) cognitive level, (2) clinical area, and (3) category of concern, which are not included in NCLEX.

The following descriptions and the five sample questions on p. 2 are presented to assist you in understanding these classifications.

Phases of the nursing process (types of behaviors of the nurse)

1. Assessment (AS). The assessment phase requires the nurse to obtain objective and subjective data from primary and secondary sources, to identify and group significant data, and to communicate this information to other members of the health team. The information necessary for making nursing decisions is obtained through assessment. Sample question 1 is an *assessment* question.
2. Analysis (AN). This phase requires the nurse to interpret data gathered during the assessment phase. A nursing diagnosis must be made, client and family needs identified, and both short-term and long-term goals set to meet the identified needs. Sample question 2 is an *analysis* question.
3. Planning (PL). The planning phase requires the nurse to design a regimen with the client and family to achieve goals set during the analysis phase. It also requires setting priorities for nursing intervention. Sample question 3 is a *planning* question.
4. Implementation (IM). The implementation phase requires the nurse to provide care designed during the planning phase. The client may be given total care or may be assisted and encouraged to perform activities of daily living or follow the regimen prescribed by the physician. Implementation also includes activities such as counseling, teaching, and supervising. Sample question 4 is an *implementation* question.
5. Evaluation (EV). This phase requires the nurse to determine the effectiveness of nursing care. The goals of care are reviewed, the client's response to intervention identified, and a consideration made as to whether the client has achieved the predetermined goals. Evaluation also includes appraisal of the client's compliance with the health plan. Sample question 5 is an *evaluation* question.

Client needs (reflect those health care needs of the client that must be addressed by the nurse)

1. Support and promotion of physiological and anatomical equilibrium (PA). Meeting this need includes reducing risks that interfere with physiological or anatomical integrity, promoting comfort and mobility, and providing basic care to assist, modify, or limit physiological and anatomical adaptations. Sample questions 1 and 5 reflect this need.
2. An environment that is safe and conducive to effective

therapeutic care (TC). The nurse must provide quality, goal-directed care that is coordinated, safe, and effective. Sample question 4 reflects this need.

3. Education and other forms of health promotion to prevent, minimize, or correct actual or potential health problems (ED). Fulfilling this need involves supporting optimal growth and development to provide for the achievement of the highest levels of functioning. This includes encouraging use of support systems and self-care directed toward promoting the prevention, recognition, and treatment of disease throughout the life cycle. Sample question 3 reflects this need.

4. Support and promotion of psychosocial and emotional equilibrium (PE). Addressing this need includes supporting individual emotional coping and adapting mechanisms to promote optimal emotional health while limiting or modifying those responses to crises that produce psychopathological consequences. Sample question 2 reflects this need.

Cognitive levels (types of intellectual processes)

1. Knowledge (KN). The knowledge level of the intellectual process requires recollection of facts about principles, theories, terms, or procedures. Knowledge questions, which require the examinee to define, identify, or select, involve the ability to recall information (a basic cognitive skill). Sample question 2 is a *knowledge* question.

2. Comprehension (CP). The comprehension level of the intellectual process requires demonstration of understanding or interpretation of the subject matter presented. It is much more than just the recall of information. The examinee is required to interpret, explain, distinguish, or predict. Sample question 1 is a *comprehension* question.

3. Application (AP). The application level of the intellectual process requires the examinee not only to know and understand information, but also apply it to a new situation. When applying comprehended information, the examinee must show, solve, modify, change, manipulate, use, demonstrate, or teach in a specific client situation. Sample question 4 is an *application* question.

4. Analysis (AN). The analysis level of the intellectual process requires the recognition of inherent structure and the relationship between component parts as well as an understanding of the underlying concepts or principles. If the examinee is required to analyze, evaluate, select, differentiate, or interpret data from a variety of sources prior to responding, the question is an analysis question. Sample question 5 is an *analysis* question.

Clinical area

1. Medicine (ME). These questions include the care of adult clients who have health problems that do not require surgical intervention or invasive techniques. Sample question 1 is a *medical* nursing question.

2. Surgery (SU). These questions include care of adult and child clients with health problems that require surgical intervention or invasive techniques. Sample question 5 is a *surgical* nursing question.

3. Obstetrics (OB). These questions include the care of

clients preparing for or experiencing childbirth. Sample question 2 is a *maternity* nursing question.

4. Pediatrics (PE). These questions include the care of clients from birth to young adulthood. Sample question 4 is a *pediatric* nursing question.

5. Psychiatry (PS). These questions include the care of clients experiencing emotional stress with or without overt psychiatric behavior in all settings. Sample question 3 is a *psychiatric* nursing question.

Category of concern (specific content within broad clinical areas)

1. Medical, surgical, and pediatric nursing. Includes cardiovascular and blood (CB); endocrine and integumentary (EI); gastrointestinal (GI); musculoskeletal and neurologic (MN); respiratory (RE); and reproductive and genitourinary (RG). Sample questions 1 and 5 reflect information related to *cardiovascular and blood* content. Sample question 4 reflects information related to *musculoskeletal and neurologic* content.

2. Obstetric nursing. Includes fertility, sterility, and family planning (FS); high-risk pregnancy (HP); prenatal period (PN); intrapartal period (IP); post-partal period (PP); and normal and high-risk neonate (NH). Sample question 2 reflects information related to *prenatal* content.

3. Psychiatric nursing. Includes mood disorders (MD); crisis situations (CS); developmental disorders throughout the life cycle (DD); personality, anxiety, somatoform, and dissociative disorders (PD); substance abuse and related disorders (SA); and schizophrenic disorders (SD). Sample question 3 reflects information related to *mood disorders*.

SAMPLE QUESTIONS:

1. Mr. Evere was admitted to the intensive care unit with a diagnosis of Adams-Stokes syndrome. Symptoms most likely include:
   ① Syncope and low ventricular rate
   ② Flushing and slurred speech
   ③ Cephalagia and blurred vision
   ④ Nausea and vertigo

2. Miss Daley has decided to go through with her pregnancy and keep her baby. Now the crisis intervention worker's primary responsibility is to:
   ① Support her for making a wise decision
   ② Make an appointment for her to see a physician for prenatal care
   ③ Explore other problems she may be experiencing
   ④ Provide information about other health resources where she may receive additional assistance

3. When monoamine oxidase (MAO) inhibitors are prescribed, the client should be cautioned against:
   ① The use of medications with an elixir base
   ② Prolonged exposure to the sun
   ③ Ingesting wines and cheeses
   ④ Engaging in active physical exercise

4. Jamey, age 4, has been hospitalized for fever of undetermined origin (FUO). He screams and becomes uncontrollable as his mother leaves after visiting hours. The best approach is to:
   ① Ignore this outburst
   ② Sit quietly at his bedside
   ③ Hold and pat him even though he struggles
   ④ Give him a favorite toy to hold

5. Following surgery, while receiving a blood transfusion, Mr. Manning develops chills and headache. The nurse's best action is to:
   ① Stop the transfusion immediately
   ② Lightly cover the client
   ③ Notify the physician STAT
   ④ Slow the blood flow to keep vein open

How to Use This Book in Studying

A. Start in one area. Study the material covered by the section. Refer to other textbooks to find additional details if you are unsure of a specific fact.

B. Answer the questions following the area. As you answer each question, write a few words about why you think that answer was correct; in other words, simply justify why you selected the answer. If you guess at an answer in this book you should make a special mark to identify it. This will permit you to recognize areas that need further review. It will also help you to see how correct your "guessing" can be. Remember on the licensing examination you should guess at answers rather than leave blank spaces since only correct answers are counted and you are not penalized for incorrect answers.

C. Record the answer by filling in the numbered circle next to the one you believe is correct.

D. Tear out the sheets with the answers for the area you are taking (pp. 532 to 704) and compare your answers with those provided. If you answered the item correctly, check your reason for selecting the answer with the rationale presented. If you answered the item incorrectly, read the rationale to determine why the one you selected was incorrect. In addition, you should review the correct answer and rationale for each item answered incorrectly. If you still do not understand your mistake, look up the theory pertaining to these questions. You should carefully review all questions and rationales for items you identified as guesses, since you did not have mastery of the material being questioned.

E. Following the correct answer you will find a letter—a, b, or c—in parentheses. These letters indicate the difficulty of the question and can serve as a guide in your studying. The letter *a* signifies that more than 75% of the graduating students in the testing group answered this question correctly; *b* signifies that between 50% and 75% answered it correctly; and *c* that 25% to 50% answered it correctly.

F. For the comprehensive examinations, in addition to the difficulty level of the question (a, b, or c), you will find a grouping of letters that classify the question according to the following six categories:
   1. Nursing process
      a. AS (assessment)
      b. AN (analysis)
      c. PL (planning)
      d. IM (implementation)
      e. EV (evaluation)
   2. Cognitive level
      a. KN (knowledge)
      b. CP (comprehension)
      c. AP (application)
      d. AN (analysis)
   3. Clinical area
      a. ME (medicine)
      b. SU (surgery)
      c. OB (obstetrics)
      d. PE (pediatrics)
      e. PS (psychiatry)
   4. Area of client needs
      a. PA (physiological and anatomical equilibrium)
      b. TC (therapeutic care)
      c. ED (education and health promotion)
      d. PE (psychosocial and emotional equilibrium)
   5. Category of concern
      a. CB (cardiovascular and blood)
      b. EI (endocrine and integumentary)
      c. GI (gastrointestinal)
      d. MN (musculoskeletal and neurologic)
      e. RE (respiratory)
      f. RG (reproductive and genitourinary)
      g. FS (fertility, sterility, and family planning)
      h. HP (high-risk pregnancy)
      i. PN (prenatal period)
      j. IP (intrapartal period)
      k. PP (postpartal period)
      l. NH (normal and high-risk neonate)
      m. MD (mood disorders)
      n. CS (crisis situations)
      o. DD (developmental disorders)
      p. PD (personality, anxiety, somatoform, and dissociative disorders)
      q. SA (substance abuse and related disorders)
      r. SD (schizophrenic disorders)

   This series of letters will always appear in the same order for each question on the comprehensive examinations.

G. A few days later, review the area again and retake the questions following it. If you miss the same questions again, you need further study of the material.

H. After you have completed the area questions, begin taking the comprehensive tests, since they will assist you in applying knowledge and principles from the specific clinical area to any nursing situation. Take each of these examinations under conditions as closely approximating those of the licensure examination as possible.
   1. Arrange a quiet, uninterrupted, 1½-hour time span for each of the comprehensive tests.
   2. Pace yourself during the testing period; allow about 1 minute per question.
   3. Do not rush.
   4. Make educated guesses.
   5. Read carefully and answer the question asked; pay attention to specific details in the question.
   6. Try putting questions and answers in your own words to test your comprehension.

I. To help analyze your mistakes on the comprehensive examinations and to provide a data base for making future study plans, two types of worksheets are included. One is designed to aid you in identifying and recording errors in the way you process information. The other is to help you identify and record gaps in knowledge. These worksheets follow the Answers and Rationales for each Comprehensive Test and are on tear-out sheets also.

J. After completing your worksheets, do the following:
   1. Use Worksheet 1 to identify the frequency with which you made particular errors. As you review material in class notes or this review book, pay special attention to correcting your most common problems.
   2. Use Worksheet 2 to identify the topics you want to review. It might be helpful to set priorities; review the most difficult topics first so that you will have time to review them more than once.

General Clues for Answering Multiple-choice Questions

On a multiple-choice test the question and possible answers are called a *test item*. The part of the item that asks the question or poses a problem is called the *stem*. All of the answers presented are called *options*. One of the options is the correct answer; the remainder are incorrect. The incorrect options are called *distractors* because their major purpose is to distract the test taker from the correct answer.

A. Read the question carefully before looking at the answers.
   1. Attempt to determine what the question is really asking; look for key words.
   2. Read each answer thoroughly and see if it completely covers the material asked by the question.
   3. Narrow the choices by immediately eliminating answers you know are incorrect.
B. Because few things in life are absolute without exceptions, avoid selecting answers that include words such as *always, never, all, every,* and *none,* since answers containing these key words are rarely correct.
C. Attempt to select the answer that is most complete and includes the other answers within it. An example might be as follows:
   1. A child's intelligence is influenced by:
      ① Heredity and environment
      ② Environment and experience
      ③ A variety of factors
      ④ Education and economic factors
   The most correct answer is 3 because it includes all the other answers.
D. Make certain that the answer you select is reasonable and obtainable under ordinary circumstances and that the action can be carried out in the given situation.
E. *Watch for grammatical inconsistencies.* If one or more of the options is not grammatically consistent with the stem, the alert test taker can identify it as a probable distractor. When the stem is in the form of an incomplete sentence, each option should complete the sentence in a grammatically correct way.
F. Avoid selecting answers that state hospital rules or regulations as a reason or rationale for action.
G. Look for answers that focus on the client or are directed toward feelings.
H. If the question asks for an immediate action or response, all the answers may be correct, so base your selection on identified priorities for action.
I. Do not select answers that contain exceptions to the general rule, controversial material, or degrading responses.
J. Reread the question if the answers do not seem to make sense, since you may have missed the words *not* or *except* in the statement.
K. Do not worry if you select the same numbered answer repeatedly, since there is usually no pattern to the answers.
L. Mark the numbered circle next to the answer you have chosen. This method of marking your answer has been used to help familiarize you with the method used on the NCLEX examination.
M. Answer every question; you are not penalized for incorrect answers.

Preparing for the Licensure Examination

A few individuals can improve their scores significantly by a highly concentrated period of study immediately before taking an examination. Most, however, profit by spreading their review over a much longer period of time, and the best time to begin studying for state boards is the first class attended.

After you have completed studying the text, you may wish to take *Mosby's AssessTest* before you take the licensing examination. The *AssessTest* is a computer-scored, multiple-choice examination designed to test nursing knowledge and evaluate your ability to apply that knowledge in clinical situations. The extensive computer analysis of your performance, which is the most outstanding feature of this test, will help you design effective and efficient plans for further study and review. Identification of your own *specific* strengths and weaknesses should eliminate much of the anxiety of deciding what material to study by giving you a sense of direction and a means of setting priorities.

Taking the Licensure Examination

The most crucial requisite for doing well on the licensure examination is a sound understanding of the subject and a high level of reading comprehension. Determination to do well and a degree of confidence will further enhance the well-prepared individual's chances of earning high scores.

At least three other requirements must be met if an individual's performance is to accurately reflect professional competence. First, the candidate must follow explicitly the directions given by the examiner and those printed at the beginning of each test, as well as any that refer to a specified group of questions. Second, the candidate must read each question carefully before deciding how to answer it. Third, the candidate must record the answers in the space and manner specified. Some candidates find it helpful to glance over a test before starting to answer questions. This enables them to answer questions in the order most efficient and comfortable for them. Others find it more efficient to go through the test answering all questions they are sure of first, then go back to the more difficult ones.

The score on each test is the number of questions answered correctly; there is no deduction for incorrect answers. You are not penalized for guessing. Do not leave an answer blank. You have a 1 in 4 (25%) chance of guessing the correct answer. Do not mark more than one answer for each question, since questions with more than one mark will be scored as incorrect.

The licensing examination is given over a 2-day period. The score is reported as pass or fail.

CHAPTER 2

Components of Nursing Practice

Conceptual Introduction
THE HEALTH-ILLNESS CONTINUUM
Introduction

A. Health is a generally accepted right; well-being is the norm toward which most governments and all health personnel direct their efforts
B. One of the primary functions of the nursing and medical professions is to help individuals, families, and groups reach the highest level of wellness of which they are capable

Definition

A. The World Health Organization states, "Health is a state of complete physical, mental, and social wellbeing and not just the absence of disease or infirmity"
B. This definition implies that there is
   1. Interaction between self and environment
   2. Preservation of structure and function
   3. Maintenance of adaptive potential
C. Significance of definition
   1. Accepted right of all rather than a privilege
   2. Reciprocal relationships between individual health and community health
   3. Increasing public expectation of government support for health services and the extent of care provided
   4. Need for nursing and medical practice to move toward maintenance and promotion of health and rehabilitation of the ill rather than merely to focus on provision of episodic care

Basic Concepts

A. Health: a continually changing phenomenon
   1. Moves on a continuum between optimal wellness (where potential is maximized and used with purpose) and death
   2. Change may be gradual or abrupt
   3. Level attainable depends on adaptive capacity, genetic and environmental factors, and life-style
      a. Fluctuates throughout life cycle
      b. Varies among individuals
   4. Individual may or may not be aware of change
   5. Person's position on the continuum determined by
      a. Ability to adapt
      b. Level of adaptation
      c. Culture's view of health
      d. Ability to carry out social, family, and job responsibilities
B. Stresses affect physical, emotional, and social health
   1. May be internal or external
   2. Can be beneficial or detrimental to life
      a. Tension is essential to life
      b. Stress of life causes wear and tear
         (1) Produces a nonspecific response that Hans Selye identifies as the general adaptation syndrome (GAS)
         (2) Three stages—alarm, resistance, and exhaustion
   3. Elicit some response from or change in the individual
   4. Vary widely for different individuals and within the same individual at different times
   5. Tolerance is individual
   6. Sources of stress
      a. Physical: thermal, acoustical
      b. Chemical: gas, hormonal, nutrient
      c. Microbiologic: viral, bacterial
      d. Physiologic: neoplasmic, hypofunctional, hyperfunctional
      e. Developmental: genetic, aging
      f. Psychologic: values, self-image
C. Rehabilitation assists people in attaining their maximum level of wellness on the continuum
   1. Particularly concerned with establishing function that is lost while expanding, maintaining, and supporting the limited remaining function
   2. Immediate or potential needs exhibited in all health problems
   3. The client is the primary rehabilitator; professional health team members assist the client and family with the process of self-rehabilitation
   4. Not an isolated process; rehabilitation involves the client, family, health team, community, and society
   5. Concerned with all levels of prevention: primary, secondary, and tertiary
   6. Health problems that cause disabilities are socially significant because of the number of people affected, economic cost and loss, distress of personal suffering, and conditions in society that increase their incidence
D. Ability to maintain and/or return to a level of health is influenced by the availability of health resources

SPONSORSHIP OF AGENCIES
Government

A. Definition: associations functioning at the international, national, state, and local levels, providing a variety of services to meet the health, education, and welfare needs of the people; these programs are funded by the government, and services are rendered by professionals
B. Examples
   1. International: World Health Organization
   2. National
      a. United States: Department of Health and Human Services, Public Health Service
      b. Canada: Department of National Health and Welfare
   3. State or provincial

a. United States: state health departments
b. Canada: provincial departments of health
4. Local: county or city department of health, fire department, police department, department of aging

Voluntary

A. Definition: organizations consisting of lay and professional persons dedicated to the prevention and solution of health problems by providing educational, research, and service programs; these agencies are dependent on voluntary donations for funds, are often concerned with specific health problems, and are national organizations that function through state or provincial and local chapters
B. Examples
1. International: Rockefeller Foundation, international branches of professional organizations
2. National: American Heart Association, American Cancer Society, National Multiple Sclerosis Society
3. State or provincial: chapters of national organizations
4. Local: branches of national voluntary organizations, community hospitals, volunteers (e.g., a league of women supporting a community hospital, a Girl Scout troop visiting a nursing home, a church group visiting an orphanage)

Proprietary

A. Definition: organizations that deliver health care in a variety of settings to meet a broad spectrum of client needs with profit for their owners as another major objective
B. Examples
1. Hospitals: Humana Corporation
2. Home care services: Upjohn Health Care Services, Olsten Health Care Services
3. Private nursing homes

TYPES OF SERVICES
Acute Care

General hospitals that provide short-term care for clients undergoing treatment for a health problem.
A. Intensive care: services and equipment to meet the needs of the acutely ill client undergoing intensive treatment for a health problem (e.g., intensive care unit, coronary care unit, burn unit, psychiatric unit)
B. Intermediate care: services for the moderately ill client overcoming a health crisis but still has special needs that cannot be adequately met in a general unit (e.g., intermediate care unit, progressive coronary care unit, isolation units)
C. Ambulatory care: admission and discharge on day of surgery; diagnostic workup is completed on an outpatient basis prior to surgery
D. Services for the client and family who need little assistance with health care but who have a need for teaching, motivation, and control over their own care; usually done on an outpatient basis because changes in reimbursement have made this in-hospital care an out-of-pocket expense

Long-term Care

Institutions that provide services over an extended period; most deal with chronic or long-term health problems.

A. Nursing homes: provide all degrees of care from skilled care to maintenance care; the Nursing Home Reform Law of 1987 has put the Skilled Nursing Facility and the Health Related Facility in the category of Nursing Home
B. Day care center: provides all degrees of care from skilled nursing care to personal care and from rehabilitation to social programs
C. Adult housing: residence where an individual goes to live; meals and recreational programs may often be supplied; however, medical and nursing supervision are generally not provided on a full-time basis
D. Rehabilitation center: institution that provides multiple services and facilities which assist a client and family to make an adjustment to living; the client can obtain an optimal level of health by developing personal abilities to their fullest potential and using the following resources
1. Medical and nursing: total health assessment and planning, physical therapy, occupational therapy, and speech therapy
2. Psychosocial: personal counseling, social service, and psychiatric service
3. Vocational: work evaluation, vocational counseling, vocational training, trial employment in sheltered workshops, terminal employment in sheltered workshops, and placement
E. Home care: comprehensive services for people who do not need to be hospitalized and yet require more care than an outpatient facility can provide (e.g., public health nurses, homemaker services, medical home care programs)

Local Support Services

Provide services for people with health needs who are living at home
A. Special services by organizations to meet specific client needs (e.g., Meals on Wheels, FISH, soup kitchens)
B. Crisis intervention groups
1. Services
a. Provide assistance for people in crises: clients' previous methods of adaptation are inadequate to meet present needs
b. The focus of some groups is specific (e.g., poison control, drug addiction centers, suicide prevention) or general (e.g., walk-in mental health clinics, hospital emergency rooms)
c. Depending on the community's needs and facilities, these services can be offered by the government (e.g., state hospitals, state health departments) or voluntary organizations (e.g., community hospitals, community drug councils)
d. Some crises intervention groups provide service over the phone (e.g., poison control, AIDS hotline, suicide prevention centers), others help those who are physically present (e.g., hospital emergency rooms, walk-in mental health clinics)
2. Success factors
a. The client or family seeking help
b. Immediate opportunity for exploring feelings
c. Assistance in investigating alternative approaches in solving the problem
d. Information about other health resources where the client may receive additional assistance

C. Self-help groups
1. Services
a. Organized by clients or their families to provide services that are not adequately supplied by previous organizations
b. Meet the needs of clients and families with chronic problems requiring intervention over an extended period of time
c. Focus of some is specific (e.g., Gamblers Anonymous); others deal with a range of problems (e.g., Association for Children with Learning Disabilities)
d. Some are nonprofit (e.g., Alcoholics Anonymous); others are profit making (e.g., Weight Watchers International)
e. Provide services to people who often are not accepted by society (e.g., a drug addict, an alcoholic, a child abuser, one who is mentally ill, obese, or brain injured)
2. Success factors
a. All members accepted as equals
b. All members have experienced similar problems
c. Dealing with behavior and changes in behavior rather than with underlying causes of the behavior
d. Ready supply of human resources available
(1) Personal resources
(2) Assistance from peers
(3) Finally, extension of self to others
e. Each member has identified the problem and wants help in meeting needs—self-motivation
f. Ritual and language specific to the group and specific to the problems
g. Leadership remains with the membership
h. Group interaction
(1) Identification with peers—sense of belonging
(2) Group expectations—discipline required of members
(3) Small steps encouraged and, when attained, reinforced by the group
i. As a member achieves success within the group, he or she often receives reinforcement from outside the group
D. Hospice: provides emotional, physical, and supportive care to the terminally ill client and significant others; may be provided on an inpatient or outpatient basis
E. Respite: care for the ill client in a health care facility or in the home to provide a temporary rest for the constant care giver

PAYMENT FOR SERVICES

A. Medicare: a federal program through the Social Security Administration that provides funding for medical and hospital services for individuals over 65 years old or disabled people
B. Medicaid: a jointly funded federal and state program to provide health insurance for those with a low income
C. Private health insurance: health insurance paid for by the employer or by the individual
D. Private funds: health care paid for by the individual without third party payment
E. Impact of federal funding
1. Government money means government regulation and control; health care system failed to recognize this fact; impact on delivery of care is still evolving
2. Reimbursement based on diagnostic related groups (DRG) instead of characteristics of the institution; this prospective-based funding resulted in an institution receiving a set amount of money for a specified period of days for a particular diagnosis; this provided an incentive for institutions to discharge clients as soon as possible
3. Private insurance companies accepted the federal guidelines for DRGs; this led to the expansion of ambulatory care and home care services

Nursing Practice and the Law— United States and Canada
TYPOLOGY OF LAWS

A. Legal systems of modern nations influenced by both Roman civil law and English common law
B. Law arises from
1. Statutory law (legislation)
a. Body of law enacted by federal, provincial, state, or local government
b. That which commands or prohibits
c. Licensing laws belong in this category
2. Common law (custom and precedent)
a. Unwritten; based on customs
b. Precedent plays large part in judge's decisions, thus giving uniformity to decisions in like situations
c. Nurses practice under common as well as statutory law
C. The British North America Act (1867) renamed the Constitution Act (1982); incorporates existing provisions of the BNA Act with a Canadian Charter of Rights and Freedoms; establishes the political and legal foundations as well as fundamental rules for Canadians to govern Canada; also gives provincial governments power in health care activities
D. The Constitution of the United States gives states the power to police the health and welfare of its citizens
E. Military law
1. Applies to nurses only in the military nurse corps
2. Applies to all citizens when martial law declared
F. Private law
1. Property law: wills, patents, copyrights, trademarks
2. Contract law: agency, conditional sales, mortgages, bail
3. Tort law: intentional aggression, negligence, strict liability, defamation, invasion of privacy
G. Public law
1. Constitutional law: government structures, federal division of powers, fundamental rights
2. Administrative law: consumer protection, social welfare
3. Criminal law: serious offenses against the individual and society
a. Felonies: more serious offenses against the individual and society
b. Misdemeanors: less serious offenses
H. Civil law: acts against individuals not covered by criminal statute; may result in a civil suit, since the act has violated civil law

TORTS AND CRIMES ESPECIALLY IMPORTANT TO NURSES

A. Torts
1. Violations of civil law
2. Failure to use care or failure to prevent injury
3. Malpractice and negligence fall into this category and are unintentional torts
   a. No precise statute describes malpractice
   b. Terms often used interchangeably, but some legal experts make a distinction between them
      (1) Malpractice: professional misconduct; negligence performed in professional practice; any unreasonable lack of skill in professional duties or illegal or immoral conduct that results in injury or death to the client/consumer
      (2) Negligence: practice without a license; measurement of negligence is "reasonableness"; involves exposure of person or property of another to unreasonable risk of injury by acts of commission or omission
4. Usual standard of conduct is that which a prudent nurse would or would not do
5. Tort different from crime, but serious tort can be tried as both civil and criminal action
6. Necessary to prove negligence—if proved, this means that the act was performed incorrectly or not at all and the nurse is responsible for injury
7. Elements essential to prove negligence: four elements of a cause of action must be present for negligence; if any element is missing, one cannot proceed or succeed with a charge of negligence; negligence is not dependent on a contract
   a. Legally recognized duty of care to protect others against unreasonable risk
   b. Failure to perform according to the established standard of conduct and care which becomes breach of duty
   c. Damage to the client which can be physical and/or mental
   d. Connection between defendant's conduct and the resulting injury referred to as "proximate cause" or "remoteness of damage"
8. Nurse responsible for own acts; if employed, employer may also be held responsible under the doctrine of *respondeat superior;* when responsibility is shared, nursing actions must lie within the scope of employment and legislation relating to nursing practice (such as Nurse Practice Acts and Standards of Nursing Practice)
9. Reasonableness and prudence in actions are usually determining factors in a judgment; increasing attention is being paid to the law governing the practice of nursing
10. Examples of malpractice/negligence include leaving sponges inside a client; causing burns from hot water bottles, heating pads, hot solutions, and electric, steam, or vapor sources; medication errors; failure to prevent falls by neglecting to raise bed or crib rails; incompetent assessment of client situations, such as ignoring complaints of chest pain leading to subsequent inappropriate actions; improper identification of clients for operative or diagnostic procedures; and carelessness in caring for a client's property, such as dentures, clothing, valuables
11. Intentional torts occur when a person does damage to another person in a willful, intentional way and without just cause and/or excuse; includes fraud and deceit, assault and battery, false imprisonment, exposure of person or body after death, eavesdropping, libel and slander (defamatory torts)
    a. Assault: mental or physical threat
       (1) Knowingly threatening or attempting to do violence to another
       (2) Forcing a medication or treatment on a person who does not want it constitutes assault so long as touching does not occur
    b. Battery: touching with or without the intent to do harm
       (1) Actually touching or wounding a person in an offensive manner
       (2) Hitting or striking a client
    c. Fraud
       (1) False presentation of facts purposefully to create deception
       (2) Presenting false credentials for purposes of entering a nursing program or gaining registration, licensure, or employment
    d. Invasion of privacy
       (1) Encroachment or trespass on another's body and/or personality includes
          (a) False imprisonment: the intentional confinement without authorization by a person who physically constricts another using force, the threat of force, or confining structures and/or clothing; even without force or malicious intent, to detain another without consent in a specified area constitutes grounds for a charge of false imprisonment; the charge is not false imprisonment if it is necessary to protect an emotionally disturbed person from harming self or others or if it is necessary to confine to defend oneself, others, or property, or to effect a lawful arrest
          (b) Exposure of a person: any unnecessary exposure or discussion of the client's case is actionable unless authorized by the client; after death, the client's right to be unobserved, excluded from unwarranted operations, and protected from unauthorized touching of the body persists
          (c) Defamation: concerns privileged communications and privacy; law grants the right of privacy to everyone; divulgence of privileged communication whether from charts, conversation, interview, or observation in a way that exposes the person to hatred, contempt, aversion, or a lowering of opinion; includes slander (oral) and libel (written, pictured, telecast), both of which are dependent on communication to a third party

B. Crimes
1. Criminal act: an act contrary to a criminal statute; in Canada, one contrary to the Criminal Code of Canada; violates societal law; includes felonies and misdemeanors
2. Criminal Code of Canada is determined by the Parliament of Canada, is applicable to all provinces and territories, and may be amended by Parliament to reflect society's changing values
3. Canadian Criminal Code and Death with Dignity
   a. Guidelines are needed to outline acceptable practices for nurses and physicians to follow in situations where intensive and resuscitative measures should not be applied
   b. CNA together with the CMA, CHA, and Canadian Bar Association (Law Reform Commission of Canada) are studying the issue of *do not resuscitate* orders
   c. Law Reform Commission (Report 28) recommends that cessation and refusal of treatment be given legal recognition in Canadian criminal law
   d. Law Reform Commission (Report 15) recommends that the Parliament of Canada adopt the following amendment to Section 28A of the Interpretation Act concerning Criteria of Death:
      (1) Death occurs with irreversible cessation of all brain function
      (2) Irreversible cessation of brain function can be determined by the prolonged absence of spontaneous circulatory and respiratory function
      (3) When detection of prolonged absence of spontaneous circulatory and respiratory function is made impossible by the use of artificial means of support, the irreversible cessation of brain function can be determined by any means recognized by the ordinary standards of current medical practice (Harvard criteria)
4. Crimes are wrongs punishable by the state, committed against the state, usually demonstrate that intent was present, and are reported by the state as the complainant
5. Commission of crime requires two fundamental factors
   a. Committing a deed contrary to criminal law
   b. Omitting an act when there is a legal obligation to perform such an act (e.g., refraining from assistance with the birth of a child if such refusal results in injury to the newborn)
6. Criminal conspiracy occurs when two or more persons agree to commit a crime
7. Giving aid to another in the commission of a crime makes the person equally guilty of the offense if awareness is present that a crime is being committed
8. Ignorance of the law is usually not an adequate defense when a crime or civil wrong is committed
9. Assault may be justified in instances of self-defense if only as much force as is absolutely necessary for self-protection is used

10. Search warrants are required before property can be searched
11. Administration of narcotics by a nurse is legal only when authorized by a physician who is legally registered under the Controlled Substances Act in the United States and the Narcotics Control Act in Canada
    a. If a nurse knowingly administers a drug that causes a major disability or death, a crime may be charged
    b. Illegal possession or sale of a controlled substance makes nurse liable, as is any citizen
12. Those involved in decisions to discontinue life-support systems may be liable to charge of murder; there is a strong movement against dramatic life-saving measures in cases of terminally ill clients; these questions are as much moral as legal; nurse should know decision must be made on knowledge; nurse is accountable; "living will" aims at giving the individual the authority to say whether life-support systems should be used at all or discontinued if in use; legality of "living will" and effectiveness of legislation permitting it are under dispute; 35 states now have legislation relating to the "living will"; states have increasingly been forced to define death, many using signs of brain death as indicator
13. In the United States, each state must define when death occurs; not all states have done so
14. Terminal Illness Protocol (1984): joint project of CNA, CHA, CMA, and Canadian Bar Association, with representation from Catholic Health Association of Canada and the Law Reform Commission of Canada; provides guidelines for resuscitative intervention for health professionals
    a. A "do not resuscitate" order must be a team decision, and the family and, if possible, the client must be included in the decision-making process
    b. A "no resuscitation" order must be recorded on the client's record

MALPRACTICE INSURANCE

A. Liability can be defined as a person's legal responsibility to be accountable for wrongful acts by making financial restitution to the party wronged
B. Malpractice insurance can be purchased from nurses' associations, bargaining organizations, and private insurance companies
C. Amount of malpractice/liability insurance is dictated by factors such as
   1. Type of nursing practiced (e.g., private practitioner, nursing instructor, acute care nursing)
   2. Increasing inclination to sue professionals, including nurses
   3. In Canada, limits of liability established in area where nursing is practiced
   4. The consumers' rights movement and increased consumer awareness
D. Employer's insurance protects the nurse while on duty in the course of employment (concept of vicarious liability, *respondeat superior*); a nurse can, however, be personally sued and held liable for negligent or malpractice actions

E. Malpractice insurance provides monetary settlement if a suit by a client is decided in favor of the client; most policies pay legal fees and costs, as well as bond for the nurse, and the cost of an appeal

F. In 1988, a professional liability protective fund operated by nurses for nurses became a reality as CNA established The Canadian Nurses Protective Fund (CNPF) designed "to protect nurses from professional liability claims and to address inequities in the present insurance system." Included is an Adjudication Committee and nurse lawyer to provide support and help with documentation.

INFORMED CONSENT

A. Purposes of informed consent
  1. Makes possible a contract between two individuals with each sharing equally
  2. Makes competent decision possible for client who has the final decision
B. Consent essential for any treatment, except in an emergency where failure to institute treatment may constitute negligence
C. In an emergency situation, two physicians may sign consent for the client when failure to intervene will cause death
D. Major question is what constitutes informed consent
  1. Elements of consent
    a. Explanation of treatment to be done
    b. Advantages and disadvantages
    c. Possible alternatives
    d. Time for decision making
    e. No undue pressure
    f. Before sedation
  2. Problems arise in determining
    a. What constitutes adequate information
    b. Who should give explanation
    c. Whether to give alternatives where one treatment is clearly preferable
    d. What constitutes mental competency in client from whom an informed consent is sought
  3. The client has a right to know, agree, or refuse
E. Nurse's responsibility is to respect rights of individual client, thus avoiding legal action
F. Nurse is a client advocate when client cannot function in this role.

THE NURSE IN THE COURTS

A. Nurse may be in court either as a witness if involved personally in a case or as an expert witness because of knowledge and expertise
B. Expert witness
  1. Not an advocate
  2. If called into court, the nurse must be
    a. Informed as to standards of care that prudent, reasonable nurses would give relative to incident in question
    b. Knowledgeable in the field specific to the incident
    c. Without opinion unless specifically asked
  3. Although a professional may elect to join in a "conspiracy of silence" when asked to testify against another professional, the basic question is ethical and concerns the willingness of the professional to deal adequately with the incompetence of another professional
  4. In some situations in Canada and in some states the Nurse Practice Act requires that the professional nurse report a colleague's incompetence
  5. The client's chart, to which nurses contribute, may be used in court, therefore placing nurses in court vicariously; notes should be accurate, complete, factual, and give evidence of knowledge and judgment

THE NURSE'S LEGAL STATUS

A. Employee
  1. Nurse acts and performs services for another and is known as *agent;* this does not eliminate the independence of the nurse in practice
  2. Contract made with the employer that sets forth the nature of the services expected, the conditions of employment, and compensation
  3. Elements of a written contract
    a. Services to be rendered
    b. Environment in which services are to be rendered
    c. Duration of contract
    d. Termination conditions
B. Collective bargaining increasingly involved in arranging contracts between employees and the employing agency
  1. Contracts binding on both parties even though individual nurse not directly involved with the deliberations; if majority of employees agree, all are bound
  2. Damages may be sought in court if contract broken
C. Independent contractor
  1. A contractor who renders direct services to clients and is in control of that service, including setting fee for service
  2. A small number of nurses setting up independent practices
  3. Joint practice is an adaptation of the independent contractor
    a. Nurse and physician practice independently and collaboratively, each rendering service to the same group of clients
    b. The client's needs determine which professional gives the service
  4. Private duty nurse is an independent contractor

THE CLIENT'S RIGHTS

A. Society is more consumer oriented and values the rights of individuals
B. Law Reform Commissions of Canada (1983) and the Manitoba Association of Rights and Liberties (1980) recommended that clients' rights be expressly recognized, but provincial governments have not done so
C. Clients have the legal right to refuse treatment (if mentally competent), to be given treatment in an emergency, to choose their own doctor, to have a proper standard of care, to execute voluntary and informed consent, to decide whether to be used for research or teaching, to be treated in confidentiality, to receive treatment free of discrimination, to have protection of personal property, and freedom to receive services in a hospital of one's choice, and the right to make a choice even if it is choosing to die rather than receive identified treatments

D. Statutory restrictions may be imposed on client's rights (e.g., rights of clients to use specific health resources) or entitlement of all citizens to receive organs for transplant.

E. National governments of both the United States and Canada, the governments of states and provinces, and various professional associations and consumer groups have attempted to educate the public concerning their rights regarding provision and delivery of health care

F. Both national governments have set stringent rules about the use of human subjects in research

G. Laws of both national governments emphasize the rights of children, the mentally disadvantaged, and the elderly to health care

H. Clients have the right to lodge complaints about a nurse and the care received when complaints are related to
1. Incompetence
2. Professional misconduct
3. Physical or mental incapacity

THE NURSE'S RIGHTS AND RESPONSIBILITIES

A. Nurses have recently been accorded certain rights by professional groups, by contracts, and by the public; those that have been suggested are
1. The right to be trusted by the public
2. The right to practice nursing in accordance with professionally defined standards
3. The right to participate in and to promote growth and direction of the profession
4. The right to intervene when necessary to protect clients
5. The right to be respected for one's knowledge, abilities, experience, and contributions
6. The right to be believed when speaking in the area of his/her expertise
7. The right to be trusted by colleagues
8. The right to give and receive support, guidance, and correction from colleagues
9. The right to be compensated fairly for services

B. Because of these rights nurses also have the responsibility to
1. Practice nursing in accordance with standards of the profession
2. Fulfill professional promises made to the public
3. Intervene to protect clients from unethical and/or illegal actions by any person delivering health care
4. Participate in and promote the growth of the profession
5. Strive constantly to increase knowledge and experience
6. Speak out accurately and honestly in one's area of expertise
7. Give to and receive guidance, support, and correction from colleagues

LEGISLATION RELATED TO NURSES

A. United States
1. Registration and licensure are used interchangeably but are not synonymous
2. Registration: entrance of name in a registry
   a. Maintained by individual states in United States
   b. Authorizes practice as a registered nurse
   c. Protects the title of registered nurse
   d. Follows automatically after licensure

3. Licensure: granting of a license after successful completion of the National Council Licensure Examination in the United States
   a. Protects the public and nursing practice; issued by individual states
   b. Mandatory licensure: all who practice nursing must be licensed; employees of federal government are not bound by state mandatory licensure laws
   c. Permissive licensure: protects the titles Reg N or RN, but does not protect the practice of nursing; the practice of nursing is not prohibited as long as the unlicensed person does not represent himself or herself as a registered nurse; thus anyone, licensed or not, may practice nursing so long as the title Reg N or RN is not used
   d. May be obtained by examination, waiver, or endorsement (reciprocity)
   e. American Nurses' Association, from the time of its inception, has seen the need for legislation to set standards for nursing
   f. First states with nurse licensing laws
      (1) North Carolina: 1903
      (2) New York: 1903
      (3) New Jersey: 1903
   g. 1952: all states and territories had nurse practice acts
   h. Early laws permissive, with New York the first state to pass a mandatory licensing law in 1938 (which, because of the war, did not become effective until 1948)
   i. All states now have mandatory laws
   j. Laws administered by a state board of nursing either as a department of state government or as an autonomous agency
   k. Definition of the practice of nursing is included in the law
   l. Many states and the professional nursing organizations are discussing legislation that would require a baccalaureate degree for eligibility for licensure as a professional nurse
   m. Renewal of licenses usually required every 2 or 3 years
   n. Different licensing laws and examinations required for practical nursing
   o. Licenses can be revoked for cause by the state board of nursing
      (1) Nursing's licensing body disciplines members of the profession of nursing according to mechanisms described in nurse practice acts
      (2) Self-regulation practices are criteria of a profession, along with autonomy and expertise

4. National Council of State Boards of Nursing, Inc. (NCSBN): separate, autonomous, nonprofit body established in 1978
   a. Membership open to any board of nursing
   b. Delegate assembly composed of one member of each board
   c. National Council Licensure Examination (NCLEX) under control of this body
   d. Executive director with office in Chicago

5. NCLEX, first administered in July 1982
   a. Criterion-referenced examination based on nursing behaviors that constitute safe and effective practice
   b. Comprehensive integrated examination divided into four sections
   c. Passing score determined by each state board
   d. Each jurisdiction agrees to adopt this examination because licensure is a state function
   e. Examination is administered by each state board of nursing two times yearly over a 2-day period

B. Canada
   1. Registration and licensure are used interchangeably but are not synonymous
   2. Registration: entrance of one's name on a register
      a. Maintained by individual provincial professional nurses associations (except in Ontario, where it is maintained by the College of Nurses, the statutory body for nurses in Ontario) after successful completion of the Canadian Nurses Association Testing Service (CNATS)
      b. Authorizes practice as a registered nurse
      c. Protects the title of registered nurse
      d. Follows automatically after licensure
      e. Beginning in 1989, feedback will be provided at no cost to all unsuccessful candidates in the CNATS nurse registration examinations, and a mechanism to evaluate this feedback process will be used
   3. Licensure: granting of a license after successful completion of the Canadian Nurses' Association Testing Service Registration Examination
      a. Mandatory licensure: all who practice nursing must be licensed; employees of the federal government are not bound by provincial mandatory licensure laws; CNA is being urged to take the position that federally-employed nurses be registered in the province/territory where they are employed
      b. CNA has publicly endorsed mandatory licensure for all nurses employed by the federal government
      c. Permissive licensure: protects the titles Reg N or RN, but does not protect the practice of nursing; the practice of nursing is not prohibited as long as the unlicensed person does not represent himself or herself as a registered nurse; thus anyone, licensed or not, may practice nursing so long as the title Reg N or RN is not used
      d. May be obtained by examination, waiver, or endorsement (reciprocity)
      e. Health Disciplines Act: (Ontario) 1975 RSO1980
         (1) Received royal assent in 1974, but not proclaimed law until July 1975
         (2) Incorporates recommendations from the Committee on the Healing Arts and the *Royal Commission Inquiry into Civil Rights*
         (3) Allows for lay representation in the professional governing council
         (4) Creates a health disciplines board to conduct hearings related to complaints and applications for licensing
         (5) Gives the Council of the College of Nurses of Ontario authority to:
            (a) Register new members and renew registration of standing members
            (b) Require nursing personnel to be registered with the College of Nurses
            (c) Discipline any person granted initial registration
            (d) Protect the titles Registered Nurse and Registered Nursing Assistant
            (e) Establish, maintain, and develop standards of knowledge, skill, and professional ethics
         (6) The Health Professions Legislation Review (1983) initiated by the government of Ontario has resulted in a draft of new legislation which is intended to regulate 25 occupational groups including the five regulated by the Health Disciplines Act (1974)
         (7) Simultaneously, the Task Force on Standards Revision (CON) completed its task and circulated to nurses registered with the CON a draft of the proposed new standards targeted for implementation in 1990
      f. Nurse practice acts
         (1) Nursing is recognized by provincial statutes (Nurses' Acts)
         (2) Purpose of registration
            (a) Registration allows for protection of the general public by distinguishing the trained nurse from the untrained nurse
            (b) Protects title of registered nurse for persons who have successfully passed registration examinations
         (3) Purposes of Nurses' Acts
            (a) In most provinces/territories the acts are tending toward a definition of legal boundaries in terms of nursing functions and toward definition of nursing practice
            (b) To provide for interprovincial registration
            (c) In some provinces to provide for the registration and licensure of nursing assistants
         (4) Enactment
            (a) First in Nova Scotia (1910), followed by Manitoba (1913), New Brunswick and Alberta (1916), Ontario (1922)
            (b) Administered by provincial associations except in Ontario, where the College of Nurses registers nurses, and in Quebec, where the Order of Nurses of the Province of Quebec licenses nurses for nursing practice
         (5) Control
            (a) In Ontario, with the Nurses' Act of 1961 amended, the College of Nurses of Ontario was established as the governing body of nursing with provision also for governing of nursing assistants (now titled Registered Nursing Assistant)
            (b) As of February 1974: only one nurses'

association had the right of appeal to a legal definition of nursing written into law; this was the Order of Nurses of Quebec

(c) Since 1986 mandatory registration has been in effect in all provinces except British Columbia, Saskatchewan, Manitoba, and Ontario

(d) These four provinces and territory have permissive registration based on approval of nursing programs and successful passing of nurse registration examination (CNATS)

(e) British Columbia nurses have submitted changes to the Registered Nurses Act to the government and are awaiting legislation; Saskatchewan nurses requested mandatory registration in 1985, and are presently studying whether discipline procedures should be in the legislation together with the scope and definition of nursing in the province; Yukon Nurses Society has been working with Yukon Territorial Government on development of legislation and regulations to govern practice and licensure of nurses in the territory by the end of 1988 (proposed Nursing Profession Act)

(f) Order of Nurses of Quebec (ONQ) L'Ordre des Infirmiers et Infirmieres du Quebec (OIIQ)

[1] February 1974: Professional Code of the Province of Quebec changed the title of Association of Nurses of the Province of Quebec (ANPQ) to Order of Nurses of Quebec (ONQ); chief purpose is protection of the public by supervising the practice of nursing and its members as legal responsibilities governed by the "Code des professions" and the "Loi sur les infirmiers et infirmieres"

[2] Passage of the Professional Code created 21 professional groups: 11 have exclusive rights to practice and 10 regulate only the title of the health worker

[3] Quebec Nurses' Act defines the profession of nursing as identification of persons' health needs, assisting with diagnosis, employing nursing interventions, and communication of health problems to clients

[4] Memberships in L'Ordre des Infirmiers et Infirmieres du Quebec (OIIQ), a professional association with unique, official status is mandatory, although OIIQ withdrew from the CNA in 1985

[5] Some Quebec nurses have joined the Yukon Nurses Society to ensure membership in the CNA and ICN

(g) Northwest Territories Registered Nurses' Association (NWTRNA)

[1] January 1975: Ordinance Respecting the Nursing Profession in the Northwest Territories approved by the Territorial Council

[2] Gave the NWTRNA authority to:
[a] Join with the Canadian Nurses' Association
[b] Grant and/or revoke certificates of registration to nurses practicing in the Northwest Territories
[c] Discipline members of the nursing profession
[d] Lay claim to being the first professional group north of the sixtieth parallel to acquire registration control over its members

[3] Major responsibilities are related to registration/licensure, defining of standards for practice, and promoting continuing nursing education

[4] Issues relate to promotion of health careers among native northerners and developing a position paper on maternal health delivery in the Northwest Territories

The Nurse's Role
MAINTENANCE OF EFFECTIVE COMMUNICATION
Introduction

A. The need to communicate is universal
B. People communicate to satisfy needs
C. Recognition of what is communicated is basic for the establishment of a therapeutic nurse-client relationship
D. Clear and accurate communication among members of the health team, including the client, is vital to support the client's welfare

Nursing Responsibilities in Promotion of Productive Communication

A. Be aware that effective communication requires skill in both sending and receiving messages
1. Verbal: words, tone of voice, etc.
2. Written
3. Nonverbal: facial expression, eye contact, body language, etc.
B. Recognize the high stress–anxiety potential of most health settings created in part by:
1. Health problem itself
2. Treatments and procedures
3. Exclusive behavior of personnel
4. Foreign environment
5. Change in life-style, body image, and self-concept
C. Recognize the intrinsic worth of each person
1. Listen, consider wishes when possible, explain when necessary
2. Avoid stereotyping, snap judgments, unjustified comparisons
3. Be nonjudgmental and nonpunitive in response and behavior
D. Be aware that each individual must be treated as a whole person

E. Recognize that all behavior has meaning and usually results from the attempt to cope with stress or anxiety
   1. Be aware of importance of value systems
   2. Be aware of significance of cultural differences
   3. Be sensitive to personal meaning of experiences to clients
   4. Recognize that giving information may not alter the client's behavior
   5. Recognize the defense mechanisms that the individual is using
   6. Recognize own anxiety and cope with it
   7. Search for patterns of adaptation on which to base action
   8. Recognize that client's previous patterns of behavior may become inadequate under stress
      a. Health problems may produce a change in family or community constellations
      b. Health problems may lead to change in self-perception and role identity
   9. Be aware that behavioral changes are possible only when the individual has other defenses to maintain equilibrium
F. Help the client to accept the health problem and its consequences
G. Identify the individual's needs and determine priority for care
H. Maintain an accepting, open environment
   1. Be permissive rather than authoritarian
   2. Identify and face problems honestly
   3. Value the expression of feelings
   4. Be nonjudgmental
I. Where possible, encourage client participation in decision making
J. Recognize the client is a unique person
   1. Use names rather than labels such as room numbers or diagnoses
   2. Maintain the client's dignity
   3. Be courteous toward the client, family, and visitors
   4. Protect the client's privacy by use of curtains, avoidance of probing
   5. Permit personal possessions where practical (e.g., own nightclothes, pictures, toys)
   6. Explain at the client's level of understanding and tolerance
   7. Encourage expression of feelings
   8. Approach the client as a person with difficulties, not as a "difficult" person
K. Support a social environment that focuses on client needs
   1. Use problem-solving techniques that focus on the client
   2. Be flexible in carrying out routines and policies
   3. Be discreet in use of power
   4. Recognize that use of medical jargon can isolate the client

RECOGNITION OF CLIENT FACTORS INFLUENCING NURSING CARE

A. Hierarchy of needs
   1. Need to survive: physiologic needs for air, food, water, etc.
   2. Need for safety and comfort: physical and psychologic security
   3. Interpersonal needs: social needs for love, acceptance, status, and recognition
   4. Intrapersonal needs: self-esteem, self-actualization
B. Developmental level
   1. Infant: must adapt to a totally new environment; the stress from this culture shock is compounded for the infant with a congenital defect
   2. Child: maturation involves physical, functional, and emotional growth; it is an ever-changing process that produces stress; disabilities will provide additional factors that may quantitatively or qualitatively affect maturation
   3. Adolescent: is experiencing a physical, psychologic, and social growth spurt; the individual is asking, "Who am I?" on the way to developing a self-image; limitations provide additional stress during identity formation
   4. Adult: is expected to be independent and productive, to provide for self and family; if one cannot assume this role totally or partially, it can cause additional stress
   5. Aged: our society tends to venerate youth and deplore old age; many elderly persons are experiencing multiple stresses (loss of loved ones, changes in usual life-style, loss of physical vigor, and, for many, the thought of approaching death) at a time when their ability to adapt is compromised by the anatomic, physiologic, and psychologic alterations that occur during the aging process
C. Type of condition affecting the client
   1. Acute illness: caused by a health problem that produces signs and symptoms abruptly, runs a short course, and from which there is usually a full recovery; an acute illness may leave an individual with a loss of a body part or function and may develop into a long-term illness
   2. Chronic illness: caused by a health problem that produces signs and symptoms over time, running a long course, and from which there is only partial recovery
      a. Exacerbation: period when a chronic illness becomes more active and there is a recurrence of pronounced signs and symptoms of the disease
      b. Remission: period when a chronic illness is controlled and signs and symptoms are reduced or not obvious
      c. Degenerative: continuous deterioration or increased impairment of a person's physical state
   3. Terminal illness: no cure possible; death is inevitable in the near future
   4. Primary health problem: original condition, developing independently of another health problem
   5. Secondary health problem: direct result of another health problem
D. Personal resources
   1. Level of self-esteem: attitude that reflects the individual's perception of self-worth; it is a personal subjective judgment of oneself
   2. Experiential background: knowledge derived from one's own actions, observations, or perceptions; maturation, culture, and environment influence the individual's experiential foundation

3. Intelligence
   a. Genetic intellectual potential
   b. Amount of formal and informal education
   c. Level of intellectual development (e.g., child versus adult)
   d. Ability to reason, conceptualize, and translate words into actions
4. Level of motivation: internal desire or incentive to accomplish something
5. Values: factors that are important to the individual
6. Religion: deep personal belief in a higher force than humanity

E. Extent of actual or perceived change in body image
1. Obvious reminder of disability to self and others
   a. Loss of a body part
   b. Need for a prosthesis (e.g., breast, leg, eye)
   c. Need for hardware (e.g., pacemaker, braces, hearing aid, wheelchair)
   d. Extent of disability or limitation
   e. Need for medication
2. Value placed on loss by self or society
   a. "No longer whole," "a cripple"
   b. Type of loss: perceptions of body part, function, or disease, as being good, pleasing, repulsive, clean, dirty, etc.
      (1) Symbols of sexuality: breast, uterus, prostate, heart
      (2) May lack social acceptability: colostomy, mental illness, incontinence, cancer, tuberculosis, AIDS, drug abuse
      (3) Impairment of senses and/or ability to communicate: laryngectomy, aphasia, deafness, blindness
      (4) Altered body image resulting from anatomic changes: amputation of limb or breast, colostomy

F. Client's and family's stage of adaptation
1. Self-protection: disbelief, denial, avoidance, and/or intellectualization; with developing awareness of implications of illness the individual defends the self further—anger, depression, and/or joking
2. With developing realization of implications of illness the individual reorganizes self-feelings and restructures relationships with family and society
3. As resolution occurs the individual begins to accept the consequences of the illness and acknowledges feelings about the self and further changes that must be made

G. Client's previous history
1. Health history
   a. Physiologic: what physical adaptations were manifested in the past
   b. Psychologic: what psychologic methods of adaptation were exhibited in the past
2. Sociocultural history
   a. Religion: particular denomination, specific belief (e.g., agnostic, atheist, "energy force")
   b. Ethnic group
   c. Occupation
   d. Economic status
   e. Family members and their personal resources
   f. Race

g. Educational background
h. Environment: urban versus rural, private home versus apartment
i. Social status
j. Life-style

USE OF THE NURSING PROCESS
Introduction

A. Basis of personalized care is planned rather than intuitive intervention
B. Most efficient way to accomplish this in a time of exploding knowledge and rapid social change is by the nursing process
   1. Theoretical framework used by the nurse
   2. Assists in solving or alleviating both simple and complex nursing problems
C. Changing, expanding, more responsible role demands knowledgeably planned, purposeful, and accountable action by nurses
D. Documentation of nursing care is done to
   1. Provide comprehensive and systematic nursing care through use of the nursing process
   2. Satisfy requirements of regulatory agencies
      a. Hospitals and nursing homes are licensed by the state in which they operate; the state sets regulations which must be met
      b. Joint Commission On Accreditation Of Health Organizations (JCAHO) accredits hospitals and some nursing homes; hospitals must be accredited by JCAHO for Medicare and Medicaid reimbursement
      c. Health Care Financing Administration (HCFA) certifies nursing homes; nursing homes must be certified by HCFA for Medicare and Medicaid reimbursement
      d. Documentation of care by staff is vital and it becomes a focal point of the accreditation/certification process
   3. Provide a legal document that reflects the care given to and the progress of the client
E. Decision making that systematically selects and uses relevant information is a requisite for individualized client care
F. Cognitive, affective, and activity components that are nursing can best be integrated by the nursing process
G. Process consists of assessing, diagnosing, planning, implementing, and evaluating a client's problem and its proposed solution via the nursing care plan; it is continuous throughout the client's stay

Steps in the Nursing Process

A. Assessment
1. Collection of personal, social, medical, and general data
   a. Sources: primary (client, family, and chart) and secondary (colleagues, Kardex, literature)
   b. Methods
      (1) Interviewing formally (nursing health history) and informally during various nurse-client interactions
      (2) Observation
      (3) Review of records

NANDA-Approved Nursing Diagnoses*

Activity intolerance
Activity intolerance, potential
Adjustment, impaired
Airway clearance, ineffective
Anxiety
Aspiration, potential for
Body image disturbance
Body temperature, altered, potential
Breast-feeding, ineffective
Breathing pattern, ineffective
Cardiac output, decreased
Communication, impaired verbal
Constipation
Constipation, colonic
Constipation, perceived
Coping, defensive
Coping, family: potential for growth
Coping, ineffective family: compromised
Coping, ineffective family: disabling
Coping, ineffective individual
Decisional conflict (specify)
Denial, ineffective
Diarrhea
Disuse syndrome, potential for
Diversional activity deficit
Dysreflexia
Family processes, altered
Fatigue
Fear
Fluid volume deficit (1)
Fluid volume deficit (2)
Fluid volume deficit, potential
Fluid volume excess
Gas exchange, impaired
Grieving, anticipatory
Grieving, dysfunctional
Growth and development, altered

Health maintenance, altered
Health seeking behaviors (specify)
Home maintenance management, impaired
Hopelessness
Hyperthermia
Hypothermia
Incontinence, bowel
Incontinence, functional
Incontinence, reflex
Incontinence, stress
Incontinence, total
Incontinence, urge
Infection, potential for
Injury, potential for
Knowledge deficit (specify)
Mobility, impaired physical
Noncompliance (specify)
Nutrition, altered: less than body requirements
Nutrition, altered: more than body requirements
Nutrition, altered: potential for more than body requirements
Oral mucous membrane, altered
Pain
Pain, chronic
Parental role conflict
Parenting, altered
Parenting, altered, potential
Personal identity disturbance
Poisoning, potential for
Post-trauma response
Powerlessness
Rape-trauma syndrome
Rape-trauma syndrome: compound reaction
Rape-trauma syndrome: silent reaction

Role performance, altered
Self care deficit, bathing/hygiene
Self care deficit, dressing/grooming
Self care deficit, feeding
Self care deficit, toileting
Self-esteem disturbance
Self-esteem, chronic low
Self-esteem, situational low
Sensory/perceptual alterations (specify) (visual, auditory, kinesthetic, gustatory, tactile, olfactory)
Sexual dysfunction
Sexuality patterns, altered
Skin integrity, impaired
Skin integrity, impaired, potential
Sleep pattern disturbance
Social interaction, impaired
Social isolation
Spiritual distress (distress of the human spirit)
Suffocation, potential for
Swallowing, impaired
Thermoregulation, ineffective
Thought processes, altered
Tissue integrity, impaired
Tissue perfusion, altered (specify type) (renal, cerebral, cardiopulmonary, gastrointestinal, peripheral)
Trauma, potential for
Unilateral neglect
Urinary elimination, altered patterns
Urinary retention
Violence, potential for: self-directed or directed at others

*Through the 8th Conference, 1988

B. Analysis
1. Classification of data: screening, organizing, and grouping significant and related information
2. Definition of client's problem: making a nursing diagnosis
   a. A nursing diagnosis is a definitive statement of the client's actual or potential difficulties, concerns, or deficits that are amenable to nursing interventions; there are two components to the statement of a nursing diagnosis
      (1) Part I: a determination of the problem (unhealthful response of client)
      (2) Part II: identification of the etiology (contributing factors)
      (3) The two parts are joined together by the phrase "related to"
   b. Development of diagnoses (see list of NANDA-Approved Nursing Diagnoses in the box on p. 16.)
      (1) Excludes all nonnursing diagnoses, for example, medical diagnoses or diagnostic tests
      (2) Excludes medical treatments as well as the nurse's problems with the client
      (3) Involves inductive and deductive reasoning
      (4) Includes both internal and external environmental stresses
      (5) Includes data that has been clustered (grouping of related data) during assessment
C. Planning: the nursing care plan, a blueprint for action
1. Previously identified nursing diagnoses are written on the care plan
2. Planned intervention may include both independent and interdependent functions of the nurse; prescriptions made by physician or allied health professionals may be included
3. New diagnoses should be noted on the nursing care plan and progress notes as they are identified
4. Client outcomes (goals of nursing intervention) are reflected in expected changes in the client
   a. Expected client outcome is written next to each nursing diagnosis on nursing care plan
   b. These outcomes must be objective, realistic, measurable, observable alterations in the client's behavior, activity, or physical state; a time period should be set for achievement of the outcome
   c. The outcome provides a standard of measure that can be used to determine if the goal toward which the client and nurse are working has been achieved
5. Nursing interventions (nursing orders) are written for each nursing diagnosis and should be specific to the stated outcome or goal; each goal may have one or more applicable interventions
D. Implementation: the actual administration of the planned nursing care
E. Evaluation and revision of nursing care plan
1. Process is ongoing throughout client's treatment/hospitalization
2. If outcome/goal is not reached in specified time, the client is reassessed to discover the reason
3. Reordering of priorities and new goal setting may be necessary

4. When diagnosis/problem is resolved, the date should be noted on care plan
F. Advantages of nursing process
1. Encourages thorough individual client assessment by nurse
2. Determines priority of care
3. Provides comprehensive and systematic nursing care planning and delivery
4. Permits independent, creative, and flexible nursing intervention
5. Facilitates team cooperation by promoting
   a. Contributions from all team members
   b. Communication among team members
   c. Coordination of care
   d. Continuity of care
6. Provides for continuous involvement and input from client
7. Facilitates the "costing-out" of nursing services and care
8. Facilitates nursing research
9. Provides accurate legal document of client care
10. Satisfies rules of regulatory agencies

QUALITY ASSURRANCE

A. Definition: a method used to ascertain the extent to which nursing practice meets particular criteria based on predetermined standards
B. Types of criteria
1. Structure criteria: include the organizational framework, level of financial support to nursing service, and physical and functional characteristics of facility
2. Process criteria: measure nursing actions used to reach expected and desired outcomes in a client
3. Outcome criteria: measure client's status on discharge against desired outcomes in clients with the same diagnosis
C. Improves nursing care by:
1. Providing accountability to the client
2. Identifying need for additional services, personnel, or equipment
3. Identifying deficiencies in policies and procedures
4. Improving interdisciplinary and intradisciplinary communication and coordination of client services
5. Promoting individual growth of staff members
6. Providing direction for development of educational programs
7. Meeting the requirements of regulatory agencies

ESTABLISHMENT OF A TEACHING-LEARNING ENVIRONMENT
Introduction

A. Teaching is communication especially structured and sequenced to produce learning
B. Learning is the activity by which knowledge, attitudes, and skills are acquired, resulting in a change in behavior
C. All problems in learning and identified knowledge deficits should be addressed when establishing the appropriate nursing diagnoses for a client
D. Goals of learning
1. Understanding or acquiring knowledge: cognitive learning (e.g., What is diabetes and how does it affect me?)

2. Feeling or developing attitudes: affective learning (e.g., What does this health problem mean to me?)
3. Doing or developing psychomotor skills: conative learning (e.g., How do I give myself an injection?)

Principles of Teaching-Learning Process and Related Nursing Approaches

A. Learning occurs best when there is a felt need or readiness to learn
   1. Identify the client's emotional or motivational readiness: is the person ready to put forth the effort necessary to learn
   2. Identify the client's experiential readiness: does the person have the necessary background of experience, skills, attitudes, and ability to learn
   3. Determine the client's level of adaptation: different teaching strategies may be necessary during the various stages of adaptation because the client is expressing denial, anger, and/or depression; once the initial defensive compensatory reactions have passed, the individual is more receptive to teaching
   4. Assess the client's level of human needs; the client whose physical and safety needs are not met will not be concerned with interpersonal and intrapersonal needs
   5. Specific signs of the client's readiness to learn
      a. The client is adapting to the initial crisis
      b. The client has a developing awareness of the health problem and its implications
      c. The client is asking direct questions
      d. The client is presenting clues that indicate indirect seeking of information
      e. The client's physical condition or behavior invites the nurse to intervene through teaching
   6. Once a need has been recognized, readiness has been determined, and the time and place are appropriate, develop a plan and teach
B. The method of presentation of material influences the client's ability to learn
   1. A tentative teaching plan should be developed with the client and/or the client's significant others and communicated to all members of the health team
   2. Information presented should be organized, accurate, and concise (e.g., simple to the complex, general to the specific)
   3. Appropriate teaching methods should be instituted
      a. Concepts are best taught with lectures, audiovisual materials, and discussion
      b. Attitudes are taught by exploring feelings, role models, discussions, and an atmosphere of acceptance
      c. Skills are taught by illustrations, models, demonstration, return demonstration, and practice
   4. Teaching tools should be used when indicated (e.g., models, filmstrips, illustrations)
   5. The client and family should be encouraged to ask questions, which should be answered directly
   6. Opportunities should be provided for evaluation
C. Learning is made easier when material to be learned is related to what the learner already knows
   1. Find out what the client knows about the problem
   2. Begin the teaching program at the client's level of understanding

3. Avoid the use of technical terminology; use simple terms or ones with which the client feels comfortable
D. Learning is purposeful; short- and long-term goals are important because they identify the behavior to be attained
   1. With the client, set short- and long-term goals
   2. Goal should meet the following criteria:
      a. Specific: state exactly what is to be accomplished
      b. Measurable: set a minimum acceptable level of performance
      c. Realistic: must be potentially achievable
E. Learning is an active process and takes place within the learner
   1. Utilize a teaching approach that includes the learner (e.g., programed instruction books, discussion, questions and answers, return demonstration)
   2. Provide opportunities for the client to practice motor skills
   3. Encourage self-directed activities
F. Every individual has capabilities and strengths (e.g., physical strengths, emotional maturity, a supportive family) that can be utilized to help the client learn
   1. Identify the client's personal resources
   2. Build on the identified strengths
   3. Utilize these personal resources when and where appropriate
G. Energy and endurance levels will affect the client's ability to learn and perform
   1. During instruction, balance teaching with sufficient rest periods
   2. Provide teaching at opportune times (e.g., earlier in the day rather than at night, after periods of rest)
   3. Present instruction in a manner the client can comprehend and at a pace that can be maintained
   4. Be flexible and adjust the plan according to the client's rest and activity needs
H. Learning does not always progress on a straight line forward and upward; the client may experience plateaus and remissions with a resulting change in adaptation and needs
   1. Accept the client's feelings regarding lack of progress
   2. Point out progress that has been made
   3. Be patient and do not cause additional stress for the learner
   4. Try alternative approaches for achieving goals
   5. Identify short-term objectives for meeting goals
   6. Alter long-term goals as necessary
I. Learning from previous experience can be transferred to new situations
   1. When teaching something new, relate the commonalities or similarities of previously learned experiences
   2. Base the plan of instructions on the foundation of the client's knowledge
   3. Once the known is reinforced, the unknown can be explored and the differences taught

Motivation

A. Definition: motivation is the process of stimulating a person to assimilate certain concepts or behavior
B. Principles of motivation and related nursing approaches

1. People are complex products of self, family, and culture; the nurse must care for the client as a unified being
   a. Respect the client as a person
   b. Accept the client's feelings without minimizing them
   c. Assist the client and family in accepting that the person's individuality and wholeness continue despite the changed physical or emotional state
   d. Involve the client in deciding what to do and how to do it
   e. The client must take precedence over the purpose of the lesson
2. Learning is fostered when the plan of instruction is designed to operate within the individual's personal attitude and value system
   a. Provide an atmosphere that allows for acceptance of differing value systems
   b. Let the client explore personal values, attitudes, and feelings concerning the health problem and its implications
   c. Explore with the family the possibilities of carrying out instruction and how to individualize it so it is acceptable and practical for the client and family
3. Motivated learner assimilates what is learned more rapidly than does one who is not motivated
   a. The client needs an opportunity to explore and discover personal learning needs and feelings concerning them
   b. Awareness of a need to know can cause mild anxiety, which in itself is motivating
   c. Motivation that is too intense may reduce the effectiveness of learning
   d. Determine the client's readiness for learning
4. Intrinsic motivation (stimulated from within the learner) is preferable to extrinsic motivation (stimulated from outside the learner)
   a. Identify factors that are essential for the individual to have a feeling of meaningful achievement (e.g., being able to care for own health needs, respect and appreciation from others, acquiring new knowledge, receiving a reward)
   b. Satisfaction with learning progress promotes additional learning; therefore design nursing care that will assist the client in attaining a feeling of meaningful achievement
   c. Encourage the client to participate as a member of the health team and to be self-directed
5. Information is learned more readily when it is relevant and meaningful to the learner
   a. Help the client interpret why the information is important and how the information gained will be useful
   b. Relate the information by building the teaching plan on the client's foundation of knowledge, experience, attitudes, and feelings
6. Learning motivated by success or rewards is preferable to learning by failure or punishment
   a. Help the client set realistic goals within the motivation zone (goals set too high may be too challenging, whereas goals set too low may lead to no action)
   b. Focus on the client's strengths and abilities rather than on failures and disabilities
   c. Select learning tasks in which the client is likely to succeed
   d. Assist the client to master or feel successful at one stage of instruction before moving on to the next
   e. Errors must be accepted as part of the learning process
   f. Tolerance for failure is best taught through providing a backlog of success that compensates for experienced failure
7. Planned reinforcement is essential for learning; operant conditioning is based on the theory that satisfaction motivates learning and that those events which occur together are associated
   a. For each client, identify and utilize factors that are stimulants or incentives for action (e.g., praise, smile, rewards, rest, specific privileges, being able to care for self)
   b. Provide visible reinforcements (e.g., progress charts, graphs)
   c. Repetition is a form of reinforcement; therefore repeated activities tend to become habitual
      (1) Provide opportunities for the client to practice old and new skills
      (2) Review information previously taught before introducing new information
   d. Involve the client in groups with people who have the same health problems but are at various stages of convalescence
      (1) To be successful, it is helpful for the client to associate with successful people
      (2) Individuals can often learn more by teaching others
8. Evaluation of performance aids in learning
   a. Purpose
      (1) To measure and interpret results with regard to what degree the set goals are being attained
      (2) To reinforce correct behavior
      (3) To help the learner realize how to change incorrect behavior
      (4) To help the teacher determine the adequacy of the teaching
   b. Together the teacher and learner should observe and evaluate the learner's response in light of the desired behavior
   c. Explain the "whys" of a good or poor evaluation
   d. Value judgments, especially "poor" or "inadequate," must relate to the performance rather than to the individual

PROVIDING LEADERSHIP
Definition

Process of influencing the actions of an individual or group toward specific goals in a particular situation

Styles of Leadership

A. Three basic styles
   1. Autocratic: leader does not seek input from the group but sets the goals, plans, makes the decisions, and evaluates the action taken

2. Democratic: leader seeks input from the group, and responsibilities for action taken are shared between the leader and the group
3. Laissez-faire: leader's input and control of the group are minimal, permitting each individual to set independent goals

B. Leadership styles influenced by the leader, the environment, and the cultural climate of the organization
C. The effective leader modifies his or her style to fit changing circumstances, problems, and people (e.g., autocratic style of leadership is appropriate in an emergency situation)

Principles of Leadership

A. Interpersonal influence is dependent upon a knowledge of human behavior and a sensitivity to others in terms of feelings, values, and problems
   1. Explore and understand attitudes, feelings, and personal values about self
   2. Project self into the place of the individuals being led
   3. Know how you appear to subordinates
B. Communication is an essential component of leadership
   1. Effective communication dependent upon use of the appropriate medium
      a. Communication may be verbal, written, and/or nonverbal
      b. Communication may be formal or informal
      c. Communication should have two directions: up and down; to and from
   2. Communication style can affect the person or persons with whom the leader communicates
      a. Meanings or ideas communicated should be received or intended without distraction
      b. People react to communication differently
      c. Written communication should be in language that is understood by the person or persons intended (e.g., ancillary personnel should have a written assignment that does not require them to make judgments)
      d. Verbal communication can be influenced by facial expressions, body movement, and tone of voice
   3. Effectiveness of communication can be influenced by inappropriate timing; the information communicated may be correct, but the time may be wrong (ascertain readiness)
C. Leader's success is influenced by how the leader's ability to respond to group needs effectively is perceived by those being led
   1. A role is composed of a number of expectations for the behavior of an individual in a specific position or status classification
      a. Any individual's role consists of a number of expectations and relationships
      b. Nurse leader, by virtue of behavior and status, can influence the perceptions of peers, clients, and colleagues
   2. Power is a leader's source of influence
   3. Power may be professional or positional
      a. *Positional power:* acquired through the position

the leader has in the hierarchy of the organization
      b. *Professional power:* acquired through the knowledge or expertise displayed by the leader and/or perceived by the followers
D. Leadership moves from one person to another as changes occur in the work situation
   1. Nurse's expertise about a specific client care problem along with the availability of other resources can place the nurse in the position of providing leadership for a group
   2. Member of another discipline may assume the role of leadership in specific situations (e.g., the physician leads the cardiac arrest team; the nurse coordinates physical rehabilitation and nutrition for the client)
E. Leadership process requires the utilization of actions associated with problem solving: decision making, relating, influencing, and facilitating
   1. Decision making requires knowledge about and skill in solving the problem; participative decision making lends itself to the quality of the decision made, improves relationships, and influences the readiness of an individual or group to accept change (e.g., the client or the family should have the opportunity to participate in the development of the client's plan of care; unit staff may decide which primary nurse or team leader should care for a newly admitted client)
   2. Effective delegation of responsibilities is inherent in effective leadership; delegation of work requires matching the task with the appropriate position (e.g., a nursing assistant should not be providing care that requires the expertise of a registered nurse; utilizing a registered nurse for housekeeping duties is wasteful)
F. Need for change should be understood by those effecting the change as well as those affected by the change
   1. Movement from goal setting to goal achievement involves change
   2. Process of changing includes communication, planning, participation, and evaluation by the individual or group affected
   3. Change is more acceptable when
      a. It has not been dictated but follows a sequence of impersonal principles
      b. Individuals or groups affected have participated in its creation
      c. It has been planned
      d. It follows a number of successful rather than unsuccessful series of changes
      e. It is initiated after other changes have been absorbed, not during the confusion of a major change
      f. It does not threaten security
G. Effective use of leadership is conducive to accomplishing the goals of the group; an evaluation process is necessary if the results of efforts to attain the goals are to be interpreted accurately
   1. Goals should be identified as short-term and long-term
   2. Evaluation process should be ongoing

3. Climate in which the evaluation process occurs influences its success

ADMINISTRATION OF MEDICATIONS
Introduction

A. Scientific age has introduced an increasing number of pharmaceuticals appropriate for relief of stress symptoms, for support of defense systems, and as adjuncts to other supplemental and curative therapies
B. Increasingly, as part of nursing care, the nurse is assuming the responsibility of administering these medications, either singly or in combinations
C. In the interest of client welfare and safety, it is imperative that the independent and collaborative responsibilities inherent in this function be understood and practiced

Basic Concepts

A. Legally, administration of medications is a dependent function requiring a physician's written order and knowledge of cause and effect
B. Legally, morally, and ethically, independent judgment is required before prescribed medications are administered
C. Certain chemical agents alter, inactivate, or potentiate other medications when mixed either prior to or after administration
D. Medications may be given for local or systemic effects
E. Pharmacologic actions of drugs tend to stimulate or depress physiologic activity
F. Medications may be given in a variety of ways, depending on factors such as the effect desired, rapidity of action desired, or the effect of the chemical on the tissues

Common Terms

A. Chemotherapy: use of drugs to destroy invading organisms or abnormal tissue in the host
B. Drug: chemical agent that interacts with living systems and is employed to prevent, diagnose, or treat disease
C. Drug legislation: laws that provide the standards for drug manufacture and distribution and protect the public against fraudulent claims about drug action (e.g., Federal Controlled Substances Act, regulations of the Federal Bureau of Narcotics and Dangerous Drugs, regulations by specific states)
D. Drug standards: criteria for drug composition established by chemical or bioassay and published in official publications (e.g., *United States Pharmacopeia, National Formulary, Pharmacopoeia Internationalis*)
E. Pharmacodynamics: biochemical and physiologic effects of drugs and their mechanisms of action on living tissue
F. Pharmacology: analysis of properties of chemicals that have a biologic action
G. Pharmacotherapeutics: planned use and evaluation of the effect of drugs employed to prevent and treat disease
H. Toxicology: analysis of poisons and poisonings caused by drugs

Terms that Describe Drug Effects

A. Adverse effect: action differing from the planned effect that is undesirable
B. Side effect: often predictable outcome that is unrelated to the primary action of the drug
C. Toxic effect: pathologic extension of the primary action of the drug
D. Cumulation: elevation of circulating levels of a drug consequent to slowing of metabolic pathways or excretory mechanisms
E. Drug dependence: driving need for continued use of a behavior- or mood-altering drug that leads to abuse
   1. Psychic dependence: craving requiring periodic or continued use of a drug for pleasure or relief of discomfort
   2. Physical dependence: appearance of characteristic symptoms when drug use is suspended or terminated (withdrawal or abstinence symptoms)
F. Hypersusceptibility: response to a drug action which is higher than that occurring when the same dosage is given to 90% of the population
G. Idiosyncrasy: unpredictable, highly individualized response; genetically conditioned enzymatic or receptor responsiveness that interferes with metabolic degradation of a drug
H. Paradoxical response: action of a drug producing a response that contrasts sharply with the usual therapeutic effect obtained with the same dosage of the drug
I. Receptor: cellular site where union between a drug and a cellular constituent produces a reversible action
J. Tolerance: lowering of effect obtained from an established dosage of a drug that necessitates raising the dosage to maintain the effect
K. Tachyphylaxis: rapidly developing tolerance to a drug
L. Drug allergy: response occurring when drugs are from protein sources or combine with body protein and induce an allergen-antibody reaction which releases vasoactive intermediates that cause fluid transudation into tissues
   1. Anaphylaxis: life-threatening episode of bronchial constriction and edema which obstruct the airway and cause generalized vasodilation that depletes circulating blood volume; occurs when a drug allergen is administered to an individual having antibodies produced by prior use of the drug
   2. Urticaria: generalized pruritic skin eruptions or giant hives; occurs when a drug is administered to an individual having antibodies produced by prior use of the drug
   3. Angioedema: fluid accumulation in periorbital, oral, and respiratory tissues with lengthening of the expiratory phase and wheezing as bronchial constriction gradually progresses; occurs when a drug is administered to an individual having antibodies produced by prior use of the drug
   4. Serum sickness: gradually emerging intermittent episodes of dyspnea, hypotension, generalized edema, joint pain, rash, swollen lymph glands; occurs 7 or more days after initial administration of a drug causing gradual low-level (titer) production of antibodies that interact with circulating drug to produce symptoms as long as the drug remains in the body
   5. Arthus reaction: localized area of tissue necrosis caused by disruption of blood supply; occurs when

spasticity, occlusion, and degeneration of blood vessels are precipitated by injection of a drug into a site having large quantities of bivalent antibodies
6. Delayed-reaction allergies: rash and fever occurring during drug therapy

Drug Actions

A. Local: drug acts at the site of application
B. Systemic: drug is distributed to selected internal receptor sites after being absorbed from tissues following administration; these routes include oral, sublingual, buccal, nasal, rectal, transdermal, parenteral (intradermal, subcutaneous, intramuscular, intravenous, intraspinal, intracardiac)

Mechanisms

A. Replacement (e.g., administration of insulin required for cellular utilization of glucose)
B. Interruption (e.g., antimetabolic drugs tricking the cell into utilizing an inactive component in building protein)
C. Potentiation (e.g., sulfonylurea group of oral hypoglycemic agents stimulating pancreatic beta cells to produce insulin)
D. Competition (e.g., antihistamine drugs competing with histamine for tissue receptor sites)

Factors Influencing Dosage-Response Relationships

A. Age, weight, sex, size, physiologic status, and genetic and environmental factors affect responses and dosage required for therapeutic effect
B. The ratio between the median toxic dose and the median effective dose (TD50/ED50) of a drug provides the therapeutic index (TI), which is used as a guide to the safe dosage range; a low TI provides a narrow margin of safety, and the client's status is monitored closely for evidence of drug-related adverse effects (e.g., antineoplastic drugs)
C. Concentration of active drug at receptors and duration of drug action are affected by
   1. Characteristics of the drug and the rate of absorption, distribution, biotransformation, and excretion
   2. Drug affinity for particular tissues, immaturity of enzymes required for metabolism of the drug, or depressed function of tissues naturally metabolizing or excreting the drug
D. Membrane barriers (e.g., placental or blood-brain) may block or selectively pass the drug from the circulating fluids to protected areas
E. Plasma protein binding of drugs maintains tissue levels by liberating the drug when stores are lowered and by slowing renal clearance until the drug is freed from binding sites

Drug Interactions

A. Drugs and foods may interact to affect the therapeutic plan adversely (e.g., ingestion of foods or vitamin preparations containing vitamin K may inhibit the hypothrombinemic effect of oral anticoagulants)
B. Drug antagonism: opposing effects of two drugs at receptor sites in body tissues
   1. Chemical antagonism: combining or binding of two drugs causing inactivation of the chemicals
   2. Pharmacologic antagonism: competition of two drugs for a receptor that may allow the weaker drug to block access by the more potent drug
   3. Physiologic antagonism: opposing action on physiologic systems that allows cancellation of action by either drug
C. Drug action summation: combined or concurrent action of drugs that increases therapeutic effects or incidence of adverse effects
   1. Synergism: interaction of drugs at common receptor sites that alters metabolism or excretion and enhances the effect of drugs
   2. Addition: action of two drugs at different receptors which produces an effect twice that possible when either drug is used alone
   3. Potentiation: intensified action occurring when two drugs are administered concurrently that is greater than when either drug is administered alone

General Information

A. Drug nomenclature
   1. Official name (generic, nonproprietary): designated title under which a drug is listed in official publications
   2. Chemical name: descriptive name identifying chemical composition and placement of atoms
   3. Trade name (brand, proprietary): manufacturer's registered and legally owned name for a drug
B. Sources of drugs
   1. Active constituents of plants: alkaloids, glycosides, gums, resins, tannins, waxes, volatile or fixed oils
   2. Animal sources of biologic products: enzymes, sera, vaccines, antitoxins, toxoids, hormones
   3. Mineral sources: iron, iodine, Epsom salt
C. Drug dosage forms
   1. Prepared by manufacturers in units for convenience of administration
   2. Forms used include capsules, extended-release capsules, tablets (enteric-coated, extended-release), troches, pills, suppositories, powders, ampules, vials, delayed-release (repository) suspensions, prefilled cartridges, liniments, lotions, creams, ointments, pastes, transdermal preparations
   3. Chemical preparations: solutions (waters, true solutions, syrups), aqueous suspensions (mixtures, emulsions, magmas, gels), spirits, elixirs, tinctures, fluid extracts, extracts

Nursing Responsibilities

A. Ascertain the presence and correctness of a physician's order
B. Know the common symbols and equivalents in the apothecary and metric systems
C. Know the common abbreviations denoting frequency and route of administration
D. Know the usual dosage of a drug, the usual route of administration, and the expected, unusual, untoward, or toxic effects of drug
E. Use independent judgment before administering a medication by assessing

1. The client's needs relative to factors such as prn medications and expected effects of the medication (e.g., diuresis or sleep)
2. Untoward or toxic manifestations of prior doses (e.g., pruritus following an antibiotic, bradycardia below 60 and visual disturbances with digoxin)
3. Compatibility of medications administered at the same time
   a. The presence of clouding or a precipitate when mixing injectables (e.g., phenobarbital [Luminal Sodium] and meperidine [Demerol])
   b. Inhibition of medication (e.g., antacids or milk given with tetracycline interferes with absorption, resulting in decreased serum levels of the antibiotic)
   c. Potentiation of another medication (e.g., ASA given when a client is receiving anticoagulants intensifies the anticoagulant effect)
4. Effects on living tissues
   a. Iron can discolor tissue and must be given through a straw in liquid form or by the Z-track method intramuscularly
   b. Abscess formation can occur when the same area is used too often for intramuscular administration; thus, rotation of site is necessary
   c. Pain, irritation, or inflammation can occur during intravenous administration and may necessitate adjustments such as greater dilution or slower flow rate

F. Help the client accept ordered medications by independent actions such as
   1. Crushing tablets that cannot be swallowed
   2. Disguising unpalatable tastes with fruit juices
   3. Reinforcing the need for medication

G. Ensure that the right medication is given to the right client at the right time in the right dose and by the right route
   1. Verify orders
   2. Read labels
   3. Calculate the dosage accurately when prescribed dose is not available
   4. Pour or draw up correct amounts
   5. Identify the client correctly by checking the arm band
   6. Prepare the client psychologically by providing explanations as needed
   7. Prepare the client physically by
      a. Positioning appropriately for oral and parenteral medications
      b. Disinfecting the skin when it is to be punctured
   8. Use clean or sterile technique as indicated by route of administration
   9. Use the route specified as appropriate for the ordered medication and dosage

H. For assistance with calculation of solutions and dosages, refer to a programed text (see Bibliography)

I. Use the appropriate technique for administration
   1. Preparations such as tablets, capsules, pills, powders, or liquids may be swallowed; in addition
      a. Tablets (e.g., nitroglycerine) may be held sublingually
      b. Powders (e.g., cromolyn sodium) may be inhaled with a Medihaler
      c. Liquids may be nebulized and inhaled or may be swabbed, sprayed, or instilled
      d. Sustained-release or enteric-coated preparations should not be crushed or broken open
      e. Suspensions should be shaken well before pouring
   2. Parenteral preparations such as ampules or vials containing the dose in solution or powder to which sterile water or saline must be added may be given in several ways
      a. Subcutaneously or hypodermically in small volume (0.5 to 2 ml)
         (1) Pinch the tissue on the outer surface of the upper arm or the anterior aspect of the thigh or the abdomen
         (2) Insert a 25- to 26-gauge needle ⅝ to 1 inch in length at a 45- to 60-degree angle, aspirate slightly, and inject the medication if there is no blood return (aspiration not indicated when heparin is administered)
         (3) Massage to increase absorption (contraindicated when giving heparin)
      b. Intramuscularly in slightly larger volume (up to 5 ml)
         (1) Spread the tissue taut or pinch if necessary
         (2) Use the upper outer quadrant of the buttock or ventral gluteal muscle, the lateral aspect of the thigh, or the deltoid area of the arm
         (3) When using the gluteal muscle, promote relaxation of the muscle whenever possible by placing the client in a prone position with toes pointing inward or on the side with the upper leg flexed
         (4) Insert a 19- to 22-gauge needle 1 to 2 inches in length at a 90-degree angle quickly and smoothly
         (5) Depth of insertion depends on factors such as weight of the client and size of the muscle used
         (6) Aspirate when the needle is in place and tissue is released (unless giving a substance such as iron-dextran [Imferon], for which it is contraindicated)
            (a) If no blood returns, continue injection
            (b) If blood is aspirated, withdraw and prepare a fresh dose
         (7) Apply pressure or massage area after injection as required (unless contraindicated, e.g., Z-track technique)
      c. Intradermally with very small volume for local effect
         (1) Use syringe with appropriate calibrations (e.g., tuberculin)
         (2) Inject at a 15-degree angle using a 26-gauge needle, ⅜ to ½ inch in length with the bevel up
      d. Piggyback administration using intravenous tubing in place
         (1) If necessary, dilute medication according to directions: add 50 to 150 ml of fluid

(2) Remove air from tubing of piggyback without losing any fluid

(3) Cleanse diaphragm on intravenous tubing already in place with alcohol

(4) Insert needle in rubber diaphragm on tubing leading from the infusion that is keeping the vein open

(5) Stop flow of or lower the primary solution below level of the piggyback

(6) Adjust rate of flow on piggyback medication to complete absorption in time designated—usually about 30 minutes

(7) Remove the piggyback and readjust flow rate

3. Transdermal preparations
   a. Medication should not be touched during preparation for administration
   b. Medication should be applied to a smooth, hairless body surface; sites should be rotated

J. Clearly and accurately record and report the administration of medications and the client's response

CHAPTER 3

Medical-Surgical Nursing

Medical-surgical nursing is concerned with those aspects of nursing care that are related to the physical and emotional needs of clients with specific types of health problems. The concepts, principles, and skills included here will assist the practitioner in all aspects of nursing care.

Medical-surgical content has been developed by using a systems approach with examples of major diseases. The areas covered include a general conceptual introduction, preoperative and postoperative care, and cardiovascular, respiratory, gastrointestinal, genitourinary, endocrine, neurologic, musculoskeletal, and integumentary systems. The format for each section follows a similar pattern, beginning with a review of anatomy and physiology, related pharmacology, and related procedures and moving into the major diseases. Etiology and pathophysiology, subjective and objective symptomatology, treatment, and the nursing process focusing on nursing diagnosis and related nursing care are included for each disease presented.

Principles Related to Needs of the Adult
THE YOUNG ADULT (25 TO 45 YEARS)
Growth and Development

A. Physiologic development
  1. Physical maturation occurs
  2. Muscle strength and coordination peak
  3. Biorhythms become established
  4. Sexuality
    a. Established sex drive remains high for men
    b. Female sex drive reaches a peak during later phase of young adulthood
    c. Physiologically optimal period for childbearing
  5. BMR decreases at rate of 2% to 4% per decade after 20 years of age
B. Psychosocial development
  1. Mental abilities reflect formal operations (see growth and development of the adolescent in pediatric nursing)
  2. Resolving the developmental crisis of intimacy versus isolation
  3. Establishing new family relationships and parenting patterns
  4. Establishing the self in, and advancing in, a chosen occupation

Health Promotion

A. Health problems
  1. Accidents—leading cause of death in the United States
  2. Periodontal disease
  3. Cancer involving the reproductive organs
  4. Hypertension
  5. Suicide
  6. Alcoholism
  7. Spouse abuse
  8. Fertility regulation
  9. Divorce
  10. Unbalanced diet
B. Nursing care
  1. Encourage attendance at safety programs to promote accident prevention (e.g., defensive driving programs)
  2. Encourage dental checkups
  3. Teach self-examination techniques and encourage regular medical checkups
  4. Promote awareness that optimal diet is essential to achieving and maintaining optimal health; encourage nutritional evaluation and consultation
  5. Teach the Dietary Goals for the United States and encourage individuals to follow the Dietary Guidelines for Americans*

    a. Dietary Goals for the United States
      (1) To avoid obesity, consume only as much energy (calories) as is expended; if overweight, decrease energy intake and increase energy expenditure.
      (2) Increase the consumption of complex carbohydrates and "naturally occurring" sugars from about 28% of energy intake to about 48% of energy intake.
      (3) Reduce the consumption of refined and processed sugars by about 45% to account for about 10% of total energy intake.
      (4) Reduce fat intake to 30% of the total calories.
      (5) Reduce saturated fat consumption to account for about 10% of total energy intake and balance that with polyunsaturated and monounsaturated fats, which should account for about 10% of energy intake each.
      (6) Reduce cholesterol consumption to about 300 mg/day.
      (7) Limit the intake of sodium by reducing the intake of salt to about 5 g/day.
    b. Dietary Guidelines for Americans
      (1) Eat a variety of foods.
      (2) Maintain ideal weight.
      (3) Avoid too much fat, saturated fat, and cholesterol.
      (4) Eat foods with adequate starch and fiber.
      (5) Avoid too much sugar.
      (6) Avoid too much sodium.
      (7) If you drink alcohol, do so in moderation.

---

*Sources: U.S. Senate Select Committee on Nutrition and Human Needs, *Dietary Goals for the United States,* ed. 2, Superintendent of Documents, Washington, DC, 1977.

U.S. Department of Agriculture, Department of Health and Human Services, *Nutrition and Your Health, Dietary Guidelines for Americans,* Superintendent of Documents, Washington, DC, 1980.

6. Increase public awareness of problems and availability of crisis counseling, support groups, and other community resources (e.g., "hot lines," Alcoholics Anonymous, family planning clinics)
7. Evaluate client's understanding of teaching

THE MIDDLE ADULT (45 TO 60 YEARS)
Growth and Development

A. Physiologic development
   1. Greater diversity in physiologic conditioning resulting from established life-style
   2. Early signs of aging (e.g., wrinkling, thinning hair, decreased muscle tone and nerve function)
   3. Decreased BMR with subsequent weight gain unless caloric intake is reduced
   4. Decreased production of sexual hormones
     a. Menopause (see maternity nursing)
     b. Male climacteric; may pass unnoticed, especially in those with high self-esteem; symptoms may include less forceful ejaculation, hot flashes, dizziness, headache, and depression
B. Psychosocial development
   1. Cognitive abilities enhanced because of motivation and past experiences
   2. Resolving developmental crisis of generativity versus stagnation
   3. Adjusting to changes in family caused by aging parents and teenage to adult children
   4. Maintaining satisfactory status of one's career
   5. Accepting physical changes associated with advancing age
   6. Developing social and civic activities that are personally satisfying

Health Promotion

A. Health problems
   1. Cardiovascular disease
   2. Presbyopia
   3. Hypertension
   4. Alcoholism
   5. Sexual dysfunction
   6. Depression
   7. Unbalanced or inadequate diet
B. Nursing care
   1. Reinforce importance of regular exercise
   2. Stress dietary changes: reduction of calories, fats and protein; increased fruits and vegetables
   3. Encourage individuals to identify new interests, and to anticipate and plan for retirement
   4. Emphasize need for regular medical evaluations as well as self-evaluations
   5. Encourage attendance at self-help groups to stop chemical dependency (e.g., smoking, alcohol)
   6. Increase awareness of the relationship between an unbalanced diet and disease
   7. Teach the Dietary Goals for the United States and encourage individuals to follow the Dietary Guidelines for Americans
   8. Evaluate client's understanding of teaching

THE OLDER ADULT (60 TO 75 YEARS)
Growth and Development

A. Physiologic development
   1. Slowing of reaction time
   2. Loss of sensory acuity
   3. Diminished muscle tone and strength
   4. Increased diversity in health status and function resulting from prior life-style and development of chronic health problems
B. Psychosocial development
   1. Cognitive abilities may be affected by cardiovascular disease
   2. Adjusting to retirement: some individuals experience a loss of self-esteem while others enjoy the freedom to explore other interests
   3. Coping with altered economic status; adjusting to fixed income
   4. Resolving death of parents and possibly spouse
   5. Accepting separation from their children and their families

Health Promotion

A. Health problems
   1. Cardiovascular disease
   2. Cancer
   3. Presbyopia
   4. Accidents
   5. Respiratory disease
   6. Sexual dysfunction
   7. Depression
   8. Unbalanced or inadequate diet
   9. Death of spouse
B. Nursing care
   1. Encourage individuals to maintain a schedule of regular medical, dental, and visual examinations to control or prevent health problems
   2. Assess living conditions for possible hazards that could cause accidents
   3. Refer widows and widowers to appropriate self-help groups as necessary
   4. Encourage individuals to anticipate and plan for retirement and to develop new interests and support systems
   5. Encourage nutritional assessment and consultation to prevent nutrient deficiencies and to provide for diet modifications with aging
   6. Teach the Dietary Goals for the United States and encourage individuals to follow the Dietary Guidelines for Americans
   7. Evaluate client's understanding of teaching

THE SENIOR ADULT (75+ YEARS)
Growth and Development

A. Physiologic development
   1. Diminished sensation and reaction time (e.g., narrowed visual field, hearing loss)
   2. Increased sensitivity to cold because of decreased subcutaneous tissue and thyroxin utilization as well as impaired circulation
   3. Decreased enzyme secretion in and motility of the GI tract
   4. Decreased glomerular filtration rate

5. Decreased cardiac output
6. Arteriosclerotic changes with diminished elasticity of blood vessels
7. Decreased lung capacity
8. Demineralization and other degenerative skeletal changes, particularly in weight-bearing bones
9. Muscle atrophy

B. Psychosocial development
1. Cognitive abilities not necessarily affected by age; but may be impaired as a result of disease, leading to diminished awareness
2. Resolving the developmental crisis of ego integrity versus despair
3. Adjusting to the death of important others
4. Adapting to decreased physical capacity and changes in body image
5. Adjusting to the economic burden of a fixed income
6. Recognizing the inevitability of death
7. Reminiscing increasingly about the past

Health Promotion

A. Health problems
1. Cardiovascular disease
2. Cataracts, glaucoma, hearing loss
3. Accidents (e.g., falls resulting in hip fractures)
4. Resistance to changes in environment
5. Respiratory disease
6. Cerebral vascular insufficiency
7. Impaired nutritional intake
8. Cancer
9. Inadequate diet

B. Nursing care
1. Encourage individuals to maintain a schedule of regular medical supervision
2. Assess the individual's ability to cope with the environment
3. Promote maximum degree of independence
4. Initiate appropriate referrals for individuals requiring assistance with activities of daily living
   a. Home health aides
   b. Day-care centers
   c. Nursing homes
   d. Acute care hospitals' outpatient services
5. Open channels of communication for reality orientation, reminiscing, and emotional support
6. Refer to social service and other channels that can provide economic assistance when necessary
7. Ensure that prosthetic devices (e.g., dentures, contact lenses, eye prosthetics, braces, limbs) fit comfortably and do not cause irritation; teach proper care of such devices
8. Encourage individuals to follow the Dietary Guidelines for Americans
9. Evaluate client's understanding of teaching

Infection
REVIEW OF PHYSIOLOGY
Resistance

A. Nonspecific resistance: that directed against all invading microbes; varies considerably from one species to another and even among individuals of same species

1. Body surface barriers
   a. Intact skin and mucosa
   b. Cilia and secretion of mucus
2. Antimicrobial secretions
   a. Oil of skin: contains fatty acids effective against many bacteria and fungi
   b. Tears: contain lysozyme, a bactericidal (gram-positive) enzyme
   c. Gastric juice: contains highly bactericidal hydrochloric acid
   d. Vaginal secretions: low pH acts to inhibit microbial growth
3. Internal antimicrobial agents
   a. Interferon: antiviral substance produced within the cells in response to a viral attack; it inhibits viral growth and multiplication
   b. Properdin: protein agent in blood that destroys certain gram-negative bacteria and viruses
   c. Lysozyme: ubiquitous; destroys mainly gram-positive bacteria
4. Phagocytosis: part of the role of the reticuloendothelial system
   a. Phagocytes: cells in the blood that ingest and destroy microbes
      (1) Microphages: polymorphonuclear leukocytes, of which the neutrophils are the most active; in the inflammatory response they pass through the intact capillary wall (diapedesis) into the intercellular area
      (2) Macrophages
         (a) Fixed (sessile) macrophages: phagocytes lining the capillary endothelium and sinuses of the liver (Kupffer cells), spleen, bone marrow, lymph nodes, and other organs where they remove microbes from the blood
         (b) Wandering macrophages (histiocytes): blood monocytes that enter the tissues (via diapedesis) and devour intercellular debris, including debilitated microphages

B. Specific resistance: that directed against a specific pathogen (foreign protein) or its toxin
1. Antigen: any substance, including allergens, that stimulates production of antibodies when introduced into the body; typically, antigens are foreign proteins, the most potent being microbial cells and their products
   a. B lymphocytes: derived from stem cells and differentiate into plasma cells in the presence of antigens; provides humoral immunity; a specific antigen provokes the production of a specific antibody (homologous antibody), which is considered to be ineffective against any other antigen
   b. T lymphocytes: derived from stem cells and are responsible for cellular immunity; involved in delayed hypersensitivity responses, graft rejection, and AIDS
   c. Memory cells: large population of antibodies that develop on first encounter with an antigen; they become somewhat dormant until stimulated by subsequent encounters with the antigen; this

phenomenon explains the dramatic rise in antibody titer following a booster shot of a vaccine (anamnestic reaction)

2. Antibody: immune substance produced by plasma cells; antibodies are gamma globulin molecules and are commonly referred to as immunoglobulin (Ig)
   a. Chemical structure: made up of four polypeptide chains in two pairs
   b. Classification: there are five major classes of antibodies
      (1) Immunoglobulin G (IgG) antibodies: most important class, making up more than 80% of the total immunoglobulins; only immunoglobulin that passes the placental barrier, providing natural passive immunity to the newborn
      (2) Immunoglobulin A (IgA) antibodies: present in blood, mucus, and human milk secretions; play an important role against respiratory pathogens
      (3) Immunoglobulin M (IgM) antibodies: first antibodies to be detected after an injection of antigen; bactericidal for gram-negative bacteria under specific conditions
      (4) Immunoglobulin D (IgD) antibodies: present in small numbers in normal individuals; specific immunologic role presently under investigation
      (5) Immunoglobulin E (IgE) antibodies: responsible for hypersensitivity and allergies; these antibodies exist tightly bound to the surface of mast cells (large basophilic connective tissue cells)
         (a) Upon introduction of their homologous antigens (allergens), they cause the mast cells to release histamine and other pharmacologic agents
         (b) Release of histamine and other pharmacologic agents causes the symptoms of hypersensitivity reactions
         (c) This process explains relief of symptoms by administration of antihistamines
3. Antigen-antibody reactions
   a. Agglutination: clumping together of cells and specific antigens by homologous antibodies called agglutinins
   b. Cytolysis: disruption or dissolution of cells (lysis) by homologous antibodies called cytolysins or lysins
   c. Opsonification: rendering of bacteria and other cells susceptible to phagocytosis by homologous antibodies called opsonins
   d. Neutralization (viral): rendering of viruses noninfective by homologous antibodies called neutralizing antibodies
   e. Neutralization (toxin): chemical neutralization of a toxin by homologous antibodies called antitoxins
   f. Precipitation: formation of an insoluble complex (precipitate) in the reaction between a soluble antigen and its homologous antibodies called precipitins

4. Complement-fixation: group of blood serum proteins needed in certain antigen-antibody reactions; both the complement and the antibody must be present for a reaction to occur

Immunity

A. Species immunity: certain species are naturally immune to specific microorganisms (e.g., humans are immune to distemper, dogs are immune to measles)
B. Active immunity: antibodies formed in the body
   1. Natural active immunity: antibodies formed by the individual during the course of the disease; in some instances the antibodies provide lifelong immunity (e.g., measles, chickenpox, yellow fever, smallpox)
   2. Artificial active immunity: use of a vaccine or toxoid to stimulate formation of homologous antibodies; revaccination (booster shots) is often needed to sustain antibody titer (anamnestic effect)
      a. Killed vaccines: antigenic preparations containing microbes grown in the laboratory separated from growth medium and killed by heat or a chemical agent; usually injected subcutaneously; less often given by intramuscular or oral routes (e.g., pertussis vaccine, typhoid vaccine)
      b. Live vaccines: antigenic preparations containing microbes weakened (attenuated) by drying, continued and prolonged passage through culture media or animals (to induce mutations), or by other means; typically such vaccines are more antigenic than killed preparations; (e.g., oral [Sabin] poliomyelitis vaccine, measles vaccine)
      c. Toxoids: antigenic preparations composed of inactivated bacterial toxins (generally an exotoxin treated with formaldehyde) (e.g., tetanus toxoids, diphtheria toxoids)
C. Passive immunity: antibodies acquired from an outside source
   1. Natural passive immunity: passage of preformed antibodies from the mother through the placenta or colostrum to the baby; therefore during the first few weeks of life the newborn is immune to certain diseases to which the mother has active immunity
   2. Artificial passive immunity: injection of antisera derived from immunized animals or humans; antisera (antiserums) provide immediate and often complete protection in susceptible exposed persons and also are of value in treatment (e.g., diphtheria antitoxin, tetanus antitoxin); individuals may be hypersensitive to certain sera such as horse serum, and pretesting for hypersensitivity must be carried out before administration

REVIEW OF MICROBIOLOGY
Pathology of Infection

A. Definition: invasion of the body by pathogenic microorganisms (pathogens) and the reaction of the tissues to their presence and to the toxins generated by them
B. Types
   1. Local, focal, or systemic
      a. Local infection: one in which etiologic agent is limited to one locality of the body, such as a boil; often a local infection may have systemic repercussions such as fever and malaise

b. Focal infection: a local infection such as an abscess from which the organisms themselves spread to other parts of body (e.g., a tooth abscess that continues to seed organisms into the blood)

c. Systemic infection: one in which the infectious agent is spread throughout the body (e.g., typhoid fever)

2. Acute or chronic
   a. Acute infection: one that develops rapidly, usually resulting in a high fever and severe sickness
   b. Chronic infection: one that develops slowly, with mild but longer-lasting symptoms; sometimes an acute infection may become chronic and vice versa

3. Primary or secondary
   a. Primary infection: initial infection, unrelated to other health problems
   b. Secondary infection: occasioned when invaders (or opportunists) take advantage of the weakened defenses resulting from the primary infection (e.g., staphylococcal pneumonia as a sequela of measles)

4. Bacteremia: presence of nonmultiplying bacteria in the blood

5. Septicemia: bacterial cells actively multiplying in the blood

6. Toxemia: presence of microbial toxins in the blood

7. Viremia: presence of viruses in the blood

C. Proof of etiology (Koch's postulates): four requirements must be fulfilled to establish a given microbe as the etiologic agent of a given disease
   1. Particular microbe must be found in every case of the particular disease
   2. Particular microbe must be isolated and grown in pure culture
   3. Particular microbe must cause particular disease when inoculated into susceptible animal
   4. Particular microbe must be recovered from inoculated animal and its identity established

D. Source and transmission of pathogens
   1. Source: ultimate source (or reservoir) of almost all pathogens is human or animal; human sources include
      a. Persons exhibiting symptoms of disease
      b. Carriers: persons who harbor a pathogen in the absence of a discernible clinical disease
         (1) Types of carriers
            (a) Healthy carriers: those who have never had the disease in question
            (b) Incubatory carriers: those in the incubation period of a disease
            (c) Chronic carriers: those who have recovered from a disease but continue to harbor pathogens
         (2) Diseases commonly spread by carriers
            (a) Typhoid fever
            (b) Diphtheria
            (c) Meningitis
            (d) Pneumonia
            (e) Dysentery

2. Transmission
   a. Direct
      (1) Body or body fluid contact
      (2) Droplets (droplet infection)
   b. Indirect
      (1) Food
      (2) Water
      (3) Air
      (4) Soil
      (5) Fomites
      (6) Vectors (insects)
         (a) Mechanical transfer: insects' feet
         (b) Biologic transfer: microbe undergoes part of its life cycle in the insect's body

3. Portals of entry and exit
   a. Portal of entry: where microbes enter the body
      (1) Nose
      (2) Mouth
      (3) Urogenital tract
      (4) Skin: wounds, abrasions, and insect bites
   b. Portal of exit: where microbes leave the body
      (1) Nose
      (2) Mouth
      (3) Feces
      (4) Urine
      (5) Vaginal discharges
      (6) Pus and exudates
      (7) Vomitus
      (8) Blood

4. Susceptible host

E. Development
   1. Definitions
      a. Pathogenicity: ability of a microbe to cause disease
      b. Virulence: degree of pathogenicity
   2. Determinants of pathogenicity
      a. Chemical products
         (1) Exotoxins: heat-labile proteins readily released from bacterial cell; most deadly of all biologic poisons (e.g., botulism, tetanus, and diphtheria)
         (2) Endotoxins: heat-stable lipopolysaccharide-protein complexes released from gram-negative bacteria; less deadly than exotoxins (e.g., typhoid fever and dysentery)
         (3) Other toxic products
            (a) Hemolysins: these destroy the red cells (erythrocytes)
            (b) Leukocidins: these destroy the white cells (leukocytes)
            (c) Coagulase: clots blood plasma
            (d) Hyaluronidase: dissolves intercellular cement
            (e) Kinases: dissolve clots or inhibit their formation
            (f) Collagenase: disintegrates collagen
      b. Cellular destruction: some microbes damage tissues and cause disease by direct mechanical injury to the cells, particularly intracellular parasites (e.g., viruses and rickettsiae)
      c. Capsules: increase virulence apparently by making microbes possessing them less vulnerable to destruction by phagocytosis

Bacteria

A. Definition: bacteria are unicellular microbes without chlorophyll
B. Some examples of medically important bacteria
  1. Eubacteriales ("true bacteria"): typically unicellular microbes having a rigid cell wall; the morphologic types are
    a. Rod-shaped bacilli: variations of the rod shape may be curved or clubbed (some of the gram-positive rods form endospores)
    b. Spherical cocci
    c. Eubacteriales are divided into five families based on shape, Gram stain, and endospore formation
      (1) Gram-positive cocci include
        (a) Diplococci: occurring predominantly in pairs (e.g., *Diplococcus pneumoniae*)
        (b) Streptococci: occurring predominantly in chains (e.g., *Streptococcus pyogenes*)
        (c) Staphylococci: occurring predominantly in grapelike bunches (e.g., *Staphylococcus aureus*)
      (2) Gram-negative cocci include *Neisseria gonorrhoeae* and *Neisseria meningitidis*
      (3) Gram-negative rods include enterobacteria such as *Escherichia, Salmonella,* and *Shigella* species
      (4) Gram-positive rods that do not produce endospores include *Corynebacterium diphtheriae*
      (5) Gram-positive rods producing endospores include *Bacillus anthracis, Clostridium botulinum,* and *Clostridium tetani*
  2. Actinomycetales (actinomycetes): moldlike microbes with elongated cells, frequently filamentous (e.g., *Mycobacterium tuberculosis* and *Mycobacterium leprae*)
  3. Spirochaetales (spirochetes): flexuous, spiral organisms (e.g., *Treponema pallidum*)
  4. Mycoplasmatales (mycoplasmas): delicate, nonmotile microbes displaying a variety of sizes and shapes
    a. Commonly referred to as pleuropneumonia-like organisms (PPLO)
    b. Mycoplasmas are the smallest organisms known that are capable of growth and reproduction outside living cells
C. Bacterial cell
  1. Size: from 0.5 to 15 mm
  2. Cell wall: gram-positive species are rich in muramic acid and low in lipids; the opposite is true of the gram-negative species
  3. Capsule: a thickened protective material (generally a polysaccharide) that is secreted by the cell, thereby protecting it from being phagocytized and increasing its virulence (e.g., *Diplococcus pneumoniae*)
  4. Spores: the inactive resistant structures into which bacterial protoplasm can transform under adverse conditions (under favorable conditions a spore germinates into an active and growing vegetative cell)
    a. The endospores are resistant to heat, desiccation, and other antimicrobial agents
    b. Spore formers *Clostridium tetani* and *Clostridium botulinum* are difficult to destroy; therefore their destruction is used to set the standards of sterilization for the hospital and food industries
  5. Flagella: organelles of locomotion possessed by all motile bacteria; some species have one flagellum (monotrichous), whereas others have flagella over their entire surface (peritrichous)
  6. Reproduction: bacteria reproduce by binary fission, an asexual process dividing the cell into new daughter cells; bacteria are also able to conjugate and exchange genetic material (recombination)
D. Growth needs
  1. Nutrition
    a. Autotrophic organisms: may do well on simple diet of carbon dioxide, inorganic salts, and water
    b. Heterotrophic organisms: demand organic nutrients
      (1) Saprophytes: derive nourishment from dead or decaying organic matter
      (2) Parasites: derive nourishment from living tissue; obligate parasites cannot be cultured except in living tissue
  2. Culturing
    a. Culture: growth of large numbers of microbes on suitable food media
    b. Culture media: food substances in or on which cultures are grown (e.g., broth, agar, milk)
    c. Colony: cluster of millions of microbes, presumably all descendants from a single bacterium, visible to naked eye
    d. Ways in which cultures are studied
      (1) Smears made and organisms studied microscopically either with or without staining
      (2) Cultural characteristics observed
        (a) Media most favorable to growth
        (b) Appearance of colonies: color, shape, and texture, whether large or small, smooth or rough, opaque or translucent
        (c) Molecular oxygen requirement: anaerobic, aerobic, or facultative
E. Biochemical reactions
  1. Fermentation: anaerobic oxidation reactions by which some organisms use carbohydrates to generate energy-rich adenosine triphosphate (ATP) molecules; various kinds of fermentation reactions are useful for identifying different groups of microorganisms
    a. Nonfermenters
    b. Fermenters that produce only acid
    c. Fermenters that produce acid and gas (e.g., *Escherichia coli,* a normal inhabitant of the intestinal tract)
    d. Lactose fermenters (e.g., *Escherichia coli* and other nonpathogens in the intestinal tract)
    e. Nonlactose fermenters (e.g., *Shigella* and *Salmonella* pathogens in the intestinal tract)
  2. Urea-splitting reaction: identifies organisms as
    a. Urease-positive organisms (contain enzyme urease, which catalyzes conversion of urea to ammonia) (e.g., *Proteus bacilli* [gram-negative, normal inhabitants of the intestinal tract])

b. Urease-negative organisms: do not contain urease so cannot convert urea to ammonia (e.g., *Salmonella* and *Shigella,* pathogens in the intestinal tract)

F. Hydrogen ion concentration (pH): majority of bacteria grow and are cultured best at a pH of about 7.5; most fungi (molds and yeasts) are cultured best at a pH of about 5

G. Oxygen utilization
  1. Obligate aerobes: organisms that cannot grow without free (molecular) oxygen
  2. Obligate anaerobes: organisms that cannot grow in the presence of free (molecular) oxygen
  3. Facultative: organisms that can grow with or without free oxygen

H. Temperature
  1. Psychrophiles: organisms growing best at low temperatures (50° to 68° F [10° to 20° C])
  2. Mesophiles: organisms growing best at "middle temperatures" (68° to 113° F [20° to 45° C]); this range includes human pathogens that have an optimum temperature of 98.6 ° F (37° C)
  3. Thermophiles: organisms growing best at high temperatures (113° to 149° F [45° to 65° C])

I. Staining: artificial coloration to facilitate visualization and identification of tissues and microorganisms
  1. Gram stain: gram-positive organisms retain the crystal violet color when treated with ethyl alcohol; gram-negative organisms are decolorized with ethyl alcohol
  2. Acid-fast stain: after being stained with carbolfuchsin, acid-fast organisms resist decolorization with dilute acid alcohol and do not take counterstain (usually methylene blue); non-acid-fast organisms decolorize and take counterstain

J. Pathogenicity: some 2,000 species of bacteria, most of which are harmless; those causing disease (pathogens) are usually heterotrophic mesophiles

Viruses

A. Definition: obligate intracellular parasite of unknown relationship to other forms of life

B. Characteristics: virions (virus particles)—range in size from 1 to 350 nanometers (nm); 1 nm equals 1 billionth of a meter or $\frac{1}{1000}$ of a millimeter; some cuboidal and others rod shaped; unlike rickettsiae and chlamydiae, composed of either ribonucleic acid (RNA) or deoxyribonucleic acid (DNA), not both

C. Classification
  1. Animal viruses: some contain RNA and others DNA; divided into 14 categories on the basis of particle size, symmetry, and nucleic acid content
  2. Plant viruses: contain RNA
  3. Bacterial viruses: most contain DNA; those which destroy bacterial cells called bacteriophages

D. Culturing: being obligate parasites, viruses demand living tissues such as embryonated hen's eggs, tissue cultures, and animal inoculation

E. Pathogenicity: viruses cause cancer in animals and Burkitt's lymphoma, mumps, rubeola, rubella, smallpox, chickenpox, herpes simplex, encephalitis, yellow fever, AIDS, and many other infections in humans

Fungi

A. Definition: higher protists; include morels, truffles, cup fungi, mildews, mushrooms, puffballs, smuts, rusts, molds, and yeasts (molds and yeasts are of medical concern)

B. Molds: fuzzy growths of interlacing filaments called hyphae
  1. Hyphae: filaments of a mold; in some species hyphae are divided by partial septa and appear to be multicellular, whereas in others they are nonseptate
  2. Mycelium: tuft of interwoven hyphae
  3. Spores: means by which molds reproduce; a single spore in the proper environment gives rise to a new mycelium; spores produced sexually and asexually

C. Yeasts: organisms that usually are single celled and usually reproduce by budding
  1. Yeast cell: round or ovoid and much larger and more complex than bacterial cell
  2. Reproduction: usually by the asexual process of budding, but many species also reproduce sexually by means of ascospores
  3. True yeasts: reproduce sexually as well as asexually (by budding); many species, such as *Saccharomyces cerevisiae* (baker's yeast), convert glucose into alcohol and carbon dioxide (alcoholic fermentation); *Candida albicans,* another type of yeast, causes "thrush" in humans (this yeast is part of the normal flora but may become an opportunistic pathogen in persons with low resistance)
  4. Pathogenicity: certain species of molds cause infection, particularly those belonging to the class Fungi Imperfecti (Deuteromycetes), which account for diseases such as athlete's foot, ringworm of the scalp and axillary regions, and systemic mycosis

PHYSICAL AND CHEMICAL CONTROL OF MICROORGANISMS
Basic Concepts

A. Disinfection: removal or destruction of pathogenic microbes

B. Sterilization: removal or destruction of all microbes

Physical Methods

A. Heat sterilization
  1. Moist heat
    a. Steam under pressure (autoclave): usually operated at 250° F (121° C) (15 lb pressure per square inch); time needed for procedure depends on material(s) being sterilized
    b. Boiling water: object(s) to be sterilized immersed in water and boiled for 15 minutes; because some spores resist boiling, this procedure is not suitable for surgical instruments
  2. Dry heat (hot-air oven)
    a. Operating temperature: 310° to 338° F (160° to 170° C) (usually for 2 hours)
    b. Items sterilized: petrolatum gauze dressings and other items that might be damaged by steam or water
  3. Pasteurization: disinfection of milk and other substances by moderate heat; pathogenic organisms

killed and microbial development considerably delayed (thus retarding spoilage)
  a. Holding method: heating to 145° F (63° C) for 30 minutes, followed by rapid cooling
  b. Flash method: heating to 161° F (71.7° C) for not less than 15 seconds, followed by rapid cooling
B. Radiation: all types of radiation injurious to microbes
  1. Gamma rays: used to sterilize food and drugs
  2. Ultraviolet light: used to inhibit the microbial population of air in operating rooms, nurseries, laboratories, school rooms, and food establishments (the disadvantage of ultraviolet light is that it has little penetration power)
C. Filtration: removal of microbes from liquids by means of porous materials (diatomaceous earth, porcelain); used to sterilize drugs, culture media, and certain other heat-sensitive substances
D. Refrigeration: low temperature inhibits microbial multiplication; used for food preservation
E. Hypertonicity: by their osmotic effects hypertonic solutions inhibit microbial multiplication (e.g., brine and syrups)
F. Desiccation (drying): removal of water; bacterial spores and certain vegetable cells are resistant to such treatment; commonly used in food preservation

Chemical Agents (for Body Surfaces and Inanimate Objects)

A. Definitions: many terms used to describe action of chemical agents on microorganisms; in actual practice such terms often have little meaning because of variables
  1. Antiseptic: inhibits microbial growth
  2. Disinfectant: destroys pathogenic microbes
  3. Germicide: destroys pathogenic microbes
  4. Bactericide: destroys bacteria
  5. Fungicide: destroys fungi
  6. Viricide: destroys viruses
B. Conditions (variables) affecting action of chemical agents
  1. Type and number of microbes: microbes respond differently to different agents; spores are resistant to most agents
  2. Concentration: typically the greater the concentration of chemical, the greater the effect
  3. Time: a certain time needed for maximum effect
  4. Temperature: a rise usually hastens action
  5. Organic matter: presence inhibits action
C. Evaluation: various tests used to evaluate antiseptics and disinfectants; all have limitations
  1. Phenol coefficient: bactericidal activity of a chemical agent in relation to the bactericidal action of phenol
  2. Culture inhibition: filter paper disks impregnated or saturated with chemical agent placed on agar plates previously inoculated with test organism; clear zone observed around disk (following incubation) if agent is inhibitory to organism (this is the same procedure used in determining the sensitivity of a culture to chemotherapeutic agents)
D. Commonly used chemical agents
  1. Ethyl alcohol (70%)
  2. Isopropyl alcohol (80%)
  3. Benzalkonium chloride (Zephiran) (1:1000)
  4. Hydrogen peroxide (3%)
  5. Silver nitrate (1%)
  6. Iodine and iodine-releasing compounds
  7. Chlorine and chlorine-releasing compounds
  8. Substituted phenols
  9. Cresols
  10. Ethylene oxide

PHARMACOLOGICAL CONTROL OF INFECTION
Definition of Terms
A. Bactericidal effect: capable of destroying bacteria at low concentrations (e.g., disrupt building of cell membrane or wall, allow leak of cytoplasm)
B. Bacteriostatic effect: slows reproduction of bacteria; natural physiologic mechanisms are required for phagocytic abolition of the bacteria
C. Superinfection: emergence of microorganism growth (e.g., yeast and fungi) when natural protective flora is destroyed by antiinfective drug
D. Bacterial resistance: a natural characteristic of an organism or one acquired by mutation preventing destruction by a drug to which it was previously susceptible

Antibiotics
A. Description
  1. Drugs derived from compounds of living origin that are used to destroy bacteria (bactericidal effect) or inhibit bacterial reproduction (bacteriostatic effect); the net result is to control infection and restore homeostasis to the human organism
  2. Available in oral, parenteral (IM, IV), and topical, including ophthalmic, preparations
B. Antibiotic sensitivity: determined by two general techniques
  1. Paper disks: multilobed disk impregnated with different antibiotics placed on surface of inoculated plate; zones of inhibition (following incubation) surround lobes containing antibiotics to which microbe is sensitive
  2. Tube dilution: antibiotic in question diluted out in growth broth and tubes then inoculated with the organisms in question; minimal inhibitory concentration (MIC) determined (following incubation) by noting minimal concentration preventing growth
C. Examples
  1. Penicillins: interfere with bacterial cell wall synthesis; broad spectrum
    a. amoxicillin (Amoxil)
    b. ampicillin (Omnipen)
    c. carbenicillin (Geopen)
    d. methicillin (Staphcillin)
    e. nafcillin sodium (Unipen)
    f. penicillin G potassium (Pentids)
    g. penicillin G procaine (Wycillin)
    h. penicillin V (V-Cillin)
  2. Cephalosporins: interfere with bacterial cell wall synthesis; broad spectrum
    a. cefazolin sodium (Ancef, Kefzol)
    b. cephalexin monohydrate (Keflex)
    c. cephalothin sodium (Keflin)

3. Erythromycins: along with similar drugs, inhibit mRNA synthesis of bacterial protein
   a. clindamycin HC1 (Cleocin)
   b. erythromycin (E-mycin)
   c. lincomycin HC1 (Lincocin)
4. Tetracyclines: inhibit bacterial protein synthesis by blocking tRNA attachment to ribosomes; broad spectrum
   a. chlortetracycline HC1 (Aureomycin)
   b. demeclocycline (Declomycin)
   c. doxycycline (Vibramycin)
   d. oxytetracycline (Terramycin)
   e. tetracycline (Achromycin, Sumycin)
5. Aminoglycocides: disrupt bacterial protein synthesis by providing a substitute for essential nucleotide required by mRNA; broad spectrum
   a. gentamicin sulfate (Garamycin)
   b. kanamycin sulfate (Kantrex)
   c. neomycin sulfate (Mycifradin)
   d. streptomycin sulfate
   e. tobramycin sulfate (Nebcin)
6. Polymyxin group: decreases bacterial cell membrane permeability
   a. colistimethate sodium (Coly-Mycin M)
   b. polymyxin B sulfate (Aerosporin)
7. Chloramphenicol: inhibits bacterial protein synthesis by interfering with mRNA activity; broad spectrum
   a. Chloromycetin
   b. Mychel

D. Major side effects
1. Depressed appetite (altered taste sensitivity)
2. Nausea, vomiting (normal flora imbalance)
3. Diarrhea (normal flora imbalance)
4. Suppressed absorption of a variety of nutrients including fat; protein; lactose; vitamins A, D, K, and B_{12}; and the minerals calcium, iron, and potassium (normal flora imbalance)
5. Increased excretion of water-soluble vitamins and minerals (normal flora imbalance)
6. Superinfection (normal flora imbalance)
7. Allergic reactions, anaphylaxis (hypersensitivity)
8. Nephrotoxicity (direct kidney toxic effect)
9. Tetracyclines
   a. Hepatotoxicity (direct liver toxic effect)
   b. Phototoxicity (degradation to toxic products by ultraviolet rays)
   c. Hyperuricemia (impaired kidney function)
   d. Enamel hypoplasia, dental caries, and bone defects in children under 8 years of age (drug binds to calcium in tissue)
10. Aminoglycosides
    a. Ototoxicity (direct auditory [8th cranial] nerve toxic effect)
    b. Leukopenia (decreased WBC synthesis)
    c. Thrombocytopenia (decreased platelet synthesis)
    d. Headache (neurotoxicity)
    e. Confusion (neurotoxicity)
    f. Peripheral neuropathy (neurotoxicity)
    g. Optic neuritis (irritation of optic [2nd cranial] nerve)
    h. Respiratory paralysis (neuromuscular blockade)

E. Nursing care
1. Assess client for history of drug allergy
2. Instruct client regarding
   a. How to take the drug (frequency, relation to meals)
   b. How to dispose of unused drugs
   c. Completing the prescribed course of therapy
   d. Symptoms of allergic response
   e. Side effects, including superinfection; suggest ingestion of yogurt or food supplements containing *Lactobacillus acidophilus* where dairy products cannot be tolerated; suggest nutritional consultation where drug therapy may impact on client's nutritional status
3. Shake liquid suspensions to thoroughly mix
4. Administer most preparations 1 hour before meals or 2 hours after meals for best absorption
5. Assess vital signs during course of therapy
6. Cephalosporins: use Clinistix or Tes-Tape for urine testing; false positive results have occurred with Clinitest, Fehling's, and Benedict's solution
7. Tetracyclines
   a. Avoid use during last half of pregnancy or by children younger than 8 years of age
   b. Assess for potentiation of oral anticoagulant effect
8. Aminoglycosides and polymyxins: assess for potentiation of neuromuscular blocking agent, general anesthetic, or parenterally administered magnesium effects
9. Chloramphenicol
   a. Assess blood work before and during therapy
   b. Assess for potentiation of phenytoin, oral antidiabetic agent, and coumarin anticoagulant effects
10. Evaluate client's response to medication and understanding of teaching

Antiviral Agents

A. Description
1. Used to provide prophylaxis when exposure to viral infection has occurred
2. Prevent entrance of the virus into host cells
3. Available in oral, parenteral (IV), and topical, including ophthalmic, preparations

B. Examples
1. acyclovir sodium (Zovirax)
2. amantadine HCl (Symmetrel)
3. idoxuridine (Stoxil)
4. methisazone (Marboran)
5. vidarabine (Vira-A)

C. Major side effects
1. CNS stimulation (direct CNS effect)
2. Orthostatic hypotension (depressed cardiovascular system)
3. Dizziness (hypotension)
4. Constipation (decreased peristalsis)
5. Nephrotoxicity (direct kidney toxic effect)
6. Local irritation (direct local tissue effect)

D. Nursing care
1. Assess vital signs during course of therapy
2. Support natural defense mechanisms of client; encourage intake of foods rich in the immune-stimu-

lating nutrients, such as vitamins A, C, and E, and the minerals selenium and zinc
3. Encourage intake of high fiber foods to reduce potential of constipation
4. Monitor disease symptoms and laboratory data
5. Evaluate client's response to medication and understanding of teaching

Sulfonamides

A. Description
1. Antiinfective drugs used primarily to treat urinary tract infections
2. Act by substituting a false metabolite for paraaminobenzoic acid (PABA) required in the bacterial synthesis of folic acid
3. Available in oral, parenteral (IM, SC, IV), and topical, including ophthalmic, preparations
B. Examples
1. succinylsulfathiazole (Sulfasuxidine)
2. sulfasalazine (Azulfidine)
3. sulfamethizole (Thiosulfil)
4. sulfamethoxazole (Gantanol)
5. sulfisoxazole (Gantrisin)
6. Combination product: sulfamethoxazole and trimethoprim (Bactrim, Septra)
C. Major side effects
1. Nausea, vomiting; decreased absorption of folacin (irritation of gastric mucosa)
2. Skin rash (hypersensitivity)
3. Malaise (decreased RBC)
4. Blood dyscrasias (decreased RBC, WBC, platelet synthesis)
5. Crystalluria (drug precipitation in acidic urine)
6. Stomatitis (GI irritation)
7. Headache (CNS effect)
8. Photosensitivity (hypersensitivity)
9. Allergic response, anaphylaxis (hypersensitivity)
D. Nursing care
1. Assess client for history of drug allergy
2. Promote increased fluid intake
3. Caution client to avoid direct exposure to sunlight
4. Assess vital signs during course of therapy
5. Maintain alkaline urine
6. Monitor blood work during therapy; potential for megaloblastic anemia due to folacin deficiency
7. Assess for potentiation of oral anticoagulant and oral hypoglycemic effects
8. Evaluate client's response to medication and understanding of teaching

Antitubercular Agents

A. Description
1. Used to treat tuberculosis
2. Administered in combination (first-line and second-line drugs) over a prolonged time period to reduce the possibility of mycobacterial drug resistance
3. Available in oral and parenteral (IM) preparations
B. Examples
1. First-line drugs
   a. ethambutol (Myambutol): interferes with mycobacterial RNA synthesis
   b. isoniazid (INH, Nydrazid): interferes with mycobacterial cell wall synthesis
   c. paraaminosalicylic acid preparations (PAS): interferes with mycobacterial folic acid synthesis
   d. rifampin (Rifadin): interferes with mycobacterial RNA synthesis
   e. streptomycin sulfate: inhibits mycobacterial protein synthesis
2. Second-line drugs: inhibit mycobacterial cell metabolism
   a. capreomycin (Capastat)
   b. cycloserine (Seromycin)
   c. ethionamide (Trecator SC)
   d. pyrazinamide (PZA)
C. Major side effects
1. Gastrointestinal irritation (direct tissue irritation)
2. Suppressed absorption of fat and B complex vitamins, especially folacin and B_{12}; depletion of vitamin B_6 by isoniazid
3. Dizziness (CNS effect)
4. CNS disturbances (direct CNS toxic effect)
5. Liver disturbances (direct liver toxic effect)
6. Blood dyscrasias (decreased RBC, WBC, platelet synthesis)
7. Streptomycin: ototoxicity (direct auditory [8th cranial] nerve toxic effect)
8. Ethambutol: visual disturbances (direct optic [2nd cranial] nerve toxic effect)
D. Nursing care
1. Support natural defense mechanisms of client; encourage intake of foods rich in the immune-stimulating nutrients such as vitamins A, C, and E, and the minerals selenium and zinc
2. Obtain cultures of all body discharge specimens
3. Monitor blood work during therapy
4. Instruct the client to take the drugs regularly as prescribed; reinforce need for medical supervision
5. Offer client emotional support during therapy
6. Utilize safety precautions (supervise ambulation) if CNS effects are manifested
7. Instruct client regarding nutritional side effects and encourage foods rich in B complex vitamins
8. Encourage client to avoid use of alcohol during therapy
9. ethambutol: encourage frequent visual exams
10. rifampin: instruct clients that body fluids may appear orange-red
11. streptomycin: encourage frequent auditory exams
12. Evaluate client's response to medication and understanding of teaching

Antifungals

A. Description
1. Used to treat systemic and localized fungal infections
2. Act to either destroy fungal cells (fungicidal) or inhibit the reproduction of fungal cells (fungistatic)
3. Available in oral, parenteral (IV), topical, vaginal, and intrathecal preparations
B. Examples
1. amphotericin B (Fungizone): disrupts fungal cell membrane permeability
2. griseofulvin (Grisactin): disrupts fungal nucleic acid synthesis

3. nystatin (Mycostatin, Nilstat): disrupts fungal cell membrane permeability
C. Major side effects
   1. Nausea, vomiting (irritation to gastric mucosa)
   2. Headache (neurotoxicity)
   3. Fever, chills (blood dyscrasias)
   4. Paresthesia (neurotoxicity)
D. Nursing care
   1. Assess vital signs during course of therapy
   2. Review proper method of application with client
   3. Amphotericin B
      a. Utilize infusion control device for IV administration
      b. Protect solution from light during IV infusion
      c. Monitor blood work during therapy; potential hypokalemia as well as increased urinary excretion of magnesium
   4. Griseofulvin
      a. Assess for antagonism of oral anticoagulant effect
      b. Instruct client to avoid direct exposure to sunlight
   5. Topical preparations
      a. Instruct client to wash drug-stained clothing with soap and water
      b. Instruct client to report signs of local irritation
   6. Evaluate client's response to medication and understanding of teaching

Antiparasitics

A. Description
   1. Used to treat parasitic diseases
   2. Act by interfering with parasite metabolism and reproduction; helminthic (pinworm and tapeworm) as well as protozoal (amebiasis and malaria) infestations respond well to this class of drugs
   3. Available in oral, parenteral (IM, SC, IV), vaginal, and rectal preparations
B. Examples
   1. Anthelmintics
      a. mebendazole (Vermox)
      b. piperazine
      c. pyrvinium pamoate (Povan)
   2. Amebicides
      a. chloroquine HCl (Aralen)
      b. emetine HCl
      c. metronidazole (Flagyl)
   3. Antimalarials
      a. chloroquine HCl (Aralen)
      b. hydroxychloroquine sulfate (Plaquenil)
      c. primaquine phosphate
      d. pyrimethamine (Daraprim)
      e. quinine sulfate
C. Major side effects
   1. Anthelmintics
      a. Gastrointestinal irritation (direct tissue irritation)
      b. CNS disturbances (neurotoxicity)
      c. Skin rash (hypersensitivity)
   2. Amebicides
      a. Gastrointestinal irritation (direct tissue irritation)
      b. Blood dyscrasias (decreased RBC, WBC, platelet synthesis)
      c. Skin rash (hypersensitivity)

d. Headache (neurotoxicity)
e. Dizziness (CNS effect)
   3. Antimalarials
      a. Nausea, vomiting (irritation to gastric mucosa)
      b. Blood dyscrasias (decreased RBC, WBC)
      c. Visual disturbances (impairment of accommodation; retinal and corneal changes)
D. Nursing care
   1. Administer drug with meals to decrease GI irritability
   2. Assess vital signs during course of therapy
   3. Monitor blood work during therapy
   4. Instruct client regarding proper hygiene to prevent spread of disease
   5. Utilize safety precautions (supervise ambulation) if CNS effects are manifested
   6. Antimalarials: encourage frequent visual exams
   7. Evaluate client's response to medication and understanding of teaching

NURSING CARE TO PREVENT INFECTION

A. Recognize chain of infection (see Source and transmission of pathogens under Pathology of infection)
   1. Microorganism or etiologic agent
   2. Source or reservoir
   3. Portal of exit from host
   4. Mode of transmission
   5. Portal of entry to body
   6. Susceptible host
B. Utilize principles of asepsis
   1. Medical asepsis
      a. Denotes absence of infectious organisms (pathogens)
      b. Limits the growth and spread of microorganisms by confining them to a specific area
      c. Contamination occurs if pathogens are transferred to a previously clean site or article
   2. Surgical asepsis
      a. Denotes absence of all microorganisms and spores
      b. Prevents microorganisms from entering a specific area
      c. Contamination occurs if a sterile article
         (1) Touches an unsterile article
         (2) Is placed beyond a one inch inside border of a sterile field
         (3) Is below waist level
         (4) Is beyond the field of vision
         (5) Rests on a wet permeable surface which enables contamination by capillary action
         (6) Is exposed to airborne microorganisms
C. Employ specific actions
   1. Limit or eliminate the microbiological agent
      a. Culture and sensitivity testing to identify the causative agent and appropriate antimicrobial therapy
      b. Disinfection and sterilization (see Physical and chemical control of microorganisms)
      c. Administration of antimicrobial agents (see Pharmacological control of infection)

Table 3-1. Isolation categories

Type of isolation (specific category)	Purpose	Example of disease or condition	Room
Strict	Prevents transmission of highly contagious or virulent infections spread by air and contact	Chickenpox; diphtheria	Private room with door closed
Contact	Prevents transmission of highly transmissible infections spread by close or direct contact, which do not warrant strict precautions	Acute respiratory infections in infants and young children; impetigo; herpes simplex; infections by multiple resistant bacteria	Private room; clients infected with same organism may share a room
Respiratory	Prevents transmission of infectious diseases over short distances via air droplets	Measles; meningitis; mumps; pneumonia; *Haemophilus* influenza (in children)	Private room; clients infected with same organism may share a room
Enteric precautions	Prevents infections transmitted by direct or indirect contact with feces	Cholera; diarrhea of an infectious cause; hepatitis A; gastroenteritis caused by highly infectious organism	Private room if client's hygiene is poor (does not wash hands, shares contaminated items); clients with same organism may share a room
Tuberculosis isolation	Special category for clients with pulmonary tuberculosis who have positive results on sputum or chest x-ray examination indicating active disease	Laryngeal tuberculosis	Private room with special ventilation preferred; door closed
Drainage/secretion precautions	Prevents infections transmitted by direct or indirect contact with purulent material or drainage from an infected body site	Abscess; burn infection; infected wound; minor infections not included in contact isolation	Private room not indicated
Universal blood and body fluid precautions*	Transmitted by direct or indirect contact with infective blood or body fluids	Acquired immune deficiency syndrome (AIDS); hepatitis B; syphilis	Private room indicated if client's hygiene is poor
Care of severely compromised clients†	Protects an uninfected client with lowered immunity and resistance from acquiring infectious organisms	Leukemia; lymphoma; aplastic anemia	Private room with door closed

From Potter PA, and Perry AG: Fundamentals of nursing, ed. 2, St. Louis, 1989, The CV Mosby Co.
*Formerly blood and body fluid precautions.
†Formerly protective or reverse isolation.

2. Prevent transmission (see Table 3-1)
   a. Employ handwashing techniques
      (1) Before client contact or procedures; after client contact; after handling contaminated material
      (2) Use friction, soap and warm water to loosen and remove microorganisms
   b. Use barriers such as gowns, gloves, and masks to protect personnel caring for infected clients or to protect susceptible clients against microbiological hazards in the environment
   c. Correctly dispose of contaminated material
      (1) Use impervious bags or double bagging technique to dispose of contaminated material
      (2) Do not recap or break needles after administering injections; use rigid container for disposal
   d. Use blood/body fluid precautions with all clients to prevent the spread of undiagnosed infections

3. Decrease host susceptibility
   a. Use hygienic practices to maintain skin and mucous membranes as first line of defense
   b. Reinforce or maintain natural protective mechanisms such as coughing, pH of secretions, resident flora
   c. Maintain nutrition and encourage rest and sleep to promote tissue repair and production of lymphocytes and antibodies
   d. Educate client about immunizations
D. Evaluate client's understanding regarding treatment, including teaching about transmission, protection of self and others, and self-care

Fluid, Electrolyte, and Acid-Base Balance
FLUID AND ELECTROLYTE BALANCE
Basic Concepts

A. Total volume of fluid and total amount of electrolytes in body normally remain relatively constant
B. Volume of blood plasma, interstitial fluid, and intracellular fluid and the concentration of electrolytes in each remain relatively constant

Gown	Gloves	Mask	Precautions
Required of all persons entering room	Required of all persons entering room	Required of all persons entering room	Discard or bag and label articles contaminated with infective materials. Send reusable articles for disinfection and sterilization.
Indicated if soiling or contact is likely	Indicated for persons touching infective material	Indicated for persons coming close to client	Discard or bag and label articles contaminated with infective material. Send reusable items for disinfection and sterilization.
Not indicated	Not indicated	Indicated for persons who come close to client	Discard or bag and label articles contaminated with infective material. Send reusable items for disinfection and sterilization. Bathroom should not be shared by clients.
Indicated if soiling is likely	Indicated when touching infective material	Not indicated	Discard or bag and label articles contaminated with infective material. Send reusable items for disinfection and sterilization. Bathroom should not be shared by clients.
Indicated only if needed to prevent gross contamination of clothing	Not indicated	Indicated only if client is coughing and does not reliably cover mouth	Articles are rarely involved in transmission of tuberculosis. Articles should be thoroughly cleansed, disinfected, or discarded.
Indicated if soiling or contact with infective material is likely	Indicated for touching infective material	Not indicated	Discard or bag and label articles contaminated with infective material. Send for disinfection or sterilization.
Indicated during procedures that are likely to generate splashes of blood or body fluids	Indicated for touching blood or body fluids, mucous membranes or nonintact skin of all clients; indicated for touching soiled items	Indicated during procedures likely to generate droplets of blood	Discard or bag and label articles contaminated with blood or body fluids. Disinfect and sterilize articles. Avoid needle stick injuries. Dispose of used needles in properly labeled, puncture-resistant container. Clean blood spills promptly with 5.25% solution of sodium hypochloride diluted 1:10 with water
Required of all persons entering room	Required of all persons entering room	Indicated for persons coming in contact with client	For open wound or burns, use sterile gloves.

C. Fluid balance and electrolyte balance are interdependent
D. Intake must equal output
E. Fluid and electrolyte balance maintained primarily by mechanisms that adjust output to intake; secondarily by mechanisms that adjust intake to output
F. Fluid balance is also maintained by a physical mechanism that controls movement of water between fluid compartments (osmosis)
G. The average adult male (68 kg) (150 lb) contains about 40 L of water, comprising 60% of his body weight; 25 L intracellular, 15 to 17 L extracellular
H. Extracellular fluid divided among
  1. Interstitial fluid: 10 to 12 L
  2. Plasma: 3 L
  3. Small fluid compartments: 1 L (e.g., cerebrospinal fluid, aqueous humor, serous and synovial fluid, lymphatic channels)
  4. Gastrointestinal tract: 1 L at any given time for all gastrointestinal organs

I. All body fluids are related and mix well with each other: plasma becomes interstitial fluid as it filters across the capillary wall; interstitial fluid can return to the capillary by osmosis or enter lymphatic channels, becoming lymph; interstitial fluid and intracellular fluid are in osmotic equilibrium across the cell membranes, regulated by the sodium ion (Na^+) concentration of interstitial fluid and the potassium ion (K^+) concentration of intracellular fluid
  1. Mechanism of fluid flow between plasma and interstitial fluid involves several forces
    a. Blood hydrostatic pressure
    b. Blood osmotic pressure
    c. Interstitial fluid hydrostatic pressure
    d. Interstitial fluid osmotic pressure
  2. Blood hydrostatic pressure, interstitial fluid osmotic pressure, and interstitial fluid hydrostatic pressure (normally a negative value) tend to move fluid out of the blood in the capillaries and into the interstitial fluid

3. Blood osmotic pressure moves fluid back into the capillary blood from the interstitial fluid
4. Starling's law of the capillaries states that equal amounts of water move back and forth between blood and interstitial fluid only when the blood hydrostatic pressure plus the interstitial fluid *osmotic* pressure equals the blood osmotic pressure; under these conditions fluid balance exists between the blood and interstitial fluid
   a. Blood gains liquid from interstitial fluid whenever the blood hydrostatic pressure plus the interstitial fluid hydrostatic pressure plus the interstitial fluid osmotic pressure is less than the blood osmotic pressure
   b. Blood loses liquid to interstitial fluid whenever blood osmotic pressure is less than blood hydrostatic pressure plus interstitial fluid hydrostatic pressure plus interstitial fluid osmotic pressure
J. Chemically, extracellular fluid and intracellular fluid are strikingly different: sodium is the main cation of extracellular fluid; potassium is the main cation of intracellular fluid; chloride is the main anion of extracellular fluid; phosphate is the main anion of intracellular fluid; protein concentration is much higher in intracellular fluid than in interstitial fluid (see Table 3-2)
K. Chemically, plasma and interstitial fluid are almost identical except that plasma contains slightly more electrolytes, considerably more proteins, somewhat more sodium, and fewer chloride ions than interstitial fluid (see Table 3-2)

Major Ions (Electrolytes)

A. Cations (+)
   1. Sodium (Na^+)
      a. Most abundant cation in extracellular fluid
      b. Sodium pump in most body cells pumps sodium out of intracellular fluid
      c. Regulates cell size by osmotically drawing water from the cells to balance flow of water into the cells due to osmotically active intracellular proteins
      d. Action potential of nervous and muscle fibers requires sodium; sodium is basic to the body's communication system

   e. Helps to regulate acid-base balance by exchanging hydrogen ions for sodium ions in the kidney tubules; excess hydrogen ions (acid) are excreted
   2. Potassium (K^+)
      a. Most abundant cation of intracellular fluid
      b. Potassium pump brings potassium into cells of the body
      c. Resting polarization and repolarization of nerve and muscle fibers depend on potassium
         (1) If potassium concentration of extracellular fluid rises above normal (hyperkalemia), the force of the contracting heart weakens; with extremely high concentrations the heart will not contract
         (2) If potassium concentration of extracellular fluid drops below normal (hypokalemia), the resting polarization in nerve and muscle fibers increases, resulting in weakness and eventual paralysis
   3. Calcium (Ca^{++})
      a. Forms salts with phosphates, carbonate, and fluoride in bones and teeth to make them hard
      b. Required for correct functioning of nerves and muscles
         (1) If calcium concentrations rise above normal levels (hypercalcemia), nervous system becomes depressed and sluggish
         (2) If calcium concentrations fall below normal levels (hypocalcemia), nervous system becomes extremely excitable, resulting in cramps and tetany
      c. Calcium is required for blood clotting, acting as a cofactor in the formation of prothrombin activator and thrombin
   4. Magnesium (Mg^{++})
      a. Cofactor for many enzymes involved in energy metabolism
      b. Normal constituent of bone
B. Anions (−)
   1. Chloride (Cl^-)
      a. Most abundant anion in extracellular fluid
      b. In great part balances sodium
      c. Major component of gastric secretions

Table 3-2. Average concentrations of major ions in extracellular and intracellular fluids (usually expressed in milliosmols per liter [mOsm/L] of H_2O)

Ion	Intracellular fluid	Extracellular fluid	
		Plasma	Interstitial
Na^+	10	144.0	137.0
K^+	141	5.0	4.7
Cl^-	4	107.0	112.7
HCO_3^-	10	27.0	28.3
Ca^{++}	0	2.5	2.4
Mg^{++}	31	1.5	1.4
$SO_4^=$	1	0.5	0.5
Phosphates ($H_2PO_4^-$; $HPO_4^=$)	11	2.0	2.0
Proteins	4	1.2	0.2

2. Bicarbonate (HCO_3^-)
   a. Part of bicarbonate buffer system
   b. Reacts with a strong acid to form carbonic acid and a basic salt, thus limiting the drop in pH
3. Phosphate ($H_2PO_4^-$ and $HPO_4^=$)
   a. Part of phosphate buffer system
   b. Functions in cellular energy metabolism: phosphate + ADP → ATP (the energy currency of the cell)
   c. Combines with calcium ions in bone, providing hardness
   d. Involved in structure of genetic material, DNA and RNA

Major Avenues by which Water Enters and Leaves the Body

A. Water enters the body through digestive tract both in liquids (drinking) and in foods (preformed water)
B. Water is formed in the body by metabolism of foods (oxidative water)
C. Water leaves the body via kidneys (as urine), intestines (with feces), and lungs and skin (insensible water losses)

Mechanisms that Maintain Total Fluid Volume

A. Osmoreceptor system
   1. Regulates water output volume to balance fluid intake volume
   2. Most important mechanism for regulation of water output, since other fluid losses through the skin, lungs, and gastrointestinal system have no feedback mechanism relative to water loss
   3. Cells in the hypothalamus synthesize ADH, which is then stored in the posterior pituitary prior to release into the circulation
   4. Osmoreceptors respond to dehydration by increasing the frequency of nerve impulses to the posterior pituitary, resulting in an increase in the amounts of ADH released; this increases water reabsorption in the kidney tubules and decreases urinary output
   5. Osmoreceptors respond to overhydration by decreasing nerve impulses to the posterior pituitary, which decreases the release of ADH, resulting in an increase in urinary output
B. Interaction of the circulatory system
   1. Regulation of blood volume (extracellular fluid volume)
   2. Increased fluid intake increases the blood volume
   3. Increased blood volume results in an increase in cardiac output, blood pressure, and therefore glomerular filtration
   4. Increased glomerular filtration results in an increase in urinary output and a decrease in blood volume
C. Regulation of fluid intake: thirst mechanism
   1. Dehydration of cells in the thirst center of the hypothalamus gives rise to thirst sensation
   2. Thirst sensations are also induced by dryness of the oral mucosa

3. Fluid intake stretches the stomach and moistens the mouth and throat; these sensations cancel thirst sensation prior to the actual hydration of body fluids
D. Various factors such as hyperventilation, hypoventilation, vomiting, diarrhea, and circulatory failure may alter the volume of fluid lost

Mechanisms that Maintain Electrolyte Concentrations

A. Aldosterone feedback mechanism
   1. Adrenal cortex secretes the steroid hormone aldosterone when extracellular fluid sodium concentrations decrease or potassium concentrations increase
   2. Aldosterone stimulates kidney tubules to reabsorb sodium; potassium reabsorption decreases as sodium reabsorption increases; sodium is salvaged while potassium is excreted
   3. This mechanism helps preserve normal sodium and potassium concentrations in extracellular fluid
   4. Secondary effects of aldosterone
      a. Chloride conserved with sodium
      b. Water conserved, since it is reabsorbed by osmosis as tubules reabsorb salt
B. Parathyroid regulation of calcium
   1. Parathyroid glands secrete parathormone when extracellular fluid calcium concentrations decrease
   2. Parathormone stimulates the release of calcium from bone, calcium reabsorption in the small intestine (vitamin D required), and calcium reabsorption in kidney tubules
   3. Increased extracellular fluid calcium concentrations result in decreased secretion of parathormone and gradual loss of excess calcium

ACID-BASE BALANCE
Basic Concepts

A. Healthy survival depends on the body's maintaining a state of acid-base balance; more specifically, healthy survival depends on the maintenance of a relatively constant, slightly alkaline pH of blood and other fluids
B. When the body is in a state of acid-base balance, it maintains a stable hydrogen ion concentration in body fluids; specifically, blood pH remains relatively constant between 7.35 and 7.45
C. The body has three devices or mechanisms for maintaining acid-base balance; named in order of the speed with which they act, they are the buffer mechanism, the respiratory mechanism, and the renal or urinary mechanisms
D. A state of uncompensated acidosis exists if blood pH decreases below 7.35
E. A state of uncompensated alkalosis exists if blood pH increases above 7.45
F. The pH of body fluids shifts from the ideal of 7.35 to 7.45 for several reasons
   1. Glucose, utilized by almost all body cells, is oxidized; as a result energy, water, and carbon dioxide are produced; the CO_2 combines with the water to produce carbonic acid (H_2CO_3)

2. Metabolism of sulfur amino acids results in formation of sulfuric acid
3. Metabolism of phospholipids and phosphoproteins results in formation of phosphoric acid
4. Muscle metabolism under anaerobic conditions produces lactic acid
5. Rapid weight loss results in extra fat metabolism, producing ketone bodies that include alpha keto acids
6. The acid produced by the normal mechanisms just mentioned requires neutralization to avoid acidosis, coma, and death

Buffer Mechanisms for Maintaining Acid-Base Balance

A. The buffer mechanism consists of chemicals called buffers, which are present in the blood and other body fluids and which combine with relatively strong acids or bases to convert them to weaker acids or bases; hence, buffers function to prevent marked changes in blood pH when either acids or bases enter the blood

B. A buffer is often referred to as a buffer pair because it consists of not one but two substances; the chief buffer pair in the blood consists of the weak acid, carbonic acid (H_2CO_3), and its basic salts, collectively called base bicarbonate ($B \cdot HCO_3$); sodium bicarbonate ($NaHCO_3$), is by far the most abundant base bicarbonate present in blood plasma

C. When the body is in a state of acid-base balance, blood contains 27 mEq base bicarbonate per liter and 1.35 mEq carbonic acid per liter; usually this is written as a ratio, referred to as the base bicarbonate/carbonic acid ratio:

$$\frac{27 \text{ mEq B·HCO}_3}{1.35 \text{ mEq H}_2\text{CO}_3} = \frac{20}{1}$$

D. Whenever the base bicarbonate/carbonic acid ratio of blood equals 20/1, blood pH equals 7.4

E. Base bicarbonate buffers nonvolatile acids that are stronger than carbonic acid; it reacts with them to convert them to carbonic acid and a basic salt

F. Some facts about the changes in capillary blood produced by the buffering of blood by base bicarbonate
1. Buffering does not prevent blood pH from decreasing, but it does prevent it from decreasing as markedly as it would without buffering
2. Buffering removes some sodium bicarbonate from blood and adds some carbonic acid to it; this necessarily decreases the base bicarbonate/carbonic acid ratio, which in turn necessarily decreases the pH of blood as it flows through capillaries (from its arterial level of about 7.4 to its venous level of about 7.38)
3. Anything that decreases the blood's base bicarbonate/carbonic acid ratio necessarily decreases blood pH and thus tends to produce acidosis; the corollary is also true; anything that increases the base bicarbonate/carbonic acid ratio necessarily increases blood pH and thus tends to produce alkalosis

G. Other buffer systems in body fluids
1. Protein buffer
   a. Most plentiful; three-fourths of all chemical buffering power lies in proteins of the body fluids
   b. Provides support to other buffering systems such as bicarbonate buffer and phosphate buffer
2. Phosphate buffer system
   a. One-sixth as concentrated as bicarbonate buffer in extracellular fluid
   b. More important in intracellular fluids, where its concentration is considerably higher
   c. Helps to buffer pH of urine in kidney tubules
3. Hemoglobin buffer system: buffers intracellular fluid of the erythrocyte

H. Bicarbonate buffer is the most important buffer in human body fluids because its components, base bicarbonate and carbonic acid, are actively and constantly regulated by the action of the respiratory and urinary systems

Respiratory Mechanism for Controlling Acid-Base Balance

A. Respiratory system controls acid-base balance by controlling rate of carbon dioxide (CO_2) exhalation from lungs; during normal body metabolism CO_2 is produced, which reacts with water to form carbonic acid, resulting in a decrease in pH (as acidity increases, pH decreases); when the respiratory system blows CO_2 out of the body, carbonic acid breaks down into CO_2 and water, resulting in an increase in pH (as acidity decreases, pH increases)

B. Respiratory acidosis
1. Conditions impairing the ability of the respiratory system to blow off CO_2 will result in a buildup of CO_2 in the body; excess CO_2 combines with water to form carbonic acid and hydrogen ions, resulting in a decrease in pH
2. Signs of respiratory acidosis include dyspnea, irritability, tachycardia, and cyanosis
3. Common causes include emphysema, pneumonia, asthmatic attack, atelectasis, pneumothorax, drug overdose

C. Respiratory alkalosis
1. Less frequently, hyperventilation blows off too much CO_2 from the body, causing an excessive breakdown of carbonic acid, resulting in an increase of pH
2. Signs of respiratory alkalosis include deep or deep and rapid breathing, light-headedness, tetany, convulsions, and unconsciousness
3. Common causes include hysteria, prolonged crying, and mechanical ventilation

D. Compensation
1. In metabolic acidosis the respiratory system compensates by hyperventilation in an attempt to blow off CO_2 and raise the pH
2. In metabolic alkalosis the respiratory system compensates by decreasing the rate and depth of breathing in an attempt to retain CO_2 and decrease the pH

Renal Mechanism for Maintaining Acid-Base Balance

A. The renal mechanism is the most effective device the body has for maintaining acid-base balance; unless it operates adequately, acid-base balance cannot be maintained

B. The renal mechanism for maintaining acid-base balance makes the urine more acidic and the blood more alkaline; this neutralizes the constant production of acid products from cells; the mechanism consists of two functions performed by the distal renal tubule cells, both of which remove hydrogen ions from blood to urine and in exchange reabsorb sodium ions from tubular urine to blood
  1. Distal tubule cells secrete hydrogen ions and reabsorb sodium ions (Fig. 3-1)
  2. Distal tubule cells form ammonia, which combines with hydrogen ions they have secreted to form ammonium ions (NH_4^+), which are excreted in the urine in exchange for sodium ions, which are reabsorbed into the blood (Fig. 3-2)
C. The distal tubule functions produce the following results
  1. They increase blood's sodium bicarbonate content and decrease its carbonic acid content, thereby increasing the base bicarbonate/carbonic acid ratio and blood pH
  2. They acidify urine (decrease urine pH)
D. Metabolic acidosis
  1. Excess acid, other than carbonic acid, which is a respiratory acid, accumulates in the body beyond the body's ability to neutralize it
  2. Signs of metabolic acidosis include weakness, malaise, headache, disorientation, deep rapid breathing, fruity odor to breath, coma

3. Common causes include diabetes mellitus, salicylate poisoning, severe diarrhea, vomiting of intestinal contents, infection
E. Metabolic alkalosis
  1. Excess base bicarbonate in the body
  2. Signs of metabolic alkalosis include muscle hypertonicity, tetany, confusion, shallow slow respirations, convulsions, coma
  3. Common causes include vomiting of stomach contents or prolonged gastric suction, excessive ingestion of alkaline drugs, potent diuretics
F. Compensation
  1. In respiratory acidosis the urinary system excretes increased hydrogen ions to compensate for the respiratory system's inability to blow off CO_2
  2. In respiratory alkalosis the urinary system may decrease excretion of hydrogen ions to compensate and maintain the body's pH in the normal range

CHEMICAL PRINCIPLES RELATED TO FLUIDS, ELECTROLYTES, ACIDS, BASES, AND SALTS
Water
General Information

A. Chemical combination of oxygen and hydrogen
B. Most abundant compound
C. Essential to life
D. Sixty percent of the average adult human body weight is water; may be as high as 80% in infants and as low as 40% to 50% in the elderly

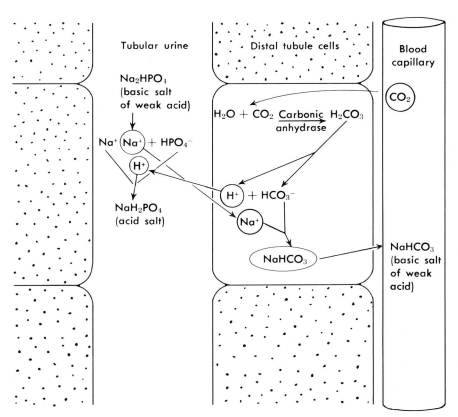

FIG. 3-1. Acidification of urine and conservation of base by the distal renal tubular excretion of hydrogen ions (H^+) from the urine and the reabsorption of sodium ions (Na^+) into the blood in exchange for the H^+ excreted into it. (From Anthony CP and Thibodeau GA: Textbook of anatomy and physiology, ed 13, St. Louis, 1989, The CV Mosby Co.)

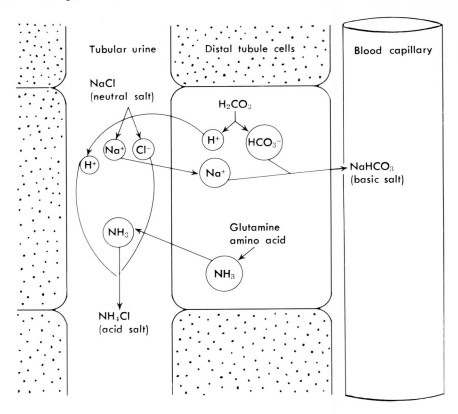

FIG. 3-2. Acidification of urine by the tubular excretion of ammonia (NH_3). An acid (glutamine) leaves the blood, enters a tubule cell, and is deaminized to form ammonia. The ammonia is excreted into the urine, where it combines with hydrogen to form the ammonium ion (NH_4^+). In exchange for NH_4^+ the tubule cell reabsorbs Na^+. (From Anthony CP and Thibodeau GA: Textbook of anatomy and physiology, ed 13, St. Louis, 1989, The CV Mosby Co.)

Physical Properties

A. Colorless, tasteless, odorless liquid
B. Exists chiefly as ice at low temperatures, liquid at moderate temperatures, and gas at elevated temperatures
   1. Water changes from liquid to solid at the freezing point (32° F [0° C])
   2. Water changes from liquid to gas at the boiling point (212° F [100° C])
   3. These transition points in the physical states of water are the basis of the Celsius temperature scale
   4. Conversion from one temperature scale to the other is accomplished by using the formula

$$°C = \frac{5}{9} (°F - 32)$$

Chemical Properties

A. Water molecule a dipolar structure; because of this molecular shape, it is an excellent solvent for ionic or slightly ionic substances
B. Water a stable compound; it dissociates very slightly to H^+ and OH^- under normal conditions
C. Electrolysis can dissociate water into its components, hydrogen and oxygen
D. Many chemical reactions need water as a solvent before they can occur
E. Process of splitting a substance with the addition of water called hydrolysis, which is the basis for the digestion of food
F. Crystals formed with water in their molecule are called hydrates

Importance

A. Necessary for life; universal solvent
B. Essential for many chemical reactions
C. Needed for digestion (hydrolysis) of food
D. Forms large percentage of plant and animal tissue
E. Necessary for circulation of blood; plasma is a water solution
F. Necessary for elimination; urine, sweat, feces contain water
G. Lubricating fluid at joints (synovial fluid) contains water
H. Water has a great capacity for absorbing heat or giving off absorbed heat; useful in ice packs, hydrotherapy, and hot compresses

Water as a Standard

A. Thermometer scales: the freezing and boiling points of water are used to standardize Celsius scale
B. Specific gravity: compares the density of a volume of water to the density of the same volume of another substance
C. Weight: 1 g is the mass of 1 ml of water at 4° C
D. Calorie: the heat needed to raise 1 g of water 1° C
E. pH: water acts as neutrality point on acid-base scale

Proteins

A. Polymers of alpha amino acids connected by peptide bonds
B. Characteristics of proteins
   1. Protein molecules are very large
   2. Proteins form colloid particles in solution
   3. Synthesis of proteins occurs in ribosomes of cell according to specific genetic patterns under direction of the nucleic acids DNA and RNA

4. Structure patterns of proteins are extremely specific; proteins differ from species to species, individual to individual, and organ to organ; this presents a problem in transplant operations
5. Proteins are the tissue builders of the body

C. Classification of proteins
1. Simple proteins: give amino acids on hydrolysis
   a. Albumins: water soluble, coagulated by heat (lactalbumin [milk], serum albumin [blood], egg white); albumin is most important in the development of the plasma colloid osmotic pressure, which helps control (through osmosis) the flow of water between the plasma and interstitial fluid; during a condition such as starvation, a fall in the albumin level of the blood results in a fall in the plasma colloid osmotic pressure; this leads to edema because less fluid is being drawn by osmosis into the capillaries from the interstitial spaces
   b. Globulins: insoluble in water, soluble in dilute salt solutions, coagulated by heat (e.g., lactoglobulin [milk], serum globulin [blood], gamma serum globulin [forms antibodies of blood])

Solutions
Basic Concepts

A. Substances that dissolve in other substances form solutions
B. A solution can be classified as a homogeneous mixture
C. Solids, liquids, and gases can be dissolved in other solids, liquids, and gases
1. Substance dissolved is called the solute
2. Substance in which the solute is dissolved is called the solvent
3. Common solution is one in which a solid, liquid, or gas is dissolved in a liquid (e.g., blood is mainly a liquid [water] containing dissolved ions, sugars, amino acids, and respiratory gases)

Factors Affecting Solubility

A. Chemical and physical nature of the solvent
B. Chemical and physical nature of the solute
C. Amount of solvent versus amount of solute
D. Temperature: warming aids some solutes (solids) to dissolve; cooling aids others (gases) to dissolve
E. Presence or absence of mixing; mixing usually speeds solution reaction
F. Pressure: especially when one of the components is a gas

Types of Solutions

A. Dilute: small amount of solute in a relatively large amount of solvent
B. Concentrated: large amount of solute in a relatively small amount of solvent
C. Unsaturated: holding less solute than is possible for it to dissolve at a certain temperature and pressure
D. Saturated: holding all the solute it can dissolve at a certain temperature and pressure
E. Supersaturated: unique case of a solution holding more solute than it normally should for a particular temperature and pressure
1. Very unstable condition
2. Excess solute easily precipitates from solution

F. Percent solution: grams of solute per gram of solution
G. Molar solution (M): number of gram-molecular weights of solute per liter of solution
H. Normal solution (N): number of gram-equivalent weights of solute per liter of solution
I. Molal solution: gram-molecular weight of solute in 1000 g of solvent

Osmosis

A. Process of selective diffusion
B. More concentrated solution is separated from a less concentrated solution by a membrane that is permeable only to the solvent: a semipermeable membrane
C. Solvent moves more rapidly from the dilute solution into the concentrated solution than in the reverse direction
D. Pressure forcing the solvent across the membrane is called osmotic pressure
E. Isotonic solutions: when the osmotic pressures of two liquids are equal, the flow of solvent is equalized and the two solutions are said to be isotonic to each other
1. Physiologic saline—0.89% NaCl in distilled water—is isotonic to blood and body tissues
2. Five percent dextrose in water is isotonic to blood and body tissues
3. When isotonic solutions are administered intravenously, the blood cells remain intact

F. Hypertonic solutions: when one solution has less osmotic pressure (is more concentrated) than another, it draws fluid from the other and is said to be hypertonic to it
G. Hypotonic solutions: when one solution has more osmotic pressure (is more dilute) than another, it forces fluid into the other and is said to be hypotonic to it
H. Both hypertonic and hypotonic types of solution may be destructive to body cells and should be used with caution in intravenous injections
I. Osmosis constantly occurs as part of the normal physiology of human beings
1. Capillary membrane: the colloid osmotic pressure of the plasma draws fluid from the tissue spaces back into the capillaries; edema results when disease states upset the normal colloid osmotic pressure (e.g., starvation, kidney disease)
2. Plasma membranes: water freely flows from interstitial fluid into intracellular fluid and vice versa, depending on the relative concentration of water in these two fluid compartments

Size of Particle of Solute Determines Type of Solution

A. Atomic, ionic, and most molecular-sized particles are extremely small: submicroscopic
1. Particles are freely dispersed by solvent
2. Particles are kept in solution by movement and attraction of solvent molecules
3. Substances of this class are called crystalloids
4. Crystalloids form true solutions
   a. Clear in appearance: particles cannot be seen
   b. Solute stays in solution as long as the solvent is not removed by evaporation or other means
   c. Solute accompanies solvent as it passes through filters and most membranes (e.g., the ions Na^+, K^+, Cl^-, HCO_3^- dissolved in plasma are in true solution)

B. Large particles of matter do not form solutions in the real sense of the term
  1. Solute particles easily settle out of solvent
  2. Solute particles can be seen by naked eye or with microscope when suspended in solvent
  3. Solute can be removed by ordinary filtration
  4. Substances of this class are called coarse suspensions (e.g., the erythrocytes are suspended in plasma and can be seen microscopically and removed by fine filters or centrifugation)
C. The colloid particle
  1. Intermediate in size between the crystalloid and the coarse suspensoid
  2. Particle much larger than the crystalloid particle although smaller than particle of coarse suspensoid; diameter of colloid around 0.0000001 to 0.00001 mm
  3. Solutions of colloids
    a. Solute particles dispersed by solvent
    b. Solution: clear, cloudy, or opalescent
    c. Show bright path of reflected light passed through the solution: Tyndall effect
    d. More stable than coarse suspensoids, less stable than true solutions
    e. With time, colloid particles will settle out
    f. Affect osmotic pressure less than do crystalloids
    g. Most of the proteins in plasma are dispersed as colloid particles
    h. Blood is classified as a colloid and a suspension
  4. Colloid particles will pass through ordinary filters but will be held back by most membranes
  5. Colloid particles carry electric charges on their surfaces: not to be confused with ionic charges
  6. Importance of colloid suspensions
    a. Proteins, fats, and many carbohydrates form molecules in the colloid size range
    b. These form colloid solutions in the cells and body fluids
    c. Protoplasm of cell itself is a colloid

Ionization
Ion

A. When an atom loses or gains an electron (electrons), it is no longer a neutral atom but a charged particle: an ion
B. The charge on this particle depends on whether electrons are lost ($+$) or gained ($-$) and the number of electrons lost or gained
C. An electron is a negative particle; the loss of 1 electron makes ion positive (less negative) by 1; with loss of 2 electrons, ion is 2^+, etc.
D. The gain of 1 electron makes ion negative by 1; with 2 electrons gained, the ion is 2^-, etc.

Ionization and Water

A. When certain compounds are placed in water, the polar water molecules dissociate the molecules of the compound into ions: a process called ionization
B. A substance that will ionize when placed in water is called an electrolyte
C. A substance that will ionize in water (an electrolyte) will allow the passage of an electric current through its solution

D. Acids, bases, and salts ionize in water and conduct an electric current

Factors Affecting Strength of Electrolytes

A. Amount of electrolyte present in solution
B. How well the electrolyte dissociates in solution: degree of ionization
  1. Weak electrolytes are substances that dissociate into ions to only a slight degree
  2. Strong electrolytes are substances that dissociate into ions to a larger degree

Bases, Acids, and Salts
Bases

A. Definition: a base is a substance that usually adds a hydroxyl ion (OH^-) to any solution in which it is placed

$$\overset{\text{in water}}{\downarrow}$$
$$NaOH \rightarrow Na^+ + OH^-$$

B. Properties of a base
  1. Bitter taste
  2. Slippery feeling
  3. Electrolyte in water
  4. Reacts with indicators, giving a base color
    a. Methyl orange: yellow
    b. Litmus: blue
    c. Phenolphthalein: red
  5. Reacts with acids to form water and a salt (neutralization)
  6. Reacts with certain metals to release hydrogen gas
  7. Combines with organic acids (fatty acids) to form soaps
  8. In high concentration destroys organic material; corrosive
C. Names and formulas of common bases
  1. Calcium hydroxide ($Ca(OH)_2$): water solution, called lime water
  2. Sodium hydroxide ($NaOH$): caustic soda
  3. Potassium hydroxide (KOH): soap making
  4. Ammonium hydroxide (NH_4OH): household cleaner
  5. Magnesium hydroxide ($Mg(OH)_2$): water solution marketed under trade name Milk of Magnesia: antacid, mild laxative
  6. Aluminum hydroxide ($Al(OH)_3$): component of antacid pills

Acids

A. Definition: an acid is ordinarily thought of as a substance that liberates an H^+ (hydrogen ion) to a solution in which it is placed

$$\overset{\text{in water}}{\downarrow}$$
$$H_2CO_3 \rightarrow H^+ + HCO_3^-$$

B. Properties of an acid
  1. Sour taste
  2. Reacts with indicators giving an acid color
    a. Methyl orange: red
    b. Litmus: red
    c. Phenolphthalein: colorless

3. Combines with certain metals, releasing hydrogen gas
4. Reacts with bases to form water and a salt (neutralization)
5. Reacts with carbonates to give carbon dioxide gas
6. Acts as an electrolyte in water
7. In high concentration destroys organic materials: corrosive

C. Names and formulas of common acids
1. Hydrochloric acid (HCl): secreted by the parietal cells of the stomach; transforms pepsinogen into pepsin, which is a protein-digesting enzyme of gastric juice
2. Nitric acid (HNO_3): used in test for proteins
3. Sulfuric Acid (H_2SO_4): in storage batteries
4. Carbonic acid (H_2CO_3)
   a. One form in which CO_2 is transported in the blood
   b. Part of the bicarbonate buffer system, which is the most important buffer system regulating the pH of body fluids
5. Boric acid (H_3BO_3): mild antiseptic
6. Acetic acid (CH_3COOH): vinegar
7. Lactic acid ($CH_3CHOHCOOH$): builds up in muscle tissue during exercise; most lactic acid is then transported to the liver via the circulatory system where it is completely oxidized into CO_2, water, and energy (as ATP)

General Considerations Concerning Acids and Bases

A. Weak acids produce few hydrogen ions in solution, whereas strong acids produce many
B. Weak bases produce few hydroxyl ions in solution, whereas strong bases produce many
C. Strong acids and bases can cause serious damage to human tissue
D. Acids and bases can be used to neutralize each other: therefore, in the event of acid or base burn, flood with water and add the opposite chemical in weak, diluted form

Salts

A. Definition: the compound (besides water) formed when an acid is neutralized by a base is a salt; e.g.,

$$HCl + KOH \rightarrow H_2O + KCl$$
Acid   Base   Water   Salt

B. Properties of a salt
1. Crystalline in nature
2. Ionic even in the dry crystal
3. Electrolyte in solution
4. "Salty" taste
C. Names and formulas of common salts
1. Sodium chloride (NaCl): salt of intercellular and extracellular spaces
2. Calcium phosphate ($Ca_3(PO_4)_2$): bone and tooth formation
3. Potassium chloride (KCl): salt of intracellular spaces
4. Calcium carbonate ($CaCO_3$): limestone
5. Barium sulfate ($BaSO_4$): when taken internally, outlines internal structures for x-ray studies

6. Silver nitrate ($AgNO_3$): antiseptic
7. Iron sulfate ($FeSO_4$): treatment of anemia
8. Sodium bicarbonate ($NaHCO_3$): antacid
9. Calcium sulfate ($CaSO_4$): hydrated form is plaster of paris (casts for broken bones)
10. Magnesium sulfate ($MgSO_4$): Epsom salt

Hydrogen Ion Concentration (pH)

A. The *p* in pH comes from the French word *puissance,* meaning power
B. The *H* in pH stands for *hydrogen*
C. Thus pH denotes the power or strength of hydrogen (ions) in a solution
D. A neutral solution has the same amount of acid-reacting ions, H^+ (actually H_3O^+), as basic-reacting ions, OH^-
E. An acid-reacting solution has more H^+ than OH^-
F. A basic-reacting solution has more OH^- than H^+
G. pH is used to represent these conditions
1. A neutral solution has a pH of 7.00
2. An acid solution would have a pH in the range from 0 to 6.99; the lower the pH, the more acid the solution
3. A basic solution would have a pH in the range from 7.01 to 14.00; the higher the pH, the more basic the solution
4. The pH of the extracellular (vascular and interstitial) fluid is in the narrow range of 7.35 to 7.45; fluctuations in pH of 0.4 unit above or below this range can result in body distress; a prolonged blood pH of 7 or less or 7.8 or more can result in death
5. Certain body fluids have a pH different from 7.4; gastric juice has a pH of 1 or 2 caused by the presence of hydrochloric acid; bile is basic; urine may be acidic or basic

NURSING CARE TO MAINTAIN FLUID AND ELECTROLYTE BALANCE

A. Assess client (see Table 3-3)
1. Monitor vital signs
2. Evaluate skin turgor, hydration, and temperature
3. Auscultate breath sounds
4. Weigh client daily
5. Monitor intake and output
6. Evaluate changes in behavior and energy level
7. Review laboratory tests
   a. Urinary specific gravity
   b. Serum pH
   c. Serum electrolytes
   d. Hematocrit
8. Determine risk factors
B. Manage fluid and electrolyte intake
1. Fluids may be encouraged to correct deficit (usually 3000 ml/day; may be restricted to prevent excess)
2. Nutritional intake can be increased or restricted to correct electrolyte disturbances
   a. Sodium: table salt, dairy products, processed meats, soup, canned foods
   b. Potassium: bananas, oranges, nuts, dark leafy greens, dried fruit
   c. Calcium: milk, cheese, yogurt

Table 3-3. Etiology, manifestations, and treatment of major fluid and electrolyte disturbances

Fluid/electrolyte imbalance	Etiology	Signs and symptoms	Treatment
Extracellular fluid deficit	Decreased fluid intake Prolonged fever Vomiting Excessive use of diuretics	Increased thirst Dry skin and mucous membranes Increased temperature Flushed skin Rapid, thready pulse Increased Hct, Na^+, and specific gravity	Administration of hypo or isotonic fluids
Extracellular fluid excess	Congestive heart failure Liver disease Malnutrition (decreased plasma protein) Renal disease Excessive parenteral fluids	Weight gain Rales Edema Ascites Confusion Weakness Decreased Hct	Administration of diuretics Fluid restriction
Hypokalemia	Diarrhea Vomiting Diabetic acidosis Diuretics Inadequate intake	Loss of muscle tone Cardiac arrhythmias Abdominal distention Vomiting Decreased serum K^+	Parenteral/oral administration of potassium supplement Increased dietary intake of potassium
Hyperkalemia	Advanced kidney disease Severe burns or tissue trauma Excessive dosages of potassium	Cardiac irregularities Weakness Diarrhea Nausea Irritability Increased serum K^+	Administration of potassium free fluids Dialysis Potassium-removing resin
Hyponatremia	Diuretics Electrolyte free IV fluids Diarrhea GI suction Excessive perspiration followed by increased water intake	Abdominal cramps Convulsions Oliguria Decreased serum Na^+ and specific gravity	Administration of IV solutions containing NaCl Administration of NaCl tablets
Hypernatremia	Diabetes insipidus Excess NaCl IV fluid intake	Dry, sticky mucous membranes Oliguria Firm tissue turgor Dry tongue Increased serum Na^+ and specific gravity	Low Na^+ diet Increased Na^+ free fluid intake
Hypocalcemia	Removal of parathyroid glands Administration of electrolyte free solutions	Tingling of extremities Tetany Cramps Convulsions	Oral/parenteral calcium replacement
Hypercalcemia	Hyperparathyroidism Prolonged immobility Excessive intake of Ca^+ or vitamin D	Flank pain (renal calculi) Deep bone pain Relaxed muscles	Correction of primary problem Increased fluid intake

3. Intravenous therapy
   a. Fluids
      (1) Dextrose in water
         (a) Provides fluid and limited calories (one liter of 5% Dextrose provides 170 calories)
         (b) Used to correct dehydration, ketosis, and hypernatremia
      (2) Dextrose in sodium chloride (NaCl): used to correct fluid loss from excessive perspiration or vomiting and to prevent alkalosis
      (3) NaCl: used to manage alkalosis, fluid loss, and adrenal cortical insufficiency
      (4) Ringer's solution
         (a) Contains Na^+, Cl^-, K^+, Ca^+
         (b) Used to correct dehydration from vomiting, diarrhea, or inadequate intake
      (5) Lactated Ringer's solution
         (a) Contains Na^+, Cl^-, K^+, Ca^+ and lactate
         (b) Lactate is metabolized by liver and forms bicarbonate (HCO_3^-)
         (c) Used to correct extracellular fluid shifts and moderate metabolic acidosis

(6) Plasma expanders
    (a) Examples include Dextran and Albumin
    (b) Used to increase blood volume in trauma or burn victims
b. Regulation of flow rate
  (1) Manual regulation of gravity flow with clamp

$$\text{Per minute drop rate} = \frac{\text{milliliters to be infused} \times \text{Drop factor (drops per 1 ml)}}{\text{Number of hours} \times 60 \text{ minutes}}$$

  (2) Use of infusion pump or controller
    (a) Drop control (follow manufacturer's instructions when setting desired rate of flow)
    (b) Volume control (follow manufacturer's instructions when setting desired volume)
c. Monitor client for complications
  (1) Infiltration
    (a) Catheter is displaced, allowing fluid to leak into tissues
    (b) Insertion site is pale, cool and edematous; flow rate decreases
    (c) IV must be removed and restarted in a new site
  (2) Phlebitis
    (a) Vein is irritated by catheter or medications
    (b) Insertion site is red, painful and warm; flow rate is decreased
    (c) IV must be removed and restarted in a new site; warm compresses are applied to inflammation
  (3) Circulatory overload
    (a) Flow rate exceeds cardiovascular system's capability to adjust to the increased fluid volume
    (b) Client exhibits dyspnea, rales, distended neck veins and increased blood pressure
    (c) Rate is decreased to keep the vein open; physician is notified and diuretics, if prescribed, are administered
4. Administer pharmacological agents
  a. Diuretics (Thiazide, potassium-sparing, loop or osmotic diuretics)
  b. Electrolyte replacement (e.g., potassium chloride, calcium gluconate)
  c. Potassium-removing resin: sodium polystyrene sulfonate (Kayexalate)

Perioperative Care
REVIEW OF PHYSICAL PRINCIPLES RELATED TO PERIOPERATIVE CARE
Electricity
Static Electricity

A. Substances can be charged by friction, whereby a negatively charged object loses negatively charged electrons which it discharges via a spark when touching an object that is a good conductor

B. Applications
  1. Removing blankets and sheets from a bed will build up electric charges through the hands that should be discharged by touching a grounded object before touching others
  2. Wool, silk, nylon, and Dacron may set off sparks caused by static electric charges and should not be used around combustible gases or monitoring equipment
  3. Electric equipment and operating room tables should be grounded to allow static charges to drain off, thus preventing sparks

Current Electricity

A. Direct current (DC): flow of electric charge in one direction only (e.g., the electric system of an automobile)
B. Alternating current (AC): electric charge moves first in one direction and then in the opposite direction, with the voltages and currents alternating back and forth (e.g., the outlets in homes and hospitals)
C. Concept of electric energy and work
  1. Potential energy per unit charge due to an electric field is called electric potential and is measured in volts (V)
  2. Rate of flow of electric charge, called current, is measured in amperes (amp); 1 amp is a current flow of 1 coulomb/second; 6.25 billion billion electrons have a negative charge of 1 coulomb
  3. Ohm's law: electric potential (volts), rate of flow of electric charge (amperes), and resistance are related; the rate of flow of charges between two points is directly proportional to the impressed voltage and inversely proportional to the resistance between the two points; thus the rate of flow of charges can be increased by either increasing the voltage or decreasing the resistance
    a. Dry fingers or hands touching an ungrounded or faulty electric source can result in a definite shock; the source touched with wet fingers or while standing in water can result in enough electric energy to be fatal
    b. As little as 0.05 amp can be fatal, and 0.1 amp is practically always fatal since the electric currents upset the natural electric rhythms of the heart and can result in fibrillation and also stop the breathing center from working
    c. The shock obtained via alternating current is not caused by electrons pouring from the socket into the body but by the powerful vibrations of electrons and ions already inside the body, which are energized via the electric field that is induced from the voltage drop at the output

Power

A. Power represents the quantity of energy used per unit of time and is expressed in watts (W)
B. The kilowatt (kW) is 1000 W; power companies compute the number of kilowatt hours of energy used for billing purposes; a kilowatt hour is the quantity of electric energy consumed in 1 hour at a rate of 1 kW

Application

A. Electronic cardiac pacemakers: battery-operated devices supplement or replace defective electric stimulation in the human heart and thus help to maintain the individual's heartbeat at a selected rate
B. Electrosurgery: an extremely high-frequency device called an oscillator is utilized to generate high temperatures in a small area to coagulate or desiccate tissue, thus preventing bleeding during surgery; electric cutting (using the oscillator) vibrates the tissues apart and simultaneously cauterizes the small blood vessels, thus preventing bleeding
C. Electronic thermometers: in these devices, temperature changes in a crystal alter the electrical resistance of the crystal; changes in an individual's temperature also alter the resistance of the crystal, allowing a certain amount of current to flow through and the amount to be read on a scale calibrated for temperature readings; these thermometers give readings more accurate than mercury thermometers in about 5 to 7 seconds
D. Electrocardiograms: these devices measure and record the electric activity of the heart as this activity is carried to the surface of the body by the ions of the body fluids; this information provides an electric picture of the heart's activity

Heat

A. Temperature can give a measure of the level of molecular thermal energy
   1. The three common measures of temperature are
      a. Celsius or centigrade
      b. Fahrenheit
      c. Absolute or Kelvin
   2. Conversions
      If
      T_f = Temperature in Fahrenheit degrees
      T_c = Temperature in Celsius degrees
      T_k = Temperature in Kelvins
      then
      $T_f = (\% \, T_c) + 32$
      $T_c = (T_f - 32) \times \%$
      $T_k = T_c + 273°$
B. The unit which expresses the quantity of thermal energy or the amount of heat that could be produced in a body is the calorie
C. The British Thermal Unit (BTU) is defined as the quantity of heat required to change the temperature of 1 lb of water 1° F
D. Specific heat is the quantity of heat per unit mass per unit temperature difference required to raise the temperature of a substance 1° C
E. Water has a high specific heat, which means that a relatively large quantity of energy must be added to water to bring about small temperature changes (e.g., a hot water bottle stays hot for a long time because water has a high specific heat)
F. Heat is used to kill all living organisms on medical instruments and other materials; dry heat at a temperature of 338° F (170° C) for 30 minutes is considered sufficient for sterilization; dry heat sterilization has an advantage over steam sterilization in that no damage is done to the fine cutting edges of surgical instruments or to ground glass surfaces

Change of State

A. Evaporation: molecules of a liquid become molecules of gas; since the most energetic molecules leave the surface of a liquid during evaporation, the average kinetic energy and temperature of the remaining liquid molecules are lower; thus evaporation causes cooling
   1. Rubbing alcohol applied to the skin will rapidly evaporate, cooling the body
   2. Sweating is an important physiologic process because evaporation helps to control body temperature
B. Boiling: evaporation occurring beneath the surface of a liquid; the gas bubbles so formed are buoyed to the liquid's surface and escape into the atmosphere; this evaporation can be speeded up by (1) adding energy to the liquid molecules so that they possess enough energy to burst out from the surface of the liquid or (2) reducing the atmospheric pressure above the liquid
   1. Autoclave: by increasing the pressure inside the autoclave (which is like a giant pressure cooker), higher water temperatures can be reached and bacteria and their spores can be readily destroyed by the steam generated; thus the autoclave sterilizes materials placed in it for specified lengths of time
   2. Distillation (all chemical and drug solutions are made in distilled water): purifying water by boiling and collecting the vapor; impurities are left behind during water evaporation

REVIEW OF PHARMACOLOGY RELATED TO PERIOPERATIVE CARE
General Anesthetics

A. Description
   1. Used in a "balanced" combination to facilitate the surgical experience by producing varying types of loss of consciousness, pain control, and skeletal muscle relaxation
   2. Act by depressing the central nervous system through the following progressive sequence
      a. Stage I: euphoria; gradual loss of consciousness
      b. Stage II: hyperexcitement; hyperactive reflexes; pupil dilation
      c. Stage III: depression of corneal reflex and pupillary response to light; absence of voluntary control; decreased muscle tone; stage of surgical anesthesia
      d. Stage IV: medullary paralysis (respiratory/cardiac failure); death
   3. General anesthetics are available in parenteral (IM, IV) and inhalation preparations; ultrashort-acting IV barbiturates are useful in the induction of anesthesia because of their ability to quickly penetrate the blood brain barrier; IV and IM nonbarbiturates produce a special type of anesthesia in which the client appears to be awake but dissociated from the environment resulting in amnesia for the surgical experience
B. Examples
   1. Inhalation anesthetics
      a. cyclopropane
      b. enflurane (Ethrane)
      c. ether

d. halothane (Fluothane)

e. methoxyflurane (Penthrane)

f. nitrous oxide

2. IV barbiturates: high lipoid affinity provides prompt effect on cerebral tissue

a. methohexital sodium (Brevital)

b. thiamylal sodium (Surital)

c. thiopental sodium (Pentothal)

3. IV and IM nonbarbiturates: induce a cataleptic state and produce amnesia for the procedure

a. ketamine HCl (Ketaject)

b. Combination product: fentanyl and droperidol (Innovar)

C. Major side effects

1. Inhalation anesthetics

a. Excitement and restlessness (initial CNS stimulation)

b. Nausea and vomiting (stimulation of chemoreceptor trigger zone in medullary vomiting center)

c. Respiratory distress (depression of medullary respiratory center)

2. IV barbiturates

a. Respiratory depression (depression of medullary respiratory center)

b. Hypotension and tachycardia (depression of cardiovascular system)

c. Laryngospasm (depression of laryngeal reflex)

3. IV and IM nonbarbiturates

a. Respiratory failure (depression of medullary respiratory center)

b. Changes in blood pressure: hypertension; hypotension (alterations in cardiovascular system)

c. Rigidity (enhancement of muscle tone)

d. Psychic disturbances (emergence reaction-recovery period)

D. Nursing care

1. Assess for allergies and other medical problems that could alter the client's response to the anesthetic agents

2. Have O_2 and emergency resuscitative equipment available

3. Assess vital signs before, during, and after anesthetic administration

4. Maintain a calm environment during induction of anesthesia

5. Utilize safety precautions with flammable agents

6. Protect client during postanesthetic period because of decreased sensory awareness

7. Judiciously administer narcotics in the initial postanesthetic period

8. Evaluate client's response to medications

Local Anesthetics

A. Description

1. Used to produce pain control without rendering the client unconscious; useful for obstetric, dental, and minor surgical procedures

2. Act in a reversible manner to block nerve impulse conduction in sensory, motor, and autonomic nerve cells by decreasing nerve membrane permeability to sodium ion influx

3. Available in topical, spinal, and nerve block preparations; epinephrine may be added to these preparations to enhance the duration of the local anesthetic effect

B. Examples

1. Topical: local infiltration of tissue

a. benzocaine

b. cocaine

c. dibucaine (Nupercaine); also used for spinal anesthesia

d. lidocaine HCl (Xylocaine); also used for nerve block

e. piperocaine HCl (Metycaine)

f. tetracaine HCl (Pontocaine); also used for spinal anesthesia and nerve block

2. Spinal: injected into the spinal subarachnoid space

a. dibucaine (Nupercaine)

b. procaine HCl (Novocain); also used for nerve block

3. Nerve block: injected at perineural site distant from desired anesthesia site

a. bupivacaine HCl (Marcaine)

b. chloroprocaine HCl (Nesacaine)

c. mepivacaine HCl (Carbocaine)

C. Major side effects

1. Allergic reactions; anaphylaxis (hypersensitivity)

2. Respiratory arrest (depression of medullary respiratory center)

3. Arrhythmias; cardiac arrest (depression of cardiovascular system)

4. Convulsions (depression of central nervous system)

5. Hypotension (depression of cardiovascular system)

D. Nursing care

1. Assess for allergies and other medical problems that could alter the client's response to the anesthetic agent

2. Have O_2 and emergency resuscitative equipment available

3. Assess vital signs before, during, and after anesthetic administration

4. Protect anesthetized body parts from mechanical and/or thermal injury

5. Maintain a calm environment while the client is anesthetized

6. Keep client flat for a specified period (usually 12 hours) after spinal anesthesia to prevent severe headache; avoid pillows

7. Utilize safety precautions (side rails up) and maintain bedrest until sensation returns to lower extremities after spinal anesthesia

8. Maintain side-lying position to prevent aspiration after general anesthesia

9. Restrict oral intake after client has had general anesthesia until ability to swallow has returned

10. Evaluate client's response to medications and understanding of teaching

Sedatives/Hypnotics

A. Description

1. Produce sedation in small doses and sleep in larger doses

2. Used for clients experiencing anxiety-related situations and insomnia
3. Act by depressing the central nervous system (CNS)
4. Available in oral, parenteral (IV, IM), and rectal preparations

B. Examples
   1. Barbiturates: depress CNS starting with diencephalon
      a. amobarbital (Amytal)
      b. butabarbital sodium (Butisol)
      c. pentobarbital sodium (Nembutal)
      d. phenobarbital (Luminal)
      e. secobarbital (Seconal)
   2. Nonbarbiturates: depress CNS and relax skeletal muscles
      a. chloral hydrate (Noctec)
      b. ethchlorvynol (Placidyl)
      c. flurazepam HCl (Dalmane)
      d. glutethimide (Doriden)
      e. methaqualone (Quaalude)
      f. methyprylon (Noludar)

C. Major side effects
   1. Drowsiness (depression of CNS)
   2. Hypotension (depression of cardiovascular system)
   3. Dizziness (hypotension)
   4. Gastrointestinal irritation (local oral effect)
   5. Skin rash (hypersensitivity)
   6. Blood disorders (hematologic alterations)
   7. Barbiturates
      a. Hangover (persistence of low barbiturate concentration in body due to decreased metabolism)
      b. Photosensitivity (hypersensitivity)
      c. Excitement in children and elderly (paradoxic reaction)

D. Nursing care
   1. Avoid administration with other CNS depressants
   2. Caution client to avoid engaging in hazardous activity; avoid concurrent use of alcohol
   3. Assess for signs of dependence
   4. Utilize safety precautions at night for hospitalized clients (side rails up)
   5. Implement supportive measures to promote sleep (back rub; warm milk)
   6. Instruct client to avoid placing medication within reach to prevent possible overdose while drowsy
   7. Monitor blood work during long-term therapy
   8. Administer controlled substances according to appropriate schedule restrictions
   9. Evaluate client's response to medication and understanding of teaching

Analgesics

A. Description
   1. Used to relieve pain
   2. Divided into two classes
      a. Nonnarcotic analgesics relieve mild to moderate pain
      b. Narcotic analgesics relieve moderate to severe pain
   3. Nonnarcotic analgesics
      a. Act by a peripheral mechanism at the level of the damaged tissue by inhibiting prostaglandin and other chemical mediator synthesis involved in the pain phenomenon
      b. Exert antipyretic activity by action on the hypothalamic heat-regulating center to reduce fever
      c. Salicylates, which belong to this class, also exert antiinflammatory and uricosuric effects
      d. Nonsalicylates, such as acetaminophen, are nonirritating to the gastrointestinal mucosa
   4. Narcotic analgesics act by blocking opioid receptors in the central nervous system, thereby altering awareness of pain
      a. Depress CNS and also produce effects on multiple body systems
      b. Produce euphoria and are addicting
   5. Available in oral, parenteral (IV, SC, IM), and rectal preparations; many combination products exist that contain both a narcotic and nonnarcotic analgesic component

B. Examples
   1. Nonnarcotic (salicylates)
      a. aspirin (ASA; Ecotrin)
      b. magnesium salicylate (Magan)
   2. Nonnarcotic (nonsalicylates)
      a. acetaminophen (Datril; Tylenol)
      b. diflunisal (Dolobid)
   3. Narcotic
      a. codeine sulfate
      b. meperidine HCl (Demerol)
      c. morphine sulfate
      d. oxycodone HCl (Percodan)
      e. pentazocine HCl (Talwin)
      f. propoxyphene HCl (Darvon)

C. Major side effects
   1. Nonnarcotic (salicylates)
      a. Gastric irritation (local oral effect)
      b. Visual disturbances (salicylism)
      c. Prolonged bleeding time (suppression of platelet aggregation)
      d. Tinnitus (early toxicity-salicylism)
   2. Nonnarcotic (nonsalicylates)
      a. Sore throat, fever (depression of WBCs)
      b. Skin rash (hypersensitivity)
      c. Hepatotoxicity (direct liver toxic effect)
   3. Narcotic
      a. Respiratory depression (depression of medullary respiratory center)
      b. Hypotension (depression of cardiovascular system)
      c. Constipation (decreased peristalsis)
      d. Euphoria (central nervous system effect)
      e. Urinary retention (increased smooth muscle tone of sphincter)
      f. Miosis (stimulation of sphincter muscle of iris)

D. Nursing care
   1. Assess for covert signs of pain
      a. Monitor vital signs
      b. Evaluate nonverbal communication (grimacing; protective motions)
   2. Administer medication before pain becomes severe

3. Administer narcotics as ordered
   a. Do not administer if respirations are less than 12 per minute
   b. Have narcotic antagonist available
   c. Observe for overdosage triad: respiratory depression, pinpoint pupils, and coma
   d. Avoid administration with CNS depressants
   e. Avoid use in head-injury clients
   f. Assess for signs of dependence
   g. Utilize safety precautions with hospitalized clients; supervise ambulation; side rails up, especially at night
   h. Note automatic stop orders
   i. Controlled substances: administer according to appropriate schedule restrictions
4. Evaluate client's response to medications and understanding of teaching

CLASSIFICATION OF SURGERY

A. Ambulatory surgery: useful in offering clients early ambulation, an active role in an individual's recovery process, and cost containment
   1. Hospital-based outpatient settings
      a. Client has diagnostic workup in hospital several days prior to surgery
      b. Client is admitted directly to the ambulatory surgical section by the perioperative nurse
      c. Client is discharged from the recovery room or clinical unit generally the same day as the surgery is performed; when complications occur, the physician must admit the client to the hospital
   2. Hospital satellite settings
      a. Client has diagnostic workup in hospital or physician's office prior to surgery
      b. Client is admitted to satellite unit and discharged from same when recovery is satisfactory
   3. Private surgical offices
      a. Surgical procedures are performed by the surgeon in a private office which has a surgical suite and surgical staff (technicians and nurses)
      b. Preoperative workup is performed by hospital, physician, or clinic prior to surgery
B. Inpatient surgical care
   1. Client is admitted to the hospital setting for surgical care
   2. Surgery may be classified as:
      a. Elective
      b. Diagnostic
      c. Urgent or emergency surgery
      d. Ablative
      e. Palliative
      f. Curative

NURSING PROCESS DURING THE PERIOPERATIVE PERIOD
Probable Nursing Diagnoses Based on Assessment

A. Potential for aspiration related to reduced level of consciousness
B. Ineffective airway clearance related to prolonged sedation
C. Ineffective breathing pattern related to incisonal pain
D. Pain related to surgical incision
E. Potential for infection related to surgical wound
F. Impaired physical mobility related to
   1. Pain
   2. Dressings
G. Potential for fluid volume deficit related to
   1. Inadequate intake
   2. Wound drainage
H. Constipation related to decreased peristalsis
I. Altered patterns of urinary elimination related to
   1. Effects of anesthesia
   2. Decreased intake
J. Potential sleep pattern disturbance related to
   1. Anxiety
   2. Pain
   3. Environmental stimuli
K. Potential hyperthermia related to inflammatory process
L. Potential for injury related to
   1. Anesthesia
   2. Sedation
M. Fear related to
   1. Surgical procedure
   2. Prognosis

Nursing Care during the Preoperative Period

A. Prior to day of surgery
   1. Allow the client time to ask questions about procedures and surgery
   2. Explain all procedures to the client and give reasons and objectives for them
   3. Determine the client's level of understanding of operative procedure to ascertain whether signature on permit represents informed consent
   4. Allow and encourage the client to ventilate feelings about diagnosis and surgery
   5. Tell the client what to expect in the operating room, recovery, and/or intensive care units if indicated
   6. Inform the client if the plan is to return him or her to other than the present room
   7. Encourage nutritional assessment so that any nutrient deficiencies can be corrected
   8. Provide a spiritual counselor if desired by the client or family
   9. Consider needs of the family when discussing surgery
   10. Teach the client the activities that will be instituted after surgery related to ventilatory function
       a. Diaphragmatic breathing
       b. Controlled coughing
       c. Deep breathing
       d. Incentive spirometry
       e. Splinting
       f. Turning
   11. Teach the client physical exercises that will be used to promote circulation after surgery
       a. Leg exercises
       b. Ambulation routines
       c. Isometric exercises
   12. Inform the client to expect some discomfort after surgery and teach the importance of requesting medication for pain

13. Make certain that history, physical examination results, recent laboratory tests, and chest x-ray report are entered on the chart
14. Inform all members of the medical team, especially the anesthesiologist, of the client's allergies and other health problems and prominently mark the chart
15. Minimize the risk of postoperative infection by proper skin preparation
    a. Bathe the evening prior to surgery with antimicrobial soap
    b. Wash skin with Betadine, hexachlorophene, or chlorhexidine as ordered
    c. Encourage repeated showers the evening prior to surgery as ordered
    d. Shampoo hair when procedure involves head, neck, or upper chest area
    e. Shave skin if ordered, however, CDC recommends hair removal only if necessary
16. Carry out ordered preoperative preparation
    a. Enemas (often until clear returns)
    b. Douches
    c. Irrigations
17. Remove nail polish from fingers and toes
18. Administer prescribed sleeping medications
    a. Sedative-hypnotics
    b. Antianxiety agents
19. Inform the client not to take anything by mouth after midnight, remove fluid, and place obvious signs at bedside
20. Evaluate client's response and revise plan as necessary

B. Day of surgery
1. In the morning, check the client's vital signs and assess overall physical status; record and report any deviations to physician
2. Check the client's medical chart to ensure that pertinent test results are present
3. Complete the preoperative checklist
4. Provide hygiene and assist client into hospital gown
5. Have the client void
6. Remove any prosthetics such as dentures and wigs
7. Apply antiembolic stockings or ace bandages as ordered
8. Arrange for insertion of any tubes as ordered
    a. Salem sump tube
    b. Nasogastric tube
    c. Indwelling urinary catheter
9. Arrange for insertion of intravenous line as ordered
10. Store any client valuables according to hospital policy
11. Make sure identification band is on client's wrist
12. Administer prescribed preoperative medications as ordered
    a. Tranquilizers
    b. Narcotic analgesics
    c. Anticholinergics
13. Put side rails up after administering medications
14. Transfer the client to a stretcher when operating room calls; fasten the stretcher strap in place before transporting

15. Consider the emotional needs of both the client and family on the day of surgery
16. Evaluate client's response and revise plan as necessary

Nursing Care during the Intraoperative Period

A. Admit to the operating room
1. Take client to a holding area outside of the operating room
2. Insert an intravenous catheter (if not already in place); usually done by the nurse or anesthesiologist
3. Transfer client to the operating room by stretcher
4. Complete checklist and allay client's anxiety
5. Apply monitoring devices as needed
6. Remember ambulatory surgical clients remain aware during most of their stay in the operating room since local anesthetics are used
7. Anesthesia is introduced by anesthesiologist to produce four stages of anesthesia
    a. Stage 1: Client becomes drowsy and loses consciousness
    b. Stage 2: Stage of excitement; muscles are tense, breathing may be irregular
    c. Stage 3: Depression of vital signs and reflexes; operation begins during this phase
    d. Stage 4: Complete respiratory depression
8. Anesthesiologist inserts an endotracheal tube or airway prior to induction of anesthesia
9. Position client for surgery
B. Operating room nurse assumes appropriate role
1. Circulating nurse—acts as an assistant to surgeon and scrub nurse
2. Scrub nurse—provides assistance in all activities that require surgical asepsis
3. Operating room nurses act as client advocates during the operative procedure

Nursing Care during the Postoperative Period

A. Immediate
1. Respiratory needs: anesthesia may result in depression of respiratory function
    a. Maintain a patent airway by keeping the artificial airway in place until gag reflex returns
    b. Position client on one side with face down and neck slightly extended to prevent aspiration and accumulation of mucus secretions
    c. Observe the rate, rhythm, symmetry of chest movement, breath sounds, and color of mucous membranes
    d. Suction artificial airway and the oral cavity as needed to remove secretions
    e. Administer oxygen as ordered
    f. Remove airway when the gag reflex has returned, suctioning prior to removal to clear mucus plugs and secretions
    g. Encourage coughing and deep breathing as soon as the client is able to cooperate
2. Circulatory needs
    a. Assess the heart rate and rhythm as well as the blood pressure at frequent intervals, approximately every 15 minutes

b. Assess peripheral circulation by noting the color, temperature, and presence of pulses to ensure tissue perfusion

c. Assess for hemorrhage by monitoring blood pressure for hypotension and observing and measuring wound drainage

d. Report signs of hemorrhage to the surgeon immediately

3. Neurological needs

a. Assess the client's level of consciousness and responses to stimuli

b. Assess pupillary and gag reflexes

c. Assess for loss or return of sensation or movement when specific areas have been surgically treated (e.g., back surgery)

d. Reorient the client to time, place, and situation

e. Call the client by name

f. Answer questions as honestly and simply as possible and avoid complicated, involved explanations

g. Expect and accept repetitious questions and give the client necessary reassurance

4. Wound care

a. Note the location of the wound and the color, odor, amount, and consistency of drainage

b. Circle drainage on the dressing to allow for more objective assessment of drainage

c. Reinforce postoperative dressings since surgeons generally perform the first dressing change

5. Care of drains and tubes

a. Maintain patency of tubing

b. Attach tubing to appropriate collection containers as ordered

c. Monitor output of drains to assess for hemorrhage

6. Fluid and electrolyte needs

a. Maintain intravenous therapy as ordered

b. Record intake and output accurately

7. Comfort needs

a. Assess the client's level of pain

b. Medicate as ordered to reduce pain and increase postoperative compliance with breathing, coughing, and activity regimens

8. Evaluate client's response and revise plan as necessary

B. Recovery for the ambulatory surgical client

1. All care included under immediate postoperative care applies to the ambulatory surgical client

2. Recovery room time is generally less for this client, since outpatient anesthesia is intended to provide for a quick recovery time and few side effects

3. When the client is responsive, encourage sips of water and ambulate to chair

4. Provide a light meal for the client when tolerated

5. When the client is stable, has retained foods, and has voided, reinforce postoperative teaching and discharge planning with client and family members; evaluate understanding of teaching

C. Recovery for the inpatient surgical client

1. Protect the client from injury by keeping under close observation, keeping side rails in place, positioning to prevent excessive pressure on body parts or on tubing, controlling restlessness and preventing the client from pulling on tubes or dressing, and making certain that all equipment is in safe working condition and properly used

2. Turn frequently and encourage deep breathing and coughing to prevent the development of atelectasis or hypostatic pneumonia

3. Perform or encourage range of motion and isometric exercises and early ambulation to prevent phlebitis, paralytic ileus, and circulatory stasis

4. Maintain patency of tubing (catheter, gastric tubes, T-tube, chest tubes, etc.) to promote drainage and maintain decompression to reduce pressure on suture line

5. Use surgical aseptic technique when changing dressings or as necessary when irrigating tubing to prevent infection

6. Monitor intake and output to prevent dehydration, fluid and electrolyte imbalance, and urinary suppression or retention

7. Observe for abdominal distention to prevent discomfort and intestinal obstruction

8. Give medication for pain as ordered to prevent discomfort and restlessness

9. Regulate IV therapy to prevent circulatory overload

10. Encourage the client to support and splint the incisional site when coughing, moving, or turning to prevent tension on the suture line

11. Position the client as required by type of surgery to prevent misalignment and prevent accumulation of fluid or blocking the drainage tubes

12. Provide emotional support; assist client to cope with changes in body image

13. Evaluate client's response and revise plan as necessary

D. Postoperative nutritional needs

1. Monitor IV therapy for water and electrolytes (oral intake needed as soon as possible for adequate nutrition)

2. Monitor hyperalimentation: parenteral nutrition of high nutrient density; solutions of amino acids, glucose, electrolytes, minerals, vitamins; usually inserted into larger veins (inferior or superior vena cava) to avoid thrombosis in peripheral veins; used in clients with major tissue trauma, injury, or extensive surgery

3. Gradually increase oral intake as permitted

a. Liquid diets

(1) Clear liquid: clear broth, bouillon, juices, plain gelatin, fruit-flavored water ices, ginger ale, coffee, tea

(2) Full liquid: may add milk and items made with milk, such as cream soups, milk drinks, sherbet, ice cream, puddings, custard

b. Soft diet: may add all soft cooked foods, such as refined cereals, pasta, rice, white bread and crackers, eggs, cheese, meat, potatoes, cooked whole vegetables, cooked fruits, few soft ripe plain fruits without membranes or skins, simple desserts

c. Light diet: same as soft with few additional whole cooked foods, light raw foods such as fruit; mainly avoid heavily seasoned or fried foods

d. Full (or general) diet: full, well-balanced diet of all foods as desired and tolerated, including a wide variety for interest and flavor

4. Provide for special nutritional needs

   a. Protein: increased need caused by protein losses and the anabolism of recovery and tissue healing; approximate requirement for adult is 1.2 to 2.0 g/kg/day; branched chain amino acid (BCAA) enriched products are available which appear to be more effective in producing a positive nitrogen balance as compared to other amino acid nutritional supports

   b. Calories: adequate amount to supply energy and spare protein for tissue building

   c. Water: adequate fluid therapy to prevent dehydration caused by large fluid losses

   d. Vitamins and minerals: need for most will be increased following surgery and the nutrition program must be designed to insure that individual requirements are met; special attention to mineral adequacy to maintain electrolyte balance is essential

     (1) Zinc

       (a) Increases the tensile strength (force needed to separate edges) of the healing wound

       (b) Supplemental dosages of 4 to 6 mg/day orally are recommended

     (2) Vitamin C

       (a) Required for collagen formation

       (b) Supplemental dosages of 500 to 1000 mg/day should be administered to promote optimal wound healing

   e. Evaluate client's response and revise plan as necessary

Neoplastic Disorders

(See related body system for specific diseases)

CLASSIFICATION OF NEOPLASMS

A. Benign neoplasia

   1. Cells adhere to each other and the growth remains circumscribed

   2. Generally not life threatening unless they occur in a restricted area (e.g., skull)

   3. Classified according to the tissue involved

     a. Adenoma—glandular tissue

     b. Leiomyoma—smooth muscle

     c. Chondroma—cartilaginous tissue

     d. Osteoma—bone osteoblast

     e. Hemangioma—blood vessels

     f. Lymphangioma—lymphatics

     g. Neurofibroma—nerve sheath

     h. Lipoma—adipose tissue

B. Malignant neoplasia

   1. Cells infiltrate surrounding tissue

   2. Cells invade other tissues and produce secondary lesions

3. May spread (metastasize by direct extension, lymphatic permeation and embolization, and diffusion of cancer cells by mechanical means)

4. Tumors are classified according to the tissue involved

   a. Adenocarcinoma—epithelial tissue

   b. Carcinoma—epithelial surface tissue

   c. Sarcoma—connective tissue

   d. Osteosarcoma—bone osteoblasts

   e. Angiosarcoma—blood vessels

   f. Lymphangiosarcoma—lymphatics

   g. Neurofibrosarcoma—nerve sheath

   h. Liposarcoma—adipose tissue

5. Tumors are often classified by a universal system of staging classification, the TNM system

   a. *T* designates a primary tumor

   b. *N* designates lymph node involvement

   c. *M* designates metastasis

   d. Numbers 0 to 4 designate degree of involvement

   e. *TIS* designates carcinoma in situ, or one which is noninfiltrating

PHARMACOLOGY RELATED TO NEOPLASTIC DISORDERS
Basic Concepts

A. Used to destroy malignant cells by interfering with reproduction of the cancer cell

B. Act at specific points in the cycle of cell division (cell-cycle specific) or at any phase of the cycle of cell division (cell-cycle nonspecific)

C. Affect any rapidly dividing cell within the body, thus having the potential for toxicity development in healthy, functional tissue (bone marrow, hair follicles, GI mucosa); to reduce the possibility of toxicity, combination therapy is often used

D. Available in oral, parenteral (IM, SC, IV), intraarterial, intrathecal, and topical preparations

Antineoplastic Drugs
Alkylating Agents

A. Cell-cycle nonspecific; attack the DNA of rapidly dividing cells

B. Examples

   1. busulfan (Myleran)

   2. chlorambucil (Leukeran)

   3. cisplatin (Platinol)

   4. cyclophosphamide (Cytoxan)

   5. lomustine (CeeNU)

   6. melphalan (Alkeran)

Antibiotics

A. Cell-cycle specific; inhibit RNA and protein synthesis of rapidly dividing tissue

B. Examples

   1. dactinomycin (Cosmegen)

   2. daunorubicin (Cerubidine)

   3. doxorubicin hydrochloride (Adriamycin)

   4. mithramycin (Mithracin)

   5. mitomycin (Mutamycin)

   6. procarbazine hydrochloride (Matulane)

Antimetabolites

A. Cell-cycle specific; inhibit protein synthesis in rapidly dividing cells during "S" phase
B. Examples
  1. azathioprine (Imuran)
  2. cytarabine (Cytosar-U)
  3. floxuridine (FUDR)
  4. fluorouracil (5-FU)
  5. hydroxyurea (Hydrea)
  6. mercaptopurine (6-MP, Purinethol)
  7. methotrexate (Mexate)

Hormones

A. Tissue-specific; inhibit RNA and protein synthesis in tissues that are dependent on the opposite (sex) hormone for development
B. Examples
  1. Androgens
  2. Estrogens (estramustine phosphate sodium [Emcyt])
  3. Progestins
  4. Steroids (prednisone [Meticorten])
  5. Other
    a. mitotane (Lysodren) cortisol antagonist
    b. tamoxifen citrate (Nolvadex) estrogen antagonist

Immune Agents

A. Involves introduction of noncancerous antigens or other agents into the body to stimulate production of lymphocytes and antibodies
B. Examples
  1. BCG vaccine (bacillus of Calmette Guerin): provides active immunity
  2. interferon alfa-2a (Roferon-a); interferon alfa-2b (Intron a)

Common Combinations of Chemotherapeutic Agents

A. ABVD
  1. doxorubicin hydrochloride (Adriamycin)
  2. bleomycin sulfate (Blenoxane)
  3. vinblastine sulfate (Velban)
  4. dacarbazine (DTIC-Dome)
B. CHOP
  1. cyclophosphamide (Cytoxan)
  2. doxorubicin hydrochloride (Adriamycin)
  3. vincristine sulfate (Oncovin)
  4. prednisone
C. CMF (may be referred to as CMFP when prednisone is included)
  1. cyclophosphamide (Cytoxan)
  2. methotrexate (Mexate)
  3. fluorouracil (5-FU)
D. COPP (may be referred to as A-COPP when doxorubicin hydrochloride [Adriamycin] is included)
  1. cyclophosphamide (Cytoxan)
  2. vincristine sulfate (Oncovin)
  3. procarbazine hydrochloride (Matulane)
  4. prednisone
E. CVP
  1. cyclophosphamide (Cytoxan)
  2. vincristine sulfate (Oncovin)
  3. prednisone
F. FAC
  1. fluorouracil (5-FU)
  2. doxorubicin hydrochloride (Adriamycin)
  3. cyclosphosphamide (Cytoxan)
G. MOPP
  1. mechlorethamine hydrochloride (Nitrogen Mustard, Mustargen)
  2. vincristine sulfate (Oncovin)
  3. procarbazine hydrochloride (Matulane)
  4. prednisone
H. VAC
  1. vincristine sulfate (Oncovin)
  2. dactinomycin (Cosmegen)
  3. cyclophosphamide (Cytoxan)

Major Side Effects

A. Anorexia, nausea, vomiting (irritation of GI tract; quick uptake by rapidly dividing alimentary tract tissue)
B. Diarrhea (irritation of GI tract; quick uptake by rapidly dividing alimentary tract tissue)
C. Bone marrow depression (quick uptake by rapidly dividing myeloid tissue)
D. Stomatitis (irritation of GI tract; quick uptake by rapidly dividing alimentary tract tissue)
E. Blood dyscrasias (bone marrow depression)
F. Alopecia (rapid uptake by rapidly dividing hair follicle cells)
G. CNS disturbances (neurotoxicity)
H. Hepatic disturbances (hepatoxicity)
I. Hyperuricemia (release of large quantities of breakdown products-uric acid)
J. Kidney failure (direct kidney toxic effect)
K. Doxorubicin: cardiac toxicity (direct cardiac toxic effect)
L. BCG: allergic reactions, anaphylaxis

RADIATION
Purpose

A. Diagnosis
B. Treatment
  1. Curative: destroys neoplasm by irradiation
  2. Palliative: shrinks neoplasm by irradiation
  3. Adjuvant: used in conjunction with chemotherapy or surgery to shrink or destroy neoplasm

Examples

A. Alpha particle: fast-moving helium nucleus
  1. Weight: 4 atomic weight units (awu)
  2. Charge: 2^+
  3. Penetration: slight
B. Beta particle: fast-moving electron
  1. Weight: practically 0 awu
  2. Charge: 1^-
  3. Penetration: moderate
C. Gamma ray: penetrating ray, similar to light ray
  1. Weight: none
  2. Charge: none
  3. Penetration: high
D. Gold (^{198}Au): ascites; pleural effusions
E. Sodium iodide (^{131}I): thyroid gland
F. Sodium phosphate (^{32}P): erythrocytes

Major Side Effects

A. Radiation sickness
B. Low-grade fever
C. Skin rash

Methods of Delivery

A. External beam radiotherapy delivers radiation to a tumor by means of an external machine (Cobalt or Linear accelerator) at a predetermined distance
B. Internal radiation therapy or brachytherapy delivers radiation by systemic, interstitial, or intracavity means
   1. Systemic involves administration by intravenous or oral routes
   2. Interstitial involves implantation of needles, wires, or seeds into the tissue
   3. Intracavity radiation involves placing an implant into a body cavity and may require a surgical procedure

Influencing Factors

A. Type of tumor
B. Location of the tumor
C. Tolerance of adjacent tissue
D. Extent of the disease process
E. Health status of the client
F. Age of the client

NURSING PROCESS FOR CLIENTS WITH NEOPLASTIC DISORDERS
Probable Nursing Diagnoses Based on Assessment

These diagnoses are related to neoplasms in general. For nursing diagnoses related to specific diseases, see the body system involved.

A. Pain related to disease process/therapeutic modalities
B. Fear related to
   1. Diagnosis
   2. Death
   3. Intractable pain
C. Altered nutrition: less than body requirements related to disease process/therapeutic modalities
D. Potential for injury related to disease process/therapeutic modalities (radiation, chemotherapy)
E. Decisional conflict (choices regarding health or death) related to
   1. Choice or continuation of treatment modality
   2. Religious, moral, or ethical beliefs
F. Fatigue related to depletion of body reserve
G. Altered oral mucous membrane, related to disease process/therapeutic modalities
H. Impaired tissue integrity related to treatment modalities
I. Powerlessness related to diagnosis/prognosis

Nursing Care for Clients with Neoplastic Disorders Receiving either Chemotherapy or Radiation

A. Review infection control guidelines with client
B. Teach client to report temperature higher than 100° F (37.7° C) to physician
C. Instruct client regarding special measures to limit infection and injury (e.g., gentle oral hygiene, prevention of pathological fractures)
D. Explain side effects that influence appearance and encourage positive adaptations (e.g., purchase of wigs, scarves)
E. Implement measures to reduce or eliminate nausea such as antiemetics, hypnosis, relaxation modalities, small frequent feedings, adjustment of meal times in relation to therapy, avoidance of spicy foods
F. Monitor blood work during therapy
G. Offer emotional support to client and family; answer questions and encourage verbalization of fears
H. Encourage conservation of client's decreasing energy
I. Support natural defense mechanisms of client; encourage intake of foods rich in the immune-stimulating nutrients, especially vitamins A, C, and E, and the mineral selenium (whole grains and seeds)
J. Encourage optimal intake of high nutrient density foods; bland or mechanical soft diet may be indicated; routinely monitor weight
K. Encourage women of childbearing age to use birth control measures while receiving therapy because of mutagenic/teratogenic effects; avoid use of birth control pill
L. Keep client well hydrated (3000 ml/24 hr); monitor intake and output
M. Assess client for pain; administer analgesics as needed; provide for client comfort
N. Encourage client to become involved in decision making; support client's decisions whenever possible even if they differ from the nurse's philosophy
O. Specific care for clients receiving chemotherapy
   1. Monitor intravenous infusion site for infiltration to prevent local tissue necrosis
   2. Institute protective isolation if WBCs are low
   3. Wear double gloves when handling urine and other excretions
   4. Observe for signs of bleeding; avoid anticoagulants because of decreased platelets
   5. Avoid skin contact with drugs during preparation for administration; wear gloves; if contact occurs, rinse area well with water
   6. Avoid use of rectal thermometers, enemas, IM injections, and razor blades because of increased bleeding tendency
   7. Monitor renal function for nephrotoxicity
   8. Monitor vital signs; monitor for cardiac toxicity
   9. Encourage client to check with physician before consuming over-the-counter (OTC) drugs, such as aspirin or alcohol
P. Specific care for client's receiving external radiation
   1. Avoid washing off the marks placed by the radiologist
   2. Instruct client to avoid creams, soaps, powders, and deodorants during the treatment periods
   3. Assess skin for erythema, dryness, burning
   4. Instruct client to wear cotton clothing which is loose fitting
   5. Protect skin from sunlight
   6. Apply a nonadherent dressing to areas of skin breakdown
Q. Specific care for clients receiving internal radiation
   1. Avoid overexposure to the client and use the principles of time, distance, and shielding
   2. Postpone routine hygiene while implant is in place

3. Ascertain if body excreta has to be placed in lead containers for disposal

R. Evaluate client's response to medication or radiation and revise plan as necessary

Emergency Situations
FIRST AID

A. Maintain or establish
   1. Airway (CPR)
   2. Breathing
   3. Circulation
B. Provide for physical safety
   1. Remove client from immediate danger
   2. Control bleeding
   3. Avoid unnecessary movement of spinal column or extremities
   4. Control pain
   5. Monitor level of consciousness
C. Establish priority for care
   1. Triage: system of client evaluation to establish priorities and assign appropriate treatment or personnel
   2. Determination of priority
      a. Emergency situations: greatest risk receives priority
      b. Major disasters: classification based on principles to benefit the largest number; those requiring highly specialized care may be given minimal or no care
D. Offering psychologic support
   1. Establish and maintain open communication with the client and family to mediate feelings of "loss of control"
   2. Allow contact between the client and family as soon as feasible

SPECIFIC EMERGENCIES

A. Circulatory
   1. See specific disease: myocardial infarction, hypertensive crisis, shock, asystole
   2. Uncontrolled hemorrhaging
      a. Stop the bleeding by direct pressure, application of a pressure dressing or ice to constrict vessels, elevation of the involved extremity, or (rarely) tourniquet application
      b. Treat for shock
B. Respiratory
   1. See specific disease: pneumothorax, pulmonary edema, pulmonary embolism, carbon monoxide poisoning, COPD, ARDS
   2. Near drowning
      a. Assessment
         (1) Possible airway obstruction from bronchospasm
         (2) Evaluation of arterial blood gases for hypoxia, hypercarbia, and acidosis
         (3) Possible pulmonary edema
            (a) *Salt water:* high osmotic pressure of aspirated water draws additional fluid into alveolar spaces from the vascular bed
            (b) *Fresh water:* removes surfactant, leading to alveolar collapse

b. Treatment and nursing care
   (1) Establish an airway and ventilate with 100% oxygen and positive pressure
   (2) Correct the acidosis
   (3) Insert a nasogastric tube to prevent aspiration of gastric contents
   (4) Treat pulmonary edema and hypothermia if present
C. Gastrointestinal (see specific diseases: perforated peptic ulcer, appendicitis, intestinal obstruction, bleeding esophageal varices associated with cirrhosis)
D. Genitourinary (see specific disease: bladder trauma)
E. Endocrine (see specific diseases: hypoglycemia, ketoacidosis, thyroid storm)
F. Neuromusculoskeletal (see specific diseases: fractures, spinal cord injury, head injury, cerebral vascular accident, myasthenic crisis)
G. Integumentary (see specific disease: burns)
H. Poisoning (see Pediatric nursing: poisoning)
I. Thermal trauma
   1. Heat stroke
      a. Risk factors: advanced age, strenuous exercise in heat, medications such as anticholinergics that interfere with sweating
      b. Signs and symptoms
         (1) Hot, dry, flushed skin progressing to pallor in the late stages of circulatory collapse
         (2) Elevation of body temperature above 40.5° C (105° F)
         (3) Complaints of dizziness, nausea, and headaches
         (4) Convulsions
         (5) Altered level of consciousness
      c. Treatment and nursing care
         (1) Rapidly reduce temperature: hypothermia blanket, cold-water baths, and enemas
         (2) Administer oxygen to meet increased metabolic demands
         (3) Institute seizure precautions
   2. Hypothermia
      a. Risk factors: exposure to cold; submersion in cold water; age (elderly and very young)
      b. Signs and symptoms
         (1) Local (frostbite): pallor, paresthesia, pain to absence of sensation of involved body part
         (2) Systemic: core temperature less than 94° F (34.4° C), weak and irregular pulse, decreased level of consciousness
      c. Treatment and nursing care
         (1) Monitor core temperature with an esophageal or rectal probe
         (2) Continually assess cardiac status, arterial blood gases, electrolytes, glucose, and BUN
         (3) Rewarm: to prevent cardiovascular collapse, core rewarming with heated oxygen and/or irrigations must precede surface rewarming
         (4) Correct fluid and electrolyte imbalances
   3. Evaluate client's response and revise plan as necessary

Circulatory System
REVIEW OF ANATOMY AND PHYSIOLOGY OF THE CIRCULATORY SYSTEM
Functions

A. Primary function: provides communication between widely separated body parts through transportation of hormones, nutrients, wastes, respiratory gases, vitamins, minerals, enzymes, water, leukocytes, antibodies, and buffers

B. Secondary functions: contributes directly or indirectly to all the body's metabolic functions: tissue perfusion with oxygen and nutrients, water balance, immunity, enzymatic reactions, and pH and temperature regulation

Structures
Blood

A. Blood components
  1. Serum: plasma with fewer or no coagulating proteins
  2. Plasma
    a. Water: 3 L in average adult; constitutes 90% of plasma
    b. Ions: see fluid and electrolytes and Table 3-4
    c. Proteins: all act as buffers; fractionated and separated from each other by electrophoretic and ultracentrifugation techniques
      (1) Albumin
        (a) Largest component of plasma proteins
        (b) Principally responsible for plasma colloid osmotic pressure (COP)

Table 3-4. Plasma constituents

Constituent	Normal concentration range
Water	Approximately 90% by volume
Ions	
Sodium (Na$^+$)	135 to 145 mEq/L
Potassium (K$^+$)	4.0 to 5.5 mEq/L
Calcium (Ca^{++})	4.5 to 5.0 mEq/L
Magnesium (Mg^{++})	1.5 to 2.5 mEq/L
Chloride (Cl$^-$)	100 to 106 mEq/L
Bicarbonate (HCO$_3^-$)	23 to 28 mEq/L
Phosphate (H$_2$PO$_4^-$; HPO$_4^-$)	1.5 to 2.5 mEq/L
Plasma proteins	
Albumin	3.5 to 5.5 g/100 ml
Globulins (alpha, beta, and gamma)	1.5 to 3.6 g/100 ml
Glucose	70 to 110 mg/100 ml
Nitrogenous substances	
Blood urea nitrogen (BUN)	5 to 25 mg/100 ml
Uric acid	2 to 8 mg/100 ml
Creatinine	0.7 to 1.5 mg/100 ml
Amino acids	0.1 to 3.0 mg/100 ml
Bilirubin	0.0 to 1.5 mg/100 ml
Lipids	
Cholesterol	120 to 220 mg/100 ml
Fatty acids	200 to 400 mg/100 ml
Triglycerides	15 to 25 mg/100 ml
Other constituents	
Respiratory gases (O$_2$ and CO$_2$)	Variable concentrations
Hormones	
Vitamins	
Enzymes	

(c) Reversibly combines with and transports certain lipids, bilirubin, thyroxin, and certain drugs, such as barbiturates
(2) Alpha and beta globulins
  (a) Help establish COP
  (b) Transport certain vitamins, iron, copper, and cortisol
  (c) Hemostasis (prothrombin and fibrinogen are in this blood fraction)
(3) Gamma globulins: antibodies
  d. Glucose: prime oxidative metabolite of body cells
3. Formed elements
  a. Erythrocytes
    (1) Shape: pliable biconcave disc that maximizes surface area proportional to volume for ease of diffusion of respiratory gases
    (2) Number: males: 4.5 to 6.2 $\times$ 10^6/mm^3; females: 4.0 to 5.5 $\times$ 10^6/mm^3
    (3) Formation: erythropoiesis
      (a) Location: red marrow of vertebrae, sternum, ribs, iliac crests, clavicles, scapulae, and skull
      (b) Maturation process: mature erythrocytes are mainly sacs of hemoglobin without a nucleus, mitochondria, ribosomes, endoplasmic reticula, or Golgi bodies; process requires folic acid and vitamin B$_{12}$; vitamin B$_{12}$ plus intrinsic factor from the parietal cells of the stomach form hemopoietic factor, which stimulates erythrocyte formation (see pernicious anemia)
      (c) Under conditions of low O$_2$ tension, liver and kidneys secrete proteins into blood that combine to form erythropoietin, which stimulates erythrocyte production
    (4) Principal component is hemoglobin
      (a) Conjugated protein: globulin plus 4 molecules of heme
      (b) Formed within the erythrocyte utilizing copper, cobalt, iron, nickel, and vitamin B$_6$
      (c) Functions to bind O$_2$ through iron in heme and CO$_2$ through globulin portion; can carry both simultaneously
    (5) Erythrocytes live for about 120 days; old or deteriorated ones are removed by reticuloendothelial cells of the liver, spleen, and bone marrow; 3.5 $\times$ 10^6 die and are replaced daily; heme is converted to bilirubin, which is excreted from the liver as part of the bile
  b. Leukocytes
    (1) Types
      (a) Granulocytes (polymorphonuclear): originate in red marrow and consist of neutrophils (50% to 70% of total), eosinophils (1% to 4% of the total), and basophils (0% to 1% of the total)

(b) Agranulocytes (mononuclear): originate in red marrow and lymphatic tissue and consist of monocytes (3% to 8% of the total), which become macrophages in tissue spaces, and lymphocytes (25% to 40% of the total)

(2) Functions

(a) Phagocytosis of bacteria by neutrophils and macrophages; phagocytosis of antibody-antigen complexes by eosinophils

(b) Antibody synthesis: B lymphocytes produce antibodies; they also become plasma cells, which produce most circulatory antibodies

(c) Destruction of transplanted tissues and cancer cells by T lymphocytes, which form in lymphoid tissue and mature in the thymus

(3) Leukocytes live for a few hours or days; some T lymphocytes live for many years and provide long-term immunity

c. Thrombocytes: anucleate cellular fragments associated with hemostasis

(1) Origin: fragmentation of megakaryocytes in bone marrow

(2) Number: 150,000 to 500,000/mm^3

(3) Function in blood coagulation

(a) Adhere to each other and to damaged areas of circulatory system to limit or prevent blood loss

(b) Release chemicals that constrict damaged blood vessels

B. Physical properties of blood

1. Volume

a. Male: 5 to 6 L; female: 4.5 to 5.5 L

b. Hematocrit: percent blood volume occupied by red cells (normal range: 36% to 45%)

2. Specific gravity (sp gr): normal range: 1.05 to 1.06

3. Viscosity: about 5.5 times as viscous as pure water

C. Blood groups

1. Names: indicate type antigens on or in red cell membrane (e.g., type A blood means that red cells have A antigens, type O that red cells have no antigens)

2. Every person's blood belongs to one of the 4 blood groups: type A, type B, type AB, or type O—and is either Rh positive or Rh negative

3. Plasma: normally contains no antibodies against antigens present on its own red cells but does contain antibodies against other A or B antigens not present on its red cells (e.g., type A plasma does not contain antibodies against A antigen but does contain antibodies against B antigen)

4. Blood does not normally contain anti-Rh antibodies; Rh-positive blood never contains them; Rh-negative blood will contain anti-Rh antibodies if the individual has been transfused with Rh-positive blood or has carried an Rh-positive fetus

5. The potential danger in transfusing blood is that the donor's blood may be agglutinated (clumped) by the recipient's antibodies

D. Hemostasis: arrest of bleeding

1. Vasoconstriction: reflex spasm in cut or ruptured vessel's smooth muscles

2. Aggregation of platelets: adhere to damaged blood vessel walls forming plugs

3. Blood coagulation (clotting): blood becomes gel as soluble fibrinogen is converted to insoluble fibrin; process brought about by at least a dozen different chemical clotting factors operating in sequence after mechanism is triggered

a. Extrinsic clotting mechanism: trigger for mechanism is blood contacting damaged tissue

b. Intrinsic clotting mechanism: trigger for mechanism is release of chemicals (platelet factors) from platelets aggregated at either the site of a wound or at a rough spot on blood vessel wall

4. Some facts about the blood proteins essential for clotting

a. Liver cells synthesize prothrombin, fibrinogen, and other clotting factors; adequate amounts of vitamin K must be present in blood for the liver to make normal amounts of prothrombin, Stuart factor (X), factor VIII, and Christmas factor (IX) (a plasma thromboplastin component [PTC])

b. Normal blood prothrombin content: 10 to 15 mg/100 ml of plasma

c. Normal blood fibrinogen content: 350 mg/100 ml of plasma

d. Both prothrombin and fibrinogen are soluble proteins normally present in blood in adequate amounts for clotting to occur at the normal rapid rate

e. Fibrin is an insoluble protein formed from the soluble protein fibrinogen, in the presence of the enzyme thrombin; fibrin appears as a tangled mass of threads having a jellylike texture; blood cells become enmeshed in these threads, and red cells give the clot its red color

5. Clinical applications

a. Hemophilia: hereditary sex-linked disease characterized by defect in clotting ability of blood caused by lack of a blood protein essential for clotting (factor VIII, or less frequently factor IX)

b. Thrombosis: partial or complete occlusion of a blood vessel, caused by presence of a stationary clot (thrombus)

c. Embolism: partial or complete occlusion of a blood vessel by a moving clot (embolus)

d. Atherosclerosis: plaques of lipoid material deposited in endothelium act as rough spots, causing platelet disintegration and thrombus formation

Heart

A. Location: in pericardial cavity within the mediastinum with apex on diaphragm and pointing to left (apical beat may be counted by placing stethoscope in fifth intercostal space on line with left midclavicular point); two-thirds of bulk of heart lies to left of midline of body, one-third to right

B. Covering: pericardium
   1. Structure
      a. Fibrous pericardium: loose-fitting, inextensible sac around heart
      b. Serous pericardium: consists of two layers
         (1) Parietal layer: lines inner surface of fibrous pericardium
         (2) Visceral layer (epicardium): adheres to outer surface of the heart; pericardial space, lying between the parietal and visceral layers, contains a few drops of lubricating pericardial fluid
   2. Function: protects heart against friction and erosion by providing well-lubricated, smooth sac in which the heart beats
C. Structure of heart
   1. Heart wall
      a. Myocardium: composed of cardiac muscle cells
      b. Endocardium: delicate endothelial lining of myocardium
      c. Cardiac skeleton: continuous dense connective tissue regions at the heart's base and in the interventricular septum serving as points of origin and insertion for cardiac muscle fibers and as supports for the heart's valves
   2. Cavities
      a. Upper two called atria
      b. Lower two called ventricles
   3. Valves and openings
      a. Openings between atria and ventricles known as atrioventricular orifices
         (1) Guarded by cuspid valves
            (a) Tricuspid on right
            (b) Mitral (bicuspid) on left
         (2) Valves consist of three parts
            (a) Flaps or cusps
            (b) Chordae tendineae
            (c) Papillary muscles
      b. Opening from right ventricle into pulmonary artery guarded by the pulmonary semilunar valve
      c. Opening from left ventricle into the aorta guarded by the aortic semilunar valve
   4. Blood supply to myocardium (heart muscle)
      a. By way of only two small vessels: the right and left coronary arteries, the first branches of the aorta
      b. Both coronary arteries send branches to both sides of the heart
      c. Right coronary branches supply right side of heart mainly but also carry some blood to the left ventricle
      d. Left coronary branches supply left side of heart mainly but also carry some blood to the right ventricle
      e. Most abundant blood supply goes to the myocardium of the left ventricle
      f. Greatest flow of blood into myocardium occurs when heart relaxes due to decreased arterial compression
      g. Relatively few anastomoses (branches from one artery to another artery) exist between the larger branches of the coronary arteries (poor collateral circulation); hence, if one of these vessels becomes occluded, little or no blood can reach the myocardial cells supplied by that vessel; deprived of an adequate blood supply, the cells soon die (myocardial infarction)
   5. Nerve supply to heart
      a. Sympathetic fibers (in cardiac nerves) and parasympathetic fibers (in the vagus nerve) form the cardiac plexuses
      b. Fibers from the cardiac plexuses terminate mainly in the sinoatrial node
      c. Sympathetic impulses tend to accelerate and strengthen heartbeat
      d. Parasympathetic (vagal) impulses slow the heartbeat
   6. Conduction system of heart
      a. Sinoatrial (SA) node: a cluster of cells located in the right atrial wall near the opening of the superior vena cava
      b. Atrioventricular (AV) node: a small mass of special conducting cells located in the base of the right atrium at the top of the interventricular septum
      c. AV bundle of His: special conducting fibers that originate in the AV node and extend by two branches down the two sides of the interventricular septum (right and left bundle branches)
      d. Purkinje fibers: special conducting fibers that extend from the AV bundles throughout the wall of the ventricles
      e. Normally a nerve impulse begins its course through the heart in the heart's own pacemaker, the SA node; it quickly spreads through both atria, via special conducting fibers, to the AV node; after a short delay at this node, the impulse is conducted by two branches of the AV bundle of His down both sides of the interventricular septum; from there, the impulse travels over Purkinje fibers to the lateral walls of the ventricles
      f. Impulse conduction through the heart generates electric currents that spread through surrounding tissues to the skin, from which visible records of conduction can be made with the electrocardiograph or oscillograph; conduction from the SA node through the atria causes atrial contraction and gives rise to the so-called P wave of the electrocardiogram; conduction from the AV node down the bundle of His and out the Purkinje fibers causes ventricular contraction and gives rise to the QRS wave; ventricular repolarization is associated with the T wave
      g. Refractory period: particularly long (¼ second) to ensure against extra beats arising as electrical energy flows around the surface of the heart; only SA node depolarizations, occurring after a refractory period, produce the next beat
D. Physiology of heart
   1. Function: to pump varying amounts of blood through the vessels as the needs of cells change

2. Cardiac cycle
   a. Consists of systole (contraction) and diastole (relaxation) of atria and of ventricles; atria contract, and as they relax ventricles contract
   b. Time required: about ⅘ second for one cardiac cycle; so 70 to 80 cycles or heartbeats per minute
3. Auscultatory events (heart sounds): first sound (I), "lub," occurs at the beginning of ventricular systole due to closing of the atrioventricular valves (tricuspid and mitral); second sound (II), "dub," occurs at the end of ventricular systole due to closing of the semilunar valves

Blood Vessels

A. Kinds
   1. Arteries: vessels that carry blood away from the heart (all arteries except pulmonary artery carry oxygenated blood); arteries branch into smaller and smaller vessels called arterioles, which branch into microscopic vessels, the capillaries
   2. Veins: vessels that carry blood toward the heart (all veins except the pulmonary veins carry deoxygenated blood); veins branch into venules, which collect blood from capillaries; veins in cranial cavity formed by dura mater are called sinuses
   3. Capillaries: microscopic vessels that carry blood from arterioles to venules; capillaries unite to form small veins or venules, which, in turn, unite to form veins; exchange of substances between blood and interstitial fluid occurs in capillaries
B. Structure of blood vessels
   1. Arteries
      a. Lining (tunica intima) of endothelium
      b. Middle coat (tunica media) of smooth muscle, elastic, and fibrous tissues; this coat permits constriction and dilation
      c. Outer coat (tunica adventitia or externa) of fibrous tissue; its firmness makes arteries stand open instead of collapsing when cut
   2. Veins
      a. Same three coats, but thinner and fewer elastic fibers
      b. Veins collapse when cut
      c. Semilunar valves present in most veins over 2 mm in diameter
   3. Capillaries
      a. Only lining coat present (intima)
      b. Wall only one cell thick
C. Fetal circulation: structures that are essential for fetal circulation but that normally cease to exist after birth
   1. Umbilical arteries: two extensions of hypogastric arteries (internal iliacs) carry fetal blood to placenta
   2. Placenta: attached to uterine wall
   3. Umbilical vein: extends from placenta back to fetus' body; returns oxygenated blood from placental to fetal circulation; two umbilical arteries and one umbilical vein constitute umbilical cord
   4. Ductus venosus: small vessel that connects umbilical vein with inferior vena cava in fetus
   5. Foramen ovale: opening in fetal heart septum between right and left atria

6. Ductus arteriosus: small vessel connecting pulmonary artery with descending thoracic aorta
7. Only two fetal blood vessels carry oxygenated blood: umbilical vein and ductus venosus; as soon as blood enters inferior vena cava from ductus venosus it becomes mixed with venous blood

Physiology of Circulation

A. Definitions
   1. Circulation: blood flow through circuit of vessels
   2. Systemic circulation: blood flow from left ventricle into aorta, other arteries, arterioles, capillaries, venules, and veins to right atrium of heart
   3. Pulmonary circulation: blood flow from right ventricle to pulmonary artery to lung arterioles, capillaries, and venules, to pulmonary veins, to left atrium
   4. Hepatic portal circulation: blood flow from capillaries, venules, and veins of stomach, intestines, spleen, pancreas, and gallbladder into portal vein, liver sinusoids, to hepatic veins, to inferior vena cava
   5. Cardiac output (CO): volume of blood pumped per minute by either ventricle; average for adult at rest; $3L/minute/m^2$body surface; cardiac output is the stroke volume (systolic discharge) times heart rate; CO increases if heart rate increases or if stroke volume increases, as by sympathetic stimulation
      a. Preload: the extent to which the left ventricle stretches at the height of diastole
      b. Afterload: force required to overcome arterial resistance and eject contents of the left ventricle during systole
B. Regulation of cardiac output
   1. Starling's law of the heart: within physiologic limits the heart, when stretched by an increased returning volume of blood, contracts more strongly and pumps out the extra returned blood; heart pumps in proportion to peripheral demand
   2. Autoregulation: volume of blood returning to heart and subsequently pumped by the heart is determined by the tissues; precapillary sphincters, which precede every capillary bed of the body, relax and permit more blood flow when O_2 tension falls; they constrict and restrict flow when O_2 tension rises
   3. Venous return: sum of all volumes of blood flowing through all capillary beds of the body; initiates Starling's law of the heart
   4. Nervous and hormonal influences on heart: physiologic limit on heart's ability to increase output as venous return increases; maximum at about 15 L/minute; sympathetic stimulation and epinephrine raise upper limit of cardiac output to 25 to 30 L/minute in normal individuals and to 35 L/minute in athletes; parasympathetic stimulation decreases heart rate and stroke volume
   5. Neural influence on veins: venous constriction due to sympathetic stimulation milks blood toward heart, increasing venous return and cardiac output
C. Principles of circulation
   1. Blood circulates because a blood pressure gradient exists in the vessels; like all fluids, blood moves from regions where its pressure is greater to re-

gions where the pressure is less; because blood pressure is highest in the left ventricle and aorta, successively lower in arteries, arterioles, capillaries, venules, veins, and lowest in the central veins (venae cavae and right atrium), blood flows through the circulatory system in this order

2. Normal range of systolic blood pressure is 100 to 139 mm Hg; consistent readings in 140s and 150s are borderline high; readings 160 and above are high; difference between systolic and diastolic pressures is the pulse pressure, normally between 30 and 40 mm Hg

3. Blood pressure normally remains relatively constant over a wide range of activities due to
   a. Neural regulation: maintains blood pressure on a minute-by-minute basis; increase in arterial pressure stimulates baroreceptors in aorta and carotid sinus, which leads to increased parasympathetic impulses to heart via vagus nerve, which slow the heart rate; a decrease in arterial pressure inhibits baroreceptors in the aorta and carotid sinus and thereby leads to decreased parasympathetic impulses and increased sympathetic impulses to the heart, which in turn cause a faster heart rate
   b. Intrinsic circulatory regulation: maintains blood pressure on an hour-to-hour basis; increased blood pressure raises the hydrostatic pressure of plasma, leading to increased filtration of plasma from circulatory system to interstitial spaces; this results in reduced venous return, decreased cardiac output, and decreased blood pressure
   c. Kidney regulation: provides long-term day-to-day regulation of blood pressure; increased blood pressure drives more blood through the kidneys, which in turn make and excrete more urine; as a result venous return, cardiac output, and blood pressure all decrease

4. Blood flow through the capillary bed: plasma filters through capillary wall at arterial end of capillary bed and becomes interstitial fluid; fluid flows over cells in capillary bed, and diffusion of nutrients and wastes occurs between fluid and cells; about half the interstitial fluid filters back into venous end of capillary bed, becoming plasma again; remaining half of interstitial fluid enters lymphatic channels along with leaked plasma proteins and returns to venous system

5. Regulation of blood flow in the circulatory system: rate of flow in liters per minute is directly proportional to blood pressure gradient and diameter of blood vessels; as pressure gradient and vessel diameter increase, flow rate increases; rate of flow is inversely proportional to blood vessel length and blood viscosity; as vessel length and blood viscosity increase, flow rate decreases; peripheral resistance refers to the combined effects of blood vessel radius and length and blood viscosity

6. Under nonpathologic conditions blood pressure remains relatively constant; since vessel length and blood viscosity are constant, the rate of flow depends almost entirely on blood vessel radius (constriction and dilation)

   a. Sympathetic discharge constricts muscular arteries and arterioles leading to the viscera, kidneys, and skin and dilates those leading to skeletal muscles
   b. Postural reflexes (baroreceptor system): arterioles are constricted when one suddenly stands after sitting or lying down; this raises blood pressure and ensures adequate perfusion of brain cells with oxygen and nutrients
   c. Sympathetic discharge constricts blood reservoirs, such as the veins, and propels blood toward the heart

D. Pulse
   1. Definition: alternate expansion and elastic recoil of blood vessel
   2. Cause: variations in pressure within vessel caused by intermittent injections of blood from heart into aorta with each ventricular contraction; pulse can be felt because of elasticity of arterial walls
   3. Pulse can be felt wherever artery lies near surface and over firm background such as bone; some of those most easily palpated are
      a. Radial artery: at wrist
      b. Temporal artery: in front of ear, or above and to outer side of eye
      c. Common carotid artery: along anterior edge of sternocleidomastoid muscle, at level of lower margin of thyroid cartilage
      d. Facial artery: at lower margin of lower jaw bone, on line with corners of mouth, in groove in mandible about one-third of way forward from angle of bone
      e. Brachial artery: at bend of the elbow, along the inner margin of the biceps muscle
      f. Posterior tibial artery: behind the medial malleolus (inner "ankle bone")
      g. Dorsalis pedis: on anterior surface of the foot, just below the bend of the ankle
   4. Venous pulse: in large veins only; produced by changes in venous pressure brought about by alternate contraction and relaxation of the atria rather than the ventricles, as in arterial pulse

Lymphatic System
Lymph Vessels

A. Structure: lymph capillaries similar to blood capillaries in structure; larger lymphatics similar to veins but are thinner walled, have more valves, and have lymph nodes in certain places along their course

B. Names: largest lymphatic known as thoracic duct; drains lymph from entire body, except upper right quadrant, into the left subclavian vein (where it joins the internal jugular); right lymphatic ducts drain lymph from the upper right quadrant into the right subclavian vein

C. Functions
   1. Lymphatics return fluid and proteins to blood from interstitial fluid; about 60% of fluid filtered out of blood capillaries returns to circulation via lymphatics rather than by osmosis into venous ends of capillaries; about 50% of total blood proteins leak out of capillaries per day; the only way these large molecules can return to blood is via lymphatics

2. Adequate lymph return is essential for maintaining homeostasis of blood proteins and therefore of blood volume
3. Interference with the return of proteins to the blood results in edema caused by the loss of protein and changes in colloid osmotic pressure

Lymph Nodes

A. Structure: lymphatic tissue, separated into compartments by fibrous partitions; afferent lymphatic vessels enter each node; one (usually) efferent vessel drains lymph out of node
B. Location: usually in clusters, some of the more important groups, from nursing viewpoint, are
   1. Submental and submaxillary groups in floor of mouth; lymph from nose, lips, and teeth drains through these nodes
   2. Superficial cervical nodes in neck, along sternocleidomastoid muscle; lymph from head and neck drains through these nodes
   3. Superficial cubital nodes at bend of elbow; lymph from hand and forearm drains through these nodes
   4. Axillary nodes in armpit; lymph from arm and upper part of the chest wall, including the breast, drains through these nodes (may be removed during mastectomy for carcinoma)
   5. Inguinal nodes in groin; lymph from the leg and external genitals drains through these nodes
C. Functions
   1. Help defend the body against injurious substances (notably, bacteria and tumor cells) by filtering them out of lymph and thereby preventing their entrance into bloodstream; leukocytes in lymph nodes destroy many of these substances by phagocytosis and antibody action
   2. Lymphatic tissue of lymph nodes carries on the process of hemopoiesis; specifically, it forms T and B lymphocytes

Lymph

A. Definition: fluid in lymphatics
B. Source: interstitial fluid that has entered the lymphatic capillaries
   1. Interstitial fluid is the fluid in the microscopic tissue spaces
   2. Interstitial fluid is formed by plasma filtering out of the blood capillaries into the tissue spaces

Spleen

A. Location: left hypochondrium, above and behind cardiac portion of the stomach
B. Structure: lymphatic tissue, similar to lymph nodes; size varies, contains numerous spaces filled with venous blood
C. Functions
   1. Defense: phagocytosis of particles such as microbes, red cell fragments, and platelets by reticuloendothelial cells of spleen (reticuloendothelial system—phagocytic cells, located mainly in the liver, spleen, bone marrow, and lymph nodes; also, macrophages of connective tissue and microglia in the brain and cord); antibody formation by plasma cells of spleen

2. Hemopoiesis: lymphatic tissue of the spleen, like that of the lymph nodes, forms lymphocytes and possibly monocytes
3. Spleen serves as blood reservoir; sympathetic stimulation causes constriction of its capsule, squeezing out an estimated 200 ml of blood into general circulation within 1 minute

REVIEW OF PHYSICAL PRINCIPLES RELATED TO THE CIRCULATORY SYSTEM
Principles of Mechanics
Newton's Laws of Motion

A. First law: a body remains at rest or in uniform motion in a straight line unless forces act on it to make it change its state of rest or uniform motion; in other words, bodies continue to do whatever they are doing unless some force acts on them
   EXAMPLE: The heart produces the force that propels the blood through the vessels; without such a force the blood would come to rest as a result of friction between the blood and the blood vessels
B. Second law: if a body is accelerated, the greater the force applied to it, the greater the acceleration; the greater the mass of the body, the more force needed to produce a desired acceleration
   EXAMPLE: In polycythemia the greater cell mass of each unit volume of blood requires greater force of cardiac contraction to produce a desired rate of blood flow
C. Third law: for every action there is an equal and opposite reaction
   EXAMPLE: As blood flows through an artery, it exerts an action force on the walls of the artery; the walls of the artery exert a reaction force on the blood, which helps to provide the pressure to keep the blood flowing

Law of Gravitation

Any two objects in the universe are attracted to each other with a force equal to the product of the masses of the two objects divided by the square of the distance between them (e.g., the greater the mass of the bodies, the greater the gravitational force; the closer they are together, the greater the gravitational force)
EXAMPLE: When a person is standing, blood tends to pool in the lower extremities, resulting in bulging of veins in lower parts of the body and requiring greater pumping force from the heart to overcome such pooling; orthostatic hypotension and recovery by the baroreceptor reflex are a direct result of gravitational forces; the evolutionary development of valves in the venous system (particularly in the legs) is due to gravitational forces

Momentum

A. Basic concept: an object's momentum is dependent on its mass and the velocity at which it is moving
   EXAMPLE: A 112.5 kg (250 lb) person in a heavy motorized wheelchair moving down a corridor at 3 mph (4.8 kph) has greater momentum than a 45 kg (100 lb) person in a light wheelchair rolling along at 5 mph (8 kph)
B. Changes in momentum: an object's momentum can be changed by applying a force to the object for a certain length of time; the greater the force applied and/or the

longer the time that the force is applied, the greater is the change in momentum of the object
EXAMPLE: During exercise, the contracting heart imparts great momentum to the blood because the force of contraction of the myocardium is great, and the duration of contraction of the myocardium is relatively long

Energy

A. Basic concept: a property that enables a body to perform work
EXAMPLE: The heart possesses energy because it is capable of doing the work of circulating the blood
B. Work: the product of the force exerted and the distance through which the force moves
EXAMPLE: The heart exerts a force that moves the blood a certain distance
C. Laws concerning energy
  1. First law of thermodynamics (law of conservation of energy): energy cannot be created or destroyed but may be transformed from one form into another
EXAMPLE: The potential energy of the ATP molecule is transformed into the kinetic energy of cardiac muscle contraction during the cardiac cycle
  2. Second law of thermodynamics: all systems in the universe have a natural tendency to become disorderly or randomized; the energy of the system continually becomes more spread out and dilute
    a. Molecules tend to move from areas where they are in high concentration to areas where they are in low concentration; this is usually stated as the law of diffusion
EXAMPLES
      (1) The diffusion of oxygen and carbon dioxide between the air sacs and capillaries of the lungs
      (2) The diffusion of water through the membrane systems of cells (osmosis)
    b. Heat always flows from a hot body into a colder one
EXAMPLES
      (1) Some of the chemical energy stored in muscles is transformed into heat when muscles contract; this heat flows from the hot body (the muscles) into cooler bodies (the surrounding tissues, including blood) and helps to maintain the human body temperature of 98.6° F (37° C)
      (2) When the human body is too hot, vasodilation occurs in the skin and heat radiates from the body into the cooler surrounding air

Efficiency

Efficiency: never total, since friction that occurs when two surfaces rub together produces resistance and heat; the greater the efficiency, the less heat produced; friction causes mechanical devices eventually to be worn away
EXAMPLE: If friction did not operate, the human heart would only have to beat once in a lifetime, since the initial force would propel the blood indefinitely through the blood vessels; friction continuously slows blood flow, and consequently the adult heart beats an average of 72 times each minute

Principles of Physical Properties of Matter
Solids

Concept of elasticity: because of external or internal stresses, solids may change their shape or size
EXAMPLE: Heart and blood vessels constantly change shape as blood pressure and degree of neural stimulation undergo change

Liquids

A. Hydrostatic pressure: force per unit area caused by the weight of the fluid on matter submerged in the fluid
EXAMPLE: The weight of blood in a capillary exerts a hydrostatic force that helps to filter the blood through the capillary wall, forming interstitial fluid
B. Pascal's principle: when pressure is applied to a fluid in a closed, nonflexible container, it is transmitted undiminished throughout all parts of the fluid and acts in all directions
EXAMPLES: In the circulatory system the pressure exerted as a result of the contracting ventricles is transmitted throughout the blood vessels of the circulatory system; this pressure is responsible for blood flow
  1. Pressure: fluid always flows from regions of higher pressure to those of lower pressure; the pressure in the human circulatory system is highest in the ventricles during systole, decreases throughout the length of the circulatory system, and is lowest in the atria; the normal pressure of blood in the circulatory system varies with age and disease
  2. Lumen of the tube: the flow of fluid through a tube is larger when the radius of the tube is larger (e.g., the degree of constriction of the arterioles for the most part determines the quantity of blood entering the capillary beds and returning to the heart)
  3. Length of the tube: the longer the tube, the less fluid flow there is through it in a unit of time; when blood circulation to the skin is greatly increased, the heart must increase its output to maintain normal circulation, since many more miles of tubing (capillaries) have been added to the system
  4. Viscosity: the molecular components of a fluid exert forces of attraction on each other; as the fluid flows along, an internal friction, caused by the molecular attractions of the fluid's components, tends to impede it; viscosity is a measure of this internal resistance to fluid flow
    a. Anemia: because of a reduced number of erythrocytes, the viscosity of the blood is decreased; therefore blood returns to the heart more rapidly, increasing cardiac output, which may overwork the heart during periods of increased exercise
    b. Polycythemia: an increased number of erythrocytes in the blood increases its viscosity; blood flows more sluggishly and the blood pressure increases to compensate
C. Capillarity: when a small-diameter tube is dipped into water or other fluid, the water will rise in the tube because of adhesion of the water molecules to the components of the glass; surface tension then causes the film of water to contract and pull itself up the tube; the water continues to rise until its weight balances the adhe-

sive force; this rise of the fluid level in a tube is called capillarity or capillary action

EXAMPLE: Capillarity draws blood into a capillary tube when a technician takes a small blood sample for various analyses

Gases

Gases are carried in the circulatory system by adhering to other molecules

Principles of Acoustics

Basic concept: sound is a wave caused by mechanical vibration that cannot occur in a vacuum; it is propagated best through solids and through liquids better than gases; it travels in waves from a vibrating source such as human vocal cords, a loudspeaker, or a dropped object

EXAMPLES

1. A very faint heartbeat can be heard only with a stethoscope or by placing the ear on the chest; even strong heartbeats cannot be heard distinctly with just the ears
2. The sound vibrations (waves) pass readily through the tissue of the human body to the surface of the skin where the stethoscope can pick them up
3. Ultrasonic fetal heart monitors can detect the fetal heart beat as early as the twelfth week of gestation
4. Echocardiography: a sound wave–constructed picture of the heart helps in the identification of cardiac diseases

Principles of Electricity
Electric Force

A. The atoms composing all matter represent an almost perfect balance of protons and electrons; the attraction of a positive proton for a negative electron (opposite charges attracting) is the electric force that also makes like charges repel each other
B. Electric forces hold atoms and molecules together and thus hold solid matter together; electric forces also provide the source for all chemical energy; the molecular rearrangements associated with cellular metabolism derive their energy from electric forces between enzymes, substrates, and cofactors

Conductors and Insulators

A. Conductors are good transferrers of electric charges and the energy they contain; copper and aluminum are good conductors and are commonly used for all electric wiring, including the electrodes for cardiac monitoring
B. Insulators: rubber and most nonmetals are good insulators, as is the connective tissue that separates the atria and ventricles of the heart and electrically insulates these regions; consequently the only way electrical energy can flow from the AV node to the ventricles is through the heart's specialized conducting system (bundle of His) in the interventricular septum
C. Water as a conductor: distilled water is a poor conductor, although tap water contains enough charged particles (ions) to make it a fairly good electric conductor; the ions (electrolytes) of body fluids make them excellent conductors of electrical energy

Application of Electricity

A. Electronic devices used in health care
   1. Electronic cardiac pacemakers: battery-operated devices supplement or replace defective electric stimulation in the human heart and thus help maintain the individual's heartbeat at a selected rate
   2. Defibrillator: electronic device that delivers electrical energy through electrodes strategically placed on an individual whose heart is in atrial or ventricular fibrillation; the use of such a device is based on the premise that the sustaining mechanism of the fibrillation process is different from the initiating mechanism; thus, if the initiating mechanism is no longer present and the sustaining mechanism is terminated by the defibrillating electric current, sinus rhythm will ensue
B. Applications to the human body: the contraction of all types of muscle is preceded by depolarization of the muscle fibers; ions carry the electric charges
   EXAMPLE: Electrocardiograms measure and record the electric activity of the heart as this activity is carried to the surface of the body by the ions of the body fluids; this information provides an electric picture of the heart's activity

Principles of Light (Electromagnetic Waves)

Basic concept: emission of high-frequency electromagnetic waves due to excitation of the orbital electrons of atoms; to excite the innermost orbital electron, considerable energy must be expended

EXAMPLE: Angiography: observation of motion picture x-ray images

REVIEW OF CHEMICAL PRINCIPLES RELATED TO THE CIRCULATORY SYSTEM
Enzymes

A. Organic catalysts that enter into reactions and are reformed at end of reaction
B. Needed in minute amounts
C. Protein in nature and inactivated by all factors that denature proteins (e.g., high temperature, changes in pH)
D. Substrate is the substance acted on by an enzyme; (e.g., carbon dioxide and water are the substrate for the enzyme carbonic anhydrase, found in the erythrocyte, which catalyzes the conversion of CO_2 and H_2O into carbonic acid)
E. Enzymes usually have ending "ase" added on to name of substrate or to action of enzyme (e.g., sucrase: enzyme hydrolyzing sucrose; lactic acid dehydrogenase: enzyme removing hydrogen from lactic acid)
F. Enzymes, being proteins, are usually quite specific in action
   1. One enzyme will usually catalyze only one reaction: substrate specificity
   2. Enzyme activity will be high at temperature specific for the enzyme and low at other temperatures: temperature specificity
   3. Enzyme activity will be high at the pH specific for the enzyme and low at other pH values: pH specificity

G. Certain inorganic ions act to speed up or slow down enzyme activity: enzyme activators and enzyme inhibitors

H. Enzymes acting within cells are called intracellular enzymes (e.g., the enzymes that bring about the breakdown of glucose and other sugars and the synthesis of carbohydrates, proteins, and nucleic acids all function within cells and are intracellular enzymes)

I. Enzymes acting outside cells are called extracellular enzymes (e.g., the digestive enzymes that are found in the mouth, stomach, and small intestine all function outside cells and are extracellular enzymes)

J. Some enzymes exist in two parts
  1. Apoenzyme: protein part of enzyme (inactive)
  2. Coenzyme: nonprotein part of enzyme (inactive)
  3. Holoenzyme: the apoenzyme and the coenzyme together (active molecule)

REVIEW OF MICROORGANISMS RELATED TO THE CIRCULATORY SYSTEM

A. *Streptococcus pyogenes:* gram-positive streptococcus; the most virulent strain (Group A beta hemolytic) causes scarlet fever, septic sore throat, tonsillitis, cellulitis, puerperal fever, erysipelas, rheumatic fever, and glomerulonephritis

B. *Streptococcus viridans:* gram-positive streptococcus; distinguishable from *S. pyogenes* by its alpha hemolysis (rather than beta) of red cells; the most common cause of subacute bacterial endocarditis

PHARMACOLOGY RELATED TO CIRCULATORY SYSTEM DISORDERS
Cardiac Glycosides

A. Description
  1. Used to improve the pumping ability of the heart, thus increasing cardiac output
  2. Produce a positive inotropic effect (increased force of contraction) by increasing permeability of cardiac muscle membranes to the calcium and sodium ions required for contraction of muscle fibrils
  3. Produce a negative chronotropic effect (decreased rate of contraction) by an action mediated through the vagus nerve which slows firing of the SA node and impulse transmission by the AV node
  4. Responsible for a diuretic effect due to increased renal blood flow
  5. Effective in the treatment of congestive heart failure and atrial flutter and fibrillation
  6. Available in oral and parenteral (IM, IV) preparations
  7. Initially, loading dose is administered to digitalize the client; after the desired effect is achieved, the dosage is lowered to a maintenance level which replaces the amount of drug metabolized and excreted each day

B. Examples
  1. digitalis
  2. digitoxin (Crystodigin)
  3. digoxin (Lanoxin)
  4. gitalin (Gitaligin)
  5. lanatoside C (Cedilanid)
  6. ouabain

C. Major side effects
  1. Nausea, vomiting, diarrhea (local oral effect-stimulates chemoreceptor zone in medulla)
  2. Anorexia (nausea and vomiting due to chemoreceptor zone stimulation)
  3. Malabsorption of all nutrients (nausea, vomiting, diarrhea)
  4. Bradycardia (increased vagal tone at AV node)
  5. Toxicity
    a. Arrhythmias (PVCs) (increased spontaneous rate of ventricular depolarization)
    b. Xanthopsia (yellow vision) (effect on visual cones)
    c. Muscle weakness (CNS effect, neurotoxicity, hypokalemia)

D. Nursing care
  1. Check apical pulse prior to administration; in the adult if pulse is below 60 or above 120, withhold dose and notify the physician
  2. Administer oral preparations with meals to reduce GI irritation
  3. Encourage intake of high nutrient density foods
  4. Assess client for signs of impending toxicity
  5. Monitor the client for hypokalemia, which potentiates the effects of digitalis
  6. Instruct the client to
    a. Count radial pulse and record prior to each administration
    b. Notify physician of occurrence of any side effects
    c. Report any changes in heart rate to physician (irregular beats; increased or decreased rate)
  7. Digoxin—monitor blood level during therapy (normal: 0.5-2.5 ng/ml)
  8. Evaluate client's response to medication and understanding of teaching

Antiarrhythmics

A. Description
  1. Used to treat abnormal variations in cardiac rate and rhythm; also used to prevent the occurrence of arrhythmias in clients with the potential for their occurrence
  2. Available in oral and parenteral (IM, IV) preparations

B. Examples
  1. disopyramide phosphate (Norpace): controls ventricular arrhythmias by decreasing the rate of diastolic depolarization
  2. lidocaine HCl: controls ventricular irritability by shortening the refractory period and suppressing ectopic foci
  3. phenytoin (Dilantin): controls atrial or ventricular arrhythmias by reducing automaticity without decreasing conduction
  4. procainamide HCl (Pronestyl): controls ventricular and atrial arrhythmias by prolonging the refractory period of the heart and slowing the conduction of cardiac impulses
  5. propranolol (Inderal): controls supraventricular arrhythmias by decreasing cardiac impulse conduction through a beta-adrenergic blocking action
  6. quinidine preparations: control atrial arrhythmias

by prolonging the effective refractory period and slowing depolarization

7. Calcium ion antagonists: control atrial arrhythmias by decreasing cardiac automaticity and impulse conduction

C. Major side effects
1. Hypotension (decreased cardiac output due to vasodilation)
2. Dizziness (hypotension)
3. Nausea, vomiting (irritation of gastric mucosa)
4. Heart block (direct cardiac toxic effect; cardiac depressant)
5. Anticholinergic effect (decreased parasympathetic stimulation)
6. Blood dyscrasias (decreased RBC, WBC, platelet synthesis)
7. Toxicity
   a. Diarrhea (GI irritation)
   b. CNS disturbances (neurotoxicity)
   c. Sensory disturbances (neurotoxicity)

D. Nursing care
1. Assess vital signs during course of therapy
2. Utilize cardiac monitoring during IV administration
3. Instruct client to
   a. Notify physician of occurrence of any side effects
   b. Report any changes in heart rate or rhythm to physician (irregular beats; increased or decreased rate)
4. Monitor blood levels during therapy
   a. quinidine (2 to 5 μg/ml)
   b. procainamide (4 to 8 μg/ml)
   c. lidocaine (2 to 5 μg/ml)
   d. phenytoin (10 to 20 μg/ml)
5. Monitor blood work during long-term therapy
6. Administer oral preparations with meals to reduce GI irritation
7. Monitor ECGs during course of therapy
8. Utilize infusion-control device for continuous IV administration
9. Utilize safety precautions (supervise ambulation, side rails up) when CNS effects are manifested
10. Evaluate client's response to medication and understanding of teaching

Cardiac Stimulants

A. Description
1. Used to increase the heart rate
2. Act by either indirect or direct mechanisms affecting the autonomic nervous system
3. Available in parenteral (IM, IV), intracardiac, and intrathecal preparations

B. Examples
1. atropine sulfate: suppresses parasympathetic nervous system control at SA and AV nodes, thus allowing heart rate to increase
2. epinephrine HCl (Adrenalin): stimulates the rate and force of cardiac contraction via the sympathetic nervous system
3. isoproterenol HCl (Isuprel): stimulates beta-adrenergic receptors of the sympathetic nervous system, thus increasing heart rate

C. Major side effects
1. Tachycardia (sympathetic stimulation)
2. Headache (dilation of cerebral vessels)
3. CNS stimulation (sympathetic stimulation)
4. Cardiac arrhythmias (cardiovascular system stimulation)
5. atropine: anticholinergic effects (dry mouth, blurred vision, urinary retention as a result of decreased parasympathetic stimulation)

D. Nursing care
1. Assess vital signs during course of therapy
2. Utilize cardiac monitoring during IV administration
3. Monitor ECG during course of therapy
4. Utilize safety precautions (side rails up) during administration
5. Evaluate client's response to medication and understanding of teaching

Coronary Vasodilators

A. Description
1. Used to decrease cardiac work and myocardial oxygen requirements by their vasodilatory action to decrease preload and decrease afterload
2. Nitrates act directly at "nitrate" receptors in smooth muscles causing relaxation of the smooth muscle (vasodilation); produces marked venodilation which decreases the preload, thus decreasing cardiac workload
3. Calcium ion antagonists inhibit the influx of the calcium ion across the cell membrane during depolarization of the cardiac and vascular smooth muscle
4. Effective in the treatment of angina pectoris
5. Available in oral, sublingual, buccal, and topical, including transdermal, preparations

B. Examples
1. Nitrates (sublingual)
   a. erythrityl tetranitrate (Cardilate)
   b. isosorbide dinitrate (Isordil, Sorbitrate)
   c. nitroglycerin
2. Nitrates (oral)
   a. isosorbide dinitrate (Isordil, Sorbitrate)
   b. erythrityl tetranitrate (Cardilate)
3. Nitrates (topical)
   a. nitroglycerin ointment
      (1) Nitro-Bid
      (2) Nitrol
   b. nitroglycerin transdermal
      (1) Nitrodisk
      (2) Nitro-Dur
      (3) Transderm-Nitro
4. Calcium-ion antagonists (calcium channel blockers)
   a. diltiazem (Cardizem)
   b. nifedipine (Procardia)
   c. verapamil (Calan, Isoptin)

C. Major side effects
1. Headache (dilation of cerebral vessels)
2. Flushing (peripheral vasodilation)
3. Orthostatic hypotension (loss of compensatory vasoconstriction with position change)
4. Tachycardia (reflex reaction to severe hypotension)
5. Dizziness (orthostatic hypotension)

D. Nursing care
   1. Assess for signs and symptoms of shock before administering; if present, withhold drug
   2. Encourage client to change positions slowly
   3. Utilize safety precautions (supervise ambulation; side rails up)
   4. Nitroglycerin: instruct client to
      a. Take sublingual preparations prior to angina-producing activities
      b. Note slight stinging, burning, tingling under the tongue; indicates potency of drug
      c. Avoid placing the drug in heat, light, moisture, or plastic; store in original amber glass container
      d. Take sublingual preparations every 5 minutes, not to exceed 3 tablets in 15 minutes for chest pain; if pain persists, go to emergency room
   5. Evaluate client's response to medication and understanding of teaching

Antihypertensives

A. Description
   1. Used to promote dilation of peripheral blood vessels, thus decreasing blood pressure and afterload
   2. Available in oral, parenteral (IM, IV), and transdermal preparations
B. Examples
   1. clonidine (Catapres): sympatholytic
   2. diazoxide (Hyperstat IV): direct smooth muscle relaxation; may promote hyperglycemia
   3. guanethidine sulfate (Ismelin): sympatholytic
   4. hydralazine HCl (Apresoline): direct smooth muscle relaxation; increases excretion of vitamin B_6
   5. methyldopa (Aldomet): sympatholytic
   6. nitroprusside sodium (Nipride): direct smooth muscle relaxation; reduces level of serum B_{12}
   7. prazosin HCl (Minipress): direct smooth muscle relaxation
   8. propranolol (Inderal): beta-adrenergic blocker (sympatholytic)
   9. reserpine (Serpasil): peripheral norepinephrine depletion
   10. captopril (Capoten): angiotensin converting enzyme (ACE) inhibitor
   11. enalapril maleate (Vasotec): ACE inhibitor
C. Major side effects
   1. Orthostatic hypotension (loss of compensatory vasoconstriction with position change)
   2. Dizziness (orthostatic hypotension)
   3. Cardiac rate alteration
      a. Bradycardia (sympatholytics) (decreased sympathetic stimulation to the heart)
      b. Tachycardia (direct relaxers) (reflex reaction to severe hypotension)
   4. Sexual disturbances (failure of erection or ejaculation due to loss of vascular tone)
   5. Blood dyscrasias (decreased RBC, WBC, platelet synthesis)
   6. Drowsiness (cerebral hypoxia)
D. Nursing care
   1. Monitor blood pressure in standing and supine positions during course of therapy

2. Instruct client to
   a. Follow a low-sodium diet
   b. Change positions slowly
   c. Continue to take medication as prescribed; therapy is usually for life
   d. Report occurrence of any side effects to physician
   e. Avoid engaging in hazardous activities when initially placed on antihypertensive drug therapy
3. Reserpine: assess client for mental depression; implement suicide precautions
4. Nitroprusside: protect IV solution from light; discard unused portions according to manufacturer's schedule
5. Assess vital signs, especially pulse, during the course of therapy
6. Encourage intake of foods high in B-complex vitamins
7. Evaluate client's response to medication and understanding of teaching

Diuretics

A. Description
   1. Used to increase urine output which reduces hypervolemia; decreases preload and afterload
   2. Interferes with sodium reabsorption in the kidney
   3. Available in oral and parenteral (IM, SC, IV) preparations
B. Examples
   1. Thiazides: interfere with sodium ion transport at loop of Henle and inhibit carbonic anhydrase activity at distal tubule sites
      a. chlorothiazide (Diuril)
      b. chlorthalidone (Hygroton)
      c. hydrochlorothiazide (HydroDIURIL)
      d. methyclothiazide (Enduron)
   2. Potassium-sparers: interfere with aldosterone-induced reabsorption of sodium ions at distal nephron sites to increase sodium chloride excretion and decrease potassium ion loss
      a. spironolactone (Aldactone)
      b. triamterine (Dyrenium)
   3. Loop diuretics: interfere with active transport of sodium ions in loop of Henle and inhibit sodium chloride and water reabsorption at proximal tubule sites
      a. ethacrynic acid (Edecrin)
      b. furosemide (Lasix)
C. Major side effects
   1. GI irritation (local oral effect)
   2. Hyponatremia (inhibition of sodium reabsorption at the kidney tubule)
   3. Orthostatic hypotension (reduced blood volume)
   4. Hyperuricemia (partial blockage of uric acid excretion)
   5. Dehydration (excessive sodium and water loss)
   6. All diuretics except potassium-sparers
      a. Hypokalemia (increased potassium excretion)
      b. Increased urinary excretion of magnesium
      c. Increased urinary excretion of zinc

7. Potassium-sparers
    a. Hyperkalemia (reabsorption of potassium at the kidney tubule)
    b. Hypomagnesemia
    c. Increased urinary excretion of calcium
D. Nursing care
    1. Maintain intake and output records
    2. Weigh daily (same time, same scale, same clothing)
    3. Administer the drug in the morning so that the maximal effect will occur during the waking hours
    4. Assess vital signs, especially pulse and blood pressure, during the course of therapy
    5. Encourage intake of foods high in calcium, magnesium, zinc, and potassium (except for potassium-sparers)
    6. Assess client for signs of fluid-electrolyte imbalance
    7. Instruct client to change positions slowly
    8. Thiazides: monitor blood sugar in diabetics; may cause hyperglycemia
    9. Be alert for signs of hypokalemia (muscle weakness, cramps)
    10. Evaluate client's response to medication and understanding of teaching

Peripheral Vasoconstrictors

A. Description
    1. Used to elevate the blood pressure
    2. Act by constriction of peripheral blood vessels through alpha-adrenergic stimulation
    3. Available in parenteral (IV) preparations
B. Examples
    1. levarterenol bitartrate (Levophed)
    2. mephentermine sulfate (Wyamine)
    3. metaraminol bitartrate (Aramine)
    4. phenylephrine HCl (Neo-Synephrine)
C. Major side effects
    1. Hypertension (compression of cerebral blood vessels)
    2. Headache (increase in blood pressure)
    3. Gastrointestinal disturbance (autonomic dysfunction)
D. Nursing care
    1. Assess vital signs during course of therapy
    2. Monitor blood pressure at frequent intervals
    3. Assess for IV infiltration; may lead to tissue necrosis
    4. Titrate IV with blood pressure to prevent hypertension
    5. Do not leave client unattended
    6. Encourage intake of high fiber foods to reduce the potential of constipation
    7. Evaluate client's response to medication and understanding of teaching

Anticoagulants

A. Description
    1. Used to prevent clot formation and clot extension
    2. Act to prevent fibrin formation by interfering with the production of various clotting factors in the coagulation process
    3. Anticoagulants available in oral and parenteral (SC, IV) preparations

B. Examples
    1. Heparin sodium: must be administered parenterally
    2. Oral anticoagulants
        a. dicumarol (Dicumarol Pulvules)
        b. warfarin sodium (Coumadin)
C. Major side effects
    1. Fever, chills (hypersensitivity)
    2. Skin rash (hypersensitivity)
    3. Hemorrhage (interference with clotting mechanisms)
    4. Diarrhea (GI irritation)
D. Nursing care
    1. Monitor blood work during course of therapy, especially coagulation studies
    2. Assess client for signs of bleeding
    3. Have appropriate antidote available
        a. Vitamin K for warfarin
        b. Protamine sulfate for heparin
    4. Avoid administration of salicylates during anticoagulant therapy
    5. Avoid IM injections of other drugs if possible
    6. Instruct client to
        a. Report any signs of bleeding to the physician immediately
        b. Carry a medical alert card
        c. Avoid use of alcohol during therapy
        d. Use an electric razor and soft toothbrush
        e. Avoid taking OTC medications containing aspirin
        f. Keep appointments for laboratory tests (coagulation studies)
        g. Eat a consistent diet of vitamin K-containing foods (leafy green vegetables)
        h. Evaluate client's response to medication and understanding of teaching

Antianemics

A. Description
    1. Used to promote RBC production
    2. Include iron-containing compounds and vitamin replacements necessary for erythrocyte formation
    3. Effective in the treatment of iron-deficiency and nutritional anemias
    4. Available in oral and parenteral (IM, SC, IV) preparations
B. Examples
    1. Iron compounds (oral)
        a. ferrocholinate (Chel-Iron)
        b. ferrous gluconate
        c. ferrous sulfate
    2. Iron compounds (parenteral)
        a. iron-dextran (Imferon)
        b. iron sorbitex (Jectofer)
    3. Vitamin replacements
        a. cyanocobalamin: Vitamin B_{12} (Rubramin)
        b. folic acid: Vitamin B_9 (Folvite)
C. Major side effects
    1. Iron replacements
        a. Nausea, vomiting (irritation of gastric mucosa)
        b. Constipation (delayed passage of iron and stool in GI tract)
        c. Black stools (presence of unabsorbed iron in stool)

d. Stained teeth (liquid preparations) (contact of liquid iron with enamel)

e. Tissue staining (injectable preparations) (leakage of iron into tissue)

2. Vitamin replacements
    a. Local irritation (local tissue effect)
    b. Allergic reactions, anaphylaxis (hypersensitivity)
    c. Diarrhea (GI irritation)

D. Nursing care
1. Iron replacements
    a. Inform client about side effects of therapy
    b. Utilize Z-track procedure for IM administration
    c. Administer liquid preparations through a straw after diluting with water or fruit juice; encourage good oral hygiene
    d. Administer oral preparations on an empty stomach if possible for optimum absorption; ascorbic acid (vitamin C) increases absorption
    e. Encourage intake of foods high in iron, vitamin B_{12}, and folacin
    f. Encourage intake of high fiber foods to reduce the potential of constipation
    g. Deferoxamine mesylate (Desferal) is the antidote for iron toxicity

2. Vitamin replacements
    a. Vitamin B_{12}: inform client that this drug cannot be administered orally; therapy is for life
    b. Folic acid: instruct client on good dietary sources of folic acid (fresh fruits, vegetables, and meats)

3. Evaluate client's response to medication and understanding of teaching

Antilipemics

A. Description
1. Used to lower serum lipid levels by reducing cholesterol or triglyceride synthesis or both
2. Available in oral preparations

B. Examples
1. cholestyramine (Questran)
2. clofibrate (Atromid-S)
3. niacin (Nicobid)
4. dextrothyroxine (Choloxin)
5. lovastatin (Mevacor)
6. colestipol hydrochloride (Colestid)
7. probucol (Lorelco)

C. Major side effects
1. Nausea, vomiting (irritation to gastric mucosa)
2. Diarrhea (GI irritation)
3. Musculoskeletal disturbances (direct musculoskeletal tissue effect)
4. Hepatic disturbances (hepatic toxicity)
5. Skin rash
6. Reduced absorption of fat and fat-soluble vitamins (A, D, E, K) as well as vitamin B_{12} and iron (except for Nicobid)
7. Niacin: flushing (transient) (vasodilation)
8. lovastatin: visual disturbances (ocular alterations)

D. Nursing care
1. Encourage the following dietary program:
    a. Low cholesterol, low fat (especially saturated)
    b. Replace vegetable oils high in PUFA with those high in MUFA such as olive, avocado
    c. Eat fish which are high in omega-3 fatty acids several times per week (salmon, tuna)
    d. Increase intake of high-fiber foods such as fruits, vegetables, cereal grains and legumes; soluble fiber is particularly effective in reducing blood lipids (oat bran, legumes)

2. Offer emotional support to client; long-term therapy may be necessary
3. Administer medications with meals to reduce GI irritation
4. Monitor serum cholesterol and triglyceride levels during therapy
5. Monitor hemoglobin and RBC levels during therapy
6. Monitor blood levels of fat-soluble vitamins during therapy
7. Monitor liver function tests during therapy
8. Cholestyramine: mix with full glass of liquid
9. Clofibrate: assess for potentiation of anticoagulant effect
10. Lovastatin: assess for visual disturbances with prolonged use
11. Evaluate client's response to medication and understanding of teaching

Thrombolytics

A. Description
1. Used to dissolve occluding thrombi in the coronary arteries
2. Act by converting plasminogen to plasmin which initiates local fibrinolysis
3. Administered intravenously or intraarterially (via cardiac catherization)
4. Initially, loading dose is administered; lower doses may be continued for 24 to 72 hours
5. Therapy must be instituted within 4 to 6 hours of the onset of the myocardial infarction

B. Examples
1. streptokinase (Streptase)
2. urokinase (Abbokinase, Win-Kinase)
3. tissue plasminogen activator (TPA)

C. Major side effects
1. Bleeding (increased fibrinolytic activity)
2. Allergic reactions (introduction of a foreign protein)
3. Low grade fever (resulting from absorption of infarcted tissue)

D. Nursing care
1. Observe for signs of bleeding
2. Monitor partial thromboplastin time (PTT) and fibrinogen concentration
3. Monitor vital signs
4. Assess for signs of allergic reactions such as chills, urticaria, pruritis, rash, and malaise
5. Keep aminocaproic acid, a fibrinolysis inhibitor, available on nursing unit
6. Evaluate client's response to medication and understanding of teaching

PROCEDURES RELATED TO THE CIRCULATORY SYSTEM
Angiography

A. Definition: an x-ray examination using contrast dye to visualize the patency of an artery
B. Nursing care
   1. Inform the client of the risks involved in this procedure (allergic reaction, embolus, cardiac arrhythmia)
   2. Administer mild sedative as ordered prior to procedure
   3. Observe the client for complications
   4. Postprocedure care involves checking the injection site for bleeding and inflammation, assessing circulatory status of the extremities, and enforcing bed rest
   5. Evaluate client's response to procedure

Angioplasty

A. Definition: Percutaneous transluminal coronary angioplasty (PTCA) is the introduction of a balloon-tipped catheter into the coronary artery to the point of stenosis to reduce or eliminate the occlusion
   1. Procedure is performed in a coronary catherization laboratory under fluoroscopy
   2. Heparin infusion is used during the procedure to prevent thrombus formation
   3. Streptokinase therapy may be combined with PTCA in some situations
B. Nursing care
   1. See care for cardiac catherization
   2. Transfer client to an institution with equipment for this procedure, if necessary
   3. Administer vasoactive drugs such as calcium-channel blockers and nitroglycerine before, during, and after this procedure, as ordered
   4. Monitor client for angina and arrhythmias
   5. Evaluate client's response to procedure

Blood Transfusion

A. Purpose
   1. Restore blood volume after hemorrhage
   2. Maintain hemoglobin levels in severe anemias
   3. Replace specific blood components
B. Nursing care
   1. Check that blood or blood components have been typed and cross matched, indicating that the blood of the donor and recipient are compatible
   2. Blood must never be administered straight from the refrigerator
   3. A baseline of the client's temperature, blood pressure, pulse, and respirations should be determined prior to administration
   4. An IV with normal saline and a blood administration set containing a filter are used to start the infusion; solutions containing glucose may cause the blood to clot in the tubing and should not be used
   5. Before starting the infusion, it is advisable for two nurses to verify the blood type, Rh factor, client and blood numbers, and expiration date
   6. The container should be inverted gently to suspend the red cells within the plasma
   7. Observe for signs of hemolytic reaction, which generally occur early in the transfusion (within the first 10 to 15 minutes)
      a. Shivering
      b. Headache
      c. Lower back pain
      d. Increased pulse and respiratory rate
      e. Hemoglobinuria
      f. Oliguria
      g. Hypotension
   8. Observe for signs of febrile reaction, which usually occur within 30 minutes
      a. Shaking
      b. Headache
      c. Elevated temperature
      d. Back pain
      e. Confusion
      f. Hematemesis
   9. Observe for allergic reaction
      a. Hives
      b. Wheezing
      c. Pruritus
      d. Joint pain
   10. If any reaction occurs
      a. Stop infusion immediately
      b. Notify the physician
      c. Maintain patency of the IV with normal saline
      d. Send blood to the laboratory
      e. Monitor vital signs frequently
      f. Send a urine specimen to the laboratory if a hemolytic reaction is suspected
   11. Evaluate client's response to procedure

Bone Marrow Aspiration

A. Definition: puncture to collect tissue from the bone marrow
   1. Sites used include the sternum, vertebral body, iliac crest, or the tibia in infants
   2. Performed to study the cells involved in blood production
B. Nursing care
   1. Obtain informed consent
   2. Attempt to allay anxiety of the client
   3. Assist the physician in maintaining a sterile field and positioning the client
   4. Send the specimen to the laboratory in a proper container with appropriate label
   5. Evaluate client's response to procedure

Cardiac Catheterization

A. Definition: introduction of a catheter into the heart via a peripheral vessel
   1. Injection of contrast material for visualization of chambers, coronary circulation, and great vessels
   2. Withdrawal of blood samples to evaluate cardiac function
   3. Measurement of pressures within chambers and blood vessels (e.g., pulmonary wedge pressure)
B. Nursing care
   1. Obtain an informed consent; the client should be aware of the purpose of and the complications possible with this procedure as well as the sensations experienced (e.g., urge to cough, nausea, heat)

2. Allow time for verbalization of fears
3. Keep the client npo for 6 to 8 hours prior to the procedure
4. Determine the presence of allergies, particularly to iodine
5. Administer sedatives as ordered prior to the procedure
6. After catheterization
   a. Monitor vital signs frequently; cardiac arrhythmias are more common during the procedure but may occur afterward
   b. Assess the puncture site for bleeding (sandbags or ice packs may be ordered if the femoral artery is used)
   c. Assess the involved extremity for signs of ischemia (e.g., absence of peripheral pulses, changes in sensation, color, and temperature)
   d. Maintain bed rest for the prescribed number of hours
7. Evaluate client's response to procedure

Cardiac Monitoring

A. Definition
   1. Electric observation of the conductivity patterns of the heart by the use of skin electrodes and a monitoring device; the heart's electric activity is conducted to the surface of the skin by the salty fluids bathing the cells and tissues
   2. Utilized in heart disease, during surgery and intrusive procedures, or when danger of arrhythmias (cardiac irregularities in rhythm) is apparent
   3. P, Q, R, S, and T segments are parts of the normal electrocardiogram (ECG); P wave represents atrial depolarization, QRS waves (QRS complex) ventricular depolarization, and T wave ventricular repolarization
B. Nursing care
   1. Explain the procedure to client and attempt to allay anxiety
   2. Prepare the skin on the chest for electrode attachment
      a. Cleanse area with alcohol swab to remove dirt and oils
      b. Shave the area to improve skin-electrode contact
   3. Place electrodes on the skin and attach to the monitor cable as indicated
      a. RA (attach to right upper chest)
      b. LA (attach to left upper chest)
      c. RA (attach to right lower chest [ground])
      d. d. LA (attach to left lower chest)
   4. Turn on the monitor scope and set the machine's sensitivity when a clear picture is obtained
   5. Observe the monitor for changes in rate and rhythm
   6. Set the alarm and readout attachment (if available) so an electric printout will be made if there is a change in cardiac activity
   7. If arrhythmia occurs, act appropriately
      a. Emergency arrhythmias require immediate intervention

b. If the arrhythmia is nonemergency, document its occurrence with a rhythm strip and notify the physician
8. Intervene immediately when life-threatening arrhythmias occur
   a. Ventricular fibrillation: repetitive rapid stimulation from ectopic ventricular foci to which the ventricles are unable to respond; ventricular contraction is replaced by uncoordinated twitching; circulation ceases, and death ensues
      (1) Defibrillate immediately
      (2) Inject lidocaine
      (3) Institute cardiopulmonary resuscitation
      (4) Document the arrhythmia and notify the physician
   b. Ventricular tachycardia: series of three or more bizarre premature ventricular beats that occur in a regular rhythm; this electric activity results in decreased cardiac output and may rapidly convert to ventricular fibrillation
      (1) Use lidocaine intravenously to convert rhythm
      (2) Be prepared to administer defibrillation and cardiopulmonary resuscitation
      (3) Document the arrhythmia and notify the physician
   c. Premature ventricular contractions (PVCs) of greater than 5 per minute: originate in the ventricles and occur before the next expected sinus beat; they can be life threatening when they occur close to the T wave, since cardiac repolarization is interfered with and ventricular fibrillation may ensue
      (1) Administer lidocaine intravenously
      (2) Document the arrhythmia and notify the physician
      (3) Long-term institution of oral antiarrhythmics may be indicated
   d. Complete heart block: occurs when there is no electric communication between the atria and ventricles and each beats independently; this activity will not provide long-term adequate circulation, and syncope, congestive failure, or cardiac arrest may ensue
      (1) Document the arrhythmia and notify the physician
      (2) Use of intravenous isoproterenol is generally indicated
      (3) Prepare for pacemaker insertion (see procedure)
   e. Asystole (cardiac standstill): occurs when there is no cardiac activity, demonstrated on the ECG tracing as a flat line; this terminates in death unless intervention is begun immediately
      (1) Institute cardiopulmonary resuscitation
      (2) Document the arrhythmia and notify the physician
      (3) Cardiac stimulants may be given via IV or intracardiac route
      (4) Pacemaker insertion may be indicated (see procedure)
9. Evaluate client's response to procedure

Cardiac Pacemaker Insertion

A. Definition: artificial pacemakers replace natural electric stimulation of the heart and are indicated in the treatment of
   1. Complete heart block: impulses generated from the SA node of the heart do not reach the ventricles; the atria and ventricles beat independently of each other
   2. Second-degree AV (atrioventricular) block: intermittent failure of impulse to reach the ventricles
   3. Adams-Stokes syndrome: a sudden drop in ventricular rate that causes syncope and temporary loss of consciousness
B. Pacemakers: involve the insertion of an electrode catheter into the right ventricle, which transmits the impulses generated by the pacing unit
   1. Demand pacemakers are most frequently used; the pacemaker will stimulate the ventricles to contract only if the client's ventricular rate falls below the rate set on the pacemaker
   2. Fixed-rate pacemakers stimulate the heart a specific amount of times per minute regardless of the client's rhythm
   3. Pacemakers may be temporary and worn externally or permanent and surgically placed under the skin
C. Nursing care
   1. Explain the procedure to the client
   2. Observe the cardiac monitor before, during, and after the procedure to verify pacemaker capture (QRS following pacemaker spike), and observe for arrhythmias
   3. Have emergency medications (e.g., lidocaine, atropine sulfate, isoproterenol) available, as well as a defibrillator
   4. Teach the client how to take pulse, to keep a diary of pulse, and to notify the physician immediately if the rate falls below that set on the pacemaker
   5. Teach the client to remain under a physician's supervision, since batteries must be replaced periodically; pacemaker function may be checked by special telephone devices
   6. Encourage the client to wear a bracelet or carry a medical alert card
   7. Teach client to avoid high magnetic fields such as airport security devices, high tension wires, and nuclear magnetic resonance (NMR); when in doubt consult physician
   8. Evaluate client's response to procedure

Cardiopulmonary Resuscitation (CPR)

A. Definition: institution of artificial ventilation and circulation with rescue breathing and external cardiac compression
B. Nursing care
   1. Ascertain the absence of spontaneous respiration and carotid pulse
   2. Call for help
   3. Place the victim on a firm surface
   4. Ventilate the lungs
      a. Straighten the airway
         (1) Head tilt maneuver
         (2) Chin tilt maneuver
         (3) Jaw thrust maneuver
      b. Pinch the nostrils
      c. Form a seal with the mouth
      d. Ventilate two times quickly
   5. Place heel of hand over lower half of body of sternum, interlock hands and compress the chest 3.8 to 5 cm (1½ to 2 inches for an adult)
   6. Maintain the ventilation/compression ratio
      a. One rescuer: two breaths after every 15 compressions (rate, 80 per minute)
      b. Two rescuers: one breath after every five compressions (rate, 80 per minute)
   7. Terminate CPR as indicated
      a. Return of cardiac rhythm and spontaneous respirations
      b. Lack of response suggestive of permanent, irreversible brain damage and death
   8. Evaluate client's response to procedure

Central Venous Pressure (CVP) Monitoring

A. Definition
   1. CVP is the right atrial pressure, which is normally 2 to 8 mm Hg
   2. A catheter is passed from the subclavian vein into the superior vena cava or right atrium
B. Nursing care
   1. Obtain informed consent
   2. Assist the physician with insertion of the catheter using surgical aseptic technique
   3. Obtain chest x-ray film after insertion to ascertain the position of the catheter
   4. Take readings as ordered
      a. Place the client in a supine position
      b. Place the stopcock of the manometer at the midaxillary line (which is approximately the level of the right atrium) and fill with fluid from line
      c. Allow fluid to enter the catheter by placing the stopcock in "off" position toward the IV bottle
      d. If the client is on a respirator, remove it during readings
   5. Record and report changes in CVP readings; often these readings are used to regulate the rate of administration of IVs (high readings are present in congestive heart failure, low readings in hypovolemia)
   6. Evaluate client's response to procedure

Exercise Stress Testing

A. Definition: assessment of cardiac function by ECG, blood pressure, and pulse rate during sustained exercise
   1. Common aerobic activities involved include walking on a treadmill or riding a stationary bicycle
   2. Cardiac workload is increased by either constant level of activity or graduating levels of difficulty to evaluate ability of the coronary circulation to supply adequate amounts of oxygen to the heart muscle when maximum heart rates are approached (depression of ST segment of ECG is one indication of myocardial hypoxia)
B. Nursing care
   1. Obtain an informed consent
   2. Attempt to allay anxiety of the client

3. Instruct the client to have only a light meal several hours prior to the test and to avoid stimulants and depressants
4. Ensure that the client does not smoke (nicotine causes peripheral vasoconstriction)
5. Ask the client to report dizziness, chest pain, dyspnea, fatigue, or nausea if experienced during the test
6. Continually observe the client, the vital signs, and the ECG during the test
7. Ensure ready access to emergency cardiac drugs and equipment (e.g., defibrillator)
8. Observe the client after the test and reinforce any medical instructions as required
9. Evaluate client's response to procedure

Nuclear Medicine Procedures

A. Multiple gated angiographic radioisotope (MUGA) scan
   1. Involves intravenous injection of a radioisotope which has an affinity for red blood cells
   2. Volume of blood pumped during one ventricular contraction is compared with the total volume in the left ventricle which yields an ejection fraction
   3. The ejection fraction gives important information on ventricular size and wall motion abnormalities
B. Thallium stress testing
   1. Intravenous injection of a radioisotope which is taken up by the heart muscle
   2. Damaged myocardial tissue takes up the isotope more slowly and retains it for a longer period
   3. The isotope is injected during and after exercise to determine myocardial perfusion
C. Pyrophosphate scan
   1. This radioisotope binds with free calcium in damaged myocardial tissue after intravenous injection
   2. Injured myocardium binds as much as 20 times more than normal tissue
   3. Test may be performed from 16 hours to 7 days after onset of symptoms
   4. Detects acute myocardial infarctions and infarct extensions
D. Nursing care
   1. Explain procedure to client
   2. Monitor client's vital signs prior to and after test
   3. Determine history of allergies and notify radiology prior to test
   4. Offer emotional support to client who may be apprehensive about test and results; allay client's fears about the use of radioactive substances
   5. Evaluate client's response to procedures

Swan-Ganz Catheter Procedure

A. Definition: catheter used to measure pulmonary capillary wedge pressure, pulmonary artery pressure, and right atrial pressure
   1. The double-lumen catheter with a balloon tip is inserted into the brachial vein and advanced through the superior vena cava, into the right atrium and ventricle, and into the pulmonary artery; the catheter is guided further until, when the balloon is inflated, it is wedged in the distal arterial branch

2. This catheter functions to yield information on the client's circulatory status, left ventricular pumping action, and vascular tone
B. Nursing care
   1. Obtain informed consent for procedure
   2. Assist the physician in inserting the catheter using surgical aseptic technique
   3. Observe the insertion site for inflammation
   4. Observe the line for patency and air bubbles
   5. Take readings with transducer at the level of the client's sternal notch
   6. Change the dressing as ordered using surgical asepsis
   7. Notify the physician if the waveform changes or pressure readings are altered
   8. Normal readings
      a. Pulmonary capillary wedge pressure: 5 to 13 mm Hg
      b. Pulmonary artery pressure
         (1) Systolic: 16 to 30 mm Hg
         (2) Diastolic: 0 to 7 mm Hg
      c. Right atrial pressure: 5 mm Hg
   9. Keep emergency medications and a defibrillator available
   10. Evaluate client's response to procedure

NURSING PROCESS FOR CLIENTS WITH CIRCULATORY SYSTEM DISORDERS
Probable Nursing Diagnoses Based on Assessment

A. Decreased cardiac output related to
   1. Excessive cardiac workload
   2. Decreased tissue perfusion
B. Altered tissue perfusion related to
   1. Decreased cardiac output
   2. Peripheral vasoconstriction or obstruction
   3. Inadequate, excessive, or inappropriate nutrition
C. Activity intolerance related to
   1. Decreased cardiac output
   2. Decreased tissue perfusion
   3. Decreased oxygen-carrying capacity of the blood
D. Ineffective individual coping related to type A personality
E. Fear related to questionable prognosis and potential disability/death
F. Personal identity disturbance related to sick role
G. Pain, related to impaired tissue perfusion
H. Sexual dysfunction related to fear, medication, and disease process
I. Fluid volume excess related to decreased cardiac output
J. Ineffective individual coping: denial, related to prognosis and disease process
K. Noncompliance (with therapeutic regimen) related to denial of diagnosis
L. Potential for injury related to diagnostic and therapeutic modalities
M. Self-care deficit (total) related to imposed restrictions
N. Fatigue related to decreased cardiac output and decreased oxygen carrying capacity of the blood
O. Potential for infection related to disease process or treatment modalities

Nursing Care For Clients With Circulatory System Disorders

(See nursing care under each specific disease)

MAJOR DISEASES
Hypertension

A. Etiology and pathophysiology
1. Hypertension increases the risk of coronary artery disease, heart failure, myocardial infarction, cerebral vascular accidents (CVAs), and renal failure
2. Essential hypertension
   a. Anxiety and other stresses are believed to play a role in releasing a pressor from kidneys that causes chronic vasoconstriction, thereby raising blood pressure
   b. Individuals with essential hypertension have difficulty handling hostile feelings, are less assertive, and have more obsessive-compulsive traits than do nonhypertensive individuals
   c. Onset is generally between 25 and 55 years of age
3. Renal hypertension
   a. Narrowing of the lumen of a renal artery as a result of atherosclerosis, causes release of renin
   b. Renin sets off series of reactions, which cause sodium retention and subsequent rise in blood pressure
   c. Onset is generally after 50 years of age
4. Malignant hypertension results from sustained hypertension of any form, which causes necrosis of the arterioles and proliferative changes of the renal arteries leading to renal failure, CVA, and heart failure, if untreated
5. Hypertensive crisis may also be caused by endocrine disorders (pheochromocytoma), increased intracranial pressure, and encephalopathy

B. Signs and symptoms
1. Subjective
   a. Headache (occipital area)
   b. Lightheadedness
   c. Tinnitus
   d. Easy fatigue
   e. Visual disturbances
   f. Palpitations
   g. Brief lapses in memory
2. Objective
   a. Blood pressure greater than 140/90 mm Hg in people younger than 50 years of age; World Health Organization defines hypertension as greater than 160/95 mm Hg
   b. Retinal changes
   c. Possible hematuria
   d. Epistaxis
   e. Cardiac hypertrophy

C. Treatment
1. Pharmacological management
   a. Diuretics
   b. Adrenergic blockers
   c. Vasodilators
   d. Peripheral adrenergic antagonists
   e. Sedatives

2. Weight reduction
3. Cessation of smoking
4. Sodium-restricted diet (1 to 3 g daily)
5. Establishment of a regular exercise program
6. Biofeedback
7. Relaxation modalities
8. Sympathectomy to dilate arteries

D. Nursing care
1. Encourage early detection by participation in community screening programs
2. Monitor vital signs with client in both upright and recumbent positions (orthostatic hypotension is a common adverse effect of antihypertensive drugs)
3. Check weight daily
4. Educate the client regarding drugs, follow-up care, activity restrictions, and diet; note that many salt substitutes contain potassium chloride rather than sodium chloride and may be permitted by the physician if client has no renal impairment (see hypertensive drugs and diuretics for additional dietary information)
5. Pay particular attention to calcium and potassium intake since hypertension has been associated with deficiencies of these minerals; monitor blood work
6. Reassure and support any expression of emotions
7. If epistaxis occurs, place an ice pack on the back of the neck, which may alleviate it; packing is sometimes required
8. Teach information related to specific medications
9. Evaluate client's response and revise plan as necessary

Arterioatherosclerosis

A. Etiology and pathophysiology
1. Deposition of fatty plaques along inner wall of the artery; most often affects the peripheral arteries, aorta, coronary arteries, and arteries supplying the brain
2. Considered to be a loss of elasticity, or "hardening," of the arteries
3. May be avoided by eating a diet low in fat and cholesterol and high in dietary fiber, exercising regularly, controlling weight, and not smoking

B. Signs and symptoms (depend on arteries affected)
1. Subjective
   a. Intermittent claudication
   b. Pain, depending on degree to which circulation is impaired
   c. Forgetfulness
2. Objective
   a. Decreased skin temperature
   b. Pallor
   c. Diminished pulsations
   d. May lead to ulcerations and gangrene
   e. Elevated serum cholesterol and lipids
   f. Objective memory loss on testing

C. Treatment
1. Drugs that cause vasodilation
2. Weight loss
3. Dietary restriction of cholesterol and fat along with increased dietary fiber

D. Nursing care
1. Evaluate all pulses, color, and temperature of involved area
2. Discourage positions that hamper circulation (e.g., cross-legged)
3. Teach the client the hazards of smoking (nicotine causes peripheral vasoconstriction)
4. Encourage the following dietary program:
   a. Low cholesterol, low fat (especially saturated)
   b. Replace vegetable oils high in polyunsaturated fatty acids (PUFA) with those high in monounsaturated fatty acids (MUFA) such as olive and avocado
   c. Eat fish which are high in omega 3 fatty acids several times per week (salmon, tuna)
   d. Increase intake of high-fiber foods such as fruits, vegetables, cereal grains, and legumes; soluble fiber is particularly effective in reducing blood lipids (oat bran, legumes)
5. Teach importance of warm clothing
6. No vigorous massages of involved area
7. Evaluate client's response and revise plan as necessary

Angina Pectoris

A. Etiology and pathophysiology
1. Commonly caused by narrowed coronary arteries (coronary artery disease)
2. Clients with aortic stenosis or extremely low pressure may also have impaired coronary artery blood flow
3. Increased metabolic demands due to strenuous exercise, emotional stress, hyperthyroidism, or severe anemia may also precipitate angina pectoris
4. When oxygen supplied by the blood cannot meet the metabolic demands of the muscle, hypoxia occurs
5. Pain is thought to be a result of anaerobic metabolic end products
B. Signs and symptoms
1. Subjective
   a. Chest pain associated with activity; generally subsides after a few minutes of rest
   b. Pain is usually substernal and can be described as "crushing" or "pressure"
   c. Pain may radiate to the left shoulder and arm, jaw, epigastric area, or right shoulder
   d. Palpitations
   e. Faintness
   f. Dyspnea
   g. Levine's sign—client clenches fist over sternum when describing discomfort
2. Objective
   a. Diaphoresis
   b. Blood pressure may be elevated
   c. Signs of underlying disease may be evident (cardiac enlargement, valvular disease, arrhythmias)
   d. ECG recordings which vary at rest and during exercise
   e. ECG often indicates a previous infarction

C. Treatment
1. Restricted activity
2. Pharmacological management
   a. Nitrates
   b. Beta-blocking agents
   c. Calcium channel-blocking agents
   d. Antilipidemics
   e. Thrombolytics
3. Weight loss
4. Oxygen therapy during attack
5. Coronary artery bypass surgery if medical regimen not successful
6. Restriction of cholesterol and fat in diet
D. Nursing care
1. Provide physical and mental rest
2. Relieve pain by administration of vasodilators
3. Assess activity tolerance
4. Discourage smoking
5. Educate the client regarding diet, medication, and activity
6. Provide necessary emotional support due to required alterations in life-style
7. Evaluate client's response and revise plan as necessary

Myocardial Infarction

A. Etiology and pathophysiology
1. Acute necrosis of part of the heart muscle caused by interruption of oxygen supply to the area, resulting in altered function and reduced cardiac output
2. Possible causes include atherosclerosis, thrombus formation, decreased blood flow, as well as client's history of smoking, obesity, high-cholesterol/low-density lipoprotein diet, and physical/emotional stress
3. May be avoided by
   a. Monitoring lipoproteins in diet
      (1) Low-density lipoprotein (LDL) carries cholesterol through the blood and deposits it in the arteries which forms plaque
      (2) Very low–density lipoprotein (VLDL) is a substance used by the liver to manufacture LDL; it is the precursor of LDL
      (3) High-density lipoprotein (HDL): protective fraction of cholesterol which draws cholesterol away from the arteries
      (4) The ratio between LDL and HDL is important as an indicator of heart disease; the higher the ratio, the greater the risk
   b. Eating a diet low in fat and cholesterol and high in dietary fiber, exercising regularly, controlling weight, and not smoking
B. Signs and symptoms
1. Subjective
   a. Sudden, severe, crushing, or viselike pain in the substernal region; may radiate to the arms, neck, and back
   b. Nausea
   c. Severe anxiety and dyspnea
2. Objective
   a. Vomiting
   b. Slight elevation of temperature

c. Changes in ECG
d. Changes in blood serum enzyme and isoenzyme levels
  (1) Creatine kinase or creatine phosphokinase (CK or CPK): elevated 3 to 6 hours after infarction, peaking at 24 hours, and returning to normal within 72 to 96 hours
  (2) CK isoenzymes or CPK isoenzymes (CK-MB or CPK-MB): elevated 4 to 6 hours after pain, peaking within 24 hours, and returning to normal within 72 hours
  (3) Lactic dehydrogenase (LDH): elevated on 1st day, reaching its peak on third to fourth day and then gradually subsiding
  (4) LDH isoenzymes: following a myocardial infarction (MI) LDH_1 is greater than LDH_2
  (5) Serum glutamic-oxaloacetic transaminase (SGOT): elevated on days 2 to 4
e. Complete blood studies, particularly white blood cells and sedimentation rate, to determine presence of inflammatory process
f. Coagulation studies: prothrombin time (PT) and partial thromboplastin time (PTT)
g. Signs of shock: cold, clammy skin; profuse diaphoresis; decreased blood pressure; rapid, thready pulse

C. Treatment
1. Admit the client to the coronary care unit
2. Morphine sulfate IV or SC to relieve pain and reduce apprehension
3. Bed rest with cardiac precautions to reduce demand for oxygen
4. Oxygen as necessary
5. Cardiac monitoring for continued surveillance of the heart's electrical activity
6. Frequent monitoring of vital signs, including temperature, pulse (apical and radial), respirations, blood pressure, intake and output
7. Pharmacologic management to stabilize client and prevent complications
  a. Nitrates
  b. Narcotic analgesics
  c. Beta-blocking agents
  d. Calcium antagonists
  e. Sedatives
  f. Hypnotics
  g. Laxatives
  h. Anticoagulants
  i. Thrombolytic agents
  j. Antiarrhythmics
  k. Potassium salts
8. IV fluids at slow rate to keep vein open for administration of medications
9. Thrombolytic therapy (streptokinase, Urokinase, TPA) may be employed to dissolve thrombi in the coronary arteries immediately after onset of infarction
10. Swan-Ganz catheter is used to monitor pressure in pulmonary artery, which reflects function of left ventricle
11. Intraortic balloon pump that inflates during diastole and deflates during systole may be used to decrease cardiac work load by decreasing afterload
12. Clear liquid diet is prescribed initially to decrease oxygen consumption, and then advanced to low sodium

D. Nursing care
1. Watch the cardiac monitor and immediately document and report changes in rate, conductivity, and rhythm
2. Observe the client for ventricular fibrillation and asystole and take appropriate life-saving actions if they occur (e.g., cardiopulmonary resuscitation, electric defibrillation)
3. Observe for other variations, such as PVCs close to a T wave, ventricular tachycardia, and atrial fibrillation; if they occur, administer prescribed medications, document the rhythm, and notify the physician
4. Observe the client's vital signs every 15 minutes until stable
5. Closely observe the client's intake and output
6. Observe for pulmonary congestion and dependent edema
7. Observe for pain and restlessness and administer medication as ordered
8. Watch for cyanosis and dyspnea and administer oxygen as necessary
9. Recognize that the client is subject to sensory overload
  a. Orient to the unit and machinery
  b. Allow the client time to express feelings and fears
10. Provide gradual increase in activity
11. Apply antiembolism stockings
12. Provide emotional support to client and family
13. Evaluate client's response and revise plan as necessary

Inflammatory Diseases of the Heart (Pericarditis, Myocarditis, Subacute Bacterial Endocarditis)

A. Etiology and pathophysiology
1. Pericarditis is an acute or chronic inflammation of the pericardium caused by bacterial or viral invasion, trauma, heart disease, an autoimmune process, collagen disease, or rheumatic fever
  a. Can result in loss of pericardial elasticity or an accumulation of fluid within the sac
  b. Heart failure or cardiac tamponade (compression of the heart due to a collection of fluid within the pericardial sac) may result
2. Myocarditis is an inflammation of the myocardium due to pericarditis, systemic infection, or allergic response
  a. The contractility of the heart is impaired due to the inflammatory process
  b. Myocardial ischemia and necrosis are critical complications
3. Subacute bacterial endocarditis is an inflammation of the inner lining of the heart and valves generally caused by *Streptococcus viridans* or other nonhemolytic streptococci spreading through the blood

to the heart from infected teeth, gums, and tonsils; structural damage to the valves may occur in a matter of days, and pump failure will ensue

B. Signs and symptoms
  1. Subjective
    a. Precordial or substernal pain
    b. Dyspnea
    c. Chills
    d. Fatigue and malaise
  2. Objective
    a. Arrhythmias
    b. Increased cardiac enzymes
    c. Fever
    d. Positive blood cultures
    e. Friction rubs evident on auscultation
C. Treatment
  1. Administer oxygen
  2. Bed rest
  3. Antibiotics to relieve underlying infection
  4. Corticosteroids
  5. Antiarrhythmics
  6. Pericardectomy (surgical removal of scar tissue and the pericardium), if indicated
D. Nursing care
  1. Carefully observe for signs of shock, heart failure, and arrhythmias
  2. Maintain a tranquil environment and help the client achieve maximum rest
  3. If surgical intervention is undertaken, care for chest tubes and follow the postoperative chest surgery routine (see Cardiac Surgery)
  4. Explain posthospitalization therapy to improve compliance (lifelong doses of penicillin prophylactically)
  5. Evaluate client's response and revise plan as necessary

Congestive Heart Failure (CHF)

A. Etiology and pathophysiology
  1. Inability of the heart to meet the demands of the body
  2. Pump failure may be caused by cardiac abnormalities or conditions that place increased demands on the heart
    a. Myocardial infarctions
    b. Valvular defects
    c. Hypertension
    d. Anemia
    e. Hyperthyroidism
    f. Obesity
    g. Circulatory overload
  3. When one side of the heart "fails," there is essentially a buildup of pressure in the vascular system feeding into that side: signs of rightsided failure will be evident in the systemic circulation, those of left-sided failure in the pulmonary system
B. Signs and symptoms
  1. Right-sided failure
    a. Subjective
      (1) Abdominal pain
      (2) Fatigue
      (3) Bloating
    b. Objective
      (1) Dependent, pitting edema; ankle edema is frequently the first sign of CHF; often subsides at night when legs are elevated
      (2) Ascites from increased pressure within the portal system
      (3) Respiratory distress
      (4) Increased CVP
      (5) Diminished urinary output
  2. Left-sided heart failure
    a. Subjective
      (1) Dyspnea from fluid within the lungs
      (2) Orthopnea
      (3) Fatigue
      (4) Paroxysmal nocturnal dyspnea
    b. Objective
      (1) Rales
      (2) Peripheral cyanosis
      (3) Cheyne-Stokes respirations
      (4) Frothy, blood-tinged sputum
C. Treatment
  1. Morphine sulfate is often given to decrease anxiety and dyspnea
  2. Oxygen is generally administered by mask or cannula; however, if acute left-sided failure exists, the client may require endotracheal intubation and placement on a ventilator
  3. Digitalis is generally prescribed to increase the efficiency of the heart's pumping action
  4. Diuretics such as furosemide (Lasix) are often ordered to remove excess fluid, thereby decreasing cardiac work load
  5. Potassium supplements are usually prescribed to prevent digitalis toxicity and hypokalemia
  6. Rotating tourniquets (dry phlebotomy) may be used to decrease venous return; generally tourniquets are applied to three of the extremities, and every 15 minutes a tourniquet is removed and rotated in a clockwise direction; when the client is stable, tourniquets are removed one at a time in 15-minute intervals
  7. A paracentesis may be performed if ascites exists and is causing respiratory distress
  8. Sodium-restricted diet
D. Nursing care
  1. Maintain the client in high-Fowler's position
  2. Elevate extremities
  3. Frequently monitor vital signs
  4. Change position frequently
  5. Monitor intake and output and daily weight
  6. Observe for electrolyte imbalances (hyponatremia, hypokalemia)
  7. Teach the client and family and provide emotional support
  8. Refer to glycoside and diuretic medications for additional nursing actions
  9. Obtain CVP readings
  10. Evaluate client's response and revise plan as necessary

Cardiac Surgery

A. May be used to
1. Correct abnormalities
   a. Mitral stenosis or regurgitation
   b. Aortic stenosis or insufficiency
   c. Coronary occlusion
   d. Ventricular aneurysm
2. Replace failing heart (cardiac transplantation)
   a. Terminal heart disease with life expectancy of less than 1 year
   b. Viral myocarditis
   c. Toxic injury to the myocardium
   d. Severe coronary artery disease
   e. Ischemic heart disease
B. Types of procedures: open or closed heart surgery (when extracorporeal circulation or the heart-lung machine is used, it is called open heart surgery; hypothermia may be used in either open or closed heart surgery to decrease the metabolic demands of the body)
1. Mitral commissurotomy or valvotomy involves splitting the joined portions of the mitral valve that are present in mitral stenosis
2. Mitral valve replacement is done for mitral insufficiency, which occurs when the mitral valve does not close properly to block the reflux of blood from the ventricle into the atrium during systole (regurgitation)
3. Coronary bypass surgery is done when severe arteriosclerotic disease causes angina pectoris; a graft or a segment of a vessel (often the saphenous vein) is anastomosed, bypassing the diseased portion of a coronary artery
4. Aneurysmectomy is done to correct a ventricular aneurysm (which occurs in approximately 10% to 30% of clients with myocardial infarction; i.e., a weakened ventricular wall balloons out, causing decreased cardiac efficiency)
5. Cardiac transplantation involves replacement of the client's diseased heart with one from a compatible donor
C. Nursing care
1. Monitor cardiac functioning
2. Evaluate vital signs, including peripheral pulses and neurologic signs
3. Monitor temperature closely
4. Maintain airway; the client will have an endotracheal tube in place postoperatively and require mechanical ventilation; suction as necessary
5. Monitor intake and output; weigh regularly
6. Assess state of hydration by frequent checks on central venous pressure (CVP) readings, electrolytes, specific gravity, and observation of the client
7. Care for chest tubes
   a. Maintain patency of tubes
   b. Avoid kinked tubing
   c. Drainage should not be more than 200 ml/hour
8. Maintain a Foley catheter in place; in addition to output, monitor specific gravity
9. Assess pain (nature, site, duration, type) and provide relief
10. Encourage coughing and deep breathing; change position frequently
11. Evaluate arterial blood gases
12. Administer parenteral therapy, including electrolytes and blood
13. Plan with the client and family for meeting both short- and long-term goals
14. Provide relief of anxiety and fear by staying with the client and explaining procedures; encourage verbalization of feelings; provide emotional support
15. Maintain protective isolation when immunosuppressants (cyclosporine and azathioprine) are used
16. Administer cardiac medications as ordered
17. Monitor client for signs of complications
    a. Hemorrhage that can lead to hypovolemia
       (1) Decreased blood pressure, increased pulse rate
       (2) Restlessness, apprehension
       (3) Lowered CVP readings
       (4) Pallor
    b. Cardiac tamponade caused by collection of fluid or blood within pericardium
       (1) Decreased arterial pressure
       (2) Elevated CVP
       (3) Rapid, thready pulse
       (4) Diminished output
    c. Congestive heart failure
       (1) Dyspnea
       (2) Elevated CVP
       (3) Tachycardia
       (4) Edema
    d. Transplant rejection
       (1) Fever
       (2) Malaise, fatigue
       (3) Signs of congestive heart failure
    e. Myocardial infarction
    f. Renal failure
    g. Embolism
    h. Psychosis resulting from an inability to cope with anxiety associated with cardiac surgery
18. Specific care for the client with a cardiac transplant
    a. Teach client not to strain for defecation, and avoid lifting or pulling for at least 8 weeks after surgery
    b. Teach client and family the importance of adhering to a sodium- and cholesterol-restricted diet (usually 2 g sodium and 300 mg cholesterol)
    c. Provide emotional support during periods of euphoria or fear
    d. Instruct client to avoid temperature extremes
    e. Tell client to report signs of respiratory infection and urinary tract infection to the physician
    f. Stress the importance of foot care and oral care
    g. Encourage client to take temperature daily and report elevations to the physician immediately
    h. Instruct client to take immunosuppressive drugs before meals diluted 1:10 in milk
    i. Inform client that frequent biopsies will be performed to identify rejection
    j. Teach client that when rejection is found to be moderate to severe, hospitalization will be necessary for intensive immunosuppressive therapy
    k. Explain that chest x-rays will be required every 2 to 6 weeks following surgery

l. Alert the client and family to signs of rejection and the need to notify the physician
   (1) Increased temperature
   (2) Increased pulse
   (3) Dependent edema
   (4) Weight gain
   (5) Malaise
   (6) Dyspnea
   (7) Confusion
19. Evaluate client's response and revise plan as necessary

Thrombophlebitis

A. Etiology and pathophysiology
   1. Thrombophlebitis is the inflammation of a vein and is associated with clot formation (thrombus)
   2. An embolus is a clot or solid particle carried by the bloodstream that may interfere with circulation to vital organs
   3. Risk factors thought to contribute to this disorder include immobilization, venous stasis, trauma to vessels, and pregnancy
   4. Surgical procedures involving the pelvic area increase the risk of phlebitis because of the vascularity of the area and subsequent vascular impairment
B. Signs and symptoms
   1. Subjective
      a. Pain on dorsiflexion of affected extremity (Homans' sign)
      b. Sometimes no signs are present until embolus is released and lodges in a vessel supplying a vital organ (e.g., pulmonary embolus)
   2. Objective
      a. Swollen limb with hard veins that are sensitive to pressure
      b. Redness and warmth of area along the vein
C. Treatment
   1. Bed rest with elastic stockings to promote venous return
   2. Warm moist heat to promote vasodilation; however, some believe this may dislodge the clot, and ice packs are ordered
   3. Elevation of extremity to reduce edema
   4. Anticoagulants to prevent recurrence of deep vein involvement
   5. Vasodilators to prevent vascular spasm
   6. Thrombolytic therapy (e.g., streptokinase) may be used to dissolve clot
   7. Transvenous filter or thrombectory
D. Nursing care
   1. Associated with medical management
      a. Observe frequently for signs of vascular impairment (e.g., pallor, cyanosis, coolness)
      b. Assist in understanding the rationale for prolonged bed rest and minimal activity
      c. Apply antiembolitic stockings or elastic bandages; remove and replace as ordered
      d. Observe and record vital signs, including peripheral pulses
      e. Instruct the client to avoid tight and constricting clothing, cigarette smoking, or maintaining one position for long periods

f. Observe for signs of pulmonary embolism (e.g., sudden pain, cyanosis, hemoptysis, shock)
      g. Evaluate client's response and revise plan as necessary
   2. Associated with surgery (in addition to those listed in 1.)
      a. Monitor for hemorrhage; notify physician if bleeding suspected
      b. Assess circulatory status of extremity
      c. Keep extremity elevated
      d. OOB as ordered; avoid prolonged hip flexion
      e. Administer ordered analgesics and anticoagulants

Varicose Veins

A. Etiology and pathophysiology
   1. The veins in the lower trunk and extremities become dilated, congested, and tortuous due to weakness of valves or loss of elasticity of vessel walls
   2. A positive Trendelenburg test is diagnostic of varicose veins: the client lies down with legs elevated until veins empty completely; the client then stands, and observation of filling of veins is made; a normal vein fills from below, whereas a varicose vein fills from above
B. Signs and symptoms
   1. Subjective
      a. Heaviness or fullness in legs
      b. Leg fatigue
      c. Leg cramping that intensifies at night
   2. Objective
      a. Positive venogram
      b. Skin discoloration, usually brown
      c. Stasis ulcer formation
C. Treatment
   1. Weight loss
   2. Avoidance of standing for prolonged periods or sitting with legs crossed
   3. Support stockings
   4. Surgical intervention involves ligation of the vein above the varicosity and removal of the involved vein; the great saphenous vein may be ligated near the femoral junction
   5. Postoperative early ambulation is essential to prevent formation of thrombi
D. Nursing care
   1. Elevate the foot of the bed for first 24 hours
   2. Observe vital signs and incisions for indications of hemorrhage
   3. Assist the client with ambulation
   4. Administer analgesics as ordered
   5. Evaluate client's response and revise plan as necessary

Peripheral Vascular Disorders (PVD)

A. Etiology and pathophysiology
   1. Reduced or occluded arterial blood flow due to atherosclerois, thrombus, or embolus
   2. Buerger's disease (thromboangiitis obliterans)
      a. Peripheral circulation impaired by inflammatory occlusions of the peripheral arteries

b. Thromboses of arteries or veins may occur

c. Incidence is highest in young adult males who smoke

3. Raynaud's disease
   a. Spasms of digital arteries thought to be caused by abnormal response of the sympathetic nervous system to cold or emotional stress; usually bilateral
   b. Primarily occurs in young females
   c. Rarely leads to gangrene

4. Raynaud's phenomenon
   a. Episodic arterial spasms of the extremities
   b. Secondary to another disease or abnormality

B. Signs and symptoms
1. Subjective
   a. Paresthesia
   b. Aching to severe pain
2. Objective
   a. Pallor or cyanosis
   b. Gangrenous ulcers (more common in Buerger's disease)
   c. Diminished pulses in Buerger's disease

C. Treatment
1. Vasodilators may be given
2. Sympathectomy to sever the sympathetic ganglia supplying the area; there is local vasodilation with improved circulation
   a. Lumbar sympathectomy deprives the leg and foot of innervation
   b. Cervicothoracic sympathectomy relieves vasospasm in the arms and hands
3. Femoropopliteal bypass grafting
   a. Saphenous vein grafting from femoral artery to the area below the obstruction
   b. Polyester fiber grafts in aortic iliac obstructions
4. Amputation if vascular supply is severely impaired
   a. Below-the-knee amputation provides the client with a more natural gait, since knee movement is maintained
   b. Above-the-knee amputation limits the client's movement, since prosthesis contains knee joint
   c. A guillotine amputation, in which the wound is left open and skin traction is applied, is performed when the area is infected, gangrenous, or extensively traumatized or if the client is a poor surgical risk
   d. A flap-type amputation is less prone to infection, since the skin covers the area and healing occurs within 2 weeks; may be above or below the knee

D. Nursing care
1. Associated with medical management
   a. Instruct the client not to smoke or wear constrictive garments
   b. Keep extremities warm; instruct the client to wear gloves when exposed to cold
   c. Protect from injury since there is decreased wound healing ability; lubricants may be applied to keep skin supple
   d. Assess color, temperature, pulses, and sensation of involved extremities

2. Associated with sympathectomy
   a. Monitor vital signs frequently, since shock can occur
   b. Change position gradually, since dizziness may be a problem
   c. Apply elastic bandages if ordered
3. Associated with femoropopliteal bypass grafting
   a. Assess circulation of involved extremity by checking pulses, color, temperature, and neurologic function
   b. Observe blood pressure frequently, since hypotension increases the possibility of thrombus formation
   c. Observe for signs of hemorrhage, including pain, change in skin color, and alteration of vital signs
   d. Ambulate as ordered; sitting should be avoided in femoropopliteal bypass surgery
4. Associated with amputation (see Amputation in Neuromusculoskeletal system)
5. Evaluate client's response and revise plan as necessary

Aneurysms

A. Etiology and pathophysiology
1. Distention at the site of a weakness in the arterial wall
   a. Saccular aneurysm: pouchlike projection at one side of the artery
   b. Fusiform aneurysm: entire circumference of the artery wall is dilated
   c. Mycotic aneurysm: tiny weaknesses in the arterial wall that result from infection
   d. Dissecting aneurysm: tear in the inner lining of an arteriosclerotic aortic wall causes blood to form a hematoma between layers of the artery, which compresses the lumen of the artery
2. Causes
   a. Congenital weakness
   b. Atherosclerosis (most common cause of both thoracic and abdominal aortic aneurysms)
   c. Syphilis
   d. Trauma
3. Represent surgical emergency if ruptured

B. Signs and symptoms
1. Thoracic aortic aneurysm
   a. Subjective
      (1) May be asymptomatic
      (2) Pain resulting from pressure against the nerves or vertebrae
      (3) Dyspnea
      (4) Dysphagia
   b. Objective
      (1) Hoarseness, aphonia from impingement on laryngeal nerve
      (2) Cough
      (3) Unequal pulses and arterial pressure in upper extremities
      (4) Trachea may be displaced from midline due to adhesions between trachea and aneurysm

2. Abdominal aortic aneurysm
   a. Subjective
      (1) May be asymptomatic
      (2) Lower back or abdominal pain (severe if aneurysm leaking)
      (3) Sensory changes in the lower extremities if aneurysm ruptures
   b. Objective
      (1) Hypertension
      (2) Pulsating abdominal mass
      (3) Mottling of the lower extremities if aneurysm ruptures
      (4) Increased abdominal girth if aneurysm ruptures
3. Dissecting aortic aneurysm
   a. Subjective
      (1) Restlessness and anxiety
      (2) Severe pain
   b. Objective
      (1) Diminished pulses
      (2) Signs of shock
C. Treatment
   1. Resection of the aneurysm and use of a Teflon or Dacron graft
   2. Surgical procedures involving the aorta would necessitate use of a heart-lung device (cardiopulmonary bypass)
   3. Medical treatment is aimed at decreasing cardiac output and blood pressure through the use of drugs
D. Nursing care
   1. Monitor the vital signs and pulses of all extremities, including the posterior tibial and dorsalis pedis
   2. Monitor central venous pressure (CVP) frequently
   3. Record intake and output, since renal failure may occur after surgery
   4. Administer narcotics as ordered to alleviate pain
   5. Apply abdominal binders to provide support when the client is coughing, deep breathing, and ambulating
   6. Prevent flexion of hip and knees to eliminate pressure on the arterial wall
   7. Apply elastic stockings and encourage dorsiflexion of the foot to help decrease the risk of thrombophlebitis
   8. Maintain patency of the nasogastric tube if present
   9. Evaluate client's response and revise plan as necessary

Shock
A. Etiology and pathophysiology
   1. Hypovolemic: occurs when there is a loss of fluid resulting in inadequate tissue perfusion; caused by
      a. Excessive bleeding
      b. Excessive diarrhea or vomiting
      c. Fluid loss from fistulas or burns
   2. Cardiogenic: occurs when pump failure causes inadequate tissue perfusion; caused by
      a. Congestive heart failure
      b. Myocardial infarction
      c. Cardiac tamponade

3. Neurogenic: caused by rapid vasodilation and subsequent pooling of blood within the peripheral vessels; caused by
   a. Spinal anesthesia
   b. Emotional tension
   c. Drugs that inhibit the sympathetic nervous system
4. Anaphylactic: due to an allergic reaction that causes a release of histamine and subsequent vasodilation
5. Septic: similar to anaphylaxis and is the body's reaction to bacterial toxins (generally gram-negative infections), which results in the leakage of plasma into tissues
B. Signs and symptoms
   1. Subjective
      a. Apprehension
      b. Restlessness
      c. Paresis of extremities
   2. Objective
      a. Weak, rapid, thready pulse
      b. Diaphoresis
      c. Cold, clammy skin
      d. Decreased blood pressure
      e. Decreased urine output
      f. Pallor
      g. Progressive loss of consciousness
      h. Lowered CVP readings
C. Treatment
   1. Aimed at correcting the underlying cause
   2. Fluid and blood replacement
   3. Oxygen therapy
   4. Vasoconstricting drugs to increase blood pressure
   5. Cardiac monitoring
   6. Cardiotonics, such as digitalis preparations, for cardiogenic shock
   7. Antihistamines for anaphylactic shock
   8. Antibiotics for septic shock based on blood cultures
   9. Elevation of lower extremities to ensure circulation to vital organs
   10. Intraaortic balloon pump may be used to aid the failing heart
D. Nursing care
   1. Keep the client warm
   2. Check vital signs and CVP frequently
   3. Monitor urine output and specific gravity
   4. Allay anxiety
   5. Carefully observe all responses to therapy
   6. Evaluate client's response and revise plan as necessary

Anemia
A. Iron deficiency anemia
   1. Etiology and pathophysiology
      a. Poor dietary habits leading to inadequate intake of iron, vitamin B_{12}, and/or folacin
      b. Iron is essential for the formation of hemoglobin and erythrocytes needed to carry oxygen to cells; B_{12} and folacin essential to erythrocyte synthesis
   2. Signs and symptoms
      a. Subjective
         (1) Fatigue
         (2) Headache
         (3) Paresthesias

b. Objective
(1) Ankle edema
(2) Dry, pale mucous membranes
(3) Pearly white sclera
(4) Decreased hemoglobin and erythrocytes
(5) Increased iron binding capacity
(6) Megaloblastic condition of blood
3. Treatment
a. Improve diet; include ascorbic acid, which stimulates iron uptake
b. Appropriate supplements of iron, vitamin B_{12}, and/or folacin
4. Nursing care
a. Teach client foods high in iron, folacin, and vitamin B_{12}
b. Teach about the side effects of medications
c. Evaluate client's understanding of teaching
B. Pernicious anemia
1. Etiology and pathophysiology
a. Lack of intrinsic factor in the stomach prevents the absorption of vitamin B_{12} in the lower portion of the ileum
b. Subsequent reduced number of erythrocytes formed, leading to anemia
2. Signs and symptoms
a. Subjective
(1) Weakness
(2) Sore mouth
(3) Paresthesias
(4) Dyspnea
b. Objective
(1) Pallor
(2) Beefy red tongue
(3) Positive Romberg test (loss of balance when eyes close)
(4) Gastric analysis: no intrinsic factor
(5) Schilling test: urine test for B_{12} absorption
3. Treatment: lifetime cyanocobalamin (B_{12}) injections
4. Nursing care
a. Explain disease process and the need for continued treatment
b. Teach family member(s) how to give IM injections or make referral to visiting nurse
c. Evaluate client's understanding of teaching
C. Aplastic anemia (hypoplastic anemia)
1. Etiology and pathophysiology
a. Bone marrow is depressed or destroyed by a chemical or drug
b. Leukopenia, thrombocytopenia, and decreased erythrocytes
2. Signs and symptoms
a. Subjective
(1) Headache
(2) Weakness
(3) Anorexia
(4) Dyspnea
b. Objective
(1) Fever
(2) Bleeding from mucous membranes
(3) Decreased leukocytes, erythrocytes, and platelets

3. Treatment
a. Identify and eliminate causative agent
b. Blood transfusions
c. Maintenance of fluid and electrolyte balance
4. Nursing care
a. Support the client and family in understanding illness
b. Prevent infection by reverse isolation
c. Evaluate client's response and revise plan as necessary

Blood Dyscrasias
A. Thrombocytopenic purpura
1. Etiology and pathophysiology: bleeding disorder of unknown origin (possibly autoimmune) in which there is a reduction of platelets
2. Signs and symptoms
a. Subjective
(1) History of epistaxis
(2) History of gum bleeding
b. Objective
(1) Low platelet count
(2) Ecchymotic areas
(3) Hemorrhagic petechiae
3. Treatment
a. Corticosteroids
b. Immunosuppressive agents
c. Splenectomy
d. Platelet transfusions
4. Nursing care
a. Prevent injury and bruises
b. Encourage client to adhere to medical regimen
c. Teach the side effects of medications, particularly proneness to infection
d. Provide postoperative care related to splenectomy
e. Evaluate client's response and revise plan as necessary
B. Polycythemia vera
1. Etiology and pathophysiology: disorder of unknown origin that results in an increased number of erythrocytes, leukocytes, and platelets
2. Signs and symptoms
a. Subjective
(1) Headache
(2) Weakness
(3) Itching
b. Objective
(1) Increased hemoglobin
(2) Purple-red complexion
(3) Dyspnea
(4) Bleeding from mucous membranes
3. Treatment
a. Phlebotomy several times yearly
b. Diet low in iron
c. Radioactive phosphorus; busulfan (Myleran)
4. Nursing care
a. Discuss diet with the client and family
b. Provide supportive care and prevent hemorrhage
c. Assist with phlebotomy
d. Evaluate client's response and revise plan as necessary

C. Agranulocytosis
1. Etiology and pathophysiology
   a. Results in a decreased number of leukocytes
   b. Thought to arise from physical agents (e.g., heavy metals) and cytotoxic drugs
2. Signs and symptoms
   a. Subjective
      (1) Fatigue
      (2) Malaise
   b. Objective
      (1) High fever
      (2) Necrotic ulcers of mucosa
      (3) Rapid weak pulse
3. Treatment
   a. Removal of causative agent
   b. Transfusions
   c. Antibiotics
4. Nursing care
   a. Prevent infection and observe for signs of infection
   b. Provide careful oral hygiene
   c. Provide for bed rest
   d. Encourage diet consisting of high nutrient density foods which are rich in vitamins and minerals
   e. Evaluate client's response and revise plan as necessary
D. Disseminated intravascular coagulation (DIC)
1. Etiology and pathophysiology
   a. Body's response to injury or disease in which microthrombi obstruct the blood supply of organs
   b. Complicated by hemorrhage at various sites throughout the body
2. Signs and symptoms
   a. Subjective
      (1) Restlessness
      (2) Anxiety
   b. Objective
      (1) Laboratory tests indicate low fibrinogen and prolonged prothrombin and partial thromboplastin times
      (2) Hemorrhage, both subcutaneous and internal
3. Treatment
   a. Goal is to relieve the underlying cause
   b. Heparin to prevent the formation of thrombi
   c. Transfusion of blood products
4. Nursing care
   a. Observe for bleeding
   b. Minimize skin punctures
   c. Prevent injury
   d. Provide emotional support
   e. Evaluate client's response and revise plan as necessary

Leukemia

A. Etiology and pathophysiology
1. Incidence highest in children ages 3 to 4; declines until age 35, at which point there is a steady increase
2. Etiology unknown, although exposure to certain toxic substances such as radiation seems to increase the incidence
3. In general, an uncontrolled proliferation of white blood cells
4. Classified according to the type of white cell affected
   a. Acute lymphocytic leukemia
      (1) Primarily occurs in children
      (2) Most favorable prognosis with chemotherapy
      (3) Results from abnormal leukocytes in blood-forming tissue
   b. Acute myelogenous leukemia
      (1) Occurs throughout life cycle
      (2) Prognosis is poor with or without chemotherapy
      (3) Results from inability of leukocytes to mature; those that do are abnormal
   c. Chronic myelogenous leukemia
      (1) Occurs after the second decade
      (2) Prognosis is poor
      (3) Results from abnormal production of granulocytic cells
   d. Chronic lymphocytic leukemia
      (1) Occurs after age 35
      (2) Life expectancy 4 to 5 years
      (3) Results from increased production of leukocytes and lymphocytes and proliferation of cells within the bone marrow, spleen, and liver
B. Signs and symptoms
1. Subjective
   a. Malaise
   b. Bone pain
2. Objective
   a. Anemia
   b. Thrombocytopenia
   c. Elevated leukocytes
   d. Decreased platelets
   e. Petechiae
   f. Gingival bleeding
C. Treatment
1. Chemotherapy
2. Transfusions of whole blood or blood fractions
3. Analgesics
4. Bone marrow transplant
D. Nursing care
1. Discuss the importance of follow-up care with the client and family
2. Provide emotional support for the client and family
3. Provide specific nursing care related to particular chemotherapeutic therapy, transfusion, or diagnostic tests
4. Evaluate client's response and revise plan as necessary

Infectious Mononucleosis

A. Etiology and pathophysiology
1. Acute infectious disease of the lymphatic system due to Epstein-Barr (EB) herpesvirus
2. Transmitted by respiratory droplets

3. Incubation period is uncertain; probably 28 to 42 days
4. Incidence highest between ages 15 and 35
5. Complications include hepatitis, ruptured spleen, pericarditis, and meningoencephalitis

B. Signs and symptoms
1. Subjective
a. Sore throat
b. Malaise
c. Stiff neck
d. Nausea
2. Objective
a. Elevated temperature
b. Enlarged, tender lymph nodes (generally, posterior cervical nodes involved first)
c. Splenomegaly in approximately 50% of clients
d. Elevated lymphocyte and monocyte counts
e. Positive heterophile antibody agglutination test

C. Treatment
1. Generally directed toward symptoms (recovery is approximately 3 weeks)
2. ASA; steroids if severely ill
3. If spleen ruptures, splenectomy and blood transfusions

D. Nursing care
1. Provide rest
2. Administer aspirin as ordered
3. Assess for signs of complications; the spleen should not be palpated once the diagnosis is made
4. Increase fluid intake
5. Support natural defense mechanisms; encourage intake of foods rich in the immune-stimulating nutrients, especially vitamins A, C, and E, and the minerals selenium and zinc
6. Evaluate client's response and revise plan as necessary

Hodgkin's Disease

A. Etiology and pathophysiology
1. Cause unknown
2. Higher incidence in males and young adults
3. Proliferation of malignant cells (Reed-Sternberg cells) within lymph nodes
4. All tissues may eventually be involved, but chiefly lymph nodes, spleen, liver, tonsils, and bone marrow
5. Classification by staging and the presence or absence of systemic symptoms

B. Signs and symptoms
1. Subjective
a. Dyspnea and dysphagia due to pressure from enlarged nodes
b. Pruritus
c. Anorexia
2. Objective
a. Enlarged lymph nodes (generally cervical nodes are involved first)
b. Diagnosis confirmed by histologic examination of a lymph node
c. Progressive anemia
d. Elevated temperature
e. Enlarged spleen and liver may occur

f. Pressure from enlarged lymph nodes may cause symptoms of edema and obstructive jaundice
g. Thrombocytopenia if spleen and bone marrow involved

C. Treatment
1. Radiotherapy
a. Vital organs must be shielded
b. Potential side effects
(1) Nausea
(2) Skin rashes
(3) Dry mouth
(4) Dysphagia
2. Surgical intervention
a. Excision of node for biopsy
b. Excision of masses to relieve pressure on other organs
c. Laparotomy or laparoscopy for determination of stage
3. Chemotherapy
a. nitrogen mustard
b. thiophosphoramide (Thiotepa)
c. chlorambucil
d. vincristine (Oncovin)
e. doxorubicin (Adriamycin)
f. prednisone
g. procarbazine hydrochloride (Matulane)
h. bleomycin (Blenoxane)
i. vinblastine sulfate (Velban)
j. dacarbazine (DTIC-Dome)
k. MOPP and ABVD protocols

D. Nursing care
1. Provide emotional support for the client and family
2. Protect from infection
3. Monitor temperature
4. Observe for signs of anemia; provide adequate rest
5. Examine sclera and skin for signs of jaundice
6. Encourage high nutrient density foods; observe for anorexia and nausea
7. Evaluate client's response and revise plan as necessary

Lymphosarcoma

A. Etiology and pathophysiology
1. Malignant tumors of the lymph nodes and lymphatic tissue
2. Gastrointestinal tract, tonsils, spleen, and liver frequently involved
3. Cause unknown; incidence is increased in clients who have immunologic disorders

B. Signs and symptoms
1. Subjective
a. Malaise
b. Lethargy
2. Objective
a. Painless lymphadenopathy
b. Fever
c. Diaphoresis
d. Weight loss
e. Decreased resistance to disease

C. Treatment similar to that for Hodgkin's disease
D. Nursing care similar to that for Hodgkin's disease

Respiratory System
REVIEW OF ANATOMY AND PHYSIOLOGY OF THE RESPIRATORY SYSTEM
Functions

A. The upper portion of the respiratory system filters, moistens, and warms air during inspiration
B.. The lower portion of the respiratory system enables the exchange of gases between blood and air to regulate serum Po_2, Pco_2, and pH

Organs
Nose

A. Structure
  1. Portions
    a. Internal: in skull, above roof of mouth
    b. External: protruding from face
  2. Cavities
    a. Divisions: right and left
    b. Meati: superior, middle, and lower; named for turbinates located above each meatus
    c. Openings
      (1) To exterior: anterior nares
      (2) To nasopharynx: posterior nares
    d. Conchae (turbinates)
      (1) Superior and middle processes of ethmoid bone; interior conchae, separate bones
      (2) Conchae partition each nasal cavity into three passageways or meati
    e. Floor: formed by palatine bones and maxillae; these also act as roof of mouth
  3. Lining: ciliated mucosa
  4. Sinuses draining into the nose (paranasal sinuses)
    a. Frontal
    b. Maxillary (antrum of Highmore)
    c. Sphenoidal
    d. Ethmoidal
B. Functions
  1. Serves as passageway for incoming and outgoing air, filtering, warming, moistening, and chemically examining it
  2. Organ of smell (olfactory receptors located in the nasal mucosa)
  3. Aids in phonation

Pharynx

A. Structure: composed of muscle with mucous lining
  1. Divisions
    a. Nasopharynx: behind the nose
    b. Oropharynx: behind the mouth
    c. Laryngopharynx: behind the larynx
  2. Openings
    a. Nasopharynx has four openings: two auditory (eustachian) tubes and two posterior nares
    b. Oropharynx has one opening: fauces, archway into mouth
    c. Laryngopharynx has two openings: into esophagus and into larynx
  3. Organs in the pharynx
    a. Nasopharynx: nasopharyngeal tonsils (adenoids) and eustachian tubes
    b. Oropharynx: palatine and lingual tonsils

B. Functions
  1. Serves as a passageway and entrance to the respiratory and digestive tracts
  2. Aids in phonation
  3. Tonsils function to destroy incoming bacteria and detoxify certain foreign proteins

Larynx

A. Location: at upper end of the trachea, just below the pharynx
B. Structure
  1. Cartilages: nine pieces arranged in a boxlike formation; thyroid cartilage is the largest (called the "Adam's apple"); epiglottis (the "lid" cartilage); cricoid (the "signet ring" cartilage)
  2. Vocal cords
    a. False cords: folds of mucous lining
    b. True cords: fibroelastic bands stretched across the hollow interior of the larynx; the paired vocal cords (folds) and the posterior arytenoid cartilages make up the glottis; the slit between the vocal cords, through which air enters and leaves the lower respiratory passages, is the rima glottidis
  3. Lining: ciliated mucosa
C. Functions
  1. Voice production: during expiration, air passing through the larynx causes the vocal cords to vibrate; short, tense cords produce a high pitch; long, relaxed cords, a low pitch
  2. Serves as part of the passageway for air and as the entrance to the lower respiratory tract

Trachea

A. Structure
  1. Walls: smooth muscle; contain C-shaped rings of cartilage at intervals; these keep the tube open at all times but do not constrict the esophagus, which is directly behind the trachea
  2. Lining: ciliated mucosa
  3. Extent: from the larynx to the bronchi; 10 to 11 cm (about 4½ inches) long
B. Function: furnishes open passageway for air going to and from lungs

Lungs

A. Structure
  1. Size: large enough to fill pleural divisions of thoracic cavity
  2. Shape: cone, base downward
  3. Location: in pleural divisions of thorax; extend from slightly above clavicle to diaphragm; base of each lung rests on diaphragm
  4. Divisions
    a. Lobes: three in the right lung, two in the left
    b. Root: consists of the primary bronchus and pulmonary artery and veins bound together by connective tissue
    c. Hilum: vertical slit on medial surface of the lung, through which root structures enter the lung
    d. Apex: pointed upper part of the lung
    e. Base: broad, inferior surface of the lung

5. Bronchial tree: consists of the following
   a. Bronchi: right and left, formed by branching of the trachea; right bronchus slightly larger and more vertical than left; each primary bronchus branches, on entering the lung, into 10 segmental bronchi in each lung; primary and segmental bronchi all contain C-shaped cartilage
   b. Bronchioles: small branches off the secondary bronchi; distinguished by lack of C-shaped cartilage and a duct diameter of about 1 mm
   c. Terminal bronchioles: last ones possess a ciliated mucosa
   d. Respiratory bronchioles: composed of cuboidal nonciliated cells
   e. Alveolar ducts: microscopic branches off bronchioles composed of a thin squamous epithelium
   f. Alveoli: microscopic sacs composed of single layer of extremely thin squamous epithelial cells; each alveolar duct terminates in cluster of alveoli, often likened to a bunch of grapes; each alveolus enveloped by network of lung capillaries
6. Covering of lung: visceral layer of pleura

B. Function: place where air and blood can come in close enough contact for rapid diffusion of gases to occur
   1. Bronchi, bronchioles, alveolar ducts: lower part of airway through which air moves into and out of alveoli
   2. Alveoli: microscopic sacs in which gases are exchanged rapidly between the air and blood; membranous walls of the millions of alveoli provide a surface area large enough and thin enough to make possible rapid gas exchange
   3. Alveolar surfaces coated with group of substances called surfactant; effect is to lower alveolar surface tension to facilitate breathing, since sacs have less tendency to collapse with their walls adhering to each other

Physiology of Respiration

A. Mechanism of inspiration
   1. Respiratory muscles contract
   2. Thorax increases in size
   3. Intrathoracic pressure decreases
   4. Lungs increase in size
   5. Intrapulmonic pressure decreases
   6. Air rushes from positive pressure in the atmosphere to negative pressure in the alveoli
   7. Inspiration is completed

B. Mechanism of expiration
   1. Respiratory muscles relax
   2. Thorax decreases in size
   3. Intrathoracic pressure increases
   4. Lungs decrease in size
   5. Intrapulmonic pressure increases
   6. Air expelled from higher pressure in the lung to lower pressure in the atmosphere
   7. Expiration is completed

C. Neural control
   1. Alveolar stretch receptors respond to inspiration (lung inflation) by sending inhibitory impulses to inspiratory neurons in brainstem; this is the Hering-Breuer inflation reflex, and it prevents lung overdistention
   2. During expiration (lung deflation) the stretch receptors no longer inhibit inspiratory neurons, and inspiration may begin again; this is the Hering-Breuer deflation reflex

D. Chemical control
   1. Blood pH: decrease in pH stimulates respiration by direct stimulation of neurons of respiratory center and indirectly by stimulation of carotid and aortic chemoreceptors
   2. Blood Pco_2: increase in arterial Pco_2 results in decrease in pH and mimics effects in no. 1 above
   3. Blood Po_2: decrease in arterial Po_2 produces effects similar to decreased blood pH
   4. Stimulation of respiratory center neurons or chemoreceptors results in hyperventilation; hypoventilation occurs when the arterial pH rises or the arterial Pco_2 falls

E. Amount of air exchanged in breathing
   1. Directly related to gas pressure gradient between atmosphere and alveoli and inversely related to resistance opposing air flow; the greater the difference between atmospheric pressure and alveolar pressure, the greater the amount of air exchanged in breathing; the greater the resistance opposing air flow to or from the lungs, the less air exchanged
   2. Measured by apparatus called a spirometer
   3. Tidal air: average amount expired after normal inspiration; approximately 500 ml
   4. Expiratory reserve volume (ERV): largest additional volume of air that can be forcibly expired after a normal inspiration and expiration; normal ERV 1000 to 1200 ml
   5. Inspiratory reserve volume (IRV): largest additional volume of air that can be forcibly inspired after a normal inspiration; normal IRV 3000 to 3300 ml
   6. Residual air: air that cannot be forcibly expired from lungs; about 1200 ml
   7. Minimal air: air that can never be removed from alveoli if they have been inflated even once, even though lungs are subjected to atmospheric pressure that squeezes part of residual air out
   8. Vital capacity: approximate capacity of lungs as measured by amount of air that can be forcibly expired after forcible inspiration; varies with size of thoracic cavity, which is determined by various factors (e.g., size of rib cage, posture, volume of blood and interstitial fluid in the lungs, size of the heart)
   9. Maximal expiratory flow rate: an individual should be able to exhale 70% of his or her vital capacity in the first second and empty more than 90% in 3 seconds; asthma and emphysema prevent such normal, forced expiratory rates; measurable with a spirometer

F. Diffusion of gases between air and blood occurs across alveolar-capillary membranes (i.e., in lungs between air in alveoli and venous blood in lung capillaries)
   1. Direction of diffusion
      a. Oxygen: net diffusion toward lower oxygen pressure gradient (i.e., from alveolar air to blood)

b. Carbon dioxide: net diffusion toward lower carbon dioxide pressure gradient (i.e., from blood to alveolar air)
2. Mechanism of oxygen diffusion (Fig. 3-3)
3. Mechanism of carbon dioxide diffusion (Fig. 3-4)
G. How blood transports oxygen
1. As solute: about 0.5 ml of oxygen is dissolved in 100 ml of blood; produces the blood Po_2 (pressure of oxygen in the blood)
2. As oxyhemoglobin: each gram of hemoglobin can combine with 1.34 ml of oxygen; hence, with normal hemoglobin content (e.g., 15 g/100 ml of blood) and 100% oxygen saturation, about 20 ml (15 × 1.34) of oxygen is transported as oxyhemoglobin
3. Various factors influence rate at which oxygen associates with hemoglobin to form oxyhemoglobin, including
a. Increasing pressure of oxygen in the blood
b. Decreasing pressure of carbon dioxide in the blood
4. Various factors influence the rate at which oxygen dissociates from hemoglobin, including
a. Decreasing pressure of oxygen in the blood
b. Increasing pressure of carbon dioxide in the blood
c. Increased blood temperature
H. How blood transports carbon dioxide
1. As solute: small amount dissolves in plasma
2. As bicarbonate ion: more than half of carbon dioxide in blood is present in the plasma as bicarbonate ion (HCO_3^-) formed by ionization of carbonic acid
3. As carbhemoglobin: less than one-third of carbon dioxide is transported in combination with hemoglobin
I. Diffusion of gases between arterial blood and tissues occurs in tissue capillaries
1. Oxygen: net diffusion of dissolved oxygen out of the blood into the tissues because of lower Po_2

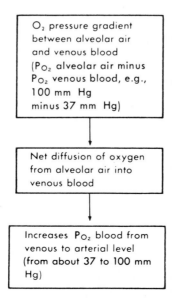

FIG. 3-3. Mechanism of oxygen diffusion.

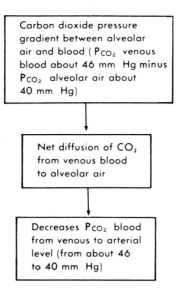

FIG. 3-4. Mechanism of carbon dioxide diffusion.

there (perhaps 30 mm Hg, compared to arterial Po_2 of 100 mm Hg); diffusion of dissolved oxygen out of the blood lowers blood Po_2 from arterial to venous level (from 100 to 40 mm Hg); decreasing Po_2 as the blood moves through tissue capillaries causes oxygen to dissociate from hemoglobin, thereby releasing more oxygen for diffusion out of the blood to the tissue cells
2. Carbon dioxide: net diffusion of carbon dioxide into the blood because of lower Pco_2 there (40 mm Hg compared with probably over 50 mm Hg in tissues); diffusion of carbon dioxide into tissue capillaries increases blood Pco_2 from arterial to venous level (from 40 to 46 mm Hg); increasing Pco_2 like decreasing Po_2 tends to accelerate oxygen dissociation from hemoglobin
J. Normal breath sounds
1. Bronchial sounds (over trachea, bronchi)
a. Result of air passing through larger airways
b. Sounds are loud, harsh, high pitched
c. Expiratory phase longer than inspiratory phase with pause in between
2. Vesicular sounds (over entire lung field except large airways)
a. Result of air moving in and out of alveoli; may reflect sound of air in larger passages that is transmitted through lung tissue
b. Sounds are quiet, low pitched
c. Inspiratory phase much longer than expiratory phase
3. Bronchovesicular sounds (near main stem bronchi)
a. Result of air moving through smaller air passages
b. Sounds are moderately pitched, breezy
c. Inspiratory and expiratory phases equal
K. Adventitious breath sounds
1. Rales (crackles)
a. Result of air passing through fluid in small airways and alveoli

b. Sound may be simulated by rubbing a few strands of hair between fingers next to ear

c. Most common during inspiratory phase

d. Associated with conditions such as COPD and pulmonary edema

2. Wheezes (sibilant rhonchi)

a. Result of air passing through narrowed small airways

b. Sounds are high pitched, musical

c. May be heard on either inspiration or expiration

d. Associated with conditions causing narrowing of airways, such as asthma, and with conditions that involve partial obstruction of airway by mucus, foreign body, or tumor

3. Sonorous rhonchi

a. Result of air passing through narrowed large airways

b. Sounds are low-pitched snores

c. Associated with same conditions as sibilant rhonchi

4. Pleural friction rub

a. Result of roughened pleural surfaces rubbing across each other

b. Sounds are crackling, grating

c. Associated with conditions causing inflammation of the pleura

REVIEW OF PHYSICAL PRINCIPLES RELATED TO THE RESPIRATORY SYSTEM
Principles of Mechanics
Law of Gravitation

EXAMPLES

1. Postural drainage: positioning the client so the throat is below level of the lungs to help drain fluid from the lungs

2. Rocking beds: abdominal viscera alternately push against and then away from the diaphragm, thus aiding in respiration

3. Position of the head postoperatively: head is placed on one side; thus, the force of gravity pulls the tongue down, breathing remains unobstructed and allows for drainage in case of vomiting

4. Use of chest tubes to restore negative pressure to intrapleural space

Momentum

EXAMPLES

1. During a cough or a sneeze, the abdominal and intercostal muscles apply a large force on the air in the lungs; the sudden opening of the vocal cords and epiglottis results in the explosive propulsion of air from the lungs; in this case momentum of the air stream is great, not because of the mass of the particles (since the molecules of gases in air are light), but because of their high velocity

2. When a person speaks, the vocal cords vibrate and in turn produce vibrations in the air molecules surrounding them; the momentum in these vibrating molecules is transferred from air molecule to air molecule all the way to the ear of the listener, where the vibrations are converted into nerve impulses that the brain interprets as sound

Energy

EXAMPLES

1. Epithelial cells of the human respiratory tract possess energy because their cilia beat back and forth and thus do the work of pushing mucus and foreign matter up toward the throat

2. Every living cell in the body possesses energy because it does work to maintain certain water and electrolyte concentrations within itself

3. The cilia exert a force that moves them through a certain distance in the fluid surrounding them

4. The cell membranes exert a force that moves ions a certain distance through the membrane

5. First Law of Thermodynamics

Principles of Physical Properties of Matter
Solids

Concept of elasticity

EXAMPLE: The elastic recoil of the lungs during quiet respiration provides the entire force necessary to effect expiration

Liquids

Surface tension: molecules of a liquid exert forces of attraction on one another; at the surface of the liquid the molecules are attracted by other molecules at the bottom and sides, but not at the top since air is there; this results in a force of contraction at the liquid surface called surface tension

EXAMPLE: The alveoli and respiratory passages of the human lungs have a mixture of surface tension–reducing substances collectively called surfactant that reduce surface tension and the pull that the water molecules would ordinarily have on each other if these surface active agents were absent; breathing is therefore much easier because of this agent

Gases

The molecules composing gases are so far apart that they do not exert any cohesive forces on each other; consequently, the gas will expand to fill any container and will exert pressure on the container because of elastic rebound of the gas molecules with the walls of the container

A. Boyle's law: at constant temperature the pressure exerted by a gas is inversely proportional to its volume; as the volume of a gas is decreased, its pressure increases, and as the volume is increased, the pressure decreases

1. Respiration: contraction and downward movements of the dome-shaped diaphragm increase the volume of the thoracic cavity containing the lungs; since the volume of air in the lungs is increased, the pressure exerted by the air is decreased; air now flows from the area of higher pressure outside the body to the area of lower pressure inside the lungs; conversely, during expiration, the upward movement of the diaphragm and the elastic recoil of the lungs themselves decrease the volume of air in the thoracic cavity and lungs as air flows out

2. Pneumothorax: opening that connects the outside air with the intrapleural space; result is that air flows into the intrapleural space; this eliminates the pressure gradient between the thoracic cavity and the atmosphere, and the lungs cannot inflate

3. Intermittent positive pressure breathing (IPPB) apparatus: special valve is operated by the individual's own respirations; on inspiration, one part of the valve opens and oxygen or a mixture of gases is forcefully pushed under greater than atmospheric pressure (positive pressure) into the lungs through a special mouthpiece or face mask

B. Dalton's law: pressure exerted (in millimeters of mercury [mm Hg]) by a gas in a mixture of gases is proportional to its percentage in the mixture; e.g., partial pressure of oxygen (O_2) in alveoli is 104 mm Hg; partial pressure of O_2 in pulmonary artery and alveolar capillaries is 40 mm Hg; therefore O_2 diffuses from alveoli air sacs into capillaries

C. Henry's law: quantity of gas dissolving in a liquid is proportional to the partial pressure of the gas at a given temperature; i.e., a person overcome by smoke inhalation or who has some obstruction to normal breathing can benefit from inhalation of either pure O_2 or a mixture of gases having a higher partial pressure of O_2 than is found in air

D. Bernoulli's principle: moving air exerts less pressure than motionless air

Principles of Light

A. X-rays use high-frequency electromagnetic waves
   EXAMPLE: The chest x-ray examination permits observation of a variety of lung disorders, such as pneumonia, tumors, and tuberculosis

B. Total internal reflection: at a certain critical angle, light between two media is not refracted (bent) through the media but is reflected back into the first medium provided the first medium is more dense than the second medium
   EXAMPLE: Fiberoptics allow illumination and visualization of trachea and bronchi (bronchoscopy); the image picked up by the lens internally reflects along fiberoptic tubing (even if bent) until it reaches the eye of the observer

REVIEW OF CHEMICAL PRINCIPLES RELATED TO THE RESPIRATORY SYSTEM

(See Fluid, electrolyte, and acid-base balance)

REVIEW OF MICROORGANISMS RELATED TO THE RESPIRATORY SYSTEM

A. Bacterial pathogens
   1. *Bordetella pertussis:* small, gram-negative coccobacillus; causes pertussis or whooping cough
   2. *Streptococcus pneumoniae:* gram-positive, encapsulated diplococcus; on the basis of the antigenic nature of the capsule there are about 100 types, the most important being Types I, II, and III; causes pneumococcal pneumonia (most commonly lobar) and often responsible for sinusitis, otitis media, and meningitis
   3. *Haemophilus influenzae:* small gram-negative, highly pleomorphic bacillus; causes acute meningitis and upper respiratory tract infections
   4. *Klebsiella pneumoniae* (Friedländer's bacillus): gram-negative, encapsulated, non-spore-forming bacillus; causes pneumonia and urinary tract infections

   5. *Mycobacterium tuberculosis* (tubercle bacillus): acid-fast actinomycete (thin, waxy rods, often bent, nonmotile, non-spore forming); causes tuberculosis
   6. *Pseudomonas aeruginosa:* gram-negative, non-spore-forming bacillus; important cause of hospital acquired infections; respiratory equipment can be source; causes pneumonia, urinary tract infections, and the sepsis that complicates severe burns

B. Rickettsial pathogen
   Coxiella burnetti: only species of rickettsiae not associated with a vector; causes Q fever, an infection clinically similar to primary atypical pneumonia

C. Viral pathogens
   1. DNA viruses
      Adenoviruses: spherical, 70 to 80 nm in diameter; cause acute respiratory tract disease, adenitis, pharyngitis, and other respiratory tract infections as well as conjunctivitis
   2. RNA viruses
      a. Coronaviruses: enveloped pleomorphic viruses; frequently associated with a mild upper respiratory tract infection
      b. Picornaviruses: spherical and 20 to 30 nm in diameter; cause poliomyelitis, Coxsackie disease, common cold, and various diseases of animals
      c. Reoviruses: double-stranded RNA virus involved in mild respiratory tract infections of humans

D. Fungal pathogen
   Histoplasma capsulatum: dimorphic fungus producing characteristic spores (chlamydospores) in infected tissue; causes histoplasmosis (a primary lung infection)

PHARMACOLOGY RELATED TO RESPIRATORY SYSTEM DISORDERS
Bronchodilators

A. Description
   1. Used to reverse bronchoconstriction, thus opening air passages in the lungs
   2. Act by
      a. Stimulating beta-adrenergic sympathetic nervous system receptors
      b. Directly relaxing bronchial smooth muscle
   3. Available in oral, parenteral (IM, SC, IV), rectal, and inhalation preparations

B. Examples
   1. Adrenergics: act at beta-adrenergic receptors in bronchus to relax smooth muscle and increase respiratory volume
      a. albuterol (Proventil)
      b. epinephrine HCl (Adrenalin; Sus-Phrine)
      c. ephedrine sulfate
      d. isoproterenol HCl (Isuprel)
      e. pseudoephedrine HCl (Sudafed)
      f. metaproterenol sulfate (Alupent)
      g. terbutaline sulfate (Brethine)
   2. Xanthines: act directly on bronchial smooth muscle, decreasing spasm and relaxing smooth muscle of the vasculature
      a. aminophylline
      b. oxtriphylline (Choledyl)
      c. theophylline (Elixophyllin; Theo-Dur)

3. Combination products
  a. Actifed
  b. Dristan
  c. Marax
  d. Sinutab
  e. Tedral
  f. Triaminic
C. Major side effects
  1. Dizziness (decrease in blood pressure)
  2. CNS stimulation (sympathetic stimulation)
  3. Palpitations (beta-adrenergic stimulation)
  4. Gastric irritation (local effect)
D. Nursing care
  1. Avoid administration to clients with hypertension, hyperthyroidism, and cardiovascular dysfunction
  2. Avoid concurrent administration of CNS stimulants (adrenergics) and bronchoconstricting agents (beta-blockers)
  3. Administer during waking hours
  4. Encourage clients to avoid smoking
  5. Assess vital signs, especially respirations
  6. Assess intake and output
  7. Administer with food
  8. Evaluate client's response to medication and understanding of teaching

Mucolytic Agents and Expectorants

A. Description
  1. Used to liquify secretions in the respiratory tract, thus promoting a productive cough
  2. Mucolytics act directly to break up mucus plugs in the tracheobronchial passages
  3. Expectorants act to liquify mucus by increasing respiratory tract secretions
  4. Mucolytic agents are available in inhalation preparations; expectorants are available in oral preparations
B. Examples
  1. Mucolytics
    a. acetylcysteine (Mucomyst)
  2. Expectorants
    a. ammonium chloride
    b. guaifenesin (Robitussin)
    c. potassium iodide (SSKI)
C. Major side effects
  1. Gastrointestinal irritation (local effect)
  2. Skin rash (hypersensitivity)
  3. Oropharyngeal irritation (mucolytics) (local effect during IPPB)
  4. Bronchospasm (mucolytics) (hypersensitivity)
D. Nursing care
  1. Promote adequate fluid intake
  2. Encourage coughing and deep breathing
  3. Avoid administering fluids immediately after taking expectorants
  4. Assess respiratory status
  5. Have suction apparatus available
  6. Evaluate client's response to medication and understanding of teaching

Antitussives

A. Description
  1. Used to suppress the cough reflex
  2. Act by inhibiting the cough reflex by either direct action on the medullary cough center or indirect action peripherally on sensory nerve endings
  3. Available in oral preparations
B. Examples
  1. Narcotic
    a. codeine
    b. hydrocodone bitartrate (Hycodan)
    c. hydromorphone HCl (Dilaudid cough syrup)
  2. Nonnarcotic
    a. benzonatate (Tessalon)
    b. dextromethorphan hydrobromide
    c. diphenhydramine HCl (Benadryl)
    d. noscapine HCl (Noscatuss)
C. Major side effects
  1. Drowsiness (CNS depression)
  2. Nausea (GI irritation)
  3. Dry mouth (anticholinergic effect of antihistamine in combination products)
D. Nursing care
  1. Provide adequate fluid intake
  2. Avoid administering fluids immediately after liquid preparations
  3. Encourage high-Fowler's position
  4. Avoid use postoperatively and in clients with head injury
  5. Administer narcotics cautiously
    a. Avoid administration with CNS depressants
    b. Caution client to avoid engaging in hazardous activity
    c. Assess for signs of dependence
  6. Evaluate client's response to medication and understanding of teaching

Narcotic Antagonists

(See Substance-use disorders in Psychiatric Nursing)
A. Description
  1. Used to reverse respiratory depression due to narcotic overdosage
  2. Act to displace narcotics at respiratory receptor sites via competitive antagonism
  3. Available in parenteral (IV, SC, IM) preparations
B. Examples
  1. levallorphan tartrate (Lorfan)
  2. nalorphine HCl (Nalline)
  3. naloxone HCl (Narcan)
C. Major side effects
  1. CNS depression (acts on opioid receptors in CNS)
  2. Nausea, vomiting
  3. Pupillary constriction
D. Nursing care
  1. Assess vital signs, especially respirations
  2. Have O_2 and emergency resuscitative equipment available
  3. Avoid use in cases of nonnarcotic respiratory depression
  4. Evaluate client's response to medication and understanding of teaching

Antihistamines

A. Description
1. Used to relieve symptoms of the common cold and allergies which are mediated by the chemical histamine
2. Act by blocking the action of histamine at receptor sites via competitive inhibition; they also exert antiemetic, anticholinergic, and CNS depressant effects
3. Available in oral and parenteral (IM, IV, SC) preparations
B. Examples
1. brompheniramine maleate (Dimetane)
2. chlorpheniramine maleate (Chlor-Trimeton)
3. diphenhydramine HCl (Benadryl)
4. promethazine HCl (Phenergan)
5. Combination products
a. Allerest
b. Drixoral
c. Ornade
d. Triaminic
C. Major side effects
1. Drowsiness (CNS depression)
2. Dizziness (CNS depression)
3. Gastrointestinal irritation (local effect)
4. Dry mouth (anticholinergic effect of decreased salivation)
5. Excitement (in children) (paradoxic effect)
D. Nursing care
1. Avoid administration with CNS depressants
2. Caution client to avoid engaging in hazardous activities
3. Administer with food or milk
4. Offer gum or hard candy
5. Evaluate client's response to medication and understanding of teaching

PROCEDURES RELATED TO THE RESPIRATORY SYSTEM
Administration of Oxygen

A. Definition
1. Administration of supplemental oxygen when the client's respiratory system is compromised and tissue hypoxia is threatened
2. May be accomplished via a catheter, cannula, mask, or tent
B. Nursing care
1. Explain the procedure to the client and family
2. Attach "no smoking" signs to door of room and instruct the client and visitors to adhere to this rule, since oxygen supports combustion
3. Assess the client's color (nail beds, general appearance) and vital signs prior to and during therapy
4. Ascertain that client does not have chronic lung disease before administering high concentrations of oxygen
5. Attach appropriate apparatus to the oxygen source and fill the humidification cannister prn with water to prevent drying of mucous membranes
6. Evaluate client's response to procedure

Arterial Blood Gases

A. Definition: measurement of arterial pH, partial pressures of oxygen and carbon dioxide, bicarbonate ion, and oxygen saturation (see acid-base balance)
B. Nursing care
1. Explain procedure to the client
2. Obtain a heparinized syringe or vacuum container tube
3. Notify the laboratory to calibrate equipment
4. Aseptically obtain approximately 3 ml of arterial blood; most common sites include the radial, brachial, and femoral arteries
5. Avoid introducing room air into the syringe, for this can alter results
6. Apply pressure over the arterial site for 5 minutes to prevent bleeding
7. Place the specimen in ice to decrease the metabolic rate of blood cells and subsequent alteration of values; transport promptly to the laboratory
8. Evaluate client's response to procedure

Bronchoscopy

A. Definition
1. Visualization of the tracheobronchial tree via a scope advanced through the mouth or nose into the bronchi
2. Procedure may be performed to remove foreign body, to remove secretions, or to obtain specimens of tissue or mucus for further study
B. Nursing care
1. Obtain an informed consent
2. Maintain the client npo prior to procedure and remove dentures and jewelry
3. Administer ordered preprocedure medications to produce sedation and decrease anxiety
4. Inform client to expect some hemoptysis after the procedure
5. Advise client to avoid coughing or clearing throat
6. Observe the client for signs of hemorrhage and/or respiratory distress
7. Monitor vital signs until stable
8. Do not allow the client to drink until the gag reflex returns
9. Evaluate client's response to procedure

Chest Tubes

A. Definition
1. Use of tubes and suction to return negative pressure to the intrapleural space
2. To drain air from the intrapleural space, the chest tube is placed in the second or third intercostal space; to drain blood or fluid, the catheter would be placed at a lower site, usually the eighth or ninth intercostal space
B. Types of drainage systems
1. One-bottle underwater system: allows air or fluid to drain from the pleural cavity by gravity via a glass rod, which extends approximately 2 cm below the surface of the water within the collection bottle
2. Two-bottle drainage system: involves one bottle that acts as a collection chamber and provides the water seal while a second bottle can be connected to a

suction apparatus; the bubbling of water within the second bottle indicates that the desired suction is maintained

3. Three-bottle system: includes one bottle that serves to collect drainage, one that acts as the water-seal chamber, and one that controls suction
4. Commercially prepared plastic unit designed for closed chest suction: combines the features of the other systems and may or may not be attached to suction (e.g., PleurEvac)

C. Nursing care

1. Ensure that the tubing is not kinked; tape all connections to prevent separation
2. Gently milk the tubing as necessary in the direction of the drainage system to maintain patency
3. Maintain the drainage system below the level of the chest
4. Turn the client frequently, making sure the chest tubes are not compressed
5. Report drainage on dressing immediately, since this is not a normal occurrence
6. Observe for fluctuation of fluid in glass tube; the level will rise on inhalation and fall on exhalation; if there are no fluctuations, either the lung has expanded fully or the chest tube is clogged
7. Palpate the area around the chest tube insertion site for subcutaneous emphysema or crepitus, which indicates that air is leaking into the subcutaneous tissue
8. Situate the drainage bottles or PleurEvac to avoid breakage
9. Place two clamps at the bedside for use if the underwater-seal bottle is broken; clamp the chest tube immediately to prevent air from entering the intrapleural space, which would cause pneumothorax to occur or extend; clamps are used judiciously and only in emergency situations
10. Encourage coughing and deep breathing every 2 hours, splinting the area as needed
11. Instruct the client to exhale or strain (Valsalva maneuver) as the tube is withdrawn by the physician; apply a gauze dressing immediately and firmly secure with tape to make an airtight dressing
12. Encourage movement of the arm on the affected side
13. Evaluate client's response to procedure

Incentive Spirometry

A. Purpose

1. Mechanical device used to maximize inspiration
2. Prevents atelectasis
3. Mobilizes secretions

B. Nursing care

1. Verify predetermined volume setting up to 5000 ml
2. Instruct client to use lips to form a seal around the mouthpiece
3. Have client inspire deeply and hold the inspiration a few seconds before forcefully expelling the air
4. Explain that the machine provides feedback only when preset volume is reached; feedback may be a light or a rising ball depending on the specific device

5. Avoid spirometry at mealtime to prevent nausea
6. Evaluate client's response to procedure

Management of Airway Obstruction

A. Suctioning of airway

1. Definition
   a. Mechanical aspiration of mucous secretions from the tracheobronchial tree by application of negative pressure
   b. Utilized to maintain a patent airway, obtain a sputum specimen, or stimulate coughing
   c. May be nasotracheal, oropharyngeal, or through an endotracheal or tracheostomy tube
2. Nursing care
   a. Maintain surgical asepsis
   b. Assess proper functioning of the equipment
   c. Hyperoxygenate client by increasing flow rate; encourage deep breathing
   d. Lubricate the suction catheter with sterile water
   e. Insert the catheter
      (1) If tracheal suction is being utilized, insert approximately 4 inches
      (2) If nasotracheal suction is being utilized, insert until the cough reflex is induced
   f. Apply no suction while the catheter is being inserted
   g. Rotate and withdraw the catheter while suction is applied; suction should not exceed 10 to 15 seconds
   h. Clear the catheter with sterile solution and encourage the client to breathe deeply
   i. If deeper suction is required, ask the client to turn his or her head to the side to permit entry of the suction catheter into the opposite bronchus
   j. Evaluate client's response to procedure; revise plan as necessary

B. Abdominal thrust (Heimlich maneuver)

1. Definition: short abrupt pressure against the abdomen (halfway between the umbilicus and xyphoid) to raise intrarespiratory pressure, which will dislodge an obstruction such as a bolus of food or a foreign body
2. Symptoms of obstruction
   a. Partial: noisy respiration, dyspnea, lightheadedness, dizziness, flushing of face, bulging of eyes, repeated coughing
   b. Total: cessation of breathing, inability to speak or cough, extension of head, facial cyanosis, bulging of eyes, panic, unconsciousness
3. Nursing care
   a. Assess client no longer than 3 to 5 seconds
      (1) Ask if client is choking
      (2) Determine if victim can speak or cough
      (3) Observe for universal choking sign (thumb and forefinger encircling throat under chin)
      (4) Assess for respirations (particularly in unconscious victim)
         (a) Observe for rise and fall of chest
         (b) Listen for escape of air from nose and mouth on expiration
         (c) Feel for flow of air from nose and mouth on expiration

b. Initiate intervention in the presence of a partial obstruction
   (1) Allow the individual's expulsive cough to dislodge the obstruction
   (2) Assess for signs of total obstruction
   (3) Remove foreign bodies coughed up into the mouth
c. Initiate intervention in the presence of a total obstruction
   (1) Open the individual's mouth and remove the obstruction if possible
   (2) Standing behind the conscious victim, encircle the hypochondrium and thrust upward and inward against the diaphragm with intertwined clenched fists
   (3) Straddling the hips of the unconscious supine victim, place the heel of one hand on the other and thrust upward and inward against the diaphragm
   (4) Repeat abdominal thrust several times (may require 6 to 10 thrusts) until foreign body is dislodged or until help arrives
   (5) Remove foreign bodies coughed up into the mouth
   (6) Assess for signs of injury to liver or spleen; there is a higher risk of this when abdominal thrusts are performed with the victim in recumbent position
   (7) If an airway cannot be established, an emergency cricothyrotomy may be necessary
d. Evaluate client's response to procedure

Mechanical Ventilation

A. Definition: use of a mechanical device to instill a mixture of air and oxygen into the lungs using positive pressure
B. Types of ventilators
   1. Volume control: delivers a preset tidal volume at various pressures
   2. Pressure control: delivers preset pressure at various volumes
C. Types of ventilation
   1. Controlled: the client receives a specified volume at a specific pressure with no triggering of the machine by the client; the nurse may have to administer drugs such as pancuronium bromide (Pavulon) or morphine to decrease the client's own respiratory response
   2. Assisted: the client triggers the machine so that the rate may vary; however, if the client has periods of apnea, the machine will take over initiation of respirations
D. Nursing care
   1. Keep the respirator at settings as ordered and notify the respiratory therapy department and the physician if distress occurs
   2. Maintain a sealed system between the respirator and the client so that volume to be delivered is kept constant and air is not lost around the tubing; this is accomplished by inflating the cuff of the endotracheal tube or tracheostomy tube to the minimum occlusive volume

   3. Perform suction as necessary, since humidified oxygen helps to liquefy secretions that must be removed
   4. Observe for signs of respiratory insufficiency, such as tachypnea, cyanosis, and changes in sensorium
   5. Ascertain blood gases as ordered to determine effectiveness of ventilation
   6. Establish a means of communication, since client will be unable to speak while on a ventilator
   7. Evaluate client's response to procedure; revise plan as necessary

Pulmonary Function Tests

A. Definition
   1. Series of tests used to detect problems in the performance capabilities of the pulmonary system
   2. A spirometer is used to measure amounts of gas exchanged between the client and the atmosphere; nose clips are used to allow only mouth breathing and prevent air leakage
   3. Measurement studies include
      a. Tidal volume: amount of air inhaled or exhaled during one respiration
      b. Vital capacity: volume of air that can be forcefully exhaled after a maximum inspiration
      c. Total lung capacity: volume of air in the lungs following a maximum inspiration
      d. Forced expiratory volume (FEV): volume of air that can be forcefully exhaled within a specific amount of time, usually 1, 2, or 3 seconds
B. Nursing care
   1. Explain procedure to the client to allay anxiety and promote compliance at time of test
   2. Notify the respiratory therapist of all medications that the client is receiving which affect respiratory function
   3. Evaluate client's response to procedure

Pulse Oximetry

A. Definition: noninvasive, continuous monitoring of arterial oxygen saturation by use of red and infrared light beams and a photodetector to determine relative light absorption
B. Nursing care
   1. Explain procedure to the client
   2. Select the appropriate transducer or sensor (adult finger or nasal transducer, neonatal foot or infant toe transducer, or pediatric finger transducer)
   3. Apply transducer to extremity and maintain at heart level; do not select an extremity which has any impediment to blood flow (blood pressure cuff or arterial line)
   4. Check the preset alarm for oxygen saturation and pulse rate
   5. Evaluate client's response to procedure

Sputum Studies

A. Definition: analysis of sputum for pathogenic bacteria or tumor cells
   1. Culture and sensitivity: identification of bacteria and appropriate antibiotic therapy; the specimen should be obtained prior to institution of antibiotic therapy

2. Acid-fast bacteria (AFB): staining technique to identify bacilli as acid fast, generally indicative of *Mycobacterium tuberculosis*
3. Cytology: microscopic examination of pulmonary epithelial cells that have sloughed off into the sputum; performed when malignancy is suspected

B. Nursing care
1. Collect specimen in the early morning before client has food or fluid; can also be obtained after an aerosol treatment
2. Have client rinse mouth with water to decrease contamination of specimen with oropharyngeal microorganisms
3. Instruct client to take several deep breaths and cough deeply to raise sputum and expectorate into a sterile specimen container; care must be taken to avoid touching the inside of the container
4. Transport specimen to laboratory promptly
5. Offer oral hygiene after collection to eliminate foul taste of sputum
6. Evaluate client's response

Thoracentesis

A. Definition
1. Surgical aseptic procedure in which the chest wall is punctured with a trocar to remove fluid or air; this is done for diagnostic purposes or to alleviate respiratory embarrassment
2. No more than 1000 ml of fluid should be removed at a time; fluid withdrawn should be sent to the laboratory for culture and sensitivity tests
3. Complications include pneumothorax from trauma to the lung and pulmonary edema as a result of sudden fluid shifts

B. Nursing care
1. Obtain an informed consent
2. Explain procedure to the client
3. Ensure that chest x-ray examination is done prior to and after the procedure
4. Assist and support the client in the sitting position
5. Set up a sterile field for the physician
6. Assess pulse and respirations prior to, during, and after the procedure
7. Inform the client not to cough during the procedure to prevent trauma to the lungs
8. After the procedure, label and send specimens for laboratory tests
9. Note and record the amount, color, and clarity of the fluid withdrawn
10. Place the client on opposite side for approximately 1 hour to prevent leakage of fluid through the thoracentesis site
11. Observe the client for coughing, bloody sputum, and rapid pulse rate and report their occurrence immediately
12. Evaluate client's response to procedure

Tracheostomy Care

A. Definition: removal of dried secretions from the cannula to maintain a patent airway, prevent infection, and prevent irritation

B. Nursing care
1. Provide tracheostomy care at least every 8 hours
2. Suction to remove secretions from the lumen of the tube (see procedure for suctioning of airways)
3. If an inner cannula is present
   a. Remove and place in a container of hydrogen peroxide and rinse with normal saline, using surgical aseptic technique
   b. Remove dried secretions within the cannula, using a sterile pipe cleaner or brush
   c. Drain excess saline before reinserting the tube, which is then locked in place
4. Clean the area around the stoma with peroxide and saline, using aseptic technique; apply antiseptic ointment if ordered
5. Change the tracheostomy string or tape, being careful not to dislodge the cannula; tie with a double knot
6. Place a tracheostomy dressing or fenestrated 4 × 4 inch (unfilled) dressing below the stoma to absorb expelled secretions
7. Humidify inhaled air mechanically or by the use of a moistened 4 × 4 inch dressing over the tracheostomy, since air is bypassing normal humidification process in the nasopharynx
8. Evaluate client's response to procedure

NURSING PROCESS FOR CLIENTS WITH RESPIRATORY SYSTEM DISORDERS
Probable Nursing Diagnoses Based on Assessment

A. Ineffective airway clearance related to
1. Improper positioning
2. Mechanical obstruction
3. Excessive secretions
B. Ineffective breathing patterns related to
1. Chemical toxicity
2. Anxiety
3. Pain
4. CNS damage
C. Impaired gas exchange related to
1. Excessive secretions
2. Loss of functioning lung tissue
3. Insufficient oxygen supply
D. Altered thought processes related to decreased cerebral oxygenation
E. Anxiety related to oxygen deprivation
F. Fear related to air hunger
G. Altered nutrition; less than body requirements, related to
1. Excessive secretions
2. Easy fatigability
H. Activity intolerance related to oxygen deprivation
I. Fatigue related to oxygen deprivation
J. Body image disturbance related to disfiguring head and neck surgery
K. Infection related to microbial invasion
L. Impaired verbal communication related to an alteration in structures necessary for speech

Nursing Care for Clients with Respiratory System Disorders

(See nursing care under each specific disease)

MAJOR DISEASES

Pulmonary Embolism and Infarction

A. Etiology and pathophysiology
1. Postoperative clients, as well as those confined to bed, are prone to venous stasis, which causes peripheral thrombus formation
2. When an embolus lodges in the pulmonary artery causing hemorrhage and necrosis of lung tissue, it is called a pulmonary infarction

B. Signs and symptoms
1. Subjective
a. Severe dyspnea that occurs suddenly
b. Anxiety
c. Restlessness
d. Sharp upper abdominal or thoracic pain
2. Objective
a. Violent coughing with hemoptysis
b. On auscultation, dullness over area of infarction
c. Increased temperature

C. Treatment
1. Anticoagulant therapy
2. Maintenance of blood pressure
3. Angiography; if the condition is severe, an embolectomy may be indicated

D. Nursing care
1. Place in the high-Fowler's position to aid respiration
2. Monitor vital signs
3. Administer medications and oxygen as ordered
4. Evaluate client's response and revise plan as necessary

Pulmonary Edema

A. Etiology and pathophysiology
1. An acute emergency condition characterized by a rapid accumulation of fluid in the alveolar spaces resulting from increased pressure within the pulmonary system
2. Possible causes include valvular disease, left ventricular failure, circulatory overload, or congestive heart disease

B. Signs and symptoms
1. Subjective
a. History of premonitory symptoms such as shortness of breath, paroxysmal nocturnal dyspnea, wheezing, and orthopnea
b. Acute anxiety, apprehension, restlessness
2. Objective
a. Rapid thready pulse
b. Pink frothy sputum
c. Elevated central venous pressure (CVP)
d. Decreased circulation time
e. Cyanosis
f. Wheezing
g. Stertorous respirations

C. Treatment
1. Medications aimed at decreasing cardiac work load and improving cardiac output, such as morphine sulfate, digitalis, diuretics, bronchodilators

2. Oxygen in high concentration or by IPPB as necessary
3. Phlebotomy to remove approximately 500 ml of blood or the application of rotating tourniquets to reduce the volume of circulating blood
4. Cardiac monitoring

D. Nursing care
1. Support client in a high-Fowler's or semi-Fowler's position
2. Observe and record vital signs and monitor cardiac activity and intake and output
3. Provide a reassuring environment to allay anxiety
4. Suction as needed to maintain a patent airway
5. Apply rotating tourniquets when ordered
a. Tourniquets are placed around extremities without completely obliterating the pulse
b. One tourniquet is released in a clockwise direction every 15 minutes; may be done manually or by an automated machine
c. Assess arterial pulses of all extremities every 15 minutes
d. When client is no longer in distress, remove tourniquets one at a time, at 15-minute intervals, to prevent sudden cardiac overload; legs are rotated off last
6. Evaluate client's response and revise plan as necessary

Pleural Effusion

A. Etiology and pathophysiology
1. Collection of fluid in the pleural space
2. Generally occurs secondary to diseases such as cancer of the lung, tuberculosis, and congestive heart failure

B. Signs and symptoms
1. Subjective
a. Pleuritic pain that is sharp and increases on inspiration
b. Dyspnea
c. Malaise
2. Objective
a. Tachycardia
b. Elevated temperature
c. Cough (may be productive or nonproductive depending on cause)
d. Decreased breath sounds
e. Chest x-ray examination shows obliteration of the angle between the ribs and diaphragm; may also reveal a mediastinal shift away from the fluid

C. Treatment
1. Thoracentesis (see procedure)
2. Treatment of underlying cause

D. Nursing care
1. Monitor vital signs, particularly temperature and respirations
2. Auscultate lung fields
3. Encourage coughing and deep breathing
4. Increase fluid intake
5. Place the client in a high-Fowler's position for maximum air exchange
6. Evaluate client's response and revise plan as necessary

Pleurisy

A. Etiology and pathophysiology
1. Inflammation of the visceral and parietal membranes, which rub together during respiration and cause pain
2. Caused by chest trauma, tuberculosis, pneumonia, or chest surgery

B. Signs and symptoms
1. Subjective
   a. Knifelike pain on inspiration
   b. Apprehension
   c. Dyspnea
2. Objective
   a. Decreased excursion of the involved chest wall
   b. Pleural friction rub discernible on auscultation of chest wall

C. Treatment
1. Treat the underlying condition
2. Analgesics for pain
3. Applications of heat or cold to thoracic area

D. Nursing care
1. Instruct the client to lie on the affected side to splint the chest wall and lessen pain on inspiration
2. Administer medications as ordered
3. Allay anxiety by checking at frequent intervals
4. Observe for signs of shock or pulmonary emboli
5. Evaluate client's response and revise plan as necessary

Empyema

A. Etiology and pathophysiology
1. Collection of pus within the thoracic cavity
2. May occur following staphylococcal pneumonia, tuberculosis, chest trauma, or surgery

B. Signs and symptoms
1. Subjective
   a. Unilateral chest pain
   b. Malaise
   c. Anorexia
   d. Dyspnea
2. Objective
   a. Chest x-ray examination shows pleural exudate
   b. Elevated temperature
   c. Cough
   d. Unequal chest expansion

C. Treatment
1. Thoracentesis to obtain a specimen of exudate to culture
2. Chest tubes inserted to drain thoracic cavity
3. Antibiotics may be instilled through the chest tube or given systemically
4. If condition is long-standing, the area of inflammation is surgically removed; this is known as decortication

D. Nursing care
1. Monitor chest tube (see procedure)
2. Provide emotional support
3. Administer antibiotics as ordered
4. Monitor vital signs, particularly temperature and character of respirations
5. Evaluate client's response and revise plan as necessary

Pneumonia

A. Etiology and pathophysiology
1. Inflammatory disease usually caused by an infectious agent (bacterial, viral, protozoan, or fungal) but may also be caused by inhalation of chemicals and aspiration of gastric contents
2. Pneumonia is commonly spread by respiratory droplets
3. Pneumococcal pneumonia, the most common type of bacterial pneumonia, occurs in winter and spring; other bacterial pneumonias include *Klebsiella pneumoniae, Haemophilus influenzae,* species of *Pseudomonas, Proteus,* and *Streptococcus,* and *Staphylococcus aureus*
4. Aspiration pneumonia occurs when gastric contents and the normal flora of the upper respiratory tract are aspirated into the lung
5. *Pneumocystis carinii* pneumonia, a rare protozoan infection, is seen in clients with impaired immune function (AIDS)

B. Signs and symptoms
1. Subjective
   a. Lassitude
   b. Chest pain that increases on inspiration
   c. Dyspnea
2. Objective
   a. Elevated temperature
   b. Increased WBC
   c. Cough
   d. Chest x-ray examination shows pulmonary infiltration
   e. Sputum production
      (1) Pneumococcal: purulent, rusty sputum
      (2) Staphylococcal: yellow, blood-streaked sputum
      (3) Klebsiella: red gelatinous sputum
      (4) Mycoplasmal: nonproductive that advances to mucoid

C. Treatment
1. If bacterial pneumonia, culture and sensitivity tests will be done on blood and sputum to determine appropriate antibiotic therapy
2. Oxygen therapy usually via nasal cannula
3. Inhalation therapy such as IPPB or the use of incentive spirometer

D. Nursing care
1. Encourage coughing and deep breathing, splinting the chest as necessary
2. Observe amount and characteristics of sputum
3. Collect sputum specimen for culture and sensitivity tests in sterile container; notify the physician if organism is resistant to the antibiotic being given
4. Increase fluid intake
5. Monitor vital signs
6. Observe for signs of respiratory distress, such as labored respirations, cool clammy skin, and cyanosis
7. Plan rest periods
8. Instruct client to cover nose and mouth when coughing
9. Evaluate client's response and revise plan as necessary

Atelectasis

A. Etiology and pathophysiology
   1. Respirations shallow and ineffective, as in postoperative clients
   2. Bronchioles obstructed by secretions, and alveoli distal to the bronchioles collapse; many small bronchioles or a stem of the bronchus may be involved
   3. Causes include compression due to large pleural effusion, empyema, or pneumothorax, obstruction of a bronchus by a tumor, and deficiency of surfactant in an infant
B. Signs and symptoms
   1. Subjective
      a. Restlessness
      b. Anxiety
   2. Objective
      a. Rapid shallow respirations
      b. Diminished breath sounds in lower lobes
      c. Productive cough
      d. Temperature elevation
C. Treatment
   1. Oxygen therapy
   2. IPPB
   3. Prophylactic antibiotics
D. Nursing care
   1. Encourage coughing and deep breathing
   2. Monitor respirations closely
   3. Auscultate breath sounds for signs of decreased ventilation
   4. Place in a high-Fowler's position; turn every 2 hours
   5. Evaluate client's response and revise plan as necessary

Sarcoidosis

A. Etiology and pathophysiology
   1. Characterized by epithelioid cell tubercles, most commonly in the lung
   2. Cause unknown, although 80% have high titers of Epstein-Barr virus
   3. Incidence is highest in blacks and young adults
B. Signs and symptoms
   1. Subjective
      a. Fatigue
      b. Malaise
      c. Dyspnea
   2. Objective
      a. Night sweats
      b. Fever
      c. Weight loss
      d. Cough
      e. Nodules of face
      f. Polyarthritis
      g. Mild anemia
      h. Elevated serum calcium
      i. Kveim test: sarcoid node antigen is injected intradermally and causes local nodular lesion in approximately 1 month
      j. Biopsy of skin, lymph node, or liver
      k. X-ray findings include bilateral hilar and paratracheal adenopathy
      l. Pulmonary function studies reveal decreased lung compliance

C. Treatment
   1. No specific treatment
   2. Corticosteroids to control symptoms
D. Nursing care
   1. Monitor temperature and other vital signs
   2. Increase fluid intake
   3. Provide frequent periods of rest
   4. Provide small nutritious meals, taking into consideration the client's preferences
   5. Evaluate client's response and revise plan as necessary

Pulmonary Tuberculosis

A. Etiology and pathophysiology
   1. Infection of lungs caused by *Mycobacterium tuberculosis,* an acid-fast bacterium
   2. Causes tubercles, fibrosis, and calcification within the lungs
   3. Tubercle bacillus may be communicated to others by means of droplet formation (inhalation), ingestion, or inoculation
   4. Predisposing factors include debilitating diseases such as alcoholism, cardiovascular disease, diabetes mellitus, and cirrhosis, as well as poor nutrition and crowded living conditions
   5. Chronic, progressive, and reinfection phase is most frequently encountered in adults and involves progression or reactivation of primary lesions after months or years of latency
   6. Swallowing infected sputum may lead to laryngeal, oropharyngeal, and intestinal tuberculosis
B. Signs and symptoms
   1. Subjective
      a. Malaise
      b. Pleuritic pain
      c. Easily fatigued
   2. Objective
      a. Fever
      b. Night sweats
      c. Cough that progressively becomes worse
      d. Hemoptysis
      e. Weight loss
      f. Chest x-ray examination to determine presence of active or calcified lesions
      g. Analysis of sputum and gastric contents for the presence of acid-fast bacilli
      h. Tuberculin testing
         (1) Examples
            (a) Tine
            (b) Heaf
            (c) Mantoux, which frequently involves the use of purified protein derivative (PPD)
         (2) Determines antibody response to the tubercle bacillus
         (3) Indicates prior exposure to bacillus, which may or may not indicate active disease state (a sudden change from negative to positive requires follow-up testing)
         (4) In each test, either old tuberculin (OT) or PPD is injected intradermally; redness and edema present 48 to 72 hours later indicate a positive finding

C. Treatment
1. Program of combined antituberculin drugs such as isoniazid, paraminosalicylic acid, streptomycin, pyrazinamide, rifampin, and ethambutol hydrochloride for 9 to 24 months
2. Bed rest until symptoms abate or therapeutic regimen is established
3. Determine whether surgical resection of the involved lobe is necessary if symptoms such as hemorrhage develop or chemotherapy is unsatisfactory
4. Provide prophylactic therapy to immediate contacts (all cases and follow-up of contacts must be reported to public health agency)
5. Have the client begin a high-carbohydrate, high-protein, high-vitamin diet with supplemental vitamin B_6

D. Nursing care
1. Teach client to provide for scheduled rest periods
2. Teach which foods to include in the diet and which are nutritious between-meal supplements
3. Teach the importance of adhering, without variation, to the drug program that has been established
4. Teach the proper techniques to prevent spread of infection
   a. Frequent hand washing
   b. Cover the mouth when coughing
   c. Proper use and disposal of tissues
   d. Proper cleansing of eating utensils and disposal of food wastes
   e. Isolation when sputum is positive for the organism
5. Encourage client to participate in developing a schedule of activities and therapy and following the schedule once established
6. Instruct client to be alert to the early symptoms of hemorrhage such as hemoptysis and to contact the physician immediately if any occur
7. Instruct client to be alert to the early symptoms of adverse drug reactions (e.g., neuritis, ringing in the ears, ataxia, dermatitis) and to contact the physician immediately if any occur
8. Encourage client to follow prescribed program for productive coughing and deep breathing
9. Instruct client to avoid any medications such as cough syrups without physician's approval
10. Explain the need and instruct client to continue follow-up care and supervision
11. Encourage client to express feelings about disease and the many ramifications (stigma, isolation, fear) it creates
12. Expect and accept client's expression of hostility and depression
13. Encourage client to limit activities until the physician gives approval for gradual increase
14. Help client plan a realistic schedule for taking the large number of necessary medications
15. Monitor client's compliance with therapeutic regimen
16. Evaluate client's response and revise plan as necessary

Chronic Obstructive Pulmonary Disease (COPD)

A. Etiology and pathophysiology
1. Group of diseases that result in an obstruction of airflow; etiology includes air pollution, smoking, chronic respiratory infections, exposure to molds and fungi, and allergic reactions
2. Types
   a. Asthma: obstruction of the bronchioles characterized by attacks that occur suddenly and last from 30 to 60 minutes; an asthmatic attack that is difficult to control is referred to as status asthmaticus
   b. Bronchitis: inflammation of the bronchial walls with hypertrophy of the mucous goblet cells; characterized by a chronic cough
   c. Emphysema: characterized by distended, inelastic, or destroyed alveoli with bronchiolar obstruction and collapse; these alterations greatly impair the diffusion of gases through the alveolocapillary membrane
3. Clients with COPD become accustomed to an elevated residual carbon dioxide level and do not respond to high CO_2 concentrations as the normal respiratory stimulant; they respond instead to a drop in oxygen concentration in the blood

B. Signs and symptoms
1. Subjective
   a. Fatigue and weakness
   b. Headache, impaired sensorium
   c. Dyspnea
2. Objective
   a. Orthopnea, expiratory wheezing, stertorous breathing sounds, cough
   b. Barrel chest, cyanosis, clubbing of fingers
   c. Distention of neck veins
   d. Edema of extremities
   e. Increased P_{CO_2} and decreased P_{O_2} of arterial blood gases
   f. Polycythemia

C. Treatment
1. Antibiotics and cortisone to prevent and reduce inflammation
2. Bronchodilators to reduce muscular spasm
3. Mucolytics and expectorants to liquefy secretions and to facilitate their removal
4. Oxygen at 2 to 3 L even if hypoxia is severe
5. Respiratory therapy program to include IPPB, postural drainage, and exercise
6. High-protein, soft diet

D. Nursing care
1. Advise the elimination of smoking and other external irritants, such as dust, as much as possible
2. Supervise client's respiratory exercises, such as pursed lip or diaphragmatic breathing
3. Teach proper use of nebulizer and other special equipment
4. Carefully observe for symptoms of carbon dioxide intoxication (CO_2 narcosis) if oxygen is being administered
5. Teach client to adjust activities to avoid overexertion

6. Teach client to avoid people with respiratory infections
7. Teach client to maintain the highest resistance possible by getting proper rest, eating proper food, dressing properly for weather conditions
8. Teach client to be alert to early symptoms of infection, hypoxia, hypercapnea, or adverse response to medications
9. Encourage client to continue with close medical supervision
10. Encourage client to express feelings about disease and therapy
11. Accept feelings about life-long restrictions in activity
12. Encourage client to take an active role in planning therapy
13. Encourage client to take medications as ordered
14. Support efforts to give up smoking by providing diversional activities such as eating hard candies
15. Encourage the family to support client's efforts to give up smoking
16. Monitor client's compliance with therapeutic regimen
17. Evaluate client's response and revise plan as necessary

Occupational Lung Disease: Silicosis (Black Lung), Asbestosis and Coal Workers' Pneumoconiosis

A. Etiology and pathophysiology
   1. Fibrotic disease of lungs caused by inhalation of inorganic dusts over long periods
   2. Common in people whose professions expose them to free silica, such as miners and sandblasters
   3. Tuberculosis a frequent complication
B. Signs and symptoms
   1. Subjective
      a. Exertional dyspnea
      b. Anxiety
   2. Objective
      a. Frequent respiratory infections
      b. Sputum may be blood streaked
      c. Cough
      d. Chest x-ray examination reveals nodular lesions and enlarged hilar nodes
      e. Biopsy to establish diagnosis
      f. Pulmonary function studies reveal decreased volume and forced vital capacity
C. Treatment
   1. Relieve cough with antitussives
   2. Prescribe medications for complications such as tuberculosis
   3. Eliminate toxic substances from the environment
   4. Administer oxygen therapy
D. Nursing care
   1. Assess the client's ability to meet oxygen needs; teach self-administration of oxygen
   2. Encourage coughing and deep breathing
   3. Involve the client and family in programs aimed at improved occupational health and safety
   4. Evaluate client's response and revise plan as necessary

Pneumothorax

A. Etiology and pathophysiology
   1. Collapse of a lung caused by disruption of the negative pressure that normally exists within the intrapleural space due to the presence of air in the pleural cavity
   2. Reduces the surface area for gaseous exchange and leads to hypoxia and retention of carbon dioxide (hypercarbia)
   3. Types
      a. Spontaneous: thought to occur when a weakened area of the lung (bleb) ruptures; air then moves from the lung to the intrapleural space causing collapse; highest incidence is in men 20 to 40 years of age
      b. Open: laceration (e.g., a stab wound) through the chest wall into the intrapleural space
      c. Hemothorax: collection of blood within the pleural cavity
      d. Hydrothorax: accumulation of fluid in the pleural cavity
      e. Tension: buildup of pressure as air accumulates within the pleural space; the pressure increase likely to induce a mediastinal shift
   4. Mediastinal shift may occur toward the uninvolved side as a result of increased pressure within the pleural space; this involves the trachea, esophagus, heart, and great vessels
B. Signs and symptoms (depend on extent of collapse)
   1. Subjective
      a. Chest pain, usually described as sharp and increasing on exertion
      b. Dyspnea
   2. Objective
      a. Rapid, shallow respirations (nonsymmetrical)
      b. Breath sounds on the affected side will be diminished or absent
      c. Chest x-ray examination will reveal extent of the pneumothorax
      d. Tachycardia
      e. Hypotension
C. Treatment
   1. Bed rest initially
   2. Analgesics
   3. Negative pressure is returned to the intrapleural space by the insertion of chest tubes attached to underwater drainage
D. Nursing care
   1. Assess respiratory status
      a. Vital signs
      b. Color
      c. Chest motion during respirations
      d. Auscultate the lung fields
   2. Maintain patency of chest tubes (see procedure)
   3. Evaluate client's response and revise plan as necessary

Chest Injuries

A. Etiology and pathophysiology
   1. Penetrating or crushing wounds of the chest wall generally caused by acts of violence (stabbing, gunshot wounds) or motor vehicle accidents

2. Flail chest: occurs when ribs are fractured in more than one area; the chest wall on the involved side becomes unstable; the portion of lung below the injury moves in the opposite direction to the remainder of the lung, which results in hypoxia

B. Signs and symptoms
  1. Subjective
    a. Dyspnea
    b. Anxiety
  2. Objective
    a. Presence of a wound with a sucking sound on inspiration
    b. Presence of cyanosis and symptoms of mild to profound shock, depending on size of wound
    c. Mediastinal shift may occur toward the unaffected side caused by the pressure exerted by a pneumothorax or hemothorax, causing a change in the site of the apical pulse and paradoxical respirations
    d. Absence of breath sounds on the affected side

C. Treatment
  1. Apply a pressure dressing over the wound
  2. Aspiration of the pleural cavity to promote lung expansion
  3. Establish a water-seal suction drainage
  4. Reduce the oxygen demand by maintaining bed rest and limitation of activity
  5. Oxygen as necessary
  6. Restore blood volume and treat shock
  7. Antibiotics and mild analgesics
  8. Respiratory therapy to promote lung expansion
  9. Volume-controlled respirator is utilized in cases of severe chest trauma

D. Nursing care
  1. Maintain chest tubes if present (see procedure)
  2. Observe client's respiratory status
  3. Encourage client to move and cough
  4. Teach client to self-splint with hands and arms
  5. Explain the purpose and functioning of chest tubes and water-seal drainage
  6. Administer oxygen and analgesics as ordered and as necessary
  7. Encourage client to follow directions of respiratory therapists (e.g., incentive spirometry, IPPB)
  8. Evaluate client's response and revise plan as necessary

Bronchogenic Carcinoma

A. Etiology and pathophysiology
  1. Carcinoma of the lungs may be primary or metastatic
  2. Etiology unknown, but is much more common in smokers than nonsmokers
  3. Incidence highest in men over the age of 40
  4. Symptoms may occur after metastasis to other organs such as the ribs, liver, adrenal glands, mediastinal organs, kidneys, and brain

B. Signs and symptoms
  1. Subjective
    a. Dyspnea
    b. Chills
    c. Fatigue
    d. Chest pain

  2. Objective
    a. Persistent cough
    b. Hemoptysis
    c. Unilateral wheeze detected by auscultation
    d. Weight loss
    e. Clubbing of fingers
    f. Pleural effusion
    g. "Coin" lesions detected by x-ray examination of the chest
    h. Cytologic test of sputum positive

C. Treatment
  1. Surgical
    a. Lobectomy: removal of one lobe of the lung when the lesion is limited to one area
    b. Wedge section: removal of a small confined lesion; may also be done for biopsy
    c. Pneumonectomy: removal of an entire lung
    d. Exploratory thoracotomy: opening of the thoracic cavity to confirm diagnosis
    e. Thoracoplasty: removal of ribs to reduce the size of the pleural cavity; may be done to prevent complications after resection of lung
  2. Radiation therapy may be used as an adjunct therapy or to alleviate symptoms of pain, dyspnea, and hemoptysis
  3. Chemotherapy (e.g., cyclophosphamide, methotrexate, vincristine)

D. Nursing care
  1. Maintain open communication between self, the client, and the family; refer to community agencies and mental health practitioner as necessary
  2. Monitor temperature and vital signs
  3. Encourage coughing and deep breathing
  4. Change position frequently; semi-Fowler's or high-Fowler's promotes greater lung expansion
  5. Provide specific care based on therapy being used
    a. Care of client with chest tubes (see procedure)
    b. Radiation therapy (see Nursing care for clients with neoplastic disorders receiving either chemotherapy or radiation)
    c. Chemotherapy (see Nursing care for clients with neoplastic disorders receiving either chemotherapy or radiation)
  6. Provide high protein, high caloric diet, and supplements
  7. Utilize interventions to manage pain: analgesics, distraction, relaxation, imagery
  8. Evaluate client's response and revise plan as necessary

Cancer of the Larynx

A. Etiology and pathophysiology
  1. Most tumors of the larynx (vocal cords, epiglottis, laryngeal cartilages, and ventricle) are squamous cell carcinoma
  2. Cigarette smoking and heavy alcohol consumption appear to be related to increased incidence
  3. More common in men 50 to 65 years of age

B. Signs and symptoms
  1. Subjective
    a. Sore throat
    b. Dyspnea
    c. Dysphagia
    d. Weakness

2. Objective
   a. Increasing hoarseness
   b. Weight loss
   c. Enlarged cervical lymph nodes
   d. Foul breath
C. Treatment
   1. Radiation therapy
   2. Chemotherapy (e.g., methotrexate, bleomycin, fluorouracil)
   3. Surgical intervention
      a. Thyrotomy: removal of tumor from the larynx via an incision through the thyroid cartilage
      b. Total laryngectomy: removal of total larynx with construction of a permanent tracheostomy
      c. Radical neck dissection (used when the tumor has metastasized into surrounding tissue and lymph nodes): removal of larynx, surrounding tissue and muscle, lymph nodes, and glands with a permanent tracheostomy
D. Nursing care of the client with a total laryngectomy
   1. Provide time to discuss the diagnosis and the ramifications of surgery
   2. Assist and encourage the client to express feelings
   3. Answer questions as thoroughly and honestly as possible
   4. Arrange for individuals with laryngectomies to visit and discuss the rehabilitative process
   5. Instruct the client as to the method of communication that will be used postoperatively (e.g., slate board and chalk, pencil and paper, sign language)
   6. Observe for obstruction of airway by mucus plugs, edema, or blood (e.g., air hunger, dyspnea, cyanosis, gurgling)
   7. Observe for signs of hemorrhage (e.g., increased pulse rate, drop in blood pressure, cold clammy skin, appearance of blood on dressing)
   8. Stay with the client but provide a bell or other system for the client to signal for help
   9. Provide, at the bedside, suction apparatus and catheters (additional laryngectomy tube and a surgical instrument set with additional hemostats should be immediately available in case the tube becomes dislodged or blocked)
   10. Suction the tracheostomy tube that is left in place for approximately 3 days (see procedure)
   11. Provide humidity to compensate for loss of normal humidification of air in the nasopharynx; later the tracheostomy may be covered with a moistened unfilled gauze pad
   12. Prevent cross infection and contamination of the wound by providing special oral hygiene, cleanliness at tracheal site, avoidance of people with respiratory infections, use of clean equipment
   13. In clients receiving radiation or chemotherapy, observe for signs of adverse reactions
   14. Expect and accept a period of mourning but prevent withdrawal from reality by
       a. Involving the client in laryngectomy care
       b. Keeping channels of communication open
       c. Supporting the client's strengths
       d. Encouraging a return to activities of daily living
       e. Allowing the client time to write responses or use sign language
   15. Encourage the client to become involved in speech therapy and realistically support efforts and gains
   16. Teach the skills necessary to handle altered body functioning
       a. Method of tracheobronchial suctioning to maintain patency of airway emphasizing pressure, depth, frequency, and safety
       b. Method of changing, cleaning, and securing the laryngectomy tube
       c. Care of skin around the opening
       d. Importance of providing humidified air for inspiration to prevent drying of secretions (can be achieved by use of moist dressing)
   17. Teach the client to avoid activities that may permit water or irritating substances to enter the trachea, since the usual defensive mechanisms (glottis and cilia) are absent; the client should avoid showers, swimming, dust, hair spray, and other volatile substances
   18. Teach the client to avoid wearing clothes with tight collars or constricting necklines
   19. Teach the client that certain other activities will be interrupted (e.g., sipping through a straw, whistling, blowing the nose)
   20. Evaluate client's response and revise plan as necessary

Adult Respiratory Distress Syndrome (ARDS)
A. Etiology and pathophysiology
   1. Respiratory failure in clients with previously healthy lungs as a complication of conditions such as trauma, aspiration, prolonged mechanical ventilation, severe infection, or open heart surgery
   2. Involves
      a. Pulmonary capillary damage with loss of fluid and interstitial edema
      b. Impaired alveolar gas exchange and tissue hypoxia due to pulmonary edema
      c. Alteration in surfactant production; collapse of alveoli
      d. Atelectasis resulting in labored and inefficient respiration
B. Signs and symptoms
   1. Subjective
      a. Restlessness
      b. Anxiety
      c. Dyspnea
   2. Objective
      a. Pco_2 initially decreased and later increased, and decreased Po_2 arterial blood gases
      b. Tachycardia
      c. Cyanosis
      d. Grunting respirations
      e. Intercostal retractions
      f. Chest x-ray reveals pulmonary edema
C. Treatment
   1. Relieve the underlying cause
   2. Mechanical ventilation
   3. Positive end expiratory pressure (PEEP): this setting on a mechanical ventilator maintains positive pressure within the lungs at the end of expiration, which increases the residual capacity, reducing hypoxia

4. Monitoring arterial blood gases
5. Corticosteroids may be used

D. Nursing care
1. Allow frequent rest periods between therapeutic interventions
2. Provide tranquil supportive environment because sedation is contraindicated due to its depressant effect on respirations
3. Observe behavioral changes and vital signs, since confusion and hypertension may indicate cerebral hypoxia
4. Auscultate breath sounds to observe for signs of pneumothorax when the client is on PEEP (lung tissue that is frail may not withstand increased intrathoracic pressure, and pneumothorax occurs)
5. Monitor arterial blood gases, as ordered; use a heparinized syringe to obtain specimen
6. Maintain a patent airway
7. Care for the client on mechanical ventilation (see procedure)
8. Measure central venous or pulmonary artery pressures
9. Evaluate client's response and revise plan as necessary

Carbon Monoxide Poisoning

A. Etiology and pathophysiology
1. Caused by inadequately vented combustion devices
2. Carbon monoxide combines with hemoglobin more readily than does oxygen, causing tissue anoxia

B. Signs and symptoms
1. Subjective
   a. Headache
   b. Faintness
   c. Vertigo
   d. Tinnitus
2. Objective
   a. Color may be normal, cyanotic, or flushed, but is usually cherry pink
   b. Paralysis
   c. Loss of consciousness
   d. ECG changes

C. Treatment
1. Administer artificial respiration
2. 100% oxygen until carboxyhemoglobin is reduced and respirations are normal
3. Administer 50% glucose or mannitol
4. Administer synthetic erythrocytes (Fluosol), which deliver oxygen to cells in the presence of carbon monoxide

D. Nursing care
1. Remove the individual from the immediate area
2. Evaluate for cardiopulmonary function
3. Institute cardiopulmonary resuscitation if necessary and maintain until additional help arrives
4. Administer oxygen if available
5. Maintain respirations with assistance if needed
6. Maintain body temperature
7. Observe vital signs, with special concern for respirations
8. Maintain oxygen flow at prescribed levels
9. Evaluate client's response and revise plan as necessary

Gastrointestinal System
REVIEW OF ANATOMY AND PHYSIOLOGY OF THE GASTROINTESTINAL SYSTEM
Functions

A. Digestion of food, essential preparation for absorption and metabolism
B. Absorption of digested food
C. Elimination of wastes of digestion

Organs
Mouth (Buccal Cavity)

A. Lips
B. Cheeks
C. Hard palate: formed by two palatine bones and palatine processes of maxillae
D. Soft palate: formed of muscle in shape of an arch that forms a partition between the mouth and nasopharynx; fauces (archway) or opening from mouth into oropharynx; uvula, conical dependent process; possesses numerous mucus-secreting glands
E. Gums (gingivae)
F. Teeth
1. Deciduous or "baby teeth": 10 in each jaw (20 in set)
2. Permanent: 16 per jaw (32 in set)
3. Eruption
   a. Deciduous: first one erupts usually at 6 months of age; rest follow at intervals of 1 or more months; however, great individual variation in time of eruption of teeth; deciduous teeth are shed between 6 and 13 years of age
   b. Permanent: usually between 6 years and about 17 years; third molars (wisdom teeth) last to erupt
G. Tongue
1. Papillae: many rough elevations on surface
2. Taste buds: specialized receptors of cranial nerves VII (facial) and IX (glossopharyngeal); located in papillae
3. Frenum (or frenulum): fold of mucous membrane that helps anchor tongue to floor of mouth
H. Tonsils: lymphatic tissue connected to the surface epithelium by a channel (crypt); produces lymphocytes; defense against infection
I. Salivary glands: produce saliva, a mixture of water, mucin, salts, enzyme (salivary amylase)
1. Parotid: below and in front of the ear
2. Submandibular: posterior part of floor of mouth
3. Sublingual: anterior part of floor of mouth, under tongue

Pharynx

(See respiratory system discussion)

Esophagus

A. Location and extent
1. Posterior to trachea; anterior to the vertebral column
2. Extends from the pharynx through an opening in the diaphragm (hiatus) to the stomach
B. Structure: collapsible muscular tube; about 25 cm (10 inches) long and 0.13 cm (0.05 inch) wide
C. Secretions and functions: secretes mucus; facilitates movement of food

Stomach

A. Size, shape, position
   1. Size: varies in different persons and according to degree of distention
   2. Shape: elongated pouch, with greater curve forming the lower left border
   3. Position: in epigastric and left hypochondriac portions of the abdominal cavity
B. Divisions
   1. Fundus: the uppermost portion of the stomach; the bulge adjacent to and extending above the esophageal opening
   2. Body: central portion
   3. Pylorus: constricted lower portion
C. Curves
   1. Lesser: upper right border
   2. Greater: lower left border
D. Sphincters
   1. Cardiac: guarding opening of the esophagus into the stomach
   2. Pyloric: guarding opening of the pylorus into the duodenum
E. Glands of the stomach: secrete gastric juice composed of mucus, hydrochloric acid, and enzymes
   1. Simple columnar epithelial cells form the surface of the gastric mucosa; goblet cells secrete mucus
   2. Millions of microscopic gastric glands embedded in gastric mucosa composed of different types of cells; mainly chief cells (zymogen cells) that secrete gastric juice enzymes, and parietal cells that secrete hydrochloric acid and intrinsic factor
F. Functions: food storage and liquefaction (chyme)

Small Intestine

A. Size: approximately 2.5 cm (1 inch) in diameter, 6.1 m (20 feet) in length when relaxed
B. Divisions
   1. Duodenum: joins pylorus of the stomach; about 25 cm (10 inches) in length; C shaped
   2. Jejunum: middle section about 2.4 m (8 feet) in length
   3. Ileum: lower section, about 3.6 m (12 feet) in length; no clear boundary between jejunum and ileum
C. Functions: digestion and absorption
D. Process: mixing movements; peristalsis; secretion of water, ions, and mucus; receives secretions from the liver, gallbladder, and pancreas

Large Intestine

A. Size: approximately 6.3 cm (2½ inches) in diameter, but only 1.5 m (5 to 6 feet) long when relaxed
B. Divisions
   1. Cecum: first 5 to 7.6 cm (2 to 3 inches)
   2. Colon
      a. Ascending: extends vertically along the right border of the abdomen up to level of the liver
      b. Transverse: extends horizontally across the abdomen, below liver and stomach and above the small intestine
      c. Descending: extends vertically down the left side of the abdomen to level of the iliac crest
      d. Sigmoid: S-shaped part of large intestine curving downward below the iliac crest to join the rectum; lower part of the sigmoid curve that joins rectum bends toward the left
   3. Rectum: last 17.7 or 20.3 cm (7 to 8 inches) of intestines
   4. Anus: terminal opening of the alimentary tract
C. Functions: water and sodium ion absorption; temporary storage of fecal matter; defecation
D. Process: weak mixing movements, mass movements, and peristalsis

Vermiform Appendix

A. Size, shape, location: about size and shape of a large angleworm; blind-end tube off the cecum just beyond the ileocecal valve; 7.6 to 10 cm (3 to 4 inches) long; 0.6 cm (¼ inch) in diameter
B. Structure: same coats as compose the intestinal wall
C. Function: part of the immune system; submucosa unique in the large size of its lymphatic nodules

Liver

A. Location and size: occupies most of the right hypochondrium and part of the epigastrium; largest gland in the body
B. Lobes: divided into thousands of lobules by blood vessels and fibrous partitions
   1. Right lobe: subdivided into two smaller lobes (caudate and quadrate) and right lobe proper
   2. Left lobe: single lobe
C. Ducts
   1. Hepatic duct: from liver
   2. Cystic duct: from gallbladder
   3. Common bile duct: formed by union of the hepatic and cystic ducts in a Y formation; drains bile into the duodenum at the hepatopancreatic papilla, surrounded by the sphincter of Oddi
D. Functions: liver is one of the most vital organs because of its role in metabolism of proteins, carbohydrates, and fats
   1. Carbohydrate metabolism by liver cells
      a. Glycogenesis: conversion of glucose to glycogen for storage
      b. Glycogenolysis: conversion of glycogen to glucose and release of glucose into the blood; epinephrine and glucagon accelerate glycogenolysis
      c. Gluconeogenesis: formation of glucose from proteins or fats; glucocorticoids (hydrocortisone, corticosterone) have an accelerating effect on gluconeogenesis
   2. Fat metabolism by liver cells
      a. Ketogenesis: occurs during accelerated fat catabolism; occurs mainly in liver cells; consists of a series of reactions by which fatty acids are broken down into molecules of acetyl CoA (Beta oxidation) which are then combined (two at a time) to form ketone bodies (acetoacetic acid, acetone, beta-hydroxybutyric acid)
      b. Fat storage
      c. Synthesis of triglycerides, phospholipids, cholesterol, and the B complex factor choline

3. Protein metabolism by liver cells
   a. Anabolism: synthesis of various proteins, notably blood proteins (e.g., prothrombin, fibrinogen, albumins, alpha and beta globulins, and clotting factors V, VII, IX, and X)
   b. Deamination: first step in protein catabolism; chemical reaction by which amino group is split off from amino acid to form ammonia and a keto acid
   c. Urea formation: liver cells convert most of the ammonia formed by deamination to urea
4. Secretes bile, substance important for emulsifying fats prior to digestion and as a vehicle for excretion of cholesterol and bile pigments
5. Detoxifies various substances (e.g., drugs, hormones)
6. Vitamin metabolism: stores vitamins A, D, K, and B_{12}; synthesizes B_3 from tryptophan

Gallbladder

A. Size, shape, location: approximately the size and shape of a small pear; lies on the undersurface of the liver
B. Structure: sac made of smooth muscle, lined with mucosa arranged in rugae (expandable longitudinal folds)
C. Functions: concentrates and stores bile

Pancreas

A. Size, shape, location: larger in men than in women, but considerable individual variation; fish shaped, with body, head, and tail; extends from the duodenal curve to the spleen
B. Structure: that of both a duct gland and a ductless gland
   1. Pancreatic cells: pour secretion (pancreatic juice) into the duct that runs length of the gland and empties into the duodenum at the hepatopancreatic papilla

2. Islands of Langerhans (or islet cells): clusters of cells not connected with pancreatic ducts; two main types of cells compose islets (namely, alpha and beta cells); constitute the endocrine gland
C. Functions
   1. Pancreatic cells connected with pancreatic ducts secrete pancreatic juice, enzymes of which help digest all three kinds of foods
   2. Islet cells constitute endocrine gland
      a. Alpha cells secrete the hormone glucagon, which accelerates liver glycogenolysis and initiates gluconeogenesis; hence, tends to increase blood glucose level
      b. Beta cells secrete insulin, one of the most important metabolic hormones, which exerts a profound influence on the metabolism of carbohydrates, proteins, and fats (Fig. 3-5)
         (1) Insulin accelerates the active transport of glucose (along with potassium and phosphate ions) through cell membranes; therefore it tends to decrease blood glucose (hypoglycemic effect) and to increase glucose utilization by the cells for either catabolism or anabolism
         (2) Insulin stimulates the production of liver cell glucokinase; therefore it promotes liver glycogenesis, another effect that tends to lower blood glucose
         (3) Insulin inhibits liver cell phosphatase and therefore inhibits liver glycogenolysis
         (4) Insulin accelerates the rate of amino acid transfer into cells, so it promotes anabolism of proteins within the cells
         (5) Insulin accelerates the rate of fatty acid transfer into cells, promotes fat anabolism (also called fat deposition or lipogenesis), and inhibits fat catabolism

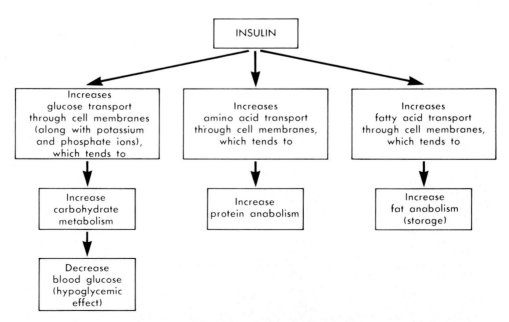

FIG. 3-5. Major insulin effects.

Digestion

A. Definition: all changes that food undergoes in the alimentary canal
B. Purpose: conversion of foods into chemical and physical forms that can be absorbed and metabolized
C. Kinds
  1. Mechanical digestion: all movements of the alimentary tract that
    a. Change physical state of foods from comparatively large solid pieces into minute dissolved particles
    b. Propel food forward along the alimentary tract, finally eliminating digestive wastes from the body
      (1) Deglutition: swallowing
      (2) Peristalsis: wormlike movements that squeeze food downward in the tract
      (3) Mass peristalsis: moving of entire intestinal contents into the sigmoid colon and rectum; usually occurs after a meal
      (4) Defecation: emptying of the rectum, so-called bowel movement
    c. Churn intestinal contents so all become well mixed with digestive juices and all parts of contents come in contact with the intestinal mucosa to facilitate absorption
  2. Chemical digestion: series of hydrolytic processes dependent on specific enzymes; hydrolysis, decomposition of complex compound into two or more simple compounds by means of chemical reaction with water
D. Control of digestive gland secretion
  1. Secretion of saliva: neural control of this reflex results from parasympathetic impulses to glands, initiated by taste, smell, and sight of food (cephalic phase of digestion)
  2. Gastric juice
    a. Neural control similar to that of salivary glands
    b. Hormonal control: partially digested proteins cause gastric mucosa to release hormone (gastrin) into blood; gastrin stimulates gastric mucosa to secrete juice with high pepsin and hydrochloric acid content
  3. Pancreatic juice
    a. Hormonal control: hydrochloric acid in chyme entering the duodenum from the stomach causes intestinal mucosa to release a hormone, secretin, into the blood; secretin stimulates pancreatic cells to secrete a juice high in sodium bicarbonate to neutralize hydrochloric acid but low in enzymes; products of protein digestion (e.g., proteoses, peptones, and amino acids) cause the intestinal mucosa to release another hormone, pancreozymin, which stimulates the pancreatic cells to secrete enzymes
    b. Neural control: reflex secretion of pancreatic juice results from parasympathetic impulses via the vagus nerve
  4. Bile
    a. Although bile is secreted continuously, secretin increases amount of bile secreted
    b. Presence of fats in the intestine causes the intestinal mucosa to release a hormone, cholecystokinin, into the blood; cholecystokinin stimulates the smooth muscle of the gallbladder to contract, ejecting bile into the duodenum
  5. Intestinal juice: control obscure but believed to be both reflexive and hormonal; food in the small intestine causes the mucosa to release hormone (enterocrinin) into blood; enterocrinin stimulates intestinal glands to secrete

Absorption

A. Definition: passage of substances through the intestinal mucosa into the blood or lymph
B. Accomplished mainly through active transport by the intestinal cells; makes it possible for both water and solutes to move through the intestinal mucosa in a direction opposite that expected in osmosis and diffusion
C. Absorption occurs in the duodenum and jejunum of the small intestine; however, absorption of alcohol, certain drugs, and some water occurs in the stomach; most water is absorbed from the large intestine
D. Absorption of protein, carbohydrate, and fat (Table 3-5)

Metabolism

A. Definition: sum of all the chemical reactions in the body
B. Catabolism
  1. Consists of a complex series of chemical reactions that take place inside the cells and yield energy, carbon dioxide, and water; about half the energy released from food molecules by catabolism is put back in storage as unstable, high-energy bonds of ATP molecules; the rest is transformed to heat; the energy in high-energy bonds of ATP can be released as rapidly as needed for cellular work
  2. Two processes involved; glycolysis and the Krebs cycle with the electron transport chain
  3. Purpose: to provide cells continually with utilizable energy
C. Anabolism
  1. Synthesis of various compounds from simpler compounds
  2. Cellular work that uses some of the energy made available by catabolism
D. Metabolism of carbohydrates
  1. Consists of the following processes:
    a. Glucose transport through cell membranes and phosphorylation
      (1) Insulin promotes this transport through cell membranes
      (2) Glucose phosphorylation: conversion of glucose to glucose-6-phosphate, catalyzed by the enzyme hexokinase (2X); insulin increases the activity of glucokinase and promotes glucose phosphorylation, which is essential prior to both glycogenesis and glucose catabolism
    b. Glycogenesis: conversion of glucose to glycogen for storage; occurs mainly in the liver and muscle cells

Table 3-5. Absorption of nutrients

Substance	Structures into which absorbed	Circulation
Protein—amino acids	Into blood in intestinal capillaries	Portal vein, liver, hepatic vein, inferior vena cava to heart, etc.
Carbohydrate—monosaccharides (glucose and fructose)	Same as amino acids	Same as amino acids
Fat—glycerol and fatty acids; fatty acids are insoluble and must first combine with bile salts to form water-soluble units called micelles	Chiefly into lymph in intestinal lacteals; some into blood	During absorption while in epithelial cells of intestinal mucosa, glycerol and fatty acids recombine and complex with protein to form microscopic particles called chylomicrons (a type of lipoprotein); lymphatics carry them by way of thoracic duct to left subclavian vein, superior vena cava, heart, etc.
Vitamins		
Fat-soluble	Same as fat	Same as fat
Water-soluble	Same as amino acid	Same as amino acid
Minerals	Same as amino acid	Same as amino acid

c. Glycogenolysis
  (1) In muscle cells glycogen is changed back to glucose-6-phosphate, which is then catabolized in the muscle cells
  (2) In liver cells glycogen is changed back to glucose; an enzyme, glucose phosphatase, is present in the liver cells and catalyzes the final step of glycogenolysis, the changing of glucose-6-phosphate to glucose; glucagon and epinephrine accelerate liver glycogenolysis
d. Glucose catabolism
  (1) Glycolysis: series of anaerobic reactions that break one glucose molecule down into two pyruvic acid molecules, with conversion of about 5% of energy stored in glucose to heat and ATP molecules
  (2) Krebs citric acid cycle with the electron transport chain: series of aerobic chemical reactions by which two pyruvic acid molecules (from one glucose molecule) are broken down to six carbon dioxide and six water molecules, with the release of some energy as heat and and some stored again in ATP; the aerobic reactions release about 95% of the energy stored in glucose, while the anaerobic reactions release only about 5%; the aerobic reactions occur in the mitochondria of cells
e. Gluconeogenesis: sequence of chemical reactions carried on in liver cells; process converts protein or fat compounds into glucose
f. Principles of normal carbohydrate metabolism
  (1) Principle of preferred energy fuel: most cells first catabolize glucose, sparing fats and proteins (muscle cells prefer fatty acids as long as adequate oxygen is available); when the glucose supply becomes inadequate, most cells (not nerve cells) next catabolize fats; nerve cells require glucose thus causing proteins to be sacrificed to provide the

amino acids needed to produce more glucose (gluconeogenesis); also small amounts of glucose can be made from the glycerol portion of fats
  (2) Principle of glycogenesis: glucose in excess of about 120 to 140 mg per 100 ml blood brought to the liver by the portal veins enters the liver cells, where it undergoes glycogenesis and is stored as glycogen
  (3) Principle of glycogenolysis: when blood glucose decreases below the midpoint of normal, liver glycogenolysis accelerates and tends to raise the blood glucose concentration back toward the midpoint of normal
  (4) Principle of gluconeogenesis: when blood glucose decreases below normal or when the amount of glucose entering the cells is inadequate, liver gluconeogenesis accelerates and tends to raise the blood glucose concentration
  (5) Principle of glucose storage as fat: when the blood insulin content is adequate, glucose in excess of the amount used for catabolism and glycogenesis is converted to fat and stored in fat depots
E. Control of metabolism: primarily by hormones
  1. Pancreatic hormones
    a. Insulin: exerts predominant control over carbohydrate metabolism but also affects protein and fat metabolism; in general, it accelerates carbohydrate metabolism by the cells, thereby decreasing blood glucose
    b. Glucagon (secreted by the alpha cells of the islands of Langerhans): primarily accelerates liver glycogenolysis but also promotes gluconeogenesis and lipolysis when blood insulin levels are low
  2. Anterior pituitary hormones
    a. Growth hormone tends to
      (1) accelerate protein anabolism; hence promotes growth of skeleton and soft tissues

(2) Accelerate fat mobilization from adipose cells, which tends to bring about a shift from the use of glucose to the use of fats for catabolism

(3) Accelerate liver gluconeogenesis from fats, which tends to increase blood glucose

(4) Stimulate glucagon secretion, which in turn stimulates liver glycogenolysis and glucose release into the blood

b. ACTH (the adrenocorticotropic hormone): stimulates the secretion of glucocorticoids by the adrenal cortex

3. Adrenal cortex hormones (glucocorticoids) mainly cortisol and corticosterone, tend to

a. Accelerate fat mobilization and catabolism, thereby promoting shift to fat catabolism from glucose catabolism whenever the latter is inadequate for energy needs

b. Accelerate tissue protein mobilization (catabolism)

c. Accelerate liver gluconeogenesis which becomes necessary to maintain blood glucose for nerve cells when carbohydrate availability is limited

4. Adrenal medulla hormones: epinephrine and norepinephrine (catecholamines) tend to accelerate both liver and muscle glycogenolysis, with release of glucose from the liver into the circulation; therefore tend to increase blood sugar

5. Male sex gland hormone: testosterone, secreted by interstitial cells of testes, tends to accelerate protein anabolism

F. Metabolic rate: calories of heat energy produced and expended per hour or per day

1. Basal metabolic rate (BMR): calories of heat produced when an individual is awake but resting in a comfortably warm environment 12 to 18 hours after the last meal

a. Factors determining basal metabolic rates

(1) Size: BMR is directly related to square meters of surface area of the body; the larger the surface area, the higher the BMR

(2) Sex: 5% to 7% higher in males than in females of the same size and age

(3) Age: BMR inversely related to age; as age increases, BMR decreases

(4) Amount of thyroid hormones secreted; thyroid hormones accelerate BMR

(5) Body temperature: BMR directly related to body temperature; 1° C increase in body temperature above normal is accompanied by about a 13% increase in BMR

(6) Miscellaneous factors such as sleep (decreases BMR), pregnancy, and emotions (increase BMR)

b. Measurement

(1) Determined by measuring the amount of oxygen inspired in a given time

(2) Reported as normal or as a definite percentage above or below normal

2. Total metabolic rate: calories of heat energy expended per day; equal to basal metabolic rate plus number of calories of energy used for muscular work, eating and digesting food, and adjusting to cool temperatures

3. Some principles about the metabolic rate and its relation to body weight

a. For body weight to remain constant (except for variations in water content) the energy balance must be maintained; body weight remains constant when energy input equals energy output

b. Whenever the energy input (food intake) is greater than the energy output (total metabolic rate), body weight increases

c. Whenever energy input (food intake) is less than the energy output (total metabolic rate), body weight decreases

REVIEW OF PHYSICAL PRINCIPLES RELATED TO THE GASTROINTESTINAL SYSTEM
Principles of Mechanics
Law of Motion

EXAMPLE: The greater the force of contraction of the intestinal wall and the more frequent the contractions, the more rapid the propulsion of food and fecal matter through digestive tract; under irritating conditions, rapid powerful peristalsis leads to abdominal cramps and diarrhea

Gravity

EXAMPLE: Colostomy irrigations and enemas

Energy

A. Potential and kinetic energy

EXAMPLE: The potential energy in glucose (food) molecules is captured in the bonds of the high-energy molecule ATP; such potential energy is released as kinetic energy when ATP powers the contraction of muscle and the beating of cilia and flagella

B. First law of thermodynamics

EXAMPLE: The energy stored in an ATP molecule exactly equals the work (of muscles, cilia, etc.) and heat energy liberated during the process

C. Second law of thermodynamics

EXAMPLE: The diffusion of nutrients and enzymes in the various digestive juices results in their collisions and chemical interactions because it is the natural tendency of molecules and systems to become more randomized

Principles of Physical Properties of Matter
Solids

EXAMPLE: The elastic properties of the connective and muscular tissues of the stomach permit distention during a meal and the consequent storage and slow digestion and absorption of food over the next several hours

Liquids

A. Pascal's principle

EXAMPLE: The voluntary contraction of muscles of the abdominal wall, such as the external and internal oblique, applies pressure on the fluids of the abdominal cavity, which is transmitted undiminished throughout the abdominopelvic cavity and aids in defecation; chronic constipation with chronic straining during defecation may predispose to hemorrhoids

B. Surface tension

EXAMPLE: Bile salts partly combine with fats and with water; this dual combination lowers the surface tension of the water molecules surrounding large fat droplets, which disperse into thousands of smaller droplets whose greater total surface area promotes more rapid hydrolysis (digestion) by pancreatic lipase

Gases

Boyle's law

EXAMPLES

1. During gastric analysis, the volume of gas in the tube is increased as the barrel of the syringe attached to the tube is pulled out; the result is a flow of gastric contents from the stomach due to the decreased pressure exerted by the gas in the tube as compared with gas pressure in the stomach
2. The same applies during paracentesis
3. During gastric gavage the process is reversed

Heat

A. Body temperature maintained by heat produced as a by-product of biochemical reactions; basal metabolic rate is a measure of heat production under specified conditions
B. The normal metabolism in each of the cells of the human body produces heat; in addition, heat is a by-product of muscular contraction

Light

A. Refraction

EXAMPLE: Total internal reflection in fiberoptics permits viewing of interior walls of stomach and intestines for diagnostic purposes such as endoscopic procedures, gastroscopy, sigmoidoscopy, and proctoscopy
B. X-rays

EXAMPLES

1. GI series and barium enemas allow visualization of the soft tissues of the upper and lower gastrointestinal tract; the barium salts coat the inner walls of the alimentary tube and absorb the x-rays striking them; as a result, the organ surfaces are outlined
2. Fluoroscopy can be considered the observation of "live" x-ray images; after the x-rays pass through the individual, they strike a fluorescent screen that absorbs them and emits visible light; with x-ray-opaque (radiopaque) chemicals the intestinal and biliary tracts can be observed

REVIEW OF CHEMICAL PRINCIPLES RELATED TO THE GASTROINTESTINAL SYSTEM
Oxidation and Reduction

A. Uniting oxygen with a substance results in oxidation
B. Uniting hydrogen with a substance results in reduction

Oxidation-Reduction Reactions in the Body

A. Important in body chemistry as a source of energy through cellular oxidation of foods in cytoplasm and mitochondria; oxidation of nutrients like glucose results in the formation of high-energy ATP molecules and heat—both useful to the body
B. Oxygen is the usual oxidizing agent in cells

C. Some forms of life (anaerobes) can use substances other than oxygen for cellular oxidation (e.g., *Clostridium perfringens* found in gangrenous tissue)

Diffusion and Osmosis

EXAMPLES

1. Diffusion of nutrients and enzymes results in the collisions necessary to promote chemical (metabolic) reactions
2. Absorption of water by osmosis occurs through the mucosa of the GI tract

Active Transport

The movement of molecules against a concentration gradient due to energy (ATP) expenditure

EXAMPLE: The absorption of most simple sugars and amino acids in the small intestine involves active transport processes

Buffers

Pairs of chemical substances that resist changes in pH

EXAMPLE: The sodium bicarbonate part of the bicarbonate buffer system secreted from the pancreas into the duodenum acts as a buffer to prevent acidification of intestinal juices due to the presence of hydrochloric acid from gastric juice

Types of Compounds
Organic Acids

$$\text{All organic acids contain the } \overset{\displaystyle O}{\underset{}{\diagup}}\!\!\overset{\|}{C}\!\!-\!\!OH \text{ (carboxyl) group}$$

EXAMPLES

1. Lactic acid: end product of anaerobic muscle metabolism; converted to pyruvic acid and oxidized completely to carbon dioxide and water aerobically
2. Citric acid: one intermediate in the Krebs citric acid cycle; cycle occurs in mitochondria as a major oxidation-reduction pathway for the generation of ATP (potential chemical energy)
3. Salicylic acid: synthesis of aspirin

Amino Acids

A. Amino acids possess two functional groups: an amine group and an acid or carboxyl group
B. Amino acids are amphoteric: act as both acids or bases; therefore proteins act as buffers in body fluids
C. Reactions of amino acids
    1. Amino acids are able to act as an acid and as a base (amphoteric character)
    2. Condense via peptide bond to form proteins
D. Essential amino acids cannot be synthesized well enough in the body to maintain health and growth and must be supplied in the food

Carbohydrates

A. Aldehyde or ketone derivatives of single oxidation of polyhydric alcohols, or compounds yielding aldehyde or ketone derivatives on hydrolysis
B. Include simple sugars, starches, celluloses, gums, and resins

C. Widespread in plant and animal tissue
D. Contain carbon, hydrogen, and oxygen; the hydrogen and oxygen are present in approximately the ratio of 2 to 1
E. Synthesis: plants synthesize carbohydrates from carbon dioxide and water with the aid of the green pigment chlorophyll (which acts as an enzyme) and solar energy
F. Classification
  1. By functional group
    a. Carbohydrates having the aldehyde group are called aldoses (e.g., glucose)
    b. Carbohydrates having the ketone group are called ketoses (e.g., fructose)
  2. By complexity of the molecule
    a. Carbohydrate having a single ketose or aldose molecule is called a monosaccharide: a simple sugar (e.g., glucose, fructose)
    b. Carbohydrate formed by combining two aldose molecules or an aldose and a ketose molecule is called a disaccharide (e.g., sucrose, lactose, maltose)
    c. Carbohydrate having more than two simple sugars joined in a molecule is called a polysaccharide (e.g., starch, glycogen)
G. Tests for glucose in urine
  1. Benedict's test and Clinitest tablets use copper ions in basic medium: show presence of sugar in urine by change in color
  2. Positive reaction gives colors from green (very little sugar) to brick red (more than 2 g sugar/100 ml urine)
  3. Iron ions and silver ions can be used instead of copper to give a test for sugar
  4. Most monosaccharides and disaccharides except sucrose are reducing sugars; therefore sucrose put into urine will not produce a reaction
H. Important carbohydrates
  1. Glycerose and dihydroxyacetone: triose intermediates in cellular metabolism of carbohydrates
  2. Ribose and deoxyribose: pentose constituents in nucleic acids
  3. Glucose (dextrose—hexose monosaccharide; a sugar found abundantly in body fluids, fruits, and vegetables; the pancreatic hormones insulin and glucagon regulate the blood glucose concentration in the normal range of 70 to 105 mg/100 ml blood; glucose is the basic food molecule that is broken down first in glycolysis (in the cytoplasm of cells) and then in the Krebs cycle (in mitochondria); the breakdown of each molecule of glucose results in the release of 38 molecules of ATP, which can be used in almost all cellular energy-requiring functions
  4. Fructose (levulose): ketose monosaccharide; found in fruits and honey, sweetest sugar known; important intermediate in cellular metabolism of carbohydrates
  5. Galactose: hexose monosaccharide; present in brain and nervous tissue
  6. Lactose (milk sugar): disaccharide of glucose and galactose molecules; bacterial fermentation of lactose to lactic acid causes milk to sour

  7. Sucrose (cane sugar): disaccharide of glucose and fructose molecules; nonreducing sugar, common table sugar used in sweetening and baking
  8. Maltose: disaccharide of two glucose molecules; found in grains and malt
  9. Starch: mixed polysaccharide of glucose molecules found in plants
    a. Amylose: straight-chained glucose polymer
    b. Amylopectin: branched-chain glucose polymer
    c. Chief food carbohydrate in human nutrition
    d. Starch polymers react with iodine to form a blue complex; used as a test for starch
      (1) Test becomes colorless as starch is hydrolyzed
      (2) Starch (blue) → amylodextrin (purple) → erythrodextrin (red) → achroodextrin (colorless) → maltose (colorless) → glucose (colorless)
  10. Glycogen: polysaccharide polymer of glucose molecules found in human and animal tissue; storage compound in the body; hydrolyzes to glucose, maintaining blood glucose levels
  11. Cellulose: polysaccharide polymer of glucose found in plants; not digestible by humans; important in the manufacture of cotton cloth, paper, and cellulose acetate synthetics
  12. Inulin: polysaccharide polymer of fructose, used in kidney function test (inulin clearance test)
  13. Agar-agar: polysaccharide polymer of galactose used as a solid medium for bacteriologic studies
  14. Hemicellulose, gums and pectin: polysaccharide polymers of glucose with high water binding capacity; have been found to be important dietary components of disease prevention and treatment programs (See Arterioatherosclerosis, Ulcerative colitis, Hemorrhoids, Diabetes mellitus and Cancer of the small and large intestine)

Lipids

A. Organic substances essentially insoluble in water but soluble in organic solvents (ether, chloroform, acetone, etc.)
B. Fatty acids: important constituents of all lipids (except sterols)
  1. Usually straight-chain carboxylic acids
  2. Naturally occurring fatty acids contain even numbers of carbon atoms
  3. Saturated fatty acids: have no double bonds (points of unsaturation) between their carbon atoms
  4. Unsaturated fatty acids: have one or more points of unsaturation between their carbon atoms
  5. Essential fatty acids: cannot be synthesized by the body; must be taken in by diet
C. Classification of lipids
  1. Simple lipids: esters of fatty acids and alcohols
    a. Fats: the alcohol of fats is the trihydric alcohol glycerol
      (1) Solid fats: fats that are solid at room temperature contain long-chain, saturated fatty acids
      (2) Liquid fats (oils): fats that are liquid at room temperature contain short-chain, unsaturated fatty acids

b. Waxes: esters of long-chained fatty acids and an alcohol other than glycerol; lanolin, a mixed wax from wool, is used in creams and salves

c. Reactions of simple lipids

   (1) Hydrolysis: splitting into fatty acid(s) and alcohol by breaking the ester bond is effected by acid, base, or enzyme action

   (2) Saponification: basic hydrolysis; soap is formed from organic salts of a fatty acid and metal ion of base

   (3) Addition: fats containing unsaturated fatty acids will form addition products at points of unsaturation

     (a) Addition of oxygen will cause fat to become rancid; antioxidants slow this reaction in packaged foods

     (b) Unsaturated oils used in paints add oxygen and oils become hard and glossy

     (c) Hydrogenation: liquid fats can form solid fats by adding in hydrogen at double bonds

2. Compound lipids: fats containing chemical substances other than fatty acids and alcohols

a. Phospholipids: contain alcohol, fatty acids, phosphoric acid, and a nitrogenous base (or inositol)

   (1) Lecithins: contain the alcohol glycerol, fatty acids, phosphoric acid, and the nitrogenous base choline; are found in brain and nervous tissue; in blood, lecithin serves to render fats soluble in plasma (a lipotropic agent)

   (2) Cephalins: similar in structure to lecithin except base is ethanolamine; important in brain and nerve tissue; help blood-clotting mechanism

   (3) Sphingomyelins: made from amino alcohol (sphingosinol), a fatty acid, phosphoric acid, and choline; important in brain and nerve tissue

b. Cardiolipids: made from unsaturated fatty acids, glycerol, and phosphoric acid; found in heart tissue

c. Glycolipids (cerebrosides) structure contains the monosaccharide galactose, amino alcohol (sphingosinol), and a fatty acid; found in brain tissue and the myelin sheaths of nerves

3. Steroids: complex monohydroxy alcohols found in plant and animal tissues—basic structure, the phenanthrine structure plus a cyclopentane ring; characteristic side chains determine specific steroids

a. Cholesterol: a sterol found in human and animal tissue, chiefly in brain and nerve tissue; an important, normal component of membranes; found in blood within a normal range of 150 to 200 mg/100 ml; high blood cholesterol seems associated with coronary thrombosis

b. Ergosterol: a plant sterol that can be converted to vitamin D by ultraviolet light

c. Bile acids: sterols that aid in digestion and absorption of fats

d. Steroid hormones: sex and adrenal gland hormones (glucocorticoids, mineralocorticoids)

e. Vitamin D: steroid helping to control calcium metabolism by regulating calcium uptake from the gastrointestinal tract

Proteins

A. Classification of proteins

1. Simple proteins: give amino acids on hydrolysis

a. Albumins: water soluble, coagulated by heat (e.g., lactalbumin [milk], serum albumin [blood], egg white); albumin is most important in the development of the plasma colloid osmotic pressure, which helps control (through osmosis) the flow of water between the plasma and interstitial fluid; during a condition such as starvation, a fall in the albumin level of the blood leads to a fall in the plasma colloid osmotic pressure; this results in edema because less fluid is drawn by osmosis into the capillaries from the interstitial spaces

b. Globulins: insoluble in water, soluble in dilute salt solutions, coagulated by heat (e.g., lactoglobulin [milk], serum globulin [blood], gamma serum globulin—forms antibodies of blood)

c. Glutenins: soluble in dilute bases or acids, insoluble in neutral solutions; coagulated by heat (e.g., glutenin [wheat])

d. Albuminoids: soluble in water (e.g., collagen [connective tissue], elastin [ligaments])

e. Histone: water soluble (e.g., globin [hemoglobin])

f. Prolamines: insoluble in water, soluble in 70% to 80% alcohol (e.g., gliadin [wheat], zein [corn])

g. Protamines: water soluble (e.g., protamine [fish spermatozoa])

2. Compound proteins: contain molecules other than amino acids

a. Chromoproteins: proteins containing a colored molecule (e.g., hemoglobin, flavoproteins)

b. Glycoproteins: proteins containing carbohydrate molecule(s) (e.g., mucopolysaccharide of synovial fluid)

c. Lipoproteins: simple proteins combined with lipid substances

   (1) Low-density lipoproteins (beta lipoproteins)

     (a) VLDL: very low–density lipoproteins which contain a high proportion of triglycerides and a small amount of protein

     (b) LDL: low-density lipoproteins which are chief carriers of cholesterol and are low in triglycerides

     (c) Contribute to atherosclerotic plaque formation

   (2) High-density lipoproteins (alpha lipoproteins)

     (a) Consist of 50% protein and 20% cholesterol

     (b) Inversely associated with coronary artery disease

d. Nucleoproteins: proteins complexed with nucleic acids (e.g., the DNA [genetic material] found in chromosomes is complexed with proteins); chromosomes are sometimes referred to as nucleoprotein structures

e. Metalloproteins: proteins containing metal ions (e.g., ferritin [iron transport compound of plasma])

f. Phosphoproteins: proteins containing the phosphoric acid radical (e.g., casein of milk)

3. Derived proteins: also called *denatured* proteins; treatment with acids, bases, heat, x-radiation, ultraviolet rays, etc. causes proteins to alter their molecular arrangements

B. Reactions of proteins

1. Amphoteric properties: like the amino acids forming them, proteins can act as an acid or a base in solution; can act as buffers

2. Hydrolysis: acid, base, or enzyme hydrolysis splits the peptide bond; yields proteose → peptones → peptides → amino acids

3. Denaturation: change in structure renders the protein less soluble, leads to coagulation of the protein

a. Heat: protein and heat → coagulated protein (e.g., cooked egg white, cooked meat)

b. Salts of heavy metals: silver, lead, mercury, etc.; taken internally, they are poison because they denature the enzymes of the cells, which are protein in nature

c. Acetone and alcohol: both harden skin proteins

d. Inorganic acids and bases: coagulate and hydrolyze proteins

e. Alkaloids and organic acids: tanning of hides, precipitation of blood proteins for clinical tests

f. Rays: x-rays, infrared rays, ultraviolet rays—long exposure can cause cataracts (precipitation of lens protein in the eye)

4. Salting out: concentrated salt solutions render soluble proteins insoluble

5. Color reactions

a. Xanthoproteic test: protein having a benzene ring (as found in the amino acids tyrosine and phenylalanine) will turn yellow on addition of concentrated nitric acid; heat and a second addition of sodium hydroxide will turn the yellow to orange

b. Millon test: protein having a phenolic ring (as found in the amino acid tyrosine) will form a red precipitate on addition of a mixture of mercuric and mercurous nitrates

c. Biuret test: test for the peptide bond; violet appears on addition of a hydroxide and dilute copper sulfate solution; negative for free amino acids (no peptide bond)

d. Hopkins-Cole test: protein that contains the indole structure (amino acid tryptophan) shows violet on addition of glyoxylic acid and concentrated sulfuric acid

e. Ninhydrin test: test for free amino acids, ninhydrin reagent gives blue color

Nucleoproteins

A. Specific proteins found in cells, made of large and complex molecules having important functions

B. Composition of nucleoproteins

1. Hydrolysis of nucleoproteins results in nucleic acids and protein

2. Hydrolysis of nucleic acid yields
   a. Phosphoric acid: H_3PO_4
   b. Pentose sugars: ribose or deoxyribose
   c. Purine or pyrimidine bases
      (1) Purine bases: adenine, guanine
      (2) Pyrimidine bases: cytosine, uracil, thymine

3. Combination of a purine or pyrimidine base with either ribose or deoxyribose forms a nucleoside

4. Addition of phosphoric acid to a nucleoside forms a nucleotide

5. Polymerization of nucleotide molecules via ester bonds yields a nucleic acid: the shape of DNA is that of a double helix

C. Two main forms of nucleic acid: RNA and DNA (ribonucleic acid and deoxyribonucleic acid)

1. RNA yields the following on hydrolysis: adenine, guanine, cytosine, uracil, ribose, phosphoric acid

2. DNA yields the following on hydrolysis: adenine, guanine, cytosine, thymine, deoxyribose, phosphoric acid

D. Role of DNA and RNA in protein synthesis

1. DNA is found chiefly in the chromatin material of interphase cells and in the chromosomes of cells in mitosis

   a. Portions of DNA molecules are the genes of classic genetics; the genetic code consists of sequences of bases (adenine, guanine, cytosine, and thymine) linearly arranged along the DNA molecule; every three bases represent a code for one amino acid (a triplet code)

   b. One enormous DNA molecule represents thousands of genes separated from each other by specific triplets (codons) representing periods or commas; i.e., the linear triplet code is punctuated so it can eventually be translated correctly on the ribosome

   c. DNA is also found in mitochondria, chloroplasts, and certain other cellular organelles (like centrioles) and is thought to play some role in their replication and metabolism

2. RNA is found both inside the nucleus and in the cytoplasm of cells

3. RNA occurs in three forms: messenger RNA (mRNA), transfer RNA (tRNA), and ribosomal RNA (rRNA)

   a. DNA transcribes its coded message of how to make proteins into mRNA; the function of mRNA is to carry this coded genetic information from the DNA in the nucleus to the ribosome in the cytoplasm where proteins can be synthesized

   b. The transcribed genetic code being carried by mRNA is translated into the synthesis of proteins on the ribosomes; these proteins then serve both structurally and enzymatically in the cell

c. tRNA molecules each carry an amino acid to the ribosome where protein synthesis is occurring; there is a specific tRNA molecule for each amino acid

d. rRNA is part of the structure of the ribosome

4. The protein difference between individuals is ultimately determined by differences in the genetic code carried by DNA; the DNA and RNA molecules are presently the only known molecules that store information and can result in the accurate transmission of genetic information from one generation of cell or organism to the next; the cellular mitotic and meiotic processes are elaborate and precise mechanisms for partitioning the genetic material appropriately between daughter cells

E. Other important related compounds
   1. ATP and ADP (adenosine triphosphate and adenosine diphosphate) are energy-storing compounds in cells
   2. NAD (nicotinamide adenine dinucleotide) and NADP (nicotinamide adenine dinucleotide phosphate) are important in hydrogen transport in the metabolism of foods

Enzymes

Hormones involved in regulating the GI tract

A. Gastrin: stimulates flow of gastric juices
B. Enterogastrone: inhibits flow of gastric juices
C. Secretin: stimulates flow of sodium bicarbonate from the pancreas to the duodenum
D. Pancreozymin: stimulates the flow of pancreatic enzymes from the pancreas to the duodenum
E. Cholecystokinin: stimulates contraction of the gallbladder
F. Enterocrinin: stimulates flow of intestinal juice

REVIEW OF MICROORGANISMS RELATED TO THE GASTROINTESTINAL SYSTEM

A. Bacterial pathogens
   1. *Brucella:* three species *(B. abortus, B. suis,* and *B. melitensis);* small, gram-negative, somewhat pleomorphic (variable shape) bacilli, cause brucellosis, an infection primarily of domestic animals (cattle, goats, swine, sheep); humans can acquire it by drinking infected milk
   2. *Escherichia coli:* small, gram-negative bacillus composing the major portion of the normal flora of the large intestine; certain strains are the most common cause of urinary tract infections and infantile diarrhea
   3. *Leptospira icterohaemorrhagiae:* long, tightly coiled spirochete similar in appearance to *Treponema pallidum;* causes infectious jaundice (Weil's disease)
   4. *Shigella:* gram-negative bacillus, similar to *Salmonella; Shigella dysenteriae* and a number of other species cause an illness known as bacillary dysentery or shigellosis
   5. *Vibrio cholerae* (formerly *V. comma*): curved, gram-negative bacillus with a single polar flagellum; causes Asiatic cholera

B. Protozoal pathogens
   1. *Balantidium coli:* ciliated protozoan; causes enteritis
   2. *Entamoeba histolytica:* an ameba; causes amebiasis (amebic dysentery)
   3. *Giardia lamblia:* flagellated protozoan; causes enteritis

C. Parasitic pathogens
   1. Nematodes (roundworms)
      a. *Ancylostoma duodenale* (hookworm): intestinal parasite similar to *Necator americanus*
      b. *Ascaris lumbricoides* (roundworm): intestinal parasite resembling the earthworm
      c. *Enterobius vermicularis* (pinworm, seatworm): small, white parasitic worm found in upper part of the large intestine; the female lays eggs in perianal area, causing irritation
      d. *Necator americanus* (The American hookworm): intestinal parasite about 1.2 cm (½ inch) long
      e. *Trichuris trichiura* (whipworm): intestinal parasite about 5 cm (2 inches) long
   2. Cestodes (tapeworm)
      a. *Diphyllobothrium latum* (fish tapeworm): large tapeworm 6.1 m (about 20 feet) long found in adult form in the intestine of cats, dogs, and humans (vertebrate and aquatic hosts in sequence)
      b. *Echinococcus granulosa* (dog tapeworm): small tapeworm of dogs; larval stage (hydatid) may develop in humans forming hydatid tumors or cysts in the liver, lungs, kidneys, and other organs
      c. *Hymenolepsis nana* (dwarf tapeworm): a species about 2.5 cm (1 inch) long, found in adult form in the intestine
      d. *Taenia marginata* (beef tapeworm): the common tapeworm of humans, a species 3.6 to 7.6 m (12 to 24 feet) long, found in adult form in the human intestine
      e. *Taenia solium* (pork tapeworm): a species 0.9 to 1.8 m (3 to 6 feet) long found in the adult form in the intestines of humans
   3. Trematodes (flukes)
      a. *Clonorchis sinensis:* one of the most common liver flukes, especially in China and Japan
      b. *Fasciola hepatica:* common liver fluke of herbivorous animals; occasionally found in the human liver
      c. *Fasciolopsis buski:* largest of the intestinal flukes
      d. *Paragonimus westermani:* lung fluke; found in cysts in the lungs, liver, abdominal cavity, and elsewhere

PHARMACOLOGY RELATED TO GASTROINTESTINAL SYSTEM DISORDERS
Antiemetics

A. Description
   1. Used to alleviate nausea and vomiting
   2. Act by
      a. Diminishing the sensitivity of the chemoreceptor trigger zone (CTZ) to irritants or
      b. Decreasing labyrinthine excitability

3. Effective in the prevention and control of eme:
   and motion sickness
4. Available in oral, parenteral (IM, IV), rectal, ar
   transdermal preparations

B. Examples
   1. Centrally acting agents
      a. benzquinamide (Emete-con)
      b. prochlorperazine (Compazine)
      c. trimethobenzamide HCl (Tigan)
   2. Agents for motion sickness control
      a. dimenhydrinate (Dramamine)
      b. meclizine HCl (Bonine)
      c. promethazine HCl (Phenergan)

C. Major side effects
   1. Drowsiness (CNS depression)
   2. Hypotension (vasodilation via central mechanism)
   3. Dry mouth (decreased salivation from anticholin-
      ergic effect)
   4. Blurred vision (pupillary dilation from anticholiner-
      gic effect)
   5. Incoordination (an extra pyramidal symptom due to
      dopamine antagonism)

D. Nursing care
   1. Observe occurrence and characteristics of vomitus
   2. Eliminate noxious substances from the diet and en-
      vironment
   3. Provide good oral hygiene
   4. Caution client to avoid engaging in hazardous activ-
      ities during therapy
   5. Offer sugar-free chewing gum or hard candy to pro-
      mote salivation
   6. Instruct client to change positions slowly
   7. Evaluate client's response to medication and under-
      standing of teaching

Anorexiants

A. Description
   1. Used to suppress the appetite
   2. Act at the hypothalamic appetite centers to suppress
      the desire for food; they generally produce CNS
      stimulation
   3. Available in oral preparations

B. Examples
   1. amphetamine sulfate (Benzedrine)
   2. benzphetamine HCl (Didrex)
   3. dextroamphetamine sulfate (Dexedrine)
   4. fenfluramine HCl (Pondimin)
   5. phenmetrazine HCl (Preludin)

C. Major side effects
   1. Nausea, vomiting (irritation of gastric mucosa)
   2. Constipation (delayed passage of stool in GI tract)
   3. Tachycardia (sympathetic stimulation)
   4. CNS stimulation (sympathetic activation)
   5. Fenfluramine: CNS depression (direct effect)

D. Nursing care
   1. Educate client regarding
      a. Drug misuse (controlled substances)
      b. Concurrent exercise and diet therapy
      c. Need for medical supervision during therapy
      d. Possibility of affecting ability to engage in haz-
         ardous activities

2. Fenfluramine: assess for history of depression, alcohol abuse, or suicidal tendencies; avoid administration in these situations
3. Evaluate client's response to medication and understanding of teaching

Antacids

A. Description
   1. Used to neutralize gastric acid
   2. Act by providing a protective coating on the stom-
      ach lining and lowering the gastric acid level which
      allows more rapid movement of stomach contents
      into the duodenum
   3. Effective in the treatment of ulcers
   4. Available in oral preparations

B. Examples
   1. aluminum carbonate gel (Basaljel)
   2. aluminum hydroxide gel (Amphojel)
   3. aluminum hydroxide with magnesium trisilicate
      (Gelusil)
   4. aluminum and magnesium hydroxides (Maalox)
   5. aluminum phosphate gel (Phosphaljel)
   6. magaldrate (Riopan)
   7. sodium bicarbonate: systemic antacid; may cause al-
      kalosis

C. Major side effects
   1. Constipation (aluminum compounds) (aluminum
      delays passage of stool in GI tract)
   2. Diarrhea (magnesium compounds) (magnesium
      stimulates peristalsis in GI tract)
   3. Alkalosis (systemic antacids) (absorption of alkaline
      compound into the circulation)
   4. Reduced absorption of calcium and iron (increase
      in gastric pH)

D. Nursing care
   1. Instruct the client regarding
      a. Overuse of antacids
      b. Need for continued supervision
      c. Dietary restrictions related to gastric distress
      d. Encourage foods high in calcium and iron
      e. Eliminating source of discomfort
   2. Caution client on a sodium-restricted diet that many
      antacids contain sodium
   3. Shake oral suspensions well prior to administration
   4. Administer with small amount of water to ensure
      passage to stomach
   5. Evaluate client's response to medication and under-
      standing of teaching

Gastrointestinal Anticholinergics

A. Description
   1. Used to alleviate pain associated with peptic ulcer
   2. Act by inhibiting smooth muscle contraction in the
      GI tract
   3. Available in oral and parenteral (IM, SC, IV) prepa-
      rations

B. Examples
   1. atropine sulfate
   2. belladonna leaf, tincture
   3. dicyclomine HCl (Bentyl)
   4. glycopyrrolate (Robinul)
   5. methantheline bromide (Banthine)
   6. propantheline bromide (Pro-Banthine)

C. Major side effects (all related to decreased parasympathetic stimulation)
   1. Abdominal distention (decreased peristalsis)
   2. Constipation (decreased peristalsis)
   3. Dry mouth (decreased salivation)
   4. Urinary retention (decreased parasympathetic stimulation)
   5. CNS disturbances (direct CNS toxic effect)
D. Nursing care
   1. Provide dietary counseling with emphasis on bland foods
   2. Offer sugar-free chewing gum or hard candy to promote salivation
   3. Evaluate client's response to medication and understanding of teaching

Gastrointestinal Antihistamines

A. Description
   1. Used to inhibit gastric acid secretion
   2. Act at the H_2-receptors of the stomach parietal cells
   3. Effective in the short-term therapy of peptic ulcer
   4. Available in oral and parenteral (IM, IV) preparations
B. Examples
   1. cimetidine (Tagamet)
   2. ranitidine (Zantac)
C. Major side effects
   1. CNS disturbances (decreased metabolism of drug because of liver or kidney impairment)
   2. Blood dyscrasias (decreased RBC, WBC, platelet synthesis)
   3. Skin rash (hypersensitivity)
   4. Reduced calcium and iron absorption (increase in gastric pH)
D. Nursing care
   1. Do not administer at same time as antacids; allow 1 to 2 hours between drugs
   2. Administer oral preparations with meals
   3. Assess for potentiation of oral anticoagulant effect
   4. Instruct client regarding dietary restrictions; also encourage foods high in calcium and iron (See Peptic ulcer for more dietary information)
   5. Evaluate client's response to medication and understanding of teaching

Antidiarrheals

A. Description
   1. Used to alleviate diarrhea
   2. Act by various mechanisms to promote the formation of a formed stool
   3. Available in oral and parenteral (IM) preparations
B. Examples
   1. Fluid adsorbants: decrease the fluid content of stool
      a. bismuth subcarbonate
      b. kaolin and pectin (Kaopectate)
   2. Enteric bacteria replacements: enhance production of lactic acid from carbohydrates in the intestinal lumen; acidity suppresses pathogenic bacterial overgrowth
      a. lactobacillus acidophilus (Bacid)
      b. lactobacillus bulgaricus (Lactinex)

   3. Motility suppressants: decrease GI tract motility so that more water will be absorbed from the large intestine
      a. diphenoxylate HCl (Lomotil)
      b. tincture of opium (Paregoric)
C. Major side effects
   1. Fluid adsorbants
      a. GI disturbances (local effect)
      b. CNS disturbances (direct CNS toxic effect)
   2. Enteric bacteria replacements
      a. Excessive flatulence (increased microbial gas production)
      b. Abdominal cramps (increased microbial gas production)
   3. Motility suppressants
      a. Urinary retention (direct parasympathetic stimulation)
      b. Tachycardia (vagolytic effect on cardiac conduction)
      c. Dry mouth (decreased salivation from anticholinergic effect)
      d. Sedation (CNS depression)
      e. Paralytic ileus (decreased peristalsis)
      f. Respiratory depression (depression of medullary respiratory center)
D. Nursing care
   1. Monitor BMs for color, characteristics, and frequency
   2. Assess for fluid/electrolyte imbalance
   3. Assess and eliminate cause of diarrhea
   4. Motility suppressants
      a. Warn client of risk of physical dependence with long-term use
      b. Offer sugar-free chewing gum and hard candy to promote salivation
      c. May interfere with ability to perform hazardous activities
   5. Evaluate client's response to medication and understanding of teaching

Cathartics/Laxatives

A. Description
   1. Used to alleviate or prevent constipation
   2. Act by various mechanisms to promote evacuation of a normal stool
   3. Available in oral and rectal preparations
B. Examples
   1. Intestinal lubricants: decrease dehydration of feces; lubricate intestinal tract
      a. mineral oil
      b. olive oil
   2. Fecal softeners: lower surface tension of feces in colon; allow water and fats to penetrate feces
      a. dioctyl calcium sulfosuccinate (Surfak)
      b. dioctyl sodium sulfosuccinate (Colace)
   3. Bulk-forming laxatives: increase bulk in intestinal lumen which stimulates propulsive movements by pressure on mucosal lining
      a. methylcellulose (Cellothyl)
      b. psyllium hydrophilic mucilloid (Metamucil)

4. Colon irritants: stimulate peristalsis by reflexive response to irritation of intestinal lumen
   a. bisacodyl (Dulcolax)
   b. cascara sagrada (Peristim)
   c. castor oil
   d. senna (Senokot)
5. Saline cathartics: increase osmotic pressure within intestine, drawing fluid from blood and bowel wall, thus increasing bulk and stimulating peristalsis
   a. effervescent sodium phosphate (Fleet Phospho-soda)
   b. magnesium citrate solution
   c. magnesium sulfate (Epsom salts)
   d. milk of magnesia
C. Major side effects
1. Laxative dependence with long-term use (loss of normal defecation mechanism)
2. GI disturbances (local effect)
3. Intestinal lubricants
   a. Inhibited absorption of fat-soluble vitamins (coat the GI mucosa prohibiting absorption of vitamins A, D, E, K)
   b. Anal leaking of oil (accumulation of lubricant near rectal sphincter)
4. Saline cathartics
   a. Dehydration (fluid volume depletion due to hypertonic state in GI tract)
   b. Hypernatremia (increased sodium absorption into circulation; loss of some fluid from vasculature)
D. Nursing care
1. Instruct the client regarding
   a. Overuse of cathartics and intestinal lubricants
   b. Increasing intake of fluids and dietary fiber
   c. Increasing activity level
   d. Compliance with bowel-retraining program
2. Monitor BMs for consistency and frequency of stool
3. Intestinal lubricants: utilize peripad to protect clothing
4. Bulk-forming laxatives: mix thoroughly in 8 oz of fluid and follow with another 8 oz of fluid to prevent obstruction
5. Administer at bedtime to promote defecation in the morning
6. Evaluate client's response to medication and understanding of teaching

Intestinal Antibiotics

(See Antibiotics—aminoglycosides in Pharmacology related to infection)

Pancreatic Enzymes

A. Description
1. Used to promote the digestion of proteins, fats, and starches
2. Act as replacements for natural endogenous pancreatic enzymes (protease, lipase, amylase)
3. Available in oral preparations
B. Examples
1. pancreatin (Viokase)
2. pancrelipase (Cotazym)

C. Major side effects
1. Nausea (GI irritation)
2. Diarrhea (GI irritation)
D. Nursing care
1. Administer with meals; teach client to take with meals
2. Avoid crushing preparations that are enteric-coated
3. Provide a balanced diet to prevent indigestion
4. Evaluate client's response to medication and understanding of teaching

PROCEDURES RELATED TO THE GASTROINTESTINAL SYSTEM
Barium Enema

A. Definition: introduction of barium, an opaque medium, into the intestines for the purpose of x-ray visualization for pathologic changes
B. Nursing care
1. Explain procedure to the client
2. Prepare the client for the procedure by
   a. Administering cathartics and/or enemas as ordered to evacuate the bowel
   b. Maintaining the client npo for 8 to 10 hours prior to the test
3. Inspect stool after the procedure for the presence of barium
4. Administer enemas and/or cathartics as ordered if the stool does not return to normal
5. Evaluate client's response to procedure

Colostomy Care

A. Definition
1. Instillation of fluid into the lower colon via a stoma on the abdominal wall to stimulate peristalsis and facilitate the expulsion of feces
2. Cleansing the colostomy stoma and collection of feces (stool consistency will depend on location of the ostomy: a colostomy of the sigmoid colon will tend to produce formed stools; a transverse colostomy will produce less formed stools)
B. Nursing care
1. Secure a physician's order
2. Irrigate the stoma at the same time each day to approximate normal bowel habits
3. Insert a well-lubricated catheter tip into the stoma approximately 7 cm in the direction of the remaining bowel (anatomy of ascending, transverse, and descending colon should be considered); as the solution is allowed to flow, the catheter may be advanced
4. Hold the irrigating container 30.5 to 45.7 cm (12 to 18 inches) above the colostomy; irrigating solution should be 105° F (40.5° C)
5. Clamp tubing or temporarily lower the container if the client complains of cramping
6. Provide privacy while waiting for fecal returns or permit the client to ambulate with the collection bag in place to further stimulate peristalsis
7. Cleanse the stoma; if excoriation occurs, a soothing ointment may be ordered
8. Apply a colostomy bag or gauze dressing (if the colostomy is well regulated)
9. Teach the client to control odor when necessary by

placing two aspirin tablets (or commercially available deodorizers) in the colostomy bag or by taking bismuth subcarbonate tablets orally to control odor
10. Evaluate client's response to procedure

Endoscopy

A. Definition: visualization of the esophagus, stomach, colon, or rectum using a hollow tube with a lighted end
   1. Gastroscopy: stomach
   2. Esophagoscopy: esophagus
   3. Sigmoidoscopy: sigmoid colon
   4. Proctoscopy: rectum
B. Nursing care
   1. Obtain an informed consent for the procedure
   2. If rectal examination is indicated, administer cleansing enemas prior to the test
   3. Restrict diet (npo) prior to procedure
   4. Following the procedure, observe for bleeding, changes in vital signs, or nausea
   5. If the throat is anesthetized (as for a gastroscopy or esophagoscopy), check for the return of gag reflex before offering oral fluids
   6. Evaluate client's response to procedure

Enemas

A. Definitions
   1. Tap water enema (TWE): introduction of water into the colon to stimulate evacuation
   2. Soapsuds enema (SSE): introduction of soapy water into the colon to stimulate peristalsis by bowel irritation; contraindicated as a preparation for an endoscopic procedure because it may alter the appearance of the mucosa
   3. Harris flush or drip: introduction of water into the colon as tolerated and subsequent repeated drainage of that water through the same tubing to facilitate passage of flatus
   4. High colonic irrigation: introduction of water into the upper portion of the colon to facilitate complete fecal evacuation
   5. Instillation: introduction of a liquid (usually mineral oil) into the colon to facilitate fecal activity through lubricating effect
B. Nursing care
   1. Explain procedure to client
   2. Provide privacy
   3. Obtain the correct solution
   4. Lubricate the tip of a rectal catheter with water-soluble jelly
   5. Insert the catheter 10 to 15 cm (4 to 6 inches) into the rectum
   6. Allow the solution to enter slowly; keep it no more than 30.5 to 45.7 cm (12 to 18 inches) above the rectum
   7. Allow ample time for client to expel the enema
   8. Observe and record the amount and consistency of returns
   9. Evaluate client's response to procedure

Gastric Analysis

A. Definition
   1. Analysis of stomach contents for the presence of abnormal constituents or lack of normal constituents

such as hydrochloric acid, blood, acid-fast bacteria, and lactic acid
   2. Acid content is elevated in ulcers, decreased in malignant conditions of the stomach, and absent in pernicious anemia
B. Nursing care
   1. Explain procedure to client
   2. Maintain the client npo prior to the test and have a nasogastric tube passed at time of procedure
   3. Administer histamine or caffeine to stimulate hydrochloric acid secretion prior to the procedure if ordered
   4. Obtain stomach contents, secure in an appropriate container, and send to laboratory
   5. Evaluate client's response to procedure

Gastrointestinal (GI) Series

A. Definition: introduction of barium, an opaque medium, into the upper GI tract via the mouth, gastrostomy tube, or nasogastric tube to visualize the area by x-ray methods
B. Nursing care
   1. Explain procedure to client
   2. Maintain the client npo after midnight
   3. Inform client that the stool will be white or pink for 24 to 72 hours after the procedure
   4. Encourage fluids and administer cathartics as ordered
   5. Evaluate client's response to procedure

Gavage (Tube Feeding)

A. Definitions
   1. Nasogastric
      a. Placement of a tube through the nose into the stomach, securing it in place with tape
      b. Prepared nutritional supplements are introduced through this tube
   2. Intestinal
      a. Placement of a tube through the nose into the small intestine, securing it in place with tape
      b. There is less likelihood of aspiration since the pyloric sphincter inhibits backflow
   3. Surgically placed feeding tubes
      a. Cervical esophagostomy: tube is sutured directly into the esophagus for clients who have had head and neck surgery
      b. Gastrostomy: tube is placed directly into the stomach through the abdominal wall and sutured in place; used for clients who require tube feeding on a long-term basis
      c. Jejunostomy: tube is inserted directly into the jejunum for clients with pathology of the upper GI tract
   4. Percutaneous endoscopic gastrostomy (PEG)
      a. Stomach is punctured during endoscopy procedure
      b. Does not require general anesthesia or laparotomy
      c. Dressing should be changed daily
      d. While associated with reduced risks, accidental removal and aspiration may still occur

B. Nursing care
  1. Nasogastric feedings
     a. Inject a small amount of air into the tube and with a stethoscope placed over the epigastric area, listen for the passage of air into the stomach
     b. Aspirate for stomach contents
     c. Place the end of the nasogastric tube in water; presence of bubbling indicates the tube is in the lungs (this method is the least reliable)
  2. Intestinal and surgically placed tubes
     a. Aspirate contents prior to instituting new feeding
     b. Withhold feeding if residual is greater than 150 ml
  3. Intermittent feeding
     a. Appropriately verify placement of tube
     b. Introduce a small amount of water first to verify the patency of the tube; the tube should not be allowed to empty during feeding so that excess air is not forced into the stomach
     c. Administer the feeding (which may be the client's normal foods blenderized) at room or body temperature slowly; observe and question the client to determine tolerance; the higher the feeding container and the larger the lumen of the feeding tube, the more rapid the flow
     d. Administer a small amount of water to clear the tube at the completion of the feeding
     e. Clamp the tubing and clean the equipment
     f. Place client in sitting position for 1 hour after feeding
  4. Continuous feeding
     a. Place prescribed feeding in gavage bag and prime tubing to prevent excess air from entering stomach
     b. Set rate of flow; rate of flow can be manually regulated by setting drops per minute or mechanically regulated by using an electric pump
     c. Appropriately verify placement of tube when adding additional fluid to a continuous feeding
     d. Flush tube intermittently with water to prevent occlusion of tube with feeding
     e. Monitor for gastric distention and aspiration; since smaller amounts of feeding are generally administered within a given time period, gastric distention and subsequent aspiration are less frequent
     f. Discard unused fluid that has been in gavage administration bag at room temperature for longer than 4 hours
  5. Care common for all clients receiving tube feedings
     a. Monitor for abdominal distension
     b. Discontinue feeding if nausea and/or vomiting occur
     c. Encourage the client to chew foods that will stimulate gastric secretions while providing psychologic comfort; chewed food may not be swallowed
     d. Provide special skin care; if the client has a tube sutured in place, the skin may become irritated from gastrointestinal enzymes; if the client has a

nasogastric tube, the skin may become excoriated at point of entry because of irritation
     e. Evaluate client's response to procedure

Ileostomy Care

A. Definition: physical care of the ileostomy stoma and surrounding skin
B. Nursing care
  1. Protect the skin from irritation, since the feces will be liquid because of the anatomic location of the stoma
  2. Explain procedure to the client and family and encourage self-care
  3. Do not irrigate the stoma
  4. Affix an appliance with an adequate seal (Karaya) to prevent accidental leakage around the stoma; the appliance is generally changed every 2 to 4 days but emptied every 6 hours
  5. Evaluate client's response to procedure

Irrigation of Nasogastric (Levin) Tube

A. Definition
  1. The Levin tube is commonly used for gastric decompression
  2. Purposes of insertion of a nasogastric tube include emptying the stomach, obtaining a specimen for diagnostic purposes, or providing a means for nourishment
  3. Irrigation is the insertion of fluid (usually normal saline) to maintain patency
B. Nursing care
  1. Check that the order for irrigations has been written by the physician
  2. Ascertain the patency of the Levin tube attached to intermittent suction by observing for drainage; nausea or abdominal discomfort may indicate that the tube is occluded
  3. Assemble equipment: 30-ml syringe or bulb syringe, irrigating solution, and basin for returning fluid
  4. Verify placement (see gavage)
  5. Instill approximately 30 ml of fluid into the tube
  6. Gently withdraw the same volume of fluid as was instilled; if the client has undergone gastric surgery, the physician will generally order instillations; in this case, irrigation fluid is instilled but not withdrawn; the amount instilled must be subtracted from total gastric output
  7. Chart the amount, color, and consistency of drainage
  8. Evaluate client's response to procedure

Paracentesis

A. Definition: surgical puncture of the peritoneal membrane of the abdominal cavity for the purpose of removing fluid
B. Nursing care
  1. Explain the procedure; obtain consent
  2. Have the client void prior to procedure
  3. Assist the client to a sitting position
  4. Observe for signs of shock; sudden fluid shifts can result in hypotension

5. Chart the amount and characteristics of fluid withdrawn
6. Apply a dry sterile dressing to the puncture site
7. Properly label the specimen if required and send to the laboratory
8. Evaluate client's response to the procedure

Parenteral Replacement Therapy

A. Definitions
   1. Peripheral parenteral nutrition (PPN)
      a. Administration of lipids and isotonic amino acid solutions through a peripheral vein
      b. Amino acid content should not exceed 4% and the dextrose content should be greater than 7%
      c. Assists in maintaining a positive nitrogen balance
   2. Total parenteral nutrition (TPN)
      a. Administration of carbohydrates, fats, and amino acids via a central vein (usually the superior vena cava)
      b. High osmolality solutions (25% dextrose) are administered in conjunction with 5% to 10% amino acids, electrolytes, minerals, and fat
      c. Assists in maintaining a positive nitrogen balance
B. Nursing care
   1. Infuse fluid through a large vein such as the subclavian because of the high osmolarity of the solution used in TPN
   2. Ensure proper placement of the tube by chest x-ray examination after insertion of a catheter; accidental pneumothorax can occur during insertion
   3. Precisely regulate the fluid infusion rate; an intravenous pump should be used if available
      a. Rapid infusion may result in movement of the fluid into an intravascular compartment; dehydration, circulatory overload, and hyperglycemia can occur
      b. Slow infusion may result in hypoglycemia, since the body adapts to the high osmolarity of this fluid by secreting more insulin; for this reason, hyperalimentation is never terminated abruptly but is gradually discontinued
   4. Use aseptic technique when handling the infusion or changing the dressing (in many institutions, only nurses specially prepared are allowed to change the dressing because of the high risk of infection)
   5. Use surgically aseptic technique when changing tubing
   6. Record daily weights and monitor urinary sugar and acetone or blood glucose levels frequently
   7. Check laboratory reports daily, especially glucose, creatine, BUN, and electrolytes
   8. Monitor temperature q4h since infection is the most common complication of hyperalimentation; if the client has a temperature elevation, order cultures of blood, urine, and sputum to rule out other sources of infection
   9. Evaluate client's response to procedure

Stool Specimens

A. Definitions
   1. Stool for guaiac (occult blood): specimen or smear of stool on a commercially prepared card is sent to the laboratory for analysis; positive results indicate the presence of blood in the stool and may suggest diverse diseases such as peptic ulcer, gastritis, gastric or colonic carcinoma, colitis, or diverticulitis
   2. Stools for O and P (ova and parasites): must be sent to the laboratory while still warm for microscopic examination
   3. Stool culture: specimen or swab of stool is sent in a sterile container for identification of abnormal bacterial growth
B. Nursing care
   1. Explain procedure to the client
   2. Collect specimen in an appropriate container
   3. Label the container with the client's name, identification number, physician, and room number
   4. Chart that the specimen was sent and any unusual assessment of the stool

NURSING PROCESS FOR CLIENTS WITH GASTROINTESTINAL SYSTEM DISORDERS
Probable Nursing Diagnoses Based on Assessment

A. Altered nutrition: more than body requirements, related to excess ingestion
B. Altered nutrition: less than body requirements, related to
   1. Anorexia
   2. Inability to ingest
   3. Malabsorption
   4. Changes in metabolism
C. Constipation related to
   1. Dietary habits
   2. Inadequate intake of fluids
   3. Inactivity
   4. Obstruction
   5. Fear of pain when defacating
D. Diarrhea related to
   1. Local inflammatory process
   2. Anxiety
   3. Food intolerance
E. Bowel incontinence related to impaired sphincter control
F. Colonic constipation related to less than adequate fiber/fluid intake
G. Perceived constipation related to personal cultural/family beliefs
H. Altered oral mucous membrane related to chemical and microbiological irritants
I. Impaired skin integrity related to irritation by intestinal enzymes
J. Potential for trauma related to mechanical devices used for irrigation
K. Potential for injury related to
   1. Hemorrhage
   2. Aspiration
L. Pain related to
   1. Pathological processes
   2. Diagnostic procedures
   3. Therapeutic modalities
M. Impaired swallowing related to obstruction in oropharyngeal and/or esophageal structures
N. Potential fluid volume deficit related to
   1. Inadequate fluid intake
   2. Increased portal hypertension resulting in ascites

O. Body image disturbance related to disease process (fluid retention or malnutrition) and/or surgical intervention
P. Social isolation related to disfiguring surgery or altered feeding patterns
Q. Fear related to diagnosis with impending death

Nursing Care For Clients With Gastrointestinal Disorders

(See nursing care under each specific disease)

MAJOR DISEASES
Stomatitis

A. Etiology and pathophysiology
1. Inflammation of the buccal mucosa because of disease, trauma, irritants, nutritional deficiencies, or medications
2. Categories
   a. Aphthous stomatitis: canker sore that can result from chronic cheek biting
   b. Herpes simplex: virus that causes vesicle formation in mouth, on lips, or on nose
   c. Vincent's angina: ulceration of the buccal membrane due to *Borrelia vincentii* (trench mouth)
   d. Thrush: fungal invasion of the mouth by *Candida albicans,* characterized by white patches
B. Signs and symptoms
1. Subjective
   a. Foul taste in the mouth
   b. Pain in the mouth
2. Objective
   a. Erythema of the mucous membranes
   b. Changes in salivation
   c. Unpleasant odor to the breath
   d. Bleeding gums in Vincent's angina
   e. White patches in thrush
C. Treatment
1. Adequate nutrition and hydration
2. Alkaline mouthwashes
3. Antifungal agents for thrush
4. Antibiotics for Vincent's angina
D. Nursing care
1. Provide mouthwashes q2h
2. Encourage foods that can be tolerated, such as soft foods, cool drinks, eggnogs
3. Promote oral hygiene; use soft toothbrush or padded tongue blade
4. Evaluate client's response and revise plan as necessary

Fracture of the Jaw

A. Etiology and pathophysiology: generally the result of trauma such as motor vehicle accidents or physical combat
B. Signs and symptoms
1. Subjective
   a. History of trauma to the face
   b. Pain in the face and jaw
2. Objective
   a. Bloody discharge from the mouth
   b. Swelling of face on the affected side
   c. Difficulty opening or closing the mouth

C. Treatment
1. Separated fragments of the broken bone are reunited and immobilized by wires and rubber bands; usually placed without surgical incision
2. Open reduction of the jaw is indicated for severely fractured or displaced bones; interosseous wiring is done
D. Nursing care
1. Postoperatively control vomiting and reduce the chance of aspiration pneumonia by positioning client on abdomen or side
2. Keep wire cutters at the bedside to release the wires and rubber bands if emesis occurs
3. Explain diet to the client and family; no solid foods are permitted; encourage high-protein liquids or blenderized soft foods
4. Stress the importance of regular oral hygiene and institute it early in the postoperative period
5. Evaluate client's response and revise plan as necessary

Cancer of the Mouth

A. Etiology and pathophysiology
1. Primarily in clients who smoke and drink alcohol in large quantities
2. Cancer of the lip, easily diagnosed; prognosis is very good; incidence highest in pipe smokers
3. Cancer of the tongue, usually occurs with cancer of the floor of the mouth; metastasis to the neck common
4. Cancer of the submaxillary glands, highly malignant and grows rapidly
B. Signs and symptoms
1. Subjective
   a. Pain not an early symptom
   b. Alterations of taste sensation
2. Objective
   a. Leukoplakia (white patches on mucosa, which are considered precancerous)
   b. Ulcerated areas in the involved structure
C. Treatment
1. Reconstructive surgery if indicated
2. Radiation or implantation of radioactive material may arrest growth of tumor
D. Nursing care
1. Maintain fluid and electrolyte balance
2. Provide for a means of communication
3. If radiation therapy is indicated, relieve dryness of the mouth by frequent mouthwashes and ample fluids
4. Consider time and distance in relation to the radioactive material when giving nursing care
5. Evaluate client's response and revise plan as necessary

Cancer of the Esophagus

A. Etiology and pathophysiology
1. Etiology unknown: occurs predominantly in persons with a history of alcohol abuse or hiatus hernia
2. Tumor may develop anywhere in the esophagus, but most commonly in the middle and lower third

B. Signs and symptoms
   1. Subjective
      a. Dysphagia
      b. Substernal pain
      c. Substernal burning after drinking hot liquids
   2. Objective
      a. Regurgitation
      b. X-ray examination of esophagus reveals irregularities of the lumen
      c. Cytologic examination of cells, obtained after esophageal lavage, reveals malignant cells
C. Treatment
   1. Surgical removal of the esophagus is the treatment of choice
      a. Esophagogastrostomy: resection of a portion of the esophagus; a portion of the bowel may be grafted between the esophagus and stomach, or the stomach may be brought up to the proximal end of the esophagus
      b. Esophagectomy: removal of part or all of the esophagus, which is replaced by a Dacron graft
      c. Gastrostomy: opening directly into the stomach in which a feeding tube is usually inserted to bypass the esophagus
   2. Radiation and/or chemotherapy may be used prior to or instead of surgery as a palliative measure
D. Nursing care
   1. Support the client and family emotionally
   2. Formulate realistic goals in planning client care
   3. Observe for respiratory distress caused by pressure of tumor on the trachea; place in a semi-Fowler's or high-Fowler's position to facilitate respirations
   4. Monitor vital signs, especially respirations
   5. Provide oral care, since dysphagia may result in increased accumulation of saliva in mouth
   6. Maintain nutritional status by providing high-protein liquids along with vitamin and mineral replacements
   7. Evaluate client's response and revise plan as necessary

Hiatal Hernia

A. Etiology and pathophysiology
   1. Portion of the stomach protruding through a hiatus (opening) in the diaphragm into the thoracic cavity
   2. May result from a congenital weakness of the diaphragm or from injury, pregnancy, or obesity
   3. Function of the cardiac sphincter is lost, gastric juices enter the esophagus, and edema and hyperemia may result
B. Signs and symptoms
   1. Subjective
      a. Substernal burning pain
      b. Heartburn after eating, which increases in the recumbent position
      c. Nocturnal dyspnea
   2. Objective
      a. GI series and endoscopy show protrusion of the stomach through the diaphragm
      b. Regurgitation

C. Treatment
   1. Small, frequent, bland feedings
   2. Antacids
   3. Surgical repair (done infrequently)
D. Nursing care
   1. Teach the client and family about the dietary regimen
   2. Encourage attempts at weight loss
   3. Avoid constricting clothing
   4. Elevate head of the bed after meals
   5. Encourage the client to eat slowly
   6. Evaluate client's response and revise plan as necessary

Gastritis

A. Etiology and pathophysiology
   1. Inflammation of the stomach; either acute or chronic
   2. May be caused by
      a. Ingestion of irritating chemicals such as aspirin and alcohol
      b. Bacterial or viral infections
      c. Allergic reactions
      d. Chronic uremia, which often leads to chronic gastritis
B. Signs and symptoms
   1. Subjective
      a. Anorexia
      b. Nausea and vomiting
      c. Epigastric fullness
   2. Objective
      a. Diarrhea and cramps if caused by an infection
      b. Dehydration
      c. Hemorrhage if aspirin or other chemicals are involved
C. Treatment
   1. Early treatment aimed at correcting the fluid and electrolyte imbalance; the client is kept npo during the acute phase of illness and then progresses to a bland diet
   2. If caused by infection, appropriate antibiotics may be given
   3. Other medications that may be prescribed include antispasmodics, anticholinergics, and antacids
D. Nursing care
   1. Observe for signs of dehydration and electrolyte imbalance
   2. Provide adequate fluid intake
   3. Alert the client to possible causes
   4. Teach the client the necessary dietary alterations, such as omission of coffee, alcohol, and spices, and maintaining a bland diet
   5. Evaluate client's response and revise plan as necessary

Peptic Ulcer

A. Etiology and pathophysiology
   1. Ulcerations of the gastrointestinal mucosa and underlying tissues caused by gastric secretions that have a low pH (acid)

2. Causes include conditions that increase the secretion of hydrochloric acid by the gastric mucosa or that decrease that tissue's resistance to the acid
   a. Zollinger-Ellison syndrome: tumors secreting gastrin, which will stimulate the production of excessive hydrochloric acid
   b. Certain drugs such as aspirin and indomethacin will decrease tissue resistance
   c. Many believe that emotional factors are strongly related to peptic ulcers; a person who is considered a perfectionist may have an increased risk of developing a peptic ulcer
3. Peptic ulcers may be present in the esophagus, stomach, or duodenum (the most common site)
4. Complications include pyloric or duodenal obstruction, hemorrhage, and perforation
B. Signs and symptoms
   1. Subjective
      a. Gnawing or burning epigastric pain that occurs 1 to 2 hours after eating and may be relieved by eructation, vomiting, food, or antacids
      b. Nausea
   2. Objective
      a. If bleeding occurs, signs of anemia will be evident; passage of tarry stools (melena) may occur
      b. Vomiting (coffee ground to port wine color if bleeding has occurred)
C. Treatment
   1. Institute measures to neutralize or buffer hydrochloric acid, inhibit acid secretion, and decrease the activity of pepsin and hydrochloric acid such as
      a. Radiation and gastric hypothermia to suppress gastric secretions
      b. Antacids to reduce acidity
      c. Diet regulation through the use of bland foods, and restriction of irritating substances such as nicotine, caffeine, alcohol, spices, and gassy foods
   2. Type and cross match so that blood will be available if gastric hemorrhage occurs
   3. Sedatives, tranquilizers, anticholinergics, and analgesics for pain and restlessness
   4. Histamine H_2 receptor antagonist to limit gastric acid secretion
   5. Antiemetics for nausea and vomiting
   6. Bed rest to reduce physical activity
   7. Encourage the client to seek counseling or psychotherapy to explore the emotional components of the illness
   8. If hemorrhage occurs, a nasogastric tube is inserted and iced saline lavages may be ordered; irrigations with medications that cause vasoconstriction to control bleeding are also used
   9. Surgical intervention
      a. Vagotomy: cutting the vagus nerve (X), which innervates the stomach, to decrease the secretion of hydrochloric acid
      b. Bilroth I: removal of the lower portion of the stomach and attachment of the remaining portion to the duodenum

c. Bilroth II: removal of the antrum and distal portion of the stomach and subsequent anastomosis of remaining section to the jejunum
d. Antrectomy: removal of the antral portion of the stomach
e. Gastrectomy: removal of 60% to 80% of the stomach
10. Common complications of partial or total gastric resection
   a. Dumping syndrome: involves the rapid passage of food from the stomach to the jejunum; the food, being hypertonic (especially if high in carbohydrates), will draw fluid from the circulating blood into the jejunum causing diaphoresis, faintness, and palpitations
   b. Hemorrhage
   c. Pneumonia
   d. Pernicious anemia
D. Nursing care
   1. Allow ample time for the client to express feelings and concerns
   2. Administer and assess effects of sedatives, antacids, anticholinergics, H_2 receptor antagonists, and dietary modifications
   3. Encourage hydration to reduce anticholinergic side effects and dilute the hydrochloric acid in the stomach
   4. Instruct client to
      a. Eat small to medium-sized meals because this helps prevent gastric distention; encourage between meal snacks to achieve adequate calories when necessary
      b. Avoid foods that increase gastric acid secretion or irritate gastric mucosa such as alcohol, caffeine-containing foods and beverages, decaffeinated coffee, red or black pepper; replace with decaffeinated soft drinks and teas; use seasonings like thyme, basil, sage, etc. to replace pepper
      c. Avoid foods that cause distress; varies for individuals but common offenders are the gas producers (legumes, carbonated beverages, the cruciferous vegetables)
      d. Eat meals in pleasant, relaxing surroundings to reduce acid secretion
      e. Administer calcium and iron supplements as ordered if client's medication increases gastric pH
   5. Refrain from administering drugs such as salicylates, phenylbutazone, steroids, and ACTH, which are normally contraindicated
   6. Observe for complications such as gastric hemorrhage, perforation, and drug toxicity
   7. Provide postoperative care after gastric resection
      a. Monitor vital signs; assess the dressing for drainage
      b. Maintain a patent nasogastric tube to the suction apparatus to prevent stress on the suture line
      c. Observe the color and amount of nasogastric drainage; excessive bleeding or the presence of bright red blood after 12 hours should be reported immediately

d. Have the client cough, deep breathe, and change position frequently to prevent the occurrence of pulmonary complications

e. Monitor intake and output

f. Apply an abdominal binder if ordered

g. Apply antiembolism stockings; have the client ambulate early to prevent vascular complications

h. To prevent dumping syndrome, instruct the client to

   (1) Eat smaller meals at more frequent intervals

   (2) Avoid high-carbohydrate intake

   (3) Consume liquids only between meals (at least 1 hour before or after meals)

   (4) Lie down or rest after eating

   (5) In severe cases, pectin or guar gum (5g dose) may be prescribed with meals; these water-soluble fibers delay gastric emptying and absorption of carbohydrates

8. Teach drug regimen and signs and symptoms of recurrence

9. Prevent recurrence by teaching client to modify dietary, working, and living patterns; maintain regularity in activities of daily living; continue medical supervision

10. Evaluate client's response and revise plan as necessary

Carcinoma of the Stomach

A. Etiology and pathophysiology

  1. Often not diagnosed until metastasis occurs; the stomach is able to accommodate to the growth of a tumor, and pain occurs late in the disease

  2. May metastasize by direct extension, lymphatics, or blood to the esophagus, spleen, pancreas, liver, or bone

  3. Heredity apparently a factor in the development of carcinoma of the stomach, as is the presence of precursors such as ulcerative disease and pernicious anemia

  4. Incidence higher in men over 40 years of age; Japan has a four times greater rate of cancer of the stomach than does the United States

B. Signs and symptoms

  1. Subjective

    a. Anorexia

    b. Nausea

    c. Belching (eructation)

    d. Heartburn

  2. Objective

    a. Weight loss

    b. Anemia

    c. Positive stools for guaiac (occult blood)

    d. Achlorhydria (absence of hydrochloric acid, determined by gastric analysis)

C. Treatment

  1. Subtotal or total gastrectomy

  2. Radiation

  3. Chemotherapy (fluorouracil is often used)

D. Nursing care

  1. Offer the client every opportunity to verbalize fears (i.e., cancer, death, family problems, self-image)

2. Postoperative care the same as nursing care after a gastric resection (see Peptic ulcer); in addition, if a total gastrectomy is performed, the chest cavity is usually entered, so the client will have chest tubes (see Pneumothorax for related nursing care)

3. Modify diet to include smaller, more frequent meals (see Peptic ulcer for more dietary information)

4. If total gastrectomy has been performed, the client will have a vitamin B_{12} deficiency (see Pernicious anemia)

5. Client may require gavage feedings via nasogastric tube or gastrostomy tube (see procedure)

6. Evaluate client's response and revise plan as necessary

Cholecystitis

A. Etiology and pathophysiology

  1. Inflammation of the gallbladder; usually caused by the presence of stones (cholelithiasis), which are composed of cholesterol, bile pigments, and calcium

  2. Diseased gallbladder is unable to contract in response to fatty foods entering the duodenum because of obstruction by calculi or edema

  3. When the common bile duct is completely obstructed, the bile is unable to pass into the duodenum and is absorbed into the blood

  4. Incidence is highest in obese women in the fourth decade

B. Signs and symptoms

  1. Subjective

    a. Indigestion after eating fatty or fried foods

    b. Pain, usually in the right upper quadrant of the abdomen, which may radiate to the back

    c. Nausea

  2. Objective

    a. Vomiting

    b. Elevated temperature and WBC

    c. Jaundice in approximately 25% of clients

    d. Diagnostic tests

      (1) Intravenous cholangiogram; clients who are allergic to the dye will complain of sensation of warmth, urticaria, nausea, and vomiting

      (2) Serum bilirubin will be elevated

      (3) Gallbladder series; approximately 6 radiopaque tablets such as Telepaque or Bilopaque are taken with water the evening before so that the gallbladder will be visible on x-ray examination

      (4) Ultrasonography to determine the presence of gallstones

C. Treatment

  1. Medical management

    a. Rest

    b. Nasogastric suctioning to reduce nausea and eliminate vomiting

    c. Narcotics to decrease pain

    d. Antispasmodics and anticholinergics to reduce spasms and contractions of the gallbladder

    e. Antibiotic therapy if infection is suspected

    f. In cases where clients are poor surgical risks, chenodiol (Chenix) is taken orally over a period

of months to dissolve radiolucent cholesterol stones, particularly if they are small
   g. Lithotripsy: ultrasonic soundwaves fragment stones to enable their passage without surgical intervention
   h. Low-fat diet to avoid stimulating the gallbladder, which constricts to excrete bile with subsequent pain; calories principally from carbohydrate foods in acute phases; if weight loss is indicated, calories may be reduced to 1000 to 1200; post-operatively clients may take fat-restricted diets initially but progress to regular diets
   2. Surgical intervention
   a. Cholecystotomy: incision into the gallbladder for the purpose of drainage
   b. Cholecystectomy: removal of the gallbladder
   c. Choledochotomy: incision into the common bile duct
D. Nursing care
   1. Teach dietary modification to achieve a low fat intake (about 25% of the kcal) because reduced bile flow will reduce fat absorption; supplementation with water miscible forms of vitamins A and E may be prescribed
   2. Relieve pain both preoperatively and postoperatively
   3. Observe for signs of bleeding (vitamin K is fat soluble and is not absorbed in the absence of bile); administer vitamin K preparations as ordered
   4. Teach the client receiving chenodiol (Chenix) that
   a. Effects will be monitored every 6 to 9 months by cholecystogram or ultrasonogram
   b. Side effects include hepatotoxicity and diarrhea
   5. Provide care following a cholecystectomy
   a. Monitor nasogastric tube attached to suction to prevent distention
       (1) Maintain patency of the tube
       (2) Assess and measure drainage
   b. Provide fluids and electrolytes via intravenous route
       (1) Monitor intake and output
       (2) Check IV site for redness, swelling, heat, or pain
   c. Keep the client in a low-Fowler's position
   d. Have the client cough and deep breathe; splint the incision (incision is high and midline, making coughing extremely uncomfortable)
   e. Provide care for the client with a T tube (if the common bile duct has been explored, a T tube is inserted to maintain patency)
       (1) Secure the drainage bag; avoid kinking of the tube
       (2) Measure drainage at least every shift; drainage during the first day may reach 500 to 1000 ml and then gradually decline
       (3) Apply protective ointments, if ordered, to prevent excoriation
       (4) When the tube is removed, usually in 7 days, observe stool for normal brown color, which indicates bile is again entering the duodenum
   6. Evaluate client's response and revise plan as necessary

Acute Pancreatitis

A. Etiology and pathophysiology
   1. May result from gallstones, alcoholism, carcinoma, or acute trauma to the pancreas or abdomen
   2. Inflammation with or without edema of pancreatic tissues, suppuration, abscess formation, hemorrhage, or necrosis, depending on the severity of the disease and the cause
B. Signs and symptoms
   1. Subjective
   a. Abrupt onset of pain in the central epigastric area that may radiate to shoulder, chest, and back described as aching, burning, stabbing, or pressing
   b. Abdominal tenderness
   c. Nausea
   2. Objective
   a. Elevated temperature
   b. Vomiting
   c. Tachycardia
   d. Changes in character of stools
   e. Hypotension
   f. Shock
   g. Grossly elevated serum amylase and lipase
   3. Severity of symptoms depends on the cause of the problem, the amount of fibrous replacement of normal duct tissue, the degree of autodigestion of the organ, the type of associated biliary disease if present, and the amount of interference in blood supply to the pancreas
   4. Symptoms may be exaggerated by the development of complications such as pseudocysts, abscesses, pancreatic fistulas, and hyperglycemia
C. Treatment
   1. Antacids to neutralize gastric secretions
   2. Barbiturates and tranquilizers to reduce emotional tension
   3. Narcotics to control pain
   4. Cardiotonics to lessen strain on the heart caused by increased metabolic demands and altered circulatory volume
   5. Bed rest to decrease metabolic demands and promote healing
   6. Nasogastric decompression to control nausea and remove gastric hydrochloric acid
   7. Diet regulated according to the client's condition: nothing by mouth; parenteral administration of fluid, electrolytes, and other nutrients; diet low in fats and proteins, with restriction of stimulants such as caffeine and alcohol
   8. Anticholinergics to suppress vagal stimulation and decrease gastric motility and duodenal spasm
   9. Antibiotics to prevent secondary infections and abscess formation
   10. Surgical intervention if the client fails to respond to medical management, develops persistent jaundice, or bleeds; type of surgery is determined by the cause (e.g., biliary tract surgery, removal of gallstones, drainage of cysts)
D. Nursing care
   1. Provide care for a client with a nasogastric tube
   a. Administer frequent, thorough mouth care

b. Apply lubricant to the external nares to prevent irritation and eventual breakdown of mucous membranes

c. Observe for electrolyte imbalances (manifested by symptoms such as tetany, irritability, jerking, muscular twitching, mental changes, and psychotic behavior)

d. Observe for signs of adynamic ileus (e.g., nausea and vomiting, abdominal distention)

2. Be alert for hyperglycemic states
3. Monitor vital signs
4. Teach importance of taking medication containing pancreatic enzymes (amylase, lipase, trypsin, etc.) with each meal to improve digestion of food
5. Encourage the adoption of a life-style that allows for emotional stability, rest, follow-up medical care
6. Use the semi-Fowler's position and encourage deep breathing and coughing to promote deeper respiration and prevent respiratory problems
7. Maintain npo during the acute stage of illness
8. Closely monitor IV feedings until oral feedings can be tolerated
9. Teach dietary modifications as required by the client's condition, usually starting with small feedings of low fat, nongas-producing liquids and progressing to a more liberalized diet which is low in fat but high in protein and carbohydrates; if fat malabsorption is severe, water-miscible forms of vitamins A and E may be necessary; daily supplements of calcium and zinc may also be needed; if insulin secretion is impaired, diabetic diet is indicated (See Diabetes mellitus for details)
10. Teach the client and family the importance of dietary discretion, especially the avoidance of alcohol, coffee, spicy foods, and heavy meals, while recognizing religious and cultural factors
11. Help the client set realistic goals for convalescent period
12. Teach the client and family about prevention of recurrences and/or control of symptoms (e.g., diet therapy, drug therapy, avoiding foods and substances such as alcohol and caffeine, regular medical supervision, rest requirements)
13. Evaluate client's response and revise plan as necessary

Cancer of the Pancreas

A. Etiology and pathophysiology
1. Malignant growth from the epithelium of the ductal system producing cells that block the ducts of the pancreas
2. Fibrosis, pancreatitis, and obstruction of the pancreas
3. Lesion tends to metastasize by direct extension to the duodenal wall, splenic flexure of the colon, posterior stomach wall, and common bile duct
4. Cause unknown

B. Signs and symptoms
1. Subjective
   a. More common in middle-aged men than women
   b. History of chronic pancreatitis, diabetes mellitus, and alcoholism is common

c. Weight loss, anxiety, depression, anorexia, and nausea

d. Severe pain present in most clients

2. Objective
   a. Jaundice
   b. Diarrhea and steatorrhea, along with clay-colored stools and dark urine
   c. In later stages usually demonstrates presence of a right upper quadrant mass
   d. Decreased serum amylase and lipase levels due to decreased secretion of enzymes
   e. Increased serum bilirubin and alkaline phosphatase levels when biliary ducts are obstructed

C. Treatment
1. Prepare for surgical intervention by ordering red blood cell and blood volume replacement and medications to correct coagulation problems and nutritional deficiencies
2. Chemotherapy and radiation when surgery is not possible to provide comfort, or in conjunction with surgery to limit metastasis
3. Medications to control diabetes if present
4. Drug therapy such as pancreatic enzymes, bile salts, and vitamin K to correct deficiencies
5. Analgesics and tranquilizers for pain
6. Surgery (the treatment of choice, although the post-surgical prognosis is grim): Whipple procedure (removal of the head of the pancreas, the duodenum, a portion of the stomach, and the common bile duct) or a cholecystojejunostomy (creation of an opening between the gallbladder and jejunum)

D. Nursing care
1. Provide emotional support for the client and family and set realistic goals in planning care
2. Administer analgesics as ordered, and as soon as needed, to promote rest and comfort
3. Use soapless bathing and antipruritic agents to relieve pruritus
4. Observe for complications such as peritonitis, gastrointestinal obstruction, jaundice, hyperglycemia, and hypotension if client has undergone surgery
5. Observe the stools for undigested fat
6. Frequently monitor the vital signs, observing for wound hemorrhage caused by coagulation deficiency
7. Administer vitamin K parenterally as ordered
8. Encourage coughing, turning, and deep breathing
9. Assist with IPPB therapy as required
10. Monitor urinary output
11. Observe for chemotherapeutic and radiation side effects (e.g., skin irritation, anorexia, nausea, vomiting)
12. Maintain skin markings of the radiation therapist
13. Support natural defense mechanisms of the client by encouraging frequent and supplemental feedings of high nutrient density foods as tolerated; stress the immune stimulating nutrients, especially vitamins A, C, and E, and the mineral selenium
14. Control nausea and vomiting before feedings, if possible
15. Administer vitamin supplements, bile salts, and pancreatic enzymes, as ordered

16. Provide oral hygiene and maintain an esthetic environment especially at mealtime
17. Evaluate client's response and revise plan as necessary

Hepatitis

A. Etiology and pathophysiology
1. Type A hepatitis (infectious hepatitis)
   a. Caused by Type A hepatitis virus (HAV)
   b. Transmitted via fecal-oral route, contact with blood, or contaminated food (e.g., shellfish)
   c. Excreted in large quantities in feces 2 weeks before and 1 week after the onset of symptoms
   d. Incubation period is 30 to 40 days
   e. Confers immunity on individual
2. Type B hepatitis (serum hepatitis)
   a. Caused by Type B hepatitis virus (HBV)
   b. Transmitted by
      (1) Contaminated blood or blood products (e.g., toothbrush, razor, needle)
      (2) Other body secretions (e.g., saliva, semen, urine)
      (3) Introduction of infectious material into eye, oral cavity, lacerations, or vagina
      (4) Contaminated needles
         (a) During administration of medication
         (b) Shared by drug users
   c. Incubation period is 40 to 180 days
3. Phases of disease
   a. Prodromal or preicteric
   b. Icteric
   c. Recovery (may take 4 months)
4. Progression to cirrhosis, hepatic coma, and death may occur, although this is rare
5. Other causes of hepatitis include chemical agents such as halothane (an anesthetic agent), carbon tetrachloride, gold compounds, and arsenic)
B. Signs and symptoms
1. Prodromal (preicteric) phase
   a. Malaise
   b. Weight loss
   c. Anorexia
   d. Symptoms of upper respiratory tract infection
   e. Intolerance for smoking
2. Icteric phase
   a. Jaundice
   b. Bile-colored urine that foams when shaken
   c. Acholic (clay-colored) stools
3. Recovery phase: easy fatiguability
C. Prevention
1. Thorough hand washing by hospital personnel
2. Utilization of disposable equipment when contact with feces, blood, or body secretions is expected
3. Careful handling of needles (dispose of needles without recapping to prevent self-injury and contamination)
4. Administration of immune serum globulin (ISG) after exposure to Type A hepatitis
5. Vaccination of individuals at risk for Type B hepatitis (vaccine developed from HB AG)
D. Treatment
1. Rest
2. Diet therapy
   a. High protein: healing of liver tissue vital; daily intake should include 1 qt milk, 2 eggs, 8 oz lean meat, fish, or cheese; total should approximate 75 to 100 g protein
   b. High carbohydrate: energy needs, restore glycogen reserves; use daily 4 servings vegetables including potato, 4 servings fruit with frequent juices, 6 to 8 servings bread or cereal; total carbohydrate should be 300 to 400 g
   c. Moderate fat: 2 to 4 tablespoons butter or fortified margarine, sufficient for making food palatable; a moderate amount of easily digestible foods such as whole milk, cream, butter, margarine, or vegetable oil is beneficial; total fat should be 100 to 150 g daily
   d. High calorie: increased energy needs for disease process and tissue regeneration and to spare protein for healing; these food amounts should provide about 2500 to 3000 calories daily
   e. Water-miscible forms of vitamins A and E should be given when steatorrhea is present; also mineral supplements of calcium and zinc
E. Nursing care
1. Encourage quiet activities
2. Attempt to stimulate the appetite
   a. Provide oral hygiene
   b. Select foods based on the client's preferences
   c. Provide a pleasant, unhurried atmosphere for eating
   d. Provide small, frequent feedings that are usually tolerated better than large meals
3. Use special precautions to prevent the spread of infectious hepatitis to others
   a. Do not cap used needles; dispose of needles by immediately placing them in hard collection containers
   b. Dispose of uneaten food and utensils by using a double-bag procedure for contaminated materials
   c. Wear gloves when handling the client's bedpan
4. Evaluate client's response and revise plan as necessary

Hepatic Cirrhosis

A. Etiology and pathophysiology
1. Irreversible fibrosis and degeneration of the liver
2. Several types of cirrhosis; Laënnec's (alcoholic cirrhosis, nutritional cirrhosis) most common
3. Incidence higher in alcoholics, who are often malnourished, and in those who have had hepatitis
4. Pressure rises in the portal system (which drains blood from the digestive organs), causing stasis and backup in digestive organs
5. As liver failure progresses, there is increased secretion of aldosterone, decreased absorption and utilization of the fat-soluble vitamins (A, D, E, K), and ineffective detoxification of protein wastes
6. Hepatic coma may result from high blood ammonia levels when the liver is unable to convert the ammonia to urea

B. Signs and symptoms
  1. Subjective
    a. Nausea
    b. Weakness, fatigue
    c. Anorexia
    d. Abdominal discomfort
  2. Objective
    a. Weight loss
    b. Ascites
    c. Esophageal varices as a result of portal hypertension
    d. Hemorrhoids
    e. Edema of extremities
    f. Hematemesis
    g. Hemorrhage due to decreased formation of prothrombin
    h. Jaundice
    i. Delirium caused by rising blood ammonia levels
    j. Elevated liver enzymes (SGOT, SGPT, LDH)
    k. Decreased serum albumin
C. Treatment
  1. Rest
  2. Restriction of alcohol intake
  3. Vitamin therapy: especially A, D, E, and K
  4. Diuretics to control ascites and edema
  5. Neomycin and lactulose may be prescribed for elevated blood ammonia levels
  6. If respiratory distress occurs as a result of ascites, a paracentesis is done; slow removal of fluid from the peritoneal cavity will relieve acute symptoms
  7. Surgical intervention for portal hypertension: a portal-caval shunt, in which the circulation from the portal vein bypasses the liver and enters the vena cava, usually decreases portal hypertension
  8. Blakemore-Sengstaken tube is utilized in the treatment of bleeding esophageal varices to apply direct pressure to the varices
  9. Dietary modification
    a. Cirrhosis
      (1) Protein according to tolerance: with increasing liver damage protein metabolism is hindered; hold to 80 to 100 g as long as tolerated; reduce as necessary
      (2) Continue high carbohydrate, moderate fat as in hepatitis to supply energy; vitamin supplements, especially B complex and water-miscible forms of vitamins A and E; mineral supplements of calcium and zinc
      (3) Low sodium: usually restricted to 500 to 1000 mg daily by eliminating salt and controlling foods processed with salt or sodium-based preservatives; sodium restriction helps to control the increasing ascites
      (4) Soft foods: if esophageal varices are present, to prevent danger of rupture and bleeding
      (5) Alcohol strictly forbidden, to avoid continued irritation and malnutrition
    b. Hepatic coma
      (1) Low protein: reduced according to tolerance, 15 to 30 g

      (2) High calories and vitamins according to need: about 1500 to 2000 calories, sufficient to prevent tissue catabolism and the liberation of additional nitrogen
      (3) Fluid carefully controlled according to output
D. Nursing care
  1. Observe the client for objective signs of disease
  2. Observe mental status, which may vary
  3. Observe for bleeding
  4. Provide special skin care and keep nails trimmed, since pruritis is associated with jaundice
  5. Maintain the client in a semi-Fowler's position to prevent ascites from causing dyspnea
  6. Monitor intake and output, abdominal girth, and daily weight to assess fluid balance
  7. Assist with paracentesis (see procedure)
  8. Provide care when a Blakemore-Sengstaken tube is in place
    a. Maintain traction once the tube is passed and the gastric balloon is inflated to ensure proper placement
    b. Maintain the esophageal balloon as it has been inflated to 30 to 35 mm Hg
    c. If ordered, deflate the balloon for a few minutes at specific intervals to prevent necrosis
    d. Irrigate with iced saline if ordered
    e. Suction orally as necessary, since the client is unable to swallow saliva
  9. Teach dietary modifications since ability of client to understand and remember instructions is often impaired due to hepatic encephalopathy
    a. Focus teaching efforts on the family
    b. Limit high protein foods
    c. Emphasize the use of carbohydrate foods such as pasta, rice, and potatoes to supply needed energy
    d. Limit salt intake
    e. Inform client that fats can be used to supply calories and improve food palatability unless steatorrhea occurs
    f. Repeat instructions to reinforce teaching
  10. Evaluate client's response and revise plan as necessary

Carcinoma of the Liver

A. Etiology and pathophysiology
  1. May be primary or metastatic carcinoma; primary carcinoma of the liver is rare
  2. Generally lethal within a few months
B. Signs and symptoms
  1. Subjective
    a. Anorexia
    b. Ache in epigastric area
  2. Objective
    a. Weight loss
    b. Anemia
C. Treatment
  1. Generally palliative
  2. Hepatic lobectomy if the tumor is confined (the liver has extraordinary regenerative capacity)
  3. Percutaneous infusions with cytotoxic agents

D. Nursing care
1. Provide comfort
2. Be available to both the client and family members to discuss their feelings
3. Provide care following hepatic surgery
   a. Maintain fluid and electrolyte balance with IV therapy
   b. Monitor intake and output
   c. Observe for signs of bleeding, hypoglycemia, and other metabolic dysfunctions resulting from impaired liver function
   d. Have the client cough, deep breathe, and change position frequently to prevent pulmonary and circulatory complications
   e. Because the thoracic cavity may be entered during surgery, be aware of the care of a client with chest tubes (see procedure for chest tubes)
4. Evaluate client's response and revise plan as necessary

Sprue

A. Etiology and pathophysiology
1. Etiology unknown; possible hereditary factor
2. Nontropical sprue similar to celiac disease in children and is characterized by intolerance to gluten, abnormalities in the structure of the small intestine, and malabsorption
3. Tropical sprue is endemic in the Indian subcontinent and the Caribbean and is thought to be due to infection rather than diet
4. Intolerance to gluten results in blunting of the intestinal villi, which reduces absorptive surface of the intestinal mucosa
B. Signs and symptoms
1. Subjective
   a. Anorexia
   b. Fatigability
2. Objective
   a. Weight loss
   b. Anemia (macrocytic)
   c. Diarrhea
   d. Steatorrhea
   e. Visualization of the small bowel demonstrates flat, blunt villi
   f. Tetany
   g. Demineralization of the skeletal system
C. Treatment
1. Tropical sprue may respond to a high-protein, normal-fat diet with supplemental vitamin B_{12}, A, D, E, K, folic acid, and iron; in addition, antibiotics such as tetracycline for at least 6 months may be helpful
2. Nontropical sprue may respond to a high-protein, normal-fat, gluten-gliadin-free diet and vitamin supplements of A, D, K, B complex, and folic acid, as well as iron and calcium
3. Whenever the disease does not respond to diet, corticosteroids may be used
4. Fluid and electrolyte imbalances must be restored
D. Nursing care
1. Teach the client and family how to modify the diet to comply with medical management

2. Instruct family that rice, corn, and soy flours should be used in place of wheat, rye, barley, and oats
3. Inform the client of the importance of reading labels, since gluten-containing grains are added to many products, and of the need to question the contents of foods in restaurants
4. Advise the client as to the importance of followup care for disease management
5. Provide an opportunity for the client and family to verbalize feelings about the illness
6. Observe the client for signs of electrolyte imbalance
7. Record weight on a regular basis
8. Evaluate client's response and revise plan as necessary

Appendicitis

A. Etiology and pathophysiology
1. Compromised circulation and inflammation of the vermiform appendix
2. Causes include obstruction by a fecalith, foreign body, or kinking
3. Inflammation may be followed by edema, necrosis, and rupture
B. Signs and symptoms
1. Subjective
   a. Anorexia
   b. Nausea
   c. Right lower quadrant pain
   d. Rebound tenderness
2. Objective
   a. Vomiting
   b. Fever
   c. Leukocytosis
C. Treatment
1. Surgical removal of the appendix without delay to decrease the chance of rupture and the risk of peritonitis
2. Prophylactic use of antibiotics postoperatively
3. Fluid and electrolyte maintenance
4. Analgesics for pain
D. Nursing care
1. Provide emotional support, since this condition is unanticipated and the individual needs to ventilate any fear of surgery
2. Monitor fluid and electrolyte balance
3. Assess the client for signs of infection
4. Encourage early ambulation, if not contraindicated by the client's condition, to prevent complications
5. Assess the client's return of bowel function
6. Evaluate client's response and revise plan as necessary

Regional Enteritis

A. Etiology and pathophysiology
1. Etiology unknown
2. Usually occurs in young adults, but can occur at any age
3. Inflammatory changes involving any part of the alimentary tract but usually demarcated segments of the small bowel

4. Ulceration of the intestinal submucosa accompanied by congestion, thickening of the small bowel, and fissure formations
5. Enlargement of regional lymph nodes
6. Fibrosis and narrowing of the intestinal wall
7. Abscesses and fistulas of the abdominal wall, bladder, and vagina

B. Signs and symptoms
   1. Subjective
      a. Pain in the lower right quadrant, cramping, and spasms
      b. Nausea
      c. Exacerbations related to emotional upsets or dietary indiscretions with milk, milk products, and fried foods
   2. Objective
      a. Borborygmus (rumbling, gurgling sound in the intestines), flatulence
      b. Weight loss
      c. Fever
      d. Electrolyte disturbance
      e. Diarrhea
      f. Gastrointestinal x-ray series to detect and outline the congested, thickened, fibrosed, and narrowed appearance of the intestinal wall; also abscesses and fistulas, partial bowel obstruction, and ulceration of the mucosa
      g. Proctosigmoidoscopy is performed to exclude other diseases, such as ulcerative colitis and diverticulitis
      h. Stools are examined for the presence of blood, fat, protein, parasites, or ova
      i. Fecal fat test is performed to determine fat content, an abnormal amount of which is significant in malabsorptive disorders or hypermotility
      j. D-Xylose tolerance test is performed to determine absorptive ability of upper intestinal tract

C. Treatment
   1. Nothing by mouth in the presence of vomiting
   2. Clear fluid diet progressing to bland low-residue, low-fat diet but increased calories, proteins, vitamins (especially vitamin K), and carbohydrates
   3. Total parenteral nutrition (TPN) may be ordered when oral intake is inadequate
   4. Medications such as
      a. Antiemetics
      b. Vitamins and minerals
      c. Anticholinergics
      d. Antidiarrheics
      e. Antiinflammatories
      f. Antiinfectives
   5. Surgery (resection of diseased part) if the client does not respond to medical therapy or if complications such as obstruction, abscesses, or fistulas occur

D. Nursing care
   1. Monitor intake and output
   2. Offer clear liquids hourly as ordered once the client ceases to experience nausea and vomiting
   3. Encourage high-calorie, high-protein, high-carbohydrate diet supplemented with vitamins and potassium as ordered

4. Assist with total parenteral nutrition (TPN) if ordered (see procedure)
5. Offer small, frequent feedings considering client preference, types of food allowed, and esthetic factors
6. Record weight daily
7. Observe for signs of complications such as elevated temperature, increasing nausea and vomiting, abdominal rigidity
8. Communicate concern and awareness regarding the client's discomfort and emotional lability during exacerbations of this chronic illness
9. Teach the client
   a. To avoid taking laxatives and salicylates that irritate the intestinal mucosa
   b. How to take antidiarrheics and mucilloid drugs effectively and the observations to make during their use
   c. Skin care if the perineal area is irritated
   d. The importance of seeking help early when exacerbations occur
10. Evaluate client's response and revise plan as necessary

Crohn's Disease

A. Etiology and pathophysiology
   1. Although the causative mechanisms are unknown, there are various theories involving genetic predisposition, autoimmune reaction, or environmental causes
   2. Cobblestone ulcerations form along the mucosal wall of the terminal ileum, cecum, and ascending colon, which form scar tissue and inhibit food and water absorption in the area
   3. Ulcerations may perforate through the intestinal wall and form fistulas with adjoining organs

B. Signs and symptoms
   1. Subjective
      a. Severe pain in the right lower quadrant
      b. Malaise
   2. Objective
      a. Moderate fever
      b. Elevated WBC
      c. Mild diarrhea with mucus but no blood
      d. Anemia

C. Treatment
   1. High-calorie, high-protein diet
   2. Vitamin supplements, including B_{12}, if a large portion of ileum is involved
   3. Medications such as
      a. Anticholinergics
      b. Analgesics
      c. Intestinal antibiotics
      d. Immunosuppressives
   4. Surgery when fistulas or intestinal obstruction occurs; the involved area of intestine is removed and the ends are anastomosed, if possible; an ostomy is indicated if large areas of intestine are involved

D. Nursing care
   1. Provide an emotionally therapeutic environment in which client can communicate concerns and stresses resulting from this illness

2. Instruct client regarding dietary restrictions and modifications (See Ulcerative Colitis)
3. Observe client for signs of fluid and electrolyte imbalances
4. Evaluate client's response and revise plan as necessary

Ulcerative Colitis

A. Etiology and pathophysiology
   1. May be caused by emotional stress, an autoimmune response, or a genetic predisposition
   2. Edema of the mucous membrane of the colon leads to bleeding and shallow ulcerations
   3. Abscess formation occurs, and the bowel wall shortens and becomes thin and fragile
   4. There is shortening of the intestinal wall, which leads to diarrhea
B. Signs and symptoms
   1. Subjective
      a. Weakness, debilitation
      b. Anorexia
      c. Nausea
   2. Objective
      a. Dehydration with poor skin turgor
      b. Passage of bloody, purulent, mucoid, watery stools
      c. Anemia
      d. Low-grade fever
C. Treatment
   1. Dietary management
      a. Diet plays a major role in the management of colitis; emphasis has changed from a low-residue diet to a more liberal diet (restricted roughage may be useful during more acute attacks of severe cramps, diarrhea, and bleeding but seems to have little effect on preventing relapses); supplementing diet with raw bran has been shown to be effective in controlling bouts of diarrhea and constipation
      b. If tolerated, unrestricted fluid intake; high-protein, high-calorie diet; avoidance of food allergens, especially milk
   2. Medications such as
      a. Antiemetics
      b. Anticholinergics
      c. Corticosteroids
      d. Antibiotics
      e. Sedatives, analgesics, and tranquilizers
      f. Antidiarrheics
   3. Replacement of fluids and electrolytes that are lost because of diarrhea
   4. A temporary ileostomy, a partial colectomy, or a total colectomy with a permanent ileostomy may be performed when
      a. No response to medical treatment is evident
      b. Course of the disease is downhill
      c. Massive hemorrhage or colonic obstruction occurs
      d. Cancer is suspected
D. Nursing care
   1. Instruct client to adhere to the following dietary program

a. Eat small, frequent feedings of high-protein, high-calorie foods (low fat helps decrease steatorrhea which is common with ileal involvement; if steatorrhea is present, water-miscible forms of vitamins A and E may be required as supplements)
b. Avoid irritating spices such as red or black pepper
c. Replace iron, calcium, and zinc losses with supplements; if there is ileal involvement, intramuscular injections of vitamin B_{12} may be prescribed monthly
d. Avoid all food allergens, especially milk (milk has been implicated as a direct cause of colitis in infants and is often associated with diarrhea in adults); milk may be reintroduced when client is relatively asymptomatic; however, lactose intolerance is common in this condition and dairy restrictions may be permanent (some lactose-intolerant individuals can manage yogurt, buttermilk, and hard cheeses; lactase enzyme preparations are available which can be added to milk products to hydrolyze lactose)
   2. Teach importance of diet in controlling and/or minimizing symptoms
   3. Involve the client in dietary selection, recognizing preferences as much as possible
   4. Initiate accurate administration and recording of fluid, electrolyte, or blood replacements as ordered by the physician
   5. Plan nursing care to allow the client complete bed rest and the maximum number of rest periods
   6. Institute comfort measures (e.g., a warm powdered bedpan, sheepskin under the buttocks, gentle thorough perineal care) as required
   7. Observe for complications such as rectal hemorrhage, fever, dehydration
   8. Allow the client and family time to verbalize feelings and participate in care
   9. If an ileostomy is performed, help the client accept the changes of body image and function involved (see Ileostomy care)
   10. Evaluate client's response and revise care as necessary

Intestinal Obstruction

A. Etiology and pathophysiology
   1. Interference with normal peristaltic movement of intestinal contents due to neurologic or mechanical impairments
   2. Causes
      a. Carcinoma of the bowel
      b. Hernias
      c. Adhesions (scar tissue that forms abnormal connections after surgery or inflammation)
      d. Intussusception (telescoping of the bowel on itself)
      e. Volvulus (twisting of the intestines)
      f. Paralytic ileus (interference with neural innervation of the intestines resulting in a decrease in or absence of peristalsis; may be caused by surgical manipulation, electrolyte imbalance, or infection)

B. Signs and symptoms
   1. Subjective
      a. Colicky abdominal pain
      b. Constipation
   2. Objective
      a. Abdominal distention
      b. Vomiting; may contain fecal matter
      c. Decreased or absent bowel sounds
      d. Signs of dehydration and electrolyte imbalance
      e. Flat plate of the abdomen shows the bowel distended with air
C. Treatment
   1. Restriction of oral intake; administration of parenteral fluid and electrolytes
   2. Surgical correction of cause (e.g., hernias, adhesions)
   3. Colostomy, cecostomy, or ileostomy as necessary
   4. Drugs such as pantothenyl alcohol (Ilopan) and neostigmine (Prostigmin) to stimulate the passage of flatus
   5. Gastric decompression by means of a nasogastric, Cantor, or Miller-Abbott tube
D. Nursing care
   1. Assess the client for dehydration and electrolyte imbalance
   2. Monitor intake and output
   3. Auscultate for bowel sounds; note the passage of flatus
   4. Administer mouth care frequently
   5. Measure abdominal girth daily to assess distention
   6. Provide special care for the client with a Miller-Abbott or Cantor tube
      a. Once the lubricated tube is inserted, position the client first on the right side, to facilitate passage of tube through the pylorus, and then in a semi-Fowler's position, to continue the gradual advance into the intestines
      b. Coil and loosely attach extra tubing to the client's gown to avoid tension against peristaltic action
      c. Irrigate as ordered to maintain patency
      d. Frequently assess placement of the tube; record the level of advancement
      e. When the tube is discontinued by the physician remove the tube gradually because it is being pulled against peristalsis
   7. Evaluate client's response and revise plan as necessary

Cancer of the Small and Large Intestines

A. Etiology and pathophysiology
   1. Cancer of the colon and rectum: can cause a narrowing of the lumen of the bowel, ulcerations, necrosis, or perforation
   2. Predisposing factors include familial polyps, chronic ulcerative colitis, and possibly bowel stasis or ingestion of food additives
   3. A high-fat, low-fiber diet has been implicated as a causative factor in colon cancer; it is thought that fat and/or bile is chemically altered by intestinal bacteria producing carcinogens which are responsible for the development of cancer; absence of dietary fiber tends to slow the passage of stool through the colon giving carcinogens more time in contact with the surface of the mucosa
   4. Cancer of the colon: more common in males, and incidence increases after 50 years of age
   5. Cancer of the small intestine: usually adenocarcinoma
B. Signs and symptoms
   1. Subjective
      a. Abdominal discomfort
      b. Weakness
   2. Objective
      a. Alterations in usual bowel function (constipation or diarrhea or alternating constipation and diarrhea)
      b. Blood in stool
      c. Distention
      d. Changes in shape of stool (pencil- or ribbon-shaped)
      e. Weight loss
      f. Secondary anemia
C. Treatment (including diagnosis)
   1. Diagnostic measures
      a. Digital examination of the rectum to detect any palpable masses
      b. Proctosigmoidoscopy to visualize the bowel directly to determine the presence of abnormalities and to perform a biopsy
      c. Stool examination to test for occult blood
      d. Cytologic examination to detect for malignant cells
      e. Hemoglobin level to detect anemia
      f. Alkaline phosphatase and SGOT levels to detect metastasis to the liver
      g. Serum carcinoembryonic antigen (CEA): measure to screen for carcinoma of the colon
   2. After diagnosis is established, the physician may prepare the client for surgery by
      a. Prescribing antibiotics to reduce bacteria in the bowel
      b. Typing and cross matching of blood for transfusions to correct the anemia
      c. Ordering vitamin supplements to improve the nutritional status
      d. Inserting a Cantor or Miller-Abbott tube with suction to decompress the colon
   3. Surgical intervention to remove the mass and restore bowel function (e.g., hemicolectomy, resection of the transverse colon, abdominal perineal resection)
   4. Radiation in nonsurgical situations in an attempt to relieve symptoms or postoperatively limit metastases
   5. Chemotherapy orally or parenterally in an attempt to reduce the lesion and limit metastases
   6. Postoperatively
      a. Antibiotic therapy to reduce infection
      b. Parenteral fluids and electrolytes to maintain balance
      c. Cholinergics to stimulate peristalsis

d. Cantor or Miller-Abbott tube clamped for regular, increasing periods and removed when the client is able to tolerate clamping and bowel sounds have returned

e. Sips of water progressing to clear liquid diet and to low-residue diet as tolerated

7. If colostomy has been performed
   a. Colostomy irrigations as required
   b. Irrigations of perineal incision if present and the application of enzymes such as streptokinase to liquefy protein matter and promote drainage

D. Nursing care
1. Observe vital signs, increasing abdominal pain, nausea, and vomiting to detect early signs of complications
2. Monitor patency of the Cantor or Miller-Abbott tube to ensure that accumulated air and fluid are decreased and distention is minimized; instill or irrigate the tube with normal saline as ordered
3. Note the character of drainage from the decompression tube
4. Implement measures for mechanical cleansing and intestinal antisepsis preoperatively (e.g., enemas, colonic irrigations, antibacterial therapy such as neomycin or sulfonamides)
5. Administer chemotherapeutic drugs if ordered and observe for significant side effects such as stomatitis (ulceration of the mouth), dehydration, nausea and vomiting, diarrhea, leukopenia
6. Administer electrolyte and parenteral fluid replacement as ordered in situations of bleeding, vomiting, and/or obstruction
7. Carefully note the client's tolerance to the introduction of oral fluids and foods while the intestinal tube is clamped
8. Teach the client and family dietary modifications, including low-residue, non-gas-forming foods, avoidance of stimulants, adequate fluid intake; diet should be as close to the client's normal as possible; encourage a positive attitude
9. Teach client the importance of diet in supporting the body's natural defense mechanisms; diet should emphasize high nutrient–density foods from the fruits, vegetables, cereal grains, and legumes groups with some lean meat, fish, and poultry; encourage client to eat as great a variety of foods as can be tolerated; vitamin and mineral supplements can be encouraged, especially the immune-stimulating factors
10. Provide colostomy care using medical aseptic technique (see procedure)
11. Recognize that the client with a colostomy may experience sadness, withdrawal, depression, and suicidal thoughts as a result of body image changes
12. Assess the client's reaction to the colostomy, recognizing that a great deal will depend on how the client sees it is affecting life-style, physical and emotional status, social and cultural background, and place and role in the family
13. Encourage involvement in colostomy care as soon as physical and emotional status permits
14. Encourage visiting by family members, stressing the client's increased need for love and acceptance

15. Recognize that the client with a cecostomy or colostomy is especially sensitive to gestures, odors, facial expressions, and the amount of attention given
16. Teach the client and family care of the colostomy, measures to facilitate acceptance and adjustment, resumption of activities, and the need for regular medical supervision
17. Teach the client that colostomy drainage can be controlled by following a regular irrigation schedule and dietary modifications
18. Arrange for follow-up care with community agencies as required (e.g., Public Health, Home Care Program, Cancer Society, ostomy resource person)
19. Evaluate client's response and revise plan as necessary

Peritonitis

A. Etiology and pathophysiology
1. Inflammation of the peritoneum
2. Generally caused by infection from perforation of GI tract or by chemical stress, as in pancreatitis

B. Signs and symptoms
1. Subjective
   a. Abdominal pain, rebound tenderness
   b. Malaise
   c. Nausea
2. Objective
   a. Muscle rigidity over the area
   b. Elevated temperature and WBC
   c. Vomiting

C. Treatment
1. Bed rest in a semi-Fowler's position to drain the area
2. Nasogastric tube attached to suction and left in place until the client passes flatus
3. Fluids and electrolytes replaced parenterally
4. Antibiotic therapy
5. Surgery to correct the cause of peritonitis (e.g., appendectomy, incision and drainage of abscesses, closure of a perforation)

D. Nursing care
1. Maintain the semi-Fowler's position to help localize infection in the pelvic area
2. Assess the client's temperature, vital signs, and pain
3. Monitor IV therapy and gastrointestinal decompression
4. Monitor intake and output
5. Auscultate for bowel sounds; note the passage of flatus
6. Evaluate client's response and revise plan as necessary

Hemorrhoids

A. Etiology and pathophysiology
1. Varicosities of the rectum that can be internal or external
2. Constipation, prolonged sitting or standing, straining at defecation, and pregnancy increase the risk of developing hemorrhoids
3. Prevention can often be achieved by high-fiber diets; soluable fibers such as pectin and guar gums are particularly effective

B. Signs and symptoms
1. Subjective
    a. Anal pain
    b. Pruritus
2. Objective
    a. Protrusion of varicosities around the anus
    b. Rectal bleeding and mucus discharge
C. Treatment
1. High-fiber diet (especially pectin containing fruits and vegetables) to prevent constipation
2. Low-roughage diet (elimination of raw fruits and vegetables) during acute exacerbations
3. Use of laxatives and stool softeners to regulate bowel habits
4. Analgesic suppositories and ointments may be prescribed in addition to sitz baths to alleviate discomfort
5. Internal hemorrhoids may be ligated with rubber bands; as necrosis occurs, the tissue sloughs off
6. Hemorrhoidectomy: surgical removal of hemorrhoids
D. Nursing care
1. Administer medication as ordered to relieve discomfort
2. Provide privacy and sufficient time for defecation
3. Educate client concerning good dietary and bowel habits
    a. Encourage generous daily intake of high-fiber foods including fresh fruits and vegetables, whole grain breads, and cereals and legumes
    b. Promote intake of at least 8 glasses of fluid per day
    c. Discourage routine use of laxatives which result in client dependency; bulking agents such as Metamucil may be prescribed
4. Assist the client with sitz baths
5. Administer cleansing enemas and prepare the perineal area preoperatively
6. Observe for rectal hemorrhage and urinary retention postoperatively
7. Administer a retention enema on the second or third postoperative day if ordered to stimulate defecation and soften the stool
8. Explain that postoperatively a small amount of bleeding with a bowel movement is normal
9. Evaluate client's response and revise plan as necessary

Hernias

A. Etiology and pathophysiology
1. Protrusion of an organ or structure through a weakening in the abdominal wall; may contain fat, intestine, or an organ, such as the bladder
2. Abdominal wall can become weakened due to a congenital or acquired defect
3. If the protruding structure can be manipulated back in place, the hernia is said to be reducible; if it cannot, it is considered incarcerated
4. Strangulation occurs when blood supply to the tissues within the hernia is disrupted; this is an emergency situation, since gangrene occurs

5. Hernias are named according to location
    a. Incisional: due to failure of fascia or muscles to heal postoperatively; intraabdominal pressure causes herniation through the scar tissue
    b. Umbilical: due to failure of the umbilicus to close at birth or to a congenital weakness of the musculature in the area; increased intraabdominal pressure due to obesity, pregnancy, or chronic cough causes herniation through the umbilicus
    c. Femoral: when a loop of intestine herniates through the femoral canal due to a weakness in the femoral ring; more common in women than men; strangulation is a common complication
    d. Inguinal: when a loop of intestine herniates through a weakened abdominal ring (frequently through the spermatic cord) into the inguinal canal; more common in men than women
B. Signs and symptoms
1. Subjective
    a. History of the appearance of swelling after lifting, coughing, or vigorous exercise
    b. Pain (may be due to irritation or strangulation)
    c. Nausea can accompany strangulation
2. Objective
    a. Swelling (lump) in the groin or umbilicus, or near an old surgical incision, that may subside when the client is in a recumbent position
    b. Vomiting and abdominal distention may develop when strangulation occurs
C. Treatment
1. Manual reduction by gently pushing the mass back into the abdominal cavity
2. When the client is a poor surgical risk, use of a truss (pad worn next to skin held in place under pressure by a belt)
3. Herniorrhaphy (surgical repair of the defect in the abdominal musculature or fascia)
4. Hernioplasty to prevent recurrence (wire, mesh, or plastic may be inserted to strengthen the abdominal wall)
D. Nursing care
1. Teach the client using a truss that it should be applied prior to getting out of bed
2. Provide care following surgery
    a. Observe the client for signs of respiratory infection; administer cough suppressants as ordered to prevent stress on the incision
    b. Instruct the client to self-splint when coughing and turning to provide incisional support
    c. When spinal or local anesthesia is used, peristalsis is not interfered with and postoperative diet can be normal; when general anesthesia is used, nasogastric decompression may be employed until peristalsis returns
    d. Administer mild cathartics as ordered to prevent straining and increased intraabdominal pressure at defecation
    e. Apply an ice bag and scrotal support with a rolled towel or suspensory if the scrotum is edematous postoperatively to reduce the edema and pain

f. Administer medication for pain as ordered when necessary

g. Instruct the client to avoid lifting or strenuous exercise on discharge until permitted by the surgeon

3. Evaluate client's response and revise plan as necessary

Anorexia Nervosa and Bulemia

(See discussion in Psychiatric Nursing)

Obesity

(See discussion in Psychiatric Nursing)

Food Poisoning

A. *Staphylococcus aureus*
   1. Etiology and pathophysiology
      a. Gram-positive *Staphylococcus* strain that clots plasma (coagulase positive); is the most virulent type and causes a variety of infections
      b. Most food poisoning resulting in GI upset occurs as a result of this bacterium
      c. Organism is found in unrefrigerated creams, mayonnaise, stuffing, meats, and fish
      d. Bacteria usually are transmitted to food on the hands of food handlers
      e. Incubation period is 1 to 6 hours after ingestion of contaminated food, with symptoms lasting 24 to 48 hours
   2. Signs and symptoms
      a. Subjective
         (1) Nausea
         (2) Malaise
         (3) Abdominal cramps and pain
      b. Objective
         (1) Diarrhea
         (2) Subnormal temperature
         (3) Vomiting
   3. Treatment
      a. Supply with adequate fluid and electrolytes orally or parenterally
      b. Bed rest
   4. Nursing care
      a. Offer fluids in small amounts as tolerated
      b. Teach the importance of eating foods that are properly prepared and stored
      c. Evaluate client's response and revise plan as necessary
B. Botulism
   1. Etiology and pathophysiology
      a. *Clostridium botulinum:* large, gram-positive bacillus; an obligate anaerobe; its exotoxin, the most powerful biologic toxic known, is responsible for botulism
      b. Organism causes the most serious, often fatal, form of food poisoning
      c. Toxins found in improperly processed foods (mostly canned foods) that have been infected with the anaerobic bacillus *Clostridium botulinum*

d. Toxins block neuromuscular transmission in cholinergic nerve fibers by possibly binding with acetylcholine

e. Incubation period usually 12 to 72 hours after ingestion of contaminated food, but may be as long as 4 to 8 days

   2. Signs and symptoms
      a. Subjective
         (1) Lassitude and fatigue
         (2) Diplopia
         (3) Weakness of muscles in the extremities
         (4) Dysphasia and dysphagia
      b. Objective
         (1) Diminished visual acuity
         (2) Loss of pupillary light reflex
         (3) Diminished gag reflex
   3. Treatment
      a. Keep the client in a darkened room
      b. IV feedings to prevent aspiration
      c. Tracheostomy and other supportive measures as necessary
      d. Cathartics and cleansing enemas to remove toxins from the body
      e. Trivalent antitoxins as necessary
   4. Nursing care
      a. Prevent aspiration pneumonia by proper positioning; keep suction equipment available at the bedside
      b. Carefully observe the client's neurologic status to determine progression of the disease
      c. Prevent contractures and emboli by the use of range-of-motion exercises
      d. Provide emotional support to the client and family in an attempt to reduce anxiety
      e. Evaluate client's response and revise plan as necessary
C. Salmonellosis
   1. Etiology and pathophysiology
      a. Many species of *Salmonella* cause a local GI infection in which organisms do not enter blood (unlike *S. typhosa* and *S. paratyphi*); such infections are referred to as salmonellosis or salmonella food poisoning
      b. Organisms found in inadequately cooked meats
      c. Multiply in the intestines, causing GI upset and infection
      d. Incubation period usually 10 to 24 hours after ingestion of contaminated food, and symptoms usually last 2 to 3 days
   2. Signs and symptoms
      a. Subjective
         (1) Nausea
         (2) Malaise
         (3) Abdominal cramps and pain
      b. Objective
         (1) Chills and fever
         (2) Vomiting
   3. Treatment
      a. Bed rest
      b. Fluid and electrolyte replacement

4. Nursing care
   a. Offer the client small amounts of fluids as tolerated
   b. Teach the client the importance of eating foods that have been cooked properly
   c. Evaluate client's response and revise plan as necessary

Genitourinary System
REVIEW OF ANATOMY AND PHYSIOLOGY OF THE GENITOURINARY SYSTEM
Urinary System
Functions

A. Secrete urine
B. Eliminate urine from body (urination, micturition, or voiding) to
   1. Excrete various normal and abnormal metabolic wastes
   2. Regulate the composition and volume of blood and regulate blood pressure; especially important in maintenance of fluid and electrolyte balance and acid-base balance (see Maintenance of fluid, electrolyte, and acid-base balance)

Organs
Kidneys

A. Gross anatomy
   1. Size, shape, and location: about 10 × 5 × 2.5 cm (4 × 2 × 1 inches); shaped like lima beans; lie against the posterior abdominal wall, behind the peritoneum at the level of the last thoracic and first three lumbar vertebrae; right kidney slightly lower than the left
   2. External structure
      a. Hilum: concave notch on the mesial surface; blood vessels, nerves, lymphatics, and ureter enter through this notch
      b. Renal capsule: protective fibrous tissue that envelops the kidney
   3. Internal structure
      a. Cortex: outer layer of the kidney substance; composed of renal corpuscles, convoluted tubules, and adjacent parts of loops of Henle
      b. Medulla: inner portion of the kidney; composed of loops of Henle and collecting tubules
      c. Pyramids: triangular wedges of medullary substance that have striped appearance and are composed of collecting tubules
      d. Columns: inward extensions of cortex between the pyramids
      e. Papillae: apices of the pyramids; collecting tubules drain into minor calyces here
      f. Calyces: bell-mouthed cups that drain the papillae; 8 to 12 minor calyces open into 2 or 3 major calyces that form the pelvis
      g. Pelvis: a small funnel tapering into the ureter and formed by union of several calyces
B. Blood flow in the kidney
   1. Kidneys receive 20% of cardiac output during rest; reduced to 2% to 4% during physical or emotional stress

2. Abdominal aorta gives rise to the renal artery, which enters the hilum of each kidney; renal artery branches into interlobar arteries which fan out into kidney cortex; smaller arterial branches form afferent arterioles, which enter glomerular capillary beds
3. Efferent arterioles leave the glomerular capillary bed forming the peritubular capillary network which then converges into progressively larger veins until the renal vein leaves the kidney

C. Nephron: anatomic and functional unit of the kidney; approximately one million per kidney
   1. Anatomy
      a. Glomerulus: cluster of capillaries invaginated into Bowman's capsule
      b. Bowman's capsule: the funnel-shaped upper end of the urinary tubules
      c. Renal corpuscle: composed of Bowman's capsule and the glomerulus invaginated into it
      d. Proximal convoluted tubule: first portion of kidney tubules
      e. Henle's loop: second portion of kidney tubules
      f. Distal convoluted tubule: third portion of kidney tubules
   2. Physiology: nephron functions via principles of filtration, reabsorption, and secretion (Fig. 3-6)
      a. Glomerulus: urine formation starts with process of filtration; water and solutes (except cellular elements of blood, albumins, fibrinogen, and other blood proteins) filter out of capillaries through glomerular-capsular membrane and into Bowman's capsule
      b. Bowman's capsule: filtrate collects here prior to flow to the tubules
      c. Tubular reabsorption and secretion: epithelial lining of tubules reabsorbs substances useful to the body and excretes, dissolved in water, all excess and waste substances; secretes electrolytes essential to acid-base balance
         (1) Proximal tubule
            (a) Reabsorption of glucose and other nutrients (e.g., vitamins and amino acids) from the tubular filtrate to the blood in the peritubular capillaries; mainly by active transport mechanisms in the tubular epithelium
            (b) Reabsorption of electrolytes from the tubule filtrate to blood in the peritubular capillaries; cations (notably sodium) are reabsorbed by active transport, stimulated by aldosterone; anions (notably chloride and bicarbonate) are reabsorbed by diffusion following cation transport
            (c) Reabsorption of about 80% of the water from the tubular filtrate to the blood in the peritubular capillaries by osmosis as a result of electrolyte reabsorption
         (2) Loop of Henle
            (a) Establishes osmotic conditions that promote water reabsorption

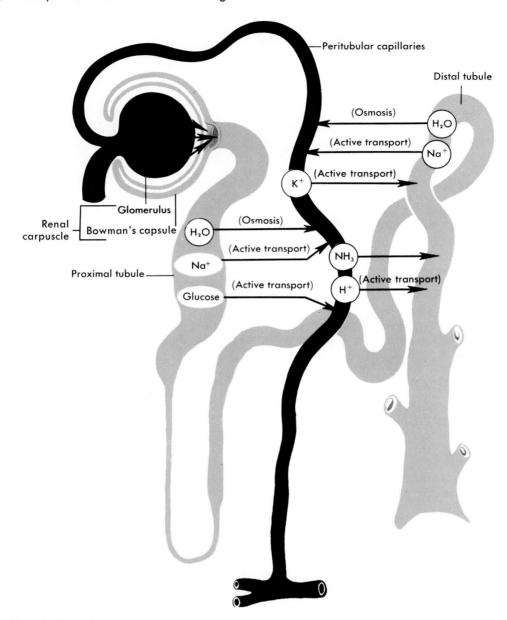

FIG. 3-6. Diagram showing glomerular filtration, tubular reabsorption, and tubular secretion—the three processes by which the kidneys secrete urine. In the proximal tubule, note that water is reabsorbed from the tubular filtrate and moves into the blood by osmosis (a passive transport mechanism) but that sodium and glucose are reabsorbed mainly by active transport mechanisms. Note also that water and sodium are reabsorbed from the distal tubule. Potassium and hydrogen ions (K^+ and H^+) and ammonia (NH_3), by contrast, are secreted into the tubule from the blood. (From Anthony CP and Thibodeau GA: Textbook of anatomy and physiology, ed 13, St. Louis, 1989, The CV Mosby Co.)

 (b) Actively transports chloride ions from the filtrate, thus passively removing sodium ions with the chloride; sodium chloride excretion results in increased osmotic force and promotes reabsorption of water in the collecting tubules

 (3) Distal tubule

  (a) Reabsorption of electrolytes, particularly sodium, under the influence of the mineralocorticoid aldosterone

  (b) Reabsorption of water into the blood by osmosis; ADH controls the amount of water osmosing out of the distal tubule, whereas amount of electrolytes reabsorbed controls the amount of osmosis out of the proximal tubule

  (c) Secretion of hydrogen, potassium, ammonia, and some other substances from the blood in the peritubular capillaries to the tubular filtrate; accomplished by active transport mechanism

D. Collecting tubules
1. Each collecting tubule receives urine from several nephrons
2. Under ADH influence, final osmotic reabsorption of most of the remaining water in urine occurs
E. Urine composition
1. Water: 1.5 L per day average
2. Urea: waste product of protein and amino acid metabolism
3. Uric acid: end product of purine metabolism or oxidation in the body
4. Creatinine: waste product of muscle metabolism
5. Ions (electrolytes): K^+, Na^+, Ca^{++}, Cl^-
6. Hormones and their breakdown products: presence of chorionic gonadotropin is the basis for a pregnancy test
7. Vitamins: particularly the water-soluble B vitamins and C
8. Drugs secreted in the urine (e.g., aspirin, penicillin, sulfa)
9. Other molecules, in low concentrations
10. Abnormal constituents: glucose, albumin, red blood cells, calculi
F. Urine volume is controlled normally by mechanisms that regulate the amount of water reabsorbed by the kidney tubules; only under abnormal conditions does the glomerular filtration rate influence urine volume
1. ADH mechanism: neurons in the hypothalamus (mainly in the supraoptic nucleus) produce the antidiuretic hormone, and the posterior pituitary gland secretes it into the blood; ADH secretion is stimulated by two conditions, an increase in the osmotic pressure of extracellular fluid or a decrease in the volume of extracellular fluid; ADH acts on distal and collecting tubules, causing more water to osmose from the tubular filtrate back into the blood; this increased water reabsorption tends to increase the total volume of body fluid by decreasing the urine volume; ADH has both a water-retaining and an antidiuretic effect
2. Aldosterone mechanism: an increase in aldosterone secretion tends to decrease urine volume by stimulating kidney tubules to reabsorb primarily more sodium and secondarily more water; thus aldosterone tends to produce sodium retention, water retention, and a low urine volume
3. Control by the amount of solutes in tubular filtrate; in general, an increase in tubular solutes causes decreased osmosis of water from proximal tubule back into blood and therefore an increase in urine volume (e.g., in diabetes, excess glucose in the tubular filtrate leads to increased urine volume [polyuria, diuresis])
4. Glomerular filtration rate normally is quite constant at about 125 ml per minute; it does not vary enough to alter volume of urine produced, but in certain pathologic conditions glomerular filtration rate may change markedly and alter urine volume (e.g., in shock the glomerular filtration decreases or even ceases, causing decreased urine volume [oliguria] or urinary suppression [anuria])

G. Control of amount of blood flow through kidneys
1. Reduced renal blood flow results in renal excretion of the hormone renin
2. Renin chemically interacts with blood proteins, producing angiotensin II
3. Angiotensin II causes vasoconstriction and aldosterone secretion, resulting in an increase in blood pressure and renal blood flow

Ureters

A. Location: behind the parietal peritoneum; extend from the kidneys to posterior part of the bladder floor
B. Structure: ureter expands as it enters the kidney to form the renal pelvis; subdivided into calyces, each of which contains renal papillae; ureter walls composed of smooth muscle with mucosa lining and fibrous outer coat
C. Function: collect urine secreted by the kidney cells and propel it to the bladder by peristaltic waves

Urinary Bladder

A. Location: behind symphysis pubis, below parietal peritoneum
B. Structure: collapsible bag of smooth muscle lined with mucosa arranged in rugae, three openings—two from ureters and one into the urethra
C. Functions
1. Reservoir for urine until sufficient amount accumulated for elimination
2. Expulsion of urine from body by way of urethra

Urethra

A. Location
1. Female: behind the symphysis pubis, in front of the vagina
2. Male: extends through the prostate gland, fibrous sheet, and penis
B. Structure: musculomembranous tube lined with mucosa; opening to exterior called urinary meatus
C. Functions
1. Female: passageway for expulsion of urine
2. Male: passageway for expulsion of both urine and semen

Reproductive System
Male Reproductive Organs
Glands

A. Main male sex glands (gonads) are the testes
1. Structure: fibrous capsule covers each testis and sends partitions into interior of gland, dividing it into lobules composed of tiny tubules called seminiferous tubules, embedded in connective tissue containing interstitial cells; ducts emerge from top of gland to enter head of epididymis
2. Location: in the scrotum, one testis in each compartment (two compartments)
3. Functions
a. Seminiferous tubules carry on spermatogenesis; that is, they form spermatozoa, the male sex cells, or gametes
b. Interstitial cells secrete testosterone, the main androgen, or male hormone

4. Structure of spermatozoon: consists of a head, middle piece, and whiplike tail that propels sperm; microscopic

B. Accessory glands
 1. Seminal vesicles
  a. Location: on posterior surface of the bladder
  b. Structure: convoluted pouches, mucous lining
  c. Function: secrete nutrient-rich fluid estimated to constitute about 30% of semen
 2. Prostate gland
  a. Location: encircles urethra just below bladder
  b. Structure: walnut-sized gland with ducts opening into urethra
  c. Function: secretes estimated 60% of semen; prostatic secretion is alkaline, which increases sperm motility; prostatic secretion contains abundance of enzyme, acid phosphatase; therefore blood level of this enzyme increases in metastasizing cancer of prostate
 3. Bulbourethral glands (Cowper's)
  a. Location: just below prostate gland
  b. Structure: small, pea-shaped structures with duct leading into urethra
  c. Function: secrete alkaline fluid that lubricates urethra prior to ejaculation

Ducts
A. Epididymis
 1. Location: lies along top and side of each testis
 2. Structure: each epididymis consists of single, tightly coiled tube enclosed in fibrous casing
 3. Function: conducts seminal fluid (semen) from testes to vas deferens; secretes small part of semen; stores semen prior to ejaculation, sperm mature during this period
B. Vas deferens (seminal ducts)
 1. Location: extend through inguinal canal into abdominal cavity, over top and down posterior surface of bladder to join ducts from seminal vesicles
 2. Structure: pair of tubes or ducts
 3. Function: conduct sperm and small amount of fluid from each epididymis to an ejaculatory duct
 4. Clinical application: vasectomy is the surgical procedure in which a short section of each vas is cut out and its separated ends tied off; as a result, sperm cannot enter the ejaculatory ducts and be ejaculated; semen from a vasectomized male contains no sperm; hence vasectomy sterilizes a man (makes him infertile); it does not render him impotent; it does, however, slightly decrease the amount of semen ejaculated
C. Ejaculatory ducts: formed by union of each vas with duct from seminal vesicle; pass through prostate gland to terminate in urethra; function: ejaculate semen into urethra
D. Urethra: described under Urinary system

Supporting Structures
A. External: scrotum and penis
 1. Scrotum: skin-covered pouch suspended from perineal region; divided into two compartments, each containing testis, epididymis, and first part of seminal duct; allows sperm to develop at 2° to 3° below the temperature of rest of body, which is ideal for sperm development
 2. Penis: made up of three cylindrical masses of erectile tissue that contain large vascular spaces; filling of these with blood causes erection of penis; two larger upper cylinders (corpora cavernosa) and one smaller lower cylinder (corpus cavernosum); the lower cylinder surrounds the urethra; glans penis: a bulging structure at distal end of the penis, over which a double fold of skin, the prepuce or foreskin, fits loosely (removed in circumcision)
B. Internal: spermatic cords are fibrous tubes located in each inguinal canal; serve as casing around each vas deferens and its accompanying blood vessels, lymphatics, and nerves

Female Reproductive Organs
Ovaries: Female Gonads
A. Location: behind and below uterine tubes, anchored to uterus and broad ligaments
B. Size and shape of large almonds
C. Microscopic structure: each ovary of the newborn female consists of several hundred thousand graffian follicles embedded in connective tissues; follicles are epithelial sacs in which ova develop; usually, between the years of menarche and menopause; one follicle matures each month, ruptures surface of the ovary, and expels its ovum into the pelvic cavity
D. Functions
 1. Oogenesis: formation of a mature ovum in a graafian follicle
 2. Ovulation: expulsion of the ovum from follicle into the pelvic cavity
 3. Secretion of female hormones: maturing follicle secretes estrogens; corpus luteum secretes progesterone and estrogens

Uterine Tubes (Fallopian Tubes, Oviducts)
A. Location: attached to upper, outer angles of uterus
B. Structure: same three coats as uterus; distal ends fimbriated and open into pelvic cavity; mucosal lining of tubes and peritoneal lining of pelvis in direct contact here (permits spread of infection from tubes to peritoneum)
C. Function: serve as ducts through which ova travel from ovaries to uterus; fertilization normally occurs in tube

Uterus
A. Location: in pelvic cavity between the bladder and rectum
B. Structure
 1. Shape and size: pear-shaped organ approximately the size of a clenched fist
 2. Divisions
  a. Body: upper and main part of the uterus; fundus, the bulging upper surface of the body
  b. Cervix: narrow, lower part of the uterus; projects into the vagina
 3. Walls: composed of smooth muscle (myometrium) lined with mucosa (endometrium)

4. Cavities
    a. Body cavity: small and triangular with three openings into it; two from uterine tubes, one into cervical canal
    b. Cervical cavity: canal with constricted opening, internal os into body cavity and another, external os, into vagina
C. Position: flexed between body and cervix portions with the body portion lying over the bladder, pointing forward and slightly upward; cervix joins the vagina at right angles; ligaments hold the uterus in position
    1. Broad ligaments (2): double fold of parietal peritoneum that forms a kind of partition across pelvic cavity, suspending uterus between its folds
    2. Uterosacral ligaments (2): foldlike extensions of peritoneum from posterior surface of uterus to sacrum, one on each side of rectum
    3. Posterior ligament (1): fold of peritoneum between posterior surface of uterus and rectum; forms deep pouch, cul-de-sac of Douglas (or rectouterine pouch); this pouch is the lowest point in the pelvic cavity and therefore the place where pus accumulates in pelvic inflammations; can be drained by posterior colpotomy (incision at top of the posterior vaginal wall)
    4. Anterior ligament (1): fold of peritoneum between uterus and bladder; forms shallow cul-de-sac
    5. Round ligaments (2): fibromuscular cords from upper, outer angles of uterus, through inguinal canals, terminating in labia majora
D. Functions
    1. Menstruation
    2. Pregnancy
    3. Labor

Vagina

A. Location: between rectum and urethra
B. Structure: collapsible, musculomembranous tube, capable of great distention; outlet to exterior covered by fold of mucous membrane called hymen
C. Functions
    1. Receives semen from the male
    2. Constitutes lower part of birth canal
    3. Acts as excretory duct for uterine secretions and menstrual flow

Vulva

Consists of numerous structures that together constitute external genitals
A. Mons veneris: hairy, skin-covered pad of fat over the symphysis pubis
B. Labia majora: hairy, skin-covered lips
C. Labia minora: small lips covered with modified skin
D. Clitoris: small mound of erectile tissue, below junction of two labia minora
E. Urinary meatus: just below clitoris; opening into urethra
F. Vaginal orifice: below urinary meatus; opening into vagina; hymen, fold of mucosa, partially closes orifice
G. Skene's glands: small mucous glands whose ducts open on each side of the urinary meatus

H. Bartholin's glands: two small, bean-shaped glands; duct from each gland opens on side of the vaginal orifice; both Bartholin's glands and Skene's glands have clinical interest because they frequently become infected (especially by gonococci)

Breasts, or Mammary Glands

A. Location: just under skin, over the pectoralis major muscles
B. Size: depends on deposits of adipose tissue rather than on amount of glandular tissue (which is approximately same in all females)
C. Structure: divided into lobes and lobules that, in turn, are composed of racemose glands; excretory duct leads from each lobe to opening in nipple; circular pigmented area, the areola, borders nipples
D. Function: secrete milk (lactation)
    1. Shedding of placenta causes marked decrease in blood levels of estrogens and progesterone, which in turn stimulates anterior pituitary to increase prolactin secretion; high blood level of prolactin stimulates alveoli of breast to secrete milk
    2. Suckling controls lactation in two ways; by acting in some way to stimulate anterior pituitary secretion of prolactin and to stimulate posterior pituitary secretion of oxytocin, which stimulates release of milk out of alveoli into ducts from which infant can remove it by suckling (letdown reflex)

Menstrual Cycle

A. Refers mainly to changes in the uterus and ovaries, which recur cyclically from the time of the menarche to the menopause
B. Length of cycle: usually 28 days, although considerable variations occur
C. Hormonal control of menstrual cycle
    1. Menses: brought on by marked decrease in blood levels of progesterone and estrogens at about cycle day 25
    2. Growth of new follicle and ovum: the low blood concentration of estrogens present for a few days before and during the menses stimulates the anterior pituitary gland to secrete follicle-stimulating hormone (FSH); the resulting high blood concentration of FSH stimulates one or more primitive graafian follicles and their ova to start growing and also stimulates the follicle cells to secrete estrogens; this leads to a high blood concentration of estrogens, which in turn has a negative feedback effect on FSH secretion by the anterior pituitary gland
    3. Endometrial thickening: in the preovulatory phase is caused by proliferation of endometrial cells stimulated by the increasing concentration of estrogens in blood; the premenstrual phase is caused partly by endometrial cell proliferation and partly by fluid retention caused by increasing progesterone concentration
    4. Ovulation: brought on by high concentrations of luteinizing hormone (LH)
    5. Postovulatory phase: increased secretion of estrogen and progesterone from corpus luteum further

prepares the uterine endometrium in event of fertilization and implantation of an ovulated egg
6. Premenstrual phase: gradual drop in level of estrogens and progesterone, leading to menses

D. Clinical applications
1. Contraceptive pills contain synthetic preparations of estrogen-like and/or progesterone-like compounds
2. Most commonly used contraceptive pills prevent pregnancy by preventing ovulation: pituitary secretion of FSH inhibited

E. Progestogen replacement provides the stimulus for desquamation of the uterine lining required for completion of the menstrual cycle or for maintenance of the uterine lining during pregnancy
1. Drugs
   a. dydrogesterone (Duphaston, Gynorest)
   b. ethisterone
   c. Hydroxyprogesterone caproate (Delalutin)
   d. medroxyprogesterone acetate (Depo-Provera, Provera)
   e. norethindrone (Norlutin)
   f. norethindrone acetate (Norlutate)
   g. progesterone (Gesterol, Lipo-Lutin, Proluton)
2. Adverse effects: initial use causes profuse vaginal flow (shedding of accumulations of endometrial tissue), spotting, irregular bleeding, nausea, lethargy, jaundice

REVIEW OF PHYSICAL PRINCIPLES RELATED TO THE GENITOURINARY SYSTEM
Principles of Mechanics
Law of Motion

Newton's law
EXAMPLES
1. Pumping action of the heart supplies hydrostatic force to filter blood in the glomerular capillary bed
2. Contraction of muscle is responsible for the force of propulsion of semen along and out the male reproductive tract

Momentum

EXAMPLE: During micturition, the walls of the urinary bladder exert a force of prolonged duration that imparts great momentum to the urine being expelled from the body

Energy

EXAMPLE: Chemical energy of ATP is used to actively transport nutrients and electrolytes from glomerular filtrate into the tubular epithelium

Principles of Physical Properties of Matter
Elasticity

EXAMPLES
1. Elastic properties of the bladder permit it to hold several hundred milliliters of urine before micturition
2. Elastic properties of uterine connective tissue partly account for the tremendous increase in size of the uterus during pregnancy

Surface Area

EXAMPLE: The proximal convoluted tubules of the nephron have a brush border consisting of numerous microvilli that have very high surface-to-volume ratio; these tiny cellular extensions greatly increase the surface area of the tubule for reabsorption of materials from the glomerular filtrate

Liquids

Pascal's principle
EXAMPLE: In conditions causing a lack of the micturition reflex, manual pressure over the bladder region will be transmitted to the urine, which results in the opening of the sphincters and the expulsion of urine from the bladder

REVIEW OF CHEMICAL PRINCIPLES RELATED TO THE GENITOURINARY SYSTEM
Urine

A. Water solution of inorganic salts and organic compounds
B. Important in excretion of wastes
C. Analysis yields information of physical condition in health and disease
D. Normal urine
1. Amount: 800 to 1800 ml/24 hours
2. Color: light yellow to dark brown, resulting from pigments (urobilin, urochrome, etc.)
3. Odor: aromatic (fresh); food and drugs alter odor
4. Sediment: varies; caused by diet and other normal changes
   a. Few blood cells
   b. Few epithelial cells
   c. Phosphates
   d. Urates
   e. Uric acid crystals
   f. Calcium oxalate
5. Specific gravity (1.005 to 1.025) varies greatly, depending on fluid intake and the quantity of solutes dissolved in the urine; the individual having diabetes insipidus may excrete 5 to 15 L of urine daily; this urine has a very low specific gravity (close to that of pure water); a person with diabetes mellitus may excrete urine of high specific gravity caused by excessive quantities of glucose dissolved in the urine
6. Reaction: usually acid (pH 4.5 to 7.5 is the normal range); alkaline immediately after a meal
7. Proteins: none; protein in the urine is usually associated with a pathologic condition although albumin traces will occasionally appear after heavy exercise or cold showers (these are of no consequence)
8. Sugar: trace to none; the presence of urinary carbohydrate is usually pathologic
9. Ketone bodies: none; ketone bodies in the urine appear in metabolic disorders
10. Indican: none; positive results indicate intestinal obstruction
11. Bile: none; positive results indicate liver or gallbladder dysfunction
12. Blood: trace to none; positive results indicate bleeding in organs of urinary system

Hormones

(See Endocrine system)

REVIEW OF MICROORGANISMS RELATED TO THE GENITOURINARY SYSTEM

A. Bacterial pathogens
1. *Enterobacter aerogenes:* small, gram-negative bacillus (morphologically indistinguishable from *Escherichia coli*); causes urinary tract infections
2. *Haemophilus ducreyi:* morphologically indistinguishable from *H. influenzae* and *H. aegyptius;* causes the venereal ulcer called chancroid (soft chancre)
3. *Neisseria gonorrhoeae:* gram-negative diplococcus; causes gonorrhea (transmitted sexually)
4. *Pseudomonas aeruginosa:* gram-negative, motile bacillus; a common secondary invader of wounds, burns, outer ear, and urinary tract; the infection characterized by blue-green pus; may be transmitted by catheters and other hospital instruments
5. *Treponema pallidum:* long, slender, highly motile spirochete; causes syphilis (transmitted sexually)
B. Protozoal pathogen *(Trichomonas vaginalis):* flagellated protozoan; causes trichomonas vaginitis (transmitted sexually)
C. Viral pathogens
1. Human immunodeficiency virus (HIV, HTLV-III, or LAV); causes acquired immunodeficiency syndrome (AIDS) (transmitted sexually and by blood)
2. *Herpesvirus hominis;* transmitted via genital or oral-genital route; causes herpes genitalis

PHARMACOLOGY RELATED TO GENITOURINARY SYSTEM DISORDERS
Urinary System
Kidney-specific Antiinfectives

A. Description
1. Used to treat local urinary tract infections
2. Exert an antibacterial effect on renal tissue, including the ureters and bladder
3. Available in oral and parenteral (IV) preparations
B. Examples
1. methanamines (Uritone, Hiprex, Mandacon)
2. nalidixic acid (NegGram)
3. nitrofurantoin (Furadantin, Macrodantin)
C. Major side effects
1. Nausea, vomiting (irritation of gastric mucosa)
2. Skin rash (hypersensitivity)
3. CNS disturbances (neurotoxicity)
4. Blood dyscrasias (decreased RBC, WBC, and platelet synthesis)
D. Nursing care
1. Administer with meals to reduce GI irritation
2. Monitor blood work, cultures, and urinary output during therapy
3. Encourage increased fluid intake
4. nalidixic acid
   a. Assess for potentiation of anticoagulant effect
   b. Utilize Clinistix or Tes-Tape for urine testing as false positives are obtained with Clinitest tablets, Fehling's, and Benedict's solutions
5. nitrofurantoins
   a. Dilute oral suspensions in milk or juice to prevent staining of teeth
   b. Instruct client that the urine will appear brown in color
6. Evaluate client's response to medication and understanding of teaching

Sulfonamides

(See Sulfonamides in Pharmacology related to infection)

Reproductive System
Estrogens

A. Description
1. Organic compounds secreted by ovarian follicles in females; responsible for triggering the proliferation phase of the menstrual cycle
2. Used to regulate menstrual disorders, uterine bleeding, and menopausal problems, as well as to treat inoperable prostatic cancer and breast cancer; also used as contraceptives alone or in combination with progestin
3. Available in oral, parenteral (IM, IV), intravaginal, and topical, including transdermal, preparations
B. Examples
1. chlorotrianisene (Tace)
2. diethylstilbestrol (DES)
3. esterified estrogens (Estratabs)
4. estradiol preparations
5. estrogenic substances, conjugated (Premarin)
6. estrone (Theelin)
C. Major side effects
1. Thrombophlebitis (increased clot formation)
2. Nausea (irritation of gastric mucosa)
3. Skin disturbances (local irritation with transdermal preparations)
4. Breast tenderness (promotion of sodium and water retention)
5. Hyperglycemia (decreased carbohydrate tolerance)
6. Males: gynecomastia, loss of libido, and testicular atrophy (hormonal imbalance related to estrogen antagonism)
7. Deficiency of one or more of the B complex vitamins may be induced with prolonged use
D. Nursing care
1. Obtain client history to assess for medical problems that may contraindicate use
2. Assess client for edema formation during therapy
3. Instruct client to
   a. Use proper procedure for application if topical or intravaginal
   b. Report unusual vaginal bleeding to physician immediately
   c. Avoid smoking during therapy
   d. Eat foods rich in the B complex vitamins daily; B complex vitamin supplements should also be considered
4. Carefully monitor blood glucose in diabetics during therapy
5. Reassure male clients that feminizing side effects will subside when therapy is completed
6. Evaluate client's response to medication and understanding of teaching

Progestins

A. Description
1. Female ovarian hormones that prepare the uterus for implantation of a fertilized ovum; essential for the maintenance of pregnancy
2. Used in the treatment of endometriosis, infertility, dysmenorrhea, and threatened abortion; also used to suppress ovulation
3. Available in oral and parenteral (IM) preparations

B. Examples
1. hydroxyprogesterone caproate (Delalutin)
2. medroxyprogesterone acetate (Provera)
3. megestrol acetate (Megace)
4. progesteron (Progestin)

C. Major side effects
1. Edema (promotion of sodium and water retention)
2. GU disturbances (renal dysfunction aggravated by fluid retention)
3. Visual disturbances (possibility of blood clots or neuro-ocular lesions)
4. Scleral jaundice (hepatic alterations)
5. Thrombophlebitis (increased clot formation)
6. Depression (CNS effect)
7. Deficiency of one or more of the B complex vitamins may be induced with prolonged use

D. Nursing care
1. Obtain client history to assess for medical problems that may contraindicate drug use
2. Assess client for edema during therapy
3. Inform significant others regarding potential for development of depression
4. Instruct client to eat foods rich in the B complex vitamins daily; B complex vitamin supplements should also be considered
5. Evaluate client's response to medication and understanding of teaching

Androgens

A. Description
1. Hormones that aid in the development of secondary sex characteristics in men and have anabolic properties, which stimulate the building and repair of body tissue
2. Used in debilitating conditions, inoperable breast cancer, and to restore hormone levels in males; also effective for treatment of fibrocytic breast disease, dysmenorrhea, and severe postpartum breast engorgement in nonnursing mothers
3. Available in oral, parenteral (IM, SC), and buccal preparations

B. Examples
1. danazol (Danocrine)
2. ethylestrenol (Maxibolin)
3. fluoxymesterone (Halotestin)
4. nandrolone phenpropionate (Durabolin)
5. norethandrolone (Nilevar)
6. testosterone preparations

C. Major side effects
1. Weight gain, edema (sodium and water retention)
2. Acne (androgen effect)
3. Changes in libido (androgen effect)
4. Hoarseness, deep voice (virilism—androgen effect)
5. Nausea, vomiting (irritation of gastric mucosa; hypercalcemia)

D. Nursing care
1. Assess for signs of virilization in females
2. Encourage a diet high in calories and proteins to aid in building body tissues
3. Encourage clients to restrict sodium intake to control edema
4. Administer with meals to reduce GI irritation
5. Monitor blood pressure during course of therapy
6. Assess for potentiation of anticoagulant effect
7. Evaluate client's response to medication and understanding of teaching

PROCEDURES RELATED TO THE GENITOURINARY SYSTEM
Common Urine Tests

A. Definition
1. Urinalysis: microscopic examination of urine for cells, as well as chemical study for pH and specific gravity
2. Culture and sensitivity tests of urine: microscopic examination of urine for bacterial growth and determination of antibiotic appropriate to control growth
3. Specific gravity: estimation of the concentration of urine relative to water; reflects concentrating ability of the kidneys; normal value of 1.005 to 1.025 depends on fluid intake and loss

B. Nursing care
1. Explain procedure to the client
2. Obtain container for the specimen
   a. For urinalysis a urine container is used
   b. For culture a sterile specimen jar is used
3. For urinalysis obtain a freshly voided specimen and place in the container
4. For culture obtain a clean-catch or midstream specimen
   a. Cleanse the outer urinary meatus with a bacteriostatic solution
   b. Instruct the client to void a small amount into a bedpan, urinal, or toilet and then stop the stream
   c. Instruct the client to continue voiding into a container without contaminating the lid or inside of the container
   d. Seal the container
5. Send the specimen to the laboratory with label indicating contents, client's name, and date
6. For specific gravity
   a. Obtain freshly voided specimen
   b. Fill specific gravity container one-half to two-thirds full with urine
   c. Place hydrometer (urinometer) in urine and spin gently
   d. Read scale at level of meniscus
7. Evaluate client's response to procedure

Cystoscopy

A. Definition
1. The visualization of the bladder wall through a tube with a fiberoptic end

2. Indicated as a diagnostic measure or as a means to enter the bladder for therapy
B. Nursing care
    1. Obtain an informed consent
    2. Maintain the client npo before the procedure (which may be done with or without general anesthesia)
    3. Provide care following the procedure
        a. Maintain the client in a comfortable state
        b. Observe the client's urine for blood and clots
        c. Ascertain that the client has voided through observation and palpation of the bladder
    4. Evaluate client's response to procedure

Intravenous Pyelography (IVP)

A. Definition: x-ray examination of the kidneys, ureters, and bladder after the injection of a contrast medium into an antecubital vein
B. Nursing care
    1. Explain procedure to the client
    2. Obtain an informed consent
    3. Administer a cathartic as ordered the evening before the test to remove feces and flatus
    4. Provide a light supper before the procedure and maintain the client npo for 6 to 8 hours prior to the test
    5. Evaluate client's response to procedure

Retention Catheter Care

A. Definition: special care to the urinary meatus and catheter to reduce the likelihood of infection
B. Nursing care
    1. Explain procedure to the client
    2. Provide privacy
    3. Gather equipment, wash hands, and don gloves
    4. Perform catheter care at least twice daily
    5. Wash the genital area well with soap and warm water and dry; uncircumcised males should have foreskin retracted to remove sebaceous secretions
    6. Use soap and water to wash encrustations from catheter (they may harbor microorganisms)
    7. Check drainage tubing at frequent intervals to assess for kinks or clogs
    8. Fasten catheter to the client's thigh to prevent tension
    9. Keep the drainage bag below bladder level without loops or kinks to ensure gravity drainage
    10. Use a syringe to remove urine if a specimen is needed; use the port site and surgical aseptic technique
    11. Empty the drainage bag at least every 8 hours and record the amount, odor, color, and consistency
    12. Change the drainage bag and catheter according to institutional policy
    13. Evaluate client's response to procedure

Urinary Catheterization

A. Definitions
    1. Sterile introduction of a catheter through the urethra to the bladder for the purpose of urine collection
    2. Intermittent catheterization is performed with a one-lumen catheter, which is removed after the bladder is drained (clients with neurogenic bladder dysfunction may be taught this procedure)
    3. Retention catheterization involves use of a catheter with an inflatable balloon around its tip to hold it in place in the bladder (Foley catheter); once inserted, it is attached to a collecting bag and thus the bladder is continually emptied by gravity
    4. Catheterization for residual urine involves the use of a straight catheter which is inserted after a client voids; the bladder should normally be empty at this time
B. Nursing care
    1. Explain procedure to the client
    2. Provide privacy
    3. Obtain equipment, including a bright light
    4. Position the female client supine with her knees flexed and abducted and the male client supine with the knees slightly abducted
    5. Wash hands, open catheterization tray, and put on sterile gloves
    6. Place the sterile fenestrated drape over the external genitalia, exposing the meatus
    7. Lubricate tip of the catheter and leave catheter on the sterile tray
    8. Saturate cotton pledgets with a suitable cleaning solution
    9. Cleanse the urinary meatus
        a. For female clients separate the labia minora with thumb and forefinger and cleanse from anterior to posterior using one pledget for each stroke (keep labia separated)
        b. For male clients hold the penis between thumb and forefinger and cleanse from meatus to shaft using one pledget for each stroke (retract foreskin during this procedure)
    10. Insert lubricated catheter into the bladder
        a. For female clients insert approximately 7.5 cm or slightly past the point at which urine returns
        b. For male clients, hold the penis perpendicular to the body and insert catheter 17 to 25 cm or slightly past the point at which urine returns
    11. Drain urine (do not exceed 750 ml); clamp catheter and notify the physician if drainage is in excess of 750 ml
        a. Intermittent catheterization: remove catheter when bladder is empty
        b. Retention catherization: inflate the balloon with sterile solution or air after the bladder is emptied and the catheter is attached to a sterile closed collection system (to reduce chance of infection)
    12. Assist the client to a comfortable position, remove equipment, and record data on appropriate records
    13. Evaluate client's response to procedure

NURSING PROCESS FOR CLIENTS WITH GENITOURINARY SYSTEM DISORDERS
Probable Nursing Diagnoses Based on Assessment

A. Altered patterns of urinary elimination related to
    1. Microbiological irritants
    2. Physical obstruction
    3. Trauma

B. Urinary retention related to physical obstruction
C. Fluid volume excess related to reduced urine output
D. Altered thought processes related to chemical toxins
E. Disturbance in body image related to
 1. Dependency on technology
 2. Ineffective coping with mutilating surgery
F. Disturbance in self-esteem related to chronic debilitation
G. Potential impaired skin integrity related to irritation by nitrogenous wastes
H. Sexual dysfunction related to
 1. Altered body image
 2. Inadequate tissue perfusion
I. Impaired physical mobility related to surgical pain and inflammation
J. Infection related to the presence of pathologic organisms
K. Pain related to
 1. Inflammation
 2. Obstruction of urine
 3. Pressure
L. Incontinence (functional, reflex, stress, total, urge) related to disease process
M. Altered role performance related to
 1. Interference with sexual functioning
 2. Infertility
N. Sensory-perceptual alteration related to chemical toxins

Nursing Care for Clients with Genitourinary System Disorders

See Nursing care under each specific disease

MAJOR DISEASES
Cystitis

A. Etiology and pathophysiology
 1. Inflammation of the bladder wall usually caused by an ascending bacterial infection *(Escherichia coli* most common)
 2. More common in females due to
  a. Shorter urethra
  b. Childbirth
  c. Anatomic position of the urethra
B. Signs and symptoms
 1. Subjective
  a. Urgency, frequency, burning, and pain on urination
  b. Nocturia
  c. Bearing down on urination
 2. Objective
  a. Pyuria and hematuria
  b. Bacterial growth evident on culture of urine
C. Treatment
 1. Chemotherapeutic and antibiotic agents (e.g., sulfonamides, penicillin, tetracycline)
 2. Antispasmodics to soothe the irritable bladder (e.g., phenazopyridine [Pyridium])
 3. Diet directed toward maintaining an acid urine (e.g., cranberry juice)
 4. Intake of additional fluids to dilute the urine
D. Nursing care
 1. Teach the client to seek medical attention at the first sign of symptoms

2. Teach the client to take medications as directed
3. Encourage the client to drink additional fluids
4. Monitor intake and output with attention to character of urine
5. Teach the client proper perineal care
6. Evaluate client's response and revise plan as necessary

Renal and Ureteral Calculi

A. Etiology and pathophysiology: formation of stones in the urinary tract; stones may be composed of calcium phosphate, uric acid, or oxalate; they tend to recur and may cause obstruction, infection, and/or hydronephrosis
B. Signs and symptoms
 1. Subjective
  a. Severe pain in kidney area radiating down the flank to the pubic area (renal colic)
  b. Frequency and urgency of urination
  c. History of prior or associated health problems (e.g., gout, parathyroidism, immobility, dehydration, urinary tract infections)
 2. Objective
  a. Diaphoresis, pallor, nausea, vomiting
  b. Hematuria; pyuria may occur if infection is present
C. Treatment
 1. Narcotics for pain
 2. Antispasmodics to reduce the renal colic
 3. Allopurinal or sulfinpyrazone to reduce uric acid excretion
 4. Antibiotics to reduce infection
 5. Monitor intake and output; forced fluids and straining of urine
 6. Diet therapy
  a. Large fluid intake to produce dilute urine
  b. Diet altered according to type of stone
   (1) Calcium stones: low-calcium diet of about 400 mg daily, achieved mainly by eliminating dairy products; if phosphate involvement, limit high-phosphorus foods—dairy products, meat; if oxalate involvement, avoid oxalate-rich foods—tea, almonds, cashews, chocolate, cocoa, beans, spinach, and rhubarb; since calcium stones have an alkaline chemistry, an acid ash diet can be used to create an acidic urinary tract, which is less conducive to their formation; stress whole grains, eggs, cranberry juice and limit milk, vegetables, and fruit
   (2) Uric acid stones: low purine (uric acid is a metabolic product of purines in the body), controlling purine foods such as meat, especially organ meats, meat extractives, and to a lesser extent plant sources (e.g., whole grains and legumes); alkaline ash, since the stone composition is acid
   (3) Cystine stones (rare): low methionine, since methionine is the essential amino acid from which the nonessential amino acid cystine is formed; controlling protein foods such as meat, milk, egg, cheese; alkaline ash, since the stone is an acid composition

7. Surgical intervention if stone is not passed or complications are present (e.g., nephrolithotomy, ureterolithotomy, cystotomy)
8. Percutaneous ultrasonic lithotripsy (PUL)
   a. Nephroscope is inserted through skin into kidney
   b. Ultrasonic waves disintegrate stones
   c. Stone fragments are removed by suction and irrigation
   d. Less traumatic alternative to conventional surgery
9. Extracorporeal shock-wave lithotripsy (ESWL)
   a. Client is immersed in water and exposed to shock waves that disintegrate stones so that they can be passed with urine; procedure is noninvasive
   b. Not widely available
D. Nursing care
   1. Administer analgesics as ordered
   2. Permit the client to set own pattern of activity
   3. Plan care to provide the client with periods of undisturbed rest
   4. Strain all urine
   5. Monitor intake and output
   6. Force fluids
   7. Administer antibiotics as ordered to prevent infection
   8. Encourage the client to accept medication for pain
   9. Provide as much privacy as possible
   10. Encourage client to remain on diet; those on calcium-restricted diet will need daily riboflavin supplement; those on an acid ash diet will need daily supplementation of vitamins C and A and folic acid
   11. Teach the client to read labels on food preparations for the presence of contraindicated additives such as calcium or phosphate
   12. Whenever possible, encourage daily weight-bearing exercise to prevent hyper-calciuria caused by release of calcium from the bones
   13. Provide care following a nephrolithotomy or percutaneous ultrasonic lithotripsy
       a. Change dressings frequently during the first 24 hours after a nephrolithotomy
       b. Maintain patency of ureteral catheter as well as urethral catheter to prevent hydronephrosis
       c. Encourage use of incentive spirometry and coughing and deep breathing to prevent atelectasis
   14. Evaluate client's response and revise plan as necessary

Hydronephrosis

A. Etiology and pathophysiology
   1. Obstruction at any point in the urinary system leading to pressure that can damage renal tissue
   2. Due to tumors, trauma, calculi, polycystic disease, congenital abnormalities, lymph enlargement, or nephrotosis (floating kidney)
B. Signs and symptoms
   1. Subjective
      a. Pain, local tenderness
      b. Dull pain in flank region or colicky pain
   2. Objective
      a. Nausea and vomiting
      b. Nocturia
C. Treatment
   1. Treat the underlying cause
   2. Promote urinary drainage with a catheter
   3. Urinary antiseptics
   4. Antispasmodics for colicky spasm
D. Nursing care
   1. Observe for signs of uremia
   2. Medicate as ordered
   3. Maintain patency of drainage tubes
   4. Evaluate client's response and revise plan as necessary

Acute Renal Failure

A. Etiology and pathophysiology
   1. Usually follows direct trauma to the kidneys or overwhelming physiologic stress (e.g., burns, septicemia, nephrotoxic drugs and chemicals, hemolytic blood transfusion reaction, severe shock, renal vascular occlusion)
   2. Sudden and almost complete loss of glomerular and/or tubular function
   3. Acute renal failure may result in death from acidosis, potassium intoxication, pulmonary edema, or infection
   4. May progress from the anuric or oliguric phase through the diuretic phase to the convalescent phase (which can take 6 to 12 months) to recovery of function
   5. May progress to chronic renal failure; chronic renal failure may develop as a separate entity and does not have to be a sequela of acute failure
B. Signs and symptoms
   1. Subjective
      a. Lethargy and drowsiness that can progress from stupor to coma
      b. Irritability and headache
      c. Circumoral numbness
      d. Tingling extremities
      e. Anorexia
   2. Objective
      a. Sudden dramatic drop in urinary output appearing a few hours after the causative event
      b. Oliguria: urinary output less than 400 ml but more than 100 ml/24 hours; anuria: urinary output less than 100 ml/24 hours
      c. Restlessness, twitching, convulsions
      d. Nausea and vomiting
      e. Skin pallor, anemia, and increased bleeding time, which can progress to epistaxis and internal hemorrhage
      f. Ammonia (urine) odor to breath and perspiration, which can progress to uremic frost on skin and pruritus
      g. Generalized edema, hypervolemia, hypertension, and increased venous pressure, which can progress to pulmonary edema and congestive heart failure
      h. In addition, respirations are deep and rapid as a compensatory response to the developing metabolic acidosis

i. Elevated serum levels of
    (1) BUN
    (2) Creatinine
    (3) Potassium
j. Decreased serum levels of
    (1) Calcium
    (2) Sodium
    (3) pH
    (4) Carbon dioxide combining power
k. Anemia
l. Albumin in urine
m. Decreased specific gravity

C. Treatment
1. Direct treatment toward correcting the underlying cause of renal failure (e.g., treat shock, eliminate drugs and toxins, treat transfusion reactions, restore integrity of urinary tract)
2. Maintain client on complete bed rest
3. Diet therapy
    a. Protein low to moderate according to tolerance: 30 to 50 g
    b. Carbohydrate relatively high for energy: 300 to 400 g
    c. Fat relatively moderate: 70 to 90 g
    d. Calories adequate for maintenance and to prevent tissue breakdown: 2000 to 2500 daily
    e. Sodium controlled according to serum levels and excretion tolerance: varying from 400 to 2000 mg
    f. Potassium controlled according to serum levels and excretion capacities: varying from 1300 to 1900 mg
    g. Water controlled according to excretion: about 800 to 1000 ml; careful intake and output records vital
    h. Calcium intake of 1000 mg/day is needed to prevent or delay progression of renal osteodystrophy, or demineralization of bone which can result from chronic acidosis and altered vitamin A metabolism; because of dietary restrictions, supplementation may be prescribed; calcium supplements, however, should not be given unless serum phosphate is under control because of risk of precipitation of calcium phosphate in the kidney
    i. Phosphorus intakes of less than 600 mg/day have been shown to delay progression of renal insufficiency; this level is usually achieved by restricting milk intake to 1 cup or less per day, avoiding soft drinks and beer, and restriction of meats, poultry, fish, eggs, and cereal grain products
    j. Renal diet is low in water-soluble vitamins, iron, and zinc, necessitating daily supplements; dialyzed clients will need daily supplements of vitamins B_6 (5-10 mg), C (70-100 mg), and folic acid (1 mg) administered following dialysis
4. Frequent monitoring of vital signs and intake and output
5. Packed cells, electrolytes, and glucose IV as necessary
6. Exchange resins to decrease serum potassium
7. Antibiotics to reduce possibility of infection

8. Peritoneal dialysis or hemodialysis
9. Surgical intervention if kidney transplant is a viable alternative

D. Nursing care
1. Monitor intake and output at frequent intervals
2. Limit fluid intake as ordered
3. Weigh the client daily
4. Observe for signs of overhydration (e.g., dependent, pitting, sacral, or periorbital edema; rales or dyspnea; headache, distended neck veins, and hypertension)
5. Observe for signs of hyperkalemia and hyponatremia
6. Administer electrolytes as ordered
7. Provide periods of undisturbed rest to conserve energy and oxygen
8. Protect client from injury caused by bleeding tendency, the possibility of convulsions, and a clouded sensorium
9. Protect client from cross infection
10. Observe for early signs and symptoms of complications (e.g., hemorrhage, convulsions, cardiac problems, pulmonary edema)
11. Provide special skin care frequently to prevent breakdown and remove uremic frost
12. Monitor vital signs and physical status at frequent intervals; record and report any deviations immediately
13. Administer antibiotics as ordered
14. Encourage intake of diet as ordered and record amount consumed
15. Allow the client as much choice as possible in the selection of food while recognizing that little variation is possible
16. Provide mouth care before, after, and between meals
17. Administer dietary and electrolyte supplements as ordered
18. Administer antiemetics to control nausea and antacids to reduce GI irritation
19. Evaluate client's response and revise plan as necessary

Chronic Renal Failure

A. Etiology and pathophysiology
1. Chronic renal failure can occur as the result of chronic kidney infections, developmental abnormalities, and vascular disorders
2. The ongoing deterioration in renal function results in uremia

B. Signs and symptoms
1. Subjective
    a. Lethargy or drowsiness
    b. Headache
2. Objective
    a. Vomiting
    b. Mental clouding
    c. Kussmaul respirations
    d. Uremic frost (powdery substance on the skin from urate wastes)
    e. Convulsions, coma, death

C. Treatment
   1. Fluid and salt restrictions
   2. Antihypertensive medications
   3. Peritoneal dialysis: warmed dialyzing solution is introduced via a catheter inserted in the peritoneal cavity; the peritoneal membrane is used as a dialyzing membrane to remove toxic substances, metabolic wastes, and excess fluid
   4. Hemodialysis: the client is attached (via a surgically created arteriovenous fistula) directly to a machine that pumps his or her blood along a semipermeable membrane; dialyzing solution is on the other side of the membrane, and osmosis of wastes, toxins, and fluid from the client occurs
   5. Diet management
      a. General protein and electrolyte control
      b. The low-protein, essential-amino-acid diet (modified Giordano-Giovannetti regimen) to sustain clients with uremia and alleviate their difficult symptoms
         (1) Very low protein (20 g); minimal essential amino acids
         (2) Controlled potassium (1500 mg); feed only essential amino acids, causing the body to use its own excess urea nitrogen to synthesize the nonessential amino acids needed for tissue protein production; foods used include 1 egg, 6 oz milk, low-protein bread, 2 to 4 fruits, and 2 to 4 vegetables from special lists to control protein and potassium
      c. See Acute renal failure for additional diet therapy information
D. Nursing care
   1. Monitor intake and output
   2. Provide skin care as needed
   3. Monitor vital signs
   4. Provide care for the client undergoing dialysis
      a. Explain the procedure and answer questions related to it
      b. Take vital signs and weigh the client before the procedure is begun
      c. Use surgical asepsis in preparation of the site (abdomen or area of fistula)
      d. Assure the client that a staff member will be present at all times
      e. If an indwelling catheter is not in place, have the client void before procedure is started
      f. Once the procedure is instituted by the physician, monitor the client's response and add dialysate as prescribed
      g. Take vs q15 min; assess for hypotension
      h. During peritoneal dialysis keep an accurate flow chart
      i. During hemodialysis watch the site for clotting; check clotting time and administer heparin as prescribed by the physician
      j. During both procedures check tubes for patency
      k. Since both procedures are long, provide back care to promote comfort and diversional activities to help pass the time

   l. Encourage client and family to seek nutritional counseling; stress importance of life-long dietary modifications
   5. Evaluate client's response and revise plan as necessary

Kidney Transplantation

A. Etiology and pathophysiology
   1. Clients with chronic renal failure who have no kidney function are candidates for transplantation
   2. Human leukocyte antigen (HLA) tests are done to decrease risk of rejection; least risk of rejection of the new kidney occurs if donor and recipient are identical twins
   3. At the time of surgery, the client's own kidney is not removed unless it is infected or enlarged
   4. New kidney is placed generally in the iliac fossa retroperitoneally, and the donor's ureter is attached to the bladder to prevent reflux of urine
B. Preoperative nursing care
   1. Prepare the client and family emotionally for the possible outcomes of surgery
   2. Explain that, postoperatively, immunosuppressive drugs and dialysis may be indicated as well as isolation to prevent infection
   3. Explain routine preoperative and postoperative procedures
   4. Evaluate client's response and revise plan as necessary
C. Postoperative nursing care
   1. Maintain patency of the drainage tubes, including the Foley catheter; gross hematuria or clots are *not* expected postoperatively
   2. Monitor fluid and electrolyte balance carefully; initial output increased because of sodium diuresis; sharp decrease may signal rejection
   3. Monitor vital signs, weight, and temperature
   4. Observe for and teach the client signs of rejection
      a. Increased serum creatinine
      b. Decreasing urinary output
      c. Malaise
      d. Fever
      e. Flank pain or tenderness
   5. Administer steroids and immunosuppressives as ordered to prevent rejection
   6. Teach the client the need for life-long immunosuppressive therapy
   7. Observe client for signs of infection
   8. Emphasize need to prevent infection by avoiding crowds and utilizing aseptic techniques
   9. Evaluate client's response and revise plan as necessary

Adenocarcinoma of the Kidneys

A. Etiology and pathophysiology
   1. Most common cancer affecting the kidneys
   2. Common sites of metastasis include lungs, liver, and long bones
   3. Incidence higher in males

B. Signs and symptoms
  1. Subjective
    a. There may be none until metastasis
    b. Dull back pain
    c. Weakness
  2. Objective
    a. Painless hematuria
    b. Enlarged kidney palpable during physical examination
    c. Elevated temperature
    d. Weight loss
    e. Anemia
C. Treatment
  1. Nephrectomy
  2. Radiation therapy if tumor is sensitive
  3. Chemotherapy
  4. Hormonal therapy with medroxyprogesterone (Provera)
D. Nursing care
  1. Monitor intake and output
  2. Increase oral fluid intake
  3. Administer analgesics as ordered to alleviate post-operative pain
  4. Encourage coughing and deep breathing while splinting the incision
  5. Examine dressing and linen under the client for drainage; a small amount of serosanguineous drainage is expected
  6. Maintain integrity of the urinary drainage system; avoid kinking of tubes
  7. Observe urine for color, amount, and any abnormal components
  8. Support natural defense mechanisms of client; encourage intake of foods rich in the immune stimulating nutrients, especially vitamins A, C, and E, and the mineral selenium
  9. Evaluate client's response and revise plan as necessary

Glomerulonephritis

A. Etiology and pathophysiology
  1. Involves damage to both kidneys resulting from filtration and trapping of antibody-antigen complexes within the glomeruli
  2. As a result, inflammatory and degenerative changes affect all renal tissue
  3. Often follows some form of streptococcal infection such as tonsillitis
  4. May be acute or chronic in nature; decreases life expectancy if progressive renal damage occurs
  5. Complications include hypertensive encephalopathy, heart failure, and infection
B. Signs and symptoms
  1. Subjective
    a. Flank pain, costovertebral tenderness
    b. Headache
    c. Malaise
    d. Dyspnea due to salt and fluid retention
    e. Weakness
    f. Visual disturbances
  2. Objective
    a. Hematuria
    b. Periorbital and facial edema
    c. Oliguria
    d. Fever
    e. Tachycardia
    f. Urine analysis reveals protein and casts
    g. Elevated plasma BUN and creatinine
    h. Anemia
C. Treatment
  1. Antibiotics such as penicillin to treat underlying infection
  2. Dietary restriction of sodium, fluids, and protein based on clinical status
  3. Diuretics and antihypertensives to control blood pressure
D. Nursing care
  1. Monitor intake and output
  2. Assess specific gravity of urine
  3. Weigh the client daily
  4. Monitor vital signs and temperature
  5. Special prophylactic skin care (these clients are prone to skin breakdown)
  6. Protect the client from infection
  7. Observe for complications such as renal failure, cardiac failure, and hypertensive encephalopathy
  8. Evaluate laboratory results (BUN, creatinine, urinalysis)
  9. Encourage continued medical supervision
  10. Refer to social service as needed; the long-term nature of the illness may create economic problems for the family
  11. Evaluate client's response and revise plan as necessary

Bladder Tumors

A. Etiology and pathophysiology
  1. Occur most frequently in men over 50 years of age
  2. Smoking, exposure to radiation, schistosomiasis, and exposure over prolonged periods to certain chemicals increase the risk of development of tumor
  3. Common sites of metastasis include lymph nodes, bone, liver, and lungs
B. Signs and symptoms
  1. Subjective
    a. Frequency and urgency of urination
    b. Dysuria
  2. Objective
    a. Direct visualization by cystoscopic examination
    b. Painless hematuria
C. Treatment
  1. Surgical intervention
    a. Resection of tumor
    b. Cystectomy (removal of the bladder); requires urinary diversion
      (1) Ureterosigmoidostomy: ureters are attached to the sigmoid colon, and urine is excreted through the rectum; these clients have constant drainage and are usually troubled by recurrent infection of the urinary tract

(2) Ileal conduit: section of the ileum is resected and attached to the ureters; one end of this ileal segment is sutured closed and the other is brought to the skin as an ileostomy to drain urine; technique most widely used to divert urine

(3) Nephrostomy: catheter is inserted into the kidney through an incision

(4) Ureterostomy: ureters are implanted in the abdominal wall to drain urine

2. Radiation therapy
3. Chemotherapy

D. Nursing care

1. Allow time for the client to verbalize fears of surgery, cancer, death, and body image alterations
2. Preoperatively, in addition to routine care and explanations, prepare the bowel by cleansing with laxatives, antibiotics, and enemas as ordered
3. Assess the color and amount of urine frequently; maintain patency of drainage system
4. Care for the client following a ureterosigmoidostomy
   a. Monitor the drainage tube, which may be in the rectum for several days
   b. After the tube in the rectum is removed, encourage the client to void frequently via the rectum to prevent complications such as reflux and absorption of urine through the intestinal wall
5. Care for the client following an ileal conduit
   a. Maintain the urinary drainage bag, which will be cemented around the stoma to collect urine
   b. After equipment is collected, remove the collection bag; use water or a commercial solvent to loosen the adhesive
   c. Hold a rolled gauze pad against the stoma to absorb urine during the procedure
   d. Cleanse the skin around the stoma and under the drainage bag with soap and water; inspect for excoriation
   e. After the skin is dry, apply skin adhesive to the area around the stoma and to the appliance
   f. Place the appliance over the stoma and secure in place by an adjustable belt
   g. Encourage self-care; teach the client to change the appliance by using a mirror
6. Expect a variety of psychologic manifestations, such as anger or depression, postoperatively
7. Arrange visit from a member of an ostomy club
8. Set realistic goals
9. Encourage fluids such as cranberry juice to keep the pH of the urine acidic and help prevent infection
10. Support natural defense mechanisms of client; encourage intake of foods rich in the immune stimulating nutrients, especially vitamins A, C, and E, and the mineral selenium
11. Evaluate client's response and revise plan as necessary

Bladder Trauma (Rupture)

A. Etiology and pathophysiology

1. Traumatic rupture of the bladder occurs following external crushing injury to the area, as in automobile accidents

2. An overdistended bladder at time of trauma increases the risk of this occurrence

B. Signs and symptoms

1. Subjective
   a. Pain
   b. Anxiety
2. Objective
   a. Oliguria or anuria
   b. Hematuria

C. Treatment

1. Exploration of the bladder to aid in diagnosing rupture
2. Surgical repair of laceration
3. Insertion of a suprapubic catheter to aid in urinary drainage (a tube inserted directly through the peritoneal cavity into the bladder to drain urine)

D. Nursing care

1. Observe vital signs for changes indicative of shock or hemorrhage
2. Observe urine for amount and color
3. Promote rest and analgesia
4. Maintain patency of catheters
5. Evaluate client's response and revise plan as necessary

Urethritis

A. Etiology and pathophysiology

1. Inflammation of the urethra caused by staphylococci, *Escherichia coli, Pseudomonas* species, and streptococci
2. Although these inflammatory symptoms are similar to gonorrheal urethritis, sexual contact is not the cause

B. Signs and symptoms

1. Subjective
   a. Burning on urination
   b. Urgency
   c. Frequency
2. Objective
   a. Purulent drainage
   b. Bacteria in urine

C. Treatment

1. Ascertain the causative organism through a culture of urine
2. Administer antibiotics
3. Hot sitz baths
4. Dilation of the urethra and subsequent instillation of antiseptic solution

D. Nursing care

1. Promote rest and comfort
2. Encourage fluid intake, especially cranberry juice since it has an acidifying effect on urine; vitamin C can also be used to acidify urine
3. Observe urine for clarity and hemorrhage
4. Evaluate client's response and revise plan as necessary

Prostatitis

A. Etiology and pathophysiology

1. Generally the result of urethritis
2. Prostate gland becomes swollen and tender

B. Signs and symptoms
  1. Subjective
     a. Difficult urination
     b. Pain
  2. Objective
     a. Fever
     b. Hematuria
C. Treatment
  1. Antibiotics or chemotherapeutics
  2. Application of heat
D. Nursing care
  1. Administer antibiotics
  2. Apply heat as ordered
     a. Sitz baths
     b. Rectal irrigations
  3. Encourage fluids
  4. Evaluate client's response and revise plan as necessary

Cancer of the Prostate

A. Etiology and pathophysiology
  1. Slow, malignant change in the prostate gland
  2. Tends to spread by direct invasion of surrounding tissues and metastases to the bony pelvis and spine
B. Signs and symptoms
  1. Subjective
     a. Frequency and urgency
     b. Difficulty initiating stream
  2. Objective
     a. Decreased force of stream
     b. Urinary retention
     c. Elevated serum acid phosphatase
     d. Enlarged hardened prostate detected by palpation
C. Treatment
  1. Type of surgical intervention depends on the extent of the lesion, the physical condition of the client, and the client's full awareness of the outcome (impotency follows radical prostatectomy)
  2. Radical prostatectomy, done by perineal or retropubic approach, removing the seminal vesicles and a portion of the bladder neck
  3. Radiation therapy alone or in conjunction with surgery may be ordered preoperatively or postoperatively to reduce the lesion and limit metastases
  4. Diethylstilbestrol (estrogen) may be ordered to reduce the size of an inoperable lesion or post operatively to limit metastases
  5. Orchiectomy may be done to limit production of testosterone
D. Nursing care
  1. Provide care similar to the client who has undergone a prostatectomy for benign prostatic hypertrophy
  2. Explain to the client that development of secondary female characteristics will occur as a result of medication and not the surgery
  3. Allow time and opportunity for the client to express concerns about impotence
  4. Support the client's male image
  5. Explain the situation to the client's family and include them in planning
  6. Assist the client and family in dealing with the diagnosis of cancer
  7. Evaluate client's response and revise plan as necessary

Epididymitis

A. Etiology and pathophysiology
  1. Acute or chronic inflammation of the epididymis
  2. Occurs as a sequela of urinary tract infections, sexually transmitted disease (STD), prostatitis
B. Signs and symptoms
  1. Subjective
     a. Chills
     b. Scrotal pain
     c. Groin pain
  2. Objective
     a. Fever
     b. Edema
     c. Elevated WBC
     d. Pyuria and bacteriuria
C. Treatment
  1. Medication to control pain, fever, and infection
  2. Scrotal support to facilitate drainage
  3. Notification of the state department of health if sexually transmitted disease is present
D. Nursing care
  1. Maintain the client in a restful state
  2. Explain the importance of good hygiene practices
  3. Encourage fluid intake
  4. Ascertain contacts if due to STD
  5. Teach the client to protect himself from contracting most STDs by use of a condom
  6. Evaluate client's response and revise plan as necessary

Benign Prostatic Hypertrophy

A. Etiology and pathophysiology
  1. Slow enlargement of the prostate gland common in men over 40 years of age
  2. Constriction of urethra and subsequent interference in urination
B. Signs and symptoms
  1. Subjective
     a. Frequency and urgency
     b. Difficulty initiating stream
  2. Objective
     a. Decreased force of stream
     b. Nocturia
     c. Total urinary retention
C. Treatment
  1. Reestablish emptying of the bladder by ordering a hot bath to induce voiding or by inserting an indwelling catheter or a cystotomy tube
  2. Urinary antiseptics and medications for reduction of pain and anxiety
  3. Have the client prepared for surgical removal of the prostate by means of a suprapubic, transurethral, perineal, or retropubic prostatectomy
  4. Postoperatively maintain drainage, force fluids, medicate for pain, administer antibiotics and stool softeners

D. Nursing care
1. Observe for or initiate measures to maintain patency of the catheter
2. Irrigate the catheter as ordered
3. Encourage increased fluid intake (2400 to 3000 ml/day)
4. Use sterile technique when necessary (e.g., insertion of the urinary catheter, irrigations, dressing changes)
5. Maintain integrity of the closed drainage systems
6. Administer antiseptics, bacteriostatics, and antibiotics as ordered
7. In acute urinary retention, decompress the bladder slowly via a Foley catheter (not more than 750 ml at a time) to prevent shock and hematuria
8. Observe for signs of hemorrhage (e.g., change in vital signs, nature of drainage, pain, symptoms of shock, frank bleeding)
9. Avoid postoperative complications by encouraging the client to deep breathe and cough and to exercise muscles in lower extremities
10. Teach the client preoperatively what can be expected postoperatively (e.g., presence of catheters, bloody drainage, bladder spasms, pain)
11. Accept and encourage the client to express concerns about sexual functioning
12. Provide as much privacy as possible
13. Administer medication for pain as ordered
14. Evaluate the client's response and revise plan as necessary

Cancer of the Cervix

A. Etiology and pathophysiology
1. Slow, malignant change in the tissue forming the neck of the uterus
2. Most common form of genital tract malignancy in women
3. High cure rate when diagnosed early
4. Tends to spread by direct invasion of surrounding tissues and metastases to the lungs, bones, and liver
5. Females exposed to diethylstilbesterol (DES) in utero have an increased risk of cervical cancer
B. Signs and symptoms
1. Subjective
   a. Back pain
   b. Leg pain
2. Objective
   a. Spotting after intercourse
   b. Vaginal discharge
   c. Lengthening of the menstrual period
   d. Papanicolaou cytologic finding of Class V is considered conclusive of cervical cancer; Papanicolaou cytologic findings of Class II, III, or IV require further studies before a conclusive diagnosis can be determined; Class I is normal
C. Treatment
1. Type of surgical intervention depends on the extent of lesion and the physical condition of the client
2. Hysterosalpingo-oophorectomy (panhysterectomy) to remove the uterus, fallopian tubes, and ovaries; in advanced lesions the parametrial tissue and lymph nodes may also be removed

3. Simple hysterectomy when preservation of ovarian function is desirable
4. Radiation therapy alone or in conjunction with surgery may be ordered to reduce the lesion and limit metastases
D. Nursing care
1. Assist the client and family in dealing with the diagnosis of cancer
2. Allow and encourage the client to express feelings and concerns about change in self-image and sexual functioning
3. Support the client's feminine image
4. Provide care for the client receiving internal radiation
   a. Explain the side effects that may occur and the procedures involved, especially the need for isolation during treatment
   b. Instruct her in maintaining proper positioning (supine and side-lying)
   c. Inspect the implant for proper position
   d. Provide low-residue diet and prevent bowel and urinary distention to avoid displacement of radioactive substance and irradiation of adjacent tissues
   e. Explain to the client and family that visitors and staff will be limited in the amount of time they can spend in the room to avoid their overexposure to radiation
   f. Utilize principles of time, distance, and shielding to minimize exposure of staff
   g. See Radiation for additional information
5. Provide care following surgery
   a. Maintain patency of the urinary catheter that was inserted prior to surgery to decompress the bladder and reduce stress on the operative site
   b. Observe for reestablishment of bowel sounds
   c. Maintain accurate intake and output
   d. Following removal of the urinary catheter, note the amount of output and pattern of voiding; catheterize for residual urine if ordered and whenever necessary for urinary retention
   e. For additional nursing responsibilities, see Postoperative care in this chapter and Nursing care for clients following hysterectomy in Maternity Nursing
6. Evaluate client's response and revise plan as necessary

Vaginitis

A. Etiology and pathophysiology
1. Trichomoniasis: overgrowth of *Trichomonas vaginalis,* which normally is present in the vagina
2. Candidiasis (moniliasis): caused by *Candida albicans,* a fungus; incidence is high in clients with diabetes mellitus and those receiving antibiotic therapy because of change in normal flora
3. Atrophic vaginitis: common in the postmenopausal period because atrophied vaginal mucosa is prone to infection
B. Signs and symptoms
1. Subjective
   a. Pruritus, burning
   b. Dyspareunia (pain with intercourse)

2. Objective
   a. Vaginal discharge
      (1) Malodorous, thin yellow discharge (trichomoniasis)
      (2) White "cheesy" discharge (moniliasis)
   b. Vaginal smear can indicate *Trichomonas vaginalis, Candida albicans,* or other microorganisms
C. Treatment
   1. Douches (acetic acid may be added)
   2. Antifungal preparations for candidiasis
      a. Nystatin (Mycostatin) vaginal suppositories
      b. Propionic acid gel inserted vaginally
      c. Gentian violet applied to vaginal mucosa and cervix
   3. Antiprotozoan preparations for trichomoniasis
      a. Metronidazole (Flagyl) tablets taken orally
      b. Aminoacridine-polyoxyethelene (Vagisec Plus) vaginal suppositories
   4. Estrogen therapy prescribed for atrophic vaginitis
D. Nursing care
   1. Advise the client to have sexual partner use a condom during coitus until vaginitis is resolved
   2. Explain that frequent douching will alter the normal pH environment of the vagina, predisposing to vaginitis
   3. Instruct the client to use tampons to prevent discharge from irritating vulvar area
   4. Administer a douche if ordered
      a. Explain procedure to the client; provide privacy
      b. Assemble equipment, including douche can, tip, bedpan, gloves, waterproof pads, and solution at 110° F (45° C) (30 ml of vinegar may be added to a liter of solution for acetic solution; alkaline solutions should never be utilized)
      c. Assist the client onto a bedpan while maintaining privacy
      d. Wearing gloves, separate the labia and insert the tip into the vagina
      e. Rotate the douche tip gently so the solution reaches all vaginal folds
      f. When all solution is used, instruct the client to bear down to expel as much remaining solution as possible; solution returns during the entire procedure
      g. Dry the perineal area gently
      h. Resterilize nondisposable equipment
   5. Instruct the client who is receiving antibiotics or having recurrent vaginal infections to include yogurt or food supplements containing *Lactobacillus acidophilus* in the diet to maintain the normal vaginal flora
   6. Evaluate client's response and revise plan as necessary

Endometriosis

A. Etiology and pathophysiology
   1. Growth of endometrial cells in areas outside the uterus
   2. Generally affects young nulliparous women
   3. Endometrial cells are stimulated by the ovarian hormones; will cause bleeding during the normal menstrual cycle
   4. Adhesions are common and may result in sterility
   5. Adenomyosis is a similar condition affecting women 40 to 50 years old in which the endometrial cells invade the muscles of the uterus
B. Signs and symptoms
   1. Subjective
      a. Lower abdominal pain beginning 2 to 7 days prior to menstruation, becoming progressively worse, and then diminishing as the menstrual flow decreases
      b. Dyspareunia
      c. Pain associated with defecation
   2. Objective
      a. Abnormal uterine bleeding (metrorrhagia, menorrhagia)
      b. Infertility
C. Treatment
   1. Hormone therapy to suppress ovulation; young married women are advised not to delay pregnancy if children are desired
   2. Surgical intervention
      a. Resection of lesions
      b. Oophorectomy, salpingectomy, and total hysterectomy if the condition is severe
D. Nursing care
   1. Provide as much privacy as possible
   2. Explain procedures to the client
   3. Ascertain the client's understanding of risks of sterility
   4. Provide the client time to talk about her feelings
   5. Administer analgesics as ordered
   6. Observe for hemorrhage (e.g., check for signs of shock, vaginal bleeding); check vaginal packing
   7. Check the client's output; make certain that the client is emptying her bladder
   8. Routine preoperative and postoperative care if surgery is necessary
   9. Evaluate client's response and revise plan as necessary

Pelvic Inflammatory Disease (PID)

A. Etiology and pathophysiology
   1. Occurs within female pelvic cavity; can affect the fallopian tubes (salpingitis), ovaries (oophoritis), peritoneum, surrounding connective tissue, and pelvic veins
   2. May be acute or chronic, bilateral or unilateral
   3. Caused by the introduction of bacteria (usually through the cervical opening) such as gonococci, streptococci, or tubercle bacilli that are transported by the blood from the lungs
   4. If untreated, can lead to adhesions and sterility
B. Signs and symptoms
   1. Subjective
      a. Severe cramping pain in lower abdomen
      b. Nausea
      c. Malaise
      d. Dysmenorrhea, dypareunia
   2. Objective
      a. Temperature elevation
      b. Foul-smelling, purulent vaginal discharge
      c. Elevated WBC

d. Cultures of vaginal discharge reveal causative organism

C. Treatment
   1. Medication to control pain and fever
   2. Specific antibiotics depending on the organism identified
   3. Identify and notify sexual contacts and the state department of health if venereal disease is present

D. Nursing care
   1. Maintain the client on bed rest in a semi-Fowler's position to localize the infection and prevent the formation of abscesses within the abdominal cavity
   2. Apply heat if ordered to the abdomen or via a douche to improve circulation
   3. Observe and record the amount and character of vaginal discharge
   4. Change perineal pads frequently using gloves; tampons should not be used
   5. Explain safety measures to prevent reinfection of the client or others; during the acute phase the client should abstain from intercourse
   6. Provide psychologic support because of the social aspects of venereal disease
   7. Evaluate client's response and revise plan as necessary

Vaginal Fistula

A. Etiology and pathophysiology
   1. Abnormal opening between two organs
   2. May be congenital or occur as a result of carcinoma or radiation therapy
   3. Types
      a. Rectovaginal: opening between the rectum and vagina
      b. Vesicovaginal fistula: opening between the bladder and vagina
      c. Ureterovaginal fistula: opening between a ureter and the vagina

B. Signs and symptoms
   1. Subjective
      a. Burning sensation
      b. Frequency of urination (if secondary urinary tract infection)
   2. Objective
      a. Discharge of urine, feces, or flatus from the vagina
      b. Excoriation of vaginal mucosa
      c. Odor

C. Treatment
   1. Dietary modification including high-protein, low-residue diet with vitamin supplement
   2. Enemas, bladder irrigations, and douches using antibiotic solutions
   3. Fistulas may be repaired surgically

D. Nursing care
   1. Provide psychologic support, since the client may be embarrassed by odor and drainage and become withdrawn
   2. Provide privacy during any treatments
   3. Change pads frequently; sitz baths and irrigations to maintain cleanliness of area

4. Observe drainage and perineum for signs of inflammation
5. Assess urine for signs of infection; maintain patency of drainage tubes
6. Monitor temperature as an indication of secondary infection
7. Evaluate client's response and revise plan as necessary

Cystocele and Rectocele

A. Etiology and pathophysiology
   1. Cystocele: herniation of the bladder into the vagina
   2. Rectocele: herniation of the rectum into the vagina
   3. Both conditions may be present at the same time and are generally associated with relaxation or injury of the pelvic muscles during childbirth

B. Signs and symptoms
   1. Subjective
      a. Feeling of fullness in vagina
      b. Constant urge to defecate
      c. Dysuria
   2. Objective
      a. Soft reducible mass evident during vaginal examination that increases when client is asked to bear down
      b. Stress incontinence
      c. Residual urine (60 ml or more after voiding)

C. Treatment
   1. Anterior colporrhaphy to correct a cystocele
   2. Posterior colporrhaphy to correct a rectocele

D. Nursing care
   1. Encourage voiding every 4 hours to prevent strain on the suture line from a distended bladder (no more than 150 ml should accumulate)
   2. If the client has difficulty voiding, insert a Foley catheter if ordered
   3. After each bowel movement and voiding, cleanse the perineum with warm normal saline and sterile cotton balls; always cleanse away from the vagina and toward the anus
   4. Administer douches if ordered; include client instruction
   5. Apply heat lamp, anesthetic spray, or ice packs if ordered to relieve discomfort
   6. Limit diet to liquids for first 5 days to avoid defecation and prevent strain on the suture line
   7. Administer medications to decrease GI motility if ordered
   8. Administer cathartics and an oil-retention enema using a thin rectal tube if prescribed
   9. Evaluate client's response and revise plan as necessary

Prolapsed Uterus

A. Etiology and pathophysiology
   1. As a result of weakness of the pelvic floor, the uterus descends into the vagina; most often associated with childbirth injury
   2. If severe, the entire uterus may protrude outside the vaginal orifice; in this case, the vagina is actually inverted; referred to as procidentia
   3. Ulcerations in procidentia increase risk of cancer

B. Signs and symptoms
  1. Subjective
    a. Heaviness within the pelvis
    b. Low back pain
    c. Incontinence
  2. Objective
    a. Mass in the lower vagina or outside the orifice
    b. Elongated cervix
    c. Urinary retention
C. Treatment
  1. Vaginal pessary to maintain the uterus in correct position
  2. Surgical intervention
    a. Suspension of the uterus and correction of retroversion
    b. Hysterectomy (if postmenopausal)
D. Nursing care
  1. Encourage the client to seek medical assistance if there is a prolapsed uterus
  2. If procidentia is present, observe for ulcerations; apply warm saline compresses or protective ointment to prevent ulceration
  3. Explain that if pessary is used, it must be taken out by the physician frequently and cleaned
  4. Observe the color, amount, and frequency of urination
  5. See Cancer of the cervix for postoperative care
  6. Evaluate client's response and revise plan as necessary

Carcinoma of the Breast

A. Etiology and pathophysiology
  1. Frequently begins as a hard, nontender, relatively fixed nodule found most often in the upper outer quadrant of the breast
  2. Metastasis by direct extension to the surrounding tissue and via lymph and blood to the axillary nodes, lungs, bone, brain, and liver
  3. Incidence increases with age and is influenced by heredity and the number of menstrual cycles a woman has had; multiparas and women with early menopause have a lower incidence, as do Japanese women
  4. Recent studies have implicated a high-fat, selenium-deficient diet as a contributing factor in development of breast cancer
  5. Paget's carcinoma is a type of breast cancer that invades the nipple and milk ducts
B. Signs and symptoms
  1. Subjective
    a. Lesion generally *non*tender
    b. Malaise in later stages
  2. Objective
    a. Dimpling of skin by lesion
    b. Inversion and discharge from nipple
    c. Changes in color of breast over lesion; in late stages skin has orange peel appearance
    d. Enlarged axillary lymph nodes
    e. Positive findings in following tests
      (1) Mammography: x-ray examination of the breast when there is an increased risk of developing breast cancer

      (2) Thermography: heat-sensing device to evaluate abnormal circulatory signs
      (3) Xerography: special x-ray plate subjected to an electric charge to image all breast tissue
      (4) Biopsy for microscopic evaluation
        (a) Aspiration of tissue by syringe
        (b) Excised tissue may be sent to the laboratory for a frozen section from which thin slices are examined
      (5) Estrogen receptor assay: if positive, indicates need for alteration of the hormonal environment by surgical or chemical means
      (6) Elevated carcinoembryonic antigen (CEA) in serum, plasma, or cerebrospinal fluid: indicative of progression of cancer, particularly of the breast, ovaries, and gastrointestinal tract; also used in detecting cancer of the prostate
C. Treatment
  1. Type of surgical and medical intervention depends on the extent of the lesion and the physical condition of the client
  2. Surgical intervention
    a. Lumpectomy: removal of the lump and a fourth to a third of the breast (only for early, minute, peripheral lesions)
    b. Simple mastectomy: removal of the breast only
    c. Radical mastectomy: removal of the breast, pectoral muscles, pectoral fascia, and nodes (pectoral, subclavicular, apical, and axillary); this procedure may be modified
    d. Breast reconstruction
    e. Oophorectomy, adrenalectomy, and/or hypophysectomy to control metastases through alteration of the endocrine environment; most successful if normal numbers of estrogen receptor sites are maintained as determined by estrogen receptor assay
  3. Radiation therapy alone or in conjunction with surgery preoperatively or postoperatively to reduce the lesion and limit metastases
  4. Corticosteroids, androgens, and antiestrogens (tamoxifen citrate) may be given to alter hormonal environment
  5. Chemotherapy
    a. Alkylating agents
      (1) cyclophosphamide (Cytoxan)
      (2) chlorambucil (Leukeran)
      (3) triethylenethiophosphoramide (Thiotepa)
    b. Antimetabolites
      (1) 5-fluorouracil (5-FU, Fluorouracil)
      (2) methotrexate (Amethopterin, MTX)
    c. Other drugs
      (1) adriamycin (Doxorubicin)
      (2) vincristine (Oncovin)
D. Nursing care
  1. Encourage and instruct the client concerning monthly breast self-examination
    a. Inspect while sitting with hands at sides and then overhead for retraction of the nipple, dimpling of skin, color change, and asymmetry
    b. Palpate the axillary and supraclavicular nodes

c. Palpate the breast tissue using a circular pattern when lying down with the arms abducted

d. Do after each menstrual cycle because premenstrual hormones can cause harmless nodules that will disappear after menses; if postmenopausal, do on the same date each month

2. Assist the client and family to cope with the diagnosis of cancer and altered body image by encouraging them to talk with staff and each other

3. Administer medication for pain as ordered

4. Listen to and accept the client's anger and depression and do not attempt to minimize it

5. Help the client identify feelings and encourage discussion of them

6. Support the client's feminine image

7. If the client is receiving cobalt therapy or antineoplastic drugs, inform, explain, and assist her to accept the side effects that may occur (e.g., nausea, vomiting, hair loss, anorexia, diarrhea, stomatitis, malaise, itching)

8. Care for the client following a mastectomy
   a. Observe for hemorrhage by checking all areas of the dressing, the drainage unit, and vital signs
   b. Maintain functioning of portable vacuum drainage unit by ensuring patency of tube, emptying when necessary, and supporting to avoid tension at site of insertion
   c. Encourage good posture and provide assistance with ambulation until the client adjusts to her altered balance
   d. Prevent or reduce lymphedema by elevating and supporting the client's hand above her elbow and the elbow above her shoulder
   e. Instruct the client who has undergone a radical mastectomy to avoid carrying heavy articles with the affected arm and to avoid cuts or bruises, having blood drawn, injections, or blood pressure readings in the affected arm because of impaired lymphatic drainage
   f. Encourage active exercises of the affected arm, beginning gradually the day after surgery if approved by the physician
      (1) Wall hand climbing
      (2) Brushing hair
      (3) Turning rope
   g. Instruct the client as to the types of prostheses and where to obtain them; cotton covered by gauze may be used to fill a client's bra until she is seen by a professional fitter
   h. Use agencies such as Reach for Recovery to help the client with physical and emotional readjustment

9. Care for client receiving radiation therapy
   a. Observe for signs of radiation burns (erythema, desquamation)
   b. Avoid removal of skin markings drawn by the radiologist
   c. Instruct her to use only ointments or emollients prescribed by the physician
   d. See Radiation for additional information

10. Support natural defense mechanisms of client; encourage intake of foods rich in the immune-stimulating nutrients, especially vitamins A, C, and E, and the mineral selenium; encourage low-fat diet

11. Evaluate client's response and revise plan as necessary

Syphilis

A. Etiology and pathophysiology
   1. Caused by spirochete *Treponema pallidum*
   2. Incubation is 10 to 90 days for primary syphilis
   3. If untreated, organism enters blood stream 6 to 8 weeks after infection (usually sexually transmitted)
   4. Latent phase begins 4 to 12 weeks after infection; client is asymptomatic
   5. Tertiary syphilis may occur 18 to 20 years later
      a. Gummas (granulomas) attack any organ and cause cardiovascular syphilis (aortitis and thoracic aortic aneurysms) and neurosyphilis
      b. During this stage it is rare for an individual to infect another; however, a fetus can be infected

B. Signs and symptoms
   1. Primary syphilis
      a. Chancre on genitalia, mouth, or anus
      b. Serous drainage from chancre
      c. Enlarged lymph nodes
      d. Positive tests for syphilis (VDRL, Kolmer, or Wasserman tests can be used)
   2. Secondary syphilis
      a. Skin lesions on palms and soles of feet
      b. Erosions of oral mucous membrane
      c. Alopecia
      d. Enlarged lymph nodes
      e. Fever
   3. Tertiary syphilis
      a. Cardiovascular changes
      b. Personality changes
      c. Ataxia
      d. Stroke
      e. Blindness

C. Treatment
   1. Penicillin
   2. Probenecid to delay excretion of penicillin
   3. Tetracycline or erthromycin if client is allergic to penicillin

D. Nursing care
   1. Provide a supportive nonjudgmental environment
   2. Encourage the use of early screening and educational programs such as STD clinics, hotlines, and workshops
   3. Explain that careful cleansing of the genitals, as well as the use of condoms, helps prevent transmission of most STDs
   4. Teach about the disease and its transmission
   5. Encourage client to identify prior contacts so they can be treated
   6. Assess genital discharge for color, amount, and consistency
   7. Explain need to complete course of antibiotic therapy
   8. Tell client to avoid any sexual activity until tests are negative

9. Encourage monogamous relationships
10. Evaluate client's response and revise plan as necessary

Gonorrhea

A. Etiology and pathophysiology
   1. Caused by *Neisseria gonorrhoeae,* a gram-negative diplococcus
   2. Penicillinase-producing *N. gonorrhoeae* is a newer strain resistant to penicillin
   3. Symptoms depend on nature of sexual contact and may appear within a few days after exposure
   4. Client may remain asymptomatic
   5. Untreated, inflammation subsides in 2 to 4 weeks but client may become a carrier
B. Signs and symptoms
   1. Subjective
      a. Lower abdominal discomfort
      b. Dysuria
      c. Urgency
      d. Joint pain
   2. Objective
      a. Purulent penile or vaginal discharge
      b. Fever
      c. Urethral or endocervical smear positive for gonococcus
      d. If untreated, complications such as sterility, urethral stricture, prostatitis, epididymitis, proctitis, and pharyngitis can occur
C. Treatment
   1. Penicillin drug of choice
   2. Tetracycline
   3. Doxycycline
   4. Spectinomycin hydrochloride
   5. Cefoxitan sodium
D. Nursing care
   1. Instruct client to wash hands to prevent conjunctivitis
   2. Make arrangements for follow-up culture 2 weeks after therapy is initiated
   3. See Syphilis for additional nursing care
   4. Evaluate client's response and revise plan as necessary

Herpes Genitalis

A. Etiology and pathophysiology
   1. Most commonly caused by Herpes simplex type II (herpesvirus hominus type II): may also be caused by type I, which is most often associated with lesions (cold sores) of the mouth
   2. Lesions occur 3 to 7 days after infection (usually by sexual contact) and may last several weeks
   3. When symptoms resolve, virus lies dormant in spinal root ganglia and is capable of repeatedly causing lesions
   4. May cause aseptic meningitis, proctitis, and prostitis
   5. Newborn may be infected during vaginal delivery
   6. Associated with higher rate of cervical cancer
   7. Transmitted only when active lesions are present

B. Signs and symptoms
   1. Subjective
      a. Anorexia
      b. Genital pain
      c. Dysuria
   2. Objective
      a. Vesicles and papules on genitalia
      b. Leukorrhea
      c. Vaginal bleeding
      d. Cultures reveal herpesvirus type II
C. Treatment
   1. No cure; acyclovir sodium (Zovirax) reduces healing time and severity of symptoms; not as effective in recurrent episodes
   2. Sedation for severe pain
   3. Alcohol may be used to dry lesions
D. Nursing care
   1. Provide emotional support to deal with incurable nature of disease
   2. Teach client regarding care of lesions with acyclovir sodium
      a. Use fingercot to apply medication
      b. Cover lesion thoroughly
   3. See Syphilis for additional nursing care
   4. Evaluate client's response and revise plan as necessary

Chlamydia

A. Etiology and pathophysiology
   1. Caused by *Chlamydia trachomatis*
   2. Most prevalent sexually transmitted disease (STD) in the United States
   3. Causes vaginitis or urethritis
B. Signs and symptoms
   1. Subjective
      a. Urgency
      b. Dysuria
      c. Pelvic discomfort
   2. Objective
      a. Positive culture
      b. Frequency
      c. Thin, white vaginal or urethral discharge
      d. Inflammation of cervix
C. Treatment
   1. Tetracycline
   2. Erythromycin
D. Nursing care
   1. See Syphilis for nursing care
   2. Evaluate client's response and revise as necessary

Acquired Immune Deficiency Syndrome (AIDS)

A. Etiology and pathophysiology
   1. Caused by human immunodeficiency virus (HIV-1 and HIV-2); previously referred to as human T-lymphotropic virus type III (HTLV-III), lymphadenopathy-associated virus (LAV) or AIDS-related virus (ARV)
   2. According to the Center for Disease Control (CDC) guidelines, the individual is considered to have AIDS when antibodies to HIV are present in the

blood and the presence of an opportunistic infection, such as *Pneumocystis carinii* pneumonia or a rare skin cancer known as Kaposi's sarcoma, has been documented

3. The individual is considered to have AIDS-related complex (ARC) when there are no opportunistic infections classically associated with AIDS, but there are symptoms such as anorexia, weight loss, decreased resistance, night sweats, and fatigue; a positive blood test for the AIDS antibody is also present
4. The individual is considered HIV positive when the blood test reveals the presence of HIV, but the individual is asymptomatic
5. Virus is present in blood, semen, vaginal secretions, saliva, tears, and cerebrospinal fluid; transmission occurs through contact with infected blood, semen, and vaginal secretions; oral secretions have been implicated
6. Once individuals are infected with HIV, whether or not they have progressed to ARC or AIDS, they are capable of transmitting the virus
7. Incubation period estimates range from 6 months to 9 years; the antibodies produced by the body can first be detected in the blood from 2 weeks to 3 months after infection; a test that detects the virus can determine its presence within 24 hours of infection
8. The virus attacks the T-lymphocytes, interfering with the client's ability to resist infections, including those infections that are considered opportunistic
9. The virus may also attack the nervous system causing HIV encephalopathy

B. Signs and symptoms
   1. Subjective
      a. Anorexia
      b. Fatigue
   2. Objective
      a. Positive test for HIV infection (antibody or virus)
      b. Night sweats
      c. Fever
      d. Enlarged lymph nodes
      e. HIV wasting syndrome, emaciation
      f. HIV encephalopathy: memory loss, lack of coordination, partial paralysis, mental deterioration
      g. Opportunistic infections
         (1) *Pneumocystis carinii* pneumonia (see Pneumonia)
         (2) Cytomegalovirus
         (3) *Candida albicans* infection of mouth or airways
         (4) Coccidioidomycosis
         (5) *Mycobacterium avium, M. kansasii,* or tuberculosis
         (6) Toxoplasmosis of the brain
      h. Kaposi's sarcoma, normally a rare skin cancer, manifested by dark purplish lesions (for additional information see Kaposi's sarcoma in Integumentary system)

C. Treatment
   1. There is no cure; prevention is the key to control
   2. Azidothymidine (AZT, Retrovir) has been successfully to interfere with the virus' ability to reproduce

3. Other drugs under investigation include suramin sodium, ribavirin, interferon A and HPA-23

D. Nursing care
   1. Use universal precautions for all clients regardless of diagnosis since virus can be transmitted before the client shows signs of disease
   2. Refer to counselor or support group
   3. Provide emotional support; client must deal with social rejection and death
   4. Protect the client from secondary infection; carefully assess for early signs
   5. Maintain body secretion precautions to prevent transmission to others
   6. Monitor client receiving Retrovir for side effects such as nervousness, anxiety, tremors, hypotension, and blood dyscrasias
   7. Teach client the importance of
      a. Informing sexual contacts of diagnosis
      b. Avoiding sexual intercourse unless using a condom
      c. Not sharing needles with other individuals
      d. Continuing medical supervision
   8. Provide high-caloric, high-protein diet to prevent weight loss
   9. Support natural defense mechanisms of client; encourage intake of foods rich in the immune-stimulating nutrients, especially vitamins A, C, and E, and the mineral selenium
   10. See Syphilis for additional nursing care
   11. Evaluate client's response and revise plan as necessary

Endocrine System
REVIEW OF ANATOMY AND PHYSIOLOGY OF THE ENDOCRINE SYSTEM
Functions

Endocrine glands secrete products called hormones, which are chemical messengers that deliver stimulatory or inhibitory signals to target cells (Table 3-6)

Glands
Thyroid Gland

A. Anatomy
   1. Soft, red-brown mass having right and left pear-shaped lobes joined by a narrow isthmus
   2. Extends from sides of cricoid and thyroid cartilages to sixth tracheal cartilage
   3. Half of glands observed have a pyramidal lobe extending upward from the isthmus

B. Actions of thyroid hormones (Table 3-7)
   1. Accelerate cellular reactions in most body cells
      a. Increase BMR
      b. Accelerate growth
      c. Alter the metabolic rate of over 100 enzyme systems by profound stimulatory effect on cellular protein synthesis
   2. Bind to nuclear and cytoplasmic receptor sites
      a. Intranuclear chromatin protein binds thyroid hormones; this stimulates cellular protein synthesis and influences growth, development, and cell differentiation
      b. Mitochondrial membranes bind thyroid hormones, which regulate energy metabolism

Table 3-6. Location and hormones of endocrine glands

Endocrine gland	Location	Hormones
Pituitary Anterior (adenohypophysis)	Cranial cavity, in sella turcica of sphenoid bone	Growth hormone (GH, somatotropin, somatropic hormone, STH)* Thyrotropin (thyroid-stimulating hormone, or TSH) Adrenocorticotropic hormone (ACTH, corticotropin)* Follicle-stimulating hormone (FSH) Luteinzing hormone (LH) in female; interstitial cell-stimulating hormone (ICSH) in male Prolactin (lactogenic hormone, luteotropin) Melanocyte-stimulating hormone (MSH) Alpha and beta lipotropins
Posterior (neurohypophysis)	In sella turcica of sphenoid bone	Antidiuretic hormone (ADH, vasopressin)† Oxytocin†
Pineal	Midbrain	Melatonin
Thyroid	Overlies thyroid cartilage below the larynx	Thyroid hormones (thyroxine and triiodothyronine), Calcitonin
Parathyroids	Usually 4 beads on posterior wall of the thyroid	Parathormone
Thymus	Root of neck and anterior thorax	Thymosin‡
Adrenals	Situated on medial anterior surface of each kidney	
Cortex		Glucocorticoids (mainly cortisol and corticosterone) Mineralocorticoids (mainly aldosterone) Sex hormones (small amounts of androgens and estrogens)
Medulla		Epinephrine (mainly) Norepinephrine
Pancreas (islets of Langerhans)	Retroperitoneal in abdominal cavity	Insulin (secreted by beta cells) Glucagon (secreted by alpha cells) Somatostatin Pancreatic polypeptide

Ovaries
    Graafian follicles
    Corpus luteum
	Pelvic cavity (female)	Estrogens (estradiol, estrone)
		Progesterone

Testes Interstitial cells of testes	Scrotum (male)	Testosterone

*Also present in placenta along with estrogens and progesterone.
†ADH and oxytocin are synthesized in the hypothalamus but are secreted by the posterior pituitary gland. Synthesis occurs in cell bodies of neurons of the supraoptic and paraventricular nuclei. From here they migrate down the neurons' axons into the posterior pituitary gland, which secretes them into the blood.
‡One of several active thymic hormones.

C. Metabolism (inactivation) of thyroid hormones
  1. Liver the principal organ regulating blood concentration of thyroid hormones; thyroxine and triiodothyronine deaminated, deiodinated, and conjugated; conjugates excreted in the bile
  2. Skeletal muscle, kidney, liver, and heart tissues deiodinate thyroid hormones; this mechanism of hormone inactivation not as important as conjugation in liver

D. Calcitonin
  1. Decreases loss of Ca^{++} from bone through inhibition of osteocytic and osteoclastic osteolysis (cAMP mechanism)
    a. Action opposite that of parathormone
    b. Some bone cells respond specifically to calcitonin; others to parathormone
  2. Decreases loss of Ca^{++} from bone and promotes hypocalcemia; this effect offsets postprandial hypercalcemia

Table 3-7. Functions of thyroid and parathyroid hormones

Hormones	Functions	Hypofunction effects	Hyperfunction effects
Thyroid hormones Thyroxine	Stimulate metabolic rate; therefore essential for normal physical and mental development	Cretinism, if occurs early in life; myxedema, if occurs in older children or adults	Hyperthyroidism
Triiodothyronine	Inhibit anterior pituitary secretion of TSH		
Thyrocalcitonin	Quickly decreases blood calcium concentration if Ca^{++} increases about 20% above normal level; presumably accelerates calcium movement from blood into bone		
Parathyroid hormone (parathormone)	Increases blood calcium concentration by accelerating following three processes: 1. Breakdown of bone with release of calcium into blood 2. Calcium absorption from intestine into blood 3. Kidney tubule reabsorption of calcium from tubular urine into blood, thereby decreasing calcium loss in urine	Decreased blood calcium (hypocalcemia), which causes increased neural excitability and tetany	Increased blood calcium (hypercalcemia), which causes decreased neural excitability and muscle weakness Bone "softening"—decalcification
	Decreases blood phosphate concentration by slowing its reabsorption by kidney tubules and thereby increasing phosphate loss in urine	Increased blood phosphorous (hyperphosphatemia)	Hypophosphatemia

Parathyroid Glands

A. Anatomy: generally four small yellow glands (but may be two to twelve); 0.6 cm (¼ inch) in diameter at their widest part; usually embedded in the capsule of the posterior part of the thyroid (but may be behind the pharynx or in the thorax with the thymus)

B. Actions of parathyroid hormones (Table 3-7)
  1. Parathormone: major sites of action are skeleton, kidneys, and intestine
    a. Bone tissue releases Ca^{++} into blood (requires active form of vitamin D)
      (1) Osteoclastic osteolysis stimulated
      (2) Osteocytic osteolysis stimulated
      (3) Enhanced rate of maturation of precursor cells into osteoclasts and osteoblasts
      (4) Inhibition of osteoblastic collagen synthesis
    b. Kidney tubule reabsorption of Ca^{++} and Mg^{++} is enhanced, which helps prevent further decreases in serum Ca^{++} levels; excretion of K^+, P^{+++}, and HCO_3^- also is enhanced; that of H^+ and NH_4^+ is decreased
    c. Parathormone, through adenylate cyclase activation, stimulates kidney's production of the enzyme that converts 25-dihydroxycholecalciferol into 1,25-hydroxycholecalciferol, which is the active form of vitamin D that works with parathormone in bone to mobilize Ca^{++}
    d. The intestinal mucosa increases its absorption of Ca^{++} and P^{+++}, with subsequent release into the blood

Testes

A. Anatomy (see Genitourinary system)

B. Actions of testicular (androgenic) hormones (Table 3-8)
  1. Major androgenic action in target tissues is stimulation of protein synthesis through enhancement of nuclear DNA and RNA

  2. Increased protein synthesis manifests itself as increased tissue growth, particularly in younger individuals; at puberty, rise in androgen level induces growth of long bones, muscular development, enlargement of the external genitalia, increased sex drive, laryngeal growth, and growth of body hair
  3. Androgens influence fetal brain development through contributing to establishment of neural pathways that help to regulate adult brain functions and behavior

C. Metabolism of androgens
  1. Liver the major site for androgen metabolism; testosterone and other androgenic steroids are enzymatically converted into other less androgenic steroids and then conjugated with glucuronic acid or sulfate
  2. The generally biologically inactive conjugates are excreted in bile and urine

Ovaries

A. Anatomy (see Genitourinary system)

B. Actions of ovarian hormones (Table 3-8)
  1. Estrogens
    a. Enter target cells, bind cycloplasmic receptors, and enter nucleus; estrogen receptor complex regulates mRNA synthesis with overall effect of stimulating cellular RNA and protein synthesis
    b. Stimulate uterine and liver lipid metabolism
    c. Stimulate long bone calcification
    d. Play a major role in the ovulatory-menstrual cycle
    e. Increased protein and lipid synthesis are manifested in the reproductive system as uterine growth
    f. Participate also in growth of pubic and axillary hair, pelvic enlargement, subcutaneous lipid distribution, growth of mammary glands, and maturation of skin (increased glandular activity)

Table 3-8. Sex hormones (ovarian and testicular)

Hormones	Functions
Estrogens (secreted by graafian follicle and corpus luteum) Estradiol Estrone Estriol	Stimulate proliferation of epithelial cells of female reproductive organs (e.g., thickening of endometrium, breast development) Stimulate uterine contractions Accelerate protein anabolism (including bone matrix synthesis) so promote growth; but also promote epiphyseal closure so limit height Mildly accelerate sodium and water reabsorption by kidney tubules; increase water content of uterus High blood estrogen concentration inhibits anterior pituitary secretion of FSH and prolactin but stimulates its secretion of LH Low blood estrogen concentration after delivery of baby stimulates anterior pituitary secretion of prolactin
Progesterone (secreted by corpus luteum and placenta)	Name "progesterone" indicates hormone's general function, "favoring pregnancy": Stimulates secretion by endometrial glands, thereby preparing endometrium for implantation of fertilized ovum Inhibits uterine contractions, thereby favoring retention of implanted embryo Promotes development of alveoli (secreting cells) of estrogen-primed breasts; necessary for lactation Protein-catabolic and salt- and water-retaining effects similar to those of corticoids but milder; increases water content of endometrium
Testosterone (secreted by interstitial cells of testes)	Growth and development of male reproductive organs; promotes "maleness" Marked stimulating effect on protein anabolism, including synthesis of bone matrix and muscular development, hence, promotes growth; however, it also tends to limit height by promoting epiphyseal closure Mild acceleration of kidney tubule reabsorption of sodium chloride and water Inhibits secretion of ICSH by anterior pituitary

2. Progesterone
  a. Increases mucus secretory activity of endometrium; such action required for implantation of young embryo
  b. Promotes growth of breasts
  c. Keeps uterine smooth muscle quiescent during pregnancy
  d. Inhibits oxytocin release by neurohypophysis (otherwise released in response to vaginal distention)
C. Metabolism of estrogens and progesterone
  1. Liver conjugates estrogens with glucuronic and sulfuric acids; the conjugates are excreted chiefly in urine
  2. Conversion of estradiol to the less active estrone in the liver; placenta also carries out this conversion
  3. Liver converts progesterone, synthesized from cholesterol in corpus luteum, placenta, and adrenals, to pregnanediol, which is then conjugated with glucuronic acid or sulfate; conjugates are excreted in urine

Adrenal Glands
A. Anatomy
  1. Wedge-shaped, flattened, yellowish structure positioned like a cap at the kidney's superior border
  2. Actually two closely associated structures: inner adrenal medulla and outer adrenal cortex; medulla and cortex each produce hormones with distinct effects on distant target structures
  3. Medulla produces two catecholamines, D-epinephrine and D-norepinephrine, in approximate ratio of 80% to 20%, respectively

4. Cortex secretes three steroid hormones in relatively large amounts: aldosterone (a mineralocorticoid), cortisol (known as hydrocortisone) and corticosterone (both glucocorticoids); also small amounts of several androgenic steroids; adrenocortical secretion is circadian, with higher levels produced during daytime; aldosterone secretion increases as sodium ions (Na^+) decrease or potassium ions (K^+) increase
B. Actions of adrenal hormones
  1. Epinephrine and norepinephine
    a. Stimulate liver and skeletal muscle to break down glycogen
    b. Increase oxygen utilization and increase carbon dioxide production
    c. Increase blood concentration of free fatty acids through stimulation of lipolysis in adipose tissue
    d. Cause constriction of nearly all blood vessels of body, thereby greatly increasing total peripheral resistance and arterial pressure
    e. Increase heart rate and force of contraction and thereby raise cardiac output
    f. Epinephrine significantly dilates bronchial smooth muscle
    g. Inhibit contractions of gastrointestinal and uterine smooth muscle
  2. Glucocorticoids and mineralocorticoids (Table 3-9)
C. Metabolism of adrenocortical steroids
  1. Liver the major organ metabolizing adrenal steroids
  2. Conjugation of steroids with glucuronic acid or sulfate produces inactive products primarily excreted in urine

Table 3-9. Functions of adrenal cortex hormones

Functions	Hypofunction effects (e.g., in Addison's disease)	Hyperfunction effects (e.g., in Cushing's syndrome)
Glucocorticoids (mainly cortisol [hydrocortisone] and corticosterone)		
In general, a normal blood concentration of glucocorticoids promotes normal metabolism of all three kinds of foods and a high blood concentration produces various stress responses		
Accelerates mobilization and catabolism of fats; i.e., causes shift from usual utilization of carbohydrates for energy to fat utilization		
Accelerates tissue protein mobilization and catabolism (tissue proteins hydrolyzed to amino acids, which enter blood and are carried to liver for deamination and gluconeogenesis)		Muscle atrophy and weakness; osteoporosis
Accelrates liver gluconeogenesis (i.e., formation of glucose from mobilized proteins [hyperglycemic effect])	Hypoglycemia	Hyperglycemia
Causes atrophy of lymphatic tissues, notably thymus and lymph nodes		Lymphocytopenia
Decreases antibody formation (immunosuppressive, antiallergic effect)		Decreased immunity Decreased allergy
Slows the proliferation of fibroblasts characteristic of inflammation (antiinflammatory effect)		Spread of infections; slower wound healing
Mild acceleration of sodium and water reabsorption and potassium excretion by kidney tubules		High blood sodium (hypernatremia); sodium retention; also water retention; low blood potassium (hypokalemia)
Decreases ACTH secretion		
Mineralocorticoids (mainly aldosterone)		
Marked acceleration of sodium and water reabsorption by kidney tubules	Low blood sodium (hyponatremia); dehydration, hypovolemia	High blood sodium (hypernatremia); water retention; edema
Marked acceleration of potassium excretion by kidney tubules	High blood potassium (hyperkalemia)	Low blood potassium (hypokalemia)

3. In liver disease, adrenal steroids increase in blood due to decreased inactivation

Pancreas

A. Anatomy (see Gastrointestinal system)
B. Actions of pancreatic hormones
  1. Regulate glucose homeostasis through action of insulin and glucagon; also secrete somatostatin and pancreatic polypeptide
  2. Insulin stimulates intracellular macromolecular syntheses, such as glycogen synthesis, protein synthesis, and lipogenesis
  3. Insulin stimulates cellular uptake of Na^+ and K^+ (latter is significant in the treatment of diabetic coma with insulin); glucose also requires K^+ supplement to offset hypokalemia
  4. Glucagon induces liver glycogenolysis similar to that produced by epinephrine, but glucagon functions at lower concentration and also does not raise blood pressure; antagonizes the glycogen synthesis stimulated by insulin
  5. Glucagon inhibits hepatic protein synthesis; this makes amino acids available for gluconeogenesis and also increases urea production

6. Glucagon stimulates hepatic ketogenesis and release of glycerol and fatty acids from adipose tissue
7. Primary target organs are muscle, liver, and adipose cells, but other tissues also affected
8. Somatostatin inhibits release of both insulin and glucagon
9. Pancreatic polypeptide increases pancreatic and gastric secretions; secreted into blood after a protein-rich meal; secretion inhibited by somatostatin

Thymus

A. Anatomy
  1. Soft, pink mass extending from lower border of thyroid to the fourth costal cartilages; great variation in size; two asymmetric lobes
  2. Large at birth; decreases in size after puberty; hardly visible beyond middle age
B. Actions of thymic hormones
  1. Regulate immunologic processes, possibly through regulation of the numbers and types of lymphoid cells; decrease in immune response; with aging, parallels thymus involution and decreasing blood concentrations of thymic hormones

Table 3-10. Functions of anterior pituitary hormones

Functions	Hyposecretion effects	Hypersecretion effects
Growth hormone (GH)		
Promotes protein anabolism (hence essential for normal growth)	Dwarfism (well-formed type) if it occurs before skeletal growth is completed	Giantism if it occurs before skeletal growth is completed
Promotes fat mobilization and catabolism (i.e., causes shift from carbohydrate catabolism to fat catabolism)	Simmonds' disease after skeletal maturity	Acromegaly if it occurs after skeletal maturity
Slows carbohydrate metabolism; has anti-insulin, hyperglycemic, diabetogenic effect (promotes glucagon secretion)		Hyperglycemia, chronic excess GH may cause diabetes mellitus
Thyroid-stimulating hormone (TSH)		
Stimulates synthesis and secretion of thyroid hormones	Hypothyroidism: cretinism in early life, myxedema in adults	Hyperthyroidism (exophthalmic goiter, various other names)
Adrenocorticotropic hormone (ACTH)		
Stimulates adrenal cortex growth and secretion of glucocorticoids; slight mineralocorticoid stimulation	Atrophy of adrenal cortex and hyposecretion (e.g., Addison's disease) Increased skin pigmentation	Hypertrophy of adrenal cortex and hypersecretion (Cushing's syndrome)
Follicle-stimulating hormone (FSH)		
Stimulates primary graafian follicle to start growing and to develop to maturity	Failure of follicle and ovum to grow and mature; sterility	
Stimulates follicle cells to secrete estrogens		
In male, FSH stimulates development of seminiferous tubules and spermatogenesis by them		
Luteinizing hormone (LH)		
Essential for bringing about complete maturation of follicle and ovum		
Required for ovulation		
Causes formation of corpus luteum in ruptured follicle following ovulation; hence the name luteinizing hormone		
Stimulates corpus luteum to secrete progesterone		
In males LH is called interstitial cell-stimulating hormone (ICSH) because it stimulates interstial cells of testes to secrete testosterone		
Prolactin		
Promotes breast development during pregnancy	Failure to lactate	
Initiates milk secretion after delivery of baby		
Stimulates progesterone secretion by corpus luteum		
Alpha and beta lipoproteins		
Cause release of lipid from adipose cells		

2. Just after birth the thymus produces specific lymphocytes that migrate to peripheral regions (e.g., lymph nodes, spleen) to provide immunologic potential

3. Thymus synthesizes hormones that regulate the rate of development of lymphoid cells, particularly T cells

Pineal Gland

A. Anatomy
   1. A firm, reddish, conical structure lying in the midbrain between the superior colliculi and attached by a short stalk to the roof of the third ventricle
   2. Composed of cords of pinealocytes (or chief cells) separated by connective tissue; septa continuous

Table 3-11. Functions of posterior pituitary hormones

Functions	Hyposecretion effects	Hypersecretion effects
Antidiuretic hormone (ADH) vasopressin Increases water reabsorption by kidney's distal and collecting tubules, thereby producing antidiuresis (less urine volume; name based on this effect) Stimulates vasoconstriction; raises blood pressure	Diuresis (polyuria); diabetes insipidus	Antidiuresis (oliguria)
Oxytocin Stimulates powerful contractions by pregnant uterus Stimulates milk ejection from alveoli (milk-secreting cells) of lactating breasts into ducts; essential before milk can be removed by suckling		
Coherin Regulates peristaltic rhythmicity in intestinal smooth muscle		
Melanocyte-stimulating hormone (MSH) Stimulates synthesis and dispersion of melanin skin, causing darkening		

with the pia mater covering the organ; cells accumulate calcareous granules (brain sand) by age 18 clearly visible at x-ray examination

B. Actions of pineal hormone
  1. Secretes melatonin
  2. Melatonin may regulate diurnal fluctuations of hypothalamic-hypophyseal hormones

Pituitary Gland

A. Anatomy
  1. Rounded body 1.2 cm (½ inch) in diameter extending downward from the floor of the brain's third ventricle by a stalk (infundibulum); supported and protected by the sella turcica of the sphenoid bone; located near the optic chiasm
  2. Composed of an anterior lobe (adenohypophysis) and a posterior lobe (neurohypophysis)
B. Actions of pituitary hormones (Tables 3-10 and 3-11)

PHARMACOLOGY RELATED TO ENDOCRINE SYSTEM DISORDERS
Antidiabetic Agents

A. Description
  1. Used to treat diabetes mellitus
  2. Classified into two types: insulin for parental use and oral hypoglycemics
  3. Insulin acts to facilitate the transport of glucose across the cell membrane and to promote glycogenesis
  4. Insulin is available in three forms: beef, pork, and human; human and purified pork insulin are less antigenic than the other forms
  5. Oral hypoglycemics stimulate pancreatic beta cells to produce insulin in clients with residual functioning cells
B. Examples
  1. Insulin: exogenous replacement of insulin hormone; parenteral administration only (see Table 3-12)

  2. Oral hypoglycemics: stimulate pancreatic beta cells to produce insulin in clients with residual functioning cells
    a. acetohexamide (Dymelor)
    b. chlorpropamide (Diabinese)
    c. glipizide (Glucotrol)
    d. glyburide (Micronase)
    e. tolazamide (Tolinase)
    f. tolbutamide (Orinase)
C. Major side effects
  1. Irritability (hypoglycemia)
  2. Confusion (hypoglycemia)
  3. Convulsions (hypoglycemia)
  4. Tachycardia (hypoglycemia)
  5. Tremor (hypoglycemia)
  6. Moist skin (hypoglycemia)
  7. Headache (hypoglycemia)
  8. Hunger (hypoglycemia)
  9. Oral hypoglycemics
    a. Skin rash (hypersensitivity)
    b. Jaundice (hepatic alterations)
    c. Pruritus (hypersensitivity)
    d. Allergic reactions (hypersensitivity)
D. Nursing care
  1. Assess client for signs of hypoglycemia
  2. Instruct client to
    a. Utilize proper medication administration procedure
    b. Comply with dietary program
    c. Avoid alcohol
    d. Utilize proper procedure for urine and/or blood testing
    e. Carry medical alert card
    f. Be prepared for hypoglycemic incidents (rapid-acting glucose solution, hard candy, orange juice)
  3. Administer insulin
    a. Administer all forms of insulin subcutaneously
    b. Use only regular insulin for IV administration

Table 3-12. Types of insulin

Insulin	Action		
	Onset (hr)	Peak (hr)	Duration (hr)
Rapid acting			
Insulin injection (regular insulin)	½ to 1	2 to 4	5 to 8
Prompt insulin zinc suspension (Semilente)	1 to 3	2 to 8	12 to 16
Intermediate acting			
Globin zinc insulin injection	2 to 3	8 to 16	18 to 24
Insulin zinc suspension (Lente)	1 to 3	8 to 12	24 to 30
Isophane insulin suspension (NPH)	3 to 4	6 to 12	24 to 30
Long acting			
Extended insulin zinc suspension (Ultralente)	4 to 6	18 to 24	34 to 36
Protamine zinc insulin suspension (PZI)	4 to 6	14 to 24	30 to 36

  c. When mixing insulins, draw regular insulin into the syringe first
  d. Rotate sites of administration
  e. Slight dosage adjustment may be necessary when switching from one form of insulin to another because of differing pharmacokinetics
 4. Offer emotional support to client; therapy is life-long
 5. Evaluate client's response to medication and understanding of teaching

Thyroid Enhancers

A. Description
 1. Used to replace thyroid hormone in clients experiencing a reduction in or absence of thyroid gland function
 2. Thyroid hormone regulates the metabolic rate of body cells, aids in growth and development of bones and teeth, and affects protein, fat, and carbohydrate metabolism
 3. Available in oral and parenteral (IV) preparations
B. Examples
 1. levothyroxine sodium (Synthroid)
 2. liothyronine sodium (Cytomel)
 3. liotrix (Euthroid, Thyrolar)
 4. thyroglobulin (Proloid)
 5. thyroid (Thyrar)
C. Major side effects
 1. Increased metabolism (increased serum T_3, T_4)
 2. Hyperactivity (increased metabolic rate)
 3. Cardiac stimulation (increased cardiac metabolism)
D. Nursing care
 1. Instruct client to
  a. Report the occurrence of any side effects to the physician immediately
  b. Take medication as scheduled at the same time each day
  c. Take radial pulse; notify physician if greater than 100 beats/minute
  d. Carry medical alert card
  e. Keep all scheduled appointments with physician; medical supervision is necessary
 2. Assess client for potentiation of anticoagulant effect
 3. Offer emotional support to client; therapy may be for life

 4. Assess client for signs of hyperthyroidism
 5. Evaluate client's response to medication and understanding of teaching

Thyroid Inhibitors

A. Description
 1. Used to treat hyperthyroidism
 2. Act by interfering with the synthesis and release of thyroid hormone; inhibit oxidation of iodides to prevent their combination with tyrosine in formation of thyroxine
 3. Available in oral and parenteral (IV) preparations
B. Examples
 1. iodine (Lugol's solution)
 2. methimazole (Tapazole)
 3. propylthiouracil (PTU)
C. Major side effects
 1. Agranulocytosis (decreased WBCs)
 2. Skin disturbances (hypersensitivity)
 3. Nausea, vomiting (irritation of gastric mucosa)
 4. Decreased metabolism (decreased production of serum T_3, T_4)
 5. Iodine: bitter taste; stains teeth (local oral effect on mucosa and teeth)
D. Nursing care
 1. Instruct client to
  a. Report the occurrence of any side effects to physician, especially sore throat and fever
  b. Avoid crowded places and potentially infectious situations
 2. Administer liquid iron preparations diluted in beverage of choice through a straw
 3. Assess client for signs of hypothyroidism
 4. Evaluate client's response to medication and understanding of teaching

Adrenocorticosteroids

A. Description
 1. Interfere with the release of factors important in producing the normal inflammatory and immune responses
 2. Increase glucose and fat formation and promote protein breakdown
 3. Available in oral, parenteral (IM, IV), inhalation, intraarticular, and topical, including ophthalmic, preparations

B. Examples
1. betamethasone preparations
2. dexamethasone (Decadron)
3. fludrocortisone acetate (Florinef Acetate)
4. hydrocortisone (Cortef)
5. hydrocortisone succinate (Solu-Cortef)
6. methylprednisolone sodium succinate (Solu-Medrol)
7. prednisone (Deltasone)
C. Major side effects
1. Cushing-like symptoms (increased glucocorticoid activity)
2. Hypertension (promotion of sodium and water retention)
3. Hyperglycemia (increased carbohydrate catabolism; gluconeogenesis)
4. CNS stimulation (CNS effect)
5. Euphoria (CNS effect)
6. GI irritation and ulcer formation (local GI effect)
7. Cataracts (hyperglycemia)
8. Hypokalemia (promotion of potassium excretion)
D. Nursing care
1. Administer oral preparations with food, milk, or antacid
2. Monitor client's weight, blood pressure, and serum electrolytes during therapy
3. Avoid placing client in potentially infectious situations
4. Assess for GI bleeding; monitor blood glucose in diabetics
5. Instruct client to
a. Avoid exposure to infections; notify physician if fever or sore throat occurs
b. Avoid using salt; encourage foods high in potassium
c. Avoid immunizations during therapy
d. Carry medical alert card
e. Avoid missing, changing, or withdrawing drug suddenly
6. Withdraw drug therapy gradually to avoid adrenal suppression
7. Evaluate client's response to medication and understanding of teaching

Antidiuretic Hormone

A. Description
1. Used in the treatment of diabetes insipidus
2. Acts to
a. Promote water reabsorption by the distal renal tubules
b. Cause vasoconstriction and increased muscle tone of the bladder, GI tract, uterus, and blood vessels
3. Available in parenteral (IM, SC) or nasal preparation
B. Examples
1. lypressin (Diapid): intranasal administration
2. vasopressin (Pitressin)
3. vasopressin tannate (Pitressin tannate)
C. Major side effects
1. Increased intestinal activity (direct peristaltic stimulant)

2. Hyponatremia (promotion of water reabsorption)
3. Pallor (hemodilution)
4. Water intoxication (promotion of water reabsorption)
5. Cardiac disturbances (fluid/electrolyte imbalance)
6. lypressin nasal irritation (local effect on nasal mucosa)
D. Nursing care
1. Assess client for signs of dehydration during therapy
2. Monitor intake and output
3. If drug is administered to improve bladder or bowel tone, assess for continence or passage of flatus
4. Assess vital signs, especially blood pressure, during course of therapy
5. Evaluate client's response to medication and understanding of teaching

PROCEDURES RELATED TO THE ENDOCRINE SYSTEM
Fingerstick for Glucose

A. Definition: capillary blood is analyzed as direct measure of blood glucose
B. Nursing care
1. Cleanse skin with antiseptic solution and allow to dry
2. Prick fingertip or earlobe with sterile needle or lancet to obtain blood specimen
3. Apply free-flowing drop of blood to glucose-sensitive reagent strip
4. Blot or wipe strip after specified interval according to manufacturer's instructions
5. Visually compare color of reagent to manufacturer's chart or use computerized blood glucose monitoring system
6. Chart results
7. Administer regular insulin coverage if ordered
8. Instruct client about individual method of self blood-glucose monitoring (BGM)
9. Evaluate client's response to procedure

Sugar and Acetone (Fractional Urine Tests)

A. Definition
1. Sugar refers to the percent of glucose in the urine as indirect measure of blood glucose
2. Acetone refers to the amount of ketones, a byproduct of fat metabolism, present in the urine
B. Nursing care
1. Obtain a recently voided specimen approximately one half hour before meals and at bedtime; a double-voided specimen would produce most accurate results (client empties bladder and one-half hour later is asked to void again)
2. Test urine with appropriate reagent (Clinitest, Ketodiastix, TestTape, Acetest)
3. Chart results
4. Administer regular insulin coverage if ordered
5. Evaluate client's response to procedure

NURSING PROCESS FOR CLIENTS WITH ENDOCRINE SYSTEM DISORDERS
Probable Nursing Diagnosis Based on Assessment

A. Activity intolerance related to decreased metabolic rate
B. Sleep pattern disturbance related to increased metabolic rate
C. Ineffective individual coping related to chronic nature of disability
D. Fluid volume excess related to electrolyte imbalance and medications
E. Fluid volume deficit related to increased urinary output
F. Altered nutrition: less than body requirements related to increased metabolic rate or altered utilization of nutrients
G. Fatigue related to decreased metabolic energy production
H. Sensory/perceptual alteration related to metabolic alteration
I. Noncompliance related to inability to accept chronic disease
J. Body image disturbance related to hormonal changes
K. Constipation related to decreased metabolic rate
L. Diarrhea related to increased metabolic rate
M. Potential for infection related to disease process

Nursing Care for Clients with Endocrine System Disorders

See Nursing care under each specific disease

MAJOR DISEASES
Hyperpituitarism

A. Etiology and pathophysiology
 1. May be due to overactivity of gland or the result of an adenoma
 2. Characterized by an excessive concentration of pituitary hormones in the blood, overactivity, and changes in the anterior lobe of the pituitary gland
 3. Two classifications
  a. Giantism: generalized increase in size, especially in children; involves the long bones
  b. Acromegaly: occurs after epiphyseal closing, with subsequent enlargement of cartilage, bone, and soft tissues of body
B. Signs and symptoms
 1. Subjective
  a. Headaches
  b. Depression
  c. Weakness
 2. Objective
  a. Increased soft tissue and bone thickness
  b. Facial features become coarse and heavy, with enlargement of lower jaw, lips, and tongue
  c. Enlarged hands and feet
  d. Increased somatotropin serum levels
  e. X-ray examination of long bones, skull (sella turcica area), and jaw demonstrates change in structure
  f. Amenorrhea
  g. Glycosuria
  h. Diabetes and hyperthyroidism may also occur

C. Treatment
 1. Medications to relieve symptoms of other endocrine imbalances resulting from pituitary hyperfunctioning
 2. Surgical intervention (hypophysectomy) or irradiation of the pituitary
D. Nursing care
 1. Help the client accept the altered body image that is irreversible
 2. Assist family to understand what the client is experiencing
 3. Help the client recognize that medical supervision will be required for life
 4. Help the client understand the basis for the change in sexual functioning
 5. Assist the client in expressing feelings
 6. Care for the client following a hypophysectomy
  a. Encourage following an established medical regimen
  b. Protect from stress situations
  c. Protect from infection
  d. Follow and maintain an established schedule for hormone replacement
  e. Follow nursing care for the client undergoing intracranial surgery
 7. Evaluate client's response and revise plan as necessary

Hypopituitarism (Simmonds' Disease)

A. Etiology and pathophysiology
 1. Total absence of pituitary hormones
 2. Occurs when there is destruction of the anterior lobe of the gland by trauma, tumor, or hemorrhage
B. Signs and symptoms
 1. Subjective
  a. Lethargy
  b. Loss of strength
  c. Decreased tolerance for cold
 2. Objective
  a. Decreased temperature
  b. Decreased blood pressure
  c. Emaciation
  d. Diminished axillary and pubic hair
C. Treatment
 1. Replace hormones
 2. If tumor is present, surgical intervention is indicated
D. Nursing care
 1. Discuss the importance of adhering to medical regimen on a long-term basis
 2. Allow the client ample time to verbalize feelings regarding the long-term nature of the disease
 3. Evaluate client's response and revise plan as necessary

Diabetes Insipidus

A. Etiology and pathophysiology
 1. Etiology unknown; but may occur as a result of head trauma or surgical ablation or irradiation of the pituitary gland or an adenoma
 2. Occurs when there is a deficiency of vasopressin (ADH), which is secreted by posterior pituitary

B. Signs and symptoms
  1. Subjective
    a. Polydipsia
    b. Craving for cold water
  2. Objective
    a. Polyuria (5 to 25 L/24 hr)
    b. Dilute urine; specific gravity 1.001 to 1.005
    c. Signs of dehydration (poor skin turgor, dry mucous membranes, elevated temperature)

C. Treatment
  1. Administer vasopressin (Pitressin Tannate), antidiuretic hormone
  2. Determine the underlying cause and attempt to treat it

D. Nursing care
  1. Weigh the client daily
  2. Carefully monitor intake and output
  3. Replace fluid by mouth or parenterally
  4. Check results of the serum electrolyte evaluation
  5. Monitor specific gravity of urine
  6. Evaluate client's response and revise plan as necessary

Hypothyroidism

A. Etiology and pathophysiology
  1. Absence or decreased production of thyroid hormone because of primary thyroid disease or response to decreased TSH
  2. Classified according to the time of life in which it occurs
    a. Cretinism: hypothyroidism in infants and young children
    b. Hypothyroidism without myxedema: mild degree of thyroid failure in older children and adults
    c. Hypothyroidism with myxedema: severe degree of thyroid failure in older individuals

B. Signs and symptoms
  1. Subjective
    a. Dull mental processes
    b. Apathy
    c. Lethargy
    d. Intolerance to cold
  2. Objective
    a. Stolid, masklike facies
    b. Increase in weight
    c. Constipation
    d. Subnormal temperature and pulse
    e. Dry, brittle hair
    f. Thickened skin
    g. Enlarged tongue; drooling
    h. Decreased BMR
    i. Decreased thyroxine (T_4) and radioactive iodine uptake
    j. Coarse, dry skin
    k. Thinning of lateral eyebrows
    l. Scalp, axilla, and pubic hair loss
    m. Diminished hearing

C. Treatment
  1. Administer thyroid hormones
  2. Maintain vital functions

D. Nursing care
  1. Explain the importance of continued use of medication
  2. Have patience with a lethargic client
  3. Teach the client and family to be alert for signs of complications
    a. Angina pectoris: chest pain, feeling of indigestion
    b. Cardiac failure: dyspnea, palpitations
    c. Myxedema coma: weakness, syncope, slow pulse rate, subnormal temperature, slow respirations, lethargy
  4. Teach the client to seek medical supervision on a regular basis and when any signs of illness develop
  5. Help the client and family recognize that client's inability to adapt to cold temperature requires additional protection and modification of outdoor activity in cold weather
  6. Teach the client to avoid constipation by the use of adequate hydration and roughage in the diet
  7. Evaluate client's response and revise plan as necessary

Hyperthyroidism (Graves' Disease, Thyrotoxicosis)

A. Etiology and pathophysiology
  1. Excessive concentration of thyroid hormones in the blood as a result of thyroid disease or increased TSH
  2. Overactivity and changes in the thyroid gland may be present
  3. May occur at periods of high physiologic and psychologic stress, although considered by some to be an autoimmune reaction
  4. The gland may also enlarge (goiter) due to decreased iodine intake; no increase in secretion of thyroid is present

B. Signs and symptoms
  1. Subjective
    a. Polyphagia
    b. Emotional lability and apprehension
    c. Heat intolerance
  2. Objective
    a. Weight loss
    b. Increased systolic blood pressure and pulse
    c. Tremors
    d. Hyperhidrosis
    e. Increased respiratory rate
    f. Exophthalmos
    g. Increased BMR
    h. Increased radioactive thyroid uptake
    i. Increased triiodothyronine (T_3), thyroxine (T_4), protein-bound iodine (PBI), and long-acting thyroid stimulator (LATS)
    j. Loose stools

C. Treatment
  1. Antithyroid medications such as propylthiouracil and methimazole (Tapazole) to block the synthesis of thyroid hormone
  2. Antithyroid medications such as iodine to reduce the vascularity of the thyroid gland

3. Radioactive iodine to destroy thyroid gland cells, thereby decreasing the production of thyroid hormone (atomic cocktail)
4. Medications to relieve the symptoms related to the increased metabolic rate (e.g., digitalis, propranolol [Inderal], phenobarbital)
5. Well-balanced, high-calorie diet with vitamin and mineral supplements
6. Surgical intervention involves a subtotal or total thyroidectomy

D. Nursing care
1. Assign the client a private room with the means for temperature control when possible; clients usually prefer a cool room
2. Provide for periods of uninterrupted rest
3. Administer medications to promote sleep
4. Use nursing measures such as warm milk, warm bath, and back rub to establish a climate for rest
5. Protect the client from stress-producing visitors
6. Provide diet high in calories, proteins, and carbohydrates with supplemental feedings between meals and at bedtime; vitamin and mineral supplements should be given as prescribed
7. Understand that the client is upset by lability of mood and exaggerated response to environmental stimuli; take time to explain disease processes involved
8. Care for the client following a thyroidectomy
   a. Observe for signs of respiratory distress and laryngeal stridor caused by tracheal edema (keep tracheotomy set available)
   b. Provide humidity with cold steam nebulizer to keep secretions moist
   c. Keep the bed in a semi-Fowler's position without pillows and teach client to support head
   d. Use a soft cervical collar if ordered to prevent unnecessary neck movement
   e. Observe dressings at the operative site and back of the neck and shoulders for signs of hemorrhage
   f. Observe for signs of thyroid storm; may result from manipulation of the gland during surgery, which releases thyroid hormone into bloodstream
      (1) High fever
      (2) Tachycardia
      (3) Irritability, delirium
      (4) Coma
   g. Notify the physician immediately if signs of thyroid storm occur
   h. Observe for signs of tetany, which can occur after accidental trauma or removal of the parathyroid glands
      (1) Numbness of extremities
      (2) Spasm of the glottis
   i. If tetany occurs, give calcium gluconate IV
   j. Evaluate client's response and revise plan as necessary

Hyperparathyroidism

A. Etiology and pathophysiology
1. Hyperfunction of the parathyroid glands; usually caused by adenoma; hypertrophy and hyperplasia of the glands may also be responsible

2. As a result the kidneys excrete excess calcium and phosphorus
3. If dietary intake is not enough to meet calcium levels demanded by high levels of parathormone, demineralization of the bone occurs

B. Signs and symptoms
1. Subjective
   a. Apathy
   b. Fatigue
   c. Muscular weakness
   d. Anorexia
   e. Emotional irritability
   f. Deep bone pain (if demineralization occurs)
   g. Constipation
2. Objective
   a. Bone cysts, pathologic fractures
   b. Renal calculi composed of calcium
   c. Pyelonephritis, renal damage, uremia
   d. Vomiting
   e. Elevated serum calcium
   f. Decreased serum phosphorus
   g. Cardiac arrhythmias

C. Treatment
1. Surgical excision of a parathyroid tumor
2. Increased fluid intake
3. Activity encouraged
4. Calcium intake restricted

D. Nursing care
1. Observe for signs of skeletal (deep bone pain, deformities) and renal (lower back pain, hematuria) involvement
2. Strain the urine, observing for stones
3. Encourage fluid intake, especially fluids like cranberry juice that acidify the urine
4. Assist the client in ambulating to help prevent demineralization
5. Monitor intake and output
6. Encourage foods such as prune juice and roughage to combat constipation
7. Instruct the client to limit intake of foods high in calcium, especially milk products
8. Provide cardiac monitoring if hypercalcemia is severe
9. If surgery is performed, provide postoperative care the same as for clients undergoing thyroidectomy (see Hyperthyroidism)
10. Evaluate client's response and revise plan as necessary

Hypoparathyroidism

A. Etiology and pathophysiology
1. Parathyroid glands may not secrete a sufficient amount of parathormone after thyroid surgery, parathyroid surgery, or x-ray therapy of the neck; idiopathic hypoparathyroidism rare
2. As levels of parathormone drop, the serum calcium also drops, causing signs of tetany; a concomitant rise in serum phosphate occurs

B. Signs and symptoms
1. Subjective
   a. Photophobia
   b. Diplopia
   c. Muscle cramps

d. Irritability
e. Dyspnea
f. Tingling of extremities
2. Objective
a. Trousseau's sign (carpopedal spasm)
b. Chvostek's sign (contraction of the facial muscle in response to tapping near the angle of the jaw)
c. Decreased serum calcium
d. Elevated serum phosphate
e. Stridor, wheezing from laryngeal spasm
f. Convulsions
g. Cataracts if the disease is chronic
h. X-ray examination reveals increased bone density
i. Cardiac arrhythmias
C. Treatment
1. Calcium chloride or calcium gluconate given IV for emergency treatment
2. Calcium salts administered orally (calcium carbonate, calcium gluconate)
3. Dihydrotachysterol to increase absorption of calcium from the GI tract
4. Calciferol (vitamin D) to help raise serum calcium levels
5. Parathormone injections
6. High-calcium, low-phosphate diet
D. Nursing care
1. Observe respiratory status and have emergency equipment available to perform a tracheostomy
2. Observe seizure precautions
3. Monitor serum calcium and phosphate levels
4. Check vital signs frequently if a history of cardiac problems is present; place on a monitor
5. Provide a calm environment free of harsh stimuli
6. Provide dietary instruction including elimination of milk, cheese, and egg yolks because of high phosphorus content
7. Evaluate client's response and revise plan as necessary

Diabetes Mellitus

A. Etiology and pathophysiology
1. Occurs when there is insufficient supply of insulin and/or cells become insulin resistant; may be due to
a. Failure in body's production
b. Blockage of insulin supply
c. Autoimmune response wherein the insulin may bind to an immune serum globulin fraction, preventing utilization
d. Excess body fat which alters glucose metabolism
2. Incidence increases with obesity, aging, and familial predisposition
3. Type I: insulin-dependent diabetes mellitus (IDDM), formerly called juvenile type; has a rapid onset and requires insulin administration
4. Type II: non-insulin dependent diabetes mellitus (NIDDM), formerly called adult onset type; over 90% of all diabetes is of this type; has a gradual onset and often can be controlled with diet; may be caused by diet high in refined carbohydrate foods which give a rapid and high rise in blood glucose

(glycemic index is high); often associated with obesity
5. Body does not have enough insulin to drive glucose into cells or to convert glucose into glycogen; cells become insensitive to insulin
a. Glucose level in the blood remains high
b. Body attempts to rid itself of excess glucose by excreting some via the kidneys
c. Osmotic force is created within the kidneys due to glucose excretion, and body fluid is lost
d. Body is unable to utilize carbohydrates properly, and fat is oxidized as a compensatory mechanism; oxidation of fats gives off ketone bodies
6. Long-term complications of diabetes include retinopathy, renal failure, peripheral neuropathy, cardiovascular and peripheral vascular diseases
B. Signs and symptoms
1. Subjective
a. Polydipsia
b. Polyphagia
c. Fatigue
d. Blurred vision from retinopathy
e. Peripheral neuropathy
2. Objective
a. Polyuria
b. Weight loss
c. Hyperglycemia: detected by fasting blood sugar, glucose tolerance test, 2-hour postprandial glucose, and glycosylated hemoglobin (provides measure of average glucose level over preceding 2 to 3 months)
d. Glycosuria
e. Peripheral vascular changes and gangrene
C. Treatment
1. Attempt to manage with life-style changes
a. Weight control: if overweight or obese, client should lose excess body fat which alters glucose metabolism (obesity leads to insulin resistance); this can be reversed by weight loss
b. Exercise: increases insulin sensitivity but must be regular; vigorous but not jarring exercise such as brisk walking, swimming, and bicycling is recommended
c. Diet: current recommendations include
(1) Calories controlled to maintain ideal body weight
(2) Stress on high-complex carbohydrate, high-fiber foods rich in water-soluble fiber (oat bran, peas, all forms of beans, pectin-rich fruits and vegetables); particular attention should be paid to the glycemic effect of foods, those with a high glycemic index should be avoided; Glycemic index refers to the effect of particular foods on blood glucose (e.g., water-insoluble fiber has little effect on blood glucose)
(3) Protein: intake should be consistent with the U.S. Dietary Guidelines, usually between 60 and 85 grams depending upon calorie intake
(4) Moderate fat intake: should not exceed 30% of daily calories (70 to 90 g/day); keep saturated fat intake low; emphasize mono- and polyunsaturated fats

(5) Dietary ratio: carbohydrate to protein to fat usually about 5:1:1

(6) Distribute food fairly evenly throughout the day in three or four meals with snacks added between as needed in accordance with total food allowance and therapy (insulin or oral hypoglycemics)

(7) Basic tools for planning diet: food exchange groups, using the exchange system of dietary control; food composition tables showing amount and type of fiber in foods; glycemic index of foods

2. Insulin administration

a. Adjusted after considering the client's physical and emotional stresses, selecting a specific type of insulin depending on the condition and needs of the client (see pharmacology section for discussion of insulin)

b. Somogyi effect: insulin-induced hypoglycemia

(1) Epinephrine is released and the blood sugar level is low

(2) Glucagon is released by alpha cells of the pancreas

(3) These reactions cause mobilization of the liver's stored glucose and iatrogenically induce hyperglycemia

(4) Somogyi phenomenon is treated by gradually lowering insulin dosage while monitoring blood glucose, particularly during the night (when hypoglycemia is most likely to occur)

c. Insulin pump

(1) Battery operated device worn on a belt or harness that delivers insulin through a needle inserted into subcutaneous tissue

(2) Small (basal) doses of regular insulin are delivered every few minutes; bolus doses (extra preset amounts) are delivered prior to meals

(3) Improves glucose control for clients with wide variations in insulin requirements as a result of irregular schedules, pregnancy, or growth requirements

(4) Insulin concentration and basal and bolus doses are programmed into computer of pump

(5) Appropriate amount of insulin for 24 hours plus priming is drawn into syringe

(6) The administration set is primed and needle inserted aseptically, usually into abdomen

3. Oral hypoglycemics for certain clients; however, these clients must have some functioning beta cells in the islets of Langerhans; more commonly prescribed for adults with late developing mild diabetes (see Pharmacology related to endocrine system disorders)

4. Other therapies include pancreas islet cell grafts, pancreas transplants, implantable insulin pumps that continually monitor blood glucose and release insulin accordingly, cyclosporine therapy to prevent beta cell destruction in insulin-dependent (Type I) diabetes

D. Nursing care

1. Assist the client to accept the diagnosis

2. Encourage the client to express feelings about illness and the necessary changes in life-style and self-image

3. Assist the client and family in understanding the disease process

4. Help the client with the administration of medication until self-administration is both physically and psychologically possible

5. Assist the client to recognize the need for continuing health supervision

6. Assist the client in recognizing the need for activities and diet that promote and maintain health

7. Teach client to

a. Test urine for sugar and acetone and interpret results; inaccurate readings may be obtained when the client is taking cephalosporins, aspirin, and ascorbic acid

b. Use blood glucose monitoring system to test blood sugar

c. Select correct testing method based on the client's medication

d. Avoid infection

e. Care for the legs, feet, and toenails properly; inspect, bathe, dry, and lubricate

f. Administer insulin by using sterile technique; rotating injection sites; measuring dosage, types, and strengths of insulin, peak action periods

g. Use dietary chart and make proper substitutions

8. Encourage the client to continue medical supervision and followup care, including visits to an eye care specialist and podiatrist

9. Teach the client and the family the signs of impending hypoglycemia (headache, nervousness, diaphoresis, rapid thready pulse, slurred speech)

10. Teach the client and family the signs of impending diabetic coma (restlessness; hot, dry, flushed skin; thirst; rapid pulse; nausea; fruity odor to breath)

11. Teach client how to use the insulin pump

a. How to insert the needle and fill the syringe; use of aseptic methods

b. When to remove the pump (e.g., before showering or sexual relations)

c. How to test capillary blood glucose levels to monitor insulin dosage at home

12. Encourage followup nutritional counseling

13. Evaluate client's response and revise plan as necessary

Diabetic Coma (Ketoacidosis)

A. Etiology and pathophysiology

1. Occurs in insulin-dependent (Type I) diabetes when there is insufficient insulin available, a systemic infection, diarrhea and vomiting, overindulgence in eating, emotional stress, injury, surgery, or pregnancy

2. Lack of insulin results in alterations of metabolism; proteins and fats are utilized; dehydration and electrolyte imbalance occur; and ketone bodies appear in the urine

B. Signs and symptoms
   1. Subjective
      a. Thirst
      b. Anorexia
      c. Drowsiness
      d. Headache
   2. Objective
      a. Vomiting
      b. Flushed appearance
      c. Lowered blood pressure
      d. Coma
      e. Sweet odor to breath
      f. Kussmaul breathing due to acidosis: very deep respirations as the body attempts to blow off CO_2
      g. Hyperglycemia
      h. Glycosuria and ketonuria
C. Treatment
   1. Insert IV to provide fluid replacement and direct access to the circulatory system, and a Foley catheter to obtain urine samples at frequent intervals
   2. Administer rapid-acting insulin
   3. Replace lost electrolytes, using blood studies to determine dosage
   4. Cardiac monitoring may be indicated if circulatory collapse is imminent
   5. Establish cause of acidosis and treat appropriately
D. Nursing care
   1. Stress adherence to dietary and therapeutic regimen to prevent occurrence
   2. Administer insulin as ordered
   3. Keep accurate records of urine and blood tests, vital signs, and fluid balance
   4. Teach the client regarding dietary habits, prevention of infection, and signs of ketoacidosis
   5. Evaluate client's response and revise plan as necessary

Hyperosmotic Hyperosmolar Nonketotic (HHNK) Coma

A. Etiology and pathophysiology
   1. Similar to ketoacidosis, but occurs in non–insulin dependent (Type II) diabetes and does not involve ketosis
   2. Precipitating factors include infection, diarrhea, and vomiting; failure to comply with dietary/medication regimen; prolonged exposure to drugs which induce hyperglycemia (e.g., steroids)
   3. High serum glucose increases osmotic pressure leading to polyuria and cellular dehydration
B. Signs and symptoms
   1. Subjective
      a. Thirst
      b. Drowsiness
      c. Confusion
   2. Objective
      a. Flushed appearance
      b. Dry, hot skin
      c. Hyperglycemia
      d. Glycosuria
C. Treatment (see Diabetic coma)
D. Nursing care (see Diabetic coma)

Insulin Coma (Insulin Shock)

A. Etiology and pathophysiology
   1. May result when a diabetic client receiving insulin therapy omits a meal, makes an error in insulin dosage, or vomits a meal; the majority of attacks occur in morning or late afternoon
   2. Occurs when blood sugar falls below 60 mg/100 ml
B. Signs and symptoms
   1. Subjective
      a. Muscular weakness
      b. Diplopia
      c. Faintness
      d. Numbness and tingling in fingers, tongue, lips
   2. Objective
      a. Diaphoresis
      b. Trembling
      c. Tachycardia
      d. Disorientation
C. Treatment
   1. Oral glucose administration if the client is alert
   2. Administration of glucagon parenterally to stimulate glucogenolysis
   3. Insertion of an IV line for access to a vein in an emergency
   4. Administration of 50% dextrose
D. Nursing care
   1. Administer medications as ordered
   2. Keep accurate record of intake and output, vital signs, and finger stick test results
   3. If ordered, give client protein or fat feeding after an easily absorbed carbohydrate meal is given
   4. Evaluate client's response and revise plan as necessary

Reactive Hypoglycemia

A. Etiology and pathophysiology
   1. Postprandial fall in blood glucose as a result of abnormal response to stimulus of food
   2. Drop in blood glucose triggers adrenergic and neurologic symptoms
B. Signs and symptoms
   1. Subjective
      a. Anxiety
      b. Irritability
      c. Weakness
      d. Fatigue
   2. Objective
      a. Hypoglycemia
      b. Pallor
      c. Diaphoresis
C. Treatment
   1. Avoidance of rapidly absorbed simple sugars
   2. Frequent meals
   3. Increased emphasis on intake of protein, complex carbohydrates, and fiber which delay gastric emptying and slow glucose absorption
D. Nursing care
   1. Help client distinguish between symptoms that are hypoglycemia-induced and those that are not
   2. Instruct client regarding dietary intake of protein, complex carbohydrates, and fiber

3. Discourage self-diagnosis; encourage medical supervision
4. Evaluate client's response and revise plan as necessary

Primary Aldosteronism (Conn's Syndrome)

A. Etiology and pathophysiology
   1. Aldosterone, a mineralocorticoid, causes the kidneys to retain sodium and excrete potassium
   2. Hypersecretion of aldosterone is usually caused by an adenoma of the adrenal cortex but may also be caused by hyperplasia or carcinoma
   3. The disease is more common in females
B. Signs and symptoms
   1. Subjective
      a. Muscle weakness
      b. Polydipsia, polyuria
      c. Paresthesia
   2. Objective
      a. Hypertension
      b. Hypokalemia
      c. Hypernatremia
      d. Elevated urinary aldosterone levels
      e. Renal damage
         (1) Proteinuria
         (2) Alkaline urine
         (3) Decreased specific gravity of urine
         (4) Pyelonephritis
C. Treatment
   1. Surgical removal of the tumor
   2. Temporary management with spironolactone
   3. Occasionally a bilateral adrenalectomy involving life-long corticosteroid therapy is necessary
D. Nursing care
   1. Monitor vital signs
   2. Observe for signs of electrolyte imbalance
   3. Provide fluids to meet excessive thirst
   4. Encourage continued medical supervision
   5. Monitor intake and output and specific gravity of urine
   6. Care for the client following a bilateral adrenalectomy
      a. Administer steroids with milk or antacid
      b. Protect the client from infection
      c. Explain drug and side effects to client
      d. Instruct the client to carry medical alert identification card
   7. Provide dietary instruction; include foods high in potassium such as orange juice and bananas while avoiding or limiting intake of foods that contain sodium
   8. Evaluate client's response and revise plan as necessary

Cushing's Syndrome

A. Etiology and pathophysiology
   1. Results from excess secretion of adrenocortical hormones
   2. Caused by hyperplasia or by a tumor of the adrenal cortex; however, the primary lesion may occur in the pituitary gland, causing excess production of ACTH
   3. Administration of excess glucocorticoids or ACTH will also cause Cushing's syndrome
B. Signs and symptoms
   1. Subjective
      a. Weakness
      b. Decreased libido
      c. Mood swings to psychosis
   2. Objective
      a. Obese trunk with relatively thin arms and legs
      b. Hypertension
      c. Moon face
      d. Buffalo hump
      e. Acne
      f. Increased susceptibility to infections
      g. Hirsutism
      h. Ecchymotic areas
      i. Purple striae on the breast and abdomen
      j. Amenorrhea
      k. Hyperglycemia
      l. Hypokalemia
      m. Elevated 17-hydroxysteroids
      n. Osteoporosis may be evident on x-ray examination
C. Treatment (aimed at correcting cause)
   1. Reduce dosage of externally administered corticoids
   2. If lesion on pituitary is causing hypersecretion of ACTH, a hypophysectomy or irradiation of the pituitary may be done
   3. Surgical excision of adrenal tumors (adrenalectomy)
   4. Potassium supplements
   5. High-protein diet with sodium restriction
D. Nursing care
   1. Monitor vital signs
   2. Protect the client from exposure to infections
   3. Collect 24-hour urine specimens for diagnostic purposes (17-ketosteroids and 17-hydroxysteroids)
   4. Encourage ventilation of feelings by the client and spouse, since changes in body image and sex drives can alter marital support
   5. Attempt to minimize stress in the environment by measures such as limiting visitors and explaining procedures carefully
   6. Monitor sugar and acetone and blood sugar
   7. Instruct client regarding diet and supplementation; encourage diet rich in nutrient-dense foods such as fruits, vegetables, whole grains, and legumes to improve and maintain nutritional status and prevent any possible drug-induced nutrient deficiencies
   8. Evaluate client's response and revise plan as necessary

Addison's Disease

A. Etiology and pathophysiology
   1. Hyposecretion of adrenocortical hormones
   2. Generally caused by destruction of the cortex or by idiopathic atrophy
B. Signs and symptoms
   1. Subjective
      a. Weakness
      b. Easy fatigue
      c. Nausea

2. Objective
   a. Increased bronze pigmentation of skin
   b. Vomiting
   c. Diarrhea
   d. Hypotension
   e. Hypoglycemia
   f. Small heart
   g. Increased plasma ACTH
   h. Decreased 17-ketosteroids and 17-hydroxy-steroids in 24-hour urines
   i. Hyponatremia
C. Treatment
   1. Replacement of hormones
      a. Glucocorticoids to correct metabolic imbalance
      b. Mineralocorticoids to correct electrolyte imbalance and hypotension
   2. High-carbohydrate, high-protein diet
   3. Special diagnostic tests to determine whether disease is caused by primary adrenocortical insufficiency or is secondary to pituitary insufficiency
      a. Eight-hour IV ACTH test to measure urinary steroid output after administration of ACTH; if output fails to rise, the problem is primary adrenocortical insufficiency (Addison's); if output rises slowly (normal response is rapid rise), the problem is secondary to pituitary insufficiency
      b. Plasma cortisol ACTH test to measure plasma cortisol level before and 30 minutes after administration of ACTH; if level fails to rise, the problem is primary adrenocortical insufficiency (Addison's); if level rises (which is also the normal response), the problem is secondary to pituitary insufficiency
      c. Thorn test to measure eosinophil count before and after administration of ACTH; if count remains the same, the problem is primary adrenocortical insufficiency (Addison's)
D. Nursing care
   1. Administer steroids as ordered
   2. Administer steroids with milk or an antacid to limit ulcerogenic factor of the drug
   3. Put the client in a private room to prevent contact with clients having infectious diseases
   4. Limit the number of visitors
   5. Monitor vital signs four times a day; be alert for elevation in temperature (infection, dehydration), alterations in pulse rate (hyperkalemia), and alterations in blood pressure
   6. Observe for signs of sodium and potassium imbalance
   7. Monitor intake and output and weigh daily
   8. Encourage diet consistent with the U.S. Dietary Goals with emphasis on diet high in nutrient-dense foods
   9. Administer antiemetics to prevent fluid and electrolyte loss by vomiting
   10. Evaluate client's response and revise plan as necessary

Pheochromocytoma

A. Etiology and pathophysiology
   1. Tumor of the adrenal medulla; usually benign
   2. Causes increased secretion of epinephrine and norepinephrine
   3. Heredity believed to be involved in the development of the tumor
B. Signs and symptoms
   1. Subjective
      a. Headache
      b. Visual disturbances
      c. Nausea
   2. Objective
      a. Hypertension and orthostatic hypotension
      b. Tachycardia
      c. Diaphoresis
      d. Increased BMR
      e. Increased urinary catecholamines
      f. Hyperglycemia
C. Treatment
   1. Surgical removal of the tumor
   2. Antihypertensive and antiarrhythmic drugs
D. Nursing care
   1. Monitor blood pressure frequently in both upright and horizontal positions (orthostatic blood pressures)
   2. Administer parenteral fluids and blood as ordered preoperatively and postoperatively to maintain blood volume
   3. Collect a 24-hour urine specimen to evaluate urinary catecholamines
   4. If bilateral adrenalectomy is performed, instruct the client regarding maintenance doses of steroids
   5. Emphasize the importance of continued medical supervision and screening for other family members
   6. Evaluate client's response and revise plan as necessary

Neuromusculoskeletal Systems
REVIEW OF ANATOMY AND PHYSIOLOGY OF THE NEUROMUSCULOSKELETAL SYSTEMS
Nervous System
Cells

Neurons (nerve cells) are basic structural and functional units; about 10 billion in the human brain
A. General properties and functions
   1. Irritability: response to stimulus
   2. Conductivity: conduct electrical energy (nerve impulse); basis for body's rapid communication and integration network
   3. Types
      a. Sensory (afferent) neurons: transmit impulses to spinal cord or brain
      b. Motoneurons (motor or efferent neurons): transmit impulses away from brain or spinal cord toward or to muscles or glands
         (1) Somatic motoneurons: transmit impulses from the cord or brainstem to skeletal muscle
         (2) Visceral or autonomic motoneurons: transmit impulses from the cord or brainstem to smooth muscle, cardiac muscle, or glands
      c. Interneurons (internuncial or intercalated neurons): transmit impulses from sensory neurons to motoneurons
   4. Neurons cannot be replaced if lost, but neuronal contents are constantly being replenished; a system

of axonal flow distributes neural components to all regions from the cell body, where most synthesis occurs

B. Structure: well suited to transmitting impulses over distances
1. Cell body contains a nucleus and other cytoplasmic organelles
2. Axon and dendrites: cellular extensions; single axon or dendrite referred to as a nerve fiber
    a. Axon: one per neuron; carries impulse away from cell body; longer and thinner than dendrites; transmits only at end where it communicates with other neurons, muscles, or glands; may be over 1 m (39 inches) in length and may communicate with 1,000 other neurons
    b. Dendrites: delicate cellular extensions carry impulses toward cell body; several per neuron; each repeatedly branches, forming complex, bushlike network around cell body; increases surface area for reception by neuron of incoming electric signals; dendrite of sensory neurons exceptional in being extremely long, extending to periphery from ganglia near brain and spinal cord
3. Supportive coverings and sheaths
    a. Myelin: multiple, dense layers of membrane wrapped around an axon or dendrite; gaps in myelin every millimeter or so along the fiber are called nodes of Ranvier; myelinated nerve fibers transmit nerve impulses more rapidly than nonmyelinated fibers of same diameter
    b. Neurilemma: sheath of cells (Schwann cells) forming an envelope around axons and some dendrites
        (1) Responsible for effective regeneration of a nerve fiber after injury in the peripheral nervous system; the neurilemma forms a cellular tube down which the regenerating fiber travels
        (2) Forms the myelin sheath
4. Neuronal cell membrane: similar in lipid content to cell membranes of all other body cells; however, specific proteins embedded in and attached to the surface of the lipid provide special characteristics; membrane proteins can be grouped into five classes
    a. Pumps: actively transport ions (notably Na^+ and K^+) between intracellular and interstitial fluid; establish ionic conditions for resting potential and nerve impulse
    b. Channels: provide selective pathways for diffusion of specific ions, as in neuronal depolarization and repolarization; channels open and close (gating mechanisms) in response to voltage changes and chemicals
    c. Receptors: depolarization and repolarization; channels provide specific binding sites for various naturally occurring transmitters and drugs
    d. Enzymes: catalyze chemical reactions on the membrane surface
    e. Structural proteins: interconnect cells to form tissues and organs; hold cell parts together
5. Synapse: point of contact between one neuron and another
    a. Typical neuron may have between 1,000 and 10,000 synapses
    b. Most often occurs between axon of one cell and dendrite of another; also commonly between axon and the cell body of another
    c. Physical gap (synaptic cleft) separates the terminal axonal branches and dendrite or cell body of the next neuron
    d. At the synapse, the axon terminals enlarge to form a terminal button, which is the information-delivering part of the synapse; some synapses are excitatory and others inhibitory
6. Neuroglia takes up most of the space in the nervous system not occupied by neurons; it supports, defends, and nourishes neurons; chief source of CNS tumors; unlike neurons, neuroglia retains the ability to divide; astrocytes, a type of neuroglia cell, provide framework of cells and fibers that suspend neurons and help provide the blood-brain barrier

Nerve Impulse

A. General considerations
1. Wave of electrical energy that flows over the surface of neurons and permits communication and integration between distant body regions
2. The larger the nerve fiber and the thicker the myelin sheath, the greater the velocity of the nerve impulse
3. Based on concentration differences between ions in the intracellular fluid of neuron and surrounding interstitial fluid
4. Ionic differences depend on ion pumps: most often studied is called sodium pump
    a. Requires ATP to work
    b. Pumps three sodium ions out of the cell in exchange for two potassium ions taken into the cell
    c. Due to action of the sodium pump, intracellular fluid is about ten times richer in potassium ions than is interstitial fluid, and interstitial fluid is about ten times richer in sodium ions than is intracellular fluid
B. Impulse generation
1. Resting potential: after the sodium pump establishes ionic gradients, some potassium diffuses out of cell through permanently open potassium channels; such potassium flow results in an excess of positive charge on the membrane's outer surface and a deficit of positive charge on the membrane's inner surface; the result is a voltage difference of 70 millivolts (mV) with the cell interior being negative; this is the resting potential
2. Action potential: change in voltage across the neuronal membrane activates (opens) specific sodium ion channels in the membrane, allowing sodium ions to enter the cell and reverse the membrane's

charge (inside becomes positive and outside becomes negative); as depolarization proceeds, the sodium channel closes and a voltage-gated potassium channel opens so that repolarization occurs with the voltage difference returning to the resting potential

3. Nerve impulse: action potential, composed of depolarization and repolarization, propagates itself down the axon or dendrite and is known as the nerve impulse

C. Basic route of impulse conduction: reflex arc
1. Description: impulse conduction
   a. Starts in receptors
   b. Continues over reflex arc(s)
   c. Terminates in effectors (muscles and glands)
   d. Results in a reflex: response by muscles or glands in which the impulse terminates; a reflex, therefore, is either contraction of muscle or secretion by gland
   e. Not all impulses result in reflexes; many are inhibited at some point along the reflex arc
2. Types of reflex arcs
   a. Two-neuron (monosynaptic) reflex arc: simplest arc possible; consists of at least one sensory neuron, one synapse, and one motor neuron (motoneuron); synapse is a region of contact between axon terminals of one neuron and dendrites or the cell body of another neuron
   b. Three-neuron arc (Fig. 3-7): consists of at least one sensory neuron, one synapse, one interneuron, one synapse, and one motoneuron

   c. Complex multisynaptic neural pathways also exist; many not yet clearly mapped
D. Conduction across synapses
1. Given synapse can transmit only one type of transmitter substance
2. There are 30 different types of neurotransmitters, including
   a. Monoamines (norepinephrine, dopamine, serotonin, acetylcholine); axons that release acetylcholine are called cholinergic; those that release norepinephrine are called adrenergic
   b. Amino acids (gamma-aminobutyric acid [GABA], glutamic acid, glycine, taurine); GABA is the most common inhibitory transmitter in the brain
   c. Neuropeptides (hormone-releasing hormones, enkephalins, and endorphins); some influence hormone levels and some influence perception and integration of pain and emotional experience
   d. Prostaglandins: high levels in brain tissue; some inhibit and some excite; may moderate the action of other transmitters by influencing the neuronal membrane
3. Overall response of the neuron: sum or average of excitatory and inhibitory inputs determines whether the cell will fire and the rate at which it will fire; the neuron is seen to be an evaluator of signals, not just a passive transmitter; the result of its evaluation is its individual rate of impulse transmission

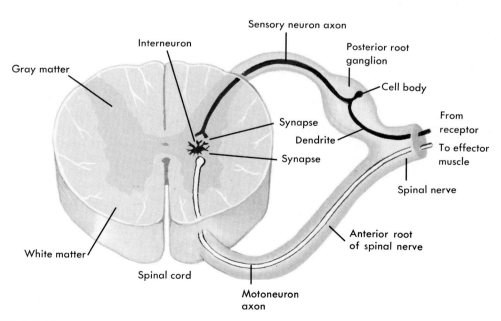

FIG. 3-7. Three-neuron ipsilateral reflex arc, consisting of an afferent (sensory) neuron, an interneuron, and an efferent (motor) neuron (motoneuron). Note the presence of two synapses in this arc: (1) between sensory neuron axon terminals and interneuron dendrites and (2) between interneuron axon terminals and motoneuron dendrites and cell bodies (located in the anterior gray matter). Nerve impulses traversing such arcs produce many spinal reflexes (e.g., withdrawing the hand from a hot object). (From Anthony CP and Thibodeau GA: Textbook of anatomy and physiology, ed 13, St. Louis, 1989, The CV Mosby Co.)

Organs of Nervous System

A. Central nervous system (CNS): spinal cord and brain
B. Peripheral nervous system (PNS): nerves and ganglia
C. Definitions
1. White matter: bundles of myelinated nerve fibers
2. Gray matter: clusters of mainly neuronal cell bodies
3. Nerves: bundles of myelinated nerve fibers located outside the CNS
4. Tracts: bundles of myelinated nerve fibers located within the CNS
5. Ganglia (singular: ganglion): microscopic structures consisting of neuron cell bodies; mainly located outside the CNS

Spinal Cord

A. Location: in the spinal cavity, from the foramen magnum to the first lumbar vertebra
B. Structure
1. Deep groove (anterior median fissure) and more shallow groove (posterior median sulcus) incompletely divide the cord into right and left symmetric halves
2. Inner core of the cord consists of gray matter shaped like a three-dimensional H
3. Long columns of white matter surround the cord's inner core of gray matter; namely, right and left anterior, lateral, and posterior columns; composed of numerous sensory and motor tracts (Fig. 3-8)
C. Functions
1. Sensory tracts conduct impulses up cord to brain; motor tracts conduct impulses down cord from brain
2. Gray matter of cord contains reflex centers for all spinal cord reflexes

Brain

A. General considerations
1. Most active of all body organs in energy consumption; has large blood supply and high oxygen consumption, which increases even further during dreaming stage of sleep
2. Unlike other cells of body, neurons can only utilize glucose for energy metabolism; therefore hypoglycemia can seriously alter brain function and lead to coma
3. Brain cells protected by the blood-brain barrier, a selective filtration system that isolates the brain from substances in the general circulation; barrier is based on the relative impermeability of blood vessels in the brain and the tight wrapping of neuroglial cells around the neurons and blood vessels of the brain; only selected brain regions designed to monitor the chemical composition of blood are not protected by the blood-brain barrier
4. Ease of drug entry into the brain depends on size and fat solubility; the smaller the molecule and the greater the fat solubility, the more easily the drug enters brain tissue
5. Overall function of the brain and spinal cord is to channel sensory input to a variety of neural structures whose analysis culminates in the convergence of impulses on various motor neurons, which effect movements of all types of muscles and activity of glands
B. Regions of brain and their functions
1. Basic tissue types
a. Gray matter: aggregations of neuron cell bodies
b. White matter: composed primarily of tracts of fibers (axons) interconnecting neurons in different regions of the CNS
2. Basic cellular types in the CNS
a. Association (intercolated) neurons: about 99.9% of all the neurons in the CNS
b. Motor neurons: several million found in the CNS
3. Gross anatomic regions
a. Hindbrain (brainstem): lowermost brain division; formed by enlargement of the spinal cord as it enters the cranial cavity
(1) Medulla: lowest portion of the hindbrain
(a) Consists mainly of white matter (sensory and motor tracts); also contains reticular formation (mixture of gray and white matter); some important reflex centers located in reticular formation: cardiac, vasomotor, respiratory, and swallowing centers
(b) Functions: contains centers for vital heart, blood vessel diameter (blood pressure), and respiratory reflexes; also centers for vomiting, coughing, swallowing, etc.; conducts impulses between the cord and brain (both sensory and motor)
(2) Pons
(a) Part of the brain located just above the medulla; consists mainly of white matter (sensory and motor tracts) interspersed with gray matter (reflex centers)
(b) Conducts impulses between the cord and various parts of the brain and contains reflex centers for cranial nerves V, VI, VII, and VIII (trigeminal, abducent, facial, and acoustic)
b. Cerebellum: dorsal appendage of the hindbrain
(1) Structure: second largest part of the human brain; surface marked with sulci (grooves) and very slightly raised, slender convolutions; internal white matter forms pattern suggestive of veins of a leaf
(2) Functions
(a) Cerebellum exerts synergic control over the skeletal muscles; this means that impulses conducted by cerebellar neurons regulate and modulate output of the somatomotor region of the neocortex, which results in coordination of skeletal muscle contractions to produce smooth, steady, and precise movements
(b) Because it coordinates skeletal muscle contractions, the cerebellum plays an essential part in producing normal postures and maintaining equilibrium
c. Midbrain: part of the brain located between the pons, which lies below it, and the diencephalon

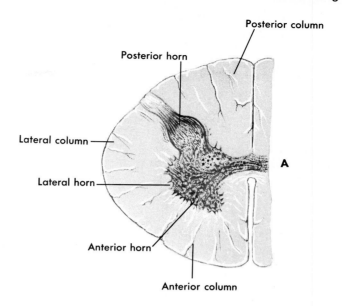

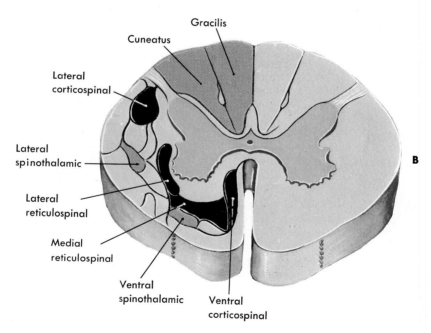

FIG. 3-8. A, Distribution of gray matter (horns) and white matter (columns) in a section of the spinal cord at the thoracic level. **B,** Location in the spinal cord of some major projection tracts. Black areas are descending motor tracts. Shaded areas are ascending sensory tracts. (From Anthony CP and Thibodeau GA: Textbook of anatomy and physiology, ed 13, St. Louis, 1989, The CV Mosby Co.)

and cerebrum, which lie above it; consists mainly of white matter (cerebral peduncles) with scattered bits of gray matter
(1) Superior and inferior colliculi (corpora quadrigemina): integrate and analyze sensory input from the ears, eyes, and various regions of the cerebral cortex; put out motor information to lower motor system

(2) Reflex centers for cranial nerves III (oculomotor) and IV (trochlear): pupillary reflexes and eye movements
(3) Pineal body: precise function unknown; may be part of endocrine system, helping to regulate secretion of gonadotropins from the hypophysis cerebri

d. Forebrain
   (1) Optic vesicles: develop into the retinas connected to base of the forebrain by their stalks, the optic nerves
   (2) Diencephalon: unpaired division of the forebrain; cerebral hemispheres diverge from this structure
       (a) Thalamus: mass of gray matter in each cerebral hemisphere
           [1] Processes incoming sensory information prior to distribution to the somatosensory cortex; crudely translates sensory impulses into sensations but does not localize them on a body region
           [2] Ventral nucleus of the thalamus processes motor information from the cerebral cortex and cerebellum and projects its analysis back to the motor cortex
           [3] Contributes to the concentrating ability by filtering out distracting sensory input
           [4] Contributes to emotional component of sensations (pleasant or unpleasant)
       (b) Hypothalamus: gray matter that forms floor of third ventricle and lower part of its lateral walls
           [1] Contains many higher autonomic reflex centers; these centers integrate autonomic functions by sending impulses to each other and to the lower autonomic centers; they form a crucial part of the neural path by which emotions and other cerebral functions can alter vital, automatic functions such as the heartbeat, blood pressure, peristalsis, and secretion by glands producing psychophysiologic diseases; neural path for psychophysiologic disease: impulses from the cerebral cortex to autonomic centers in the hypothalamus, to lower autonomic centers in the brainstem and cord, to visceral effectors (e.g., heart, smooth muscle, glands)
           [2] Helps control the anterior pituitary gland; certain neurons in the hypothalamus secrete neuropeptides into the pituitary portal veins, which transport them to the anterior pituitary gland where they influence secretion of various important hormones; e.g., TRH and LH-RH regulate the pituitary secretions of TSH and gonadotropic hormones respectively
           [3] Neurons in the supraoptic nucleus of the hypothalamus synthesize ADH and oxytocin; from the cell bodies of these neurons, ADH and oxytocin are transmitted down their axons into the posterior pituitary gland, from which they are released into the blood; in short, hypothalamic neurons make ADH and oxytocin, but the posterior pituitary gland secretes them
           [4] Certain hypothalamic neurons serve as an appetite center and others function as a satiety center; together these centers regulate appetite and food intake
           [5] Certain hypothalamic neurons serve as heat-regulating centers by relaying impulses to lower autonomic centers for vasoconstriction, vasodilation, and sweating, and to somatic centers for shivering
           [6] Maintains waking state; constitutes part of the arousal or alerting neural pathway
       (c) Corpus callosum: mass of white matter (nerve tracts) that interconnects the two cerebral hemispheres
       (d) Optic chiasm: the point of crossing over (decussation [X, Latin *decem*]) of optic nerve fibers from the nasal half of each retina to the opposite side where they join optic nerve fibers from the lateral half of the other eye's retina to form the optic tracts
   (3) Paired cerebral hemispheres (telencephalon): longitudinal fissure divides the cerebrum into two hemispheres connected only by the corpus callosum; each cerebral hemisphere divided by fissures into four major lobes: frontal, parietal, temporal, occipital; also contains deeper regions of gray matter and fiber tracts
       (a) Cerebral cortex is outer layer of gray matter forming folds (convolutions) composed of hills (gyri) and valleys (sulci)
       (b) Frontal lobes
           [1] Abstract thinking, sense of humor, and uniqueness of personality
           [2] Contraction of skeletal muscles and synchronization of muscular movements
           [3] Exert control over hypothalamus; influence basic biorhythms
           [4] Control muscular movements necessary for speech; found only in one cerebral hemisphere
       (c) Parietal lobes
           [1] Translate nerve impulses into sensations (e.g., touch, temperature)
           [2] Interpret sensations; provide appreciation of size, shape, texture, and weight
           [3] Sense of taste

(d) Temporal lobes
  [1] Translate nerve impulses into sensations of sound and interpret sounds
  [2] Sense of smell
  [3] Control behavior patterns
(e) Occipital area
  [1] Translates nerve impulse into sights and interprets sights
  [2] Provides appreciation of size, shape, and color
(f) Angular gyrus: analysis and integration of sights, sounds, and somatic sensations
(g) Amygdala: controls patterns of emotional behavior
(h) Corpus striatum: helps regulate muscle contraction and emotional reactions
(i) Cerebral tracts: bundles of axons compose the white matter in the interior of the cerebrum; ascending projection tracts transmit impulses toward the cerebral cortex; descending projection tracts transmit impulses from cerebral cortex; commissural tracts transmit from one hemisphere to the other; association tracts transmit from one convolution to another in the same hemisphere

4. Brain and spinal cord coverings
  a. Bony: vertebrae around the cord; cranial bones around the brain
  b. Membranous: called meninges; consist of three layers
    (1) Dura mater: white fibrous tissue, outer layer
    (2) Arachnoid membrane: cobwebby middle layer
    (3) Pia mater: innermost layer; adheres to outer surface of the cord and brain; contains blood vessels

5. Cord and brain fluid spaces
  a. Subarachnoid space around the cord and extending beyond the cord into the fourth and fifth lumbar vertebrae
  b. Subarachnoid space around the brain
  c. Central canal inside the cord
  d. Ventricles and cerebral aqueduct inside the brain; four cavities
    (1) First and second (lateral) ventricles: large cavities, one in each cerebral hemisphere
    (2) Third ventricle: vertical slit in the cerebrum beneath the corpus callosum and longitudinal fissure
    (3) Fourth ventricle: diamond-shaped space between the cerebellum and medulla and pons; expansion of the central canal of the cord

6. Formation and circulation of the cerebrospinal fluid (CSF)
  a. Formed by plasma filtering from the network of capillaries (choroid plexus) in each ventricle; active transport of plasma also involved
  b. Circulates from the lateral ventricles to the third ventricle, cerebral aqueduct, fourth ventricle, central canal of the cord, and the subarachnoid space of the cord and brain; returns to blood via venous sinuses of the brain

Cranial Nerves: 12 Pairs

See Table 3-13

Spinal Nerves: 31 Pairs

A. Each nerve attaches to the cord by two short roots, anterior and posterior; the posterior roots are marked by a swelling, the spinal ganglion
B. Branches of the spinal nerves form plexuses or intricate networks of fibers (e.g., brachial plexus), from which nerves emerge to supply various parts of the skin, mucosa, and skeletal muscles
C. All spinal nerves are mixed nerves composed of both sensory dendrites and motor axons; they function in both sensations and movements
D. Nerve consists of bundles of nerve fibers (axons and dendrites) supported by connective tissue

Sensorineural Pathways: Conduction

A. Sensory pathways to the cerebral cortex from the periphery consist of relays of at least 3 neurons, which are identified by Roman numerals
  1. Sensory neuron I: conducts from the periphery to the cord or to the brainstem
  2. Sensory neuron II: conducts from the cord or brainstem to the thalamus
  3. Sensory neuron III: conducts from the thalamus to the somatosensory area of the cerebral cortex
B. Crude awareness of sensations occurs when impulses reach the thalamus
C. Full consciousness of sensations with accurate localization and discrimination of fine details occurs when impulses reach the cerebral cortex
D. Most sensory neuron II axons decussate; so one side of the brain registers most of the sensations for the opposite side of the body
E. Principle of divergence applies to the sensorineural pathways; each sensory neuron synapses with many neurons, and therefore impulses may diverge from any sensory neuron and be conducted to many brain regions, including the cerebellum, reticular formation, and also more directly the motor neurons
F. Impulses that produce pain and an awareness of temperature are conducted up the cord to the thalamus by the lateral spinothalamic tracts
G. Impulses that produce touch and pressure sensations are conducted up the cord to the thalamus by the following two pathways:
  1. Impulses that result in discriminating touch and pressure sensations (e.g., stereognosis, precise localization, vibratory sense) are conducted by the tracts of the posterior white columns of the cord to the medulla and from there are transferred to the thalamus
  2. Impulses that result in crude touch and pressure sensations are conducted up the cord to the thalamus by fibers of the ventral spinothalamic tracts

Table 3-13. Distribution and function of cranial nerve pairs

Name and number	Distribution	Function
Olfactory (I)	Nasal mucosa, high up along the septum especially	Sense of smell (sensory only)
Optic (II)	Retina of eyeball	Vision (sensory only)
Oculomotor (III)	Extrinsic muscles of eyeball, except superior oblique and external rectus; also intrinsic eye muscles (iris and ciliary)	Eye movements; constriction of pupil and bulging of lens, which together produce accommodation for near vision
Trochlear (IV), smallest cranial nerve	Superior oblique muscle of eye	Eye movements
Trigeminal (V) (or trifacial), largest cranial nerve	Sensory fibers to skin and mucosa of head and to teeth; muscles of mastication (sensory and motor fibers)	Sensation in head and face; chewing movements
Abducent (VI)	External rectus muscle of eye	Abduction of eye
Facial (VII)	Muscles of facial expression; taste buds of anterior two thirds of tongue; motor fibers to submaxillary and sublingual salivary glands	Facial expressions; taste; secretion of saliva
Acoustic (VIII) (vestibulocochlear)	Inner ear	Hearing and equilibrium (sensory only)
Glossopharyngeal (IX)	Posterior third of tongue; mucosa and muscles of pharynx; parotid gland; carotid sinus and body	Taste and other sensations of tongue; secretion of saliva; swallowing movements; function in reflex arcs for control of blood pressure and respiration
Vagus (X) (or pneumogastric)	Mucosa and muscles of pharynx, larynx, trachea, bronchi, esophagus; thoracic and abdominal viscera	Sensations and movements of organs supplied; for example, slows heart, increases peristalsis and gastric and pancreatic secretion; voice production
Spinal accessory (XI)	Certain neck and shoulder muscles (muscles of larynx, sternocleidomastoid, trapezius)	Shoulder movements; turns head; voice production; muscle sense
Hypoglossal (XII)	Tongue muscles	Tongue movements, as in talking; muscle sense

Note: The first letters of the words in the following sentence are the first letters of the names of the cranial nerves, and many generations of anatomy students have used it as an aid to memorizing the names: "On Old Olympus' Towering Tops, A Finn And German Viewed Some Hops." (There are several slightly different versions of this mnemonic.)

H. Sensory impulses that result in conscious proprioception or kinesthesia (sense of position or movement of body parts) are conducted over the same pathway as are impulses that result in discriminating touch and pressure sensations

I. Sensory impulses, in addition, are also conducted to the cerebral cortex via complex multineuron pathways known as the reticular activating system; spinoreticular tracts relay sensory impulses up the cord to the brainstem reticular gray matter, and from there other neurons relay them to the hypothalamus, thalamus, and probably other parts of the brain, then finally to the cerebral cortex; conduction by the reticular activating system is essential for producing and maintaining consciousness; presumably, general anesthetics produce unconsciousness by inhibiting conduction by the reticular activating system; conversely, amphetamines and norepinephrine are thought to produce wakefulness by stimulating the reticular activating system

Motoneural Pathways to Skeletal Muscles

A. Principle of the final common path: the final common path for impulse conduction to skeletal muscles consists of anterior horn neurons (i.e., motoneurons whose dendrites and cell bodies lie in the anterior gray columns of the cord and whose axons extend out through the anterior roots of spinal nerves and their branches to terminate in skeletal muscles); besides being referred to as the final common path and as anterior horn cells, these neurons are also called lower motoneurons, somatic motoneurons, and lower motor system

B. Principle of convergence: axons of many neurons converge on (i.e., synapse with) each anterior horn motoneuron

C. Motor pathways from the cerebral cortex to anterior horn cells are classified according to the route by which the fibers enter the cord

1. Pyramidal tracts (corticospinal tracts): axons of neurons whose dendrites and cell bodies lie in the cerebral cortex; axons descend from cortex through internal capsule, pyramids of medulla, and spinal cord; a few of these axons synapse with anterior horn cells, but most of them synapse with internuncial neurons that synapse with anterior horn cells; conduction by pyramidal tracts is necessary for willed movements to occur; hence one cause of paralysis is interruption of pyramidal tract conduction

2. Extrapyramidal tracts: all tracts that conduct between the motor cortex and the anterior horn cells, except the pyramidal tracts; upper extrapyramidal tracts relay impulses between the cortex, basal ganglia, thalamus, and brainstem; reticulospinal tracts

(the main lower extrapyramidal tracts) relay impulses from the brainstem to the anterior horn cells in the cord; impulse conduction via extrapyramidal tracts is essential for producing large, automatic movements (e.g., walking, swimming) and for producing facial expressions and movements that characterize many emotions

D. Motor conduction pathway from the primary motor area of the cerebral cortex to skeletal muscles via pyramidal tracts consists of a two-neuron relay; an upper motoneuron conducts impulses from cerebrum to cord and a lower motoneuron (anterior horn cell) conducts from cord to skeletal muscle (Fig. 3-9)

E. Motor conduction pathway from the cerebral cortex via the extrapyramidal tracts consists of complex multineuron relays; several upper motoneurons relay impulses through the basal ganglia, thalamus, and brain stem down the cord to the lower motoneuron

F. Motor pathways from the cerebral cortex to anterior horn cells classified according to their influence on anterior horn cells as follows:

1. Facilitatory tracts: conduct impulses that have a facilitating or stimulating effect on anterior horn cells; main facilitatory tracts are the pyramidal tracts and the facilitatory reticulospinal tracts

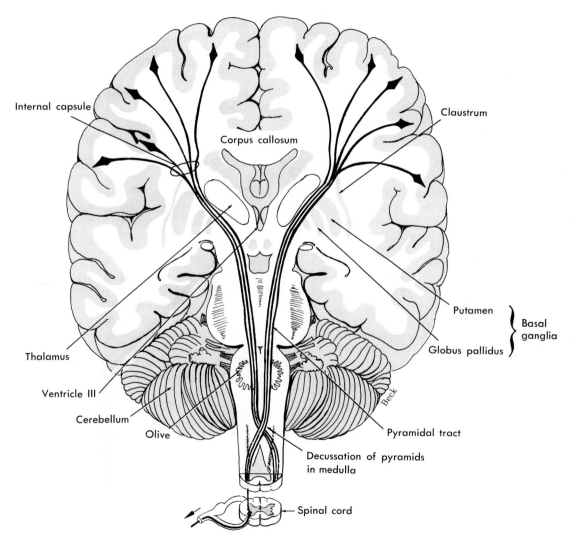

FIG. 3-9. Cross pyramidal (lateral corticospinal) tracts, the main motor tracts of the body. Axons that compose the pyramidal tracts come from neuron cell bodies in the cerebral cortex. After they descend through the internal capsule of the cerebrum and the white matter of the brainstem, about three/fourths of the fibers decussate—cross over from one side to the other—in the medulla, as shown here. Then they continue downward in the lateral corticospinal tract on the opposite side of the cord. Each lateral corticospinal tract, therefore, conducts motor impulses from one side of the brain to skeletal muscles on the opposite side of the body. (From Anthony CP and Thibodeau GA: Textbook of anatomy and physiology, ed 13, St. Louis, 1989, The CV Mosby Co.)

2. Inhibitory tracts: conduct impulses that have an inhibiting effect on anterior horn cells; main inhibitory tracts are the inhibitory reticulospinal tracts; interruption of inhibitory reticulospinal tracts results in spasticity and rigidity

G. Ratio of facilitatory and inhibitory impulses impinging on anterior horn cells determines their activity (whether they are facilitated, stimulated, or inhibited)

Autonomic Nervous System

A. Definition: division of the nervous system that conducts impulses from the brainstem or cord out to visceral effectors: cardiac muscle, smooth muscle, and glandular tissue

B. Divisions: consists of two divisions: the sympathetic (thoracolumbar) system and the parasympathetic (craniosacral) system
   1. Sympathetic system
      a. Sympathetic ganglia: two chains of 21 or 22 ganglia located immediately in front of the spinal column, one chain to the right, one to the left
      b. Collateral ganglia: located a short distance from the cord (e.g., celiac ganglia [solar plexus], superior and inferior mesenteric ganglia)
      c. Sympathetic nerves: (e.g., splanchnic nerves, cardiac nerves)
   2. Parasympathetic system
      a. Parasympathetic ganglia: located some distance from the spinal column, in or near the visceral effectors (e.g., ciliary ganglion in posterior part of the orbit, near the iris and ciliary muscle)
      b. Parasympathetic nerves: (e.g., vagus nerve, called the great parasympathetic nerve of the body)

C. Neurons
   1. Preganglionic sympathetic neurons: dendrites and cell bodies lie in the lateral gray columns of thoracic and lumbar segments of the cord; their axons conduct from the cord to the sympathetic ganglia or the collateral ganglia (see D,3 which follows)
   2. Postganglionic sympathetic neurons: dendrites and cell bodies lie in the sympathetic ganglia or the collateral ganglia; their axons conduct to visceral effectors
   3. Preganglionic parasympathetic neurons: dendrites and cell bodies of some of these neurons lie in gray matter of the brain stem; others exit at sacral segments of the cord; conduct impulses from the brain stem or cord to the parasympathetic ganglia (see D,3 which follows)
   4. Postganglionic parasympathetic neurons: dendrites and cell bodies lie in the parasympathetic ganglia; their axons conduct to visceral effectors (see D,3 which follows)

D. Some principles about the autonomic nervous system
   1. Dual autonomic innervation: both sympathetic and parasympathetic fibers supply most visceral effectors
   2. Single autonomic innervation: only sympathetic fibers supply sweat glands and probably the smooth muscles of hairs and of most blood vessels; preganglionic sympathetic fibers terminate in adrenal medulla (not postganglionic fibers as in other glands)
   3. Autonomic chemical transmitters: all preganglionic axons are cholinergic fibers, as are most (or perhaps all) parasympathetic postganglionic axons and a few sympathetic postganglionic axons (to sweat glands, external genitalia, and smooth muscle in walls of blood vessels located in skeletal muscles); sympathetic postganglionic axons are the only adrenergic (i.e., norepinephrine-releasing) fibers; but, as just mentioned, a few of them are cholinergic
   4. Autonomic antagonism and summation: sympathetic and parasympathetic impulses tend to produce opposite effects; the algebraic sum of two opposing tendencies determines the response made by dually innervated visceral effectors (Table 3-14)
   5. Principle of parasympathetic dominance of the digestive tract: normally, parasympathetic impulses to digestive tract glands and smooth muscle dominate over sympathetic impulses to these effectors; the dominance of parasympathetic impulses promotes digestive gland secretion, peristalsis, and defecation
   6. Principle of sympathetic dominance in stress situations: under conditions of stress, sympathetic impulses to the visceral effectors usually increase greatly and dominate over parasympathetic impulses; however, in some individuals under stress, parasympathetic impulses via the vagus nerve to glands and smooth muscle of the stomach greatly increase, causing increased hydrochloric acid secretion and increased gastric motility; this can eventually cause peptic ulcer, a condition that may aptly be called the great parasympathetic stress disease
   7. In general, when the sympathetic system dominates control of visceral effectors, it causes them to function in ways that enable the body to expend maximum energy as is necessary in strenuous exercise and other types of stress (see Table 3-14 for sympathetic action on specific visceral effectors)
   8. Principle of nonautonomy: the autonomic nervous system is neither anatomically nor physiologically independent of rest of the nervous system; all parts of nervous system work together as a single functional unit; i.e., dendrites and cells of all preganglionic neurons in gray matter of the brainstem or cord (lower autonomic centers) are influenced by impulses conducted to them from higher autonomic centers, notably the hypothalamus
   9. Importance of autonomic nervous system: plays a major role in maintaining physiologic balance; under usual conditions, autonomic impulses regulate activities of the visceral effectors so they maintain or quickly restore this balance; under highly stressful conditions, problems may occur

Sense Organs

Millions of receptors distributed widely throughout the skin and mucosa; muscles, tendons, joints, and viscera are sense organs of body (Table 3-15)

A. General considerations
   1. Receptors monitor internal and external environment
   2. Stimuli are interpreted and converted to nerve impulses, which are conducted through sensory neurons to the brain

Table 3-14. Autonomic functions

Visceral effector	Effect of sympathetic stimulation (neurotransmitter, norepinephrine unless otherwise stated)	Effect of parasympathetic stimulation (neurotransmitter, acetylcholine)
Heart	Increased rate and strength of heartbeat (beta receptors)	Decreased rate and strength of heartbeat
Smooth muscle of blood vessels		
Skin blood vessels	Constriction (alpha receptors)	No parasympathetic fibers
Skeletal muscle blood vessels	Dilation (beta receptors)	No parasympathetic fibers
Coronary blood vessels	Dilation (beta receptors)	No parasympathetic fibers
Abdominal blood vessels	Constriction (alpha receptors)	No parasympathetic fibers
Blood vessels of external genitals	Ejaculation (contraction of smooth muscle in male ducts, e.g., epididymis and vas deferens)	Dilation of blood vessels causing erection in male
Smooth muscle of hollow organs and sphincters		
Bronchi	Dilation (beta receptors)	Constriction
Digestive tract, except sphincters	Decreased peristalsis (beta receptors)	Increased peristalsis
Sphincters of digestive tract	Contraction (alpha receptors)	Relaxation
Urinary bladder	Relaxation (beta receptors)	Contraction
Urinary sphincters	Contraction (alpha receptors)	Relaxation
Eye		
Iris	Contraction of radial muscle; dilated pupil	Contraction of circular muscle; constricted pupil
Ciliary	Relaxation; accommodates for far vision	Contraction; accommodates for near vision
Hairs (pilomotor muscles)	Contraction produces goose pimples, or piloerection (alpha receptors)	No parasympathetic fibers
Glands		
Sweat	Increased sweat (neurotransmitter, acetylcholine)	No parasympathetic fibers
Digestive (salivary, gastric, etc.)	Decreased secretion of saliva; not known for others	Increased secretion of saliva
Pancreas, including islets	Decreased secretion	Increased secretion of pancreatic juice and insulin
Liver	Increased glycogenolysis (beta receptors); increases blood sugar level	No parasympathetic fibers
Adrenal medulla*	Increased epinephrine secretion	No parasympathetic fibers

From Anthony CP and Thibodeau GA: Textbook of anatomy and physiology, ed. 11, St. Louis, 1983, The CV Mosby Co.
*Sympathetic preganglionic axons terminate in contact with secreting cells of the adrenal medulla. Thus the adrenal medulla functions (to quote a descriptive phrase) as a "giant sympathetic postganglionic neuron."

Table 3-15. Receptors

Kinds	Locations	Stimulated by	Functions
Exteroceptors	Skin, mucosa, ear, eye	Changes in external environment (e.g., pressure, heat, cold, light waves, sound waves)	Initiate reflexes Initiate sensations of many kinds (e.g., pressure, heat, cold, pain, vision, hearing)
Visceroceptors (interoceptors)	Viscera	Changes in internal environment (e.g., pressure, chemical)	Initiate reflexes Initiate sensations of many kinds (e.g., hunger, sex, nausea, pressure)
Proprioceptors	Muscles, tendons, joints, semicircular canals of inner ear	Pressure changes	Initiate reflexes Initiate muscle sense, or sense of position and movement of parts; also called kinesthesia

3. Receptors' degrees of depolarization depend on the strength of the stimulus; the variable degree of depolarization is called the generator potential
4. Generator potential determines the frequency of nerve impulses sent to the CNS by afferent nerve fibers attached to receptors
5. Most receptors display sensory adaptation: steady and prolonged stimulus results in a steady decrease in strength of generator potential

B. Types of receptors
   1. Exteroceptors of skin and mucosa: consist of receptors for spinal or cranial nerve branches; different types of receptors for different sensations such as heat, cold, pain, touch, and pressure
   2. Proprioceptors of muscles, tendons, and joints: stretching of muscles or tendons during movements initiates stretch reflexes
   3. Visceroceptors: pressoreceptors (baroreceptors) respond to stretch in walls of the aorta and carotid arteries, providing the brain with information on blood pressure; oxygen chemoreceptors in the aortic and carotid bodies monitor O_2 levels; carbon dioxide chemoreceptors in the respiratory center (in medulla) help control the rate and depth of respirations
   4. Taste
      a. Taste buds consist of groups of receptor cells bundled together with sensory hairs protruding from a pore in the taste bud and connected to the facial and glossopharyngeal nerves (VII and IX)
      b. Respond to chemicals: sweet at tongue tip; sour and salt at tip and sides; bitter at back; receptors for bitter most sensitive
      c. Olfaction intimately involved in the sense of taste
   5. Olfaction
      a. Receptors in epithelium of the nasal mucosa
      b. Odors sensed as chemicals interact with receptor sites on sensory hairs of olfactory cells
      c. Olfactory neural pathways utilize cranial nerve I
   6. Sight
      a. Coats of the eyeball
         (1) Outer: sclera proper and cornea
         (2) Middle: choroid proper, ciliary body, suspensory ligament holding lens, and iris
         (3) Inner: retina

   b. Cavities and humors of the eyeball
      (1) Anterior cavity with an anterior and posterior chamber; both contain aqueous humor
      (2) Posterior cavity has no divisions; contains vitreous humor
   c. Muscles of the eye (Table 3-16)
   d. Refractory media of the eye
      (1) Cornea
      (2) Aqueous humor
      (3) Crystalline lens (has greatest refractive power)
      (4) Vitreous humor
   e. Accessory structures of the eye
      (1) Eyebrows and lashes
      (2) Eyelids or palpebrae: lined with mucous membrane (conjunctiva) that continues over surface of eyeball; corners of eyes, where upper and lower lids join, called inner and outer canthi
      (3) Lacrimal apparatus: lacrimal glands, ducts, sacs, and nasolacrimal ducts
   f. Physiology of vision
      (1) Formation of an image on the retina, accomplished by
         (a) Refraction: bending of light rays as they pass through the eye
         (b) Accommodation: bulging of the lens for viewing near objects
         (c) Constriction of pupils: occurs simultaneously with accommodation and in bright light
         (d) Convergence of the eyes for near objects so light rays from the object may fall on corresponding points of two retinas; necessary for single binocular vision
      (2) Stimulation of the retina: dim light causes breakdown of the chemical rhodopsin present in rods, thereby initiating impulse conduction by the rods; bright light causes breakdown of chemicals in the cones; rods considered receptors for night vision, cones receptors for daylight and color vision
      (3) Most cones concentrated in small region of the retina called fovea centralis; provides sharpest color vision

Table 3-16. Eye muscles

Location	Kind of muscle	Names	Functions
Extrinsic—attached to outside of eyeball and to bones of orbit	Skeletal (voluntary, striated)	Superior rectus Inferior rectus Lateral rectus Medial rectus Superior oblique Inferior oblique	Move eyeball in various directions
Intrinsic—within eyeball	Visceral (involuntary, smooth)	Iris	Regulate size of pupil
		Ciliary muscle	Control shape of lens, making possible accommodation for near and far objects

(4) Conduction to visual area in occipital lobe of cerebral cortex by fibers of optic nerves and optic tracts
7. Hearing
   a. External ear: consists of the auricle (or pinna), external acoustic meatus (ear opening), and external auditory canal
   b. Middle ear: separated from the external ear by the tympanic membrane; middle ear contains auditory ossicles (malleus, incus, stapes) and openings from the auditory (eustachian) tubes, mastoid cells, external ear, and internal ear; auditory tube is collapsible and lined with mucosa and extends from the nasopharynx to the middle ear; equalizes pressure on both sides of eardrum, as when tubes open during yawning, swallowing, or sucking
   c. Inner ear (or labyrinth): composed of a bony labyrinth that has a membranous labyrinth inside it; parts of the inner ear
     (1) Bony vestibule: contains the membranous utricle and saccule, each of which in turn contains a sense organ called the macula; vestibular nerve (branch of eighth cranial [acoustic or vestibulocochlear] nerve) supplies the maculae acusticae; these sense organs give information about equilibrium, position of the head, and acceleration and deceleration
     (2) Bony semicircular canals: contain the membranous semicircular canals in which are located the crista ampullaris, the sense organ for sensations of equilibrium and head movements; vestibular nerve supplies the crista as well as the macula
     (3) Bony cochlea: contains the membranous cochlear duct in which is located the organ of Corti, the hearing sense organ; cochlear nerve (branch of eighth cranial nerve) supplies the organ of Corti
   d. Physiology of hearing
     (1) Sound waves moving through the air enter the ear canal and move down it to strike against the tympanic membrane, causing it to vibrate
     (2) Vibrations of the tympanic membrane move the malleus, whose handle is attached to the membrane
     (3) Movement of the malleus moves the incus, to which the head of the malleus attaches
     (4) Incus attaches to the stapes; so, as the incus moves, it moves the stapes against the oval window, into which it fits; as the stapes presses inwardly on the perilymph around the cochlear duct, it starts a ripple in the perilymph
     (5) Movement of the perilymph is transmitted to the endolymph inside the cochlear duct and stimulates the organ of Corti, which projects into the endolymph

     (6) Cochlear nerve conducts impulses from the organ of Corti to the brain; hearing occurs when impulses reach the auditory area in the temporal lobe of the cerebral cortex

Muscular System

A. Functions
  1. Movement
  2. Posture
  3. Heat production: metabolism in muscle cells produces relatively large share of body heat
B. Types of muscles and neural control
  1. Striated: controlled by voluntary nervous system via somatic motoneurons in spinal and some cranial nerves
  2. Smooth: controlled by autonomic nervous system via autonomic motoneurons in autonomic, spinal, and some cranial nerves; not under voluntary control (with rare exceptions)
  3. Cardiac: control is identical to that of smooth muscle
C. Anatomy of skeletal muscle as a whole
  1. Typically spindle shaped; composed of long muscle cells referred to as muscle fibers; invested by coating of fibrous connective tissue (fascia), which binds muscle to surrounding tissues
  2. Arranged in bundles or fasciculi; each muscle contains several fasciculi
  3. Contains rich blood supply; numerous capillary beds provide nutrients to and remove wastes from muscle
  4. Characteristics of individual skeletal muscle fibers
    a. Generally long and spindle shaped
    b. Multinucleate; called a syncytium
    c. Cell membrane called sarcolemma; endoplasmic reticulum called sarcoplasmic reticulum; mitochondria may be referred to as sarcosomes
    d. Contain myofibrils specialized for contraction; composed of two types of protein myofilaments, actin and myosin
D. Neuromuscular junction
  1. Axon terminal forms junction with the sarcolemma of muscle fiber; tiny synaptic cleft separates the presynaptic membrane (axon) from postsynaptic membrane (sarcolemma)
  2. Axon terminals contain tiny sacs, synaptic vesicles; these contain the neurotransmitter acetylcholine
  3. When a nerve impulse reaches the axon terminal, acetylcholine is released from synaptic vesicles into synaptic cleft; acetylcholine diffuses across synaptic cleft and attaches to receptor sites on sarcolemma; receptor sites are attached to channels in the membrane; when acetylcholine binds to the receptor site, a channel opens and sodium and potassium ions flow down their concentration gradients; the sarcolemma is depolarized, and electrical energy flows into the muscle fiber.
  4. The enzyme cholinesterase, found in the synaptic cleft, inactivates acetylcholine; additional stimulation of muscle requires release of more acetylcholine

E. Muscle fiber contraction
  1. Electrical energy flows deep into muscle fiber along transverse intracellular tubules associated with sarcoplasmic reticulum
  2. Calcium ions released by flow of electrical energy inactivate troponin, which normally blocks the interaction between actin and myosin
  3. Myosin releases and uses energy from ATP to cause actin to slide along myosin filaments (contraction); cessation of impulses leaves actin and myosin in a relaxed unassociated phase
  4. Energy for contraction: immediate energy is ATP; creatine phosphate, a high-energy molecule stored in abundance in muscle, replenishes supply of ATP as needed; the ultimate source of energy is glucose and fatty acids oxidized aerobically to carbon dioxide and water, with the release of energy
  5. Anaerobic breakdown of glucose during prolonged and vigorous muscle contraction results in lactic acid buildup associated with fatigue and an aching feeling; this oxygen debt is paid off during rest, when oxygen is plentiful
F. Basic principles of skeletal muscle action
  1. Skeletal muscles contract only if stimulated; a skeletal muscle and its motor nerve function as a physiologic unit (motor unit); either is useless without the other's functioning; for this reason anything that prevents impulse conduction to a skeletal muscle paralyzes the muscle
  2. Most skeletal muscles attach to at least two bones; as a muscle contracts and pulls on its bones, it mobilizes the bone that moves most easily; the bone that moves is called the muscle's insertion bone, and that which remains stationary is its origin bone
  3. Bones serve as levers, and joints as fulcrums of these levers; a muscle's contraction exerts a pulling force on its insertion bone at the point where it inserts, pulling that point nearer the muscle's origin bone
  4. Skeletal muscles almost always act in groups rather than singly; members of groups are classified as follows:
    a. Prime movers: muscle or muscles whose contraction actually produces the movement
    b. Synergists: muscles that contract at the same time as the prime mover, helping it produce the movement or stabilizing the part (i.e., holding it steady) so the prime mover can produce a more effective movement
    c. Antagonists: muscles that relax while the prime mover is contracting (exception: antagonist contracts at the same time as the prime mover when a part needs to be held rigid, as the knee joint does in standing); antagonists are usually located directly opposite the bones they move; e.g., muscle that flexes the lower arm lies on anterior surface of the upper arm bone, whereas that which extends the lower arm lies on posterior surface of the upper arm
  5. Body of a muscle usually does not lie over the part moved by the muscle; instead it lies above or below, or anterior or posterior to, the part; thus the body of a muscle that moves the lower arm will not be located in the lower arm but in the upper arm; e.g., biceps and triceps brachii muscles
  6. Contraction of a skeletal muscle either shortens the muscle, producing movement, or increases the tension (tone) in the muscle; contractions are classified according to whether they produce movement or increase muscle tone as follows:
    a. Tonic contractions: produce muscle tone; do not shorten the muscle so do not produce movements; only a few fibers contract at one time, and this produces a moderate degree of muscle tone; in the healthy, awake body all muscles exhibit tone
    b. Isometric contractions: increase the degree of muscle tone; do not shorten the muscle so do not produce movements; daily repetition of isometric contractions gradually increases muscle strength
    c. Isotonic contractions: the muscle shortens, thereby producing movement; all movements are the result of isotonic contractions
G. Origins, insertions, and functions of main skeletal muscles grouped according to functions (Table 3-17)
H. Weak places in abdominal wall where hernias may occur
  1. Inguinal rings: right and left internal, right and left external
  2. Femoral rings: right and left
  3. Umbilicus
I. Metabolism of skeletal muscle
  1. Hypertrophy is physical enlargement of the muscle due to the addition of more myofibrils to muscle fibers, making them swell; muscle fibers do not divide to produce new fibers
  2. Atrophy is reduction in size of muscle due to decrease in number of myofibrils in muscle fiber
  3. Treppe (staircase phenomenon): when a muscle has contracted a few times, subsequent contractions are more powerful; may be related to the release of increased quantities of calcium ions from sarcoplasmic reticulum after the first few contractions
  4. Shivering: rapid, repeating, involuntary skeletal muscle contractions; caused by hypothalamic temperature regulating center; makes use of inefficiency of muscle contraction (i.e., most of the energy of ATP is converted to heat; a smaller part goes into the mechanical motion of contraction)
  5. Rigor mortis: ATP must combine with myosin to effect release of actin from myosin, which permits relaxation; after death, ATP is depleted from muscle fibers, and actin and myosin strongly associate, producing rigor mortis; subsequent bacterial decomposition of muscle proteins brings about relaxation; body enters rigor state about 24 hours after death and comes out of rigor about 24 hours later
J. Bursae
  1. Definition: small sacs lined with synovial membrane and containing synovial fluid
  2. Locations: wherever pressure is exerted over moving parts
    a. Between skin and bone
    b. Between tendons and bone
    c. Between muscles or ligaments and bone

3. Names of bursae that frequently become inflamed (bursitis)
   a. Subacromial: between the acromion and the capsule of the shoulder joint
   b. Olecranon: between the olecranon process of the ulna and the skin; inflammation called student's elbow
   c. Prepatellar: between the patella and the skin; inflammation called housemaid's knee
4. Function: act as cushions, relieving pressure between moving parts

K. Tendon sheaths
   1. Definition and location: tube-shaped structures that enclose certain tendons, notably those of wrist and ankle; made of connective tissue lined with synovial membrane
   2. Function: facilitate gliding movements of tendon

Skeletal System

A. Functions
   1. Furnishes supporting framework
   2. Affords protection for the viscera, brain, and hemopoietic system
   3. Provides levers for the muscles to pull on to produce movements
   4. Hemopoiesis by red bone marrow: formation of all kinds of blood cells; note that some lymphocytes and monocytes are formed in lymphatic tissue
   5. Mineral storage: calcium, phosphorus (in the form of phosphates), and sodium are stored in bone

B. Nature of bone substance
   1. Organic matter: makes up about 33% of bone by weight
      a. Cells
         (1) Osteoblasts: bone-producing cells
         (2) Osteoclasts: bone-dissolving cells
         (3) Osteocytes: former osteoblasts embedded in and maintaining bone substance
      b. Collagen: collagen fibers make up about 97% of organic matter of bone; give bone tough and somewhat flexible quality; responsible for high tensile strength of bone
      c. Polysaccharides: part of ground substance of bone consists of polysaccharides such as hyaluronic acid and sialic acid
      d. Protein: polysaccharide complexes such as chondroitin sulfate are part of ground substance of bone
   2. Inorganic matter: makes up about 67% of bone by weight
      a. Apatite salts: apatite, a complex ion composed of calcium and phosphates, forms hydroxyapatite, carbonate apatite, and fluoride apatite; makes bone hard and is responsible for the high compressional strength of bone
      b. Magnesium and sodium ions are part of bone matrix
      c. Certain radioactive isotopes accumulate in bone (e.g., strontium 90, calcium 45, phosphorus 32, plutonium 259); may increase likelihood of bone tumors and leukemia

C. Bone formation
   1. Intramembranous ossification: fibrous membranes composing certain parts of fetal skeleton, such as skull bones and lower jaw, are converted to bone
   2. Endochondral ossification: conversion of cartilage bone models into actual bone in fetus; most of fetal skeletal system ossifies by endochondral ossification
   3. Ossification: end result of either intramembranous or endochondral ossification is the same, cancellous (spongy) bone; the denser type of bone substance, compact bone, forms later in development through conversion of selected regions of cancellous bone into compact bone
      a. Distribution of cancellous and compact bone
         (1) Outer surface of all bones, except at joints, composed of compact bone
         (2) Interior of short, flat, and irregular bones (all bones except long bones) composed of cancellous bone; epiphyses of long bones composed of cancellous bone in their interior
         (3) Diaphyses of long bones hollow; walls of diaphysis composed of compact bone
      b. Ossification process
         (1) Formation of bone matrix (the intercellular substance of bone), made up of collagen fibers and a cementlike ground substance composed of polysaccharides and protein-polysaccharide complexes; the osteoblasts (bone-forming cells) synthesize collagen and cement substance from proteins provided by the diet; vitamin C promotes the formation of bone matrix; exercise and estrogens act to stimulate osteoblasts to form bone matrix
         (2) Calcification of bone matrix: calcium salts deposited in the bone matrix; vitamin D promotes calcification by stimulating calcium uptake in small intestine
      c. Bone growth
         (1) In length: by continual thickening of epiphyseal cartilage followed by ossification; as long as bone growth continues, epiphyseal cartilage grows faster than it can be replaced by bone; therefore line of cartilage persists between diaphysis and epiphyses and can be seen on x-ray film; during adolescence cartilage is completely transformed into bone, at which time bone growth is complete
         (2) In diameter: osteoclasts destroy bone surrounding the medullary cavity, thereby enlarging the cavity; at the same time, osteoblasts add new bone around outer surface of the bone; bones may thicken throughout life, depending on the stresses placed on the bone; the more prolonged the stress (walking, running, weight lifting), the thicker the bones become (within physiologic limits)

Table 3-17. Origins, insertions, and functions of main skeletal muscles

Part of body moved	Movement	Muscle	Origin	Insertion
Upper arm	Flexion	Pectoralis major	Clavicle (medial half) Sternum Costal cartilages of true ribs	Humerus (greater tubercle)
	Extension	Latissimus dorsi	Vertebrae (lower thoracic, lumbar, and sacral) Ilium (crest) Lumbodorsal fascia	Humerus (intertubercular groove)
	Abduction	Deltoid	Clavicle Scapula (spine and acromion)	Humerus (lateral side on deltoid tubercle)
	Adduction	Latissimus dorsi contracting with pectoralis major	See above (Latissimus dorsi) See above (Pectoralis major)	Humerus (greater tubercle) Humerus (intertubercular groove)
Shoulder	Shrugging, elevating	Trapezius	Occipital bone Vertebrae (cervical and thoracic)	Scapula (spine and acromion) Clavicle
	Lowering	Pectoralis minor Serratus anterior	Ribs (second to fifth) Ribs (upper 8 or 9)	Scapula (coracoid) Scapula (anterior surface)
Lower arm	Flexion With forearm supinated	Biceps brachii	Scapula (supraglenoid tuberosity) Scapula (coracoid)	Radius (tubercle at proximal end)
	With forearm pronated	Brachialis	Humerus (distal half, anterior surface)	Ulna (front of cornoid process)
	With forearm semisupinated or semipronated	Brachioradialis	Humerus (above lateral epicondyle)	Radius (styloid process)
	Extension	Triceps brachii	Scapula (infraglenoid tuberosity) Humerus (posterior surface—lateral head above radial groove; medial head, below)	Ulna (olecranon process)
Thigh	Flexion	Iliopsoas (iliacus and psoas major)	Ilium (iliac fossa) Vertebrae (bodies of twelfth thoracic to fifth lumbar)	Femur (small trochanter)
		Rectus femoris	Ilium and anterior inferior iliac spine	Tibia (by way of patellar tendon)
	Extension	Gluteus maximus	Ilium (crest and posterior surface) Sacrum and coccyx (posterior surface)	Femur (gluteal tuberosity) Iliotibial tract
		Hamstring group (see below)	Ischium (tuberosity) Femur (linea aspera)	Fibula (head of) Tibia (lateral condyle, medial condyle, and medial surface)
	Abduction	Gluteus medius and minimus	Ilium (lateral surface)	Femur (greater trochanter)
		Tensor fasciae latae	Ilium (anterior part of crest)	Iliotibial tract
	Adduction	Adductor group Brevis Longus Magnus	Pubic bone	Femur (linea aspera)
Lower leg	Flexion	Hamstring group Biceps femoris Semitendinosus Semimembranosus	Ischium (tuberosity) Femur (linea aspera)	Fibula (head of) Tibia (lateral condyle, medial condyle, and medial surface)
		Gastrocnemius	Femur (condyles)	Tarsal bone (calcaneus by way of tendo calcaneus)

Table 3-17. Origins, insertions, and functions of main skeletal muscles—cont'd

Part of body moved	Movement	Muscle	Origin	Insertion
Lower leg— cont'd	Extension	Quadriceps femoris group	Ilium (anterior inferior spine)	Tibia (by way of patellar tendon)
		Rectus femoris Vastus lateralis Vastus medialis Vastus intermedius	Femur (linea aspera and anterior surface)	
Foot	Flexion (dorsiflexion)	Tibialis anterior	Tibia (lateral condyle)	First cuneiform tarsal Base of first metatarsal
	Extension (plantar flexion)	Gastrocnemius	Femur (condyles)	Calcaneus (by way of tendo calcaneus)
		Soleus	Tibia	Same as gastrocnemius, but underneath
Head	Flexion	Sternocleidomastoid	Sternum Clavicle	Temporal bone (mastoid process)
	Extension	Trapezius	Vertebrae (cervical) Scapula (spine and acromion) Clavicle	Occiput
Abdominal wall	Compress abdominal cavity; therefore assists in straining, defecation, forced expiration, childbirth, posture, etc.	External oblique	Ribs (lower 8)	Innominate bone (iliac crest and pubis by way of inguinal ligament) Linea alba
		Internal oblique	Innominate bone (iliac crest, inguinal ligament) Lumbodorsal fascia	Ribs (lower 3) Pubic bone Linea alba
		Transversus	Ribs (lower 6) Innominate bone (iliac crest, inguinal ligament) Lumbodorsal fascia	Pubic bone Linea alba
		Rectus abdominis	Innominate bone (pubic bone and symphysis pubis)	Ribs (costal cartilage of fifth, sixth, seventh)
Chest wall	Elevate ribs, thereby enlarging anteroposterior and anterolateral dimensions of chest and causing inspiration	External intercostals	Ribs (lower border of all but twelfth)	Ribs (upper border of rib below origin)
	Depress ribs	Internal intercostals	Ribs (inner surface, upper border of all except first)	Ribs (lower border of rib above origin)
	Pull floor of thorax downward, thereby enlarging vertical dimension of chest and causing inspiration	Diaphragm	Lower circumference of rib cage	Central tendon of diaphragm
Trunk	Flexion	Iliopsoas	Femur (small trochanter)	Ilium Vertebrae (bodies of twelfth thoracic to fifth lumbar)
	Extension	Sacrospinalis Iliocostalis (lateral) Longissimus (medial)	Vertebrae (posterior surface of sacrum, spinous processes of lumbar, and last 2 thoracic) Ilium (posterior part of crest)	Ribs (lower 6) Vertebrae (transverse processes of thoracic) Ribs Vertebrae (spines of thoracic)
		Quadratus lumborum	Ilium (posterior part of crest) Vertebrae (lower 3 lumbar)	Ribs (twelfth) Vertebrae (transverse processes of first 4 lumbar)

4. Nutrients required for growth, maintenance, and re-modeling of bone
   a. Vitamin A: promotes chondrocyte function and synthesis of lysosomal enzymes for osteoclast activity
   b. Vitamin C: promotes synthesis of collagen
   c. Vitamin D: promotes calcium and phosphorus absorption
   d. Calcium: needed to form calcium phosphate and hydroxyapatite
   e. Magnesium: important enzyme activator in the mineralization process
   f. Phosphorus: needed to form calcium phosphate and hydroxyapatite
D. Structure of long bones (Fig. 3-10)
E. Names and numbers of bones (Table 3-18)
F. Joints
   1. Synarthrotic: generally nonmovable joints; also called fibrous joints; no joint cavity or capsule; joining bones held together by fibrous tissue
      a. Sutures: bind skull bones together
      b. Syndesmoses: bind tibia and fibula; also the diaphyses of the radius and ulna
   2. Amphiarthrotic: slightly movable joints; also called cartilaginous joints: no joint cavity or capsule; joining bones held together by cartilage and ligaments
      a. Symphyses: disc of cartilage between bones, as between vertebrae or at the pubic symphysis

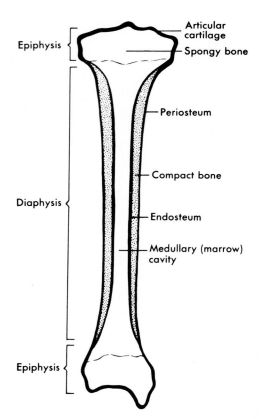

Epiphysis
Articular cartilage
Spongy bone
Periosteum
Compact bone
Diaphysis
Endosteum
Medullary (marrow) cavity
Epiphysis

FIG. 3-10. Diagram to show the structure of a long bone as seen in longitudinal section. (From Anthony CP and Thibodeau, GA: Textbook of anatomy and physiology, ed 13, St. Louis, 1989, The CV Mosby Co.)

b. Synchondroses: costal cartilages bind ribs to the sternum
3. Diarthrotic: freely movable joints; the joint cavity or space between articular surfaces of two bones is lined by a thin layer of hyaline cartilage covering the articular surfaces of the joining bones; the bones are held together by a fibrous capsule lined with synovial membrane and ligaments; may be ball and socket (as in hip), hinge (as in elbow), condyloid (as at wrist), pivot, gliding, or saddle
   a. Kinds of movement possible at diarthrotic joints
      (1) Flexion: bending one bone on another; (e.g., bending forearm on upper arm)
      (2) Extension: stretching one bone away from another (e.g., straightening lower arm out from a flexed position)
      (3) Abduction: moving bone away from body's midline (e.g., moving arms straight out from sides)
      (4) Adduction: moving bone back toward the body's midline (e.g., bringing arms back to sides of body from an outstretched, or abducted, position)
      (5) Rotation: pivoting bone on its axis (e.g., partial rotation such as turning the head from side to side)
      (6) Circumduction: describing surface of a cone with the moving part (e.g., moving arm around so the hand describes a circle)
      (7) Supination: forearm movement turning the palm forward
      (8) Pronation: forearm movement turning the back of the hand forward
      (9) Inversion: ankle movement turning the sole of the foot inward
      (10) Eversion: ankle movement turning the sole outward
      (11) Protraction: moving a part, such as the lower jaw, forward
      (12) Retraction: pulling a part back; opposite of protraction
      (13) Plantar flexion: pointing the toes (as a ballerina) away from the body
      (14) Dorsiflexion: pointing toes toward the body
G. Differences between male and female skeletons
   1. Male skeleton larger and heavier than female skeleton
   2. Male pelvis deep and funnel shaped with narrow pubic arch; female pelvis shallow, broad, and flaring with wider pubic arch
H. Age changes in skeleton
   1. From infancy to adulthood, not only do bones grow but their relative sizes change as well; the head becomes proportionately smaller, the pelvis relatively larger, the legs proportionately longer, etc.
   2. From young adulthood to old age, bone margins and projections change gradually; bone piles up along them (marginal lipping and spurs), thereby restricting movement; such continuing growth is due, in part, to stimulation of somatotrophic hormone

Table 3-18. Bones of the body

Part of body	Name of bone	Number	Description
1. Axial skeleton			
a. Skull*			
(1) Cranium	1. Frontal	1	1. Forehead bone
	2. Parietal	2	2. Bulging bones that form top sides of cranium
	3. Temporal	2	3. Form lower sides of cranium and part of cranial floor
	4. Occipital	1	4. Forms posterior part of cranial floor and walls
	5. Sphenoid	1	5. Forms mid portion of cranial floor
	6. Ethmoid	1	6. Composes part of anterior portion of cranial floor; lies anterior to sphenoid, posterior to nasal bones
(2) Face	1. Nasal	2	1. Form upper part of bridge of nose
	2. Maxillary	2	2. Upper jaw bones
	3. Zygomatic (malar)	2	3. Cheek bones
	4. Mandible	1	4. Lower jaw bone
	5. Lacrimal	2	5. Fingernail-shaped bones posterior and lateral to nasal bones, in medial wall of orbit
	6. Palatine	2	6. Form posterior part of hard palate
	7. Inferior conchae (turbinates)	2	7. Thin scroll of bone along inner surface of side wall of nasal cavity
	8. Vomer	1	8. Lower, posterior part of nasal septum
(3) Ear ossicles	1. Malleus (hammer)	2	Tiny bones in middle ear in temporal bone; resemble, respectively, miniature hammer, anvil, and stirrup
	2. Incus (anvil)	2	
	3. Stapes (stirrup)	2	
b. Hyoid bone		1	U-shaped bone in neck between mandible and upper part of larynx; only bone in body that forms no joints with any other bones
c. Vertebral column	1. Cervical vertebrae	7	1. Upper seven vertebrae
	2. Thoracic vertebrae	12	2. Next twelve vertebrae; ribs attached to these
	3. Lumbar vertebrae	5	3. Next five vertebrae, located in "small" of back
	4. Sacrum	1	4. In embryo, five separate vertebrae, but fused in adult into one wedge-shaped bone
	5. Coccyx	1	5. In embryo, four or five separate vertebrae, but fused in adult into one bone
d. Ribs and sternum	1. True ribs	7 pairs	1. Upper seven pairs fastened to sternum by costal cartilages
	2. False ribs	5 pairs	2. Do not attach to sternum directly; upper three pairs of false ribs attached by means of costal cartilage of seventh ribs; last two pairs not attached at all and therefore called "floating" ribs
	3. Sternum	1	3. Breast bone
2. Appendicular skeleton			
a. Upper extremities	1. Clavicle	2	1. Collar bone; shoulder girdle fastened to axial skeleton by articulation of clavicle with sternum
	2. Scapula	2	2. Shoulder blade
	3. Humerus	2	3. Long bone of upper arm
	4. Radius	2	4. Thumb side of forearm
	5. Ulna	2	5. Little finger side of forearm
	6. Carpals	16	6. Wrist bones; arranged in two rows at proximal end of hand
	7. Metacarpals	10	7. Long bones; form framework of palm of hand
	8. Phalanges	28	8. Miniature long bones of fingers; three in each finger, two in each thumb
b. Lower extremities	1. Os coxae, or pelvic bone	2	1. Large hip bones; lower extremities attached to axial skeleton by articulation of pelvic bones with sacrum
	2. Femur	2	2. Thigh bone
	3. Patella	2	3. Kneecap
	4. Tibia	2	4. Shin bone
	5. Fibula	2	5. Long, slender bone of lateral side of lower leg
	6. Tarsals	14	6. "Ankle" bones; form heel and proximal end of foot
	7. Metatarsals	10	7. Long bones of feet
	8. Phalanges	28	8. Miniature long bones of toes
	TOTAL	206†	

*Paranasal sinuses—holes in frontal, sphenoidal, maxillary, and ethmoid bones reduce weight of skull, serve as resonating chambers in speech, produce mucus, and often become inflamed due to allergic responses and viral or bacterial infection.
†Sesamoid bones (rounded bones found in various tendons) have not been counted except for patellae, which are largest sesamoid bones; number of these bones varies greatly between individuals. Wormian bones (small islets of bone in some cranial sutures) have not been counted because of variability of occurrence.

3. Osteoporosis may occur in postmenopausal women; related to decreased estrogen production, lack of exercise that stresses skeleton, and inadequate intake of calcium, magnesium, and vitamins A, C, and D
I. Repair of skeleton
    1. When bone is fractured, connective tissue called a callus grows into and around the broken region
    2. Macrophages reabsorb dead and damaged cells
    3. Osteoclasts dissolve bone fragments
    4. Osteoblasts produce new bone substance and fuse bone together
    5. Final bone shape slowly remodeled; the complete process takes several months; much slower than epithelial tissue, which has a higher metabolic rate and richer blood supply

REVIEW OF PHYSICAL PRINCIPLES RELATED TO THE NEUROMUSCULOSKELETAL SYSTEMS
Principles of Mechanics
A. Applications of energy laws—machines: apart from friction, the work output of a machine is equal to the work input to the machine; the first law of thermodynamics indicates that energy cannot be created or destroyed; a machine can multiply force, that is, provide a mechanical advantage, but at the expense of distance
    1. Lever: rigid bar that moves about a fixed point known as the fulcrum; a small force is applied through a large distance and the other end of the lever exerts a large force over a small distance; the musculoskeletal system operates through lever systems
        a. First-class lever: fulcrum between resistance and effort (e.g., scissors, hemostat, bending head backward or forward)
        b. Second-class lever: resistance between fulcrum and effort (e.g., wheelbarrow, oxygen tank carrier)
        c. Third-class lever: effort between resistance and fulcrum (e.g., forceps, bending over and using your back muscles to lift an object with your hips acting as the fulcrum; swinging the arm when using a tennis racquet)
    2. Pulleys: can multiply force at the expense of distance; the use of a number of pulleys together, as in a block and tackle, provides a mechanical advantage equal to the number of ropes excluding the pull rope; thus a block and tackle with two ropes gives a mechanical advantage of 2; a 100-lb weight can be lifted by application of a force of 50 lb (e.g., traction, lifting heavy objects like engines; pulleys used to change direction of a force); used in traction to apply tension in back injuries
B. Center of gravity
    1. Position in a body where all the weight is considered to be located; sphere, such as a rubber ball, has its center of gravity in its center
    2. Object is stable (will not topple over) as long as a line dropped from its center of gravity to the ground is within the base of the object; in a human the center of gravity is in the pelvic cavity, and for

upright balance the line drawn from this point to the ground must fall somewhere between the legs
        a. When lifting a client, the back should be kept straight to keep torque at a minimum; in addition, when bending over, the body's center of gravity shifts from a stable position between the legs to an unstable position outside the legs; the back muscles must then work even harder to prevent the body from toppling over
        b. When walking and carrying a load, the load should be carried as close to the body (center of gravity) as possible to maintain balance and to avoid strain

Principles of Physical Properties of Matter
A. Pascal's principle: when pressure is applied to a fluid in a closed, nonflexible container, it is transmitted undiminished throughout all parts of the fluid and acts in all directions
    EXAMPLE: Cerebrospinal fluid: abnormal increase of pressure on this fluid is transmitted to all parts of the central nervous system containing the fluid
    1. Brain tumor: mass of tissue displaces fluid and increases the pressure of the cerebrospinal fluid
    2. Hydrocephalus: blockage in the canal of Sylvius or overactivity of the choroid plexuses results in a tremendous collection of fluid and increased pressure
B. Electromagnetic radiation
    1. X-ray
    EXAMPLE: Pneumoencephalogram: ventricles of the brain can be imaged radiographically if the cerebrospinal fluid of the ventricles is temporarily replaced by air; as x-rays pass through the brain, the ventricles are outlined; the picture obtained is called a pneumoencephalogram
    2. Radiation hazards: individuals working with x-rays should leave the room, stand behind a lead shield, or wear a lead apron when activating the x-ray machine, since there is some scattering of radiation in all directions even though the x-ray beam is aimed at a particular area; film badges (photographic film) should be worn when working near sources of radiation to provide a record of the individual's overall exposure to the radiation
C. Sound: mechanical vibration; cannot occur in a vacuum; propagated best through solids, and through liquids better than gases; travels in waves from vibrating source such as vocal cords, loudspeaker, or dropped object
    1. Properties of waves
        a. Transverse waves: particles of the medium vibrate at right angles to the direction of the wave (e.g., waves on the surface of liquids and all electromagnetic waves [light, infrared, and ultraviolet])
        b. Longitudinal waves: particles of the medium vibrate back and forth along the same direction as the wave (e.g., sound waves)
        c. Frequency: number of complete vibrations (or waves) generated or moving along per second; units of frequency are cycles per second or a hertz (Hz)

d. Passage of a wave through a medium (gas, liquid, solid, or plasma) is actually the passage of a disturbance in the medium, not a flowing of the medium itself; the wave represents sequential vibration or swinging of the molecules of the medium from the vibrating source to the ears

e. Refraction of sound waves: sound travels faster in warm air than in cool air; in warm air the average kinetic energy of the air molecules is higher than in cool air and the wave can be propagated more quickly

f. Reflection of sound waves: many solid objects reflect sound waves from their surfaces resulting in an echo; a reverberation is a series of echoes

g. Energy of sound waves: all waves possess energy but to differing degrees; ultraviolet waves and gamma radiation possess high energy, whereas sound waves possess little energy; the structure of the ear reflects the need to amplify the relatively weak energy of sound waves into more energetic waves capable of stimulating the liquid-filled organ of hearing, the cochlea in the inner ear

h. Velocity of sound: frequency of the wave multiplied by the length of the wave; the velocity of sound waves varies with the nature and temperature of the medium; since light travels much faster than sound, lightning is seen before thunder is heard

2. Interpretation of sounds

a. Loudness: neurologic or psychologic interpretation of intensity; although the exact relationship is complex, one could say that the greater the intensity of the sound waves stimulating the organ of Corti, the greater will be the size of nerve impulses reaching the auditory centers of the brain and the louder the sound seems to be

(1) Noise level is measured in decibels (dB); a normal conversation is about 65 dB, amplified rock music about 120 dB, and the sound of a nearby jet airplane about 140 dB; the decibel scale is logarithmic so that 120 dB is 1 million times more intense than 60 dB

(2) Excessive noise can result in hearing loss at certain frequencies of sound; noise levels of about 85 dB and over can damage the organ of Corti; damage increases with the length and intensity of noise and is irreversible

(3) Doppler effect: when a vibrating source and a receiver of sound move toward each other, the pitch or frequency of the sound produced by the source becomes higher; as the vibrating source and the receiver move away from each other, the frequency of the sound becomes lower

(4) Speech audiometry: this technique detects the threshold of hearing of actual speech for individuals by presenting groups of two-syllable words at successively lower levels until the person fails to hear; these data are presented as a speech reception threshold (SRT) in decibels; phonetically balanced single-syllable words can also be presented; these words represent a frequency of sounds of speech that approximates a typical conversation; the percentage of words repeated correctly is the Davis Social Adequacy Index (SAI); a score of 94% to 100% is considered normal

b. Pitch: corresponds to frequency; the higher the frequency, the higher the pitch of the sound

(1) Humans can potentially hear sounds whose frequencies range from 16 to 20,000 Hz; with increasing age, the upper range decreases slightly, which presents no problem in hearing speech, since speech falls in the range of 85 to 1,050 Hz

(2) Audiometers are capable of electronically producing sounds at a variety of frequencies as well as intensities and are used to measure hearing loss

c. Quality: people have different and distinct qualities or timbres to their voices; similarly, the sounds of different musical instruments are easily recognized; a musical sound or a voice rarely represents a pure tone but usually many frequencies occurring simultaneously

d. Ultrasonic sound: vibrational frequencies exceeding the upper level of human hearing (20,000 Hz)

(1) Can be used in cleaning metal parts; the high-frequency vibrations shake the solution and produce bubbles that help in the cleaning process

(2) Low-intensity ultrasonic waves have been used to treat arthritis and bursitis, to break kidney stones, and to help dissolve scars

(3) Ultrasonic dental drills can quickly drill into teeth without the pain associated with tooth vibrations, which stimulate the nerve of the tooth

(4) Sonograms are pictures of the body derived through differential reflection or transmission of sound waves

e. Deafness: condition wherein sound vibrations are not transmitted to the brain for interpretation

(1) Perforation or tear of the tympanic membrane

(2) Inflexibility of the three middle ear bones or ossicles; vibrations are thus only poorly transmitted to the oval window

(3) Otosclerosis: abnormal bone formation over the oval window immobilizes the stapes

(a) Surgery can remove the abnormal bony tissue in the early stages of the disease

(b) In later stages the stapes may be removed and a prosthesis implanted

(c) If the oval window is ossified, a new opening in the cochlea is made to replace the oval window (fenestration)

(d) Bone-conduction hearing aids can essentially bypass the middle ear

(4) Deafness caused by auditory nerve damage; the nerve cannot be regenerated nor can hearing be helped by hearing aids

   f. Hearing aids: electronic devices that amplify sounds and assist partially deaf persons to hear; a miniature microphone picks up the sound, sends it to an amplifier and then to a miniature loudspeaker fitted in or behind the ear

     (1) Air-conduction type sends an amplified sound wave into the ear, thus utilizing the person's own middle ear

     (2) Bone-conduction type bypasses the middle ear and transmits amplified vibrations to the skull bones, which in turn produce vibrations in the inner ear

D. Light
1. Basic concepts
   a. Visible light is a type of electromagnetic radiation; all electromagnetic radiation consists of oscillating electric and magnetic fields that come into existence because of the vibrations of electrically charged particles

   b. All types of electromagnetic radiation have the same electric and magnetic nature and travel at the same constant velocity: 186,000 miles per second (speed of light)

   c. Electromagnetic spectrum varies from extremely long AM and FM radio waves measured in miles to very short gamma and cosmic rays measured in tenths of picometer

   d. Product of the frequency of vibration and the wavelength is constant (the velocity of light); the lower the frequency of vibration of the wave, the longer will be the wavelength, and the higher the frequency, the shorter the wavelength

   e. The higher the frequency (or the shorter the wavelength) of electromagnetic radiation, the greater will be the energy content of the radiation

2. Wavelengths of electromagnetic radiation
   a. Wavelengths can be measured in millimicrons or Angstrom units

     (1) A millimicron is one thousandth of a micron; a micron is one millionth of a meter (39 inches)

     (2) An Angstrom unit is one tenth of a millimicron

   b. Wavelengths of visible light possess just the right amount of vibrational energy to excite the photoreceptor cells (rods and cones) of the retina

   c. Different wavelengths of light are bent or refracted to slightly different degrees and appear to the eyes and brain as different colors; this principle of dispersion is responsible for a rainbow

   d. Emission of light: atoms can be excited by absorbing energy that causes orbiting electrons to jump to higher energy levels within the atom; as the electrons fall back to their lower (more stable) energy levels (deexcitation), the energy of excitation is released and may appear as visible

light (e.g., advertising signs, mercury vapor street lamps)

     (1) Characteristic pattern of wavelengths of light (a discontinuous spectrum) is emitted from every element in the vapor state; this pattern is best seen by means of a spectroscope

     (2) Fluorescence: property of absorbing radiation of one frequency and emitting radiation of a lower frequency and energy; a substance is said to be fluorescent if it emits visible light when energized or bombarded with ultraviolet (UV) light; high-intensity fluorescent light bulbs have been used to treat jaundice in newborn infants; the excess bilirubin in the blood, which is responsible for the jaundice, is oxidized by exposure to the bright light as blood passes through the vessels of the thin skin

     (3) Phosphorescence: atoms of a phosphorescent substance become deexcited a relatively long time after being excited; the phosphorescent atoms in the dial of a luminous clock are excited during the day by the visible light striking them; the dial then glows throughout the night as billions of excited atoms gradually become deexcited, releasing their energy as visible light

3. Laser
   a. Acronym for light amplification by stimulated emission of radiation; a laser produces monochromatic coherent light, which means that the light waves are all of the same frequency, are all in phase with each other (peak with peak, trough with trough), and are all traveling in the same direction; in coherent light, millions of light waves become additive and form a single, concentrated beam of light that travels in a straight line without spreading out and that can be precisely focused on minute areas

   b. As coherent light leaves the laser (one type of laser uses a ruby crystal), it can be utilized for a variety of purposes

     (1) Eye surgery: energy in the coherent light produced by a laser is used to fuse minute areas of the retina to the surrounding choroid coat; an ophthalmoscope is used to focus the coherent light precisely on specific, tiny areas of the retina; a detached retina can thus be reattached, and the fusion points are so tiny that there is no apparent loss of light-sensitive retinal tissue; the machine used in this type of surgery is called a photocoagulator and uses a ruby laser

     (2) Cancer therapy: laser has been used in the selective treatment of pigmented skin cancers, which apparently absorb the light more readily than do surrounding, less pigmented, normal tissues

4. Color
   a. Perception of color is the result of the translation and interpretation of certain nerve impulses in the brain that come from the retina; the fre-

quency of light determines the color that is seen; the lowest frequency stimulating the retina is red, the highest is violet, in between are all the colors of nature

b. Objects may appear to be colored because they emit electromagnetic radiation that falls within the visible range; may also appear colored not because they emit light, but because of selective reflection

c. Color mixing
   (1) Red, green, and blue are the additive primaries; any color in the spectrum can be obtained with the proper blend of these three; equal amounts of the three produce white light
   (2) Magenta, yellow, and cyan (turquoise) are the subtractive primaries; any color in the spectrum can be obtained using the proper blend of these three; they are sometimes loosely called red, yellow, and blue
   (3) Complementary colors are any two colors that, when added together, produce white: red and cyan, magenta and green, and yellow and blue

d. Perception of color is believed to depend on the cones of the retina, which are located most densely at the part of the retina called the fovea centralis; one type of cone detects red, another detects green, and another blue; it is generally thought that the brain blends nerve impulses from these three types of cones to produce our perception of all the colors of nature
   (1) Faulty color vision is thought to be caused by cones that are either missing or not functioning properly; red-green color blindness is the most common type and is a genetically inherited trait that causes individuals to see red and green objects as shades of gray; more men are affected than women, since the trait appears to be sex linked
   (2) Color and emotion: even though red light has a lower frequency and therefore less energy than a quantum of blue light, the human mind generally associates red with warmth, excitement, and mental stimulation, and blue with coolness and calmness; for many individuals the color of an object or a room determines to a great extent whether they will keep and use the object or stay in the room; thus color has a physical basis in the electromagnetic radiation but involves complex interpretation by the human mind

5. Reflection and refraction
   a. General principles
      (1) Source of light: sun the primary outdoor source; incandescent and fluorescent bulbs are indoor sources
      (2) Most objects visible because they reflect light emitted from various sources
      (3) Pane of glass is transparent if it allows light to pass through it in straight lines
      (4) Thin cloth window shade or a piece of paper is translucent if it allows light to pass through it in a diffused manner so objects cannot be seen; in hospitals, shades or blinds diffuse light and cut down on harsh glare
      (5) Heavy pair of curtains is opaque if light cannot pass through it
      (6) Light traveling in any single medium travels in straight lines; each straight line called a ray
   b. Reflection
      (1) When light strikes a surface off which it can reflect, the angle of incidence equals the angle of reflection as measured from the normal (a line perpendicular to the plane of the reflecting surface)
         (a) When successive elevations of any surface are less than about one fourth the wavelength of the incident light, the light reflected from the surface travels mainly in one direction and the surface is polished
         (b) Light reflected from rougher surfaces travels in many directions and is diffusely reflected; it is easier to read a page of text printed on paper that provides a more diffuse than polished reflection, since glare is eliminated
         (c) The word *ambulance* is often printed backward on the front of these vehicles so that motorists seeing the lettering via reflected light through their rearview mirrors will be able to read the lettering correctly
      (2) Virtual images: as light reflects off a mirror, the angles of incidence and reflection are equal; the reflected rays of light appear to come from a point behind the mirror; because the light rays do not actually come from this point, the image is referred to as a virtual image as opposed to a real image; the virtual image of a plane mirror is as far behind the mirror as the object is in front of the mirror
   c. Refraction
      (1) Refraction: bending of an oblique ray of light as it travels from one transparent medium into another; refraction is caused by the change in velocity of light as it passes through the medium
      (2) Index of refraction: average speed of light varies in different, transparent media; the average speed of light in water is only 75% of its average speed in a vacuum; the average speed in a diamond is 41% of its average speed in a vacuum; the index of refraction is a measure of how much the average speed of light differs from its speed in a vacuum; index of refraction equals the speed of light in a vacuum divided by its speed in a me-

dium; the higher the index of refraction, the slower the speed of light through the medium

EXAMPLES

1. Thermometer or syringe half immersed in a beaker of water appears to be bent at the point of immersion
2. Object in water appears to be nearer the surface than it actually is; thus it seems larger because it is magnified
3. Mirage: average speed of light is slightly greater in hot air than in cool air; on a hot paved road or a desert the light reflected from an object is refracted upward, away from the hot surface and may then produce an upside-down virtual image to an individual some distance away; the wet shimmering look of a hot road is refracted light from the sky reaching a motorist's eye after passing through hot air layers
4. Total internal reflection: at a certain critical angle, light between two media is not refracted (or bent) but is reflected back into the first medium provided the first medium has a higher index of refraction than the second medium
   a. This phenomenon permits viewing of the interior walls of the stomach, intestines, and blood vessels
   b. Dentist's flashlight will "curve" the light (via total internal reflection) to the appropriate part of an individual's mouth
   c. Total internal reflection via the paired prisms in a pair of binoculars permits higher magnifications in a short optic tube

6. Diffraction

Bending of light or any type of electromagnetic wave around corners; the longer the wavelength of electromagnetic radiation, the larger the object that it can be bent around

EXAMPLES

1. AM radio waves, some of which are over 3 miles long, easily bend around objects, thereby allowing AM broadcasts to come in clearly even in cities having many tall buildings and mountainous regions
2. FM radio waves, which are from 9 to 12 feet long, cannot easily bend around large objects; consequently, a specific location in a city or suburban area with large obstructing objects can determine the quality of the reception of FM broadcasts
3. Some spectrophotometers used in certain laboratory analyses of blood and urine rely on diffraction gratings to disperse white light into its component wavelengths and to utilize these specific wavelengths in the analytic procedure

4. X-ray diffraction: because of their very short wavelengths, x-rays diffract around the atoms in large molecules and produce diffraction patterns on photographic plates; analyses of these patterns can reveal the details of the arrangement of the atoms in a molecule; used in DNA analysis

7. Polarization

Certain naturally occurring crystals, like tourmaline and herapathite, absorb light waves striking them in all planes but one; the light transmitted through and emerging from the crystal vibrates in only one plane; this is called plane-polarized light

EXAMPLES

1. Polaroid filters contain a material, like herpathite or certain synthetic molecules, that will permit only light vibrating in a single plane to pass through; when used in sunglasses, they cut down on glare and eye strain; much of the light reflected from nonmetallic surfaces, such as water, glass, or roadways, is already polarized because these surfaces tend to transmit light waves perpendicular to their surfaces and to reflect light waves parallel to their surfaces; when this polarized light strikes the Polaroid filters in the sunglasses, many of the light waves are absorbed; thus fewer waves are transmitted and the harsh glare is reduced
2. Polarizing filters for cameras cut down on glare in photographs and also have the effect of deepening the blue color of the sky
3. Polarizing microscopes are used in research laboratories to analyze the molecular structure of many substances

8. Lenses
   a. Refraction of light through transparent glass (or quartz or fluorite) lenses is of great practical importance; magnification of objects is possible using simple lenses as well as groups of lenses arranged in telescopes and microscopes; the principal axis of a lens is the line joining the two points that represent the centers of curvature of the curved surfaces of a given lens
   b. Convex lenses (converging or positive lenses) converge light rays passing through them; concave lenses (diverging or negative lenses) diverge light rays passing through them
   c. When light rays parallel with the principal axis pass through a converging lens, they converge on the focal point; parallel light rays which are not parallel with the principal axis converge in a series of points above and below the focal point, making up the focal plane
      (1) Converging lens will magnify an object (acting as a simple magnifying glass) if it is held inside the focal point of the lens; the image is enlarged, right side up and virtual; this means that the image only appears to exist but has no physical reality

(2) When an object is placed outside the focal point of a converging lens, a real, inverted image is obtained that can be focused on a screen; whenever a real image is formed, the object and image are on opposite sides of the lens

EXAMPLES
1. Motion pictures utilize converging lenses, and the movie screen is the plane where light rays are converged; slide projectors also operate under the same principle
2. In cameras the film is flattened out and placed in the focal plane of the camera's lens; in popular single-lens reflex (SLR) cameras a mirror diverts the light to a prism, which erects the image, allowing the viewer to see exactly what will be focused on the film; when the shutter button is pushed and the mirror flips out of the way, light is focused on and exposes the photographic film
3. Diverging lenses used alone produce smaller, virtual images; they are used on some cameras (not SLR cameras) as "finders," since the virtual image seen approximates the proportions of the photograph; whenever a virtual image is formed, the object and the image are on the same side of the lens
4. Lens defects: distortions in an image produced by a given lens are called aberrations; combining a number of lenses as a system can usually minimize aberrations; this is the reason that microscopes and telescopes employ compound lenses in their construction
   a. Spherical aberration: unsharp (uncrisp) images are formed because light refracted from the outer edges of the lens is focused at a point slightly different from the point at which light refracted from more central areas of the lens is focused
      (1) In cameras and microscopes this is corrected by using more than one lens and also by using diaphragms to cover the outer regions of the lens
      (2) In the human eye the iris is generally contracted to varying degrees and acts, in effect, like a diaphragm to block light from being refracted through the outer regions of the lens
   b. Chromatic aberration: each wavelength of visible light refracts through lenses at different angles; thus each wavelength (color) of white light is brought to focus at a slightly different point; the result of this is that objects take on colors that they do not possess; this is corrected in cameras, microscopes, and telescopes by using combinations of simple lenses made of different types of glass called achromatic lenses; in the human eye, vision is sharpest when the pupil is the smallest; cutting down on light moving through the periphery of the lens minimizes chromatic as well as spherical aberration
   c. Astigmatism: human eye astigmatism is a type of abberration caused by the surface of the cornea possessing irregular curves; since the cornea in

addition to the lens is important in refracting (focusing) light on the retina, the result of astigmatism is blurred vision, which can be corrected by using lenses that have variable curvature to compensate for the irregular curvature of the cornea
5. Focusing: camera focuses on objects at varying distances by changing the distance between the lens and the film; the human eye focuses on objects at varying distances by changing the degree of curvature of the lens; this ability of the human eye to change the focal length of the lens is called accommodation; whereas the cornea, aqueous humor, and vitreous humor all help to focus light on the retina, only the crystalline lens is able to accommodate; the muscle responsible for accommodation is the ciliary body; when the ciliary body contracts, the suspensory ligaments loosen and the lens rounds out and is in position for focusing on near objects; when the ciliary body relaxes, the suspensory ligaments pull the lens into a flattened position, which allows for focusing on distant objects; the limit for accommodation is represented by the near point; objects closer to the eye than the near point (about 15 cm [6 inches] from the surface of a normal eye) cannot be clearly focused on the retina
   a. Emmetropia: normal refractive state of the eye
   b. Ametropia: any abnormality in refractive ability of the eye
      (1) Myopia: eye focuses light anterior to the retina (somewhere in the vitreous humor); from this abnormal focal point, light rays diverge and produce a blurred image on the retina; however, if objects are held about 2.5 cm (1 inch) from the eye, they will focus on the retina; for this reason, myopia is also called near-sightedness; glasses containing diverging lenses correct this condition
      (2) Hyperopia: eye focuses light posterior to the retina; thus a circle of not-yet-converged light strikes the retina, producing a blurred image; hyperopia is also called far-sightedness and can be corrected using glasses containing converging lenses
   c. Contact lenses: thin lenses that are molded to the shape of the outer surface of the cornea; this can correct near-sightedness, far-sightedness, and astigmatism; the lens is applied to the surface of the eye using a saline solution that helps adhere the lens to the eye's surface
6. Eye examination with the ophthalmoscope and the retinoscope
   a. Ophthalmoscope: permits visualization of the interior of the eye; thus the examiner can study a client's vision with this instrument; light shone into an eye with normal refractive ability will be focused on the retina and reflected back to the examiner's eye; persons with myopia or hyperopia will not converge the light on the retina, and the examiner will not clearly see the eye's interior; then by using lenses of varying refractive abilities the examiner can compensate for

the person's abnormal refraction, study the interior of the eye, and determine the state of vision

b. Retinoscope: permits diagnosis and evaluation of the refractive state of the eye; a beam of light shone into the eye is reflected from the retina as it leaves the pupil; by observing its distribution as it leaves the pupil, the examiner can determine the refractive error in the eye

7. Binocular vision: visual fields of the two human eyes overlap; while each eye sees some areas of the environment that the other eye cannot see, both eyes also see large areas in common; the human brain interprets these overlapping fields in terms of depth; the environment appears in three dimensions, as opposed to the visual effect of a movie projected on a flat screen; the blind spot of the right eye can be seen by the left eye and vice versa; therefore no gaps in the field of vision exist

REVIEW OF CHEMICAL PRINCIPLES RELATED TO THE NEUROMUSCULOSKELETAL SYSTEMS
Amines

A. Organic compounds containing an amino group (NH_2) that can be considered derivatives of ammonia
B. Reactions of the amines
   1. Basic, in water solution
   2. Like a base with acids, forming complex ions
C. Important amines
   1. Monoamines such as norepinephrine, dopamine, serotonin, acetylcholine, and histamine serve as transmitter chemicals in the nervous system
   2. Amino acids such as gamma-aminobutyric acid (GABA) and glycine act as inhibitors; glutamic acid has an excitatory influence on the nervous system

Lipids

Phospholipids, lecithin, cephalins, and sphingomyelins are important components of nerve membranes and sheaths

Proteins

Actin, myosin, and troponin are important in muscle contraction

Group I A Alkali Metals

A. Sodium: in the extracellular fluid these ions are responsible for action potentials of nervous and muscular tissue; after some stimulus, it is the diffusion of Na^+ from the interstitial fluid into the intracellular fluid of neurons and muscle fibers that brings about depolarization; thus sodium ions are basic to the functioning of the body's communication system, the nervous system, and all muscular movements
B. Potassium
   1. Resting polarization of neurons, all types of muscle fibers (e.g., smooth, cardiac, striated), and most cells of the body is caused by the continual diffusion of K^+ from the intracellular fluid to the interstitial fluid; similarly, repolarization of neurons and muscle fibers is caused by the outward diffusion of K^+ to the interstitial fluid from the intracellular fluid

   2. Several important cellular enzymes functioning in glucose and amino acid metabolism require K^+ as a cofactor

Group II A Alkali Earth Metals

A. Magnesium
   1. Activator for many enzymes
   2. Present in bones
B. Calcium
   1. Gives hardness to bones and teeth by forming phosphate, carbonate, and fluoride salts
   2. Important in muscle contraction; ATP must combine with Ca^{++} before its energy can be used to slide actin and myosin filaments together
   3. Extracellular Ca^{++} concentration must be precisely regulated (through the parathyroid glands) for normal body functioning; hypocalcemia can result in tetany; hypercalcemia can result in depression of the nervous system
C. Strontium
   1. May substitute for calcium in body
   2. Radioactive isotope (strontium 90) can be a health hazard, forming pockets of radiation in tissues

Group VII A Halogens

Fluorine: prevents tooth decay when added to water supply

Group I B

A. Silver: filling for teeth, surgical mending of bone, photography
B. Gold: filling for teeth

REVIEW OF MICROORGANISMS RELATED TO THE NEUROMUSCULOSKELETAL SYSTEMS

A. Bacterial pathogens
   1. *Clostridium tetani:* large, gram-positive, motile bacillus forming large terminal spores; like all clostridia, it is an obligate anaerobe; causes tetanus (lockjaw)
   2. *Haemophilus aegyptius* (Koch-Weeks bacillus): indistinguishable morphologically from *Haemophilus influenzae;* causes a common conjunctivitis called pinkeye
   3. *Neisseria meningitidis:* gram-negative diplococcus; causes epidemic (meningococcic) meningitis
B. DNA viruses: herpetoviruses; spherical and 150 to 200 nm in diameter; cause herpes simplex, varicella (chickenpox), herpes zoster (shingles), infectious mononucleosis, and cytomegalic inclusion disease
C. RNA viruses: togaviruses; spherical and 40 to 60 nm in diameter; mostly borne by mosquitoes and ticks; cause eastern equine encephalomyelitis, western equine encephalomyelitis, Venezuelan equine encephalomyelitis, and a number of other infections
D. Fungal pathogen: *Cryptococcus neoformans*—pathogenic yeast with a characteristic large capsule around the cell; causes cryptococcosis (torulosis, European blastomycosis), a serious infection involving the lungs and central nervous system

E. Protozoa: *Trypanosoma*—flagellated ribbonlike protozoa; *T. gambiense* and *T. rhodesience* cause African sleeping sickness (transmitted by tsetse flies) and *T. cruzi* causes South American trypanosomiasis or Chagas' disease (transmitted by reduviid bugs)

F. Worm: *Trichinella spiralis*—one of smallest parasitic nematodes (about 1.5 mm in length), causes trichinosis (muscle infestation with trichina)

PHARMACOLOGY RELATED TO NEUROMUSCULOSKELETAL SYSTEMS DISORDERS
Anticonvulsants

A. Description
1. Used to decrease the occurrence, frequency, and/or severity of convulsive episodes; end result of anticonvulsant therapy is the control of seizures
2. Act by modifying bioelectric activity at subcortical and cortical sites by stabilizing the nerve cell membrane and/or raising the seizure threshold to incoming stimuli
3. Available in oral and parenteral (IM, IV) preparations

B. Examples
1. Grand mal seizure control
   a. carbamazepine (Tegretol): also used for psychomotor seizures
   b. diazepam (Valium): used IV for status epilepticus
   c. phenytoin (Dilantin): also used for psychomotor seizures
   d. phenobarbital (Luminal)
   e. magnesium sulfate
2. Petit mal seizure control
   a. ethasuximide (Zarontin)
   b. methsuximide (Celontin)
   c. paramethadione (Paradione)
   d. trimethadione (Tridione)

C. Major side effects
1. Dizziness, drowsiness (CNS depression)
2. Nausea, vomiting (irritation of gastric mucosa)
3. Skin rash (hypersensitivity)
4. Blood dyscrasias (decreased RBC, WBC, platelet synthesis)
5. Phenytoin
   a. Ataxia (neurotoxicity)
   b. Gingival hyperplasia (gum irritation leading to tissue overgrowth)
   c. Hirsutism (virilism)
   d. Hypotension (decreased atrial and ventricular conduction)

D. Nursing care
1. Administer with food to reduce GI irritation
2. Provide care for the client having a seizure
   a. Maintain airway; place in side-lying position after seizure
   b. Protect client from injury
   c. Assess the type and duration of seizure
3. Instruct client to
   a. Avoid alcohol and other CNS depressants
   b. Notify physician if fever, sore throat, or skin rash develops
   c. Carry medical alert card

4. Teach client receiving barbiturates to
   a. Avoid engaging in hazardous activities
   b. Assess for cardiac and respiratory depression
5. Care for the client receiving phenytoin (Dilantin)
   a. Provide oral hygiene; inspect oral mucosa for infection
   b. Avoid mixing with other IV infusions
   c. Assess for potentiation of anticoagulant effect
   d. Assess urine; drug may discolor urine pink to red-brown
   e. Assess for therapeutic blood levels (10 to 20 mcg/ml)
6. Encourage diet rich in nutrient-dense foods such as fruits, vegetables, whole grains, and legumes to improve and maintain nutritional status and prevent possible drug-induced nutrient deficiencies
7. Evaluate client's response to medication and understanding of teaching

Osmotic Diuretics

A. Description
1. Reduce cerebral edema and intraocular pressure by increasing the osmotic pressure within the vasculature, thus causing fluid to leave the tissues and be excreted in the urine
2. Used to treat increased intracranial pressure
3. Available in parenteral (IV) preparations

B. Examples
1. mannitol (Osmitrol)
2. urea (Ureaphil)

C. Major side effects
1. Headache (dehydration)
2. Nausea (fluid and electrolyte imbalance)
3. Chills (fluid and electrolyte imbalance)
4. Rebound edema when discontinued (fluid and electrolyte imbalance)
5. Fluid/electrolyte imbalances (hyponatremia, hypokalemia) (promotion of sodium and potassium excretion)

D. Nursing care
1. Monitor intake and output during therapy
2. Avoid administration in clients with congestive heart failure or impaired renal function
3. Elevate head of bed during therapy
4. Monitor daily weight and serum electrolytes during course of therapy
5. Assess client for signs of increased intracranial pressure (decreasing pulse rate, widening pulse pressure, increasing systolic pressure, unequal pupils, change in level of consciousness)
6. Evaluate client's response to medication and understanding of teaching

Calcium Enhancers

A. Description
1. Used to restore calcium ion balance
2. Serum calcium concentration is increased through
   a. Direct calcium ion replacement
   b. Vitamin D replacement, which improves the absorption of calcium from the intestines
3. Available in oral and parenteral (IM, IV) preparations

B. Examples
  1. Calcium ion replacement
    a. calcium chloride: IV administration only
    b. calcium gluconate
    c. calcium carbonate (Os-Cal)
  2. Vitamin D replacement
    a. calcitriol (Rocaltrol)
    b. cholecalciferol (Calciferol)
    c. dihydrotachysterol (Hytakerol)
C. Major side effects
  1. Nausea, vomiting (hypercalcemia)
  2. Constipation (increased serum calcium delays passage of stool in GI tract)
  3. Renal calculi (hypercalcemia)
  4. Muscle flaccidity (hypercalcemia)
  5. Calcium preparations: cardiac disturbances (stimulation of cardiac conduction)
  6. Vitamin D: dry mouth; metallic taste (early vitamin D toxicity associated with hypercalcemia)
D. Nursing care
  1. Assess client for signs of tetany and hypercalcemia
  2. Encourage increased fluid intake and acid ash diet to reduce potential of renal calculi and constipation; stress vitamin D and calcium-rich foods such as eggs, cheese, whole grain cereals, and cranberries; limit milk, fruits, and vegetables
  3. Monitor serum electrolytes during course of therapy
  4. Calcium preparations: assess for potentiation of digitalis effect
  5. Evaluate client's response to medication and understanding of teaching

Antiparkinson Agents

A. Description
  1. Anticholinergic drugs act at central sites to inhibit cerebral motor impulses and to block efferent impulses that cause rigidity of the musculature
  2. Levodopa preparations and others supply or cause the release of dopamine required for norepinephrine synthesis and maintenance of the neurohormonal balance at subcortical, cortical, and reticular sites that control motor function
  3. Used to control the symptoms of Parkinson's disease
  4. Available in oral and parenteral (IM, IV) preparations
B. Examples
  1. Anticholinergic drugs
    a. benztropine mesylate (Cogentin)
    b. ethopropazine HCl (Parsidol)
    c. trihexyphenidyl HCl (Artane)
  2. Other drugs
    a. amantadine HCl (Symmetrel)
    b. levodopa (Dopar, Larodopa)
C. Major side effects
  1. Anticholinergic drugs (decrease parasympathetic stimulation)
    a. Dry mouth (decreased salivation)
    b. Blurred vision (pupillary dilation)
    c. Constipation (decreased peristalsis)
    d. Urinary retention (decreased muscle tone)

  2. Other drugs
    a. Orthostatic hypotension (loss of compensatory vasoconstriction with position change)
    b. Ataxia (neurotoxicity)
    c. CNS disturbances and emotional disturbances (CNS effect)
    d. Nausea, vomiting (irritation of gastric mucosa)
D. Nursing care
  1. Instruct client to
    a. Avoid discontinuing drug suddenly
    b. Understand that treatment controls symptoms but is not a cure
    c. Keep all scheduled appointments; medical supervision is necessary
  2. Offer emotional support to client at this time; therapy is usually for life
  3. Care for the client receiving anticholinergic drugs
    a. Offer sugar-free chewing gum and hard candy to increase salivation
    b. May interfere with ability to perform potentially hazardous activities
  4. Care for the client receiving levodopa
    a. Eliminate vitamin B_6 from diet
    b. Inform client regarding dosage and "holiday" periods
  5. Encourage diet rich in nutrient-dense foods such as fruits, vegetables, whole grains, and legumes to improve and maintain nutritional status and prevent possible drug-induced nutrient deficiencies; clients taking levodopa should limit intake of foods high in vitamin B_6 (for example, pork, glandular meats, lamb, veal, legumes, potatoes, oatmeal, wheat germ, and bananas
  6. Evaluate client's response to medication and understanding of teaching

Cholinesterase Inhibitors

A. Description
  1. Used to diagnose and treat myasthenia gravis
  2. Act by
    a. Preventing enzymatic breakdown of acetylcholine at nerve endings, thus allowing accumulation of the neurotransmitter
    b. Improving the strength of contraction in all muscles, including those involved with the process of respiration
  3. Available in oral and parenteral (IM, IV) preparations
B. Examples
  1. ambenonium chloride (Mytelase)
  2. edrophonium chloride (Tensilon): for diagnostic purposes
  3. neostigmine bromide (Prostigmin)
  4. pyridostigmine bromide (Mestinon)
C. Major side effects
  1. Nausea, vomiting (irritation of gastric mucosa)
  2. Diarrhea (increased peristalsis)
  3. Hypersalivation (increased parasympathetic stimulation)
  4. Muscle cramps (increased skeletal muscle contraction)
  5. CNS disturbances (CNS effect)

6. Acute toxicity: pulmonary edema and respiratory failure (bronchial constriction)

D. Nursing care
1. Monitor client closely; dosage is adjusted according to needs
2. Have atropine sulfate available for treatment of overdosage
3. Administer medications exactly according to schedule
4. Administer with food to reduce GI irritation
5. Instruct client to
   a. Carry a medical alert card
   b. Take medication before meals to improve chewing and swallowing
   c. Encourage diet rich in nutrient-dense foods such as fruits, vegetables, whole grains, and legumes to improve and maintain nutritional status and prevent possible drug-induced nutrient deficiencies
6. Evaluate client's response to medication and understanding of teaching

Skeletal Muscle Relaxants

A. Description
1. Used to relieve inappropriate and abnormal muscle contraction.
2. Central agents act by CNS depression to bring about relaxation of voluntary muscles
3. Peripheral agents block nerve impulse conduction at the myoneural junction
4. Available in oral and parenteral (IM, IV) preparations

B. Examples
1. Central agents
   a. carisoprodol (Soma)
   b. chlorzoxazone (Paraflex)
   c. cyclobenzapine (Flexeril)
   d. diazepam (Valium)
   e. methocarbamol (Robaxin)
   f. orphenadrine (Norflex)
2. Peripheral agents
   a. gallamine triethiodide (Flaxedil)
   b. pancuronium bromide (Pavulon)
   c. succinylcholine chloride (Anectine)
   d. tubocurarine chloride

C. Major side effects
1. Central agents
   a. Dizziness, drowsiness (CNS depression)
   b. Nausea (irritation of gastric mucosa)
   c. Headache (central antimuscarinic effect)
   d. CNS disturbances (direct CNS effect)
   e. Tachycardia (brain stem stimulation)
2. Peripheral agents
   a. Hypotension (increased vagal stimulation; increased release of histamine; ganglionic blockade)
   b. Respiratory depression (neuromuscular blockade)
   c. Arrhythmias (increased vagal stimulation)

D. Nursing care
1. Provide care for the client receiving central agents
   a. Utilize safety precautions (supervise ambulation; side rails up) during initial therapy
   b. Instruct client to
      (1) Avoid concurrent use of alcohol and other CNS depressants
      (2) Avoid engaging in potentially hazardous activities
2. Provide care for the client receiving peripheral agents
   a. Have O$_2$ and emergency resuscitative equipment available
   b. Assess vital signs before, during, and after administration
   c. Administer under direct medical supervision
3. Encourage diet rich in nutrient-dense foods such as fruits, vegetables, whole grains, and legumes to improve and maintain nutritional status and prevent possible drug-induced nutrient deficiencies
4. Evaluate client's response to medication and understanding of teaching

Nonsteroidal Antiinflammatory Drugs (NSAIDs)

A. Description
1. Used to alleviate the inflammation and subsequent discomfort of rheumatoid conditions
2. Act by interfering with prostaglandin synthesis in the body
3. Available in oral preparations

B. Examples
1. ibuprofen (Motrin)
2. indomethacin (Indocin)
3. naproxen (Naprosyn)
4. phenylbutazone (Butazolidin)
5. piroxicam (Feldene)
6. salicylates (ASA)
7. sulindac (Clinoril)

C. Major side effects
1. GI irritation (local effect)
2. Skin rash (hypersensitivity)
3. Blood dyscrasias (decreased RBC, WBC, platelet synthesis)
4. CNS disturbances (neurotoxicity)
5. Indomethacin: drowsiness (CNS effect)

D. Nursing care
1. Administer with meals to reduce GI irritation
2. Evaluate client's response to drug therapy
3. Monitor blood work during therapy
4. Assess vital signs during course of therapy
5. Instruct client to report the occurrence of any side effects to the physician
6. Inform client taking Indomethacin that it may interfere with ability to engage in hazardous activities
7. Encourage diet rich in nutrient-dense foods such as fruits, vegetables, whole grains, and legumes to improve and maintain nutritional status and prevent possible drug-induced nutrient deficiencies
8. Evaluate client's response to medication and understanding of teaching

Antigout Agents

A. Description
1. Used to prevent and arrest gout attacks which are due to high levels of uric acid in the blood

2. Act by
   a. Increasing the excretion of uric acid (uricosuric agent)
   b. Decreasing uric acid formation by the body
3. Available in oral and parenteral (IV) preparations

B. Examples
   1. allopurinol (Zyloprim): blocks formation of uric acid within the body
   2. colchicine: decreases uric acid crystal deposits by inhibiting lactic acid production by leukocytes; used for acute attacks
   3. probenecid (Benemid): prevents formation of tophi by inhibiting the reabsorption of uric acid by the kidneys

C. Major side effects
   1. Nausea, vomiting (irritation of gastric mucosa)
   2. Blood dyscrasias (decreased RBC, WBC, and platelet synthesis)
   3. Liver damage (hepatotoxicity)
   4. Skin rash (hypersensitivity)

D. Nursing care
   1. Administer antiinflammatory drugs (Prednisone, Indocin) in addition to drugs that will lower serum uric acid during the acute phase
   2. Increase fluids to discourage the formation of renal calculi
   3. Encourage weight reduction
   4. Monitor serum urate levels to determine effectiveness of treatment
   5. Administer with meals to reduce GI irritation
   6. Instruct client to avoid high purine foods such as organ meats, anchovies, sardines, and shellfish; encourage diet rich in nutrient-dense foods such as fruits, vegetables, and whole grains as well as milk, cheese, and eggs; teach Dietary Goals for the United States and importance of preventing drug-induced nutrient deficiencies with improved diet
   7. Monitor blood work during therapy
   8. Evaluate client's response to medication and understanding of teaching

Ophthalmic Agents

A. Description
   1. Used to treat conditions affecting the eyes
   2. Produce effects ranging from antibiotic to antiinflammatory; play significant roles in medical and surgical diagnosis and treatment
   3. Available in a variety of topical preparations; drugs having a systemic action are available in oral and parenteral (IM, IV) preparations

B. Examples
   1. Miotics: constrict the pupil, pulling the iris away from the filtration angle and improving outflow of aqueous humor
      a. carbachol
      b. physostigmine
      c. pilocarpine HCl
      d. trimolol maleate (Timoptic)
   2. Anticholinergics: dilate the pupil (mydriasis) by relaxing the ciliary muscle and the sphincter muscle

of the iris; paralyze accommodation (cycloplegia); thus facilitating eye examination
      a. atropine sulfate
      b. cyclopentolate (Cyclogyl)
      c. homatropine HBr
      d. scopolamine HBr
      e. tropicamide (Mydriacyl)
   3. Mydriatics: dilate pupil (mydriasis) by causing contraction of the dilator muscle of iris with minimal effect on ciliary muscle, which lessens the effect on accommodation
      a. hydroxyamphetamine (Paredrine)
      b. phenylephrine HCl (Neo-Synephrine)
   4. Carbonic anhydrase inhibitors: decrease inflow of aqueous humor in control of intraocular pressure
      a. acetazolamide (Diamox)
      b. dichlorphenamide (Daranide, Oratrol)
      c. ethoxzolamide (Cardrase, Ethamide)
      d. methazolamide (Neptazane)
   5. Osmotic agents: administered systemically to decrease blood osmolality, which mobilizes fluid from the eye to reduce volume of intraocular fluid
      a. glycerin (Glycerol, Osmoglyn)
      b. mannitol (Osmitrol)
      c. urea (Urevert)

C. Major side effects
   1. Miotics
      a. Twitching of eyelids (increased cholinergic stimulation)
      b. Brow ache (increased cholinergic stimulation)
      c. Headache (vasodilation)
      d. Conjunctival pain (irritation of conjunctiva)
      e. Contact dermatitis (local irritation)
   2. Anticholinergics (decreased parasympathetic stimulation)
      a. Dry mouth (decreased salivation)
      b. Flushing, fever (CNS effect)
      c. Blurred vision (pupillary dilation)
      d. Skin rash (hypersensitivity)
      e. Tachycardia (decreased vagal stimulation)
      f. Ataxia (CNS effect)
   3. Mydriatics
      a. Brow ache (vasoconstrictor effect)
      b. Headache (vasoconstrictor effect)
      c. Blurred vision (pupillary dilation)
      d. Tachycardia (increased sympathetic stimulation)
      e. Hypertension (vasoconstrictor effect)
   4. Carbonic anhydrase inhibitors
      a. Diuresis (increased excretion of sodium and water in renal tubule)
      b. Paresthesia (fluid-electrolyte imbalance)
      c. Nausea, vomiting (GI irritation)
      d. CNS disturbances (CNS effect)
   5. Osmotic agents
      a. Headache (cerebral dehydration)
      b. Nausea, vomiting (fluid-electrolyte imbalance)

D. Nursing care
   1. Instruct client regarding
      a. Effects of drug prior to administration
      b. Proper method of application
      c. Need for medical supervision during therapy

2. Provide care for the client receiving mydriatics
   a. Caution client that vision will be blurred temporarily
   b. Advise client that sunglasses will relieve photophobia
   c. Have client avoid engaging in hazardous activities
3. Assess for occurrence of side effects and/or worsening of condition
4. Encourage diet rich in nutrient-dense foods such as fruits, vegetables, whole grains, and legumes to improve and maintain nutritional status and prevent possible drug-induced nutrient deficiencies
5. Evaluate client's response to medication and understanding of teaching

PROCEDURES RELATED TO THE NEUROMUSCULOSKELETAL SYSTEMS
Arthroscopic Examination

A. Definition: direct visualization of a joint with a fiberoptic scope inserted through a small skin incision
B. Purposes
   1. Allow for evaluation of changes in joint structures
   2. Permit removal of torn cartilage and repair of torn ligaments
   3. Reduce period required for rehabilitation because adjacent muscles and ligaments are not disrupted
C. Nursing care
   1. Explain procedure to client and obtain consent
   2. Maintain sterile technique when changing postoperative dressing
   3. Apply prescribed ace bandages to minimize swelling and stabilize joint
   4. Maintain limb in position as ordered
   5. Assist client with ambulation as ordered
   6. Evaluate client's response to procedure

Bárány's Caloric Test

A. Definition
   1. Used to assess vestibular labyrinthine function
   2. Warm or cold water is instilled rapidly into the auditory canal, causing motion of the endolymph within the semicircular canals and normally resulting in vertigo, nystagmus, and nausea
   3. Eyes deviate toward the stimulated ear if cold water is used and away if warm water is used
B. Nursing care
   1. Explain procedure to the client
   2. Assemble equipment for the procedure
   3. Assist the physician and support the client during irrigation
   4. Observe and record reaction of the client
   5. Evaluate client's response to procedure

Computerized Axial Tomography (CT or CAT Scan)

A. Definition
   1. Cross-sectional visualization of the brain determined by computer analysis of relative tissue density as an x-ray beam passes through

2. Provides valuable information about location and extent of tumors, infarcted areas, atrophy, and vascular lesions
3. May be done with or without intravenous injection of dye for contrast enhancement
B. Nursing care
   1. Explain procedure; inform the client that it will be necessary to lie still and that the equipment is complex but will cause no pain or discomfort
   2. If the facility is small, arrange transportation to a larger facility that has the required equipment
   3. Evaluate for possible allergy to iodine, a component of the contrast material
   4. Withhold food for approximately 4 hours prior to testing; dye may cause nausea in sensitive patients
   5. Remove wigs, clips, and pins prior to the test
   6. Evaluate client's response to procedure

Cerebral Angiography

A. Definition: visualization of the cerebral vasculature with a contrast dye and x-ray projection
B. Nursing care (see Angiography under Procedures related to the circulatory system)

Continuous Passive Motion Devices (CPM)

A. Definition: a machine that provides for passive range of motion
B. Purposes
   1. Move joint without weight bearing or straining muscles following orthopedic surgery
   2. Stimulate regeneration of articular tissues
   3. Enhance joint mobility
C. Nursing care
   1. Adjust device according to length of client's extremity (the thigh and lower leg are measured for the CPM of the hip and knee)
   2. Set foot cradle at the angle ordered by the physician
   3. Set flexion, extension, and speed dials as ordered by the physician; these are generally increased gradually as tolerated to maximize mobility
   4. Demonstrate use of control cord to client
   5. Align extremity in padded CPM device
   6. Evaluate client's response to procedure

Electroencephalography (EEG)

A. Definition
   1. Measurement and recording of electrical activity of the brain in the form of waves
   2. Provides information about seizure disorders, local tumors, infections of the central nervous system, and chemical toxicity
   3. May be done at the bedside with portable equipment but generally is done in a special room to decrease distractions and interference
   4. The client may be asked to hyperventilate, or flashing lights may be utilized to trigger any abnormal wave pattern
B. Nursing care
   1. Explain procedure; common misconceptions include fear of receiving electrical shock and fear that personal thoughts will be revealed

2. Provide the client with a normal meal to avoid hypoglycemia; stimulants such as coffee or tea and depressants are withheld because of their effect on the EEG; withhold anticonvulsants as ordered
3. Shampoo hair after the test to remove collodion, the conducting jelly
4. Evaluate client's response to procedure

Electromyography (EMG)

A. Definition
   1. Measurement and recording of the electrical activity of specific muscles into which needle electrodes have been inserted
   2. In addition to providing information about primary muscle disease, it helps differentiate between motor symptoms that are secondary to neurologic disturbances; contraindicated in clients with arrythmias
B. Nursing care
   1. Explain procedure to the client
   2. Evaluate client's response to procedure

Instillation of Eye Medications

A. Purpose: to provide therapeutic effect of medication ordered
B. Nursing care
   1. Explain procedure to the client
   2. Position the client with the head slightly backward
   3. Pull lower eyelid down and place ointment or solution in the center of the cul-de-sac of the eye that is to be medicated (check order: OD—right eye, OU—both eyes, OS—left eye)
   4. Allow the client to close the eyes gently and instruct that they should not be rubbed
   5. Record administration of medication appropriately
   6. Evaluate client's response to procedure

Irrigations of the Ear

A. Definition
   1. Introduction of fluid into the external auditory canal
   2. Usually done for cleansing purposes but can be used to apply antiseptic solutions
B. Nursing care
   1. Explain procedure to the client
   2. Assemble equipment: irrigating solution, sterile irrigating syringe, cotton balls, cotton-tipped applicators, towel
   3. Assist the client to sitting position with the head tilted to affected side to facilitate drainage
   4. Gently pull up and back on the external ear of an adult, down and forward on a child, to straighten the canal
   5. Direct solution into the canal without exerting excessive force; collect returns in a basin
   6. Dry the outer ear and have client lie on the affected side
   7. Record the procedure, type of drainage, etc.
   8. Evaluate client's response to procedure

Lumbar Puncture

A. Definition: involves the introduction of a needle into the subarachnoid space, usually between L_3 and L_4 or L_4

and L_5, to prevent injury to the spinal cord above this level
B. Purposes
   1. Withdrawal of spinal fluid for diagnostic purposes or to reduce spinal pressure (normal is 70 to 200 mm H_2O)
   2. Measurement of spinal pressure (Queckenstedt test involves compression of the jugular veins; normally pressure will rise; but if blockage exists, pressure will not change)
   3. Injection of air or dye for diagnostic x-ray examination
   4. Injection of medication such as anesthetics
C. Nursing care
   1. Explain procedure to the client and obtain a signed consent
   2. Set up a sterile field
   3. Assist the client into a position that will enlarge the opening between the vertebrae
      a. Lying on side with feet drawn up and head lowered to chest; back near edge of mattress
      b. Sitting over side of bed, leaning on overbed table, feet supported on a stool
   4. Observe for signs of shock, such as tachycardia, diaphoresis, and pallor
   5. After procedure assist the client into a recumbent position; the client should remain recumbent up to 24 hours, depending on the physician's orders
   6. Label specimens and send to laboratory
   7. Note color and amount of spinal fluid, as well as the client's condition, and record
   8. Administer fluids unless contraindicated
   9. Evaluate client's response to procedure

Mobility: Use of Braces or Splints

A. Purposes
   1. Support and protect weakened muscles
   2. Prevent and correct anatomic deformities
   3. Aid in controlling involuntary muscle movements
   4. Immobilize and protect a diseased or injured joint
   5. Provide for improvement of function
B. Nursing care
   1. Keep equipment in good repair (e.g., oil joints, replace straps when worn, wash with saddle soap)
   2. Provide adequate shoes (e.g., keep in good repair, heels low and wide, high top to hold the heel in the shoe)
   3. Examine the skin daily for evidence of breakdown at pressure points
   4. Check alignment of the braces (e.g., leg braces: joints should coincide with body joints; back brace: upright bars in center of back, brace should grip the pelvis and trochanter firmly, lacing should begin from the bottom)
   5. Evaluate client's response to procedure

Mobility: Use of a Cane

A. Purposes
   1. Improve stability of the client with a lower limb disability
   2. Maintain balance
   3. Prevent further injury

4. Provide security while developing confidence in ambulating
5. Relieve pressure on weight-bearing joints
6. Assist in increasing speed of ambulation with less fatigue
7. Provide for greater mobility and independence

B. Nursing care
   1. Ascertain that the client is able to bear weight on the affected extremity
   2. Ensure that the client is able to use the upper extremity opposite the affected lower extremity
   3. Measure to determine the length of cane required
      a. Highest point should be about level with the greater trochanter
      b. Handpiece should allow 30 degrees of flexion at the elbow with the wrist held in extension
   4. Explain the proper techniques in using a cane
      a. Hold in the hand opposite the affected extremity
      b. Advance the cane and the affected extremity simultaneously, and then the unaffected leg
      c. Keep the cane close to the body
      d. When climbing, step up with the unaffected extremity and then place the cane and the affected lower extremity on the step; when descending, reverse the procedure
   5. Observe for incorrect use of the cane
      a. Leaning the body over the cane
      b. Shortening the stride on the unaffected side
      c. Inability to develop a normal walking pattern
      d. Persistence of the abnormal gait pattern after the cane is no longer needed
   6. Evaluate client's response to procedure

Mobility: Crutch Walking

A. Purposes
   1. Support body weight, assist weak muscles, and provide joint stability
   2. Relieve pain
   3. Prevent further injury and provide for improvement of function
   4. Allow for greater independence

B. Nursing care
   1. Ensure proper fit of crutches by measuring the distance from the anterior fold of the axilla to a point 15 cm (6 inches) out from the heel
      a. Axillary bars must be 5 cm (2 inches) below the axillae and should be padded
      b. Hand bars should allow almost complete extension of the arm with the elbow flexed about 30 degrees when the client places weight on the hands
      c. Rubber crutch tips should be in good condition, about 5.1 to 7.6 cm (2 to 3 inches) in height, with a circumference of 3.8 to 4.4 cm (1½ to 1¾ inches)
   2. Assist in use of proper technique, depending on ability to bear weight and to take steps with either one or both of the lower extremities
      a. Four-point alternate crutch gait
         (1) Right crutch, left foot, left crutch, right foot
         (2) Equal but partial weight bearing on each limb

   (3) Slow but stable gait; there are always three points of support on the floor
   (4) The client must be able to manipulate both extremities and get one foot ahead of the other (e.g., persons with polio, arthritis, cerebral palsy)

   b. Two-point alternate crutch gait
      (1) Right crutch and left foot simultaneously
      (2) There are always two points of support on the floor
      (3) This is a more rapid version of the four-point gait and requires more balance and strength (e.g., a bilateral amputee)

   c. Three-point gait
      (1) Advance both crutches and the weaker lower extremity simultaneously, then the stronger lower extremity
      (2) Fairly rapid gait, but requires more balance and strength in the arms and the good lower extremity
      (3) Used when one leg can support the whole body weight and the other cannot take full weight-bearing (e.g., a client with a fractured hip)

   d. Swing crutch gaits
      (1) Swing-to gait
         (a) Place both crutches forward, lift and swing the body *up* to the crutches, then place crutches in front of the body and continue
         (b) There are always two points of support on the floor
         (c) This technique is indicated for anyone with adequate power in the upper arms
      (2) Swing-through gait
         (a) Place both crutches forward, lift and swing the body *through* the crutches, then place crutches in front of the body and continue
         (b) Very difficult gait, because as the client swings through the crutches it necessitates rolling the pelvis forward and arching the back to get the center of gravity in front of the hips
         (c) Indicated for the client who has power in the trunk and upper extremities, excellent balance, self-confidence, and a dash of daring (e.g., a bilateral amputee, a paraplegic with braces)

   e. Tripod crutch gaits
      (1) Tripod alternate gait
         (a) Right crutch, left crutch, drag the body and legs forward
         (b) The client constantly maintains a tripod position: both crutches are held fairly widespread out front while both feet are held together in the back
         (c) Necessary for the individual who cannot place one extremity ahead of the other (e.g., a person with flaccid paralysis from poliomyelitis, one with spinal cord injuries)

(2) Tripod simultaneous gait
  (a) Place both crutches forward, drag the body and legs forward
  (b) Because the tripod must have a large base, the client's body must be inclined forward sufficiently to keep the center of gravity in front of the hips
3. Observe for incorrect use of crutches
  a. Using the body in poor mechanical fashion
  b. Hiking hips with abduction gait (common in amputees)
  c. Lifting crutches while still bearing down on them
  d. Walking on ball of foot with foot turned outward and flexion at hip or knee level
  e. Hunching shoulders (crutches usually too long) or stooping with shoulders (crutches usually too short)
  f. Looking downward while ambulating
  g. Bearing weight under arms; should be avoided to prevent injury to the nerves in the brachial plexus; damage to these nerves can cause paralysis and is known as crutch palsy
4. Evaluate client's response to procedure

Mobility: Transfer of Clients

A. Definitions
  1. Methods of moving a client from one surface to another (e.g., bed to wheelchair, wheelchair to commode)
  2. Weight-bearing transfers: by clients who have at least one stable lower extremity (e.g., hemiplegics, clients who have undergone a unilateral lower extremity amputation, clients with a fractured hip)
  3. Non-weight-bearing transfers: by clients who do not have a stable lower extremity (e.g., paraplegics not wearing braces, clients with double lower extremity amputations)
B. Nursing care
  1. Assess the client's abilities (e.g., sitting tolerance, balance, weight-bearing potential, strength, motivation, understanding of principles of transfer)
  2. Identify need for and selection of assistive devices (e.g., slide board, trapeze, wheelchair with a removable arm, hydraulic lift)
  3. Select most appropriate transfer method and teach and assist the client with this new technique
  4. Provide for client safety (e.g., encourage use of low-heeled shoes, lock wheelchair brakes during transfer, remove hazards [scatter rugs, slippery floors, stepstools], ensure adequate assistance)
  5. Communicate individualized transfer techniques by instructing the client and family and informing the entire health team
  6. Consider the client's abilities and disabilities when deciding appropriate transfer technique and need for assistive devices (e.g., hemiplegia: place the wheelchair on the side opposite the affected extremities; paraplegia: may use trapeze, slide board, or wheelchair with removable arm)
  7. Maintain correct proximity and visual relationship of wheelchair to the bed (e.g., paraplegia: place the wheelchair lateral or perpendicular to the bed; hemiplegia: place the wheelchair at a 30-degree angle to the bed on the unaffected side)
  8. Evaluate client's response to procedure

Mobility: Use of a Walker

A. Purposes
  1. Maintain balance
  2. Provide additional support because of wide area of contact with floor
  3. Allow for some ambulatory independence
B. Nursing care
  1. Assist in selecting a walker
    a. Device should not be used unless the client will never be able to ambulate with a cane or crutches
    b. Measurements for a walker are the same as for a cane
    c. The client must have strong elbow extensors and shoulder depressors and partial strength in the hands and the wrist muscles
    d. The client needs maximum support to ensure security and enhance confidence
    e. Device is ordinarily limited to the home because it cannot be used on steps
  2. Assist in ambulating with the walker
    a. Lift the device off the floor and place forward a short distance, then advance between the walker
    b. Two-wheeled walkers: raise back legs of the device off the floor, roll walker forward, then advance to it
    c. Four-wheeled walkers: push device forward on floor and then walk to it
  3. Observe for incorrect use of the walker
    a. Keeping arms rigid and swinging through to counterbalance the position of the lower extremity
    b. Tending to lean forward with abnormal flexion at the hips
    c. Tending to step forward with the good leg and shuffle the affected leg up to the bar
  4. Evaluate client's response to procedure

Mobility: Use of a Wheelchair

The client is propelled or propels himself or herself on wheels or casters in a sitting position
A. Purposes
  1. Support the body
  2. Decrease cardiac workload
  3. Promote independence and stimulate activities
  4. Provide mobility for those who cannot ambulate or those who can ambulate but whose ambulation is unsteady, unsafe, or too strenuous
B. Nursing care
  1. Instruct the client that prolonged sitting in one position can cause flexion contractures of the hips and knees and ischial decubiti (encourage the client to change body positions and to use padded cushions and exercises such as push-ups every hour to relieve pressure)
  2. Ensure that specific devices necessary for client safety (e.g., wheel brakes, arm locks, seat belts, swing foot rests) are in operating condition

3. Alert the wheelchair-bound client to the accessories that meet the client's specific needs (e.g., removable arms, lap boards, knobs on the handrims, extra long leg panels, battery or motor propulsion)
4. Evaluate client's response to procedure

Myelography

A. Definition: visualization of the spinal canal after it has been injected with radiopaque dye
B. Nursing care
   1. Explain procedure to the client and obtain a signed consent
   2. Maintain the npo status prior to the test
   3. Remove dentures and metal objects
   4. Administer a sedative as ordered prior to the procedure
   5. Care for the client following the procedure
      a. Observe for neurologic signs
      b. Keep the client in a recumbent position for 24 hours
      c. Encourage fluid intake
   6. Evaluate client's response to procedure

Neurologic Assessment

A. Definition: systematic evaluation of the cranial nerves, motor and sensory functioning, and mental status to detect neurologic abnormalities
   1. Critical aspects of a complete neurologic assessment are generally extracted and compose a "neuro checklist," which is used when the nature of the situation does not warrant complete evaluation
   2. See Review of anatomy and physiology of the neuromusculoskeletal systems
B. Nursing care
   1. Perform assessment as dictated by the client's needs
      a. Cranial nerves
         (1) Olfactory (I): ability to identify familiar odors such as mint or alcohol with eyes closed and one nostril occluded at a time
         (2) Optic (II): visual acuity measured by use of Snellen chart or by gross estimation with reading material; gross comparison of visual fields with those of examiner; color perception
         (3) Oculomotor (III), trochlear (IV), and abducent (VI): ability of the pupils to react equally to light and to accommodate to varying distances; normal range of extraocular movement (EOM) evaluated by asking the client to follow a finger or object with the eyes; should also include assessment for nystagmus (jerking motion of eyes) particularly when eyes are directed laterally
         (4) Trigeminal (V): sensations of the face evaluated by lightly stroking cotton across forehead, chin, and cheeks while the client's eyes are closed; ability to clench the teeth (jaw closure)
         (5) Facial (VII): symmetry of the facial muscles as the client speaks or is asked to make faces
         (6) Acoustic or vestibulocochlear (VIII): hearing acuity determined by a watch tick or whis-

pered numbers; Weber test may be performed by holding the stem of a vibrating tuning fork at midline of the skull (should be heard equally in both ears)
         (7) Glossopharyngeal (IX) and vagus (X): uvula should hang in midline; swallow and gag reflexes should be intact
         (8) Spinal accessory (XI): symmetrical ability to turn the head or shrug the shoulders against counterforce of the examiner's hands
         (9) Hypoglossal (XII): ability to protrude the tongue without deviation to left or right, and without tremors
      b. Motor function (including cerebellar function)
         (1) Balance
            (a) Observation of gait
            (b) Romberg test: positive if the client fails to maintain an upright position with feet together when the eyes are closed
         (2) Coordination: ability to touch the finger to the nose when arms are extended or to perform similar tasks smoothly
         (3) Muscle strength: evaluated by having the client move major muscle groups against opposition supplied by the examiner
      c. Sensory function: bilateral testing of the response to light touch with cotton, superficial pinprick, vibration of a tuning fork
      d. Mental status of cerebral functioning
         (1) Level of consciousness: determined by the response to stimuli (e.g., verbal or physical); a client may be in any state, ranging from alert to comatose
         (2) Orientation to person, place, and time: determined by general conversation and direct questioning
         (3) Judgment, memory, and ability to perform simple calculations
         (4) Appropriateness of behavior and mood
      e. Reflexes
         (1) Deep tendon (biceps, triceps, patellar, Achilles reflexes) with a reflex hammer; classification from 0 (absent) to 4 + (signifying hyperactive)
         (2) Plantar: plantar flexion of the foot when the sole is stroked firmly with a hard object such as a tongue blade; abnormal adult response (dorsiflexion of the foot and fanning of the toes) is described as a positive Babinski and is indicative of corticospinal tract disease
   2. Accurately record findings
   3. Report any deviations that warrant immediate treatment
   4. Explain and reassure the client when the examination must be repeated frequently (e.g., after head trauma)
   5. Evaluate client's response to procedure

Nuclear Magnetic Resonance Imaging (NMRI)

A. Definition
   1. This procedure utilizes magnetism and radio waves to produce images of cross sections of the body

2. The NMRI machine registers the existence of odd-numbered atoms in the cross sections of the body, yielding data about the chemical makeup of the tissues
3. NMRI can produce accurate images of blood vessels, bone marrow, gray and white brain matter, the spinal cord, the globe of the eye, the heart, abdominal structures, and breast tissue, and can monitor blood velocity

B. Nursing care
  1. Assess ability to withstand confining surroundings, since client must remain in the tunnel-like machine for up to 90 minutes
  2. Instruct client to toilet prior to test, since this will be impossible during the procedure
  3. Advise client to remove jewelry, clothing with metal fasteners, dentures, and glasses prior to entering scanner
  4. Since this procedure is contraindicated for certain clients, before the test assess for
    a. Metal prostheses, such as orthopedic screws, since the magnetic force can dislodge the devices
    b. Pacemakers, since the scanner deactivates pacemaker
    c. Arrhythmias, because the magnetic field can affect the conduction system of the heart
    d. Unstable medical conditions, since their condition cannot be monitored during the test
  5. Evaluate client's response to procedure

Positron Emission Tomography (PET Scan)

A. Definition
  1. This test registers glucose metabolism in a cross section of the brain; glucose metabolism increases in areas of the brain that are active
  2. Utilized to diagnose Alzheimer's disease, depression, dementia, and brain tumors

B. Nursing care
  1. Instruct client to abstain from alcohol, tobacco, and caffeine 24 hours prior to test
  2. Allow client to eat a meal 3 hours prior to test; diabetic clients should have a dose of long-acting insulin prior to this meal
  3. Provide tranquil environment since anxiety can affect test results
  4. Instruct client about what to expect during test
    a. Two IVs will be utilized: one for drawing blood samples and one for infusing the radioactive oxyglucose
    b. Arm with IV that will be used to draw glucose samples must be kept in a "hot box" during procedure; this shunts arterial blood into veins to allow collection of a specimen that contains both venous and arterial blood
    c. The scan will take 60 to 90 minutes and client must remain still
    d. A blindfold will be applied and cotton plugs placed in the ears during the test
  5. Following test, encourage client to void to clear radioactive isotope from the body
  6. Evaluate client's response to procedure

Special Beds for Positioning Clients

A. Devices and their purposes
  1. Stryker or Foster frames: allow for horizontal turning of the client
  2. CircOlectric bed: allows for vertical turning; the client can be placed in a variety of positions (Trendelenburg, prone, standing, supine); one nurse can turn the client, with the electric motor providing the power; attachments permit application of traction and other accessories
  3. Clinitron bed: uses flow of temperature-controlled air through small ceramic spheres to evenly distribute client's weight, reducing pressure and friction
  4. Flexicare bed: uses an automatic airbag system that adjusts to individual's weight and activity to evenly distribute client's weight, reducing pressure and friction
  5. Purposes
    a. Hyperextension
    b. Immobilization
    c. Correction of deformities
    d. Facilitation of turning
    e. Relief of pressure and friction
    f. Promotion of body functions (circulation, respiration, elimination)

B. Nursing care
  1. Turn the client all in one piece
  2. Since frames are narrow, for safety purposes do not permit the client to sit up, roll over, or reach out to the side; do not place extremely obese and disoriented clients on a frame
  3. Since only the prone and supine and, on the CircOlectric bed, vertical positions can be used, strict attention must be paid to prevention of decubiti
  4. Before releasing pivot pins, secure all bolts and straps to ensure client safety
  5. When turning the CircOlectric bed, do so slowly so that the client's cerebral circulation can adjust to the new position; observe for signs of hypotension
  6. Turn client before turning off Clinitron bed when providing care
  7. Call company representative for regular servicing of bed
  8. Evaluate client's response to procedure

NURSING PROCESS FOR CLIENTS WITH NEUROMUSCULOSKELETAL SYSTEM DISORDERS
Probable Nursing Diagnoses Based on Assessment

A. Potential for aspiration related to reduced level of consciousness
B. Ineffective thermoregulation related to head trauma
C. Dysreflexia related to spinal cord injury T7 or above
D. Potential for disuse syndrome related to immobilization/pain
E. Altered thought processes related to brain injury
F. Impaired swallowing related to paralysis
G. Sexual dysfunction related to actual or perceived limitation imposed by disease and/or therapy
H. Potential for impaired skin integrity related to immobility

I. Deficit in diversional activity related to
   1. Long-term hospitalization
   2. Bed rest
   3. Impaired sensory function
J. Constipation related to
   1. Immobility
   2. Loss of ennervation
K. Bowel incontinence related to
   1. Impaired neuromuscular control
   2. Impaired thought processes
L. Reflex incontinence related to impaired neuromuscular control
M. Disturbance in body image related to actual change in function
N. Situational low self-esteem related to actual change in function
O. Altered nutrition: less than body requirements, related to inability to ingest
P. Self-care deficit (bathing/hygiene, dressing/grooming, feeding, toileting) related to
   1. Neuromuscular impairment
   2. Cognitive impairment
   3. Musculoskeletal impairment
Q. Impaired verbal communication related to
   1. Impaired articulation
   2. Disorientation
R. Potential for injury related to
   1. Cognitive impairment
   2. Sensory impairment
   3. Neuromuscular impairment
S. Impaired physical mobility related to
   1. Inability to purposefully move
   2. Impaired coordination
   3. Limited range of motion
   4. Imposed restrictions
T. Altered role performance related to interruption of neuromuscular functioning

Nursing Care for Clients with Neuromusculoskeletal System Disorders

See Nursing care under each specific disease

MAJOR DISEASES
Migraine Headache

A. Etiology and pathophysiology
   1. Caused by constriction and then dilation of the cerebral arteries
   2. Individuals who have migraines are frequently described as perfectionists, inflexible, and ambitious
   3. Incidence higher in females
B. Signs and symptoms
   1. Subjective
      a. Severe throbbing pain, often in temporal or supraorbital area, that lasts several hours to a day
      b. Fatigue and irritability may precede headache
      c. Nausea
      d. Visual disturbances
   2. Objective
      a. Pallor
      b. Vomiting

C. Treatment
   1. Methysergide maleate (Sansert) to prevent attacks; should not be continued for more than 6 to 12 months consecutively; then, should be omitted for a few months before it is resumed
   2. Ergotamine tartrate (Glynergen) or ergotamine with caffeine (Cafergot) to relieve migraines
   3. Elimination of factors (physical, psychologic, environmental) that precipitate illness
D. Nursing care
   1. Assist the client in identifying situations that seem to precipitate attacks
   2. Support the client in modification of life-style and development of insight
   3. Provide a dark, quiet environment when migraine begins
   4. Provide care for the nauseated client
      a. Administer an antiemetic if ordered
      b. Offer small, frequent sips of fluid as tolerated
      c. Assist with mouth care
   5. Evaluate client's response and revise plan as necessary

Head Injuries

A. Etiology and pathophysiology
   1. Result from trauma, frequently seen after motor vehicle accidents
   2. Fractures
      a. Linear: simple break in the bone
      b. Depressed: break that results in fragments of bone penetrating the brain tissue
   3. Hemorrhages
      a. Epidural: hematoma forms between the dura and the skull; may result from a laceration of the middle meningeal artery
      b. Subdural: hematoma forms between the dura and arachnoid layers; generally follows venous damage
   4. Concussion: temporary disruption of synaptic activity
   5. Contusions: bruising of brain tissue, with slight bleeding of small cerebral vessels into surrounding tissues
B. Signs and symptoms
   1. Subjective
      a. Lethargy
      b. Indifference to surroundings
   2. Objective
      a. Signs of increased intracranial pressure (see brain surgery)
      b. Lack of orientation to time and place
      c. Paresthesia
      d. Labored respirations
      e. Positive Babinski sign (stroking bottom of the foot causes dorsiflexion of the toes)
      f. Coma
      g. Dilation and fixation of pupils
C. Treatment
   1. Control seizures with anticonvulsants
   2. Maintain adequate fluid and electrolyte balance
   3. Surgical intervention in cases of depressed skull fractures or hematomas

D. Nursing care
 1. Observe for signs of increased intracranial pressure (see brain surgery); institute neural checks every 15 minutes for several hours, progressing to every hour and then every 4 hours
 2. Maintain airway
 3. Perform neurological assessment (See procedure)
 4. Institute seizure precautions; administer anticonvulsants if ordered
 5. Provide care for the unconscious client
    a. Observe for changes in vital signs and neurologic status (Use Glasgow Coma Scale [GCS])
    b. Keep the client's head slightly elevated to reduce venous pressure within the cranial cavity
    c. Maintain the airway by suctioning as necessary; use an airway or endotracheal tube
    d. Provide sterile tracheostomy care as well as frequent oral hygiene
    e. Position the client to prevent pressure areas from forming decubiti
    f. Maintain adequate fluid balance
    g. Evaluate the client's level of consciousness at frequent intervals
    h. If the client's eyes remain open, protect the corneas with moistened pads, mineral oil, or ointment as ordered
    i. Protect the client during seizures
    j. Provide auditory and tactile stimulation
 6. Support natural defense mechanisms; encourage diet emphasis of nutrient-dense foods, especially those rich in the immune-stimulating nutrients selenium and vitamins A, C, and E
 7. If surgery is indicated, see care of the client undergoing brain surgery
 8. Evaluate client's response and revise plan as necessary

Brain Tumor

A. Etiology and pathophysiology
 1. Either benign or malignant; they require intervention, since the skull cannot accommodate the increasing size of the tumor, and intracranial pressure rises
 2. Classified according to tissue of origin
    a. Meningioma: occurs outside the brain from the covering meninges
    b. Acoustic neuroma and optic nerve spongioblastoma polare: occur from the cranial nerves
    c. Gliomas: originate in neural tissue
    d. Hemangioblastomas: occur from within blood vessels
B. Signs and symptoms
 1. Subjective
    a. Headache that increases with stooping
    b. Lethargy
 2. Objective
    a. Vomiting
    b. Papilledema (noted on ophthalmoscopy)
    c. Abnormal brain waves on the EEG
 3. Symptoms may vary depending on location of tumor
    a. Frontal lobe: personality changes, focal seizures, blurred vision, hemiparesis, aphasia

b. Temporal lobe: seizures, headache, papilledema, aphasia
    c. Parietal lobe: jacksonian convulsions, visual loss
    d. Occipital region: focal seizures, visual hallucinations
    e. Cerebellar region: loss of coordination, papilledema
C. Treatment
 1. Radiation therapy or chemotherapy for inaccessible tumors
 2. Brain surgery for complete removal of the lesion if location and extension into surrounding tissues permit
 3. Steroids, anticonvulsives, and osmotic diuretics to control symptoms
 4. Laser therapy to eradicate treatable lesions
D. Nursing care
 1. Give emotional support to the client undergoing palliative procedures
 2. Maintain the client as comfortably as possible with analgesics and antiemetics as ordered
 3. Provide care for the client requiring brain surgery
    a. Obtain consent for surgery and removal of hair (save the hair)
    b. After surgery keep the client's head elevated 30 cm (12 inches) to aid drainage
    c. Observe for return of cough and swallowing reflexes
    d. Assess the client's level of consciousness and neurologic status for changes
    e. Utilize hypothermia as ordered if the client is febrile; fever increases metabolic needs of the brain
    f. Observe dressings for CSF leakage or hemorrhage
    g. Maintain accurate intake and output records
    h. Observe for signs of increased intracranial pressure
       (1) Restlessness
       (2) Weakness or paralysis
       (3) Increased systolic pressure; widening pulse pressure
       (4) Decreased pulse
       (5) Pupillary dilation
 4. Evaluate client's response and revise plan as necessary

Brain Abscess

A. Etiology and pathophysiology
 1. Occurs when there is an infection in another region of the body that spreads to the brain or after a penetrating head wound
 2. Results from invasion of the brain causing formation and collection of exudate within the brain tissue
B. Signs and symptoms
 1. Subjective
    a. Malaise
    b. Headache
    c. Anorexia
 2. Objective
    a. Fever
    b. Vomiting
    c. Weight loss

C. Treatment
  1. Large doses of antibiotics
  2. In severe cases, a craniotomy may be performed to allow removal of the abscess

D. Nursing care
  1. Observe for changes in vital signs or neurologic responses
  2. Encourage nutrient-dense diet to compensate for antibiotic impact on nutritional status (See Pharmacology related to infection)
  3. See care of the client undergoing brain surgery
  4. Evaluate client's response and revise plan as necessary

Cerebral Aneurysm

A. Etiology and pathophysiology
  1. Sac formed by dilation of the walls of an artery within the cranial cavity
  2. May be the result of a congenital weakness in the vessel, trauma, or arteriosclerosis
  3. Symptoms occur when the aneurysm compresses nearby nerves or when it ruptures

B. Signs and symptoms
  1. Subjective
    a. Unilateral headache
    b. Pain in the eye
    c. Diplopia
    d. Tinnitus
  2. Objective
    a. Rigidity of the back of the neck and spine
    b. Ptosis of the eyelid
    c. Hemiparesis

C. Treatment
  1. Attempt to keep the client hypotensive, usually with rauwolfia alkaloids
  2. If there is a stalk connecting the aneurysm, clips may be inserted surgically to cut off blood supply to the aneurysm permanently

D. Nursing care
  1. See care of the client undergoing brain surgery
  2. See Head injuries for care of the unconscious client

Cerebral Hemorrhage

A. Etiology and pathophysiology
  1. Result of arteriosclerosis, trauma, hemorrhagic disorder, brain tumor, or ruptured aneurysm
  2. May occur in various areas of the brain
    a. Subarachnoid hemorrhage: generally from a congenital aneurysm near the circle of Willis
    b. Intracerebral hemorrhage: generally occurs because of hypertension, although may result from various disorders; the bleeding is usually located in the basal ganglia
    c. Subdural hemorrhage: generally involves a bridging vein, and therefore more time may pass before a hematoma is formed

B. Signs and symptoms
  1. Subjective
    a. Headache
    b. Dizziness

  2. Objective
    a. Convulsions
    b. Hemiplegia
    c. Unconsciousness
    d. Right-sided hemiplegia usually accompanied by aphasia

C. Treatment
  1. Complete bed rest
  2. Steroids, stool softeners, anticonvulsants, analgesics, aminocaproic acid (Amicar) by continuous IV drip to inhibit fibrinolysis
  3. Surgical intervention if indicated

D. Nursing care
  (See Head injuries for care of the unconscious client and Nursing care under Cerebral vascular accident)

Cerebral Vascular Accident (CVA or Stroke)

A. Etiology and pathophysiology
  1. Term applied to destruction (infarction) of brain cells caused by a reduction in the oxygen supply
  2. Caused by a sudden or gradual interruption in the blood supply following an intracerebral hemorrhage, blockage of vessels by thrombi or emboli, or vascular insufficiency
  3. Symptoms depend on the area of the brain involved and extent of damage
  4. Conditions that predispose to a CVA include cerebral arteriosclerosis, syphilis, dehydration, trauma, and hypertension
  5. Transient ischemic attacks (TIA) may also occur without causing permanent damage; these usually last only a few minutes
  6. Incidence increases with age

B. Signs and symptoms
  1. Subjective
    a. Syncope
    b. Changes in level of consciousness
    c. Transient paresthesias
    d. Headache
    e. Mood swings
  2. Objective
    a. Convulsions
    b. Nuchal rigidity (if caused by subarachnoid or intracerebral hemorrhage)
    c. Hemiplegia on side opposite the lesion
    d. Aphasia: brain unable to fulfill its communicative functions because of damage to its input, integrative, or output centers; a disturbance of language function that may involve impairment of the ability to read, write, speak, or interpret messages
      (1) Expressive aphasia: difficulty making thoughts known to others; speaking and writing is most affected
      (2) Receptive aphasia: difficulty understanding what others are trying to communicate; interpretation of speech and reading is most affected
      (3) Expressive-receptive aphasia: equal difficulty with speaking, writing, interpreting speech, and reading

e. Alterations in reflexes

f. Functional disorders of the bladder and bowel

g. CSF is bloody if cerebral or subarachnoid hemorrhage is present

h. Abnormal EEG

i. Cerebral angiography may reveal vascular abnormalities such as aneurysms, narrowing, or occlusions

j. If increased intracranial pressure exists, as with hemorrhage, elevated blood pressure and bounding pulse

C. Treatment

1. Complete bed rest with sedation as needed

2. Maintenance of nutrition, by the parenteral route or nasogastric feedings, if the client is unable to swallow

3. Anticoagulant therapy

4. Antihypertensive agents if indicated

5. Surgical intervention

   a. To relieve pressure and control bleeding if hemorrhage is present

   b. Carotid endarterectomy to improve cerebral blood flow when carotid arteries are narrowed by arteriosclerotic patches, may be done on a client in stable condition

D. Nursing care

1. Assess respiratory functioning (vital signs, type and rate of respirations, color, blood gases, etc.)

2. Observe for level of consciousness

3. Monitor vital signs

4. Observe for signs of increasing intracranial pressure

5. Assess swallowing and gag reflexes

6. Maintain patency of the airway by positioning, suctioning, and inserting an artificial airway

7. Provide for drainage and expansion of lungs by placing client in a low semi-Fowler's position with the head turned to the side

8. Provide oxygen as necessary

9. Provide frequent oral hygiene

10. Encourage the client to breathe deeply and cough; administer intermittent positive pressure if necessary

11. Provide elastic stockings for both legs

12. Provide for frequent nursing observations, since the client may be unable to signal for assistance

13. Prevent decubiti

    a. Provide special care to the back and bony prominences; keep the client clean and dry

    b. Relieve pressure by use of mechanical and supportive devices

    c. Turn the client every 2 hours

    d. Provide adequate hydration to maintain skin turgor

14. Prevent muscle atrophy and contractures

    a. Provide for active and passive range of motion and other exercises

    b. Use footboards and other devices to prevent footdrop, flexion of fingers, abduction of hips, adduction of shoulders and arms

15. Encourage the aphasic client to communicate

    a. Be aware of own reactions to the speech difficulty

    b. Evaluate extent of the client's ability to understand and express self at a simple level

    c. Include the health team, especially the speech therapist, in planning care

    d. Involve the family as much as possible

    e. Convey that there is a problem with communication, not with intelligence

    f. Try to eliminate anxiety and tension related to communication attempts (e.g., be consistent, give the client time to respond, employ a calm, accepting, and deliberate manner)

    g. Help the client set attainable goals

    h. Stimulate communication without pushing to point of frustration

    i. Keep distractions at a minimum, since they interfere with the reception and integration of messages (e.g., one-to-one conversations rather than group conversations, shut off the radio when speaking)

    j. Speak slowly, clearly, and in short sentences and do not raise voice

    k. Use alternate means of communication (e.g., gestures, writing, picture board)

    l. Involve the client in social interactions (e.g., encourage socialization, do not anticipate all needs, ask questions and expect answers, do not ignore the client in group conversations)

    m. Make a definite transition between tasks to prevent or reduce confusion

    n. Be alert for clues and gestures when speech is garbled (e.g., continue to listen, nod, and make occasional neutral statements, let the client know when you cannot understand)

    o. Provide for periodic reevaluation to demonstrate the effect and nature of progress to the client and health team

16. Attempt to prevent fecal impaction and/or urinary tract problems

    a. Provide adequate fluid intake

    b. Provide a diet with enough roughage for sufficient quantity of bowel content and proper consistency for evacuation

    c. Avoid preoccupation with elimination

    d. Avoid the overt encouragement of incontinence (e.g., through the routine use of diapers, Chux, and other depersonalizing devices)

    e. Stimulate normal elimination by exercise and activity

    f. Help the client develop regular bowel and bladder patterns

    g. Respect the individual (e.g., provide for privacy, individuality of routine, avoidance of delay); encourage the client to make decisions

    h. Utilize physical and psychologic techniques to stimulate elimination (e.g., running water, place the client's hands in warm water, place the client in as normal a position as possible for elimination)

i. Create an environment that keeps sensory monotony to a minimum (e.g., orient to time and place, use a radio and television selectively, increase the client's social contacts, provide visual stimuli, extend environment beyond the client's room)

j. Provide for self-esteem (e.g., encourage the client to wear own clothes, do self-care activities, make decisions)

k. Accept and explore the client's feelings of fear, anger, and depression; a disabled person has few avenues by which to express anger; incontinence is often used in this manner

17. Keep the side rails in place or use safety straps
18. Provide the client with tube feedings if swallowing and gag reflexes are depressed or absent
19. Provide food in a form that is easily swallowed; encourage intake of nutrient-dense foods; when client is capable of chewing, introduce dietary fiber to promote normal bowel function
20. Assist with feeding (e.g., use a padded spoon handle; feed on the unaffected side of mouth; feed in as close to a sitting position as possible)
21. Provide realistic encouragement and praise
22. Accept mood swings and emotional outbursts
23. Assist the client and family to set realistic goals
24. Help the client to adjust to change in body image and altered self-concept
25. See Head injuries for care of the unconscious client
26. Evaluate client's response and revise plan as necessary

Epilepsy (Convulsive Disorders)

A. Etiology and pathophysiology
1. Abnormal discharge of electric impulses by the nerve cells in the brain from idiopathic or secondary causes resulting in the typical manifestation of seizures
2. Onset of idiopathic epilepsy generally before age 30
3. Other conditions associated with seizures include brain tumor, CVA, hypoglycemia, and head trauma
4. Types of seizures
   a. Generalized motor seizures (grand mal): aura, loss of consciousness, tonic and clonic movements, interruption of respirations, loss of bladder and bowel control
   b. Petit mal seizures: brief transient loss of consciousness with or without minor motor movements of eyes, head, or extremities
   c. Jacksonian seizures (focal-motor seizures): disturbed sensations and interrupted motor functioning, beginning in a somewhat localized area of the body and progressing to other parts of the body; the areas affected by the seizure usually reflect the area of the brain involved
   d. Psychomotor seizures: characterized by a transient clouding of consciousness, behavioral alterations, and changes in affect and perception; may become violent and engage in antisocial activity
   e. Status epilepticus: continuous convulsion that may completely exhaust the client and lead to death

B. Signs and symptoms (grand mal seizures)
1. Subjective
   a. Aura or warning sensation such as seeing spots or feeling dizzy often precedes a grand mal seizure
   b. Loss of consciousness during seizure
   c. Lethargy often follows return to consciousness
   d. Dyspnea
2. Objective
   a. Pupils become fixed and dilated
   b. Often the client cries out as seizure begins or as air is exhaled forcefully
   c. Tonic and clonic movement of the muscles
   d. Incontinence
   e. Abnormal EEG

C. Treatment
1. Anticonvulsant therapy continued throughout life
   a. Phenytoin sodium (Dilantin), mephenytoin (Mesantoin) and primidone (Mysoline) often used to control grand mal seizures
   b. Trimethadione (Tridione), phensuximide (Milontin), and ethosuximide (Zarontin) to control petit mal seizures
   c. Diazepam (Valium) given IV to treat status epilepticus
2. Sedatives (e.g., phenobarbital) used to reduce emotional stress
3. Operant conditioning is also used experimentally

D. Nursing care
1. Assist the client to identify the aura
2. Help the client prepare and provide some protection before the seizure develops
3. Provide protection for the client during and after the seizure by maintaining and protecting from injury; nothing should be forced into a client's mouth when teeth are firmly clenched, since this may cause the tongue to occlude the airway or may loosen teeth
4. Encourage the client to carry and wear a medical alert tag
5. Encourage the client to take medications even when seizure free
6. Help the client plan a schedule that provides for adequate rest and a reduction of stress
7. Instruct the client to refrain from excessive use of alcohol, since it is contraindicated with the medications
8. Observe and teach the client and family to observe the aura, initial point of seizure, type of seizure, level of consciousness, loss of control of bladder and bowel, progression of seizure, and postseizure condition
9. Encourage the client to express feelings about illness and the necessary changes in life-style and self-image
10. Assist the client and family to accept the diagnosis and develop some understanding of the disease process
11. Help the client understand that medication must be taken continuously for the remainder of life
12. Refer the client for job counseling as needed
13. Encourage the client and family to attend meetings of the local epilepsy association

14. Refer the client for genetic counseling if appropriate (age of client, cause of seizures)
15. Encourage diet rich in nutrient-dense foods such as fruits, vegetables, whole grains, and legumes to improve and maintain nutritional status and prevent possible drug-induced nutrient deficiencies
16. Evaluate client's response and revise plan as necessary

Mononeuritis and Polyneuritis

A. Etiology and pathophysiology
1. May involve only one nerve (mononeuritis) or several nerves (polyneuritis)
2. Mononeuritis occurs when there is trauma to the trunk of a nerve, such as from pressure of a tumor, dislocation of a joint, or infection; the nerve involved near the area of injury becomes part of the scar tissue or callus of bone
3. Polyneuritis occurs when there is a deficiency of thiamine (e.g., alcoholism) and subsequent disturbances in metabolism of nerve tissue
B. Signs and symptoms
1. Subjective
a. Pain which increases after any body movement that stretches nerve involved
b. Burning pain along the injured nerve in mononeuritis
2. Objective
a. Swelling over the affected nerve in mononeuritis
b. Paresis or paralysis of the affected limb in polyneuritis
C. Treatment
1. Mononeuritis
a. Sympathetic nerve block
b. Physical therapy
c. Analgesics
2. Polyneuritis
a. Thiamine replacement
b. Bed rest
c. Analgesics
D. Nursing care
1. Administer pain medications as ordered
2. Provide emotional support for the client during the course of hospitalization
3. Encourage diet rich in nutrient-dense foods such as fruits, vegetables, whole grains, and legumes to improve and maintain nutritional status and prevent possible drug-induced nutrient deficiencies
4. Evaluate client's response and revise plan as necessary

Bell's Palsy

A. Etiology and pathophysiology
1. Paralysis that occurs on one side of the face as a result of an inflamed seventh cranial (facial) nerve; generally lasts only 2 to 8 weeks but may last longer in older clients
2. May follow trauma or exposure to the elements
3. Most common between ages 20 and 50 years
B. Signs and symptoms
1. Subjective
a. Facial pain
b. Difficulty eating
2. Objective
a. Distortion of face
b. Speech difficulty
c. Diminished blink reflex
d. Increased lacrimation
C. Treatment
1. Prednisone therapy
2. Heat, massage, and electric stimulation are used to maintain circulation and muscle tone
3. Prevention of corneal irritation with eyedrops and the use of a protective eye shield
D. Nursing care
1. Explain to the client in most cases recovery occurs within 2 to 8 weeks
2. Assess blink reflex and the client's ability to close the eye
3. Keep the face warm
4. Teach the client to massage the face gently and perform simple exercises such as blowing
5. Encourage ventilation of feelings, since self-image will be affected
6. Encourage diet rich in nutrient-dense foods such as fruits, vegetables, whole grains, and legumes to improve and maintain nutritional status and compensate for nutrient interactions of corticosteroid medications
7. Evaluate client's response and revise plan as necessary

Trigeminal Neuralgia (Tic Douloureux)

A. Etiology and pathophysiology
1. Disorder of the fifth cranial (trigeminal) nerve characterized by excruciating knifelike pain along the branches of the nerve
2. Etiology unknown
3. Incidence higher in women of middle and older age
B. Signs and symptoms
1. Subjective
a. Burning or knifelike pain lasting 1 to 15 minutes, usually over the lip or chin and in teeth
b. Pain precipitated by stimulation of trigger zones during activities such as brushing hair and eating or when sitting in a cold draft
2. Objective
a. Sudden closure of an eye
b. Twitching of the mouth
C. Treatment
1. Carbamazepine (Tegretol) to relieve and prevent pain
2. Antiepileptic drugs
3. Injection of alcohol into the ganglion to relieve pain for several months or years until nerve regenerates
4. Surgical intervention involves sectioning the sensory root of the nerve, which will cause loss of all sensation in the area supplied by the nerve
D. Nursing care
1. Prevent factors that can trigger an attack
a. Avoid foods that are too hot or cold
b. Use cotton pads to gently wash the client's face
c. Avoid jarring the bed
d. Keep the room free of drafts

2. Provide teaching to clients who have had surgery
   a. Inspection of the eye for foreign bodies, which the client will not be able to feel, should be done several times a day
   b. Warm normal saline irrigation of the affected eye two or three times a day is helpful in preventing a corneal infection
   c. Dental checkups every 6 months, since dental caries will not produce pain
3. Evaluate client's response and revise plan as necessary

Paralysis Agitans (Parkinson's Disease)

A. Etiology and pathophysiology
   1. Progressive disorder in which there is a destruction of nerve cells in the basal ganglia of the brain, which results in a generalized degeneration of muscular function
   2. Suspected causes include neuromuscular imbalance (dopamine and acetylcholine), unknown virus, cerebral vascular disease, and chemical or physical trauma
B. Signs and symptoms
   1. Subjective
      a. Mild diffuse muscular pain
      b. Feelings of stiffness and rigidity, particularly of large joints
      c. Defects in judgment and emotional lability may be present, but intelligence is usually not impaired
      d. Sensitivity to heat
   2. Objective
      a. Increased difficulty in performing usual activities such as writing, dressing, and eating
      b. Generalized tremor commonly accompanied by "pill-rolling" movements of the thumb against the fingers; tremors usually reduced by intentional movements
      c. Various disorders of locomotion (e.g., bent posture, difficulty in rising from a sitting position, shuffling propulsive gait, loss of rhythmic arm swing when walking)
      d. Masklike facial expression with unblinking eyes
      e. Low-pitched, slow, poorly modulated, poorly articulated speech
      f. Drooling because of difficulty in swallowing saliva
      g. Various autonomic symptoms (e.g., lacrimation, constipation, incontinence, decreased sexual capacity, excessive perspiration)
C. Treatment
   1. Medical regimen is palliative rather than curative
   2. Levodopa may be utilized to alleviate dopamine deficiency and decrease dyskinesia and rigidity
   3. Anticholinergic agents that counteract the action of acetylcholine in the central nervous system
   4. Medications to relieve related symptoms (e.g., antispasmodics, antihistamines, analgesics, sedatives)
   5. Physiotherapy to reduce rigidity of muscles and prevent contractures
   6. Surgical intervention using alcohol, freezing (cryosurgery), electric cautery, ultrasound, etc. to destroy the globus pallidus (to relieve rigidity), and/or the thalamus (to relieve tremor) portions of the brain

D. Nursing care
   1. Provide a safe environment
   2. Teach the client or family to cut food into small bite-size pieces to prevent choking
   3. Teach the client activities to limit postural deformities (e.g., use firm mattress without a pillow, periodically lie prone, keep head and neck as erect as possible, consciously think about posture when walking)
   4. Teach the client activities to maintain gait as normal as possible (e.g., clasp hands behind the back when walking, exercise with stationary bicycle, use low-heeled shoes)
   5. Teach and encourage daily physical therapy to limit rigidity and prevent contractures (e.g., warms baths, passive and active exercises)
   6. Attempt to administer care when the client is able to accept it emotionally and avoid rushing the client, since he or she is unable to function under pressure
   7. Encourage the client to continue taking medications even though results may be minimal
   8. Encourage diet rich in nutrient-dense foods such as fruits, vegetables, whole grains, and legumes to improve and maintain nutritional status and prevent possible drug-induced nutrient deficiencies
   9. Teach clients taking levodopa to limit intake of foods high in vitamin B_6, such as pork, glandular meats, lamb, veal, legumes, potatoes, oatmeal, wheat germ, and bananas
   10. Provide small, frequent meals prepared so they can be easily masticated
   11. Encourage an adequate intake of roughage and fluids to avoid constipation
   12. Encourage small intake of alcohol, since it promotes relaxation and reduces rigidity
   13. Suction when necessary to maintain an adequate airway (usually advanced stages)
   14. Administer medications as ordered
   15. Evaluate client's response and revise plan as necessary

Multiple Sclerosis, Disseminated Sclerosis

A. Etiology and pathophysiology
   1. Chronic, debilitating, progressive disease with periods of remission and exacerbation characterized by randomly scattered patches of demyelination in the brain stem, cerebrum, cerebellum, and spinal cord
   2. Cause unknown
   3. Onset in early adult life
B. Signs and symptoms
   1. Subjective
      a. Paresthesia
      b. Altered position sense
      c. Dysphagia
      d. Ataxia
      e. Weakness
      f. Diplopia
      g. Inappropriate emotional affect (euphoria occurs in later stages)
   2. Objective
      a. Nystagmus
      b. Intention tremors

c. Slurred speech
d. Spastic paralysis
e. Increased deep tendon reflexes
f. Pallor of optic discs evident on examination with ophthalmoscope
g. Increased gamma globulin levels in the CSF
C. Treatment
1. Generally palliative
2. Corticosteroids
3. Physiotherapy, rehabilitation, and psychotherapy
D. Nursing care
1. Encourage the client to use supportive devices to maintain ambulation
2. Provide active and passive range of motion and other exercises
3. Teach the client to use assistive devices in carrying out activities of daily living
4. Assist the family to understand why the client should be permitted and encouraged to be active
5. Assist the client and family to plan and implement a bowel and bladder regimen
6. Explain the disease process to both the client and the family in understandable terms
7. Do not encourage false hopes during periods of remission
8. Spend time listening to both the client and the family and encourage them to ventilate feelings
9. Attempt to refer the client and family to the National Multiple Sclerosis Society
10. Encourage the client to seek counseling and rehabilitation
11. Explain to the client and family that mood swings and emotional alterations are part of the disease process
12. Help the client reestablish a realistic self-image
13. Teach the client to compensate for problems with gait (walk with feet farther apart to broaden base of support, use low-heeled shoes) and provide assistive devices when necessary (tripod cane, walker, wheelchair)
14. Teach the client to compensate for loss of sensation by using a thermometer to test water temperature, avoiding constricting stockings, using protective clothing in cold weather, changing position frequently
15. Teach the client to compensate for difficulty in swallowing by taking small bites, chewing well, using a straw with liquids, using foods of more solid consistency
16. Provide a diet rich in nutrient-dense foods such as fruits, vegetables, whole grains, and legumes to improve and maintain nutritional status and compensate for nutrient interactions of corticosteroid medications
17. Provide care to prevent decubiti and contractures
a. Provide special skin care to prevent the formation of decubiti; turn frequently
b. Provide special attention to joints and attempt to prevent dysfunctional contractures; provide range-of-motion exercises
18. Evaluate client's response and revise plan as necessary

Myasthenia Gravis

A. Etiology and pathophysiology
1. Neuromuscular disorder in which there is a disturbance in the transmission of impulses at the myoneural junction
2. Dysfunction thought to be caused by rapid breakdown or insufficient supply of acetylcholine at the junction
3. Highest incidence in young adult females
4. Myasthenic crisis refers to the sudden inability to swallow or maintain respirations due to weakness of the muscles of respiration
B. Signs and symptoms
1. Subjective
a. Extreme muscle weakness, which becomes progressively worse as the muscle is used but disappears with rest
b. Dysphagia (difficulty chewing)
c. Diplopia
d. Dysarthria (difficulty speaking)
2. Objective
a. Ptosis of the lid
b. Weak voice
c. Myasthenic smile (snarling, nasal smile)
d. Strabismus
e. Diagnostic measures include administration of neostigmine (Prostigmin) subcutaneously or IV administration of edrophonium (Tensilon) to provide spontaneous relief of symptoms; edrophonium is also used to distinguish myasthenic crisis from cholinergic crisis (toxic effects of excessive neostigmine)
C. Treatment
1. Specific medications that block the action of cholinesterase at the myoneural junction
a. neostigmine (Prostigmin)
b. pyridostigmine bromide (Mestinon)
c. ambenonium chloride (Mytelase)
2. X-ray therapy of the thymus may cause partial remission
3. Corticosteroids or ACTH
4. Tracheostomy with mechanical ventilation is often necessary in myasthenic crisis
D. Nursing care
1. Administer medications on strict time schedule to prevent onset of symptoms; instruct the client and family to do the same
2. Observe for signs of dyspnea, dysphagia, and dysarthria, which may indicate myasthenic crisis
3. Have an emergency tracheostomy set at bedside
4. Plan activity to avoid fatigue based on the individual's tolerance
5. Instruct the client to avoid people with upper respiratory tract infections, since pneumonia may develop as a result of fatigued respiratory muscles
6. Encourage the client to carry a medical alert card or identification stating condition
7. Do not administer morphine to clients receiving anticholinesterases, since these drugs potentiate the effects of morphine and may cause respiratory depression

8. Provide emotional support and close contact with the client to allay anxiety
9. Administer tube feedings when necessary if the client has difficulty swallowing so that aspiration will not occur
10. In severe instances anticipate all needs, since the client is too weak to turn, drink, or even request assistance
11. Evaluate client's response and revise plan as necessary

Guillain-Barré Syndrome

A. Etiology and pathophysiology
 1. Cause unknown; thought to be linked to swine flu–like virus
 2. Changes in the motor cells of the spinal cord and medulla with areas of demyelination
 3. Most common in young adults
B. Signs and symptoms
 1. Subjective
  a. Generalized weakness
  b. Paresthesia
 2. Objective
  a. Paralysis begins in lower extremities; ascends within the body, usually 24 to 72 hours
  b. Respiratory paralysis
  c. Hypertension, tachycardia, and low-grade fever
C. Treatment
 1. Steroids
 2. Support vital functions (similar to that for poliomyelitis)
D. Nursing care
 1. Monitor vital signs and vital capacity
 2. Suction, provide fluid replacement therapy, and monitor functioning of the respirator as required
 3. Provide emotional support to the client and family because of the severity and lengthy convalescent period

Amyotrophic Lateral Sclerosis (ALS)

A. Etiology and pathophysiology
 1. Cause unknown
 2. Progressive degenerative process involving the spinal, corticobulbar, and lower motor neurons, with subsequent atrophic and spastic changes in the cranial as well as the spinal nerves
 3. Occurs more frequently in men than in women
B. Signs and symptoms
 1. Subjective
  a. Muscular weakness
  b. Malaise
 2. Objective
  a. Irregular spasmodic twitching in small muscle groups (fasciculations)
  b. Difficulty in chewing, swallowing, speaking
  c. Outbursts of laughter or crying
C. Treatment
 1. Physiotherapy may be helpful in relieving spasticity
 2. Support respiratory functions
D. Nursing care
 1. Provide emotional support for the client and family
 2. Encourage range-of-motion exercises

3. Support natural defense mechanisms; encourage a diet consisting of high nutrient-dense foods, especially those rich in the immune-stimulating nutrients selenium and vitamins A, C, and E
4. Teach the avoidance of situations that may contribute to infection
5. Evaluate client's response and revise plan as necessary

Poliomyelitis

A. Etiology and pathophysiology
 1. Invasion of the lymph system by the poliovirus through the pharynx, with eventual spread to the lymph nodes, circulatory system, and nervous system
 2. Virus causes inflammation and necrosis of the cells, with resultant paralysis
 3. When it occurs in spinal cord, the anterior horn cells are affected; bulbar poliomyelitis involves the cranial nerves, and encephalitic poliomyelitis the cerebrum
 4. Incubation period 5 to 12 days
B. Signs and symptoms
 1. Subjective
  a. Fatigue
  b. Headache
  c. Muscular pain, especially in head and back
 2. Objective
  a. Flaccid paralysis
  b. Absent deep tendon reflexes
  c. Increased spinal fluid pressure
  d. Poliovirus in stool, throat secretions, blood, or spinal fluid
  e. Fever
  f. Respiratory paralysis may occur
C. Treatment
 1. Strict bed rest
 2. Support vital functions
  a. Tracheostomy
  b. Fluid replacement
  c. Urinary drainage
 3. Antibiotics
D. Nursing care
 1. Stress the importance of immunization as a way to prevent disease
 2. Carefully observe vital signs and vital capacity
 3. Maintain body alignment
 4. Allow the client time to verbalize feelings; realize that respiratory paralysis may make this difficult, which can be frustrating for the client
 5. Evaluate client's response and revise plan as necessary

Huntington's Chorea

A. Etiology and pathophysiology
 1. Inherited disorder, considered autosomal dominant
 2. Progressive atrophy of the basal ganglia and some portions of the cerebral cortex
 3. Appears during the middle adult years
B. Signs and symptoms
 1. Subjective
  a. Memory loss
  b. Disorientation
  c. Eventual dementia

2. Objective
   a. Uncontrolled jerky movements of the extremities or trunk
   b. Disorganized gait
   c. Uncontrolled periods of anger
   d. Hesitant or explosive patterns of speech
   e. Grimacing facial movements
C. Treatment
   1. Control of jerky movements with haloperidol, fluphenazine, or L-dopa
   2. Symptoms are treated as they occur
D. Nursing care
   1. Provide emotional support for client and family
   2. Provide for safety
   3. Utilize community agencies to provide situational support
   4. Evaluate client's response and revise plan as necessary

Rheumatoid Arthritis

A. Etiology and pathophysiology
   1. Chronic disease characterized by inflammatory changes in the body's connective tissue particularly areas that have a cavity and easily moving surfaces
   2. Cause unknown, although theories include autoimmunity, heredity, and psychophysiologic factors
B. Signs and symptoms
   1. Subjective
      a. Fatigue
      b. Malaise
      c. Joint pain
      d. Muscle stiffness after periods of inactivity
      e. Paresthesia
   2. Objective
      a. Anemia
      b. Weight loss
      c. Joint deformity as demonstrated by x-ray examination
      d. Subcutaneous nodules
      e. Elevated sedimentation rate
      f. Presence of rheumatoid factors in serum identified by latex fixation test
C. Treatment
   1. Corticosteroids, antiinflammatories, analgesics, immunosuppressive drugs
   2. Physiotherapy to minimize deformities
   3. Surgical intervention to remove severely damaged joints (e.g., hip replacement)
   4. Paraffin dips of affected extremity for relief of joint pain by providing uniform heat
D. Nursing care
   1. Administer analgesics and other medications as ordered
   2. Teach the client to take medications as ordered
   3. Apply heat and cold as ordered; heat paraffin to 125° to 129° F (52° to 54° C)
   4. Promote rest and position to ease joint pains
   5. Provide for range-of-motion exercises up to the point of pain, recognizing that some discomfort is always present
   6. Encourage the client to verbalize feelings
   7. Set realistic goals, focusing on strengths

8. Encourage use of supportive devices to help client conserve energy and maintain independence
9. For nursing care of the client following hip replacement, see Fractured hip
10. Encourage diet rich in nutrient-dense foods such as fruits, vegetables, whole grains, and legumes to improve and maintain nutritional status and compensate for nutrient interactions of corticosteroid and other treatment medications
11. Evaluate client's response and revise plan as necessary

Osteoarthritis

A. Etiology and pathophysiology
   1. Etiology is unknown, but predisposing factors include obesity, aging, and joint trauma
   2. A degeneration and atrophy of the cartilages and calcification of the ligaments
B. Signs and symptoms
   1. Subjective
      a. Pain after exercise
      b. Stiffness of joints
   2. Objective
      a. Heberden's nodes symmetrically occurring on fingers (bony extensions)
      b. Decreased range of motion
C. Treatment
   1. Weight reduction in instances of obesity
   2. Local heat to affected joints
   3. Medications to reduce symptoms, such as analgesics, antiinflammatory agents, and steroids
   4. Exercise of affected extremities
   5. Surgical intervention
      a. Synovectomy: removal of the enlarged synovial membrane before bone and cartilage destruction occurs
      b. Arthrodesis: fusion of a joint performed when the joint surfaces are severely damaged; this leaves the client with no range of motion of the affected joint
      c. Reconstructive surgery: replacement of a badly damaged joint with a prosthetic device (see hip replacement)
D. Nursing care
   1. Assist client in activities that require using affected joints; allow for rest periods
   2. Attempt to relieve the client's discomfort by the use of medications or the application of heat as ordered
   3. Allow client ample time to verbalize feelings regarding limited motion and changes in life-style
   4. Encourage diet rich in nutrient-dense foods such as fruits, vegetables, whole grains, and legumes to improve and maintain nutritional status and compensate for nutrient interactions of corticosteroid and other treatment medications
   5. Evaluate client's response and revise plan as necessary

Gouty Arthritis (Gout)

A. Etiology and pathophysiology
   1. Disorder in purine metabolism that leads to high levels of uric acid in the blood and the deposition

of uric acid crystals (tophi) in tissues, especially joints; followed by an inflammatory response

2. Incidence highest in males; a familial tendency has been demonstrated

3. Renal urate lithiasis (kidney stones) may result from precipitation of uric acid in the presence of a low urinary pH

B. Signs and symptoms
1. Subjective
   a. Sudden onset of asymmetric joint pain usually in the metatarsophalangeal joint of the great toe
   b. Local pruritus
   c. Malaise
   d. Headache
   e. Anorexia
2. Objective
   a. Elevated serum uric acid
   b. Signs of inflammation of joint including swelling, heat, and redness
   c. Tophi in outer ear, hands, and feet

C. Treatment
1. Administration of antiinflammatory and uricosuric (antigout) agents (see Pharmacology)
2. Alkaline-ash diet to increase the pH of urine to discourage precipitation of uric acid and enhance the action of drugs such as probenicid (Benemid)
3. Elimination of foods high in purines
4. Weight loss is encouraged if indicated

D. Nursing care
1. Assess joint pain, motion, and appearance
2. Administer antiinflammatory agents such as phenylbutazone (Butazolidin), oxyphenbutazone (Tandearil), or indomethacin (Indocin) with antacids or milk to help prevent peptic ulcers; observe therapeutic response
3. Carefully align joints so they are slightly flexed during acute stage; encourage regular exercise, which is important for long-term management
4. Use a bed cradle during the acute phase to keep pressure of sheets off joints
5. Increase fluid intake to 2000 to 3000 ml daily to prevent formation of calculi
6. Instruct client to avoid high-purine foods such as organ meats, anchovies, sardines, and shellfish; encourage diet rich in nutrient-dense foods of the fruit, vegetable, and whole-grain groups as well as milk, cheese, and eggs; teach Dietary Goals for the United States and importance of preventing drug-induced nutrient deficiencies with improved diet
7. Provide education regarding drug therapy and avoidance of excess alcohol intake
8. Evaluate client's response and revise plan as necessary

Osteomyelitis

A. Etiology and pathophysiology
1. Occurs as the result of bacterial invasion of the bone by *Staphylococcus aureus,* streptococcal organisms, *Escherichia coli,* or *Salmonella* organisms
2. Infection of the bone results from trauma or systemic infection and involves the entire bone and surrounding soft tissue

B. Signs and symptoms
1. Subjective
   a. Pain and tenderness of the bone
   b. Malaise
   c. Difficulty in weight-bearing
2. Objective
   a. Fever
   b. Swelling over the affected bone
   c. Signs of sepsis

C. Treatment
1. Antibiotic therapy
2. Incision and drainage of a bone abscess
3. Sequestrectomy: surgical removal of the dead infected bone and cartilage

D. Nursing care
1. Administer pain medications and antibiotics as ordered
2. Use surgical aseptic technique when changing dressings
3. Maintain functional body alignment and promote comfort
4. Utilize room deodorizer if a foul odor is apparent
5. Allow the client ample time to express feelings about long-term hospitalization
6. Encourage nutrient-dense diet to compensate for antibiotic impact on nutritional status (See Pharmacology related to infection)
7. Evaluate client's response and revise plan as necessary

Osteoporosis

A. Etiology and pathophysiology
1. Decrease in bone substance so the bone can no longer maintain the skeletal structure
2. Most commonly affects the vertebrae, pelvis and femur
3. Related factors include menopause, aging, inactivity, insufficient calcium intake or absorption, hyperparathyroidism, acromegaly, Cushing's syndrome, and hyperthyroidism

B. Signs and symptoms
1. Subjective
   a. Backache
   b. Difficulty maintaining balance
2. Objective
   a. Decreased height resulting from compression of the vertebrae
   b. X-ray examination reveals a demineralization of bone and compression of the vertebrae

C. Treatment
1. Planned program of exercise
2. Estrogen therapy to decrease bone reabsorption
3. High-protein, high-calcium diet with vitamin D supplement
4. Support for the spine (e.g., corset, Taylor brace)
5. Treatment of underlying disorder vital to halt the process

D. Nursing care
1. Encourage active exercise and assist with passive exercises
2. Instruct the client about proper body mechanics

3. Encourage diet rich in nutrient-dense foods such as fruits, vegetables, whole grains, and legumes to improve and maintain nutritional status; special emphasis should be placed on foods that will supply nutrients needed for mineralization of bone (vitamins A, C, and D, and the minerals calcium, magnesium, and phosphorus)
4. Consider safety factors associated with instability; a cane or walker may be necessary for ambulation
5. Provide rest periods to prevent fatigue
6. Encourage fluids in acute osteoporosis to discourage the formation of renal calculi
7. Evaluate client's response and revise plan as necessary

Osteogenic Sarcoma

A. Etiology and pathophysiology
1. Malignant bone tumor that usually begins in the long bones, especially around the knee
2. Metastasis to the lungs common and occurs early; prognosis is poor
3. Highest incidence between 20 and 30 years of age
B. Signs and symptoms
1. Subjective
a. Pain
b. Limited motion
c. Malaise
2. Objective
a. Local swelling
b. Weight loss
c. Anemia
d. Elevated serum alkaline phosphatase
e. Fever
f. Microscopic evaluation of biopsy reveals neoplastic cells
C. Treatment
1. Amputation of limb or resection of tumor
2. Chemotherapy
3. Radiation
D. Nursing care
1. Be available for the client and family to discuss fears, concerns, and treatment
2. Support natural defense mechanisms; encourage a diet of nutrient-dense foods, especially those rich in the immune-stimulating nutrients selenium and vitamins A, C, and E, as well as protein
3. Administer special nursing care following surgery (see Amputation)
4. Administer analgesics and antiemetics as needed
5. Provide special care if the client is receiving radiation therapy
a. Observe the skin for breakdown
b. Do not wash off port marks
c. Avoid use of powders and ointments that contain metals
d. See Radiation for additional information
6. Evaluate client's response and revise plan as necessary

Multiple Myeloma

A. Etiology and pathophysiology
1. Cause unknown, although genetic and viral factors are being closely considered

2. Malignant overgrowth of plasma cells and malignant tumor growth in bone and bone marrow
3. Occurs primarily in middle-aged men
B. Signs and symptoms
1. Subjective
a. Bone pain
b. Progressive weakness
c. Low back pain
2. Objective
a. Anemia
b. Cachexia
c. Idiopathic bone fractures
d. Macroglobulinemia
e. Platelet deficiency with resultant bleeding tendency
f. Punched-out appearance of the bones at x-ray examination
g. Presence of Bence Jones protein in urine
C. Treatment
1. Chemotherapeutic agents, especially melphalan (Alkeran)
2. Radiation therapy
3. Analgesics and narcotics for pain
4. Supportive therapy such as transfusions as indicated
D. Nursing care
1. Carefully ambulate the client to prevent pneumonia and reduce pathologic fractures
2. Allow the client ample time to express feelings about the disease and related therapies
3. Allow the client to participate in planning nursing care to aid in self-esteem and promote a feeling of self-control
4. Support natural defense mechanisms; encourage diet high in nutrient-dense foods, especially those rich in the immune-stimulating nutrients selenium and vitamins A, C, and E, as well as protein
5. Evaluate client's response and revise plan as necessary

Intractable Pain

A. Etiology and pathophysiology
1. Pain not relieved by conventional treatment
2. Causes include cancer, neuralgia, tic douloureux, and ischemia
B. Signs and symptoms
1. Subjective
a. Pain
b. Fatigue
c. Irritability
2. Objective
a. Evidence of a related disease process
b. Pallor
C. Treatment
1. Surgical intervention
a. Rhizotomy: posterior spinal nerve root is resected between the ganglion and the cord, resulting in permanent loss of sensation; the anterior root may be cut to alleviate painful muscle spasm
b. Cordotomy: to alleviate intractable pain in the trunk or lower extremities; the transmission of pain and temperature sensation is interrupted by

creation of a lesion in the ascending tracts, percutaneously using an electrode or surgically via laminectomy

   c. Sympathectomy: to control pain of vascular disturbances and phantom limb pain (see procedures related to gastrointestinal disorders)

2. Acupuncture therapy
3. Biofeedback helps the client develop control over anxiety and physiologic function
4. Electronic stimulation may alter the electric potential of the nerve to prevent complete depolarization or block the transmission of pain sensations to the brain
   a. Percutaneous stimulator: electrodes applied over the painful area or along the nerve pathway
   b. Dorsal column stimulator and peripheral nerve implant: involve direct attachment of an electrode to the sensory nerve; a transmitter attached to the electrode is carried by the client so electric stimulation can be administered as needed

D. Nursing care
1. Assess pain, including location, duration, type, and severity
2. Eliminate factors from the environment that seem to intensify pain
3. Support the client and family, since the client frequently will withdraw
4. Educate the client and family about treatments available and the potential side effects
5. Provide postoperative care
   a. Nursing care for a client undergoing a cordotomy or rhizotomy or implantation of a dorsal column stimulator (see Ruptured nucleus pulposus)
   b. Neurologically assess the extremities for movement, sensation, and skin temperature
   c. Carefully inspect skin, since the client will not feel pain of ulceration
   d. Instruct the client to avoid extreme environmental conditions and the use of heating pads and to check the temperature of bath water, since temperature sensitivity is absent
6. Evaluate client's response and revise plan as necessary

Ruptured Nucleus Pulposus ("Slipped Disc," Herniation of an Intervertebral Disc)

A. Etiology and pathophysiology
1. Involves protrusion of the nucleus pulposus into the spinal canal with subsequent compression of the cord or nerve roots; usually occurs as a result of trauma
2. Most common site is lumbosacral area (between L_4 and L_5), but herniation can also occur in the cervical region (between C_5 and C_6 or C_6 and C_7)

B. Signs and symptoms
1. Subjective
   a. Lumbosacral disc
     (1) Acute pain in lower back, radiating across the buttock and down the leg (sciatic pain)
     (2) Pain when raising the unflexed leg on the affected side (Lasègue's sign)
     (3) Weakness of the foot

   b. Cervical disc
     (1) Neck pain that may radiate down arm to the hand
     (2) Weakness of the affected upper extremity

2. Objective
   a. Straightening of the normal lumbar curve with scoliosis away from the affected side (lumbosacral disc)
   b. Atrophy of the biceps and triceps may be present (cervical disc)
   c. Elevated CSF protein
   d. Myelogram shows impingement on the spinal cord
   e. Electromyography (EMG) can help localize the site of a herniated disc

C. Treatment
1. Bed rest with traction to the lower extremities (lumbosacral disc) or cervical traction (cervical disc)
2. Back brace or support; cervical collar
3. Local application of heat
4. Muscle relaxant
5. Surgical intervention
   a. Laminectomy: excision of the ruptured portion of the nucleus pulposus through an opening created by removal of part of the vertebra
   b. Discectomy: entire disc and cartilaginous plate are removed
   c. Laminotomy: inscision into the lamina
   d. Spinal fusion: if three or more discs are involved, the affected vertebrae are permanently fused to stabilize the spine

D. Nursing care
1. Administer analgesics and other medications as ordered
2. Use a firm mattress and bed board under the client
3. Make certain that traction and/or braces are correctly applied and maintained and that weights hang freely
4. Use the fracture bedpan to avoid lifting of hips
5. Give frequent and extensive back care to relax muscles and promote circulation
6. Support body alignment at all times
7. Use log-rolling method to turn the client (instruct the client to fold arms across the chest, bend the knee on the side opposite the direction of the turn, and then roll over)
8. Increase fluid intake and encourage diet rich in nutrient-dense foods such as fruits, vegetables, whole grains, and legumes to improve and maintain nutritional status as well as prevent constipation; if necessary use stool softeners to prevent straining
9. Keep the client flat for 24 hours and encourage fluids to limit headache after a myelogram is done
10. Provide special care for the client undergoing a laminectomy
   a. Explain that pain may persist postoperatively for some time because of edema
   b. Place the bedside table, phone, and call bell within reach to prevent twisting
   c. Observe the dressing for hemorrhage and leakage of spinal fluid; notify the physician immediately if either occurs

d. Observe for inadequate ventilation, especially in clients who have undergone a cervical laminectomy
e. Assess the client for changes in neurologic functioning
11. Allow the client to be dependent, but foster independence
12. Encourage the client to express feelings about altered functioning and self-image
13. Encourage the client to verbalize fears about the present condition and future disability
14. Teach the client to use proper body mechanics to prevent subsequent injury
15. Evaluate client's response and revise plan as necessary

Fractures

A. Etiology and pathophysiology
   1. Breaks in the continuity of bone, usually accompanied by localized tissue response and muscle spasm
   2. Cause usually trauma, but pathologic fractures may occur as a result of osteoporosis, multiple myeloma, or bone tumors, which weaken bone structure
   3. Types
      a. Complete fracture: bone completely separated into two parts; may be transverse or spiral
      b. Incomplete fracture: only part of the bone broken
      c. Comminuted fracture: bone broken into several fragments
      d. Greenstick fracture: splintering on one side of the bone, with bending of the other side; occurs only in pliable bones, usually in children
      e. Simple (closed) fracture: bone broken but no break in the skin
      f. Compound (open) fracture: break in the skin at the time of fracture with or without protrusion of the bone
   4. Stages of healing include formation of a hematoma followed by cellular proliferation and callus formation by the osteoblasts; finally ossification and remodeling of the callus
B. Signs and symptoms
   1. Subjective
      a. Pain aggravated by motion
      b. Tenderness
   2. Objective
      a. Loss of motion
      b. Edema
      c. Crepitus (grating sound heard when fractured limb is moved)
      d. Ecchymosis
      e. X-ray examination reveals break in continuity of bone
C. Treatment
   1. Traction may be used to reduce the fracture or to maintain alignment of bone fragments until healing occurs
      a. Skin traction: weights attached to adhesive, which is applied to the skin
         (1) Buck's extension: exerts a straight pull on a limb; often used temporarily to immobilize the leg when a client fractures a hip

(2) Bryant's traction: both lower limbs extended vertically; used to align fractured femurs in young children
(3) Russell traction: lower leg is supported in a hammock, which is attached to rope and pulleys on a Balkan frame; used to treat fractures of the femur (the foot of the bed is usually elevated for countertraction)
      b. Skeletal traction applied to the bone
         (1) Steinmann pin or Kirschner wire may be inserted through the bone and skin; weights are then attached to a spreader, which is attached to both ends of the pin or wire (this may be used in conjunction with a cast)
         (2) Crutchfield tongs are inserted into the skull and weights are attached to immobilize the client with a cervical fracture in a position of hyperextension
   2. Surgical intervention to align the bone (open reduction), often with plates and screws to hold fracture in alignment
   3. Manipulation to reduce fracture (closed reduction)
   4. Application of cast to maintain alignment and immobilize limb
D. Nursing care
   1. Provide emergency care
      a. Evaluate the client's general physical condition
      b. Treat for shock
      c. Splint extremity in position found before moving the client; consider all suspected fractures to be fractures until x-ray films are available
      d. Cover open wound with sterile dressing if available
   2. Observe for signs of emboli (fat or blood clot): severe chest pain, dyspnea, pallor, diaphoresis
   3. Provide special care for a client with a cast
      a. Observe for signs of circulatory impairment: change in skin temperature or color, numbness or tingling, unrelieved pain, decrease in pedal pulse, prolonged blanching of toes after compression
      b. Protect the cast from damage until dry by elevating it on a pillow; handle with palms of hands only
      c. Promote drying of the cast by leaving it uncovered; a hair dryer or light may be used with care to prevent burning
      d. Maintain bed rest until the cast is dry and ambulation is permitted
      e. Observe for signs of hemorrhage and measure extent of drainage on cast when present
      f. Observe for irritation caused by rough cast edges, and pad as necessary for comfort and to prevent soiling
      g. Observe for swelling and notify the physician if necessary
      h. Administer analgesics judiciously and report unrelieved pain
      i. Observe for signs of infection (e.g., elevated temperature, odor from cast, swelling)
   4. Provide special care for a client in traction
      a. Check that weights are hanging freely and that the affected limb is not resting against the bed; countertraction may be necessary to prevent this

by raising the foot of the bed (Russell traction and Buck's extension) or head of the bed (cervical traction)

b. Maintain in proper alignment

c. Observe for foot-drop in clients with Russell traction or Buck's extension, since this may be indicative of nerve damage

d. Observe for signs of thrombophlebitis; this is a more common complication of Russell traction because there is pressure on the popliteal space in addition to the stress of immobility

e. Provide careful skin care

f. Observe skin for irritation and observe site of insertion of skeletal traction for signs of infection

g. Use aseptic technique when cleansing the site of insertion of skeletal traction (frequently an antiseptic ointment is also ordered)

5. Encourage high-protein, high-vitamin diet to promote healing; high-calcium diet is not recommended for the client confined to prolonged bed rest, since decalcification of the bone will continue until activity is restored, and a high calcium intake could lead to formation of renal calculi

6. Encourage fluids to help prevent complications of constipation, renal calculi, and urinary tract infection

7. Teach isometric exercises to promote muscle tone

8. Teach appropriate crutch-walking technique; non-weight-bearing (three-point swing-through); weight-bearing (four-point) progressing to use of cane (see procedures)

9. Evaluate client's response and revise plan as necessary

Fractured Hip

A. Etiology and pathophysiology
 1. Fractures of the head or neck of the femur (intracapsular fracture) or trochanteric area (extracapsular fracture)
 2. Incidence highest in elderly females due to osteoporosis

B. Signs and symptoms
 1. Subjective
  a. Pain
  b. Changes in sensation
 2. Objective
  a. Affected leg appears shorter
  b. External rotation of the affected limb
  c. X-ray examination reveals lack of continuity of the bone

C. Treatment
 1. Buck's extension or Russell traction as a temporary measure to relieve the pain of muscle spasm or if surgery is contraindicated
 2. Closed reduction with a hip spica cast in fractures of the intertrochanteric region
 3. Open reduction and internal fixation
  a. Austin Moore prosthesis
  b. Thompson prosthesis
  c. Smith-Petersen nail
  d. Jewett nail

D. Nursing care
 1. See nursing care under Fractures
 2. Encourage the use of a trapeze to facilitate movement
 3. Use the fracture pan for elimination
 4. Provide postoperative care
  a. Inspect dressing and linen for bleeding
  b. Use a trochanter roll to prevent external rotation of legs
  c. Do not turn client on the operated side unless specifically ordered
  d. Use pillows or abductor pillow to maintain the legs in slight abduction; after hip replacement it prevents dislodging of the prosthesis
  e. Encourage quadriceps setting exercises
  f. Assist the client to ambulate—first using a walker, progressing to three-point crutch walking, and then to total weight-bearing using a cane to provide stability
  g. Avoid flexing the hips of a client with a total-hip replacement; assist to a lounge chair position when permitted to sit
 5. Evaluate client's response and revise plan as necessary

Spinal Cord Injury

A. Etiology and pathophysiology
 1. Sudden impingements on the spinal cord as a result of trauma
 2. Fractures of the vertebrae can cut, compress, or completely sever the spinal cord if the client is not positioned and moved correctly at the scene of an accident; the symptoms depend on the location (lumbar, thoracic, cervical) and extent of the damage (complete transection, partial transection, compression) and may be temporary or permanent; the sensation and mobility of areas that are supplied by nerves below the level of the lesion are lost

B. Signs and symptoms
 1. Subjective
  a. Loss of sensation below the level of the injury
  b. Inability to move
 2. Objective
  a. Early symptoms of spinal shock
   (1) Absence of reflexes below the level of the lesion
   (2) Flaccid paralysis (immobility accompanied by weak, soft, flabby muscles) below the level of injury
   (3) Hypotonia caused by disruption of neural impulses results in bowel and bladder distention
   (4) Inability to perspire in affected parts
   (5) Hypotension
  b. Later symptoms of spinal cord injury
   (1) Reflex hyperexcitability (spastic paralysis): muscles below the site of injury become spastic and hyperreflexic
   (2) State of diminished reflex excitability (flaccid paralysis) below the site of injury follows the state of reflex hyperexcitability

in all instances of total cord damage and may occur in some instances of partial cord damage

(3) In total cord damage, since both upper and lower motoneurons are destroyed, the symptoms depend totally on the location of the injury; loss of motor and sensory function present at this time is usually permanent

(a) Sacral region: paralysis (usually flaccid type) of the lower extremities (paraplegia) accompanied by atonic (autonomous) bladder and bowel with impairment of sphincter control

(b) Lumbar region: paralysis of the lower extremities that may extend to the pelvic region (usually flaccid type) accompanied by a spastic (automatic) bladder and loss of bladder and anal sphincter control

(c) Thoracic region: same symptoms as in the lumbar region except extends to the trunk below level of the diaphragm

(d) Cervical region: same symptoms as in the thoracic region except extends from the neck down and includes paralysis of all extremities (quadriplegia); if injury is above C_4, respirations are depressed

(4) In partial cord damage either the upper or the lower motoneurons, or both, may be destroyed; therefore the symptoms depend not only on the location but also on the type of neurons involved; destruction of lower motoneurons will result in atrophy and flaccid paralysis of the involved muscles, whereas destruction of upper motoneurons causes spasticity

C. Treatment
  1. Neurologic assessment
  2. Maintain vertebral alignment by use of the following:
    a. Bed rest with supportive devices (bed board, sand bags, etc.)
    b. Bed rest with total immobilization (see procedures): Stryker frame, CircOlectric bed
    c. Traction (skeletal or skin traction): e.g., Crutchfield tongs, Buck's extension
    d. Corsets, braces, and other devices when mobility is permitted
  3. Surgery to reduce pain or pressure and/or stabilize the spine (e.g., laminectomy, spinal fusion)
  4. Mechanical ventilation as needed
  5. Temperature control via hypothermia or tepid baths
  6. Extensive rehabilitation therapy
D. Nursing care
  1. Maintain frequent observation of respiratory and neurologic functioning
  2. Maintain spinal alignment at all times; when turning, use the log-rolling method and make certain enough help is available to move the client as a single unit
  3. Check safety locks on Stryker frames and CircOlectric beds before turning
  4. Maintain surgical asepsis for the client with Crutchfield tongs or spinal surgery
  5. Provide special skin care to back and bony prominences
  6. Maintain body parts in a functional position; prevent dysfunctional contractures
  7. Institute active and passive range-of-motion exercises as soon as approved by physician
  8. Provide the client with simple explanations
  9. Encourage the client to verbalize and accept that hostility will surface
  10. Stay with the client when possible to provide assurance
  11. Allow the client to be independent when possible
  12. Include the client in decision-making process
  13. Help the client to adjust to changes in body image and altered self-concept
  14. Accept periods of depression that occur
  15. Allow the client time to reorganize life-style
  16. Set realistic short-term goals so the client can achieve some success
  17. Test the temperature of bath water to avoid burns; teach the client to test water temperature in any water-related activity
  18. Avoid bumps and bruises when involved in activities; utilize techniques to prevent pressure and examine skin for signs of pressure from positioning, braces, or splints
  19. Use a footboard to stimulate pressure sensation and proprioception
  20. Provide an opportunity for the client to touch, grasp, and manipulate objects of different sizes, weights, and textures to stimulate tactile sensation
  21. Encourage the client to be aware of all body segments: look at both extremities, comb both sides of the hair, shave both sides of the chin, put makeup on both sides of the face
  22. Protect the affected limbs by proper positioning during transfer; use a sling when indicated
  23. Teach the client to use the unaffected extremities to manipulate, move, and stabilize the affected ones
  24. Attempt to reestablish a scheduled pattern of bowel function
    a. Understand what the individual's bowel functioning means to the client and family
    b. Involve the client, family, and entire health team in the development of a plan of care
    c. Review the client's bowel habits prior to illness as well as the current pattern of elimination
    d. Provide a diet with bowel-stimulating properties; emphasis should be placed on fruits, vegetables, cereal grains, and legumes since these are rich sources of dietary fiber
    e. Encourage sufficient fluid intake: 2000 to 3000 ml per day
    f. Encourage the client to be as active as possible to develop the tone and strength of the muscles that can be used

g. Establish a specific and definite time for the bowel movement; regularity is the most important aspect of bowel reeducation
  (1) Depends on the client's schedule
  (2) Depends on the client's past pattern
  (3) Consider scheduling evacuation after a meal to utilize the gastrocolic reflex (peristaltic wave in the colon induced by entrance of food into a fasting stomach)
h. Determine if the client is aware of the need to defecate (e.g., feeling of fullness or pressure in the rectum, flatus, borborygmus)
i. Provide privacy during toileting activities
j. Encourage the client to assume a position most near the physiologic position for defecation (sitting the client up frequently assists in preparing for this)
k. Utilize assistive measures to induce defecation by
  (1) Teaching the client to bear down and contract abdominal muscles (the Valsalva maneuver should be avoided by people with cardiac problems)
  (2) Teaching the client to lean forward to increase intraabdominal pressure by compressing the abdomen against the thighs
  (3) Digital stimulation
  (4) Using suppository if necessary
  (5) Using enemas only as a last resort
l. Provide for adaptation of equipment as necessary (e.g., elevated toilet seat, grab bars, padded backrest)
m. Teach the family the bowel training program

25. Attempt to reestablish bladder function
  a. Determine the type of bladder problem
    (1) Neurogenic bladder: any disturbance in bladder functioning caused by a lesion of the nervous system
    (2) Spastic bladder (reflex or autonomous): disorder caused by a lesion of the spinal cord above the bladder reflex center, in the conus medullaris; there is a loss of conscious sensation and cerebral motor control; the bladder empties automatically when the detrusor muscle is sufficiently stretched (about 500 ml)
    (3) Flaccid bladder (atonic, nonreflex, or autonomous): disorder caused by a lesion of the spinal cord at the level of the sacral conus or below; the bladder continues to fill, becomes distended, and periodically overflows; the bladder muscle does not contract forcefully and therefore does not empty except with a conscious effort
  b. Understand what the individual's bladder functioning means to the client and family
  c. Involve the client, family, and entire health team in the development of a plan of care
  d. Review the client's bladder habits prior to illness as well as the current pattern of elimination
  e. Encourage activity
  f. Encourage sufficient fluid intake
    (1) 3000 to 5000 ml per 24-hour period
    (2) Glass of water with each attempt to void
    (3) Reduce the amount of fluid as the day progresses and restrict fluid after 6 PM to limit the amount of urine in the bladder during the night
  g. Provide for privacy during toileting activities
  h. Encourage the client to assume as normal a position as possible for voiding
  i. Establish a voiding schedule
    (1) Begin trial voiding at the time the client is most often incontinent
    (2) Attempt voiding every 2 hours all day and two to three times during the night
    (3) Time intervals between voiding should be shorter in the morning than later in the day
    (4) As the client's ability to maintain control improves, lengthen the time between attempts at voiding
    (5) Time of intervals is not as important as regularity
  j. Determine whether the client is aware of need or act of urination (e.g., fullness or pressure, flushing, chilling, goose pimples, cold sweats)
  k. Utilize assistive measures to induce urination by teaching the client to
    (1) Use the Credé maneuver: manual expression of the urine from the bladder with moderate external pressure, downward and backward, from the umbilicus to over the suprapubic area
    (2) Bend forward to increase intraabdominal pressure
    (3) Stimulate "trigger points": areas that, for the individual, will instigate urination (e.g., stroke the thigh, pull pubic hair, touch meatus)
  l. Record intake, output, voiding times, and times of incontinence
  m. Provide for adaptive equipment as necessary (e.g., elevated toilet seats, commode, urinals, drainage systems)
  n. Teach the family the bladder training program

26. Evaluate client's response and revise plan as necessary

Amputation

A. Necessitated by
  1. Malignant tumor
  2. Trauma
  3. Acute arterial insufficiency
B. Preoperative preparation
  1. Initiation of exercises to strengthen muscles of extremities in preparation for crutch walking
  2. Coughing and deep breathing exercises
  3. Emotional support for anticipated alteration in body image
C. Types of procedures
  1. Below-the-knee amputation (BKA) common in peripheral vascular disease; facilitates successful adaptation to prosthesis because of retained knee function

2. Above-the-knee amputation (AKA) necessitated by trauma or extensive disease
3. Upper extremity amputation usually necessitated by severe trauma, malignant tumors, or congenital malformation

D. Postoperative nursing care
1. Monitor vital signs and stump dressing for signs of hemorrhage
2. Place tourniquet at bed side for use only if hemorrhage is life-threatening
3. Elevate stump for 12 to 24 hours to decrease edema; remove pillow after this time to prevent contractures
4. Provide stump care
   a. Keep bandaged to shrink and shape stump in preparation for prosthesis
   b. When wound is healed, wash stump daily, avoiding the use of oils which may cause maceration
   c. Apply pressure to end of stump with progressively firmer surfaces to toughen stump
   d. Encourage client to move the stump
   e. Place the client with a lower extremity amputation in a prone position twice daily to stretch the flexor muscles and prevent hip flexion contractures
5. Teach client about phantom limb sensation
   a. Phantom limb: physiologic reaction of the nerves in the stump causing an unpleasant feeling that the limb is still there; this response may or may not be precipitated by a psychologic overlay
   b. Phantom limb pain: when the unpleasant feelings become painful or disagreeable
   c. Characteristics of phantom limb: sensations may be constant or intermittent, and of varying severity
   d. Institute care that may help relieve phantom limb phenomenon: have the client look at the stump or close eyes and put the stump through range of motion as if the full limb were still there; if the client continues to have severe pain of long duration, the medical therapy may include
      (1) Injecting the nerve endings in the stump with alcohol to give temporary relief
      (2) Surgical revision of the stump
6. Consider the special needs related to an upper extremity amputation
   a. Mastery of an upper extremity prosthesis is more complex than that of a lower extremity prosthesis
   b. The client must do bilateral shoulder exercises to prepare for fitting the prosthesis
   c. The artificial arm cannot be used above the head or behind the back because of the harnessing
   d. No artificial hand can duplicate all the fine movements of the fingers and thumb of the normal hand, although the development of electronic limbs does not negate this possibility for the future
   e. There is a loss of sensory feedback; therefore the client must use visual control at all times (a blind person could not adequately use a functional prosthesis)

7. Support client through fitting, application, and utilization of prosthesis
8. Encourage family to participate in care
9. Allow client to express emotional reactions
10. Evaluate client's response and revise plan as necessary

Anterior Segment Disorders of the Eye

A. Etiology and pathophysiology
1. Conjunctivitis: inflammation of the conjunctiva; can result from invasion by organisms, allergens, or irritants
2. Blepharitis: inflammation of the lid margins; classified as staphylococcal or seborrheic
3. Keratitis: inflammation of the cornea due to invasion of an organism
4. Uveitis: an inflammation of the iris, ciliary body, and/or the choroid
5. Pterygium: segment of thickened conjunctiva that can extend over the cornea
6. Trachoma: viral infection of the lids and conjunctiva that can result in corneal ulceration and blindness
7. Chalazion: sterile cyst of the meibomian gland that causes inflammation of the lid; cyst remains when the inflammation subsides
8. Hordeolum: infection of a follicle of the eyelash commonly caused by staphylococcal organisms

B. Signs and symptoms
1. Subjective
   a. Photophobia (keratitis, uveitis)
   b. Blurred vision (keratitis, uveitis, trachoma)
   c. Pain (keratitis, uveitis)
   d. Burning and itching of eyes (conjunctivitis, blepharitis, hordeolum)
2. Objective
   a. Scaling and crust formation of lids (conjunctivitis, blepharitis, keratitis, uveitus)
   b. Swelling and redness (conjunctivitis, blepharitis, keratitis, uveitis, hordeolum)
   c. Tearing (keratitis)
   d. Ciliary injection (uveitis)
   e. Purulent drainage (conjunctivitis)

C. Treatment
1. Conjunctivitis, blepharitis, hordeolum
   a. Antibiotic ointments
   b. Warm compresses
2. Keratitis
   a. Culture analysis to determine causative organism
   b. Topical steroids and antibiotics
   c. If the cornea is badly damaged, corneal transplant
3. Uveitis
   a. Mydriatics to keep the iris at rest
   b. Topical steroids and antibiotics
   c. Dark glasses
4. Pterygium: surgical removal
5. Trachoma: oral antibiotics, usually tetracycline, for 3 to 5 weeks
6. Chalazion: usually surgical excision of cyst

D. Nursing care
1. Instruct the client on proper care of the eyes (hand washing, avoidance of rubbing)

2. Administer antibiotic ointment and instruct client in its use
3. Apply soaks as ordered
4. Prepare the client for surgery, if indicated
5. Provide care for the client who has undergone a corneal transplant (keratoplasty)
   a. Maintain bed rest for 1 or 2 days with the eyes bandaged
   b. Explain the importance of avoiding the Valsalva maneuver during healing
   c. Explain that healing may take up to 6 months because the circulatory supply of the cornea is decreased
6. Evaluate the client's response and revise plan as necessary

Tumors of the Eye

A. Etiology and pathophysiology
  1. May be benign or malignant; can form in or metastasize to the eye
  2. Retinoblastoma, a congenital malignant neoplasm found in children; spreads easily by extension to the brain
  3. Melanoma common in the iris and choroid; grows slowly but metastasizes to the liver and lungs
B. Signs and symptoms
  1. Subjective
     a. Headache
     b. Visual complaints
  2. Objective
     a. Increased injection of the conjunctiva
     b. Decreased vision
     c. In retinoblastoma, white pupillary reflex, strabismus, retinal detachment
C. Treatment
  1. Chemotherapy
  2. Radiation therapy
  3. Enucleation (surgical removal of the eye)
D. Nursing care
  1. Support the client and family as they attempt to cope with the diagnosis
  2. Observe for side effects of medical therapy and attempt to limit their effects
  3. Provide care for the client who has undergone an enucleation
     a. Maintain pressure dressings on the eye for 1 or 2 days to minimize hemorrhage
     b. Watch for signs of meningitis, which occurs as a complication, including headache or pain on the operative side
     c. Explain that monocularity results in the loss of depth perception, and activities that require this should be performed cautiously
     d. Explain that the artificial eye may be inserted when healing is complete, usually 6 to 8 weeks; support adaptation to changes in body image
  4. Support natural defense mechanisms; encourage intake of nutrient-dense foods, especially those rich in the immune-stimulating mineral selenium and vitamins A, C, and E, as well as protein
  5. Evaluate client's response and revise plan as necessary

Cataract

A. Etiology and pathophysiology
  1. Opacity of the crystalline lens or its capsule
  2. Results from injury, exposure to heat, heredity, aging, or congenital factors that cause a diminution of sight
B. Signs and symptoms
  1. Subjective
     a. Distortion of vision (e.g., haziness, cloudiness, diplopia)
     b. Photophobia
  2. Objective
     a. Progressive loss of vision
     b. Usual black pupil appears clouded, progressing to milky white appearance
C. Treatment
  1. Corrective lenses until the cataract matures enough for removal
  2. Surgical intervention to remove the opaque lens
     a. Preoperative preparation with mydriatics and ophthalmic antibiotics
     b. Antiemetics, analgesics, and stool softeners postoperatively
     c. Corrective lenses (contact lenses or glasses)
        (1) Contacts fitted approximately 3 months postoperatively
        (2) Temporary eyeglasses given soon after discharge, with the final prescription several weeks later
  3. Insertion of a lens implant sometimes at the time of surgery
D. Nursing care
  1. Instruct the client to prevent pressure on eyes by
     a. Not touching or rubbing the eyes
     b. Not closing the eyes tightly
     c. Avoiding coughing, sneezing, or bending from the waist (teach the client to open the mouth when coughing)
     d. Lying on the back or the nonoperated side
     e. Avoiding rapid head movements
     f. Avoiding straining at stool
  2. Instruct the client to request prescribed analgesics and antiemetics as required
  3. Administer stool softeners
  4. Provide side rails to help in turning and preventing falls
  5. Assist the client with ambulation because of distortions in depth perception and extremely blurred vision
  6. Provide an easily accessible call bell
  7. Reduce the amount of light and encourage the use of sunglasses when the eye patch is removed
  8. Provide a quiet environment to promote rest
  9. Avoid substances that might precipitate coughing or sneezing (e.g., pepper, talcum powder)
  10. Observe for signs of increased intraocular pressure (e.g., pain, restlessness, increased pulse rate)
  11. Observe for signs of infection (e.g., pain, changes in vital signs)
  12. Encourage deep breathing

13. Explain that depth perception will be altered but assure client that the corrective lenses will help to compensate for this distortion
14. Evaluate client's response and revise plan as necessary

Angle Closure Glaucoma

A. Etiology and pathophysiology
   1. Condition in which the pressure within the eyeball is higher than normal
   2. Closed angle of the drainage system of the canal of Schlemm prevents aqueous from reaching the lymph drainage spaces called the trabecular meshwork
B. Signs and symptoms
   1. Subjective
      a. Nausea
      b. Halos around lights
      c. Malaise
   2. Objective
      a. Gradual loss of peripheral vision
      b. Increased intraocular pressure (24 to 32 mm Hg) as measured with a tonometer
      c. Steamy cornea
      d. Conjunctival injection
C. Treatment
   1. Lowering the intraocular pressure with miotics or carbonic anhydrase inhibitors
   2. Surgical intervention to facilitate drainage of the aqueous humor is called an iridectomy; a surgical incision is made through the cornea to remove a portion of the iris to facilitate aqueous drainage
D. Nursing care
   1. Explain the importance of continued use of eye medications as ordered
   2. Explain the need for continued medical supervision for observation of intraocular pressure to ensure control of the disorder
   3. Teach the client to avoid exertion, stooping, heavy lifting, or wearing constricting clothing, since these increase intraocular pressure
   4. Evaluate client's response and revise plan as necessary

Detached Retina

A. Etiology and pathophysiology
   1. May result from trauma, the aging process, or cataract surgery; also seen in cases of myopia
   2. Retina separates from the choroid, and vitreous humor seeps behind the retina
B. Signs and symptoms
   1. Subjective
      a. Flashes of light
      b. Floaters
      c. Sensation of a veil in the line of sight
   2. Objective
      a. Retinal separation noted on ophthalmoscopy
      b. Assessment of visual loss
C. Treatment
   1. Bed rest, with the area of detachment in a dependent position to promote healing
   2. Tranquilizers to promote rest and reduce anxiety

3. Surgical intervention
   a. Cryosurgery: supercooled probe causes retinal scarring and healing of area
   b. Photocoagulation: laser beam through the pupil produces a retinal burn, which causes scarring of the involved area
   c. Scleral buckling: shortening of the sclera to force the choroid closer to the retina
D. Nursing care
   1. Keep the client on bed rest in position as ordered
   2. Provide the client with a call bell and answer promptly
   3. Observe for signs of hemorrhage postoperatively (severe pain, restlessness)
   4. Diminish lights in the room
   5. Explain that return to a sedentary occupation may occur in approximately 3 weeks and to a more active job in 6 to 8 weeks
   6. Evaluate client's response and revise plan as necessary

Macular Degeneration

A. Etiology and pathophysiology
   1. Growth of new blood vessels into the area of central retinal vision (macula) that obscures central vision
   2. Etiology is unknown but it is believed to be a vascular response, since the macula is normally devoid of vessels
   3. It is the leading cause of newly diagnosed legal blindness in persons over 65 in the United States
B. Signs and symptoms
   1. Subjective
      a. Distortion of straight lines
      b. Scotoma or intermittent blurring of central vision that worsens over time
   2. Objective
      a. Ophthalmoscopic examination reveals vessels on the macula
C. Treatment
   1. Laser photocoagulation in 10% of client's in early stage
   2. Steroid therapy
   3. Vitamin therapy, including zinc, has had questionable results
D. Nursing care
   1. Provide emotional support for client and family
   2. Institute safety measures to prevent injury
   3. Provide information related to medical management
   4. Evaluate client's response and revise plan as necessary

Chronic Otitis Media

A. Etiology and pathophysiology
   1. Chronic inflammatory disease of the middle ear; usually begins in childhood
   2. Related to perforation of the eardrum; may be associated with mastoiditis
B. Signs and symptoms
   1. Subjective
      a. Hearing loss
      b. Feeling of fullness within the ear

2. Objective
   a. Drainage from the ear that may be foul smelling
   b. Perforation of the eardrum apparent during examination with an otoscope
   c. Presence of cholesteatoma (epidermal inclusion cyst)
C. Treatment
   1. Systemic antibiotics
   2. Antibiotic eardrops
   3. Gentle irrigations to cleanse the ear
   4. Treatment of upper respiratory tract infection
D. Nursing care
   1. Instill antibiotics as prescribed
   2. Instruct the client to report headache or stiff neck immediately, since this may indicate complications of meningitis
   3. Evaluate client's response and revise plan as necessary

Mastoiditis

A. Etiology and pathophysiology
   1. Disease of the mastoid process; may be acute or chronic
   2. Generally occurs secondary to otitis media
   3. Disruption of the intercellular construction of the bone; suppurative mastoiditis
B. Signs and symptoms
   1. Subjective
      a. Tenderness over the mastoid process
      b. Headache and ear pain
   2. Objective
      a. Drainage from the ear
      b. Elevated temperature
C. Treatment
   1. Antibiotics: eardrops or systemic
   2. Cleansing of the ear
   3. Surgical intervention
      a. Mastoidectomy (radical or modified)
      b. Tympanoplasty
D. Nursing care
   1. Instruct the client to seek treatment for any ear infections
   2. Provide care associated with mastoidectomy
      a. Cleanse the postauricular area preoperatively
      b. Postoperatively reinforce the dressing over drain site from the mastoid
      c. Observe for facial paralysis and report, since this may indicate damage to facial nerve
      d. Utilize safety precautions such as side rails to prevent injury to the client who is experiencing vertigo
   3. Evaluate client's response and revise plan as necessary

Otosclerosis

A. Etiology and pathophysiology
   1. Fixation of the stapes, preventing transmission of auditory vibrations to the inner ear (conduction deafness)
   2. Cause unknown, but incidence higher in females; heredity a factor
B. Signs and symptoms
   1. Subjective
      a. Loss of hearing
      b. Ringing or buzzing in the ears
   2. Objective
      a. Use of a tuning fork shows bone conduction better than air conduction (Rinne test)
      b. Presence of spongy bone in the labyrinth
C. Treatment
   1. Hearing aids to amplify sound
   2. Stapedectomy: removal of the diseased portion of the stapes, and replacement with a prosthetic implant to conduct vibrations from the middle to inner ear
D. Nursing care
   1. Position postoperatively according to the physician's preference
      a. Lying on the operated side facilitates drainage
      b. Lying on the nonoperated side helps prevent displacement of the graft
   2. Instruct the client to alter position gradually to prevent vertigo
   3. Question the client about pain, headache, vertigo, or unusual sensations in ear and report
   4. Instruct the client to avoid sneezing and blowing nose, swimming, showers, and flying until permitted by the physician; if the client must sneeze, instruct to keep the mouth open to equalize pressure in the ear
   5. Explain that because of edema from surgery and the presence of packing, hearing will be diminished but will improve
   6. Evaluate client's response and revise plan as necessary

Ménière's Disease

A. Etiology and pathophysiology
   1. Chronic disease of the inner ear causing severe vertigo
   2. Cause unknown, but follows infections of the middle ear or trauma
   3. Incidence highest in males between the ages of 40 and 60 years
B. Signs and symptoms
   1. Subjective
      a. Vertigo
      b. Nausea
      c. Headache
      d. Sensitivity to loud sounds
      e. Sensory hearing loss, usually unilateral
      f. Tinnitus
   2. Objective
      a. Vomiting
      b. Diaphoresis
      c. Nystagmus during attacks
      d. Bárány's caloric test (reveals diminished or absent response)
      e. Weber test and auditory testing document hearing loss
C. Treatment
   1. Diuretics
   2. Antihistamines

3. Surgical destruction of the labyrinth or vestibular nerve, which will cause deafness in that ear
4. Salt-free diet combined with administration of ammonium chloride

D. Nursing care
1. Support emotionally
2. To prevent the onset of symptoms, encourage the client not to move rapidly
3. Protect from injury during attack; use side rails; encourage the client to lie down during an attack
4. Instruct the client to pull off the road if driving when an attack occurs
5. Care for the client following a total labyrinthectomy
   a. Maintain bed rest in the presence of severe vertigo
   b. Instruct the client to avoid sudden movements
   c. Explain that Bell's palsy may occur postoperatively but will subside within a few months
6. Encourage diet rich in nutrient-dense foods such as fruits, vegetables, whole grains, and legumes to improve and maintain nutritional status and prevent possible drug-induced nutrient deficiencies; foods high in salt such as salted meats and fish, cheese, condensed milk, carrots, and spinach should be avoided
7. Evaluate client's response and revise plan as necessary

Integumentary System
REVIEW OF ANATOMY AND PHYSIOLOGY OF THE INTEGUMENTARY SYSTEM
Functions

A. Prevents loss of body fluids
B. Protects deeper tissues from pathogenic organisms, noxious chemicals, and short wavelength ultraviolet radiation
C. Helps regulate body temperature
D. Provides location for sensory reception of touch, pressure, temperature, pain, wetness, tickle, etc.
E. Assists in vitamin D synthesis
F. Plays a minor excretory role

Anatomy

A. Epidermis: contains no blood or lymphatic vessels; cells nourished by diffusion from underlying dermal papillae
1. Layers from the dermis outward
   a. Stratum germinativum: cell layers undergoing mitosis; gradually pushed to surface to replace those exfoliated
   b. Stratum granulosum: granule-filled cells in several layers; contain keratohyalin, intermediate in keratin formation; most free nerve endings of epidermis are here; contains epidermal pigment
   c. Stratum lucidum: translucent layers; nails are outgrowths of this layer
   d. Stratum corneum: upper horny layer of flat, dead cells that exfoliate rapidly, taking bacterial flora with them; responsible for variations in skin thickness
2. Melanocytes of the lower epidermis produce melanin, which colors skin

3. Exceptional epidermal regions
   a. Conjunctiva: epidermis so thin it is transparent
   b. Lips: epidermis very thin and highly vascular, which accounts for redness

B. Dermis
1. Extremely vascular fabric of collagen and elastic fibers woven to provide strength and flexibility
2. Upper papillary layer joined to epidermis by upward projecting papillae; vascular loops in papillae nourish overlying epidermis; contain abundant touch receptors; double-row papillae in finger pads and palms and soles give great strength against shearing stress, provide fingerprint pattern as unique arrangement of ridges projected to epidermal surface, and allow hands and feet to grip surfaces
3. Deeper reticular layer contains loose arrangement of connective tissue gradually merging with subcutaneous fatty layer (superficial fascia)
4. Skin stretched beyond certain limits (e.g., during pregnancy) may rupture dermal collagen and elastic fibers; consequent scar tissue repair produces striae gravidarum

C. Glands
1. Eccrine: tubular coiled glands deep in dermis; duct rises straight through dermis and spirals through epidermis, opening in sweat pore on crest of skin ridges; secretes clear fluid
2. Apocrine: scent glands; very large branched tubular glands found in the axillary, mammary, and genital areas that produce an originally odorless secretion rapidly metabolized by bacteria to produce typical body odors
3. Ceruminous: wax glands in external auditory canal; large branched glands frequently opening into hair sheaths along with sebaceous glands
4. Sebaceous: small saclike glands lacking innervation, usually forming close to hairs and opening into upper portion of hair follicle; form independent of hairs at corners of mouth and in eyelids as meibomian glands; absent on palms and soles, accounting for wrinkling of these areas after lengthy immersion in water
5. Mammary: milk-secreting, compound tubular alveolar glands developing to full extent only during pregnancy

D. Hair
1. Long strands of tightly compacted and cemented, dead and keratinized cells sheathed in hair follicles (tubes of epidermal cells plunged obliquely into dermis surrounded by dermal connective tissue sheath)
2. About the same number of follicles in males and females; hormones stimulate differential growth
3. Determines appearance; round (straight hair); ribbon shaped (kinky hair); alternately round and oval (wavy hair)
4. Arrector pili (smooth muscle) attached at one end to connective sheath in middle of the hair follicle and at other end to the dermal papillary region of the dermis; on contraction, elevates hair and surrounding skin but depresses skin overlying the der-

mal papillary attachment point; result is "goose-flesh"; such contraction also stimulates sebaceous gland secretion

Tissue Repair

A. Inflammation
1. Vascular changes: initially there is vasoconstriction (5 to 10 minutes); vessel walls lined with leukocytes (margination); then vasodilation with increased blood flow and increased vessel permeability (effects of histamine from mast cells, kinins, and prostaglandins); lymphatics become plugged with fibrin to wall off damaged area
2. Polymorphonuclear and mononuclear leukocytes leave the vessels (diapedesis) and phagocytize foreign substances
3. Chronic inflammation: longer-lived mononuclear leukocytes (macrophages) predominate, and fibroblasts deposit a wall of collagen around each group of macrophages and foreign substances; stage of granuloma formation
B. Fibroplasia
1. Epithelization: epithelial cells of the epidermis begin to cover tissue defect through migration of basal cells across wound defect with continued mitosis in intact epithelium
2. Deep in the wound, fibroblasts synthesize collagen and ground substance; process begins about fourth or fifth day and continues for 2 to 4 weeks
3. Capillaries regenerate by endothelial budding; tissue becomes red
4. Fibrin plugs are lysed
C. Scar maturation
1. Collagen fibers rearranged into a stronger, more organized pattern
2. Scar remodels, sometimes for months and years due to collagen turnover; if collagen synthesis exceeds breakdown, a hypertrophic scar or keloid forms; if collagen breakdown exceeds synthesis, scar gradually softens and fades
3. Wound contracture: contraction of wound margins begins about 5 days after injury; caused by fibroblast migration into the wound along the lines of fibrin strands initially deposited in the wound; assists in closing the defect but may also result in contractures that can be debilitating

REVIEW OF PHYSICAL PRINCIPLES RELATED TO THE INTEGUMENTARY SYSTEM
Principle of Mechanics

Friction: epidermal ridges resulting from upthrusting dermal papillae provide palms of hands, fingers, and soles of feet with friction surfaces for grasping and walking

Principle of Physical Properties of Matter

Elasticity: molecular structure of elastin, a protein, permits stretching of skin under tension and the ability to snap back to its original shape when tension is relieved; less elastic properties of collagen give skin its strength to resist tearing and shearing forces

Principles of Heat

A. Conduction: heat brought to the dermis by blood passes through the epidermis; allows for elimination of excess heat
B. Evaporation: sweat evaporating cools the body surface and acts to drain heat from the body interior

Principle of Light

Radiation absorption
A. Ultraviolet absorption by melanin protects the skin and underlying structures from damage
B. Quantity and degree of dispersed melanin, which absorbs visible light wavelengths differently, produces different skin colors

REVIEW OF CHEMICAL PRINCIPLES RELATED TO THE INTEGUMENTARY SYSTEM
Solutions (Solubility)

A. Fat-soluble substances have a greater tendency to penetrate skin than do water-soluble substances
Example: Oleoresins of poison ivy, fat-soluble vitamins (A, D, E), and insecticides are absorbed, whereas water is repelled
B. Fat-soluble (oily) substances secreted by the meibomian glands (modified sebaceous glands) of the eyelids, which are not capable of mixing with water; act as barriers to prevent tears from constantly flooding over lower eyelid

Water

Dehydration of epidermal cells leaves water-insoluble keratin impregnated in surface and corneum providing a water-resistant protective barrier

PHARMACOLOGY RELATED TO INTEGUMENTARY SYSTEM DISORDERS
Antibiotics and Antifungals

See Pharmacology related to infection

Pediculocides/Scabicides

A. Description
1. Used to destroy parasitic arthropods
2. Act at the parasite's nerve cell membrane to produce death of the organism
3. Available in topical preparations
B. Examples
1. benzyl benzoate lotion (Scabanca)
2. crotamiton (Eurax)
3. gamma benzene hexachloride (Kwell)
4. malathion (Prioderm lotion)
C. Major side effects
1. Skin irritation (hypersensitivity)
2. Contact dermatitis (local irritation)
D. Nursing care
1. Inspect skin, particularly the scalp, for scabies and pediculosis before and after treatment
2. Use gown, gloves, and cap to prevent spread of parasitic arthropods
3. Keep linen of an infected client separate and sterilized to prevent reinfection
4. Assess for skin irritation during therapy

5. Assess source of infection; provide client and family education
6. Avoid drug contact with the eyes and mucous membranes
7. Evaluate client's response to medication and understanding of teaching

Topical Antiinfectives

A. Description
    1. Agents that act on the bacterial cell wall or alter cellular function to produce bactericidal effects
    2. Available in topical preparations
B. Examples
    1. silver sulfadiazine (Silvadene)
    2. Mafenide acetate (Sulfamylon)
    3. Silver nitrate 0.5% solution
C. Major side effects
    1. Silver sulfadiazine: skin irritation; hemolysis in clients with G-6-PD deficiency
    2. Mafenide acetate: metabolic acidosis; burning sensation when first applied
    3. Silver nitrate: electrolyte imbalance; brown/black discoloration produced on contact
D. Nursing care
    1. Adhere to strict surgical asepsis
    2. Assess burns and the client's general condition during therapy
    3. Provide comprehensive nursing burn care; offer emotional support
    4. Cleanse and debride prior to application
    5. Apply prescribed medications
        a. Silver sulfadiazine
            (1) Apply to a thickness of ¹⁄₁₆ inch
            (2) Monitor G-6-PD level before initiation of treatment
        b. Mafenide acetate: assess client for signs of acidosis during course of therapy
        c. Silver nitrate
            (1) Apply dressings soaked in silver nitrate
            (2) Avoid contact with the drug
            (3) Assess for signs of electrolyte imbalance during course of therapy
    6. Evaluate client's response to medication and understanding of teaching

Antipruritics

A. Description
    1. Used to relieve itching and promote comfort
    2. Act by inhibiting sensory nerve impulse conduction at the local site and by exerting a local anesthetic effect
    3. Available in topical preparations
B. Examples
    1. benzocaine (Anbesol, Solarcaine)
    2. lidocaine HCl (Xylocaine)
    3. phenol
    4. pramoxine HCl (Tronolane)
    5. tars
    6. tetracaine HCl (Pontocaine)
C. Major side effects
    1. Skin irritation (hypersensitivity)
    2. Contact dermatitis (local irritation)

D. Nursing care
    1. Assess the lesion, including location and size
    2. Assess for local irritation during course of therapy
    3. Question client regarding relief obtained from treatment
    4. Discourage client from scratching; keep nails well trimmed
    5. Advise medical follow-up, since these medications provide only temporary relief of symptoms
    6. Evaluate client's response to medication and understanding of teaching

Antiinflammatory Agents

A. Description
    1. Reduce signs of inflammation
    2. Produce vasoconstriction, which decreases swelling and pruritis
    3. Available in topical preparations
B. Examples
    1. betamethasone (Celestone)
    2. betamethasone valerate (Valisone)
    3. dexamethasone (Decaderm; Hexadrol)
    4. fluocinonide (Lidex)
    5. hydrocortisone (Acticort)
    6. triamcinolone acetonide (Aristocort, Kenalog, Trimalone)
C. Major side effects
    1. Skin irritation (hypersensitivity)
    2. Contact dermatitis (local irritation)
    3. Adrenal insufficiency if absorbed systemically (suppression of hypothalamic-pituitary-adrenal axis)
D. Nursing care
    1. Assess lesions for color, location, and size
    2. Protect skin from scratching or rubbing
    3. Use appropriate topical agent
        a. Lotions: axillae; groin
        b. Creams: draining lesions
        c. Ointments: dry lesions
    4. Avoid contact with eyes
    5. Cleanse skin before application
    6. Utilize occlusive dressings if ordered
    7. Assess client for signs of sensitivity during course of therapy
    8. Evaluate client's response to medication and understanding of teaching

Dermal Agent

A. Description
    1. Inhibits keratinization and sebaceous gland function to improve cystic acne and reduce sebum excretion
    2. Available preparation: oral
B. Example
    1. Isotretinoin (Accutane)
C. Major side effects
    1. Visual disturbances (corneal opacities)
    2. Decreased night vision (vitamin A toxicity—effect on visual rods)
    3. Papilledema, headache (pseudotumor cerebri)
    4. Hepatic dysfunction (hepatotoxicity)
    5. Cheilitis (vitamin A toxicity)

6. Pruritis, skin fragility (dryness)
7. Hypertriglyceridemia (increased plasma triglycerides)

D. Nursing care
1. Assess visual and hepatic status prior to administration
2. Monitor blood lipids prior to and during therapy
3. Instruct client to:
   a. Avoid pregnancy during and for 1 month after therapy
   b. Use contraception
   c. Avoid vitamin A supplements
   d. Side effects are reversible when therapy is discontinued
4. Evaluate client's response to medication and understanding of teaching

PROCEDURES RELATED TO THE INTEGUMENTARY SYSTEM
Biopsy

A. Definition: a sample of tissue generally 3 mm or more is removed by use of a sharp, circular punch; when more tissue is needed, a wedge is excised through an incision
B. Nursing care
1. Offer emotional support to client
2. Assist the physician and help to maintain strict surgical aseptic technique
3. Place specimen in appropriate container and send to pathology laboratory for analysis
4. Use surgically aseptic technique when dressing wound at biopsy site
5. Evaluate client's response to procedure

Cultures of the Skin

A. Definition
1. To determine the presence of fungi on the skin, the skin is covered with a 10% potassium hydroxide solution prior to scraping for microscopic examination
2. To determine bacterial infection of the skin, adequate tissue sampling is obtained using a sterile applicator or swab
3. Organisms obtained from the skin are observed in the laboratory so that identification may be made
B. Nursing care
1. Explain procedure to client
2. Allay anxiety and offer reassurance
3. Obtain samples using surgically aseptic technique prior to instituting antibiotic therapy
4. Notify physician of results so that appropriate therapy may be instituted
5. Evaluate client's response to procedure

Skin Grafts

A. Definition
1. Covering of denuded tissue with skin to prevent infection and loss of body fluids, promote healing, and prevent contractures
2. Applied between the fifth and twenty-first day, depending on extent of the burn

3. Types of skin grafts
   a. Xenografts: skin from animals, usually pigs (porcine xenograft)
   b. Homografts: skin from another person
   c. Autografts: skin from another part of the client's body
      (1) Mesh graft: machine used to mesh skin obtained from a donor site so it can be stretched to cover a larger area of burn
      (2) Postage stamp graft: earlier method of accomplishing the same goal as a mesh graft; a small amount of skin is used to cover a larger area; the donor skin is cut into small pieces and applied to the burn
      (3) Sheet grafting: large strips of skin placed over the burn as close together as possible
B. Nursing care
1. Explain procedure; obtain a written consent
2. Prepare the donor site carefully
3. Postoperatively keep donor sites (which are covered with a nonadherent dressing and wrapped in an absorbent gauze) dry using a heating lamp or hair dryer as ordered; remove absorbent gauze as ordered; nonadherent dressing will separate as healing occurs
4. Monitor the grafts which are generally left with a light pressure dressing for approximately 3 days; after the graft has "taken," roll cotton-tipped applicators gently over the graft to remove underlying exudate; allowed to remain, exudate could promote infection, which could prevent the graft from adhering
5. Observe for foul-smelling drainage, temperature elevation, and other signs of infection
6. Evaluate client's response to procedure

Wood's Light Examination

A. Definition: the skin is viewed under ultraviolet light through special glass (Wood's glass) to identify superficial infections of the skin
B. Nursing care
1. Explain procedure to client
2. Reassure client that procedure is noninvasive and painless
3. Evaluate client's response to procedure

NURSING PROCESS FOR CLIENTS WITH INTEGUMENTARY SYSTEM DISORDERS
Probable Nursing Diagnoses Based on Assessment

A. Impaired skin integrity related to disruption of the skin surface
B. Potential for infection related to disruption of the skin surface
C. Potential for injury related to
   1. Altered mobility
   2. Pain
D. Fluid volume excess related to
   1. Response to stress
   2. Disease process
   3. Therapeutic modalities

E. Fluid volume deficit related to
   1. Excess loss via skin or kidney
   2. Fluid shift into interstitial spaces
F. Ineffective thermoregulation related to interrupted skin integrity
G. Impaired physical mobility related to
   1. Pain
   2. Contractures
   3. Scar tissue
H. Pain related to irritation/exposure of nerve endings
I. Altered peripheral tissue perfusion related to interrupted skin integrity
J. Disturbance in body image related to altered appearance

Nursing Care for Clients with Integumentary System Disorders

See Nursing care under each specific disease

MAJOR DISEASES
Primary Skin Lesions

A. Macule: flat circumscribed area from 1 to several centimeters in size, without elevation (freckle, flat pigmented moles)
B. Papule: raised circumscribed area less than 1 cm in size (acne)
C. Nodule: raised solid mass that extends into the dermis and is 1 to 2 cm in size (pigmented nevi)
D. Tumor: solid raised mass that extends into the dermis and is over 2 cm in size (dermatofibroma)
E. Wheal: flattened collection of fluid 1 mm to several centimeters in size (mosquito bites)
F. Vesicle: raised collection of fluid less than 1 cm in size (chickenpox, herpes simplex)
G. Bulla: fluid-filled vesicle over 1 cm in size (second-degree burn, pemphigus)
H. Pustule: vesicle or bulla filled with pus, 1 mm to 1 cm in size (acne vulgaris)
I. Cyst: mass of fluid-filled tissue that extends to the subcutaneous tissues or dermis, over 1 cm in size (epidermoid cyst)

Secondary Skin Lesions

A. Fissure: a linear crack in the skin (athlete's foot)
B. Erosion: nonbleeding loss of superficial dermis (chickenpox rupture)
C. Ulcer: deep loss of skin surface which may bleed (stasis ulcer)
D. Crust: dried residue from blood or pus (impetigo)
E. Scale: flake of exfoliated epidermis (dandruff)

Burns

A. Etiology and pathophysiology
   1. Thermal, radiation, and chemical burns: cause cell destruction and result in depletion of fluid and electrolytes
   2. Extent of the fluid and electrolyte loss directly related to extent and degree of the burn
      a. First degree (also known as partial thickness): erythema, edema, and pain; fluid loss slight, especially if less than 15% of body surface is involved
      b. Second degree (also known as deep dermal): erythema, pain, vesicles, with oozing; fluid loss slight to moderate, especially if less than 15% of the body surface is involved
      c. Third degree (also known as full thickness): charred or pearly white, dry skin, absence of pain; fluid loss usually severe, especially if more than 2% of the body surface is involved
   3. Classification of second- and third-degree burns
      a. Minor burns: no involvement of hands, face, or genitalia; total burn area does not exceed 15%, and third-degree burns do not exceed 2% of body area
      b. Major burns: involvement of 15% to 30% of body; but third-degree burns do not exceed 10% of body area
      c. Critical burns: involvement exceeds 30% of body surface; this classification is also used if the client has a preexisting chronic health problem, is under 18 months or over 50 years of age, or has additional injuries
   4. Pulmonary injury should be suspected if two of the following factors are present and expected if three or all four are present
      a. Hair in nostrils singed
      b. The client was trapped in a closed space
      c. Face, nose, and lips burned
      d. Initial blood sample contains carboxyhemoglobin
   5. Extent of trauma can be estimated by rule of nines or other burn area chart
   6. Curling's ulcer may occur after a burn
      a. The client may complain of gastric discomfort, or there may be profuse bleeding
      b. Usually occurs by end of the first week after a burn
      c. Treatment essentially the same as for a gastric ulcer; however, mortality following surgical repair is high because of the client's debilitated state
B. Signs and symptoms
   1. Subjective
      a. Extreme anxiety
      b. Restlessness
      c. Pain, severity depending on the type of burn
      d. Paresthesia
      e. Disorientation
   2. Objective
      a. Changes in appearance of skin indicate degree of burn (see etiology and pathophysiology)
      b. Hematuria; blood hemolysis with subsequent rise in plasma hemoglobin may occur with third-degree burns
      c. Elevated hematocrit as a result of fluid loss
      d. Electrolyte imbalance
      e. Presence of symptoms of hypovolemic shock caused by circulatory failure resulting from seepage of water, plasma, proteins, and electrolytes into burned area
      f. Presence of symptoms of neurogenic shock (symptoms similar to hypovolemic shock) caused by the fright, terror, hysteria, and pain involved in the situation
      g. Disorientation and confusion may be present

C. Treatment
1. Tetanus toxoid immediately
2. IV replacement therapy at a rate of 250 ml per hour to achieve an intake of between 6000 and 7000 ml for the first 24 hours (half of total IV solutions will be an electrolyte solution such as Ringer's lactate and half will be plasma or plasma substitute)
3. Reduction of total IV solutions during second 24 hours depending on the urinary output, blood work, and central venous pressure
4. Foley catheter; monitor the urinary output and specific gravity hourly to observe kidney functioning and determine fluid replacement
5. Insert a central venous pressure (CVP) line and take an hourly reading to monitor circulating fluid volume
6. Vital signs monitored every 15 minutes
7. Serum electrolytes and blood gases to observe for levels and assist in deciding replacement therapy
8. IPPB and continuous oxygen to assist with respirations
9. Tracheostomy if laryngeal edema occurs
10. Reverse isolation
11. Permit nothing by mouth except mineral water for first 24 to 48 hours; allow clear liquids as tolerated after 2 days; then place on high-protein, high-carbohydrate, high-fat, high-vitamin diet as tolerated
12. Daily Hubbard tank baths after the fifth day; use antibiotic ointment and Kling dressing
13. Intervene surgically to perform debridement and skin grafting (see Procedures), promote healing, and limit contractures
14. Mechanical debridement (wet to dry dressings) or enzymatic debridement (e.g., Travase ointment) may be used
15. IV and topical antibiotics to limit infection (Keflin and penicillin intravenously; Sulfamylon ointment; gentamicin; silver nitrate solution; and silver sulfadiazine)
16. Narcotics to reduce pain and sedatives to decrease anxiety, given IV or orally due to decreased muscle absorption
D. Nursing care
1. Observe vital signs, central venous pressure, intake and output, and specific gravity as ordered; notify the physician if deviations occur or if output falls below 30 ml or rises above 50 ml per hour
2. Maintain patency of the Foley catheter to ascertain the correct information regarding fluid balance
3. Make certain that blood electrolyte and gas tests are performed and results are available
4. Administer fluid and electrolytes as ordered
5. Observe for signs of electrolyte imbalance (calcium, potassium, and sodium) and metabolic acidosis
6. Observe for signs of tracheal edema (dyspnea, stridor)
7. Elevate head of the bed
8. Encourage to cough and deep breathe
9. Maintain reverse isolation to prevent infection of burned areas
10. Use sterile technique (irrigating drainage tubes, dressings, and bed linens)
11. Administer tetanus toxoid as ordered
12. Administer IV and topical antibiotics as ordered
13. Observe for signs of infection (rising temperature and white blood cell count, odor)
14. Support the joints and extremities in a functional position
15. Support the client while turning
16. Keep room temperature warm and humidity high
17. Observe for symptoms of stress ulcer; give ordered drugs to decrease or neutralize HCl
18. Provide small, frequent feedings; diet should be high in protein, carbohydrate, vitamins, and minerals, moderate in fat, with adequate calories for protein sparing
19. Give medication for pain as ordered and particularly before dressing change
20. Expect the client to express negative feelings about burns, and accept it
21. Explain need for staff wearing gowns and masks
22. Give realistic reassurance
23. Evaluate client's response and revise plan as necessary

Acne Vulgaris

A. Etiology and pathophysiology
1. Hormonal activity produces hyperkeratosis of the follicular orifices, leading to blockage of secretions and the subsequent formation of fatty plugs known as blackheads (comedones)
2. When a blackhead (comedo) forms, the sebaceous gland involved becomes hypertrophic and infected
3. Cysts and nodules form, leaving scars
4. Most common among adolescents
B. Signs and symptoms
1. Subjective
a. Pain when sebaceous glands become infected
b. Depression
2. Objective
a. Blackheads on skin (open comedones)
b. Whiteheads on skin (closed comedones)
C. Treatment
1. Mechanical removal with a comedo extractor
2. Abrasive cleaners, astringents, and bacteriostatic creams
3. Ultraviolet light as a peeling agent
4. Cryotherapy to produce desquamation of skin
5. Oral administration of antibiotics such as tetracycline
6. Intralesional injections of corticosteroids
7. Dermabrasion to improve the scars but not to cure the condition
a. Instrument that functions at a high speed with a cylinder of wire or sandpaper at its end
b. Epidermis and some dermis are removed at high points of the scars so they do not appear as deep
c. Local anesthesia for treatment of small areas; general is indicated for large areas
D. Nursing care
1. Promote good hygienic care when instructing how to wash areas and apply topical medications
2. Discuss the use of water-base cosmetics to prevent clogging of pores

3. Instruct the client how to take medications
4. Emphasize importance of diet which should be high in fruits, vegetables, whole grains, and legumes and low in fats and animal foods; vitamin A is essential to promote proper epidermal function and status
5. Provide postoperative care following dermabrasion
   a. Apply ointment to lubricate skin and remove crust from area
   b. Observe serum draining from the area and report copious amounts of drainage to the surgeon
   c. Explain that the feeling of being sunburned is normal after dermabrasion
6. Evaluate client's response and revise plan as necessary

Contact Dermatitis

A. Etiology and pathophysiology
   1. Results from contact with a substance that reacts with the protein in the skin to form an antigen in a sensitized client
   2. Antigen causes proliferation of lymphocytes, and the interaction of these factors causes eczematous changes
   3. Common causes: poison ivy, hair dye containing paraphenylenediamine, benzocaine, soaps, cements, insecticides, rubber compounds
B. Signs and symptoms
   1. Subjective
      a. Discomfort
      b. Pruritus
   2. Objective
      a. Erythema at the point of contact
      b. Vesicles and papules
      c. Edema
      d. Thickening of the skin and scaling
C. Treatment
   1. Identification of the allergen through patch testing; a suspected allergen is applied to the unbroken skin; the skin is observed for erythema, papules, and vesicles in 24 to 48 hours
   2. Antihistamines, antipruritics
   3. Topical corticosteroids
D. Nursing care
   1. Instruct the client to avoid situations or substances that involve the identified allergen
   2. Maintain cool environment, provide tepid baths, and trim finger nails to help control injury from scratching
   3. Provide diversional activities
   4. If topical corticosteroids are ordered, apply occlusive plastic dressing (Saran Wrap) over the ointment or lotion as ordered
   5. Evaluate client's response and revise plan as necessary

Cellulitus

A. Etiology and pathophysiology
   1. Infection of upper layers of the dermis and subcutaneous tissue
   2. Usually caused by streptococcal or staphylococcal organisms
   3. Spreads along connective tissue planes

B. Signs and symptoms
   1. Subjective
      a. Pain
      b. Itching
   2. Objective
      a. Swelling
      b. Redness
      c. Warmth
      d. Leukocytosis
C. Treatment
   1. IV, IM, or oral antibiotic therapy following cultures of the area
   2. Rest with elevation of extremity
   3. Hot compresses
D. Nursing care
   1. Use proper aseptic technique when cleaning area
   2. Use isolation precautions if necessary; see Infection for additional information
   3. Andminister analgesics as ordered
   4. Evaluate client's response and revise plan as necessary

Psoriasis

A. Etiology and pathophysiology
   1. Inflammatory disease that may be acute or chronic
   2. Genetic predisposition is thought to be a factor
   3. Uncommon in blacks
   4. Injury to the skin and psychologic stress appear to be factors in flare-ups
B. Signs and symptoms
   1. Subjective
      a. Mild pruritus (severe if in skin folds)
      b. If psoriatic arthritis is present, joint pain and stiffness
   2. Objective
      a. Bright red, well-demarcated plaque covered with silvery scales, usually on knees, elbows, and scalp
      b. Stippling and thickening of the nails
      c. Inflammatory changes of the joints if psoriatic arthritis is present
      d. Uric acid levels may be elevated
C. Treatment
   1. Exposure to solar or ultraviolet irradiation
   2. Application of coal tar ointment or antiinflammatory topical agents
   3. Systemic corticosteroid therapy may be used in severe cases
   4. Methotrexate may also be used for severe psoriasis
   5. Exposure to black light combined with oral administration of methoxsalen useful in treatment of intractable cases
D. Nursing care
   1. Encourage ventilation of feelings about changes in body image; show acceptance
   2. Assess lesions and the response to therapy
   3. Determine factors linked to flare-ups; the client may need help coping with stressful situations
   4. Instruct the client to use a soft brush to remove scales when bathing
   5. If occlusive dressings are ordered with topical ointment, use Saran Wrap, plastic bags, or rubber gloves

6. Encourage diet rich in nutrient-dense foods such as fruits, vegetables, whole grains, and legumes to improve and maintain nutritional status and prevent possible drug-induced nutrient deficiencies; vitamin A is essential to promote improved epidermal status
7. Evaluate client's response and revise plan as necessary

Pemphigus

A. Etiology and pathophysiology
   1. Potentially fatal skin disease
   2. Occurs only in adults
   3. Cause unknown
B. Signs and symptoms
   1. Subjective
      a. Debilitation
      b. Malaise
      c. Pain associated with lesions
   2. Objective
      a. Bullae on normal skin and mucosa
      b. Separation of epidermis caused by rubbing skin (Nikolsky's sign)
      c. Acantholysis (changes in intercellular connections of the epidermis) evident on microscopic examination
      d. Leukocytosis, eosinophilia
      e. Foul-smelling discharge
C. Treatment
   1. Oral corticosteroids
   2. Antibiotics for secondary infections
   3. Topical treatment for relief of symptoms
      a. Potassium permanganate baths
      b. Oatmeal baths
D. Nursing care
   1. Administer steroids with antacid or milk to prevent gastric irritation (see Pharmacology)
   2. Monitor intake and output (NaCl and fluid are lost through the skin)
   3. Test urinary sugar and acetone levels, since the client is receiving large doses of corticosteroids
   4. Protect from infection
   5. Watch for signs of infection such as elevated temperature and WBC
   6. Provide oral hygiene and increased fluid intake to soothe oral lesions
   7. Encourage ventilation of feelings; clients are often discouraged and depressed
   8. Encourage diet rich in nutrient-dense foods such as fruits, vegetables, whole grains, and legumes to improve and maintain nutritional status and compensate for nutrient interactions of corticosteroid and other treatment medications; vitamin A is essential to promote improved epidermal status
   9. Evaluate client's response and revise plan as necessary

Cancer of the Skin

A. Etiology and pathophysiology
   1. Most common cancer; however, early detection and slow progression make the cure rate high
   2. Exposure to the sun, irritating chemicals, and chronic friction implicated; more common in persons with fair complexions
   3. Types
      a. Basal cell carcinoma: generally located on the face and appears as a waxy nodule that may have telangiectasias visible; the most common type of skin cancer, but metastasis is rare
      b. Squamous cell carcinoma: develops rapidly and may metastasize through local lymph nodes; may develop secondarily to precancerous lesions such as keratosis and leukoplakia and is found most frequently on upper extremities and face, which are exposed to the sun; it appears as a small red nodular lesion
      c. Malignant melanoma: most serious type and arises from the pigment producing melanocytes; the color of the lesion may vary greatly (white, flesh, gray, brown, blue, black); changes in size, color, sensation, or characteristics of a mole suggest the possibility of malignant melanoma; metastasis via blood can be extensive
B. Signs and symptoms
   1. Subjective
      a. Pruritus may or may not be present
      b. Localized soreness
   2. Objective
      a. Change in color, size, or shape of preexisting lesion
      b. Oozing, bleeding, or crusting
      c. Biopsy of tumor reveals type of cancer
      d. Lymphadenopathy if metastasis has occurred
C. Treatment
   1. Surgical excision of the lesion and surrounding tissue
   2. Chemosurgery, which involves the use of zinc chloride to fix the cells before they are dissected
   3. Cryosurgery utilizing liquid nitrogen to destroy the tumor cells by freezing
   4. Radiation (malignant melanoma does not respond well to this mode of treatment)
   5. Chemotherapy
   6. Nonspecific immunostimulants such as BCG vaccine
D. Nursing care
   1. Assess skin lesions
   2. Instruct the client to examine moles for changes and have those subject to chronic irritation (bra or belt line) removed
   3. Encourage limitation of exposure to sun
   4. Emphasize continued medical supervision
   5. Use surgical aseptic technique when caring for surgical site
   6. Encourage verbalization; maintain a therapeutic environment
   7. Provide care to the client receiving radiation
      a. Observe skin for local reaction
      b. Avoid use of ointments or powders containing metals
   8. Provide care related to specific chemotherapeutic agents (see Pharmacology related to neoplastic disorders)

9. Support natural defense mechanisms of client; encourage intake of nutrient-dense foods with emphasis on fruits, vegetables, whole grains, and legumes, especially those high in the immune-stimulating nutrients selenium and vitamins A, C, and E; Beta-carotene has been associated with prevention of skin cancer
10. Evaluate client's response and revise plan as necessary

Herpes Zoster (Shingles)

A. Etiology and pathophysiology
1. Acute viral infection of nerve structures caused by the varicella-zoster virus
2. Inflammation occurs along the pathway of one or more peripheral sensory nerves
3. Occurs in clients who have not had chickenpox and are exposed to an affected individual
4. May frequently occur with other debilitating illness; (e.g., tuberculosis, Hodgkin's disease)
B. Signs and symptoms
1. Subjective
a. Malaise
b. Headache
c. Pain
d. Paresthesias
2. Objective
a. Painful, pruritic vesicles arranged along the pathway of the involved nerves
b. Stains made from lesion exudate isolate the organism
C. Treatment
1. Medications for pain, relaxation, itching, and preventing secondary infection
2. Control of pain by blocking the nerve through injection of drugs such as lidocaine or applying medication such as triamcinolone (Kenalog)
3. Antiinflammatory drugs such as systemic steroids or Kenalog ointment to decrease inflammation
D. Nursing care
1. Administer analgesics and other medications as ordered
2. Reduce itching and protect lesions from air by the application of salves, ointments, lotions, and sterile dressings as ordered
3. Protect from pressure by use of air mattress, bed cradle, and light loose clothing (avoid synthetic and woolen materials and use cotton fabrics)
4. Use aseptic technique when caring for a client with open lesions
5. Administer antibiotics as ordered
6. Encourage client to avoid scratching and to use gloves at night to limit the possibility of accidental scratching
7. Assist the client to understand the basis for the rash and the itch
8. Allay fears that may be based on old wives' tales about shingles
9. Encourage the client to express feelings
10. Encourage diet rich in nutrient-dense foods such as fruits, vegetables, whole grains, and legumes to improve and maintain nutritional status and prevent

possible drug-induced nutrient deficiencies; encourage intake of vitamin C because it has been reported to stimulate the immune response to viral infection by increasing interferon, which limits viral reproduction in early stages
11. Evaluate client's response and revise plan as necessary

Systemic Lupus Erythematosus (SLE)

A. Etiology and pathophysiology
1. Origin unknown; affects the connective tissue and is thought to be due to a defect in the body's immunologic mechanisms or to genetic predisposition
2. Fibrinoid deposits in blood vessels, among collagen fibers, and on organs
3. Necrosis of the glomerular capillaries, inflammation of cerebral and ocular blood vessels, necrosis of lymph nodes, vasculitis of the GI tract and pleura, and degeneration of the basal layer of skin
B. Signs and symptoms
1. Subjective
a. Malaise
b. Photosensitivity
c. Joint pain
2. Objective
a. Fever
b. Butterfly erythema on the face
c. Erythema of palms
d. Positive LE prep
C. Treatment
1. Corticosteroids and analgesics to reduce pain and inflammation
2. Supportive therapy as major organs become affected (heart, kidneys, CNS, GI tract)
D. Nursing care
1. Administer medications and observe for side effects
2. Help the client and family cope with severity of the disease as well as its poor prognosis
3. Encourage diet rich in nutrient-dense foods such as fruits, vegetables, whole grains, and legumes to improve and maintain nutritional status and compensate for nutrient interactions of corticosteroid and other treatment medications; emphasize vitamin C since it is essential in the biosynthesis of collagen, and large doses have been found to increase total collagen synthesis
4. Evaluate client's response and revise plan as necessary

Polyarteritis Nodosa

A. Etiology and pathophysiology
1. Cause unknown; occurs primarily in women in midlife
2. Collagen disease that causes inflammation and necrosis of small and medium-sized arteries
3. When healing of the arteries occurs, there is a thickening of the walls with subsequent circulatory impairment
4. Common areas involved are the kidneys, heart, liver, and GI tract

B. Signs and symptoms
   1. Subjective
      a. Malaise
      b. Weakness
      c. Severe abdominal pain, muscle aches
   2. Objective
      a. Weight loss
      b. Low-grade fever
      c. Bloody diarrhea
      d. Proteinuria if kidneys are affected
      e. Positive rheumatoid factor (RF) and elevated sedimentation rate
C. Treatment
   1. Corticosteroids and analgesics to control pain and inflammation
   2. Balanced diet to combat weight loss
D. Nursing care
   1. Provide relief of symptomatic pain
   2. Provide emotional support for both the client and the family because of the poor prognosis
   3. Evaluate client's response and revise plan as necessary

Progressive Systemic Sclerosis (Scleroderma)

A. Etiology and pathophysiology
   1. Thought to be caused by an autoimmune defect; occurs in women more frequently than in men
   2. Systemic disease that causes fibrotic changes in connective tissue throughout the body
   3. May involve the skin, synovial membranes, esophagus, heart, lungs, kidneys, or GI tract
B. Signs and symptoms
   1. Subjective
      a. Articular pain
      b. Muscle weakness
   2. Objective
      a. Masklike hard skin that eventually adheres to underlying structures
      b. Telangiectases on the lips, fingers, face, and tongue
      c. Dysphagia
      d. Restriction of body motion as the disease progresses
      e. Positive LE prep, elevated gamma globulin levels, false-positive test for syphilis
C. Treatment
   1. Corticosteroids
   2. Salicylates or analgesics for joint pain
   3. Physical therapy
   4. Skin care to prevent decubitus formation
D. Nursing care
   1. Support the client and family emotionally; there is no cure at present
   2. Administer medications as ordered
   3. Encourage the client to exercise actively
   4. Observe vital signs, urinary output, and vital capacity for changes in function of vital organs
   5. Evaluate client's response and revise plan as necessary

Kaposi's Sarcoma

A. Etiology and pathophysiology
   1. Cause is unknown: occurs in individuals with a compromised immune system; often occurs in individuals with AIDS
   2. Lesions generally begin in the epidermis and extend into the dermis
   3. The lesions most commonly begin on the dorsum of the foot and between the toes
   4. There are four classifications of lesions
      a. Nodular: found on the extremities and slow growing
      b. Florid: very rapid growing and ulcerated
      c. Infiltrate: penetrating deeper structures, including bone
      d. Lymphadenopathic: disseminated type, rare, generally found in children
   5. Involvement of GI, bone, and lung are common
B. Signs and symptoms
   1. Subjective
      a. Pain
      b. Tenderness
   2. Objective
      a. Edema of lower extremities
      b. Lesions on skin
C. Treatment
   1. Radiation may be used alone or in conjunction with chemotherapy
   2. Chemotherapeutic treatment may be administered intravenously, intraarterially, or intralesionally
   3. Immunotherapy may be employed to stabilize the immune system
D. Nursing care
   1. Provide for pain relief
   2. Provide emotional support
   3. Utilize precautions to maximize skin integrity including a diet high in vitamin A and foods that are of high nutrient density
   4. Institute protective isolation if client is severely immune depressed; utilize body fluid precautions if client has AIDS
   5. Evaluate client's response and revise plan as necessary

Infectious Diseases

See Infection for additional information

NURSING PROCESS FOR CLIENTS WITH INFECTIOUS DISEASES
Probable Nursing Diagnoses Based on Assessment

A. Infection related to exposure to causative organism
B. Hyperthermia related to pyrogenic activity
C. Fluid volume deficit related to
   1. Diaphoresis/fever
   2. Diarrhea
   3. Decreased intake
D. Altered nutrition: less than body requirements related to decreased intake
E. Impaired skin integrity related to disease process

F. Social isolation related to imposed isolation precautions
G. Disturbance in body image related to altered body appearance
H. Diarrhea related to increased peristalsis and altered gastrointestinal flora
I. Fatigue related to increased metabolic rate and decreased oxygen carrying capacity of blood
J. Altered peripheral tissue perfusion related to interrupted skin integrity
K. Pain related to inflammatory response
L. Disturbance in self-esteem related to contagious nature of illness

Nursing Care for Clients with Infectious Diseases

See Nursing care under each specific disease

MAJOR DISEASES
Gas Gangrene

A. Etiology and pathophysiology
  1. Caused by an anaerobic gram-positive clostridium *(Clostridium perfringens, C. novyi)* that enters through a deep wound
  2. Usually occurs 2 to 5 days after injury
  3. Bacilli colonize in muscle tissue surrounding the wound
B. Signs and symptoms
  1. Subjective
    a. Pain
    b. Apprehension
    c. Anorexia
  2. Objective
    a. Bronzed or blackened wound tissue
    b. Crepitus
    c. Sweetish-smelling exudate
    d. Necrosis of muscle tissues
    e. Presence of clostridia on culture
    f. Pallor
    g. Diarrhea
    h. Vomiting
    i. Temperature elevation (may be slight)
    j. Anemia
C. Treatment
  1. Multiple incisions for decompression and drainage
  2. Extirpation and debridement of involved tissue with copious irrigations
  3. Penicillin G, tetracycline, chloramphenicol, or erythromycin, depending on drug sensitivity
  4. Amputation
  5. Hyperbaric oxygenation
  6. Whole blood, packed erythrocytes, or plasma transfusions to combat hemolysis and profound anemia
  7. Antitoxin therapy may be started
D. Nursing care
  1. Prevent infection whenever the wound is near the rectum, since the organism is found in feces
  2. Utilize wound and skin precautions
  3. Monitor fluid and electrolyte balance
  4. Check cardiovascular status frequently to determine complications

5. Instruct client regarding side effects of medications and importance of diet to support immune system (see Pharmacological control of infection)
6. Evaluate client's response and revise plan as necessary

Hansen's Disease (Leprosy)

A. Etiology and pathophysiology
  1. Thought to be transmitted by direct contact with the acid-fast bacillus *Mycobacterium leprae*
  2. Bacillus causes lesions of the peripheral nervous system that extend to and destroy nearby skin tissues
B. Signs and symptoms
  1. Subjective: loss of sensation
  2. Objective: painless, colorless, or red-brown macules and papules, nodules, sores, and ulcers
C. Treatment
  1. Sulfone drugs
  2. Reconstructive surgery
D. Nursing care
  1. Provide emotional support for the client and the family, allowing ample time for verbalization of feelings
  2. Maintain mobility of the client with decreased use of painful extremities
  3. Encourage case-finding examinations of all family members and friends; assure them that the disease has a very low incidence of communicability
  4. Evaluate client's response and revise plan as necessary

Toxoplasmosis

A. Etiology and pathophysiology
  1. Caused by protozoan *(Toxoplasma gondii),* a parasite of warm-blooded animals
  2. Contracted by eating raw meat containing cysts or by exposure to contaminated cat feces
  3. Disease can be transmitted to fetus through placental circulation causing death or congenital anomalies, even though mother may be asymptomatic
B. Signs and symptoms
  1. Subjective
    a. Malaise
    b. Fatigue
  2. Objective
    a. Fever
    b. Lymphadenopathy
C. Treatment
  1. Usually no treatment required for adults
  2. Pregnant women and immunosuppressed clients may be treated with pyrimethamine, trisulfapyrimidine, and sulfadiazene
D. Nursing care
  1. Provide emotional support to pregnant clients
  2. Caution pregnant clients to avoid cleaning cat litter pans or gardening where they may be exposed to cat feces
  3. Teach client about proper handling and storage of meat, washing fruits and vegetables, and care of cat litter

4. Encourage a diet rich in nutrient-dense foods
5. Evaluate client's response and revise plan as necessary

Malaria

A. Etiology and pathophysiology
   1. Caused by a protozoon *(Plasmodium falciparum, P. vivax, P. ovale, P. malariae)* that enters during a bite by an infected *Anopheles* mosquito, through the use of dirty needles, or by a transfusion from an infected donor
   2. When the parasite enters the bloodstream, it invades the red blood cells; destruction of red blood cells, blockage of capillaries, and irreversible damage to the spleen and liver may follow
   3. Rare complications is "blackwater fever"; name derived from the fact that there is intravascular hemolysis and hemoglobinuria
   4. Individuals with the sickle cell trait have natural resistance to malaria
B. Signs and symptoms
   1. Subjective
      a. Malaise
      b. Headache
      c. Muscle aches
      d. Chills
      e. Thirst
   2. Objective
      a. High fever
      b. Anemia
      c. Enlarged spleen
      d. Dehydration
      e. Renal failure
C. Treatment
   1. Antimalarial drugs (see chemoprophylaxis under nursing care)
   2. Aspirin
D. Nursing care
   1. Monitor fluid and electrolyte balance
   2. Utilize blood and body fluid precautions
   3. Use sprays and wear protective clothing to prevent mosquito bites
   4. Use therapeutic measures such as sponges to decrease the fever; maintain hydration
   5. Maintain bed rest until the fever and other symptoms have ceased
   6. Assist with dialysis and monitor blood transfusions as needed when blackwater fever is present
   7. Teach preventive measures
      a. Avoid stagnant pools
      b. Initiate chemoprophylaxis 1 week prior to visiting infested areas and regularly while in the area: pyrimethamine, proguanil hydrochloride, chloroquine diphosphate, or amodiaquine dihydrochloride
   8. Support natural defense mechanisms of client; encourage intake of nutrient-dense foods with emphasis on fruits, vegetables, whole grains, and legumes, especially those high in the immune-stimulating nutrients selenium and vitamins A, C, and E
   9. Evaluate client's response and revise plan as necessary

Rabies (Hydrophobia)

A. Etiology and pathophysiology
   1. Caused by a virus found in the saliva of an infected animal and usually spread by bite; the animal can be a carrier and not be ill with the disease
   2. Incubation period 30 to 50 days in bites of the upper parts of the body, 4 months in bites of the lower parts
   3. Bites are usually unprovoked; suspected animals are observed for 10 days
   4. Negri bodies (round objects) found in the brain tissue of infected animals
   5. Virus affects the CNS; may cause punctate hemorrhages and neuronal destruction
B. Signs and symptoms
   1. Subjective
      a. Anxiety
      b. Depression, malaise, lethargy
      c. Irritability
      d. Headaches
      e. Stiff neck
      f. Anorexia, nausea
      g. Photophobia
      h. Respiratory difficulty such as wheezing, hyperventilation, and dyspnea
      i. Thirst
      j. Paresthesia or pain near the bite or in the bitten extremity
   2. Objective
      a. Severe difficulty swallowing
      b. Excessive salivation
      c. Choking
      d. Aerophobia
      e. Apnea
      f. Paralysis
      g. Coma
      h. Cardiac arrhythmias
C. Treatment
   1. Cleansing of the wound with aqueous benzalkonium chloride
   2. Tracheostomy if respiratory embarrassment severe
   3. Human rabies immune globulin for passive immunity; dose given in the buttock; wound is bathed with the drug
   4. Human diploid cell vaccine is used to induce active immunity; treatment consists of five doses over 4 weeks followed by a sixth dose after 2 months; duck embryo rabies vaccine (DEV) was formerly used requiring a total of 23 doses administered subcutaneously
   5. Sedative or anesthetics as necessary; phenytoin (Dilantin) used for seizures
D. Nursing care
   1. Maintain strict isolation technique
   2. Monitor blood gases, fluid and electrolyte balance, and electrocardiograms
   3. Keep the room dark and quiet to prevent agitation
   4. Monitor the tracheostomy and the need for suctioning
   5. Prevent drafts, which may result in spasms

6. Allow the family and client to verbalize their feelings
7. Evaluate client's response and revise plan as necessary

Rocky Mountain Spotted Fever

A. Etiology and pathophysiology
   1. Contamination of an individual by a tick infected with *Rickettsia rickettsii* (through bite or contamination by a crushed tick on the fingers or in the eye); there may or may not be a history of tickbite
   2. Sudden onset, with an incubation period of 3 to 17 days
   3. Organism attacks endothelial cells and extends into the vessel walls, causing thrombi, inflammation, and necrosis
B. Signs and symptoms
   1. Subjective
      a. Malaise
      b. Insomnia
      c. Headache
      d. Anorexia
      e. Photophobia
      f. Joint and muscle discomfort
   2. Objective
      a. Fever
      b. Rash (rose-colored macules)
      c. Subcutaneous hemorrhage
      d. Necrosis
      e. Enlarged spleen
      f. Hearing loss
      g. Hypotension
      h. Circulatory collapse
C. Treatment
   1. Prompt recognition and treatment vital
   2. Tetracycline or chloramphenicol therapy continued until the client is afebrile for 3 to 5 days
   3. Treatment of symptoms and complications as they develop
D. Nursing care
   1. Assure the family that the client's disturbed emotional responses are associated with the disease
   2. Monitor symptoms to determine progression of the disease
   3. Assess the cardiovascular status to determine developing circulatory collapse
   4. Reassure that hearing loss will last only several weeks
   5. Teach prevention such as wearing tick repellents and checking pants legs and animals for the presence of ticks
   6. Teach all individuals to kill ticks with a tweezer to prevent contamination of fingers
   7. Evaluate client's response and revise plan as necessary

Lyme Disease

A. Etiology and pathophysiology
   1. Caused by spirochete bacteria, *Borrelia bergdorferi*
   2. Disease is most often carried by mice, deer, or raccoons; cats, dogs, and horses may also be carriers
   3. Transmitted by carrier tick that acquired bacterium from infected host (Deer tick, Western black-legged tick, or Lone Star tick)
   4. Most common in coastal areas during June and July, but tick is active from April to October
   5. Infectious organism can survive in host 10 years or more
   6. Initial rash and flu-like symptoms; later neuromusculoskeletal symptoms
   7. Named for mysterious 1972 outbreak of arthritis in Lyme, Connecticut
B. Signs and symptoms
   1. Subjective
      a. Chills
      b. Muscle aches
      c. Joint pain
      d. Headache
      e. Dizziness
      f. Stiff neck
   2. Objective
      a. Fever
      b. Red-ringed, circular rash
      c. Blood work positive for causative bacterium
      d. Swollen joints
      e. Lack of coordination
      f. Facial palsy
      g. Paralysis
      h. Dementia
C. Treatment
   1. Antibiotics such as penicillin and tetracycline
   2. Symptomatic treatment
D. Nursing care
   1. Question clients with arthritic symptoms about possible exposure
   2. Teach clients to
      a. Avoid tall grass
      b. Use chemical repellents
      c. Wear light colors to enhance tick identification
      d. Wear long sleeves and pants tucked in high boots when walking in areas with tick infestation
      e. Shower and inspect skin
      f. Remove ticks with tweezers, grasping close to skin to avoid breaking mouth parts
   3. Evaluate client's response to treatment and understanding of teaching and revise plan as necessary

Tetanus (Lockjaw)

A. Etiology and pathophysiology
   1. Caused by the anaerobic bacillus *Clostridium tetani,* which is transmitted through an open wound
   2. Symptoms from 2 days to 3 weeks after exposure to the bacillus
   3. Toxins from the bacillus invade the nervous tissue, and the motor and sensory nerves become hypersensitive, resulting in prolonged contractions and respiratory failure
B. Signs and symptoms
   1. Subjective
      a. Irritability
      b. Restlessness

2. Objective
   a. Muscle rigidity
   b. Local or general spastic contractions of the voluntary muscles
   c. Trismus (spasm of the masticatory muscles)
   d. Spasms of the respiratory tract
   e. Convulsions
C. Treatment
   1. Tetanus immune globulin, (TIG) to provide temporary passive immunity
   2. Maintain adequate pulmonary ventilation
   3. Debridement of the wound to allow exposure to air
   4. Control of muscle spasms
   5. Penicillin G to limit secondary infection
   6. Maintain fluid balance and nutrition
   7. Diazepam and barbiturates to sedate the client and limit spasms
   8. Once symptoms develop, specific therapy is ineffective; therefore institution of supportive therapy is necessary until toxins are reduced by time
D. Nursing care
   1. Prevent the disease through immunization with tetanus toxoid to provide active immunity; prophylaxis in suspect injuries
   2. Maintain a quiet environment to decrease stimuli, which may result in convulsions
   3. Frequently assess respiratory status; administer oxygen as needed
   4. Frequently suction the airway to maintain patency and promote ventilation; keep an endotracheal tube and tracheostomy set at the bedside
   5. Allow the client and family to verbalize fears and feelings
   6. Evaluate client's response and revise plan as necessary

Typhoid Fever

A. Etiology and pathophysiology
   1. Caused by the bacterium *Salmonella typhi,* which can be carried in human feces and transmitted through sewage, flies, and shellfish
   2. Incubation period 3 to 20 days
   3. Bacterium invades the GI tract and localizes in lymph tissue of the intestinal wall (Peyer's patches); these areas may become thrombosed and tissue sloughs off, leaving ulcers
   4. Hemorrhage, peritonitis, perforation, and hepatitis are serious complications
B. Signs and symptoms
   1. Subjective
      a. Headaches
      b. Drowsiness
   2. Objective
      a. Fever
      b. Bradycardia
      c. Rose-colored papules on the abdomen
      d. Enlarged spleen
      e. Enlarged liver
      f. Delirium

   g. Constipation during the early stage; diarrhea during the late stage
C. Treatment
   1. Chloramphenicol or sulfamethoxazole and trimethoprim
   2. Corticosteroids the first 4 to 5 days of treatment
D. Nursing care
   1. Encourage a diet rich in nutrient-density foods and high caloric foods
   2. Employ methods to decrease the fever
   3. Monitor fluid and electrolytes to prevent imbalance
   4. Maintain enteric precautions and isolation technique
   5. Utilize high-fiber diet, stool softeners, enemas, or mild laxatives, as ordered, to limit constipation
   6. Educate the public to prevent disease through proper sewage treatment
   7. Encourage vaccination programs with booster injections every 3 years in endemic areas
   8. Allow the client and family ample time to verbalize emotional reactions and concerns resulting from the illness
   9. Evaluate client's response and revise plan as necessary

Medical-Surgical Nursing Review Questions
The Circulatory System

Situation: Mrs. Hollens, age 30 and a chemist, is the mother of two young children. For the past few months she has noticed that she tires easily, has painless swelling of the lymph nodes, and has been running a low-grade fever with excessive diaphoresis at night. She also has anorexia with loss of weight. She does not recall having had any serious illness except that once during the winter she experienced what she believed was a viral infection. On her admission to the hospital the physician ordered a complete medical examination for Mrs. Hollens. On the basis of diagnostic tests, Mrs. Hollens is said to have Hodgkin's disease. Questions 1 through 5 refer to this situation.

1. The lymph nodes usually affected first are the:
   ① Inguinal
   ② Axillary
   ③ Cervical
   ④ Mediastinal
2. The highest incidence of Hodgkin's disease is in:
   ① Children
   ② Young adults
   ③ Middle-aged persons
   ④ Elderly persons
3. Which of the following would the nurse expect Mrs. Hollens to develop as a result of whole-body irradiation? Increased:
   ① Red blood cell production
   ② Susceptibility to infection
   ③ Tendency for pathologic fractures
   ④ Blood viscosity

4. Whole-body irradiation injures or destroys bone marrow, making it unable to function normally. As a result, the nurse would expect Mrs. Hollens to develop:
   ① Decreased number of erythrocytes
   ② Decreased susceptibility to infections
   ③ Increased tendency for fractures
   ④ Increased blood viscosity

5. The apparent paradox of radiation being a known cancer-inducing agent as well as a widely used therapy for cancer is clarified when one considers the:
   ① Extent of the body irradiated
   ② Nutritional environment of the cells
   ③ Dosage of radiation utilized
   ④ Physical condition of the client

Situation: Mrs. Johnson, a 64-year-old housewife, is admitted to the hospital with a diagnosis of hypertension. Questions 6 through 14 refer to this situation.

6. Mrs. Johnson is receiving methyldopa hydrochloride (Aldomet) intravenously for control of hypertension. Her blood pressure, before the infusion started, was 150/90. Fifteen minutes after the infusion is started her blood pressure rises to 180/100. The response to the drug would be described as a(n):
   ① Synergistic response
   ② Individual hypersusceptibility
   ③ Allergic response
   ④ Paradoxical response

7. To assess the effectiveness of Aldomet in lowering blood pressure levels, the nurse would take Mrs. Johnson's pulse and blood pressure:
   ① Thirty minutes after giving the drug
   ② Immediately after she gets out of bed
   ③ After she has been supine for 5 minutes
   ④ Prior to giving the drug

8. Mrs. Johnson's serum potassium level is low and she is placed on a cardiac monitor. She is to receive 40 mEq potassium chloride in 1000 ml of 5% dextrose in water IV. The nurse analyzes the monitor pattern to obtain a baseline for evaluating progress. The monitor pattern would show:
   ① Shortening of the QRS complex
   ② Elevation of the ST segment
   ③ Increased deflection of the Q wave
   ④ Lowering of the T wave

9. Mrs. Johnson's IV medication inadvertently runs in rapidly. The physician prescribes insulin added to a 10% dextrose in water solution. The rationale for the prescription is:
   ① Glucose and insulin increase the metabolic rate and accelerate potassium excretion
   ② Potassium moves into body cells with glucose and insulin
   ③ Increased potassium causes a temporary slowing of pancreatic production of insulin
   ④ Increased insulin accelerates excretion of glucose and potassium

10. Mrs. Johnson's condition has improved, and methyldopa (Aldomet) is being given orally. When explaining why orthostatic hypotension occurs, the nurse should base the response on knowledge that the drug causes vasodilation by:
    ① Depleting acetylcholine
    ② Decreasing adrenal release of epinephrine
    ③ Stimulating histamine release
    ④ Interrupting norepinephrine release

11. When discussing the plan for taking Aldomet at home, the nurse would tell Mrs. Johnson that orthostatic hypotension may be modified by:
    ① Lying down for 30 minutes after taking the drug
    ② Avoiding tasks that require high energy expenditures
    ③ Wearing support hose continuously
    ④ Sitting on the edge of the bed a short time before arising

12. The primary cause of essential hypertension is:
    ① Generalized arteriosclerosis
    ② Unresolved grief
    ③ Kidney failure
    ④ Unexpressed rage

13. Which mechanism mediates long-term (day-to-day, week-to-week) blood pressure regulation?
    ① Fight or flight response
    ② Adjustment of urinary output
    ③ Nervous system baroreceptors
    ④ Capillary fluid shifts

14. Mrs. Johnson's medication is changed to propranolol hydrochloride (Inderal). She should be told she might:
    ① Experience dizziness with strenuous activity
    ② Have a flushing sensation for a few minutes after taking the drug
    ③ Notice acceleration of the heart rate after eating a heavy meal
    ④ Have pounding of the heart for a few minutes after taking the drug

Situation: Mr. Evere, a 69-year-old retired musician, was admitted to the intensive care unit with a diagnosis of Adams-Stokes syndrome. Questions 15 through 20 refer to this situation.

15. Mr. Evere's symptoms most likely include:
    ① Syncope and low ventricular rate
    ② Flushing and slurred speech
    ③ Cephalalgia and blurred vision
    ④ Nausea and vertigo

16. Mr. Evere is having a pacemaker inserted. The nurse observing the cardiac monitor should be aware that the lethal arrhythmia that often requires immediate intervention by the nurse is:
    ① Atrial fibrillation
    ② Auricular flutter
    ③ Second-degree heart block
    ④ Ventricular fibrillation

17. To evaluate the effectiveness of Mr. Evere's pacemaker, the nurse ensures that his pulse remains:
    ① Equal to the pacemaker
    ② In a regular rhythm
    ③ Palpable at distant sites
    ④ Above the demand rate

18. The nurse notes Mr. Evere's pulse pressure is decreasing. Pulse pressure is the:
    ① Difference between the apical and radial rates
    ② Force exerted against an arterial wall
    ③ Degree of ventricular contraction in relation to output
    ④ Difference between systolic and diastolic readings

19. The physician suspects cardiogenic shock. Shock is:
    ① A failure of peripheral circulation
    ② An irreversible phenomenon
    ③ Always caused by decreased blood volume
    ④ A fleeting reaction to tissue injury
20. The physical law explaining the greatly increased venous return accompanying mild vasoconstriction underlies the use of:
    ① Adrenaline in treating shock
    ② Rotating tourniquets in pulmonary edema
    ③ Sympathectomy in treating hypertension
    ④ Digoxin to increase cardiac output

Situation: Mr. Topper, age 72, is admitted with cerebral arteriosclerosis, complicated by polycythemia vera. He has had transient periods of weakness and confusion. When his symptoms subside, Mr. Topper requests that he be discharged because he has been cured. Questions 21 through 27 refer to this situation.

21. When explaining why Mr. Topper is not being discharged, the nurse should be aware that arteriosclerosis of blood vessels leading to the brain may not become evident until there is an extremely severe blockage or until a stroke occurs because of collateral blood circulation supplied through the:
    ① Hypothalamic-hypophyseal portal system
    ② The bicarotid trunk
    ③ Circle of Willis
    ④ Jugular vessels
22. Mr. Topper finally understands that his risk of suffering a CVA is high if left untreated. The increased tendency toward coronary and cerebral thromboses seen in individuals with polycythemia vera is attributable to the:
    ① Elevated blood pressure
    ② Immaturity of red blood cells
    ③ Fragility of the cells
    ④ Increased viscosity
23. In general, the higher the red blood cell count:
    ① The greater the blood viscosity
    ② The higher the blood pH
    ③ The less it contributes to immunity
    ④ The lower the hematocrit
24. The physician prescribes heparin q6h for Mr. Topper. The response that indicates that heparin anticoagulant therapy has been effective is:
    ① APT twice normal value
    ② Decreased viscosity of the blood
    ③ Absence of ecchymotic areas
    ④ Reduction of confusion and weakness
25. Once stabilized Mr. Topper is scheduled for an endarterectomy. After an endarterectomy the nurse should plan to observe Mr. Topper for change in:
    ① Bowel habits
    ② Skin color
    ③ Tissue turgor
    ④ Appetite
26. After surgery the physician prescribes albumin IV. An important function of the albumin of the blood is:
    ① Red blood cell formation
    ② The activation of white blood cells
    ③ Blood clotting
    ④ The development of the colloid osmotic pressure

27. The capillary endothelium is a selectively permeable membrane. Which of the following molecules cannot easily pass through it?
    ① O_2 and CO_2
    ② Plasma proteins
    ③ Glucose, O_2, and CO_2
    ④ Ions, amino acids, and water

Situation: Mrs. Harvey has an acute episode of right-sided heart failure and is receiving furosemide (Lasix). Questions 28 through 34 refer to this situation.

28. The physician has prescribed aspirin for her arthritic pain. When Mrs. Harvey asks why she is not receiving the same aspirin dosage she usually takes, the nurse's response would be based on knowledge that:
    ① Aspirin in large doses after an acute stress episode increases the bleeding potential
    ② Use of furosemide and aspirin concomitantly increases formation of uric acid crystals in the nephron
    ③ Competition for renal excretion sites by the drugs causes increased serum levels of aspirin
    ④ Aspirin accelerates metabolism of furosemide and decreases the diuretic effect
29. The symptoms that Mrs. Harvey most likely displayed on admission are:
    ① Dyspnea, edema, fatigue
    ② Weakness, palpitations, nausea
    ③ Fatigue, vertigo, and headache
    ④ A feeling of distress when breathing
30. Mrs. Harvey has edema during the day and it disappears at night. The client states it is not painful and is located in the lower extremities. The nurse should suspect:
    ① Pulmonary edema
    ② Right-sided heart failure
    ③ Myocardial infarction
    ④ Lung disease
31. Pitting edema in the lower extremities occurs with this problem because of the:
    ① Increase in tissue colloid osmotic pressure
    ② Increase in the tissue hydrostatic pressure at the arterial end of the capillary bed
    ③ Decrease in the plasma colloid osmotic pressure
    ④ Increase in the plasma hydrostatic pressure at the venous end of the capillary beds
32. The nurse can best assess the degree of edema in an extremity by:
    ① Checking for pitting
    ② Weighing the client
    ③ Measuring the affected area
    ④ Observing intake and output
33. The nurse notes that Mrs. Harvey's abdomen is distended. The nurse should realize that the client with congestive heart failure develops ascites because of:
    ① Increased pressure within the circulatory system
    ② Rapid diffusion of solutes and solvents into plasma
    ③ Rapid osmosis from tissue spaces to cells
    ④ Loss of cellular constituents in blood

34. Mrs. Harvey's condition worsens. The physician has ordered CVP readings q2h. Which of the following is true of CVP?
    ① A high reading may be indicative of dehydration
    ② A normal reading is 60 to 120 mm of water
    ③ The zero point of the manometer is level with the midaxilla
    ④ The client must be kept flat in bed while the catheter is in place

Situation: Mr. Green, age 37, is admitted with a gangrenous lesion of his right great toe. He has a history of thromboangiitis obliterans (Buerger's disease). Questions 35 through 39 refer to this situation.

35. Common symptoms of Buerger's disease are:
    ① Burning pain precipitated by cold exposure, fatigue, blanching of skin
    ② Easy fatigue of part, continuous claudication
    ③ General blanching of skin, intermittent claudication
    ④ Intermittent claudication, burning pain after exposure to cold

36. Mr Green is instructed to stop smoking because the nicotine:
    ① Dilates the peripheral vessels, causing a reflex constriction of visceral vessels
    ② Constricts the peripheral vessels and increases the force of flow
    ③ Constricts the collateral circulation, dilating the superficial vessels
    ④ Constricts the superficial vessels, dilating the deep vessels

37. In chronic occulsive arterial disease the precipitating cause for ulceration and gangrenous lesions often is:
    ① Poor hygiene
    ② Stimulants such as coffee, tea, or cola drinks
    ③ Emotional stress
    ④ Trauma from mechanical, chemical, or thermal sources

38. Mr. Green becomes openly hostile when he learns that amputation is being considered. The best indication that the nurse's interaction has been therapeutic would be:
    ① An increase in physical activity
    ② An absence of further outbursts
    ③ A relaxation of tensed muscles
    ④ A denial that further discussion is necessary

39. The physician performs a bilateral lumbar sympathectomy. After surgery the nurse notes a sudden drop in blood pressure but no evidence of bleeding. This is most likely due to:
    ① The after effects of anesthesia
    ② A reallocation of the blood supply
    ③ An inadequate fluid intake
    ④ An increased level of epinephrine

Situation: Mr. Wolfsmith, a 46-year-old executive, is admitted with chest pain and shortness of breath. A diagnosis of myocardial infarction is made. Questions 40 through 47 refer to this situation.

40. Mr. Wolfsmith is placed in the CCU, where the nurse will observe for one of the more common complications of myocardial infarction, which is:
    ① Cardiac arrhythmia
    ② Anaphylactic shock
    ③ Cardiac enlargement
    ④ Hypokalemia

41. To ascertain Mr. Wolfsmith's diagnosis, tests for which the nurse would prepare him include:
    ① Paul-Bunnell, serum potassium
    ② LDH, CPK, SGOT
    ③ Sedimentation rate, SGPT
    ④ Serum calcium, APPT

42. Mr. Wolfsmith is in the coronary unit on a cardiac monitor. The nurse observes ventricular irritability on the screen. The medication that might be administered for this would be:
    ① Digoxin (Lanoxin)
    ② Lidocaine
    ③ Furosemide (Lasix)
    ④ Levarterenol bitartrate (Levophed)

43. The nurse observes Mr. Wolfsmith's monitor and identifies asystole. This arrhythmia requires nursing attention because the heart is:
    ① Beating very rapidly
    ② Not beating
    ③ Beating irregularly
    ④ Beating slowly

44. A cardiac arrest code is called for Mr. Wolfsmith. During a cardiac arrest, the nurse and the arrest team must keep in mind the:
    ① Time the client is anoxic
    ② Heart rate of the client before arrest
    ③ Age of the client
    ④ Emergency medications available

45. When it is discovered that Mr. Wolfsmith has no carotid pulse or respirations, the nurse:
    ① Clears the airway
    ② Gives four full lung inflations
    ③ Compresses the lower sternum 15 times
    ④ Checks for a radial pulse

46. The nurse performing cardiac compression on Mr. Wolfsmith is aware that it is essential to exert a vertical downward pressure, which depresses the lower sternum at least:
    ① 1.3 to 2 cm (½ to ¾ inch)
    ② 2 to 2.5 cm (¾ to 1 inch)
    ③ 2.5 to 4 cm (1 to 1½ inches)
    ④ 4 to 5 cm (1½ to 2 inches)

47. A sample of Mr. Wolfsmith's arterial blood is drawn for assessing acidosis. A normal pH for arterial blood would be:
    ① 7.0
    ② 7.30
    ③ 7.42
    ④ 7.50

Situation: Mr. Everett has been admitted to the CCU with a tentative diagnosis of bundle branch block. Questions 48 through 52 refer to this situation.

48. When observing the client's cardiac monitor, the nurse would expect:
    ① Absence of P waves
    ② Widening of QRS complex to 0.12 second or greater
    ③ Inverted T waves following each QRS complex
    ④ Sagging ST segment

49. The physician has scheduled Mr. Everett for a pacemaker insertion. The pacing catheter will be inserted into a large vein such as the subclavian and advanced so that the electrode is positioned in the:
    ① Superior vena cava
    ② Left atrium
    ③ Right ventricle
    ④ SA node

50. The nurse realizes that a pacemaker is used in some clients to serve the function normally performed by the:
    ① Accelerator nerves to the heart
    ② AV node
    ③ Bundle of His
    ④ SA node

51. While the pacemaker catheter is being inserted, Mr. Everett's heart rate drops to 38. Which of the following drugs might the nurse expect the physician to order?
    ① Digoxin (Lanoxin)
    ② Lidocaine (Xylocaine)
    ③ Atropine sulfate
    ④ Procainamide (Pronestyl)

52. The physician has inserted a permanent demand pacemaker. In client teaching, the nurse should:
    ① Instruct the client to sleep on two pillows
    ② Inform the client that the pacemaker will function continuously at a set rate
    ③ Instruct the client to take his pulse daily and keep accurate records
    ④ Encourage the client to reduce his former level of activity

Situation: Mr. McNabb, a 65-year-old self-employed grocer, is admitted to the hospital with congestive heart failure and pulmonary edema. His treatment includes oxygen by mask, digoxin, chlorothiazide (Diuril), and a low-sodium diet. He is dyspneic, apprehensive, and restless. Questions 53 through 60 refer to this situation.

53. Mr. McNabb would be most comfortable with the oxygen set at:
    ① 12 to 14 L
    ② 5 to 7 L
    ③ 2 to 4 L
    ④ 16 to 18 L

54. Safety precautions are especially important in Mr. McNabb's room because oxygen:
    ① Is flammable
    ② Has unstable properties
    ③ Increases apprehension
    ④ Supports combustion

55. The nurse attempts to allay Mr. McNabb's anxiety, since restlessness:
    ① Decreases the amount of oxygen available
    ② Interferes with normal respiration
    ③ Increases the cardiac workload
    ④ Produces elevation in temperature

56. When instituting oxygen therapy, the nurse recognizes that the method of oxygen administration least likely to increase apprehension in the client is:
    ① Catheter
    ② Cannula
    ③ Tent
    ④ Mask

57. After receiving a sedative, Mr. McNabb says to the nurse, "I guess you are too busy to stay with me." The best response in this circumstance is:
    ① "I have to see other clients."
    ② "The medication will help you rest soon."
    ③ "I have to go now but I will come back in 10 minutes."
    ④ "You will feel better; I will adjust your oxygen mask."

58. Before giving Mr. McNabb digoxin, the nurse should measure the:
    ① Radial pulse in one arm
    ② Apical heart rate
    ③ Radial pulse in both arms
    ④ Difference between apical and radial pulses

59. In charting notes describing Mr. McNabb's heart rate, the nurse uses the term bradycardia. This describes:
    ① A grossly irregular-heartbeat
    ② A heart rate of over 90 per minute
    ③ A heartbeat that has regular "skipped" beats
    ④ A heart rate of under 60 per minute

60. In addition to its cardiotonic action, the digitalis preparations also promote diuresis. As a result, Mr. McNabb can be seriously depleted of:
    ① Calcium
    ② Phosphate
    ③ Potassium
    ④ Sodium

Situation: Miss Fleming, a 35-year-old executive secretary, is hospitalized for treatment of hypertension. Her orders include bed rest with bathroom privileges, low-sodium diet, reserpine (Serpasil), and chlordiazepoxide (Librium). She has been active in both her business and social life, usually having a cocktail before dinner and smoking a pack of cigarettes daily. Miss Fleming expresses disgust for her regimen and dissatisfaction with the nursing care. Questions 61 through 67 refer to this situation.

61. Miss Fleming's behavior is probably a manifestation of her:
    ① Denial of illness
    ② Response to cerebral anoxia
    ③ Reaction to hypertensive medications
    ④ Fear of the health problem

62. The nurse should administer the Librium as ordered because it:
    ① Promotes rest
    ② Induces sleep
    ③ Produces hypotension
    ④ Reduces hostility

63. Miss Fleming has been receiving Librium, 10 mg qid, for the past 5 days. The nurse should question giving the medication if the client exhibits:
    ① Muscle twitching
    ② Blurred vision
    ③ Hypotension
    ④ Extreme drowsiness

64. Miss Fleming is receiving Serpasil because it is an effective:
    ① Diuretic
    ② Hypnotic
    ③ Antihypertensive
    ④ Tranquilizer

65. To avoid an error of parallax when taking a client's blood pressure, the nurse should:
    1. Use a narrow cuff
    2. Stand close to the manometer
    3. Elevate the client's arm on a pillow
    4. Read at eye level

66. Miss Fleming has been told she must stop smoking and eliminate her predinner cocktail. The nurse discovers a pack of cigarettes in Miss Fleming's bathrobe. The best course of action to take at this time is to:
    1. Report the situation to the head nurse
    2. Let the client know they were found
    3. Discard them and say nothing to her
    4. Call the physician and request directions

67. When Miss Fleming is being overtly verbally hostile, the most appropriate nursing response is:
    1. Reasonable exploration of situation
    2. Complete withdrawal from her behavior
    3. Silent acceptance of her behavior
    4. Verbal defense of the nurse's position

Situation: Mrs. Campenella, an 80-year-old widow, is admitted with congestive heart failure and pulmonary edema. Questions 68 through 72 refer to this situation.

68. To help alleviate Mrs. Campenella's distress, the nurse should:
    1. Elevate the lower extremities
    2. Place the client in orthopneic position
    3. Encourage frequent coughing
    4. Prepare for modified postural drainage

69. When a client is admitted to the coronary care unit with a diagnosis of acute pulmonary edema, the nurse should be prepared for:
    1. Postural drainage
    2. Inhalation therapy
    3. Rotating tourniquets
    4. Wet phlebotomy

70. Mrs. Campenella is receiving furosemide (Lasix) and digoxin. Nursing care for her includes observation for symptoms of electrolyte depletion caused by:
    1. Sodium restriction
    2. Inadequate oral intake
    3. Continuous dyspnea
    4. Diuretic therapy

71. To help assess Mrs. Campenella's condition, a CVP catheter is inserted. In taking a central venous pressure reading the nurse should place the client:
    1. Horizontal
    2. In a low-Fowler's position
    3. Side lying, on affected side
    4. Side lying, opposite to manometer

72. Since Mrs. Campenella will be staying with her daughter for the summer, the nurse suggests that her room be air conditioned. This is because:
    1. The internal body temperature drops below 98.6° F (37° C)
    2. The heart is relieved of the strain of pumping blood through many miles of blood vessels in the skin
    3. The increased circulation in the skin causes excess body heat to radiate away
    4. The increased circulation in the skin gives the heart the exercise it needs

Situation: Mr. Rush is admitted to the coronary care unit with atrial fibrillation and a rapid ventricular response. The nurse prepares for cardioversion. Questions 73 through 79 refer to this situation.

73. Cardioversion is a procedure used to convert certain arrhythmias to normal rhythm. In addition to atrial fibrillation, which of the following arrhythmias is an indication for cardioversion?
    1. Ventricular fibrillation
    2. Premature ventricular contractions
    3. Ventricular tachycardia
    4. Ventricular standstill

74. When ventricular fibrillation occurs in a coronary care unit, the first person reaching the client should:
    1. Initiate cardiopulmonary resuscitation
    2. Defibrillate the client
    3. Administer sodium bicarbonate intravenously
    4. Administer oxygen

75. To overcome the potential danger of inducing ventricular fibrillation during cardioversion, the nurse should ensure that:
    1. The energy level is set at its maximum level
    2. The synchronizer switch is in the "on" position
    3. The skin electrodes are applied after the T wave
    4. The alarm system of the cardiac monitor is functioning simultaneously

76. The portion of the cardiac monitor that is related to the alarm system for extremes in the heart rate is called the:
    1. Oscilloscope
    2. Voltmeter
    3. Pacemaker
    4. Synchronizer

77. Cardioversion is only temporarily successful. Mr. Rush again develops atrial fibrillation. The physician has prescribed quinidine sulfate (Quinicardine) and digoxin (Lanoxin). The nurse should understand that the goal of the drug therapy plan is to:
    1. Decrease atrial irritability and slow transmission of impulses through the AV node
    2. Stimulate SA node control of conduction and shorten the refractory period of atrial tissue
    3. Suppress irritability of atrial and ventricular myocardial tissue
    4. Slow SA node firing rate and decrease irritability of the atrial myocardial tissue

78. When taking Mr. Rush's apical pulse the nurse should place the stethoscope:
    1. Between the sixth and seventh ribs at the left midaxillary line
    2. Between the third and fourth ribs and to the left of the sternum
    3. In the fifth intercostal space along the left midclavicular line
    4. Just to the left of the median point of the sternum

79. Mr. Rush is receiving digoxin (Lanoxin). Because he will continue taking the drug after discharge, the nurse should be primarily concerned with:
    1. Taking his apical pulse before drug administration and teaching him how to count his pulse rate
    2. Observing him for return of normal cardiac conduction patterns and for adverse effects of the drug

③ Observing him for changes in cardiac rhythm and planning activity at home based on his tolerance

④ Monitoring vital signs and encouraging gradual increase in activities of daily living

Situation: Mrs. Franklin, age 33, is a known epileptic whose seizures are controlled by phenytoin. She is receiving IV heparin sodium and oral warfarin sodium (Coumadin) concurrently for a partial occlusion of the left common carotid artery. Questions 80 through 84 refer to this situation.

80. Mrs. Franklin expresses concern about why she needs both heparin and Coumadin. The nurse's explanation is based on knowledge that the plan:
① Immediately provides maximum protection against clot formation
② Allows clot dissolution and prevents new clot formation
③ Permits the administration of smaller doses of each drug
④ Provides anticoagulant intravenously until the oral drug reaches its peak effect

81. After Mrs. Franklin has received IV heparin sodium for 3 days, the drug is discontinued. The nurse continues to observe her closely during the early days of treatment with Coumadin because:
① Coumadin action is greater in clients with epilepsy
② Seizures increase the metabolic degradation rate of Coumadin
③ Coumadin affects the metabolism of phenytoin
④ Phenytoin increases the clotting potential

82. Mrs. Franklin is being discharged from the hospital at the end of the week. When discussing problems that relate to adverse effects of Coumadin, the nurse will tell her to consult with the physician if she experiences the problem of:
① Increased transient ischemic attacks
② Excess menstrual flow
③ Swelling of ankles
④ Decreased ability to concentrate

83. Mrs Franklin's prothrombin levels have been somewhat unstable when checked in the clinic laboratory. The nurse interviews her to identify factors contributing to the problem. The first question asked deals with her:
① Intake of vitamin tablets or capsules
② Use of sleeping medications
③ Use of analgesics
④ Compliance with the plan for taking Coumadin

84. Mrs. Franklin calls the clinic nurse after her weekly prothrombin test to find out if her oral anticoagulant dosage is to be changed. She mentions that her sleeping medication, secobarbital sodium (Seconal), is gone but she plans to get more when she comes for her appointment in 3 days. The nurse tells her to come for a refill today because:
① Absence of sleep may precipitate seizures
② Discontinuance of the drug may affect the prothrombin level
③ She may have withdrawal symptoms because she has been taking the drug for 3 weeks
④ Control is dependent on the combined action of phenytoin (Dilantin) and the barbiturate

Situation: Mrs. Oliver is hospitalized with coronary heart disease. She is receiving IV fluids, her vital signs are checked q4h, and bed rest and medications, including digitalis and a sedative, are prescribed. She does not seem to be acutely ill, but her prognosis is guarded. Questions 85 through 92 refer to this situation.

85. The nurse who has been caring for Mrs. Oliver for several days notes cyanosis and a change in respiration. The nurse starts oxygen administration immediately. Which of the following statements is correct?
① Oxygen had not been ordered and therefore should not be administered
② The physician should have been called for an order before oxygen was begun
③ The symptoms were too vague for the nurse to diagnose a need for oxygen
④ The nurse's observations were sufficient to begin administration of oxygen

86. Mrs. Oliver asks what the coronary arteries have to do with her angina. In determining the answer, the nurse should take into consideration that the coronary arteries:
① Carry reduced-oxygen-content blood to the lungs
② Carry blood from the aorta to the myocardium
③ Supply blood to the endocardium
④ Carry high-oxygen-content blood from the lungs toward the heart

87. After activity Mrs. Oliver states she has anginal pain. The nurse should realize that angina pectoris is a sign of:
① Myocardial ischemia
② Myocardial infarction
③ Coronary thrombosis
④ Mitral insufficiency

88. Mrs. Oliver's condition improves. Nitroglycerin is prescribed for anginal pain prn. When teaching Mrs. Oliver how to use nitroglycerin, the nurse tells her to place 1 tablet under her tongue when she has pain and to repeat the dose in 5 minutes if pain persists. The nurse should also tell her to:
① Place 2 tablets under her tongue when intense pain occurs
② Place 1 tablet under her tongue 3 minutes before activity and repeat the dose in 5 minutes if pain occurs
③ Swallow 1 tablet and place 1 tablet under her tongue when pain is intense
④ Place 1 tablet under her tongue when pain occurs and use an additional tablet after the attack to prevent recurrence

89. The nurse would tell Mrs. Oliver that she should suspect her nitroglycerin tablets have lost their potency when:
① Slight tingling is absent when the tablet is placed under her tongue
② Onset of relief is delayed but the duration of relief is unchanged
③ Pain occurs even after taking the tablet prophylactically to prevent its onset
④ Pain is unrelieved but facial flushing is increased

90. Evaluation of the effectiveness of cardiac nitrates is based on:
    ① Relief of anginal pain
    ② A decrease in blood pressure
    ③ Improved cardiac output
    ④ Dilation of superficial blood vessels

91. In addition to a decreased apical rate, which one of the following symptoms would the nurse teach Mrs. Oliver to be alert for as an indication to withhold the digitalis?
    ① Decreased urinary output
    ② Singultus
    ③ Chest pain
    ④ Blurred vision

92. When discharged, Mrs. Oliver will continue to take a diuretic and digitalis. The nurse reviewing Mrs. Oliver's diet would be especially careful to look for adequate sources of potassium because:
    ① Under conditions of hyperglycemia digitalis exerts toxic effects on the heart
    ② Potassium is a necessary ion for normal body function
    ③ Under conditions of hypokalemia, digitalis exerts toxic effects on the heart
    ④ Potassium is a cofactor for several important enzymes

Situation: Mrs. Jesse, age 45, is scheduled for cardiac surgery. Questions 93 through 97 refer to this situation.

93. Prior to surgery a cardiac catheterization is performed. Blood samples from the right atrium, right ventricle, and pulmonary artery are analyzed for their oxygen content. Normally:
    ① The samples all contain about the same amount of oxygen
    ② All contain less CO_2 than does pulmonary vein blood
    ③ Pulmonary artery blood contains more oxygen than the other samples
    ④ All contain more oxygen than does pulmonary vein blood

94. During surgery a Swan-Ganz catheter is inserted to give the medical team information on:
    ① Stroke volume
    ② Left-sided heart failure
    ③ Venous pressure
    ④ Cardiac output

95. Mrs. Jesse is manifesting a diminished urine output after cardiac surgery. Her serum potassium level is elevated and the physician has prescribed polystyrene sodium sulfonate (Kayexalate) and sorbitol orally. This drug combination will:
    ① Remove potassium ions from serum and provide carbohydrate for nutrition
    ② Stimulate transfer of potassium ions and increase coupling with the resin
    ③ Allow exchange of sodium ions for potassium ions and increase intestinal water content
    ④ Increase solubility of polystyrene sodium sulfonate and facilitate its absorption

96. The physician prescribes prophylactic administration of penicillin. Mrs. Jesse has an anaphylactic reaction within the first half hour after an IV infusion containing the penicillin is started. Problems occurring during an anaphylactic reaction are the result of:
    ① Decreased cardiac output and dilation of major blood vessels
    ② Bronchial constriction and decreased peripheral resistance
    ③ Respiratory depression and cardiac standstill
    ④ Constriction of capillaries and decreased cardiac output

97. Occurrence of an anaphylactic reaction after receiving penicillin indicates that Mrs. Jesse has:
    ① An acquired atopic sensitization
    ② Passive immunity to the penicillin allergen
    ③ Antibodies to penicillin acquired after prior use of the drug
    ④ Developed potent bivalent antibodies when the IV administration was started

Situation: Mrs. Arthur, a 42-year-old woman with a history of hypertension, is admitted with weakness, exertional dyspnea, and jaundice. Questions 98 through 100 refer to this situation.

98. In addition to a CBC, a serum bilirubin is performed. A bilirubin level above 2 mg/100 ml blood volume could be indicative of:
    ① Hemolytic anemia
    ② Low oxygen-carrying capacity of erythrocytes
    ③ Pernicious anemia
    ④ Decreased rate of red cell destruction

99. The nurse questions Mrs. Arthur about the medications she takes routinely. In light of her symptoms, the nurse should be most concerned about her taking:
    ① Chlordiazepoxide (Librium) 10 mg qid
    ② Multivitamin with iron daily
    ③ Methyldopa (Aldomet) 250 mg bid
    ④ Aspirin 10 grains just prior to admission

100. The physician performs a bone marrow aspiration. Immediately after the procedure, the nurse should:
    ① Briefly apply pressure over the aspiration site
    ② Position Mrs. Arthur on the affected side
    ③ Cleanse the site with an antiseptic solution
    ④ Begin frequent monitoring of vital signs

---

101. Prolonged anemia or polycythemia may eventually place strain on a client's heart. The concept underlying this strain is:
    ① Pressure
    ② Surface tension
    ③ Viscosity
    ④ Temperature

102. Prompt treatment is most essential for a client with:
    ① Head injury
    ② Ventricular fibrillation
    ③ Penetrating abdominal wound
    ④ Fractured femur

103. The protein of blood involved with immune responses is:
    ① Hemoglobin
    ② Albumin

③ Globulin
④ Thrombin

104. Fragments of cells in the bloodstream that break down on exposure to injured tissue and begin the chain reaction leading to a blood clot are known as:
① Red blood cells
② Platelets
③ Leukocytes
④ Erythrocytes

105. With respect to human blood cells, sodium chloride solution of 0.85% strength is:
① Isotonic
② Hypertonic
③ Hypotonic
④ Isomeric

106. Prolonged bed rest after surgery appears to promote hemostasis, particularly in the deep veins of the calves. The most likely pathologic result of such hemostasis may be thrombus formation and:
① Cerebral embolism
② Dry gangrene of a limb
③ Pulmonary embolism
④ Coronary occlusion

107. A pulmonary embolism is a most unlikely complication in the postoperative period following:
① Prostatectomy
② Hysterectomy
③ Saphenous vein ligation
④ Appendectomy

108. Thromboplastin is found in:
① Plasma
② Erythrocytes
③ Platelets
④ Bile

109. When blood clots, the soluble substance that becomes an insoluble gel is:
① Fibrin
② Fibrinogen
③ Prothrombin
④ Thrombin

110. An ion that acts as a catalyst in blood clotting is:
① Fe^{+++}
② Ca^{++}
③ F^-
④ Cl^-

111. Pulmonary edema is most likely to occur in an individual with:
① Mitral stenosis
② Calcification and incomplete closure of the tricuspid valve
③ Severe arteriosclerosis of the coronary arteries
④ Pulmonary valve stenosis

The Respiratory System

Situation: Mr. Josh is admitted with a diagnosis of possible tuberculosis or pneumonia. Several diagnostic tests are performed. Questions 112 through 119 refer to this situation.

112. As a general rule, the test most valuable in the selection of an antibiotic is the:
① Susceptibility test
② Tissue culture test
③ Serologic test
④ Sensitivity test of organism

113. Acid-fast rods found in sputum are presumed to be:
① Influenza virus
② *Bordetella pertussis*
③ Diphtheria bacillus
④ *Mycobacterium tuberculosis*

114. As a result of pulmonary tuberculosis, Mr. Josh has a decreased surface area for gaseous exchange in his lungs. Oxygen and carbon dioxide are exchanged in the lungs by:
① Active transport
② Diffusion
③ Filtration
④ Osmosis

115. Mr. Josh says the physician told him his tidal volume is slightly diminished and asks the nurse what this means. The nurse explains that tidal air is the amount of air:
① Exhaled normally after a normal inspiration
② Exhaled forcibly after a normal expiration
③ Forcibly inspired over and above a normal inspiration
④ Trapped in the alveoli that cannot be exhaled

116. Before discontinuing respiratory isolation for Mr. Josh, the nurse must determine that:
① He no longer has the disease
② His tuberculin skin test is negative
③ No acid-fast bacteria are in his sputum
④ His temperature has returned to normal

117. Mr. Josh has been receiving streptomycin sulfate daily for 1 week. He is being discharged and the physician plans to have him come to the clinic for administration of the drug twice a week. The spaced dosage is planned to:
① Increase compliance with the therapy plan
② Lessen risk of adverse effects of the drug on neural tissue
③ Minimize disruption of the rest hours required for recovery
④ Lessen tissue trauma from injections while resistance is low

118. Vitamin B_6 is given with isoniazid (INH) because it:
① Improves the nutritional status of the client
② Enhances tuberculostatic effect of isoniazid
③ Provides the vitamin when isoniazid is interfering with natural vitamin synthesis
④ Accelerates destruction of remaining organisms after inhibition of their reproduction by isoniazid

119. After Mr. Josh has been receiving streptomycin sulfate for 2 weeks, he states that he is "walking like a drunken seaman." The nurse withholds the drug and promptly reports the problem to the physician because the signs may be a result of drug effect on the:
① Cerebellar tissue
② Peripheral motor end-plates
③ Vestibular branch of the eighth cranial nerve
④ Internal capsule and pyramidal tracts

Situation: Mr. Arlo has come to the emergency room with shortness of breath, which occurred suddenly while he was getting dressed. He also has a history of emphysema. The physician diagnoses a spontaneous pneumothorax. Questions 120 through 129 refer to this situation.

120. The probable cause of a spontaneous pneumothorax is:
    ① Rupture of a subpleural bleb
    ② Pleural friction rub
    ③ Tracheoesophageal fistula
    ④ Puncture wound of the chest wall

121. Besides dyspnea, which of the following symptoms is generally associated with a spontaneous pneumothorax?
    ① Increased chest motion
    ② Unilateral chest pain
    ③ Hematemesis
    ④ Mediastinal shift toward the involved side

122. Air rushes into the alveoli as a result of:
    ① The rising pressure in the alveoli
    ② The rising pressure in the pleura
    ③ The lowered pressure in the chest cavity
    ④ The relaxation of the diaphragm

123. Mr. Arlo questions the nurse as to what has happened to his lung. The nurse bases the explanation on the understanding that:
    ① The heart and great vessels shift to the affected side
    ② There is a greater negative pressure within the chest cavity
    ③ Inspired air will move from the lung into the pleural space
    ④ The other lung will collapse if not treated immediately

124. If Mr. Arlo has suffered a complete pneumothorax, there is danger of a mediastinal shift. If such a shift occurs, it may lead to:
    ① Increased volume of the unaffected lung
    ② Infection of the subpleural lining
    ③ Rupture of the pericardium or aorta
    ④ Decreased filling of the right heart

125. Mr. Arlo becomes extremely drowsy; his pulse and respirations increase. The nurse should suspect:
    ① Elevated Po_2
    ② Respiratory alkalosis
    ③ Hypercapnia
    ④ Hypokalemia

126. In addition to calling the physician, the nurse should:
    ① Place the client on his unaffected side
    ② Administer 60% O_2 via Ventimask
    ③ Prepare for IV administration of electrolytes
    ④ Give 2 L O_2 per minute via nasal cannula

127. The physician inserts a chest tube in the right side and attaches it to a two-bottle closed-drainage system. In caring for Mr. Arlo, the nurse should:
    ① Administer morphine sulfate, since he will be agitated
    ② Apply a thoracic binder to prevent tension on the tube
    ③ Clamp the tubing to prevent a rapid decline in pressure
    ④ Observe for fluid fluctuations in the underwater glass tube

128. Complete lung expansion before the removal of chest tubes is evaluated by:
    ① Absence of additional drainage
    ② A decrease in adventitious sounds
    ③ Return of normal tidal volume
    ④ Comparison of chest radiographs

129. Mr. Arlo is scheduled for a pulmonary function test. The nurse explains that during the test the respiratory therapist will ask him to breathe normally in order to measure his:
    ① Vital capacity
    ② Tidal volume
    ③ Inspiratory reserve
    ④ Expiratory reserve

Situation: Mr. Psanka is admitted from the emergency room in acute respiratory distress resulting from an asthmatic attack. Questions 130 through 136 refer to this situation.

130. In which position should the nurse place Mr. Psanka to facilitate maximum air exchange?
    ① High Fowler's
    ② Semi-Fowler's
    ③ Orthopneic
    ④ Supine with pillows

131. Inhalation of isoproterenol (Isuprel), 1:200 prn, is prescribed to:
    ① Increase bronchial secretions
    ② Decrease blood pressure
    ③ Produce sedation
    ④ Relax bronchial spasm

132. During therapy with isoproterenol Mr. Psanka complains of palpitation, chest pain, and a throbbing headache. In view of these symptoms, which of the following statements represents the most appropriate nursing action?
    ① Reassure Mr. Psanka that these effects are temporary and will subside as he becomes accustomed to the drug
    ② Withhold the drug until additional orders are obtained from the physician
    ③ Tell him not to worry; he is experiencing expected side effects from the medicine
    ④ Ask him to relax; then instruct him to breathe slowly and deeply for several minutes

133. Mr. Psanka's pulmonary function studies are abnormal. The nurse should realize that one of the most common complications of chronic asthma is:
    ① Atelectasis
    ② Emphysema
    ③ Pneumothorax
    ④ Pulmonary fibrosis

134. Emphysema causes a failure in oxygen supply because of:
    ① Infectious obstructions
    ② Respiratory muscle paralysis
    ③ Pleural effusion
    ④ Loss of aerating surface

135. When the alveoli lose their normal elasticity, the nurse teaches Mr. Psanka exercises that lead to effective use of the diaphragm because:
    ① Mr. Psanka has an increase in the vital capacity of his lungs

② The residual capacity of the lungs has been increased

③ Inspiration has been markedly prolonged and difficult

④ Abdominal breathing is an effective compensatory mechanism that is spontaneously initiated

136. Respiratory acidosis may occur as a result of a long-term problem in oxygen maintenance when:
① The carbon dioxide is not excreted
② Any localized tissue necrosis occurs as a result of poor oxygen supply to the area
③ Hyperventilation occurs, even if the cause is not physiologic
④ There is a loss of carbon dioxide from the body's buffer pool

Situation: Mr. Rogers, with a long history of emphysema, is now terminally ill with cancer of the esophagus. His plan of care includes a soft diet, modified postural drainage, and IPPB treatments bid. He is weak, dyspneic, emaciated, and apathetic. Questions 137 through 143 refer to this situation.

137. Nursing care plans for Mr. Rogers should give priority to:
① Diet and nutrition
② Hygiene and comfort
③ Body mechanics and posture
④ Intake and output

138. Mr. Rogers expresses aversion to his meals and eats only small amounts. The nurse should provide:
① Only foods he likes in small portions
② Supplementary vitamins to stimulate appetite
③ Nourishment between meals
④ Small portions more frequently

139. The term used to describe Mr. Rogers' response to food most accurately is:
① Anorexia
② Anoxia
③ Apathy
④ Dysphagia

140. To obtain maximum benefits after postural drainage, Mr. Rogers should be:
① Placed in a sitting position to provide drainage
② Encouraged to cough deeply
③ Placed on an IPPB machine
④ Encouraged to rest for 30 minutes before coughing

141. Mr. Rogers' pain and dyspnea are increasing in severity. The physician has ordered 100 mg meperidine q4h and oxygen prn. In preparing Mr. Rogers' medication, the nurse should know that meperidine is commonly available for administration as:
① Darvon
② Doriden
③ Demerol
④ Narcan

142. The nurse administers nasal oxygen at 2 L/minute. The nurse should observe Mr. Rogers closely for:
① Hyperemia and increased respirations
② Cyanosis and lethargy
③ Anxiety and tachycardia
④ Drowsiness and decreased respirations

143. Mr. Rogers has a 44-year-old wife, a 16-year-old daughter in high school, and a 20-year-old son in college. They visit him frequently. In view of Mr. Rogers' extreme weakness and dyspnea, nursing care plans should include:
① Limiting family visiting hours to the evening before sleep
② Allowing self-activity whenever possible
③ Encouraging family to feed and assist him
④ Planning all necessary care at one time with long rests in between

Situation: Mr. Lange, a 36-year-old delicatessen clerk, is admitted with a pulmonary embolism. Questions 144 through 148 refer to this situation.

144. Mr. Lange is receiving an anticoagulant for a pulmonary embolism. Which of the following drugs is contraindicated for clients receiving anticoagulants?
① Isoxsuprine (Vasodilan)
② Chloral hydrate
③ Chlorpromazine (Thorazine)
④ Aspirin

145. Which of the following actions would the nurse initiate with Mr. Lange as a measure to prevent further emboli?
① Encourage deep breathing and coughing
② Use of the knee gatch when positioning the client
③ Limit the fluid intake of the immobilized client
④ Encourage him to move his legs while confined to bed

146. The nursing care plan should include observations of Mr. Lange for:
① Headache
② Epistaxis
③ Nausea
④ Chest pain

147. Mr. Lange begins to expectorate blood. The nurse describes this episode as:
① Hematuria
② Hematemesis
③ Hematoma
④ Hemoptysis

148. Mr. Lange becomes dyspneic. In which position should the nurse place him?
① Trendelenburg
② Sims
③ Orthopneic
④ Supine

Situation: Mr. Arnold is admitted to the CCU with a diagnosis of acute pulmonary edema. The physician has ordered rotating tourniquets. Questions 149 through 155 refer to this sitation.

149. When rotating tourniquets are used, the nurse should remember that:
① The automatic tourniquets occlude arterial blood flow
② The tourniquets are simultaneously applied to four limbs
③ The tourniquets are rotated every 15 minutes
④ The tourniquets are rotated two at a time

150. The rotating tourniquet technique is effective for:
    ① Decreasing arterial flow of blood to the body
    ② Restricting visceral flow in the internal body cavities
    ③ Decreasing venous flow of blood to the heart
    ④ Increasing the flow of blood through the capillaries

151. Mr. Arnold's respirations are rapid and he appears extremely anxious. The nurse should be aware that the medication most frequently used to relieve anxiety and apprehension in the client with pulmonary edema is:
    ① Hydroxyzine (Atarax)
    ② Sodium phenobarbital
    ③ Chloral hydrate
    ④ Morphine sulfate

152. An example of a rapidly acting diuretic that can be administered intravenously to clients with acute pulmonary edema is:
    ① Spironolactone
    ② Ethacrynic acid
    ③ Chlorothiazide
    ④ Chlorthalidone

153. Mr. Arnold is receiving aminophylline intravenously to relieve pulmonary edema. The nurse should observe him for:
    ① Decreased pulse rate
    ② Decreased urinary output
    ③ Hypotension
    ④ Visual disturbances

154. Mr. Arnold's condition worsens; he is intubated and placed on a mechanical ventilator. Central venous pressure must be monitored. In caring for Mr. Arnold, the nurse understands that:
    ① The client should not be taken off the ventilator for the central venous pressure readings
    ② The fluid level in the manometer fluctuates with each respiration
    ③ Blood should not be easily aspirated from the central venous pressure line
    ④ The zero mark on the manometer should be at the level of the diaphragm

155. The physician orders an IV digitalis preparation. Which of the following preparations is only administered intravenously?
    ① Digoxin
    ② Gitalin
    ③ Deslanoside
    ④ Digitalis leaf

Situation: Mr. Singer, age 68, is admitted with severe dyspnea and hemoptysis. Cancer of the lung is suspected and he is scheduled for a bronchoscopy. Questions 156 through 165 refer to this situation.

156. To prevent laryngeal edema after the procedure, the intervention most frequently used is the:
    ① Administration of lidocaine (Xylocaine)
    ② Utilization of a cool mist vaporizer
    ③ Provision of ice chips to suck on
    ④ Ensurance of a liberal fluid intake

157. Mr. Singer develops pleural effusion. This is most likely the result of:
    ① Irritation from the bronchoscopy
    ② Extension of cancerous lesions
    ③ Inadequate chest expansion
    ④ Excessive fluid intake

158. A thoracentesis is performed. Following the procedure it is most important for the nurse to observe Mr. Singer for:
    ① Increased breath sounds
    ② Expectoration of blood
    ③ Periods of confusion
    ④ Decreased respiratory rate

159. Mr. Singer is receiving prednisone and other chemotherapeutic agents and is placed in protective isolation. The administration of corticosteroids to control the symptoms of one disease can cause infections because of all the following *except:*
    ① Interference with the inflammatory response of the body
    ② Prevention of the production of leukocytes
    ③ Promotion of the growth and spread of enteric viruses
    ④ Stoppage of antibody production in lymphatic tissue

160. During Mr. Singer's chemotherapeutic course, he may develop soreness in the mouth and anus because:
    ① The side effects of the chemotherapeutic agents tend to concentrate in these body areas
    ② The entire GI tract is involved because of the direct irritating effects of chemotherapy
    ③ These tissues are poorly nourished because the client is anorectic
    ④ These tissues normally divide rapidly and are damaged by the chemotherapeutic agent

161. In caring for Mr. Singer the nurse realizes that sink faucets in his room are considered contaminated because:
    ① They are not in sterile areas
    ② Water encourages bacterial growth
    ③ They are opened with dirty hands
    ④ Large numbers of people use them

162. On one occasion Mr. Singer says to the nurse, "If I could just be free of pain for a few days, I might be able to eat more and regain strength." In reference to the stages of dying, the client indicates:
    ① Rationalization
    ② Frustration
    ③ Bargaining
    ④ Depression

163. When Mr. Singer reaches the point of acceptance in the stages of dying, it may be manifested in his behavior by:
    ① Euphoria
    ② Detachment
    ③ Apathy
    ④ Emotionalism

164. Mr. Singer drank 7½ oz of orange juice, 6 oz of tea, and 8 oz of eggnog. The calculated intake would be:
    ① 515 ml
    ② 645 ml
    ③ 625 ml
    ④ 585 ml

165. The best nursing approach in dealing with Mr. Singer is to:
    ① Ignore his behavior
    ② Point out the reality of the situation
    ③ Join him, since denial is his only defense
    ④ Recognize and accept the behavior at this point

166. A rocking bed promotes circulation and breathing through the principle of:
① Centrifugal force
② Inertia
③ Momentum
④ Gravity

167. The efficacy of the abdominal-thoracic thrust (Heimlich maneuver) to expel a foreign object in the larynx demonstrates the gas volume related to the individual's:
① Vital capacity
② Residual volume
③ Tidal volume
④ Inspiratory reserve volume

168. A client who undergoes a submucosal resection should be observed carefully for:
① Occipital headache
② Periorbital crepitus
③ Spitting up or vomiting of blood
④ White areas of healing sublingually

169. The usual stimulant for the respiratory center is:
① Calcium ions
② Carbon dioxide
③ Lactic acid
④ Oxygen

170. Oxygen dissociation from hemoglobin and therefore oxygen delivery to the tissues are accelerated by:
① A decreasing oxygen pressure in the blood
② A decreasing oxygen pressure and/or an increasing carbon dioxide pressure in the blood
③ An increasing oxygen pressure and/or a decreasing carbon dioxide pressure in the blood
④ An increasing carbon dioxide pressure in the blood

171. The poisonous nature of carbon monoxide (CO) results from:
① Its preferential combination with hemoglobin
② Its tendency to block CO_2 transport
③ Its inhibitory effect on vasodilation
④ The bubbles it tends to form in blood plasma

172. With an oxygen debt, muscle shows:
① High levels of calcium
② Low levels of lactic acid
③ High levels of glycogen
④ Low levels of ATP

173. Two body systems that interact with the bicarbonate buffer system to preserve the normal body fluid pH of 7.4 are the:
① Respiratory and urinary systems
② Muscular and endocrine systems
③ Skeletal and nervous systems
④ Circulatory and urinary systems

174. If breathing is deliberately stopped by a person:
① The individual will soon die of suffocation
② Rising oxygen concentrations will stimulate the breathing center
③ Accumulated CO_2 will force resumption of breathing
④ Increased N_2 concentration will have a toxic effect

175. A nurse will use an Ambu bag in the intensive care unit when:
① The client is in ventricular fibrillation
② A surgical incision with copious drainage is present
③ Respiratory output must be monitored at intervals
④ There is respiratory arrest

176. In suctioning a client with a tracheostomy the nurse must remember that it is important to:
① Initiate suction as the catheter is being withdrawn slowly
② Insert catheter until cough reflex is stimulated
③ Untie the neck tapes while cleansing the skin edge of the wound
④ Remove the inner cannula before inserting the suction catheter

177. Cutting the left phrenic nerve results in:
① Relief of pain in the left side of the chest
② Paralysis of the left side of the diaphragm
③ Collapse of the right lung
④ Paralysis of the diaphragm on the opposite side

The Gastrointestinal System

Situation: Mrs. Graham has a diagnosis of possible bowel obstruction. She complains of nausea, is vomiting dark bile material, and has severe crampy, intermittent, abdominal pain. Her physician suspects the bowel obstruction is caused by an intussusception. Questions 178 through 184 refer to this situation.

178. An intussusception is:
① Kinking of the bowel onto itself
② Telescoping of a proximal loop of bowel into a distal loop
③ A band of connective tissue compressing the bowel
④ A protrusion of an organ or part of an organ through the wall that contains it

179. A flat plate radiograph of the abdomen is ordered. The nurse recognizes that the client should receive:
① Nothing by mouth for 8 hours
② A low soapsuds enema
③ No special preparation
④ A laxative the evening before the x-ray film is taken

180. Surgery is performed; Mrs. Graham is found to have a perforated appendix with localized peritonitis rather than an intussusception. In view of this finding, the nurse should position Mrs. Graham postoperatively in the:
① Semi-Fowler's position
② Trendelenburg position
③ Sims' position
④ Dorsal recumbent position

181. Four days after surgery Mrs. Graham has not passed any flatus and there are no bowel sounds. Despite the fact that her abdomen has become more distended, she feels little discomfort. Paralytic ileus is suspected. In this condition there is an interference caused by:
① Impaired blood supply
② Impaired neural functioning
③ Perforation of the bowel wall
④ Obstruction of the bowel lumen

182. Mrs. Graham is convalescing from abdominal surgery when she develops thrombophlebitis. Which of the following signs would indicate this complication to the nurse?
① Severe pain on extension of an extremity
② Pitting edema of the lower extremities
③ Intermittent claudication
④ Warm, tender area on the leg

183. Mrs. Graham is receiving Dicumarol, a coumarin derivative. Which of the following tests would be most specific for calculating daily dosage of anticoagulant?
    ① Prothrombin time
    ② Clotting time
    ③ Bleeding time
    ④ Sedimentation rate

184. Which of the following drugs would the nurse expect the physician to order if symptoms of Dicumarol overdose are observed?
    ① Iron-dextran (Imferon)
    ② Heparin
    ③ Vitamin K
    ④ Protamine sufate

Situation: Mrs. McCann, a 93-year-old widow, has been admitted to the hospital from a nursing home. She has been complaining of severe lower abdominal pain, anorexia, nausea, and vomiting for the past 24 hours. History and physical examination reveal a thin, elderly white woman in remarkably good physical and mental condition except for the present complaints. The most likely cause of Mrs. McCann's illness is thought to be sigmoid diverticulitis. After the appropriate diagnostic workup and preparation for surgery, an exploratory laparotomy is performed. Surgery comfirms the admitting diagnosis but also reveals a large silent giant ulcer in the stomach, which requires a subtotal gastrectomy (Billroth I). Mrs. McCann does well after surgery but on the fifth postoperative day develops severe abdominal pain with distended abdomen, a markedly elevated WBC, and temperature of 103° F (39.5° C) rectally. She is taken to the OR once again, where plication for a leak in the duodenostomy is performed. Questions 185 through 190 refer to this situation.

185. The primary reason for performing surgery in the first instance is most likely that
    ① Diverticulitis in some instances is difficult to differentiate from carcinoma except surgically
    ② The symptoms exhibited by the client on admission were serious
    ③ The complication—perforation—had occurred with resultant abscess formation or generalized peritonitis
    ④ Surgery is usually indicated for clients with a diagnosis of diverticulitis

186. One of the major problems after this type of surgery is the prevention of pulmonary complications. The nurse can best achieve this by:
    ① Encouraging deep breathing and coughing to counteract voluntary diaphragm splinting
    ② Promoting frequent turning, moving, and deep breathing to mobilize bronchial secretions
    ③ Ambulating to increase respiratory exchange
    ④ Administering IPPB every 4 hours

187. A gastrectomy following severe stomach ulceration may eventually be associated with pernicious anemia because:
    ① Vitamin B_{12} is only absorbed in the stomach
    ② The stomach parietal cells secrete the intrinsic factor
    ③ The hemopoietic factor is secreted in the stomach
    ④ Chief cells in the stomach secrete the extrinsic factor

188. In caring for a client with a nasogastric tube attached to suction, the nurse should:
    ① Irrigate the tube with physiologic saline
    ② Allow the client to have small chips of ice or sips of water unless nauseated
    ③ Use sterile technique in irrigating the tube
    ④ Withdraw the tube quickly when decompression is terminated

189. Because Mrs. McCann's skin is extremely dry, flaky, wrinkled, sagging, and sallow, an important nursing measure is to:
    ① Avoid daily bathing but use emollients
    ② Bathe her once or twice a week and use emollients
    ③ Bathe when necessary and use emollients
    ④ Use emollients for skin care

190. The wisest guideline for Mrs. McCann's diet would be:
    ① No oral feedings for a prolonged period
    ② Gradual resumption of small, easily digested feedings
    ③ At her age allow anything she wants at any time
    ④ Give nothing by mouth and depend on IV feedings indefinitely

Situation: Mr. Weinberg is admitted to the hospital with cirrhosis of the liver and malnutrition. Questions 191 through 196 refer to this situation.

191. Mr. Weinberg begins to develop slurred speech, confusion, drowsiness, and tremors. With these symptoms his diet would be limited to:
    ① 20 g protein, 2000 calories
    ② 80 g protein, 1000 calories
    ③ 100 g protein, 2500 calories
    ④ 150 g protein, 1200 calories

192. Mr. Weinberg has a swollen appearance as a result of the edema and ascites. The ascites is caused by:
    ① Portal hypertension
    ② Kidney malfunction
    ③ Decreased production of potassium
    ④ Diminished plasma protein

193. The symptoms of portal hypertension are largely caused by:
    ① Infection of the liver parenchyma
    ② Fatty degeneration of Kupffer cells
    ③ Obstruction of the portal circulation
    ④ Obstruction of the cystic and hepatic ducts

194. What complication is most likely to occur when a client has portal hypertension?
    ① Perforation of the duodenum
    ② Hemorrhage from esophageal varices
    ③ Liver abscess
    ④ Intestinal obstruction

195. Mr. Weinberg's long-standing poor nutrition, especially his deficiency of protein, has led to:
    ① Fat accumulation in the liver tissue
    ② Coagulation of blood in microcirculation
    ③ Tissue anabolism and positive nitrogen balance
    ④ Decreased bile in the blood

196. The nurse expects weight loss in a client receiving IV administration of 5% dextrose in water due to:
    ① Insufficient carbohydrate intake
    ② Lack of protein supplementation
    ③ Insufficient intake of water-soluble vitamins
    ④ Increased concentration of electrolytes in cells

Situation: Mrs. Smith, a 45-year-old, rather obese mother of five children, is admitted to the emergency room complaining of nausea, belching, gas, and right upper quadrant pain that was not relieved by taking Alka-Seltzer. She states that she has had attacks for the past several years, especially after eating fatty or fried foods. After a series of diagnostic tests, the client is prepared for surgery. A cholecystectomy and choledochotomy are performed. Mrs. Smith is reluctant to cough or move. Questions 197 through 203 refer to this situation.

197. Mrs. Smith experienced discomfort after ingesting fatty foods because:
    ① The liver was manufacturing inadequate bile
    ② Fatty foods are hard to digest
    ③ Obstruction of the common bile duct prevented emptying of the bile into the intestine
    ④ She did not eliminate fatty foods from her diet

198. A client with obstruction of the common bile duct may show a prolonged bleeding and clotting time because:
    ① The extrinsic factor is not absorbed
    ② Vitamin K is not absorbed
    ③ The ionized calcium level falls
    ④ Bilirubin accumulates in the plasma

199. Cholecystography was performed to:
    ① Detect obstruction at the ampulla of Vater
    ② Observe patency of the common bile duct
    ③ Determine the concentration ability of the gallbladder
    ④ Distinguish stone formation from other types of obstruction

200. Mrs. Smith had an interference in bile utilization caused by cholecystitis. The ejection of bile into the alimentary tract is controlled by which of the following hormones?
    ① Cholecystokinin
    ② Secretin
    ③ Gastrin
    ④ Enterocrinin

201. Mrs. Smith has a Penrose drain inserted. The nurse caring for her in the recovery room notices that the dressing has become soiled with a brownish red fluid. The nurse should:
    ① Change the dressing
    ② Reinforce the dressing
    ③ Apply an abdominal binder
    ④ Remove the tape and apply Montgomery straps

202. Postoperatively Mrs. Smith suddenly complains of numbness in the right leg and a "funny feeling" in the toes. The nurse should first:
    ① Elevate the legs and tell her to stay in bed
    ② Rub her legs to start circulation and place a warm blanket on her
    ③ Tell her she has been staying in bed too much and encourage ambulation
    ④ Tell her to remain in bed and notify the physician

203. When Mrs. Smith is able to eat solid food, which of the following special diets should be ordered?
    ① High in protein and calories to promote wound healing

② Low in fat to avoid painful contractions in the wound area
    ③ Low in protein and carbohydrate to avoid excess calories and help her lose weight
    ④ High in fat and carbohydrate to meet energy demands

Situation: Dr. Grove, a single, 25-year-old professor of mathematics at a major university, is hospitalized for bleeding gastric ulcers. A conservative regimen is being followed at present. At an early age it became apparent that Dr. Grove was a genius. His capabilities were encouraged to develop to their fullest potential by his mother. He graduated from high school summa cum laude at the age of 13 and at the age of 19 had received a Ph.D. degree in mathematics. Dr. Grove lives at home with his aging mother. Questions 204 through 208 refer to this situation.

204. Dr. Grove describes his pain as:
    ① A dull ache radiating to the left side
    ② An intermittent colicky flank pain
    ③ A generalized abdominal pain intensified by moving
    ④ A gnawing sensation relieved by food

205. Analysis of factors resulting in psychologic conflict for Dr. Grove reveals:
    ① An unconscious need to be dependent
    ② The drive to excel in whatever he does
    ③ Conversion of emotional tension due to chronic repressed hostility
    ④ Many feelings that are deep in the unconscious

206. Despite initiation of therapy, Dr. Grove continues to be apprehensive and restless. Nursing action should include:
    ① Telling him everything will be all right
    ② Administering antibiotics as ordered
    ③ Explaining the importance of rest
    ④ Administering sedatives as ordered

207. What is the basic goal underlying Dr. Grove's conservative regimen?
    ① To increase roughage and bulk
    ② To eliminate chemical, mechanical, and thermal irritation
    ③ To provide optimum amounts of all nutrients
    ④ To provide psychologic support by offering a wide variety of foods

208. If Dr. Grove has lost enough blood to develop a mild anemia, he would probably be treated with:
    ① Dextran
    ② Cari-Tab Softabs
    ③ Salts of iron
    ④ Vitamin B_{12}

Situation: Mr. Ergotano, 50 years old, recently came from Italy with his wife to visit with American relatives. While here, he is admitted to the hospital complaining of anorexia, loss of weight, abdominal distention, and passage of abnormal stools. The most likely diagnosis on the basis of history and physical examination is cancer of the stomach or malabsorption syndrome. Neither Mr. Ergotano nor his wife speaks any English. Their trip to America was sponsored by relatives. Questions 209 through 216 refer to this situation.

209. To determine the correct diagnosis, extensive diagnostic studies are performed. Tests in connection with cancer of the stomach include:
   ① X-ray examination
   ② CBC
   ③ Thorn test
   ④ Gastroscopy

210. Mr. Ergotano appears frightened and Mrs. Ergotano is near hysteria. Identifying their emotional state and being able to communicate with only rudimentary sign language, the nurse should:
   ① Give them a booklet with Italian translations of English medical terms
   ② Call an Italian-speaking employee from another part of the hospital when necessary
   ③ Reduce communication to the bare essentials
   ④ Permit an American relative to stay with Mr. and Mrs. Erogotano at all times

211. An IV of 1000 ml 5% dextrose in water each shift is started on admission to correct fluid imbalance. The infusion set delivers 10 drops per milliliter. To regulate the rate of flow so that the solution would be infused over an 8-hour period, the nurse should set the rate of flow at:
   ① 160 drops per minute
   ② 60 drops per minute
   ③ 20 drops per minute
   ④ 40 drops per minute

212. Later the physician changes the order to keep vein open. What is the longest possible period of time that one bottle of 1000 ml of 5% dextrose in water to keep a vein open can be infused without producing untoward effects?
   ① 6 hours
   ② 12 hours
   ③ 18 hours
   ④ 24 hours

213. Differential diagnosis establishes that Mr. Ergotano has nontropical sprue. Striking clinical improvement is noted after administration of:
   ① A gluten-free diet
   ② Folic acid
   ③ Corticotropin
   ④ Vitamin B_{12}

214. Because malabsorption syndrome seems to be present, a trial period on a sprue diet is ordered for Mr. Ergotano. He is not allowed to have:
   ① Wheat, rye, or oats
   ② Rice or corn
   ③ Milk or cheese
   ④ Fruit or fruit juices

215. A typical food combination served to Mr. Ergotano on this diet would be:
   ① Creamed turkey on toast, rice, green peas, milk
   ② Roast beef, baked potato, carrots, tea
   ③ Cheese omelet, noodles, green beans, coffee
   ④ Baked chicken, mashed potatoes with gravy, zucchini, Postum

216. Since Mr. Ergotano's nutritional status is poor, the nurse should:
   ① Encourage meats at mealtime and high protein snacks
   ② Keep him npo, since food precipitates diarrhea
   ③ Allow whatever foods he will eat from the diet
   ④ Institute IV therapy to improve hydration

Situation: Mr. Gray is admitted to the hospital with extensive carcinoma of the descending portion of the colon with metastasis to the lymph nodes. Questions 217 through 224 refer to this situation.

217. The operative procedure that would probably be performed is a(an):
   ① Cecostomy
   ② Ileostomy
   ③ Colectomy
   ④ Colostomy

218. The nurse administers neomycin sulfate to Mr. Gray preoperatively to:
   ① Decrease the possibility of postoperative urinary tract infection
   ② Increase the production of vitamin K
   ③ Destroy intestinal bacteria
   ④ Decrease the incidence of any secondary infection

219. The nurse protects the skin surrounding the colostomy opening by using:
   ① Petroleum jelly
   ② Alcohol
   ③ Aluminum paste
   ④ Mineral oil

220. After surgery Mr. Gray asks what effect the surgery will have on his sexual relationships. The nurse should tell him that:
   ① Sexual relationships must be curtailed
   ② He should tell his partner about his surgery prior to sexual activity
   ③ He will be able to resume normal sexual relationships
   ④ The surgery will temporarily decrease his sexual impulses

221. In teaching Mr. Gray to care for the colostomy, the nurse should advise him to irrigate it at the same time every day and to choose a time:
   ① When he can be assured of uninterrupted bathroom use at home
   ② That approximates his usual daily time for elimination
   ③ About halfway between the two largest meals of the day
   ④ About 1 hour before breakfast

222. If, during the colostomy irrigation, Mr. Gray complains of abdominal cramps, the nurse should:
   ① Lower the container of fluid
   ② Discontinue the irrigation
   ③ Clamp the catheter for a few minutes
   ④ Advance the catheter about 2.5 cm (1 inch)

223. When performing the colostomy irrigation, the nurse inserts the catheter into the stoma:
① 5 cm (2 inches)
② 10 cm (4 inches)
③ 15 cm (6 inches)
④ 20 cm (8 inches)
224. When teaching Mr. Gray to irrigate his colostomy, the nurse indicates that the distance of the container above the stoma should be no more than:
① 45 cm (18 inches)
② 15 cm (6 inches)
③ 25 cm (10 inches)
④ 30 cm (12 inches)

Situation: Mr. Fink, a soft drink vendor, enters the hospital with diarrhea, anorexia, weight loss, and abdominal cramps. A tentative diagnosis of colitis has been made. He is scheduled for a sigmoidoscopy and barium enema. Questions 225 through 232 refer to this situation.

225. In eliciting a health history the nurse bases the interview on the knowledge that colitis is commonly associated with:
① Chemical stress
② Endocrine stress
③ Psychologic stress
④ Physiologic stress
226. The symptoms of fluid and electrolyte imbalance caused by Mr. Fink's condition that the nurse should report immediately are:
① Extreme muscle weakness and tachycardia
② Development of tetany with muscle spasms
③ Nausea, vomiting, and leg and stomach cramps
④ Skin rash, diarrhea, and diplopia
227. Specific nursing responsibility in preparing Mr. Fink for his diagnostic procedures includes:
① Administering soapsuds enemas until clear
② Giving castor oil the afternoon before
③ Withholding food and fluid for 8 hours
④ Ensuring his understanding of what is to happen
228. Prior to the barium enema, Mr. Fink is to receive an enema. When receiving the enema, Mr. Fink should be positioned in the:
① Sims' position
② Knee-chest position
③ Mid-Fowler's position
④ Back lying position
229. The maximum safe height at which the container of fluid can be held when administering an enema is:
① 30 cm (12 inches)
② 37 cm (15 inches)
③ 45 cm (18 inches)
④ 66 cm (26 inches)
230. During administration of the enema Mr. Fink complains of intestinal cramps. The nurse should:
① Give at a slower rate
② Lower the height of the container
③ Stop until cramps are gone
④ Discontinue the procedure
231. The visualization of the GI tract after a barium enema is made possible by:
① The high x-ray absorbing properties of barium
② Barium physically coloring the intestinal wall

③ The high x-ray transmitting properties of barium
④ The chemical interaction between barium and the electrolytes
232. To decrease GI irritability, the nurse should teach Mr. Fink to minimize use of:
① Triglycerides and amino acids
② Milk products and cola drinks
③ Table salt and rice products
④ Sugar products and proteins

Situation: Mrs. Smith is admitted to the hospital with an acute attack of ulcerative colitis. She has been very worried about her two small children and calls her mother frequently for help. She recently pleaded with her mother to come and live with them. Mr. Smith objects to this, goes out alone quite often, and does not seem to take an interest in the children. Questions 233 through 239 refer to this situation.

233. The nurse will understand the emotional aspects of these disorders more readily by recognizing the stress functions of the:
① Cerebral cortex and thyroid gland
② Sympathetic nervous system and pancreas
③ Autonomic nervous system and adrenal glands
④ Central nervous system and hypothalamus
234. To give complete nursing care to Mrs. Smith, the nurse should:
① Understand the client's emotional conflict
② Recognize his or her own feelings toward this client
③ Talk with the client's husband and mother
④ Develop rapport with the client's physician
235. The nurse recognizes that the prognosis for Mrs. Smith will remain guarded until:
① A surgical procedure is performed to remove the somatic factor
② Her husband accepts her desire to have her mother move in with them
③ Her emotional conflicts are resolved
④ She reaches her 40s and endocrine activity is decreased
236. The symptoms that the nurse should expect when assessing Mrs. Smith on admission are:
① Diarrhea, anorexia, weight loss, abdominal cramps, anemia
② Anemia, hemoptysis, weight loss, abdominal cramps
③ Fever, anemia, nausea and vomiting, leukopenia, diarrhea
④ Leukocytosis, anorexia, weight loss
237. The physician orders daily stool examinations. Mrs. Smith is also scheduled for a sigmoidoscopy and barium enema. Stool examinations are ordered to determine:
① Culture and sensitivity
② Occult blood and organisms
③ Ova and parasites
④ Fat and undigested food
238. A serious complication of this disease is:
① Hemorrhage
② Perforation
③ Obstruction
④ Ileus

239. Mrs. Smith's initial hospital diet is residue free during the acute stage. Which food combination should the nurse indicate as the best choice for her?
    ① Cream soup and crackers, omelet, mashed potatoes, roll, orange juice, coffee
    ② Stewed chicken, baked potato with butter, strained peas, white bread, plain cake, milk
    ③ Baked fish, macaroni with cheese, strained carrots, fruit gelatin, milk
    ④ Lean roast beef, buttered white rice with egg slices, white bread with butter and jelly, tea with sugar

Situation: Mrs. Carter, the mother of two children, has infectious hepatitis. Questions 240 through 242 refer to this situation.

240. Mrs. Carter's children are being given gamma globulin to provide passive immunity, which:
    ① Stimulates production of short-lived antibodies
    ② Stimulates the lymphatic system to produce large numbers of antibodies
    ③ Provides antibodies that neutralize the antigen
    ④ Accelerates antigen-antibody union at hepatic sites
241. The physician has prescribed phenobarbital sodium (Luminal) for Mrs. Carter. The nurse tells Mrs. Carter to contact the physician if she notices:
    ① Decreased tolerance to common foods, constipation
    ② Diarrhea, rash on the upper part of her body
    ③ Anal pruritus, orthostatic hypotension
    ④ Loss of appetite, persistent lethargy
242. When caring for Mrs. Carter the nurse should take special precautions to:
    ① Use caution when bringing food tray to client
    ② Wear mask and gown before entering the room
    ③ Use gloves when removing the client's bedpan
    ④ Prevent droplet spread of infection

Situation: Mr. Brown is admitted to the hospital with delirium tremens. His physician prescribes bed rest, and he is receiving paraldehyde, thiamine chloride, and nicotinic acid. Questions 243 through 247 refer to this situation.

243. On Mr. Brown's admission, the nurse should assign him to a:
    ① One-bed room next to the bathroom
    ② Two-bed room at the quiet end of the unit
    ③ One-bed room next to the nurses' station
    ④ Two-bed room next to the nurses' station
244. The nurse understands that paraldehyde is given to combat which of Mr. Brown's problems?
    ① Fluid and electrolyte
    ② Detoxification from alcohol
    ③ Emotional
    ④ Motor and sensory
245. When Mr. Brown is able to eat, the diet ordered for him is:
    ① High protein, low carbohydrate, low fat
    ② Protein to tolerance, moderate fat, high calorie, high vitamin, soft
    ③ High carbohydrate, low saturated fat, 1800 calories
    ④ Low protein, high carbohydrate, high fat, soft

246. A high-calorie diet fortified with vitamins will prevent damage to which organ that detoxifies alcohol?
    ① Kidneys
    ② Liver
    ③ Pancreas
    ④ Adrenals
247. Mr. Brown requires thiamine chloride and nicotinic acid because these vitamins are needed for the maintenance of:
    ① Good circulation
    ② The nervous system
    ③ Prothrombin formation
    ④ Elimination

Situation: Mrs. Green underwent a cholecystectomy. Questions 248 through 252 refer to this situation.

248. When changing Mrs. Green's dressing, the nurse is careful not to introduce microorganisms into the surgical incision. This is an example of what kind of asepsis?
    ① Concurrent
    ② Medical
    ③ Wound
    ④ Surgical
249. Signs of obstructive jaundice include:
    ① Dark-colored urine, clay-colored stools, itchy skin
    ② Straw-colored urine, putty-colored stools, yellow sclerae
    ③ Inadequate absorption of fat-soluble vitamin K
    ④ Light amber urine, dark brown stools, yellow skin
250. To promote healing of the large incision, Mrs. Green's physician would order daily doses of which of these vitamins?
    ① Ascorbic acid
    ② Mephyton
    ③ Vitamin B_{12} complex
    ④ Vitamin A
251. Mrs. Green is prone to upper respiratory tract complications because of:
    ① Lowering of resistance due to bile in the blood
    ② Invasion of bloodstream by infection from the biliary tract
    ③ Proximity of the incision to the diaphragm
    ④ Length of time required for the surgery
252. Because vitamin A is fat soluble, it requires a helping agent for absorption. This agent is:
    ① Lipase
    ② Amylase
    ③ Hydrochloric acid
    ④ Bile

Situation: Mrs. Thomas, 62 years of age, is admitted to the hospital complaining of nausea, vomiting, weight loss of 20 pounds in 2 months, and periods of constipation and diarrhea. A diagnosis of carcinoma of the colon is made. Questions 253 through 259 refer to this situation.

253. A sigmoidoscopy is performed as a diagnostic measure. The nurse should place Mrs. Thomas in which position for this examination?
    ① Prone
    ② Lithotomy
    ③ Sims'
    ④ Knee-chest

254. As part of the preparation of Mrs. Thomas for the sigmoidoscopy, the nurse should:
① Withhold all fluids and foods for 24 hours before the examination
② Explain to the client that a chalklike substance will have to be swallowed
③ Administer an enema the morning of the examination
④ Provide a container for collection of a stool specimen

255. During the preoperative shaving preparation Mrs. Thomas starts to cry and says, "I'm sorry you have to do this messy thing for me." The choice response for a nurse at this time is:
① "I don't mind it."
② "Nurses get used to this."
③ "This is part of my job."
④ "You are upset."

256. Neomycin is especially useful prior to colon surgery because:
① It is effective against many organisms
② It acts systemically without delay
③ It will not affect the kidneys
④ It is poorly absorbed from the GI tract

257. The physician performs a colostomy. Postoperative nursing care should include:
① Having her change her own dressing
② Keeping the skin around the stoma clean and dry
③ Limiting fluid intake
④ Withholding all fluids for 72 hours

258. A person who has a permanent colostomy:
① Needs special clothing
② Has to limit activities
③ Will have to dilate the stoma periodically
④ Needs to be on a bland, low-residue diet

259. When at home, Mrs. Thomas' diet should be:
① As close to normal as possible
② Rich in protein
③ Low in fiber content
④ High in carbohydrate

Situation: Mrs. Eve, a 40-year-old housewife, is admitted to the hospital with a history of vomiting, tarry stools, ascites, and longstanding poor nutrition due to excessive alcohol intake. Her admitting diagnosis is bleeding esophageal varices. After emergency treatment the plan of therapy involves preparing Mrs. Eve for a portal-caval anastomosis. Questions 260 through 267 refer to this situation.

260. The pathophysiologic problem in cirrhosis of the liver causing esophageal varices is:
① Dilated veins and varicosities
② Portal hypertension
③ Ascites and edema
④ Loss of regeneration

261. Which of the following medical treatments would be unrelated to the control of hemorrhage?
① Aminocaproic acid (Amicar)
② Balloon tamponade
③ Gastric suctioning
④ Iced lavage

262. Neomycin may be administered to prevent formation of:
① Urea
② Ammonia
③ Bile
④ Hemoglobin

263. If intubation is favored, the type of tube most likely to be used is:
① Sengstaken-Blakemore
② Miller-Abbott
③ Andersen
④ Levin

264. Characteristic signs that are a direct result of liver insufficiency may include:
① Anuria
② Fetor hepaticus
③ Globus hystericus
④ Blepharospasm

265. In an effort to prevent hepatic coma, it may become necessary to:
① Eliminate protein from the diet
② Eliminate carbohydrate from the diet
③ Give Fleet enemas
④ Prepare for emergency surgery

266. When Mrs. Eve is able to eat, the most therapeutic diet would be:
① High protein, low carbohydrate, low fat
② Low sodium, protein to tolerance, moderate fat, high calorie, high vitamin, soft
③ High carbohydrate, low saturated fat, 1200 calories
④ Low protein, low carbohydrate, high fat, soft

267. Mrs. Eve begins to develop slurred speech, confusion, drowsiness, and a flapping tremor. With these evidences of impending hepatic coma, her diet would probably be changed to:
① 20 g protein, 2000 calories
② 70 g protein, 1200 calories
③ 80 g protein, 2500 calories
④ 100 g protein, 1500 calories

Situation: Mr. Smith, a 36-year-old father of two children, is admitted to the hospital after an episode of vomiting "coffee-ground" material. The tentative diagnosis is peptic ulcer. Questions 268 through 274 refer to this situation.

268. Most peptic ulcers occurring in the stomach are in the:
① Pyloric portion
② Body of the stomach
③ Cardiac portion
④ Esophageal junction

269. The physician orders propantheline (Pro-Banthine) for Mr. Smith. Pro-Banthine is an anticholinergic drug whose main action is to:
① Neutralize gastric acidity
② Increase gastric motility
③ Reduce the pH of gastric contents
④ Delay gastric emptying

270. Mr. Smith does not respond to conservative therapy, and a vagotomy and partial gastrectomy are scheduled. Mr. Smith is returned to the unit from the recovery room with IV solutions running and a nasogas-

tric tube in place. Later that evening the nurse notes that there has been no nasogastric drainage for ½ hour. Physician's orders state: "Irrigate nasogastric tube prn." The nurse should insert:
  ① 30 ml of normal saline and withdraw slowly
  ② 15 ml of distilled water and disconnect suction for 30 minutes
  ③ 20 ml of air and clamp off suction for 1 hour
  ④ 50 ml of saline and increase pressure of suction

271. A vagotomy is performed to:
  ① Increase heart rate
  ② Hasten gastric emptying
  ③ Eliminate pain sensation
  ④ Decrease secretions in the stomach

272. Intravenous orders for Mr. Smith state that he is to receive 1000 ml of fluid every 8 hours. If the equipment delivers 15 drops/minute, the nurse should regulate the flow at approximately:
  ① 60 drops/min
  ② 15 drops/min
  ③ 23 drops/min
  ④ 31 drops/min

273. When preparing an IV piggyback medication for Mr. Smith, the nurse is aware that it is essential to:
  ① Rotate the bag after adding the medication
  ② Use strict sterile technique
  ③ Use exactly 100 ml fluid to mix medication
  ④ Change needle prior to adding medication

274. During the convalescent period the nurse sets up a health teaching program designed specifically to meet Mr. Smith's needs. This plan would include:
  ① A thorough explanation of the dumping syndrome and how to limit or prevent it
  ② A warning to avoid all gas-forming foods
  ③ Encouragement to resume his previous eating habits as soon as possible
  ④ An explanation of the therapeutic effect of a high-roughage diet

Situation: Mrs. Simone is admitted to the unit with a diagnosis of liver cirrhosis and hepatic coma. Questions 275 through 279 refer to this situation.

275. One classic sign of hepatic coma is:
  ① Elevated cholesterol
  ② Bile-colored stools
  ③ Flapping hand tremors
  ④ Depressed muscle reflexes

276. Considering the diagnosis, the nurse should assess Mrs. Simone for:
  ① Uremic frost
  ② Urticaria
  ③ Hemangioma
  ④ Icterus

277. The ascites seen in cirrhosis is in part due to:
  ① Increased plasma colloid osmotic pressure due to excessive liver growth and metabolism
  ② The escape of lymph into the abdominal cavity directly from the inflamed liver sinusoid
  ③ Compression of the portal veins with resultant increased backpressure in the portal venous system
  ④ The decreased levels of ADH and aldosterone due to increasing metabolic activity in the liver

278. Liver cirrhosis may promote varicose veins because of:
  ① Toxic irritating products released into the blood from the diseased organs
  ② Increased plasma hydrostatic pressure in veins of the extremities
  ③ Decreased plasma protein concentration resulting in pooling of blood in the venous system
  ④ Ballooning of the vein walls due to decreased venous pressure and incompetent valves

279. The laboratory test which would indicate that the liver is compromised and neomycin enemas might be helpful would be:
  ① Culture and sensitivity
  ② Serum glutamic-pyruvic transaminase
  ③ White blood count
  ④ Ammonia level

Situation: Mrs. Evans, a 60-year-old homemaker, is admitted because of possible intestinal obstruction. A Cantor tube has been inserted and attached to suction. Questions 280 through 285 refer to this situation.

280. A serious danger to which Mrs. Evans is exposed because of intestinal suction is excessive loss of:
  ① Protein enzymes
  ② Energy carbohydrates
  ③ Water and electrolytes
  ④ Vitamins and minerals

281. Critical assessment of Mrs. Evans includes observation for:
  ① Dehydration
  ② Excessive salivation
  ③ Edema
  ④ Belching

282. The solution of choice used to maintain patency of the Cantor tube is:
  ① Hypertonic glucose
  ② Isotonic saline
  ③ Hypotonic saline
  ④ Sterile water

283. Mrs. Evans is scheduled for a colostomy after diagnostic workup. Her anxiety is overt and realistic. The most effective way to help Mrs. Evans at this point is to:
  ① Encourage her to express her feelings
  ② Reassure her that many people cope with this problem
  ③ Explain the procedure and postoperative course
  ④ Administer a sedative and tell her to rest

284. The primary step toward long-range goals in Mrs. Evans' rehabilitation is her:
  ① Mastery of techniques of colostomy care
  ② Readiness to accept her altered body function
  ③ Knowledge of the necessary dietary modifications
  ④ Awareness of available community resources

285. Mrs. Evans has a transverse colostomy. When inserting a catheter, the nurse should:
  ① Use an oil-base lubricant
  ② Direct it toward the client's right side
  ③ Apply gentle but continuous force
  ④ Instruct her to bear down

Situation: Mr. Olgen has been diagnosed with cancer of the liver. He is in a debilitated state and is admitted for palliative treatment. Questions 286 through 290 refer to this situation.

286. On admission the objective information that would be most helpful for future monitoring of Mr. Olgen's condition would be:
① Pain description
② Diet history
③ Present weight
④ Bowel sounds

287. Mr. Olgen is to have gastric gavage. When the gavage tube is inserted the nurse should place him in the:
① High-Fowler's position
② Mid-Fowler's position
③ Low-Fowler's position
④ Supine position

288. The nurse recognizes that the main role of the liver in relation to fat metabolism is:
① The production of phospholipids
② Oxidizing fatty acids to produce energy
③ Converting fat to lipoproteins for rapid transport out into the body
④ Storing fat for energy reserves

289. The nurse expects Mr. Olgen to complain of fatigue since a readily available form of energy, although limited in amount, is stored in the liver by conversion of glucose to:
① Glycogen
② Glycerol
③ Tissue fat
④ Amino acids

290. The nurse would also expect Mr. Olgen to have difficulty digesting fatty foods since the liver is involved in the production of:
① Lipase
② Amylase
③ Bile
④ Cholesterol

Situation: Mrs. Jery, a 43-year-old divorced housewife, is admitted to the hospital with cancer of the tongue. Questions 291 through 293 refer to this situation.

291. When assessing Mrs. Jery, the nurse should expect to find:
① Halitosis
② Bleeding gums
③ Substernal pain
④ Leukoplakia

292. The nurse recognizes that Mrs. Jery may have developed this health problem due to her tendency to:
① Chew gum
② Drink excessive alcohol
③ Bite her nails
④ Have poor dental habits

293. The intake and output for Mrs. Jery for an 8-hour period is:
8 AM: IV with D5W running and 900 ml left in bottle
8:30 AM: 150 ml urine voided
9 AM to 3 PM: q3h intervals 200 ml gastric tube formula and 50 ml H$_2$O; no aspirate obtained until final feeding; 25 ml at this time

8 AM to 4 PM: vitamin solution, 10 ml q4h
1 PM: 220 ml voided
3:15 PM: 235 ml voided
4 PM: IV with 550 ml left in bottle
The nurse calculates the intake and output as:
① Intake, 930 ml; output, 650 ml
② Intake, 1050 ml; output, 680 ml
③ Intake, 1080 ml; output, 595 ml
④ Intake, 1130 ml; output, 630 ml

Situation: Jenny Worth, 18 years old, is admitted with an acute onset of right lower quadrant pain. Appendicitis is suspected. Questions 294 through 300 refer to this situation.

294. To determine the etiology of her pain, Jenny should be assessed for:
① Increased lower bowel motility
② Rebound tenderness
③ Gastric hyperacidity
④ Urinary retention

295. Jenny is diagnosed as having acute appendicitis. This condition is primarily associated with:
① Poor dietary habits
② Infection of the bowel
③ Compromised circulation of the appendix
④ Hypertension and resultant edema

296. Jenny has an appendectomy and develops peritonitis. The nurse should assess her for an elevated temperature and:
① Extreme hunger
② Local muscular rigidity
③ Urinary retention
④ Hyperactivity

297. Jenny is to have an enema to reduce flatus. The rectal catheter should be inserted:
① 5 cm (2 inches)
② 10 cm (4 inches)
③ 15 cm (6 inches)
④ 20 cm (8 inches)

298. The physician has ordered a rectal tube to help relieve abdominal distention. To achieve maximum effectiveness the nurse should leave it in place:
① 15 minutes
② 30 minutes
③ 45 minutes
④ 60 minutes

299. While helping Jenny reestablish her regular pattern of defecation, the nurse should base the teaching on the principle that:
① The gastrocolic reflex initiates peristalsis
② Inactivity produces muscle atonia
③ Increased fluid promotes ease of evacuation
④ Increased potassium is needed for normal neuromuscular irritability

300. The nurse teaches Jenny to include more bulk in her diet. The nurse recognizes that the action of bulk to promote defecation is a consequence of the:
① Irritating effect of fiber on the bowel wall
② Tendency of smooth muscle to contract when stretched
③ Direct chemical stimulation of the colonic musculature
④ Action of the multiflora of the large intestine

Situation: Mr. Robert, a 34-year-old professor, enters the hospital for a hemorrhoidectomy. Questions 301 through 303 refer to this situation.

301. The nurse should assess the area for the presence of:
① Pruritus
② Rectal bleeding
③ Anal stenosis
④ Flatulence

302. Postoperative care for Mr. Robert should include:
① Administration of enemas to promote defecation
② Occlusive dressings to the area
③ Administration of laxatives and stool softeners
④ Encouraging showers when needed

303. Mr. Robert asks what caused this problem to occur. The nurse explains that it generally results from:
① Eating spicy foods
② Poor bowel control
③ Hypertension
④ Constipation

---

304. The portal vein can be identified as the one that:
① Brings blood away from the liver
② Brings venous blood from the intestinal wall to the liver
③ Enters the superior vena cava from the cranium
④ Is located superficially on the anteromedial surface of the thigh

305. An attack of pancreatitis can be precipitated by heavy drinking because:
① Alcohol promotes the formation of calculi in the cystic duct
② The pancreas is stimulated to secrete more insulin than it can immediately produce
③ The alcohol alters the composition of enzymes so they are capable of damaging the pancreas
④ Alcohol increases enzyme secretion and pancreatic duct pressure and causes backflow of enzymes into the pancreas

306. A vitamin necessary for the synthesis of prothrombin by the liver is:
① Vitamin K
② Vitamin B_{12}
③ Vitamin D
④ Vitamin C

307. Jaundiced clients are susceptible to postoperative hemorrhage because their blood does not clot normally due to the fact that:
① Excess bile salts in blood inactivate prothrombinase and prevent formation of thrombin from prothrombin
② Excess bile salts in blood inhibit liver synthesis of prothrombin
③ Excess bile salts in blood inhibit synthesis of vitamin K and prothrombin in the liver
④ Lack of bile in intestines causes inadequate vitamin K absorption, which causes inadequate prothrombin synthesis by liver

308. Miss McGill was admitted to the hospital for diagnostic tests, which included blood and stool. The blood samples were drawn by the laboratory technician. She was told that a stool specimen was necessary.

However, she was not told a total specimen was necessary and she saved only a small amount. When it was noted that a whole specimen was not available, the test was cancelled. This necessitated an additional day in the hospital. Miss McGill was very disturbed and insisted on not paying for the additional day because of the error. In situations such as this:
① The order for a total specimen should have been written by the physician
② A full explanation of tests or treatments is the right of the client and the nurse was negligent
③ Tests do go wrong, and hospital personnel are not responsible unless there is gross negligence
④ The client is responsible for the hospital bill and must pay

309. Clients with fractured mandibles usually have them immobilized with wires. The life-threatening problem that can develop postoperatively is:
① Vomiting
② Infection
③ Osteomyelitis
④ Bronchospasm

310. Energy stored as ATP, ADP, and other high-energy compounds is formed chiefly by:
① Oxidation of glucose
② Hydrolysis of fats
③ Respiration
④ Peptidation

311. An adult intolerance to milk, found mostly in black populations, is caused by a genetic deficiency of the enzyme:
① Sucrase
② Lactase
③ Maltase
④ Amylase

312. One of the main functions of bile is to:
① Produce an acid condition
② Provide vitamins
③ Emulsify fats
④ Split protein

313. An anaerobic spore-forming rod that produces an exotoxin in canned food is:
① *Salmonella typhosa*
② *Clostridium botulinum*
③ *Clostridium tetani*
④ *Escherichia coli*

314. Carbohydrates provide one of the main fuel sources for energy. The carbohydrate food that provides the quickest source of energy would be:
① A slice of bread
② A glass of orange juice
③ A glass of milk
④ Chocolate candy bar

315. Phospho-Soda is classified as a:
① Bulk-forming cathartic
② Saline cathartic
③ Emollient cathartic
④ Stimulant cathartic

316. The end products of protein digestion—amino acids (the "building blocks")—are absorbed from the small intestine by:
① Simple diffusion because of their small size
② Active transport with aid of vitamin B_6 (pyridoxine)

③ Osmosis caused by their greater concentration in the intestinal lumen

④ Filtration according to the osmotic pressure direction

317. A complete protein, a food protein of high biologic value, is one that contains:
① All 22 of the amino acids in sufficient quantity to meet human requirements
② All 8 of the essential amino acids in correct proportion to meet human needs
③ The 8 essential amino acids in any proportion, since the body can always fill in the difference needed
④ Most of the 22 amino acids from which the body will make additional amounts of the 8 essential amino acids needed

318. Twenty-two amino acids are involved in total body metabolism building and rebuilding various tissues. Of these, 8 are essential amino acids. This means that:
① The body cannot synthesize these 8 amino acids and thus they must be obtained from the diet
② These 8 amino acids are essential in body processes and the remaining 14 are not
③ These 8 amino acids can be made by the body because they are essential to life
④ After synthesizing these 8 amino acids, the body uses them in key processes essential for growth

319. The most important method of preventing amebic dysentery is:
① Proper pasteurization of milk
② Killing biting gnats
③ Proper sewage disposal
④ Tick control

320. Excessive loss of gastric juice caused by gastric lavage or prolonged vomiting can lead to:
① Acidosis
② Alkalosis
③ Loss of osmotic pressure of the blood
④ Loss of oxygen from the blood

321. Mrs. Aster is diagnosed as having a hiatus hernia. She tells the nurse she is having difficulty sleeping at night. Appropriate intervention would be:
① Suggesting a large glass of milk before retiring
② Eliminating carbohydrates from the diet
③ Sleeping on two or three pillows
④ Administering antacids such as sodium bicarbonate

322. Which of the following statements are true about the sources of vitamin K?
① Vitamin K is found in a wide variety of foods, so there is no danger of deficiency
② Vitamin K can easily be absorbed without assistance, so all that is consumed is absorbed
③ Vitamin K is rarely found in dietary food sources, so a natural deficiency can easily occur
④ Almost all vitamin K sufficient for metabolic needs is produced by intestinal bacteria

323. Prophylaxis for serum hepatitis includes:
① Enteric precautions applied to infected individuals
② Screening of blood donors
③ Case finding and treatment of infection
④ Client isolation

324. In the client with serum hepatitis the earliest indication of parenchymal damage to the liver usually is:
① Elevation in transaminase
② Rise in bilirubin
③ Alteration in proteins
④ Rise in alkaline phosphatase

325. The chief complaint in a client with Vincent's angina is:
① Chest pain
② Shortness of breath
③ Bleeding and ulcerations in mouth
④ Shoulder discomfort

326. After undergoing surgery for removal of impacted molars, the client should be instructed to notify the physician if there is:
① Pain and swelling after 1 week
② Tenderness in the mouth when chewing
③ Pain associated with swallowing
④ Foul odor to the breath

327. Vitamin C in human nutrition is related to tissue integrity and hemorrhagic disease. It controls such disorders by:
① Preserving the structural integrity of tissue by protecting the lipid matrix of cell walls from peroxidation
② Preventing tissue hemorrhage by providing essential blood clotting materials
③ Facilitating adequate absorption of calcium and phosphorus for bone formation to prevent bleeding in the joints
④ Strengthening capillary walls and structural tissue by depositing cementing material to build collagen from ground substance and thus prevent tissue hemorrhage

328. The main function of adipose tissue in fat metabolism is synthesizing and:
① Using lipoproteins for fat transport
② Storing triglycerides for energy reserves
③ Regulating cholesterol production
④ Releasing glucose for energy

329. Many vitamins and minerals regulate the chemical changes of cell metabolism by acting in a coenzyme role. This means that the vitamin or mineral:
① Is not a part of the enzyme controlling a particular reaction
② May be a necessary catalyst present for the reaction to proceed
③ Forms a new compound by a series of complex changes
④ Prevents unnecessary reactions by neutralizing the controlling enzyme

330. Because fat is insoluble in water, it cannot travel freely in the blood. Therefore the main type of compound formed to serve as a vehicle of transport is:
① Triglyceride
② Plasma protein
③ Phospholipid
④ Lipoprotein

331. The food group lowest in natural sodium is:
① Meat
② Milk
③ Vegetables
④ Fruits

332. The terms *saturated* and *unsaturated,* when used in reference to fats, indicate degrees of:
    1. Color
    2. Taste
    3. Hardness
    4. Digestability

333. When the transport fat compounds accumulate in abnormal levels in the blood, the diet may be modified as one effort to control them. The foods most affected by such diet therapy would be:
    1. Vegetable oils
    2. Fruits
    3. Grains
    4. Animal fats

334. The breakdown of triglyceride molecules can be expected to produce:
    1. Urea nitrogen
    2. Amino acids
    3. Simple sugars
    4. Fatty acids

335. Cholesterol is important in the human body for:
    1. Bone formation
    2. Blood clotting
    3. Cellular membrane structure
    4. Muscle contraction

336. Cholesterol is frequently discussed in relation to atherosclerosis. It is a substance that:
    1. All persons would be better off without because it causes the disease process
    2. Circulates in the blood, the level of which responds usually to dietary substitutions of unsaturated fats for saturated fats
    3. Is found in many foods, both plant and animal sources
    4. May be controlled entirely by eliminating food sources

337. In caring for the client with an ileostomy the nurse would:
    1. Expect the stoma to start draining on the third postoperative day
    2. Explain that the drainage can be controlled with daily irrigations
    3. Anticipate that emotional stress can increase intestinal peristalsis
    4. Encourage the client to eat foods high in residue

338. If the ileum is removed surgically, the individual may suffer from anemia because:
    1. The hemopoietic factor is absorbed only in the terminal ileum
    2. Folic acid is absorbed only in the terminal ileum
    3. Iron absorption is dependent on simultaneous bile salt absorption in the terminal ileum
    4. The trace elements copper, cobalt, and nickel, required for hemoglobin synthesis, occur only in the ileum

339. Which of the following types of sports should a client with an ileostomy avoid?
    1. Track events
    2. Swimming
    3. Skiing
    4. Football

340. Advocating megadoses of vitamin A must be questioned because:
    1. The vitamin cannot be stored, and the excess amount would saturate the general body tissues
    2. The vitamin is highly toxic even in small amounts
    3. The liver has a great storage capacity for the vitamin, even to toxic amounts
    4. Although the body's requirement for the vitamin is very large, the cells can synthesize more as needed

341. GI bleeding can be treated medically by infusing medication through an intravenous line. The drug commonly used for this purpose is:
    1. Phytonadione (Aquamephyton)
    2. Neostigmine (Prostigmin)
    3. Propantheline (Pro-Banthine)
    4. Vasopressin (Pitressin)

342. A client who may develop pernicious anemia is one who has:
    1. Diabetes
    2. Had a gastrectomy
    3. Hemorrhaged
    4. Poor dietary habits

343. An antrectomy would most likely be done for a client with a diagnosis of:
    1. Trigeminal neuralgia
    2. Otosclerosis
    3. Gastric ulcers
    4. Cataracts

344. Surgery may be needed to excise a pseudocyst of the pancreas. A pseudocyst of the pancreas:
    1. Is filled with pancreatic enzymes
    2. Contains necrotic tissue and blood
    3. Is a pouch of undigested food particles
    4. Is generally a malignant growth

345. A hormone that stimulates the flow of pancreatic juice is:
    1. Cholecystokinin
    2. Enterocrinin
    3. Enterogastrone
    4. Pancreozymin

346. The major digestive changes in fat are accomplished in the small intestine by a lipase from the pancreas. This enzymatic activity:
    1. Easily breaks down all the dietary fat to fatty acids and glycerol
    2. Splits off all the fatty acids in only about 25% of the total dietary fat consumed
    3. Synthesizes new triglycerides from the dietary fat consumed
    4. Emulsifies the fat globules and reduces their surface tension

347. Secretin and pancreozymin are hormones secreted by the:
    1. Duodenum
    2. Pancreas
    3. Adrenals
    4. Liver

348. When cardiovascular disease is a concern, reduction of the saturated fat in an ulcer diet may be desired and substitutes made of polyunsaturated fat. Which of the following foods would be contraindicated?

① Whole milk
② Special soft margarine
③ Corn oil
④ Fish

349. In teaching a client with a cardiac problem who is on a high-unsaturated fatty acid diet, the nurse should stress the importance of increasing the intake of:
① Liver and other glandular organ meats
② Enriched whole milk
③ Red meats, such as beef
④ Vegetable oils, such as corn oil

350. Vitamin K is essential for normal blood clotting because it promotes:
① Ionization of blood calcium
② Platelet aggregation
③ Fibrinogen formation by liver
④ Prothrombin formation by liver

351. Most of the work of changing raw fuel forms of carbohydrates to the refined usable fuel glucose is accomplished by enzymes located in the:
① Mouth
② Stomach mucosa
③ Small intestine
④ Large intestine

The Genitourinary System

Situation: Mr. Piter has developed acute renal failure and uremia. Questions 352 through 357 refer to this situation.

352. Metabolic acidosis develops in renal failure as a result of:
① Depression of respiratory rate by metabolic wastes causing carbon dioxide retention
② Inability of renal tubules to secrete hydrogen ions and conserve bicarbonate
③ Inability of renal tubules to reabsorb water to achieve dilution of the acid contents of the blood
④ Impaired glomerular filtration causing retention of sodium and metabolic waste products

353. Of the following, which is most important in maintaining the fluid and electrolyte balance of the body?
① Urinary system
② Respiratory system
③ Antidiuretic hormone (ADH)
④ Aldosterone

354. Mr. Piter is to receive a modified Giordano-Giovannetti dietary regimen. This diet is based on the principles that:
① A high-protein intake ensures an adequate daily supply of all amino acids to compensate for losses
② Essential and nonessential amino acids are necessary in the diet to supply materials for tissue protein synthesis
③ Urea nitrogen cannot be used to synthesize amino acids in the body, so all the nitrogen for amino acid synthesis must come from the dietary protein
④ If the diet is low in protein and supplies only essential amino acids, the body will use the excess urea nitrogen to synthesize the nonessential amino acids needed for tissue protein production

355. Mr. Piter complains of tingling of the fingers and toes and muscle twitching. This is caused by:
① Acidosis
② Potassium retention
③ Calcium depletion
④ Sodium chloride depletion

356. Mr. Piter becomes confused and irritable. The nurse realizes that this behavior may be caused by:
① An elevated BUN
② Hypernatremia
③ Limited fluid intake
④ Hyperkalemia

357. To gain access to a vein and an artery, an external shunt may be given to clients who require hemodialysis. The most serious problem with an external shunt is:
① Clot formation
② Septicemia
③ Sclerosis of vessels
④ Exsanguination

Situation: Mr. Carson is hospitalized with severe right flank pain, general weakness, and fever. He has a history of recurrent urinary tract infection, and the formation of renal calculi is suspected. The physician orders a 200 mg calcium diet for 3 days to be monitored with urinary calcium tests. Questions 358 through 364 refer to this situation.

358. In caring for clients with renal calculi, the most important nursing action is to:
① Record blood pressure
② Strain all urine
③ Limit fluids at night
④ Administer analgesics every 3 hours

359. Background knowledge that helps the nurse understand the reasons for this strict 200 mg calcium diet is:
① Excessive calcium intake has little influence on renal stone formation
② The thyroid hormone controls the serum levels of calcium and phosphorus
③ If calcium excretion is lowered on the test diet, hyperparathyroidism can be identified as the cause of the calculi
④ If calcium excretion is still elevated on the test diet, dietary influences can be ruled out

360. Mr. Carson's calcium balance studies following his test diet are negative. His diet order is increased to 400 mg calcium—a general low-calcium diet level. The foods permitted on his diet would include:
① Vanilla ice cream with chocolate syrup and nuts
② Salmon loaf with cheese sauce
③ Chocolate pudding
④ Roast beef with baked potato

361. The name of the procedure for the removal of a urinary bladder stone is:
① Cystolithiasis
② Cystolithectomy
③ Cystometry
④ Cystoextraction

362. Diet therapy for renal calculi of calcium phosphate composition would probably be:
    ① High calcium and phosphorus, alkaline ash
    ② High calcium and phosphorus, acid ash
    ③ Low purine and phosphorus, alkaline ash
    ④ Low calcium and phosphorus, acid ash
363. Mr. Carson will be taking sulfisoxazole (Gantrisin) at home. The nurse instructs him to:
    ① Measure and record urine output
    ② Strain urine for crystals and stones
    ③ Maintain the exact time schedule for drug taking
    ④ Stop the drug if his urinary output increases
364. If Mr. Carson's renal stones had been of calcium oxalate composition, he probably would have been placed on a diet:
    ① Low in calcium and oxalate, acid ash
    ② Low in calcium and oxalate, alkaline ash
    ③ Low in methionine, acid ash
    ④ Low in purines, alkaline ash

Situation: Mrs. Virginia Wolfsmith is admitted to the hospital with a diagnosis of left hydronephrosis. She is scheduled for a left nephrectomy. Questions 365 through 369 refer to this situation.

365. The physician orders meperidine (Demerol), 50 mg, and atropine, gr ¹⁄₁₅₀ IM, preoperatively for Mrs. Wolfsmith before the nephrectomy. Knowing that these two drugs are compatible and available in multidose vials, the nurse would *best* administer them by:
    ① Drawing each up in a separate syringe
    ② Drawing up saline to dilute both drugs
    ③ Drawing up the atropine and then the Demerol in the same syringe
    ④ Drawing up Demerol and then atropine in the same syringe
366. After the nephrectomy Mrs. Wolfsmith arrives in the recovery room with a plastic airway in place. In observing the client for signs of hemorrhage, the nurse must be certain to:
    ① Keep her nail beds in view at all times
    ② Report any increase in blood pressure immediately
    ③ Observe her for hemoptysis when suctioning
    ④ Turn her to observe her dressings
367. In the recovery room, while caring for Mrs. Wolfsmith who has received a general anesthesic, the nurse should notify the physician if:
    ① The client pushes out the airway
    ② The respirations are regular but shallow
    ③ The systolic blood pressure drops from 130 to 100 mm Hg
    ④ The client has snoring respirations
368. During the immediate postoperative period the nurse should give the highest priority to:
    ① Checking vital signs every 15 minutes
    ② Maintaining a patent airway
    ③ Recording intake and output
    ④ Observing for hemorrhage
369. The most *inaccurate* method to estimate Mrs. Wolfsmith's drainage postoperatively would be by:
    ① Counting saturated 4 × 4 gauze pads
    ② Measuring drainage that has seeped through the dressing
    ③ Wringing saturated 4 × 4 pads into a graduated container
    ④ Weighing saturated dressings

Situation: Miss Stewart was admitted to the hospital with complaints of hematuria, frequency, urgency, and pain on urination. She stated that she has had this problem for several days. Questions 370 through 372 refer to this situation.

370. The admitting diagnosis would most likely be:
    ① Cystitis
    ② Pyelitis
    ③ Nephrosis
    ④ Pyelonephritis
371. Miss Stewart is receiving methenamine mandelate (Mandelamine) and ammonium chloride. The primary reason for administering the two drugs concurrently is that ammonium chloride:
    ① Improves methanamine mandelate's effect on bacteria by acidifying the urine
    ② Promotes healing of irritated bladder mucosa
    ③ Interacts with methenamine mandelate to decrease crystal and stone formation
    ④ Decreases bladder irritation by acidifying the urine
372. Miss Stewart has a higher risk of developing cystitis than does a man. This is due to:
    ① Hormonal secretions
    ② Length of the urethra
    ③ Juxtaposition of the bladder
    ④ Altered urinary pH

Situation: Miss Jenner has chronic renal failure. Questions 373 through 377 refer to this situation.

373. Miss Jenner is not responding to treatment. Dialysis may be performed to remove waste products from the blood. The main indication for dialysis is:
    ① Increase in blood pressure
    ② High and rising potassium levels
    ③ Ascites
    ④ Acidosis
374. The artificial kidney machine primarily makes use of the physical principle of:
    ① Filtration
    ② Osmosis
    ③ Diffusion
    ④ Dialysis
375. Miss Jenner, who is receiving hemodialysis for chronic renal failure, is especially prone to develop:
    ① Peritonitis
    ② Renal calculi
    ③ Bladder infection
    ④ Serum hepatitis
376. In caring for Miss Jenner, who has had an arteriovenous shunt inserted for hemodialysis, the nurse should:
    ① Notify the physician if a bruit is heard in the cannula
    ② Use strict aseptic technique when giving shunt care
    ③ Cover the entire cannula with an elastic bandage
    ④ Take the blood pressure every 4 hours from the arm that contains the shunt

377. A nurse working in a hemodialysis unit runs a high risk of developing:
① Type A viral hepatitis
② Infectious hepatitis
③ Type B viral hepatitis
④ Hemolytic hepatitis

Situation: Mr. Lambert, a 54-year-old engineer, is admitted to the hospital with the medical diagnosis of renal calculi. Questions 378 through 382 refer to this situation.

378. The nurse would expect Mr. Lambert to complain of:
① Frequency and urgency on urination
② Dry, itchy skin and pyuria
③ Pain radiating from kidney to shoulder
④ Irritability and twitching

379. A routine urinalysis is ordered for Mr. Lambert. If the specimen cannot be sent immediately to the laboratory, the nurse should:
① Discard and collect a new specimen later
② Store on "dirty" side of utility room
③ Refrigerate the specimen
④ Take no special action

380. The physician orders a 24-hour urine test for Mr. Lambert. The nurse should:
① Weigh him before starting
② Check if any preservatives are needed
③ Place the collection jar in ice
④ Check intake and output

381. Mr. Lambert has surgery under spinal anesthesia to remove the stone. Postural changes immediately after spinal anesthesia may result in hypotension because there is:
① Dilation of capacitance vessels
② Decreased response of baroreceptors
③ Interruption of cardiac accelerator pathways
④ Decreased strength of cardiac contractions

382. The pathology report states that Mr. Lambert's stone is composed of uric acid. The nurse should instruct him to avoid:
① Milk and fruit
② Eggs and cheese
③ Organ meats and extracts
④ Red meats and vegetables

Situation: Mr. Hurt, 40 years old, is admitted to the hospital with urethritis. Questions 383 through 386 refer to this situation.

383. Prior to initiating treatment orders, the nurse should plan to:
① Prepare for urinary catheterization
② Start a 24-hour urine collection
③ Administer an oil-retention enema
④ Obtain a urine specimen for culture and sensitivity

384. Each specimen of urine should be assessed for:
① Specific gravity
② Clarity
③ Sugar and acetone
④ Viscosity

385. Mr. Hurt is to have his urethra dilated by the physician. The nurse understands that the structure that encircles the male urethra is the:
① Bulbourethral gland
② Epididymis

③ Prostate gland
④ Seminal vesicle

386. Mr. Hurt takes chlorothiazide (Diuril) at home and continues to take it in the hospital. He asks what this drug actually does. The nurse explains that the planned therapeutic effect of the drug is to:
① Decrease the amount of fluid reabsorption in Henle's loop
② Increase the excretion of sodium and chloride
③ Decrease the reabsorption of potassium
④ Increase the glomerular filtration rate

Situation: Mr. Carpenter, a 60-year-old laborer, is admitted to the hospital with the complaint of dysuria. Questions 387 through 391 refer to this situation.

387. A cystoscopy is performed and a tumor is visualized and biopsied. The activity most often associated with bladder tumors is:
① Jogging 3 miles a day
② Working with a jackhammer every day
③ Smoking two packs of cigarettes a day
④ Drinking three cans of cola a day

388. Mr. Carpenter has been diagnosed as having bladder cancer and a cystectomy and ileal conduit are planned. Preoperatively, the nurse plans to:
① Provide cleansing enemas and laxatives
② Limit fluid intake for 24 hours
③ Teach muscle-tightening exercises
④ Teach procedure for irrigation of the stoma

389. The nurse recognizes that the major disadvantage of an ileal conduit is that:
① Stool continuously oozes from it
② Absorption of nutrients is diminished
③ Peristalsis is greatly decreased
④ Urine drains from it continuously

390. Mr. Carpenter is receiving a form of folic acid intramuscularly during intraarterial chemotherapy with methotrexate. The drug is being administered intramuscularly to:
① Provide levels of folic acid required by blood-forming organs
② Provide the metabolite required for destruction of cancer cells
③ Provide folic acid, which acts synergistically with antineoplastic drugs to destroy cancer cells
④ Increase production of phagocytic cells required to remove debris liberated by disintegrating cancer cells

391. The physician orders antibiotic therapy for Mr. Carpenter because chemotherapeutic agents destroy rapidly growing cells in the:
① Blood
② Lymph
③ Liver
④ Bone marrow

392. The body fluids that make up 40% to 50% of the total body weight are:
① Intracellular
② Extracellular
③ Intravascular
④ Interstitial

393. Which of the following statements correctly compares blood plasma and interstitial fluid?
    ① Both contain the same kinds of ions
    ② Plasma contains slightly more of each kind of ion than does interstitial fluid
    ③ Plasma exerts lower osmotic pressure than does interstitial fluid
    ④ The main cation in plasma is sodium, whereas the main cation in interstitial fluid is potassium

394. To better understand fluid balance the nurse needs to recognize that:
    ① Glomerular filtration occurs in the glomeruli which are small arteries in the kidneys
    ② The volume of urine secreted is regulated mainly by mechanisms that control the glomerular filtration rate
    ③ An increase in the hydrostatic pressure in Bowman's capsule tends to increase the glomerular filtration rate
    ④ A decrease in blood protein concentration tends to increase the glomerular filtration rate

395. A palliative method of urinary divergence sometimes used for clients with advanced kidney disease is:
    ① Ileostomy
    ② Nephrostomy
    ③ Cecostomy
    ④ Ureterostomy

396. A solution containing 1 gram-equivalent weight of solute in 1 L of solution is called:
    ① An isotonic solution
    ② A normal solution
    ③ A molar solution
    ④ A saturated solution

397. The reabsorption of water from glomerular filtrate (in the kidney tubules), the flow of water between the intracellular and interstitial compartments, and the exchange of fluid between plasma and interstitial fluid spaces are caused by:
    ① Dialysis
    ② Active transport
    ③ Osmosis
    ④ Diffusion

398. Ammonia is excreted by the kidney to help maintain:
    ① Low bacterial levels in the urine
    ② Osmotic pressure of the blood
    ③ Acid-base balance of the body
    ④ Normal red blood cell production

399. The client with unresolved edema is most likely to develop:
    ① Thrombus formation
    ② Tissue ischemia
    ③ Proteinemia
    ④ Contractures

400. The mercurial diuretics alter active transport systems in the kidney tubules, resulting in increased excretion of sodium and, secondarily, water. The principle explaining the secondary water loss (diuresis) is:
    ① Osmosis
    ② Diffusion
    ③ Filtration
    ④ Active transport

401. Women are more susceptible to urinary tract infections because of:
    ① Poor hygienic practices
    ② Length of the urethra
    ③ Continuity of the mucous membrane
    ④ Inadequate fluid intake

402. Severe albuminuria may cause edema because of the:
    ① Rise in plasma hydrostatic pressure
    ② Fall in plasma colloid osmotic pressure
    ③ Fall in tissue hydrostatic pressure
    ④ Rise in tissue colloid osmotic pressure

403. The percentage of water in the average adult human body is:
    ① 80%
    ② 60%
    ③ 40%
    ④ 20%

404. The receptors for the regulation of body water through detection of osmotic pressure are located in the:
    ① Hypothalamus
    ② Neurohypophysis
    ③ Kidney tubules
    ④ Blood

405. The major role in maintaining fluid balance in the body is performed by the:
    ① Heart
    ② Kidneys
    ③ Liver
    ④ Lungs

406. The weight of extracellular body fluid is approximately 20% of the total body weight of an average individual. The component of the extracellular fluid that contributes the greatest portion to this amount is the:
    ① Interstitial fluid
    ② Plasma fluid
    ③ Fluid in body secretions
    ④ Fluid in dense tissue

407. The most important electrolyte of intracellular fluid is:
    ① Calcium
    ② Sodium
    ③ Potassium
    ④ Chloride

The Reproductive System

Situation: Walter Sams, a 75-year-old man, enters the hospital with benign prostatic hypertrophy for further tests and a prostatectomy. Questions 408 through 412 refer to this situation.

408. The nurse insists that a medication for sleep be taken at 9 PM even though the client tells her he never went to sleep this early and would like the medication delayed. Later the client awakens and is confused. He tries to get out of bed and in so doing falls, fracturing his hip. Legally:

① Hospital policy requires that sleep medications be given at 9 PM and *respondeat superior* applies

② Client's rights have precedence over hospital policy or physician's orders

③ The time the medication was given has nothing to do with the confusion

④ When the physician orders a medication, it must be given at the scheduled time unless the nursing supervisor authorizes differently

409. The definitive diagnosis of benign prostatic hypertrophy is arrived at by:
① Biopsy of prostatic tissue
② Pap smear of prostatic fluid
③ Rectal examination
④ Serum phosphatase studies

410. The tests that might be ordered to estimate the effect of Mr. Sams' illness on his kidneys are:
① PSP, urea clearance, urine concentration
② Sulkowitch, catecholamines, urine dilution
③ Bence Jones protein, urine concentration, albumin
④ Microscopic porphyrins, urinalysis

411. While caring for Mr. Sams, the nurse is aware that benign prostatic hypertrophy (BPH):
① Usually becomes malignant
② Predisposes to hydronephrosis
③ Is a congenital abnormality
④ Causes an elevated acid phosphatase

412. Mr. Sams had a suprapubic prostatectomy with continuous bladder irrigations. When caring for a client with a continuous bladder irrigation, the nurse should:
① Measure urinary specific gravity
② Record hourly outputs
③ Include irrigating solution on intake and output records
④ Exclude irrigating solution from any 24-hour urine tests ordered

Situation: Mrs. Garvin is admitted for treatment of cancer of the cervix. Questions 413 through 417 refer to this situation.

413. An early symptom of cancer of the cervix that should have brought Mrs. Garvin to the gynecologist is:
① Bloody spotting after intercourse
② Foul-smelling discharge
③ Abdominal heaviness
④ Pressure on the bladder

414. Mrs. Garvin is to have a radium implant. When caring for Mrs. Garvin, the nurse should:
① Spend as much time with the client as possible
② Have the client void q2h
③ Use rubber gloves when giving the client a bath
④ Maintain the client in isolation

415. Radium is stored in lead containers because:
① Chemical heat is produced when radium disintegrates
② The lead absorbs the harmful radiations
③ Radium is a heavy substance
④ Lead prevents disintegration of the radium

416. In caring for Mrs. Garvin after the radium implant, the nurse would:

① Collect and store urine for examination by nuclear medicine
② Wear a lead apron when giving care
③ Restrict visitors to a 10-minute stay
④ Avoid giving IM injections into the gluteal muscle

417. Before discharge the nurse would explain to Mrs. Garvin the importance of:
① Eating a diet high in fat
② Taking daily multivitamin supplements
③ Returning for medical follow-up care
④ Limiting daily fluid intake

Situation: Mrs. Row is seen at the gynecology clinic because of profuse vaginal discharge, pruritus, and burning. A smear for microscopic examination is taken and reveals the presence of *Trichomonas vaginalis*. Questions 418 through 420 refer to this situation.

418. The organism that causes a trichomonal infection is a:
① Fungus
② Yeast
③ Spirochete
④ Protozoon

419. The nurse would expect Mrs. Row's physician to order douches with:
① Physiologic saline to decrease the pH of the vagina
② Vinegar to decrease the pH of the vagina
③ Sodium bicarbonate to increase the pH of the vagina
④ Tap water to increase the pH of the vagina

420. The oral drug that is most likely to be prescribed for treatment of *Trichomonas vaginalis* is:
① Gentian violet
② Pencillin
③ Metronidazole (Flagyl)
④ Nystatin

Situation: Mrs. Butler had a radical mastectomy and will start chemotherapy while hospitalized. Questions 421 through 423 refer to this situation.

421. The nurse is aware that many of the chemotherapeutic agents cause:
① Increased hemoglobin count and hematocrit
② Bone marrow depression
③ Decreased sedimentation rate
④ Leukocytosis

422. Mrs. Butler's pathology report shows metastatic adenocarcinoma. She is to receive doxorubicin (Adriamycin), which modifies the growth of cancer cells by:
① Preventing folic acid synthesis
② Changing the osmotic gradient in the cell
③ Inhibiting RNA synthesis by binding DNA
④ Increasing the permeability of the cell wall

423. Because of problems occurring in 80% of the clients receiving Adriamycin, the nurse will observe Mrs. Butler for evidence of:
① Nausea and vomiting, tachycardia
② Hair loss, erythema of the oral mucosa
③ Decreased appetite, necrosis at the IV site
④ Low blood pressure, decreased vital capacity

Situation: Joan Yeats, 16 years of age, comes to the clinic because of severe burning on urination, persistent vaginal discharge, and irritation of the vulva. On examination, the vulva and vagina appear red and irritated and there is profuse greenish-yellow discharge. A cervical culture and smear are taken. The smear reveals a gonorrheal infection. Questions 424 through 428 refer to this situation.

424. The causative organism of gonorrhea is:
① *Treponema pallidum*
② *Neisseria gonorrhoeae*
③ *Staphylococcus* organism
④ Döderlien's bacillus

425. The nurse understands that gonorrhea is highly infectious and:
① Is easily cured
② Can produce sterility
③ Occurs very rarely
④ Is limited to the external genitalia

426. In relation to the public health implications of this condition, the nurse would be most interested in:
① The reasons for Joan's promiscuity
② Interviewing Joan's parents to find out how she got this infection
③ Finding Joan's contacts
④ Instructing Joan in birth control measures

427. The drug of choice for the treatment of gonorrhea is:
① Penicillin
② Actinomycin
③ Chloramphenicol
④ Colistin

428. The nurse tells Joan that the drug therapy can be expected to:
① Cure the infection
② Prevent complications
③ Control its transmission
④ Reverse pathologic changes

Situation: Mr. Amond, age 84, is admitted to the hospital with the following signs and symptoms: severe dyspnea; marked generalized edema of lower extremities, penis, scrotum, back, and abdomen; confusion and irritability. He complains of frequent low back pain. Three months earlier he had been hospitalized for acute urinary retention, at which time a transurethral prostatectomy (TURP) was done, followed by bilateral orchidectomy and radiation therapy when the pathology report revealed carcinoma of the prostate. Laboratory findings indicate markedly elevated chemistries. Corticosteroids are currently being administered. Questions 429 through 435 refer to this situation.

429. In cancer of the prostate it is possible to follow the course of the disease through the study of:
① Serum acid phosphatase
② Creatinine
③ Blood urea nitrogen
④ Nonprotein nitrogen

430. Bladder irritability may follow radiation therapy. A sign of this complication would probably be:
① Polyuria
② Dribbling
③ Hematuria
④ Dysuria

431. Mr. Amond requests the urinal at frequent intervals but either does not void or voids in very small amounts. This is most likely due to:
① Renal failure
② Edema
③ Retention
④ Suppression

432. A urinary retention catheter is inserted. If Mr. Amond complains of persistent discomfort in the bladder and urethra, the nurse should first:
① Check the patency of the catheter
② Notify the physician at once
③ Milk the tubing gently
④ Irrigate the catheter with prescribed solutions

433. The nurse can best prevent the contamination from retention catheters by:
① Forcing fluids
② Cleansing around the meatus periodically
③ Perineal cleansing
④ Irrigating the catheter

434. A Foley catheter operates by the principle of:
① Inertia
② Diffusion
③ Osmosis
④ Gravity

435. Mr. Amond experiences difficulty in voiding after the catheter is removed. This is probably related to:
① Interruption in normal voiding habits
② Nervous tension
③ Remaining effects of anesthetics
④ Toxic symptoms from chemotherapy

Situation: Mrs. Vale is 42 years old and the mother of two children, ages 3 and 7. She is admitted to the hospital because of spotting between menstrual periods. The bleeding increases during intercourse and when straining at defecation. Her admission diagnosis is possible cervical polyps, and she is scheduled for a dilation and curettage (D & C) and polypectomy. The nurse admitting her notes that she is pale, wringing her hands, and unable to sit still but not speaking unless asked a direct question. From these observations the nurse deduces that Mrs. Vale is very anxious. Questions 436 through 441 refer to this situation.

436. To help Mrs. Vale express her anxieties, the best approach for the nurse to use would be to:
① Tell Mrs. Vale that there is no need to worry; a polypectomy and a D & C are considered minor surgery
② Say, "I can tell that something is troubling you. It might help to talk about it."
③ Tell Mrs. Vale that it is normal for her to be anxious; everybody is fearful, even though there is no reason to worry
④ Ask, "What are you really upset about, Mrs. Vale?"

437. Mrs. Vale finally tells the nurse that she believes she has cancer because the physician told her that he would have to remove the polyps and wait for laboratory reports. The best response of the nurse would be:
① "No operation is done without specimens being sent to the laboratory; that's strictly routine."
② "Of course you don't have cancer; polyps are always benign. The laboratory report is simple routine."

③ "Worrying today is not going to help you at all. It will only interfere with your rest, and you need to be relaxed for the surgery."

④ "It is very upsetting to have to wait for a laboratory report. It might help you to know that most of the time polyps are not cancerous."

438. The nurse knows that cervical polyps:
① Are usually benign, but curettage of the uterus is always done to rule out malignancy
② Are usually malignant, and curettage is always done
③ Do not cause bleeding until they are malignant
④ Are frequently the precursors of uterine cancer

439. Following surgery the laboratory reports reveal a stage 0 lesion. According to the International Federation of Gynecology and Obstetrics, stage 0 is indicative of:
① Carcinoma in situ
② Carcinoma strictly confined to cervix
③ Early stromal invasion
④ Parametrial involvement

440. The most common site for cancer cell growth in the cervix is at the:
① Internal os and endocervical glands
② External os and regional nodes
③ Columnosquamous junction of the internal and external ossa
④ Junction of the cervix and lower uterine segment

441. After her discharge from the hospital, Mrs. Vale is asked to return in 1 month for an excisional conization of the cervix or a hysterectomy. This is done because:
① Mrs. Vale is anxious about her condition and needs time to make her decision
② Cervical cancer is slow growing so there is no need to hurry
③ In the preinvasive stage the prognosis is excellent if treatment is performed
④ This time is needed to rule out pregnancy

Situation: Mrs. Prior, 35 years of age, had her third baby 6 months ago and is returning for a routine gynecologic examination. The doctor finds a small erosion of the cervix. He cauterizes the area and tells her to douche once daily with 3 tablespoons of vinegar to 2 quarts of water. Questions 442 through 446 refer to this situation.

442. Erosions of the cervix are common when:
① There has been a long labor
② The cervix stretches during delivery and there is an unhealed laceration
③ The cervix is not dilated completely and delivery occurs
④ The normal acidity of the vagina is altered

443. Douches are ordered for Mrs. Prior primarily to:
① Keep the vaginal canal clean and free of bacteria
② Promote healing by heat and elimination of sloughed tissue
③ Promote healing by altering the pH of the vagina
④ Make her comfortable

444. When receiving a douche, the best position for Mrs. Prior to assume would be the:
① Knee-chest
② Sims

③ Dorsal
④ Fowler's

445. Mrs. Prior should be instructed to direct the douche nozzle:
① Downward
② Upward
③ Downward and backward
④ Backward and upward

446. Early treatment of cervical erosion is performed specifically to prevent:
① Infections of the reproductive system
② Cancer of the cervix
③ Metrorrhagia
④ Further erosions from occurring

Situation: Mr. Neil has undergone a transurethral resection and returns to the unit with an indwelling urinary catheter. Questions 447 through 449 refer to this situation.

447. When irrigating Mr. Neil's catheter, the nurse should:
① Use medically clean technique
② Instill the solution under pressure
③ Heat irrigating solution to 100° F
④ Allow the solution to flow out by gravity

448. The solution of choice for maintaining patency of an indwelling catheter is:
① Isotonic saline
② Hypotonic saline
③ Sterile water
④ Genitourinary irrigating solution

449. When irrigating Mr. Neil's catheter the nurse should:
① Instill the fluid under pressure
② Obtain and use sterile equipment
③ Aspirate to ensure return flow
④ Warm the solution to body temperature

Situation: Mrs. Gorham, a 56-year-old woman, is admitted for repair of a cystocele and rectocele. She has nine children: three are married, two are away at college, and four are still at home. The youngest child is 17 years old. Her husband is a Civil Service worker. Questions 450 through 453 refer to this situation.

450. In taking the health history, the nurse would expect Mrs. Gorham to report the occurrence of:
① Sporadic bleeding accompanied by abdominal pain
② Stress incontinence, feeling of low abdominal pressure
③ Heavy leukorrhea, pruritus
④ Change in acidity level of the ragina, leukorrhea, spotting

451. Rectocele and cystocele are usually due to:
① Relaxation of musculature of the pelvic floor
② Injury during childbirth
③ Infection of the bladder
④ Trauma in repair of an episiotomy or laceration

452. Based on Mrs. Gorham's age and parity, the nurse expects the surgery done will most likely be:
① Insertion of a pessary
② Abdominal hysterectomy
③ Vaginal hysterectomy
④ Colporrhaphy

453. Mrs. Gorham returns from the operating room with a Foley catheter in place. The primary reason for the catheter is to prevent:
    ① Retention
    ② Discomfort
    ③ Pressure on the suture line
    ④ Loss of bladder tone

Situation: Mrs. Elliot is a 52-year-old woman admitted to the hospital with the diagnosis of cancer of the cervix. She is scheduled for a hysterectomy and insertion of radium. She returns to the floor from the recovery room with a Foley catheter in place and vaginal packing. The packing is to be removed in 24 hours. Questions 454 through 457 refer to this situation.

454. The nurse checking the perineum finds the packing protruding from the vagina. The immediate action to take is to report this situation to the physician at once because the:
    ① Packing is radioactive
    ② Purpose of the packing is to increase the distance between the insert and the rectum and/or bladder
    ③ Packing must be removed
    ④ Purpose of the packing is to prevent bleeding

455. In caring for Mrs. Elliot the nurse should:
    ① Use disposable sheets and towels to prevent exposure of laundry personnel
    ② Limit Mrs. Elliot's activity so as not to dislodge the radium insert
    ③ Wear a lead-lined apron while administering any care
    ④ Spend time with Mrs. Elliot to alleviate her anxiety

456. Which symptoms observed by the nurse following radium insertion are indicative of a radium reaction?
    ① Nausea and vomiting
    ② Pain and elevation of temperature
    ③ Restlessness and irritability
    ④ Vaginal discharge

457. Safety precautions the nurse should employ when the radium is being removed include:
    ① Ensuring that lead aprons and long forceps are available for use
    ② Cleaning radium carefully in ether or alcohol using long forceps
    ③ Charting the date and hour of removal and the total time of treatment
    ④ Handling the radium carefully wearing foil-lined rubber gloves

Situation: Mrs. Dreck is admitted with a history of abdominal pain, chills, nausea, and a purulent vaginal discharge. She is diagnosed as having pelvic inflammatory disease. There is also a history of exposure to syphilis. Questions 458 through 462 refer to this situation.

458. The nurse should assist Mrs. Dreck to the:
    ① Sims' position
    ② Fowler's position
    ③ Lithotomy position
    ④ Supine position with knees flexed

459. Mrs. Dreck menstruates regularly every 30 days. Her last menses started on January 1. She will most probably ovulate again on:
    ① January 5
    ② January 15
    ③ January 17
    ④ January 28

460. The incubation period for syphilis is about:
    ① 72 hours
    ② 1 week
    ③ 2 months
    ④ 2 to 6 weeks

461. The most sensitive and reliable treponemal antibody test for syphilis is the:
    ① Wasserman test
    ② VDRL test
    ③ Kahn test
    ④ FTA-ABS test

462. Syphilis is not considered contagious in the:
    ① Primary stage
    ② Tertiary stage
    ③ Secondary stage
    ④ Incubation stage

Situation: Mrs. Uri is 45 years old. She has three children ages 12, 9, and 5 years. She is admitted to the hospital with complaints of severe metrorrhagia and menorrhagia of 1 year's duration. She was found to have a submucous myoma 6 months ago and has been carefully examined monthly. On the last examination, a week ago, the myoma was found to have grown appreciably, and she was told that a hysterectomy was necessary. Questions 463 through 466 refer to this situation.

463. The term *metrorrhagia* refers to:
    ① Periods of bleeding in between menstrual periods
    ② Severe bleeding during each menstrual period
    ③ Presence of occult blood in vaginal discharge
    ④ Spotting or staining at time of ovulation

464. Mrs. Uri expresses concern about having a hysterectomy done at her age because she has heard from friends that she will undergo severe symptoms of menopause after surgery. Based on Mrs. Uri's knowledge, the most appropriate response for the nurse would be:
    ① "This is something that does occur in older women on occasion, but you don't have to worry about it."
    ② "It's too bad you did not discuss this with your doctor. I really can't give you any kind of information about this."
    ③ "You were misinformed. This never happens following this type of surgery. Your friend probably had a different diagnosis."
    ④ "Some women occasionally experience exaggerated symptoms of menopause. This is usually transitory, since the ovaries are mainly responsible for maintenance of the hormone balance."

465. Mrs. Uri wants to know if it would be wise for her to take hormones right away to prevent symptoms. The most appropriate response should be:
    ① "It is best to wait; you may not have any symptoms at all."
    ② "You have to wait until symptoms are severe; otherwise, hormones will have no effect."

③ "This is something you should discuss with your physician, since it is important for him to know how you feel and what your concerns are."

④ "Isn't it comforting to know that hormones are available if you should need them?"

466. Mrs. Uri, when being prepared for the night, starts to sob a little and says, "I told my husband today that after this operation I will only be half a woman. He reassured me, but I know that was just a front." The most appropriate response would be:
① "You feel this operation will have an effect on how your husband feels about you as his wife?"
② "You know of course that this is silly. I wish you would not worry about such irrelevant things. The main thing is that you have to get well quickly."
③ "It must be frightening to know that your husband rejects you as a woman."
④ "I think I'll call your physician. He might want to postpone the operation until you and your husband have adjusted better to the outcomes of a hysterectomy."

Situation: Mrs. Warren, a 64-year-old housewife, is admitted for surgery for a prolapsed uterus. Questions 467 through 469 refer to this situation.

467. The physician informs the nurse that Mrs. Warren has severe procidentia (prolapse of uterus). The nurse plans to assess this area for:
① Exudate
② Ulcerations
③ Vaginal discharge
④ Swelling

468. Mrs. Warren is scheduled for a vaginoplasty. Preoperatively the nurse may expect to:
① Encourage ambulation
② Manipulate the procidentia
③ Apply warm compresses
④ Elevate the foot of the bed

469. While Mrs. Warren is recovering from general anesthesia, the nurse should position her:
① On her left side
② In the Trendelenburg position
③ In bed with her head elevated
④ Flat on her back

470. During the ovulation phase of the menstrual cycle, ovulation is caused by secretion of:
① Follicle-stimulating hormone
② Luteinizing hormone
③ Estrogen
④ Progesterone

471. The large amount of progesterone secreted during the secretory phase of the menstrual cycle is responsible for:
① Sustaining the thick endometrium of the uterus
② The regulation of menstruation
③ The onset of ovulation
④ The incidence of capillary fragility

472. The hormones responsible for the proliferation phase of menstruation are:
① Luteinizing hormone and progesterone
② Follicle-stimulating hormone and estrogen
③ Lactogenic hormone and progesterone
④ Luteinizing hormone and estrogen

473. Eve is 15 years old and has complained of persistent dysmenorrhea. The nurse should encourage her to:
① Practice relaxation of abdominal muscles
② Have a gynecologic exam
③ Maintain daily activities
④ Eat a nutritious diet containing iron

474. The main blood supply to the uterus is directly from the:
① Uterine and ovarian arteries
② Uterine and hypogastric arteries
③ Ovarian arteries and the aorta
④ Aorta and the hypogastric arteries

475. The hormones responsible for the menstrual cycle are:
① Estrogen and progesterone
② Gonadotropins
③ Gonadotropins and estrogen
④ Gonadotropins, estrogen, and progesterone

476. A disease that can arise from normal microbial flora, especially after prolonged antibiotic therapy, is:
① Candidiasis
② Scarlet fever
③ Q fever
④ Herpes zoster

477. Gram-negative diplococci found in a vaginal smear are presumed to be:
① Gonococci
② Meningococci
③ Pneumococci
④ *Treponema pallidum*

478. The test that the physician might perform to determine the underlying cause of uterine pain is:
① Endometrial smear
② Laparoscopy
③ Tubal insufflation
④ Estradiol level

479. When counseling a client after a vasectomy, the nurse should advise him that:
① It requires at least 10 ejaculations to clear the tract of sperm
② Recanalization of the vas deferens is impossible
③ Unprotected coitus is possible within a week to 10 days
④ Some impotency is to be expected for several weeks

480. Torsion of the testes requires immediate surgical correction because:
① Irreversible damage occurs after a few hours
② There is no other way to control the pain
③ Swelling is excessive and the testicle may rupture
④ The reduction in testicular blood flow leads to rapid death of sperm

481. Spermatogenesis occurs:
① During embryonic development
② Immediately following birth
③ At the time of puberty
④ At any time following birth

482. The testes are suspended in the scrotum to:
    ① Facilitate the passage of sperm through the urethra
    ② Protect the sperm from the acidity of urine
    ③ Protect the sperm from high abdominal temperatures
    ④ Facilitate their maturation during embryonic development

483. When a young woman complains of especially severe abdominal cramps for 1 or 2 days each month at the time of menstruation, the nurse should suspect:
    ① Hypocalcemia
    ② Hyperglycemia
    ③ Hypernatremia
    ④ Hypokalemia

484. The term *condylomata acuminata* refers to:
    ① Venereal warts
    ② Cancer of epididymis
    ③ Herpes zoster
    ④ Scabies

485. A disease produced by a gram-negative diplococcus that generally invades the urogenital tract is:
    ① Cholera
    ② Syphilis
    ③ Gonorrhea
    ④ Chancroid

486. Acute salpingitis is most commonly the result of:
    ① Abortion
    ② Gonorrhea
    ③ Hydatidiform mole
    ④ Syphilis

487. Clients who develop general paresis as a complication of syphilis are usually treated with:
    ① Behavior modification
    ② Major tranquilizers
    ③ Penicillin
    ④ Electroconvulsive therapy

The Endocrine System

Situation: Dr. Kinsey was found in a coma in his room at the large hospital where he had begun his residency. There was a strong odor of acetone on his breath. He is married and 28 years of age. His wife, Jane, states that he is a diabetic and recently switched to Orinase on his own instead of taking insulin as prescribed. Health records submitted did not reveal that Dr. Kinsey had diabetes mellitus. Emergency measures were instituted immediately. Questions 488 through 497 refer to this situation.

488. Oral hypoglycemic agents may be used for diabetic clients with:
    ① Ketosis or impending coma
    ② Mature onset (noninsulin dependent)
    ③ Juvenile onset (insulin dependent)
    ④ Obesity

489. Dr. Kinsey has most likely omitted pertinent information from his health record because:
    ① Physicians with diabetes are not accepted for residency in many hospitals
    ② He is unable to handle the psychologic stress related to alterations in body functioning

③ He needs assistance in developing a more favorable adaptation to this stress
④ Diabetics often have lapses of memory

490. Diabetic coma results from an excess accumulation in the blood of:
    ① Nitrogen from protein catabolism, causing ammonia intoxication
    ② Ketones from rapid fat breakdown, causing acidosis
    ③ Glucose from rapid carbohydrate metabolism, causing drowsiness
    ④ Sodium bicarbonate, causing alkalosis

491. The most common cause of diabetic ketoacidosis is:
    ① Presence of infection
    ② Increased insulin dose
    ③ Inadequate food intake
    ④ Emotional stress

492. Early treatment of diabetic acidosis will include administration of:
    ① Potassium
    ② IV fluids
    ③ NPH insulin
    ④ Sodium polystyrene sulfonate (Kayexalate)

493. As Dr. Kinsey recovers from this episode:
    ① The precipitating cause of the coma must be investigated to prevent a recurrence
    ② The cause of his condition should be reviewed with him so he understands how to avoid a recurrence
    ③ Teaching will be necessary to help him accept his disease
    ④ He will need assistance in obtaining a clear conception of the general character of diabetes

494. When glucagon is administered for reversal of the hypoglycemic state, it acts by:
    ① Liberating glucose from hepatic stores of glycogen
    ② Competing for insulin and blocking its action at tissue sites
    ③ Providing a glucose substitute for rapid replacement of deficits
    ④ Supplying glycogen to the brain and other vital organs

495. An independent nursing action which should be included in the plan of care for Dr. Kinsey is:
    ① Regulating insulin dosage according to the amount of ketones found in the urine
    ② Withholding glucose in any form until the ketoacidosis is corrected
    ③ Observing for signs of hypoglycemia
    ④ Giving fruit juices, broth, and milk as soon as he is able to take fluids orally

496. The nurse suspects hypokalemia when it is observed that Dr. Kinsey has:
    ① Edema, bounding pulse, confusion
    ② Apathy, weakness, abdominal distention
    ③ Sunken eyeballs, Kussmaul breathing, thirst
    ④ Spasms, diarrhea, irregular pulse rate

497. Important to both Dr. Kinsey and his wife, Jane, is an understanding that his diet for management of his diabetes:
    ① Is based on nutritional requirements that are the same for all clients
    ② Can be planned around a wide variety of commonly used foods

③ Should be rigidly controlled to avoid similar emergencies

④ Must not include combination dishes and processed foods, since they have too many variable seasonings

Situation: Mrs. Thompson, age 39, was admitted to the hospital with a diagnosis of Addison's disease. She exhibited the following signs and symptoms: muscular weakness, anorexia, emaciation, GI distress, generalized dark pigmentation, hypotension, hypoglycemia, low sodium and high potassium levels, and a loss of libido. Questions 498 through 505 refer to this situation.

498. The hypotension can be explained by the fact that Addison's disease involves a disturbance in the production of:
① Glucocorticoids
② Androgens
③ Mineralocorticoids
④ Estrogens

499. The nurse should observe Mrs. Thompson closely for signs of infectious complications because there is a disturbance of function in the:
① Proinflammatory effect
② Antiinflammatory effect
③ Metabolic effect
④ Electrolytic effect

500. The emaciation, muscular weakness, and fatigue are due to disturbance of function in:
① Protein anabolic effect
② Electrolytic effect
③ Diurnal effect
④ Masculinizing effect

501. An important aspect of nursing care specific for Mrs. Thompson is:
① Encouraging exercise
② Providing a variety of diversional activities
③ Permitting as much activity as the client desires
④ Protecting from exertion

502. Therapy for Mrs. Thompson is aimed chiefly at:
① Restoring electrolyte balance
② Improving carbohydrate metabolism
③ Increasing lymphoid tissue
④ Increasing eosinophils

503. Mrs. Thompson's treatment includes a high-protein, high-calorie diet with extra salt. As a means of encouraging her to eat, the nurse explains the reasons for this diet therapy as:
① Extra salt is needed to replace the amount being lost due to lack of sufficient aldosterone to conserve sodium
② Increased vitamins are needed to supply energy to help her regain lost weight
③ Increased protein is needed to heal the adrenal tissue and thus cure the disease
④ Increased amounts of potassium are needed to replace renal losses

504. Prior to discharge the physician prescribes hydrocortisone, 10 mg tid, and fludrocortisone, 0.1 mg qd. The nurse expects hydrocortisone to:
① Prevent hypoglycemia and permit Mrs. Thompson to respond to stress

② Increase amounts of angiotensin II to raise Mrs. Thompson's blood pressure
③ Control excessive loss of potassium salts
④ Decrease cardiac arrhythmias and dyspnea

505. The nurse should teach Mrs. Thompson to consult her physician immediately if she experiences the side effects related to fludrocortisone therapy, namely:
① Fatigue, particularly in the afternoon
② Increased frequency of urination
③ Rapid weight gain and dependent edema
④ Unpredictable changes in mood

Situation: Mr. Sohl, age 52, develops symptoms of diabetes insipidus following head trauma. Questions 506 through 510 refer to this situation.

506. The assessment of Mr. Sohl that would be most indicative of diabetes insipidus is:
① Decreased serum osmolality
② Increased blood glucose
③ Low urinary specific gravity
④ Elevation of blood pressure

507. The nurse administers vasopressin tannate intramuscularly. To evaluate the effectiveness of the drug the nurse should monitor Mr. Sohl's:
① Intake and output
② Pulse rate
③ Fractional urines
④ Arterial blood pH

508. In order to understand diabetes insipidus, the nurse must be aware that an antidiuretic substance important for maintaining fluid balance is secreted by the:
① Anterior pituitary
② Adrenal cortex
③ Adrenal medulla
④ Posterior pituitary

509. This diagnosis means that Mr. Sohl is lacking the antidiuretic hormone (ADH). Normally as this hormone increases:
① Glomerular filtration tends to decrease
② Tubular reabsorption of potassium and water increases
③ Tubular reabsorption of sodium and water increases
④ Urine concentration tends to decrease

510. Normally the antidiuretic hormone (ADH) influences kidney function by stimulating the:
① Glomerulus to control the quantity of fluid passing through it
② Glomerulus to withhold the proteins from the urine
③ Nephron tubules to reabsorb water
④ Nephron tubules to reabsorb glucose

Situation: Mr. Ambro, age 34, is brought to the hospital in a coma. It is discovered that he is diabetic. He is given an IV containing insulin, glucose, and potassium. A retention catheter is inserted. Questions 511 through 517 refer to this situation.

511. A client with untreated diabetes may lapse into a coma because of acidosis. This acidosis is directly caused by an increased concentration in the blood of:
① Glucose
② Lactic acid
③ Glutamic acid
④ Alpha-keto acids

512. The IV solution prescribed contains potassium because potassium ions in the extracellular fluid must be replenished since they:
    ① Are carried with glucose to the kidneys and excreted in the urine in increased amounts
    ② Enter the intracellular fluid because of the generalized anabolism induced by insulin and glucose
    ③ Are rapidly lost from the body by copious diaphoresis present during coma
    ④ Are quickly used up during the rapid series of catabolic reactions stimulated by insulin and glucose

513. A fractional urine specimen should be removed from Mr. Ambro's retention catheter by:
    ① Cleansing the drainage valve and removing from the collection bag
    ② Disconnecting and draining into a clean catheter
    ③ Wiping the catheter with alcohol and draining into a sterile test tube
    ④ Using a sterile syringe to remove from a clamped, cleansed catheter

514. Mr. Ambro has a hypoglycemic reaction to the insulin. The assessments that are indicative of this response include:
    ① Pallor, perspiration, tremors
    ② Excessive thirst, dry hot skin
    ③ Anorexia, glycosuria, tachycardia
    ④ Fruity odor to breath, acetonuria

515. In an emergency the rapid adjustments made by the body are associated with the increased activity of the:
    ① Pituitary gland
    ② Thyroid gland
    ③ Adrenal gland
    ④ Pancreas gland

516. The nursing intervention that would most likely relieve the symptoms associated with Mr. Ambro's hypoglycemic reaction include:
    ① Withholding subsequent dose of insulin
    ② Providing a snack of cheese and crackers
    ③ Administering 5% dextrose solution IV
    ④ Giving 8 oz of fruit juice or soda

517. The best indication that Mr. Ambro is successfully managing his disease after discharge is:
    ① His statement that he is complying with insulin orders
    ② A stabilization of his serum glucose
    ③ A reduction in his excess body weight
    ④ His evident knowledge of his disease

Situation: Mrs. Louis is admitted to the hospital with the diagnosis of Cushing's syndrome. Questions 518 through 523 refer to this situation.

518. The nurse understands that the cause of Cushing's syndrome is most commonly:
    ① Deprivation of adrenocortical hormones
    ② Insufficient ACTH production
    ③ Hyperplasia of the adrenal cortex
    ④ Pituitary hypoplasia

519. Glucocorticoids and mineralocorticoids are secreted by the:
    ① Pancreas
    ② Hypophysis cerebri
    ③ Adrenal glands
    ④ Gonads

520. When assessing Mrs. Louis the nurse would expect to observe:
    ① "Buffalo hump" and hypertension
    ② Dehydration and menorrhagia
    ③ Pitting edema and frequent colds
    ④ Migraine headache and dysmenorrhea

521. A bilateral adrenalectomy is scheduled. Prior to surgery, steroids are administered to Mrs. Louis. The nurse understands the reason for this is to:
    ① Compensate for sudden lack of these hormones following surgery
    ② Increase the inflammatory action to promote scar formation
    ③ Foster accumulation of glycogen in the liver
    ④ Facilitate urinary excretion of salt and water following surgery

522. The medication the nurse would expect to administer to Mrs. Louis on the day of surgery and in the immediate postoperative period is:
    ① Regular insulin
    ② ACTH
    ③ Hydrocortisone succinate (Solu-Cortef)
    ④ Pituitary extract (Pituitrin)

523. An adrenalectomy is performed. Postoperatively, until regulated by steroid therapy, Mrs. Louis may show symptoms of:
    ① Hyperglycemia
    ② Sodium retention
    ③ Potassium excretion
    ④ Hypotension

Situation: Alice, a 45-year-old college student, is admitted to the hospital for diabetic acidosis. Questions 524 through 530 refer to this situation.

524. The cause of Alice's symptoms is a:
    ① Sudden increase in the concentration of cholesterol in the extracellular compartment
    ② Physiologic phenomenon following the ingestion of too much highly acidic food
    ③ Rise in the pH of the blood to a point above 7.5
    ④ Decrease in the pH of the blood to a point below 7.3

525. Several laboratory tests are done. Alice's symptoms lead the nurse to expect the blood test to reveal:
    ① Low sugar, decreased acidity, low CO_2 combining power
    ② Elevated sugar, normal acidity, high CO_2 combining power
    ③ Elevated sugar, increased acidity, low CO_2 combining power
    ④ Low sugar, increased acidity, high CO_2 combining power

526. The type of insulin that will be used during the emergency treatment of the acidosis and until Alice is eating regularly is:
    ① Isophane insulin suspension (NPH insulin)
    ② Insulin injection (regular insulin)
    ③ Insulin zinc suspension (lente insulin)
    ④ Protamine zinc insulin suspension

527. After blood studies and observation of urinary volume, the physician orders potassium chloride, 20 mEq, to be added to the IV solution. The primary purpose for administering this drug to Alice is:
    ① Replacement of potassium deficit
    ② Treatment of hyperpnea

③ Prevention of flaccid paralysis
④ Treatment of cardiac arrhythmias

528. The nurse should recognize that Alice needs further teaching when, reviewing the dietary exchange system, she states that:
① 1 scoop ice milk = 1 slice bread
② 1 oz cheese = 1 cup milk
③ 1 egg = 1 oz meat
④ 1 slice bacon = 2 Tbsp cream

529. Alice and her family members should be taught the use of glucagon. The primary use of glucagon is to treat:
① Diabetic acidosis
② Insulin-induced hypoglycemia
③ Idiosyncratic reactions to insulin
④ Hyperinsulin secretion related to neoplasm

530. Alice's nursing plan includes that before discharge she will know how to give herself insulin, adjust the dosage, understand her diet, and test her blood for glucose. She progresses well and is discharged 10 days following admission. Legally:
① The physician was responsible and the nurse should have cleared the care with him
② The nurse was properly functioning as a health teacher
③ The visiting nurse should do health teaching in the home
④ A family member also should have been taught to administer the insulin

Situation: Mr. Pierce, a client who has acromegaly and diabetes mellitus, has had a hypophysectomy. Questions 531 through 535 refer to this situation.

531. Acromegaly is produced by an oversecretion of:
① Growth hormone
② Thyroid hormone
③ Thyroid-stimulating hormone
④ Testosterone

532. The nurse recognizes that Mr. Pierce needs further teaching about his condition after the hypophysectomy when he states, "I know I will:
① Be sterile for the rest of my life."
② Have to take cortisone (or similar preparation) for the rest of my life."
③ Have to take thyroxin (or similar preparation) for the rest of my life."
④ Require larger doses of insulin than I did preoperatively."

533. Increased blood concentration of cortisol (hydroxycortisone):
① Decreases the anterior pituitary secretion of ACTH
② Makes the body less able to resist stress successfully
③ Tends to accelerate wound healing
④ Tends to decrease liver gluconeogenesis

534. Following the hypophysectomy the nurse should observe Mr. Pierce for signs of:
① Urinary retention
② Bleeding at suture site
③ Increased intracranial pressure
④ Respiratory distress

535. The nurse knows that most of the hormones present in the body at any given time were secreted from the endocrine glands:
① 24 hours ago
② 4 to 6 hours ago
③ More than 72 hours ago
④ 8 to 12 hours ago

Situation: Mrs. Green, a known diabetic, has been admitted to the hospital in diabetic acidosis. Blood gases are determined immediately. Questions 536 through 542 refer to this situation.

536. Mrs. Green is in a state of uncompensated acidosis. The nurse would expect her arterial blood pH to be approximately:
① 6.9
② 7.2
③ 7.45
④ 7.48

537. Larger than normal amounts of acetoacetic acid have been entering Mrs. Green's blood as one of the indirect results of her insulin deficiency. Like lactic acid and other nonvolatile acids, acetoacetic acid is buffered in the blood chiefly by:
① Carbon dioxide
② Potassium salt of hemoglobin
③ Sodium bicarbonate
④ Sodium chloride

538. As a result of excessive acetoacetic acid:
① Mrs. Green's blood pH remains unchanged
② Mrs. Green's blood pH increases slightly
③ The carbonic acid content of Mrs. Green's blood remains unchanged
④ The sodium bicarbonate content of Mrs. Green's blood decreases and its carbonic acid content increases

539. The insulin given to Mrs. Green in this emergency would be:
① Protamine zinc
② Globulin
③ NPH
④ Regular

540. Initially, when the acidosis is controlled, NPH insulin, 40 units each morning, is prescribed for Mrs. Green. NPH insulin (100 U = 1 ml) is available. To give 40 units, using a regular syringe, the nurse should withdraw:
① 6 minims
② 12 minims
③ 20 minims
④ 40 minims

541. The nurse knows that glucagon is given with 50% dextrose in the treatment of hypoglycemia because it:
① Provides more storage of glucose
② Increases blood sugar levels
③ Stimulates release of insulin
④ Inhibits glycogenesis

542. When Mrs. Green is discharged, she is receiving isophane insulin suspension (NPH) daily and also is receiving insulin injection (regular insulin) when her

blood sugar is positive. In instructing Mrs. Green the nurse should teach her to:
1. Mix the insulins in any required dosage in the same syringe
2. Give the insulins separately unless the ratio of dosage is greater than 1:1
3. Give the insulins in the same syringe when the ratio is 1:1
4. Administer the insulins in separate syringes using different sites for injection

Situation: Mrs. McNeer has been diagnosed as having Graves' disease. Radioactive iodine is prescribed to decrease the activity of the thyroid, but this therapy is unsuccessful. Questions 543 through 551 refer to this situation.

543. The nurse knows that after radioactive iodine Mrs. McNeer is:
1. Not radioactive and can be handled as any other individual
2. Highly radioactive and should be isolated as much as possible
3. Mildly radioactive and should be treated with standard precautions
4. Not radioactive but may still transmit some dangerous radiations and must be treated with precautions

544. After this therapy Mrs. McNeer would probably be placed on a:
1. High-calorie diet with supplementary feeding
2. High-roughage diet with supplementary nourishment
3. Regular diet with nourishment between meals
4. Soft, easily digested, nourishing diet

545. The nurse, recognizing the need to decrease the size and vascularity of the thyroid gland prior to surgery, would expect the physician to order:
1. Propylthiouracil
2. Liothyronine sodium (Cytomel)
3. Lugol's iodine solution
4. Potassium permanganate

546. To evaluate possible laryngeal nerve injury following a thyroidectomy, the nurse should, on an hourly basis:
1. Swab the client's throat to test gag reflex
2. Ask the client to swallow
3. Ask the client to speak
4. Have the client hum a familiar tune

547. While taking Mrs. McNeer's blood pressure the nurse notices she is pale and has spasms of her hand. The nurse prepares for replacement of:
1. Potassium chloride
2. Magnesium
3. Calcium
4. Bicarbonate

548. The nurse suspects accidental removal of the parathyroids, which causes:
1. Tetany and death
2. Adrenocortical stimulation
3. Myxedema
4. Hypovolemic shock

549. Calcium is required because parathormone is the hormone that tends to:
1. Accelerate bone breakdown with release of calcium into the blood
2. Decrease blood calcium concentration and relieve tetany
3. Increase blood phosphate concentration and decrease calcium levels
4. Increase calcium absorption into bone and remove calcium from the blood

550. The two interbalanced regulatory agents that control overall calcium balance in the body are:
1. Vitamin A and thyroid hormone
2. Ascorbic acid and growth hormone
3. Phosphorus and ACTH
4. Vitamin D and parathyroid hormone

551. The hormone that tends to decrease calcium concentration in the blood is:
1. Aldosterone
2. Thyrocalcitonin
3. Parathyroid hormone
4. Thyroid hormone

Situation: Mr. Jackson, 47 years old, is admitted with a diagnosis of primary hyperparathyroidism as a result of a malignant neoplasm. Questions 552 through 555 refer to this situation.

552. When assessing for complications of hyperparathyroidism, the nurse should monitor Mr. Jackson for:
1. Tetany
2. Seizure disorder
3. Bone destruction
4. Graves' disease

553. The nursing action that should be included in Mr. Jackson's plan of care is the:
1. Maintenance of absolute bed rest
2. Ensurance of a large fluid intake
3. Institution of seizure precautions
4. Provision of a high-calcium diet

554. Following a parathyroidectomy, Mr. Jackson has abnormally low blood levels of triidothyronine (T_3) and thyroxine (T_4). Underproduction of thyroxin produces:
1. Myxedema
2. Acromegaly
3. Cushing's disease
4. Graves' disease

555. As a result of the low levels of T_3 and T_4, the nurse should expect Mr. Jackson to exhibit signs of:
1. Cold intolerance
2. Irritability
3. Profuse diaphoresis
4. Tachycardia

556. The gland which regulates the rate of oxygenation in all the body cells is the:
1. Pituitary gland
2. Thyroid gland
3. Adrenal gland
4. Pancreas gland

557. Glucose is an important molecule to a cell because this molecule is primarily used for:
① The building of cell membranes
② The synthesis of proteins
③ Extraction of energy
④ Building the genetic material

558. The source of glucose for maintaining blood glucose at normal levels at all times is:
① Ingested food
② Intestinal hydrolysis
③ Liver glycogen
④ Gluconeogenesis

559. The fuel glucose is delivered to the cells by the blood for production of energy. The hormone controlling use of glucose by the cell is:
① Thyroxine
② Growth hormone
③ Adrenal steroids
④ Insulin

560. When teaching a client about an oral hypoglycemic medication, the nurse should emphasize the significance of:
① Manifestations of toxicity
② Untoward reactions
③ Taking it regularly and on time
④ Increasing dosage when necessary

561. Ketone bodies appear in the blood and urine when fats are being oxidized in great amounts. This condition is associated with:
① Starvation
② Alcoholism
③ Positive nitrogen balance
④ Bone healing

The Neuromusculoskeletal Systems

Situation: Mr. Saul, a 68-year-old retired civil service employee, is admitted to the hospital via the emergency service. He was found unconscious 30 minutes prior to admission. The physical examination reveals right hemiplegia. Tentative diagnosis is cerebral vascular accident. Questions 562 through 568 refer to this situation.

562. In observing Mr. Saul the nurse should check for signs of increased intracranial pressure. Of the following combinations of symptoms the most indicative of increased intracranial pressure is:
① Slow bounding pulse, rising blood pressure, elevated temperature, stupor
② Rapid weak pulse, fall in blood pressure, low temperature, restlessness
③ Weak rapid pulse, normal blood pressure, intermittent fever, lethargy
④ Slow bounding pulse, fall in blood pressure, temperature below 97° F (36° C), stupor

563. Since Mr. Saul is unconscious, the nurse should expect him to be:
① Unable to react to painful stimuli
② Incontinent of urine and feces

③ Incapable of spontaneous motion
④ Incapable of hearing

564. Mr. Saul regains consciousness and has expressive aphasia. As a part of the long-range planning, the nurse would:
① Help the family to accept the fact that Mr. Saul cannot participate in verbal communication
② Wait for Mr. Saul to state his needs verbally regardless of how long it may take
③ Provide positive feedback when he uses a word correctly
④ Suggest that he get help at home because his disability is permanent

565. Urinary retention and overflow, a frequent problem of a client after a stroke, is evidenced by:
① Decrease in total amount of urine voided
② Frequency from inability to empty bladder
③ Continual incontinence
④ Oliguria and edema

566. In encouraging hospitalized clients to void the most basic method for the nurse to employ is:
① Having the client listen to running water
② Warming a bedpan
③ Placing the client's hands in warm water
④ Providing privacy

567. Once stable, Mr. Saul is transferred to a rehabilitation unit. A basic concept about rehabilitation is:
① Rehabilitation is a specialty area with unique methods for meeting the client's needs
② Rehabilitation is unnecessary for clients returning to their usual activities following hospitalization
③ Rehabilitation needs, immediate or potential, are exhibited by all clients with a health problem
④ Rehabilitation needs are best met by the client's family and community resources

568. Mr. Saul is placed into a whirlpool tub for range of motion exercises. Rehabilitating exercises carried out under water use:
① Water pressure
② Water vapor
③ Water's buoyant force
④ Water temperature

Situation: Ellen Smith, a 76-year-old woman, is admitted to the rehabilitation unit following a stroke. She is bedridden and aphasic. The morning after her admission the physician orders an indwelling catheter, since she has been incontinent during the night. Questions 569 to 575 refer to this situation.

569. It is learned from the daughter that her mother had not been incontinent while at home, and she insisted that the nurse had failed to communicate with her mother. This is an example of:
① Treatment without consent of the client, which is an invasion of rights
② A catheter inserted for the client's benefit
③ Inability to obtain consent for treatment because the client was aphasic
④ A treatment that does not need special consent

570. Mrs. Smith has left hemiplegia. The nurse contributes to Mrs. Smith's rehabilitation by:
    ① Making a referral to the physical therapist
    ② Not moving the affected arm and leg unless necessary
    ③ Beginning active exercises
    ④ Positioning Mrs. Smith to prevent deformity and decubiti

571. The nurse can best prevent footdrop in a client for whom bed rest has been prescribed by the use of:
    ① Boards
    ② Blocks
    ③ Cradles
    ④ Sandbags

572. Mrs. Smith's emotional responses to her illness would probably be determined by:
    ① Her premorbid personality
    ② The location of her lesion
    ③ The care she is receiving
    ④ Her ability to understand her illness

573. Mrs. Smith's position should be changed:
    ① Every hour
    ② Every 2 hours
    ③ Every 4 hours
    ④ Every 6 hours

574. In aiding Mrs. Smith to develop independence, the nurse should:
    ① Demonstrate ways she can regain independence in activities
    ② Reinforce success in tasks accomplished
    ③ Establish long-range goals for the client
    ④ Point out her errors in performance

575. For optimum nutrition the nurse may find that Mrs. Smith needs assistance with her eating. To accomplish this goal, the nurse should:
    ① Encourage her to participate in the feeding process
    ② Feed Mrs. Smith to conserve her energy
    ③ Feed her rapidly before she tires
    ④ Have her daughter feed her every meal

Situation: Mrs. Scully, a small 78-year-old woman, fell in her back-yard. X-ray films were taken, and the attending surgeon told Mrs. Scully that she had fractured her hip (fractured neck of the femur). She was admitted to the hospital, and Buck's extension was applied to her limb. The following day she was given a general anesthetic, the fracture was reduced, and a Smith-Petersen nail inserted. Questions 576 through 581 refer to this situation.

576. When Mrs. Scully is helped from the bed to a chair after the nailing of her hip, the nurse encourages her to stand on her good leg before sitting in a chair (no weight-bearing on the involved limb). This is important because:
    ① There is usually insufficient help to lift her from bed to chair
    ② This will help maintain strength in her good limb
    ③ This is the quickest method of getting her to and from the bed
    ④ There is less danger of injuring her hip

577. When Mrs. Scully is in the side-lying position, the nurse ensures that she has a firm pillow placed between her thighs and that the entire length of her upper limb is supported. The most important reason for this is to:
    ① Prevent strain on the fracture site
    ② Make the client more comfortable
    ③ Prevent flexion contractures of the hip joint
    ④ Prevent skin surfaces from rubbing together

578. When teaching crutch walking, the nurse instructs Mrs. Scully to place weight on:
    ① The axillary region
    ② Palms of the hands and axillary region
    ③ Palms of the hands
    ④ Both extremities, with partial weight-bearing

579. Aseptic necrosis of the head of the femur occurs. The nurse should be aware that this is caused by:
    ① Infection at the site of the wound
    ② Immobilization after reduction of the fracture
    ③ Loss of blood supply to head of the femur
    ④ Weight-bearing before fracture is healed

580. Contractures that develop most frequently after fracture of the hip are:
    ① Hyperextension of the knee joint, with footdrop deformity
    ② Internal rotation with abduction
    ③ Flexion and adduction of the hip, with flexion of the knee
    ④ External rotation with abduction

581. Intramedullary nailing is used in the treatment of:
    ① Fracture of the shaft of the femur
    ② Fracture of the neck of the femur
    ③ Slipped epiphysis of the femur
    ④ Intertrochanteric fracture of the femur

Situation: Mrs. Olin, a 38-year-old schoolteacher with rheumatoid arthritis, is admitted to the hospital with severe pain and swelling of the joints in both hands. Questions 582 through 587 refer to this situation.

582. Mrs. Olin's condition would indicate that a primary consideration in her care is:
    ① Motivation
    ② Education
    ③ Comfort
    ④ Surgery

583. The laboratory test or procedure that the nurse would use in reference to the diagnosis of arthritis is:
    ① Latex agglutination
    ② Pancreatic lipase
    ③ Bence Jones protein
    ④ Alkaline phosphatase

584. Mrs. Olin must be protected against injury to the joints. Therefore, therapeutic exercise by the nurse should be:
    ① Passive
    ② Avoided
    ③ Preceded by heat
    ④ Active assistive

585. In helping Mrs. Olin toward self-reliance and independence the nurse should approach the problem with:
    ① A positive attitude toward the eventual outcome
    ② The understanding that little can be accomplished

③ A feeling that Mrs. Olin should be placed in an extended care facility

④ Limited objectives

586. Through motivation and teaching, Mrs. Olin may:
① Learn to perform most activities of daily living
② Become vocationally employed
③ Ambulate with crutches
④ Be transferred to a halfway house

587. It would be unusual if long-term therapy for Mrs. Olin included:
① Range-of-motion exercises
② Braces
③ Massage
④ Conductive heat

Situation: Mr. Smith is a 60-year-old man who is admitted to the hospital with a diagnosis of idiopathic trigeminal neuralgia (tic douloureux). Questions 588 through 594 refer to this situation.

588. In planning the nursing care for Mr. Smith, the nurse should specifically:
① Emphasize the importance of brushing teeth
② Be alert to prevent dehydration or starvation
③ Initiate exercises of the jaw and facial muscles
④ Apply iced compresses to the affected area

589. The nurse would expect Mr. Smith to exhibit:
① Uncontrollable tremors of the eyelid
② Excruciating facial and head pain
③ Unilateral muscle weakness
④ Multiple petechiae

590. The nurse would also expect Mr. Smith to demonstrate:
① Exhaustion and fatigue due to extreme pain
② Excessive talkativeness due to apprehension
③ Hyperactivity due to medications received
④ Prolonged periods of sleep due to anxiety

591. In planning care for Mr. Smith, the nurse should:
① Avoid walking swiftly past the client
② Discontinue oral hygiene temporarily
③ Massage both sides of the face frequently
④ Keep the client in the prone position

592. Mr. Smith tells the nurse he is taking all four of the medications listed. The nurse should be aware that the medication used to treat trigeminal neuralgia is:
① Carbamazepine (Tegretol)
② Allopurinol (Zyloprim)
③ Morphine sulfate
④ Ascorbic acid

593. Surgery, with severing of the nerve, is performed. An unusual occurrence after surgery would be the:
① Development of herpes simplex
② Recurrence of the pain, which will gradually decrease over time
③ Development of a crawling or tingling sensation in the area
④ Loss of muscle power in the area

594. In discharge planning for Mr. Smith, the nurse should counsel the client to:
① Perform facial exercises
② Have regular dental checkups
③ Avoid stressful situations
④ Chew food on the affected side

Situation: Mr. Davis is a 55-year-old man who has had a cerebral vascular accident. He has right-sided paralysis, dysphagia, and dysarthria. His nursing care includes frequent monitoring of vital signs. Questions 595 through 601 refer to this situation.

595. Mr. Davis' temperature should be taken:
① Orally
② In the groin
③ Rectally
④ In the axilla

596. Mr. Davis is experiencing difficulty in:
① Swallowing
② Focusing
③ Writing
④ Understanding

597. Mr. Davis' dysarthria requires initial provision for:
① Routine hygienic needs
② Prevention of aspiration
③ Effective communication
④ Liquid formula diet

598. Blood pressure should not be taken on Mr. Davis' right arm because circulatory impairment may:
① Precipitate the formation of a thrombus
② Hinder restoration of function
③ Produce inaccurate readings
④ Cause excessive pressure on the brachial artery

599. Three days after admission Mr. Davis has a nasogastric tube inserted and is prescribed a liquid formula diet six times daily. For the first day the amount of liquid administered at one time should not exceed:
① 150 ml
② 250 ml
③ 350 ml
④ 450 ml

600. The formula temperature most compatible for administration of the tube feeding is:
① 77° F (25° C)
② Body
③ Room
④ 108° F (42° C)

601. The nurse should administer the tube feeding slowly to reduce the hazard of:
① Indigestion
② Regurgitation
③ Flatulence
④ Distention

Situation: Mr. Bloom, a 56-year-old baker, was admitted to the hospital 5 weeks ago with a fractured skull and concussion. Two weeks after admission he exhibited evidence of increasing intracranial pressure. Questions 602 through 607 refer to this situation.

602. Mr. Bloom has been receiving dexamethasone (Decadron) during the past 3 weeks for control of cerebral edema. The planned effect of the drug is to:
① Increase fluid removal from the tissues
② Reduce CSF secretion by the choroid plexus
③ Increase elasticity of the ventricle walls
④ Suppress production of antibodies

603. While Mr. Bloom is receiving dexamethasone (Decadron) the nurse is testing his blood for glucose every 4 hours because the drug:
    ① Lowers the renal threshold for glucose
    ② Mobilizes liver stores of glycogen
    ③ Accelerates protein breakdown and liberates excess glycogen
    ④ Has a glucose component, which raises the blood sugar level

604. Mr. Bloom has been taking Maalox while he is receiving dexamethasone. The antacid is prescribed because dexamethasone is a drug that:
    ① Irritates the gastric mucosa
    ② Stimulates gastric production of hydrochloric acid
    ③ Increases gastric acidity and slows emptying time
    ④ Increases pepsin-induced erosion of the gastric mucosa

605. Mr. Bloom has several loose bowel movements and the physician changes his antacid prescription to Amphojel. The change is made because:
    ① Maalox and dexamethasone act synergistically to increase fluid content of the intestine
    ② Amphojel increases the bulk of feces and slows peristalsis
    ③ Amphojel neutralizes larger amounts of the hydrochloric acid that causes diarrhea
    ④ Maalox contains a magnesium component that stimulates peristalsis

606. Mr. Bloom complains about the chalky taste of Amphojel. He states that he would rather take bicarbonate of soda as he does at home. The nurse tells him it is not advisable to take bicarbonate of soda regularly. This statement is based on knowledge that bicarbonate of soda:
    ① Causes distention by producing carbon dioxide in the stomach
    ② Is absorbed from the stomach, and the sodium component causes ankle edema
    ③ Is absorbed from the stomach and may cause alkalosis
    ④ Causes rebound hyperacidity after initial neutralization of hydrochloric acid

607. The physician states that he plans to reduce Mr. Bloom's dexamethasone dosage gradually and to continue him on a lower maintenance dosage during the next few weeks. The nurse explains to Mr. Bloom that the reason for the gradual dosage reduction is to allow:
    ① Production of adrenocorticotropic hormone (ACTH)
    ② Return of cortisone production by the adrenal glands
    ③ Time to observe for return of increased intracranial pressure
    ④ Building of glycogen and protein stores in liver and muscle

Situation: Mrs. Pring, a 34-year-old mother of five children, has been diagnosed as having rheumatoid arthritis. Mrs. Pring is being admitted to the hospital because of a recent flare-up of symptoms. She has been taking aspirin and steroids for the past year. Questions 608 through 611 refer to this situation.

608. Daily blood work is ordered for Mrs. Pring during the first 3 days of her hospitalization. The symptom that may indicate a complication of the prolonged use of these medications is:
    ① Elevated sedimentation rate
    ② Leukepenia
    ③ Elevated C-reactive protein
    ④ Hypochromic, normocytic anemia

609. While taking a nursing history from Mrs. Pring, the nurse promotes communication by:
    ① Asking questions that can be answered by a simple "yes" or "no"
    ② Telling Mrs. Pring there is no cause for alarm
    ③ Asking "why" and "how" questions
    ④ Using broad, open-ended statements

610. Mrs. Pring questions the nurse as to the source of her disease. The nurse is aware that this is a disease of:
    ① Bones
    ② Joints
    ③ Purine metabolism
    ④ Connective tissue

611. Gold salts may be used to treat rheumatoid arthritis. A serious side effect of this drug is:
    ① Cardiac decompensation
    ② Kidney damage
    ③ Persistent nausea
    ④ Pulmonary emboli

Situation: Mrs. Grey is a 45-year-old woman who has been admitted to the hospital with a diagnosis of open-angle chronic glaucoma. Questions 612 through 619 refer to this situation.

612. The first symptom Mrs. Grey is most likely to exhibit is:
    ① A sudden, complete loss of vision
    ② Impairment of peripheral vision
    ③ Sudden attacks of acute pain
    ④ Constant blurred vision

613. The nurse explains to Mrs. Grey that the chief aim of medical treatment in chronic glaucoma is:
    ① Controlling intraocular pressure
    ② Dilating the pupil to allow for an increase in the visual field
    ③ Allowing for healing process by resting the eye
    ④ Preventing secondary infections that may add to the visual problem

614. When the ciliary muscles contract:
    ① They bring about convergence of both eyes
    ② They close the eyelids
    ③ They focus the lens on distant objects
    ④ They focus the lens on near objects

615. The nurse would recognize that Mrs. Grey needs further teaching when she states, "It would be dangerous for me to:
    ① Use any sedatives."
    ② Release my emotions by crying."
    ③ Use atropine in any form."
    ④ Become constipated."

616. Mrs. Grey should be advised to:
    ① Use eyewashes on a regular basis
    ② Use laxatives daily
    ③ Keep an extra supply of eye medication on hand
    ④ Have prescriptions filled when necessary

617. Drugs instilled in the eye are administered by the method known as:
① Topical
② Intraocular
③ Injection
④ Insufflation

618. A systemic drug that may be prescribed to produce diuresis and inhibit formation of aqueous humor is:
① Acetazolamide (Diamox)
② Bendroflumethiazide (Naturetin)
③ Chlorothiazide (Diuril)
④ Demecarium bromide (Humorsol)

619. If Mrs. Grey develops an inflammatory reaction in the eye the drug that will probably be prescribed is:
① Nitrofurazone (Furacin)
② Sulfisoxazole (Gantrisin)
③ Neomycin
④ Cortisone

Situation: Mrs. O'Reilly, 62 years of age, has been admitted to the hospital after having had a cerebral vascular accident resulting in left hemiplegia. Questions 620 through 627 refer to this situation.

620. The nurse identifies left hemiplegia by the following observations:
① Paralysis of the left lower extremity
② Paralysis of the left arm, left leg, and left side of the face
③ Paralysis of the left arm and left side of the face
④ Paralysis of the left arm, left leg, and right side of the face

621. When the nurse brings in the dinner tray, Mrs. O'Reilly is staring blankly at the wall and states that she feels like half a person. Specific nursing care of Mrs. O'Reilly should be directed at:
① Including her in all decisions
② Helping her explore her feelings
③ Distracting her from self-pity
④ Preventing contractures and decubiti

622. Mrs. O'Reilly has been incontinent of feces. When establishing a bowel training program, the nurse must remember that the most important factor is the:
① Client's previous habits in the area of diet and use of laxatives
② Timing of elimination to take advantage of the gastrocolic reflex
③ Use of medication to induce elimination
④ Planning with the client a definite time for attempted evacuations

623. Developing independence is a primary goal for Mrs. O'Reilly. The nurse plans to achieve this by:
① Demonstrating ways she can regain independence
② Establishing long-range goals for the client
③ Reinforcing success in tasks accomplished
④ Pointing out her errors and helping her correct them

624. Mrs. O'Reilly's daughter threatens to sue when her mother develops a large decubitus ulcer after she insisted on lying on her back for long periods. She is very upset and blames the nurses. The decision in this suit would take into consideration the fact that:
① The nurse should uphold the client's right not to be moved

② Decubitus ulcers frequently occur in immobilized clients
③ Clients should be turned at least every 2 hours
④ Nurses are not responsible to the client's family

625. The drug most likely to be used to treat Mrs. O'Reilly's decubitus ulcer is:
① Chymotrypsin
② Hyaluronidase (Wydase)
③ Penicillinase
④ Dextranomer (Debrisan)

626. The nurse suspects Mrs. O'Reilly has become impacted when she states:
① "I don't have much of an appetite."
② "I have a lot of gas pains."
③ "I feel like I have to go and just can't."
④ "I haven't had a bowel movement for 2 days."

627. The assessment by the nurse that is a further indication of the probable presence of a fecal impaction is:
① Tympanites
② Decreased number of bowel movements
③ Fecal liquid seepage
④ Bright red blood in the stool

Situation: Mr. Ray, a 67-year-old retired plumber, falls and is unable to get up. His daughter calls an ambulance, and he is brought to the emergency room, where it is found that he has a fracture of the neck of the left femur. Mr. Ray is admitted to the orthopedic unit, put in Buck's extension, and prepared for surgery the next day. Questions 628 through 633 refer to this situation.

628. On examination of Mr. Ray, the nurse would expect to find:
① Shortening of the affected extremity with internal rotation
② Shortening of the affected extremity with external rotation
③ Abduction with external rotation
④ Adduction with internal rotation

629. The nurse should know that, following a fracture of the neck of the femur, the desirable position for the limb is:
① External rotation with flexion of the knee and hip
② External rotation with extension of the knee and hip
③ Internal rotation with extension of the knee
④ Internal rotation with flexion of the hip and knee

630. The nurse should explain to Mr. Ray that the chief reason for applying Buck's extension is to:
① Help reduce the fracture and to relieve muscle spasm and pain
② Keep him from turning and moving in bed
③ Prevent contractures from developing
④ Maintain the limb in a position of external rotation

631. Part of the nursing care of Mr. Ray is assessment of peripheral pulses. The important characteristics when assessing the peripheral pulses are:
① Contractility and rate
② Color of skin and rhythm
③ Amplitude and symmetry
④ Local temperature and visible pulsations

632. When Mr. Ray is ready to walk with crutches after the hip pinning, he will probably be taught:
① Four-point crutch walking
② Two-point crutch walking
③ Swing-through gait
④ Three-point crutch walking

633. The principle that the nurse should use in teaching Mr. Ray the four-point gait once bone regrowth has occurred is:
① Most of weight should be supported by the axillae
② Elbows should be maintained in rigid extension
③ The client must be able to bear weight on both legs
④ The affected extremity should be kept about 15 cm (6 inches) off the ground

Situation: Mrs. Newt, a 35-year-old housewife and the mother of five young children, ages 6 months to 15 years, is involved in a serious auto accident on the highway when her car skids on the wet pavement, striking the concrete partition. She is taken to a hospital, where it is determined that she has multiple trauma, possible fractured skull, fractures of the fifth and sixth cervical and the tenth, eleventh, and twelfth thoracic vertebrae, as well as a ruptured spleen and hematuria. Questions 634 through 640 refer to this situation.

634. A splenectomy was necessary because:
① The spleen is a highly vascular organ
② Rupture of the spleen is frequently associated with diseases of the liver and blood
③ The spleen is the largest lymphoid organ in the body
④ An enlarged spleen causes such discomfort or disability as to justify its removal

635. Because of the nature of the particular surgery, in the immediate postoperative period the nurse should observe Mrs. Newt for:
① Hemorrhage, abdominal distention
② Peritonitis, pulmonary complications
③ Shock, infection
④ Intestinal obstruction, bleeding

636. When planning care for Mrs. Newt, the nurse should:
① Observe her for signs of brain injury
② Place her in Trendelenburg position if in shock
③ Check for hemorrhaging from oral cavity
④ Observe for decreased intracranial pressure and temperature

637. Following surgery the nurse should observe Mrs. Newt for the depletion of the electrolyte:
① Sodium
② Calcium
③ Chloride
④ Potassium

638. The nurse can expect Mrs. Newt to complain of:
① Excessively moist respirations
② Pain on inspiration
③ Shortness of breath
④ Pain on expiration

639. Since Mrs. Newt has hematuria, the nurse should observe her for:
① Diarrhea
② Symptoms of peritonitis
③ Gross blood in the urine
④ Acetone in urine

640. Hematuria in this instance probably means that there has been injury to the:
① Kidneys
② Ureters
③ Bladder
④ Urethra

Situation: Mrs. Smith is admitted with a diagnosis of partial occlusion of the left common carotid artery. She is an epileptic and has been taking phenytoin (Dilantin) for 10 years. Questions 641 through 645 refer to this situation.

641. In planning her care it is most important that the nurse:
① Place an airway, suction, and restraints at her bedside
② Ask her to remove her dental bridge and eyeglasses
③ Obtain a history of seizure incidence
④ Observe her for evidence of increased restlessness and agitation

642. Mrs. Smith is scheduled for an arteriogram at 10 AM and is to have nothing by mouth before the test. Her phenytoin (Dilantin) is scheduled for administration at 9 AM. The nurse should:
① Administer the drug with 30 ml of water at 9 AM
② Give the same dosage of the drug rectally
③ Omit the 9 AM dose of the drug
④ Ask the physician if the drug can be given IV

643. Mrs. Smith is scheduled to receive phenytoin (Dilantin), 100 mg, orally at 6 PM. She is having difficulty swallowing capsules since the arteriogram. The nurse should:
① Open the capsule and sprinkle the powder in a cup of water
② Give her 4 ml of phenytoin suspension containing 125 mg/5 ml
③ Obtain a change in the prescribed administration route to allow IM administration
④ Insert a rectal suppository containing 100 mg phenytoin

644. The nursing history indicates that Mrs. Smith neglects her personal hygiene. The nurse plans health teaching and emphasizes meticulous oral hygiene because phenytoin (Dilantin):
① Causes hypertrophy of the gums
② Irritates the gingiva and destroys tooth enamel
③ Increases alkalinity of the oral secretions
④ Increases plaque and bacterial growth at the gum lines

645. Mrs. Smith will receive folic acid at home. The most likely reason for continuing the drug is:
① Folic acid will prevent neuropathy caused by phenytoin
② Folic acid improves absorption of iron from foods
③ Folic acid content of common foods is inadequate to meet her needs
④ Phenytoin inhibits folic acid absorption from foods

Situation: Mrs. Burt is unconscious when admitted to the hospital. Questions 646 through 652 refer to this situation.

646. The fact that Mrs. Burt cannot close her right eye can be explained by nonconduction of the:
    ① Second cranial nerve
    ② Third cranial nerve
    ③ Fourth cranial nerve
    ④ Seventh cranial nerve

647. Mrs. Burt's dilated right pupil can be explained by nonconduction of the:
    ① Second cranial nerve
    ② Third cranial nerve
    ③ Fourth cranial nerve
    ④ Seventh cranial nerve

648. Mrs. Burt's mouth is drawn over to the left. This suggests nonconduction by the:
    ① Left facial nerve
    ② Right facial nerve
    ③ Left abducent nerve
    ④ Right trigeminal nerve

649. Tendon reflexes, for example, the knee-jerk on the right side of Mrs. Burt's body, are found to be exaggerated. Therefore the nurse is aware that impulses are still being conducted by the:
    ① Anterior horn neurons
    ② Basal ganglia
    ③ Pyramidal tracts
    ④ Upper motoneurons

650. When Mrs. Burt regains consciousness, she has a spastic paralysis of the right side of her body. Spasticity results from nonconduction by certain:
    ① Extrapyramidal pathways
    ② Lower motoneurons
    ③ Spinothalamic tract fibers
    ④ Pyramidal tract fibers

651. Mrs. Burt's physician performs a lumbar puncture. To do this procedure, he inserts a needle into the:
    ① Aqueduct of Sylvius
    ② Foramen ovale
    ③ Subarachnoid space
    ④ Pia mater

652. Impulses initiated by stimulation of pain receptors are conducted by the:
    ① Lateral spinothalamic tracts
    ② Posterior white columns
    ③ Reticulospinal tracts
    ④ Ventral spinothalamic tracts

Situation: Mrs. Purcell is a 72-year-old woman with Parkinson's disease. Questions 653 through 657 refer to this situation.

653. This disease is caused by:
    ① Disintegration of the myelin sheath
    ② Degeneration of neurons of the basal ganglia
    ③ Decreased acetylcholine levels at synapses
    ④ Degeneration of the corpora quadrigemini

654. The nurse would expect Mrs. Purcell to exhibit:
    ① Grand mal seizures
    ② Decreased intelligence
    ③ A flattened affect
    ④ Changes in pain tolerance

655. Levodopa is prescribed for Mrs. Purcell. The nurse should know that this drug:
    ① Is poorly absorbed if given with meals
    ② May cause a side effect of orthostatic hypotension
    ③ Must be monitored by weekly laboratory tests
    ④ Causes an initial euphoria followed by depression

656. Levodopa appears to be useful in treating Parkinson's disease because it can:
    ① Replace the dopamine in the brain cells
    ② Cause regeneration of injured thalamic cells
    ③ Increase acetylcholine production
    ④ Improve myelination of neurons

657. Coordination of skeletal muscles and equilibrium are controlled by the:
    ① Medulla oblongata
    ② Hypothalamus
    ③ Cerebellum
    ④ Thalamus

Situation: Mr. Blake is a 68-year-old retired widower who lives alone. He has a 10-year history of arthritis and has just been admitted to the hospital in an acute episode. Questions 658 through 662 refer to this situation.

658. In planning the nursing care for Mr. Blake, the nurse would take into consideration the fact that:
    ① If redness and swelling of a joint occur, they signify irreversible damage
    ② Bony ankylosis of the joint is irreversible and causes immobility
    ③ Inflammation of the synovial membrane will rarely occur
    ④ Complete immobility is desired during the acute phase of inflammation

659. A regimen of rest, exercise, and physical therapy will:
    ① Help prevent the crippling effects of the disease
    ② Prevent arthritic pain
    ③ Provide for the return of joint motion after prolonged loss
    ④ Halt the inflammatory process

660. The occurrence of a chronic illness that limits major activity is:
    ① Present to the same degree in every age group
    ② Greatest in children because of the prevalence of congenital defects
    ③ Greatest in the older age group
    ④ Greatest in the middle years of life

661. Mr. Blake reports that over the years the following diet suggestions have been given him for his arthritis. Of the following recommendations for his daily diet, the nurse should reinforce his use of:
    ① Yogurt and blackstrap molasses
    ② Wheat germ and yeast
    ③ A variety of meats, fruits, vegetables, milk, cereal grains
    ④ Multiple vitamin supplements in large doses

662. The nurse understands the joints that would most likely be involved in a client with osteoarthritis are the:
    ① Fingers and metacarpals
    ② Hips and knees
    ③ Ankles and metatarsals
    ④ Cervical spine and shoulders

Situation: Following a car accident Harry Martin, a 26-year-old high school math teacher, is diagnosed as having quadriplegia. He is critically ill and needs specific services and equipment; therefore he is admitted to the hospital's intensive care unit. Questions 663 through 667 refer to this situation.

663. Harry is placed on a Stryker frame because it:
    ① Allows horizontal turning of the client
    ② Promotes body functions
    ③ Allows vertical turning of the client
    ④ Helps prevent deformities

664. Before releasing the pivot pins and turning the Stryker frame, the nurse should:
    ① Tell the client to hold on to the bottom part of the frame
    ② Observe the client for signs of hypotension
    ③ Secure all bolts and straps to ensure client safety
    ④ Get another nurse, since this procedure requires two people

665. Two weeks after his accident Harry's physical condition has stabilized. He is overcoming his initial health crisis but still has special needs that could not be met on a general unit; therefore Harry is transferred to the intermediate care unit. Progressive client care means:
    ① Providing specialized nursing care using an episodic approach
    ② Utilizing a variety of services and facilities to provide specialized care, depending on a client's individual needs
    ③ Transferring clients from an area of greater intensive care to an area of lesser intensive care
    ④ Providing total nursing care by using the latest techniques and technology

666. Three weeks after his injury Harry is placed on a tilt table for 1 hour while the head of the table is elevated to a 20-degree angle. Each day the angle is gradually increased. The tilt table is used to:
    ① Facilitate turning
    ② Prevent pressure sores
    ③ Promote hyperextension of the spine
    ④ Prevent loss of calcium from the bones

667. The majority of clients with quadriplegia are taught to use wheelchairs because:
    ① They usually are not and never will be functional walkers
    ② It assists them in overcoming orthostatic hypotension
    ③ Their lower extremities are paralyzed but they have the strength in the upper extremities for self-propulsion
    ④ It prepares them for bracing and crutch walking

Situation: Mr. Greene, a 56-year-old married construction worker, has been in the hospital for 2 weeks with a diagnosis of cerebral thrombosis. His symptoms include aphasia, right-sided paresis, and loss of the gag reflex. Questions 668 through 673 refer to this situation.

668. Due to the location of the lesion, Mr. Greene has expressive aphasia. As part of the long-range planning, the nurse should:

① Help the family to accept the fact that Mr. Greene cannot be verbally communicated with
② Wait for Mr. Greene to verbalize his needs regardless of how long it may take
③ Begin associating words with physical objects
④ Help Mr. Greene accept this disability as permanent

669. Since Mr. Greene was comatose on admission, the nurse would expect him to:
    ① Be unresponsive to painful stimuli
    ② Be incontinent
    ③ Respond with purposeful motions
    ④ Have twitching or picking motions

670. Since one of the primary nursing objectives is maintenance of the airway, the nurse should initially place Mr. Greene in the:
    ① Sims' position
    ② Prone position
    ③ Semi-Fowler's position
    ④ Orthopneic or Fowler's position

671. Mr. Greene is still confined to bed rest, and, even though his physician has not ordered physical therapy for him, the nurse should institute:
    ① Active exercises of all extremities
    ② Passive range of motion exercises
    ③ Light weight-lifting exercises of the right side
    ④ Exercises that would actively capitalize on returning muscle function

672. Mr. Greene's wife insists on doing everything for him when she visits. After she leaves, Mr. Greene seems to be quite depressed. The nurse should assume that:
    ① Mr. Greene feels guilty about being a burden to his wife
    ② This depression is a natural outcome of his illness
    ③ Mr. Greene feels the loss of his independence
    ④ Mr. Greene is losing faith in the future

673. Mrs. Greene seems unable to accept the idea that her husband must be encouraged to do things for himself. The nurse may be able to work around these feelings by:
    ① Telling Mrs. Greene to let her husband do things for himself
    ② Letting Mrs. Greene know that the nursing staff has full responsibility for Mr. Greene's activities
    ③ Letting Mrs. Greene assume the responsibility as she sees fit
    ④ Asking Mrs. Greene for her assistance in planning the activities most helpful to Mr. Greene

Situation: Mr. Brown suffered severe head injuries in an automobile accident. Questions 674 through 681 refer to this situation.

674. Because Mr. Brown is still unconscious when placed on a stretcher to be moved from the emergency room to the intensive care unit, the nurse makes sure his arms do not hang down over the edge of the cart. By taking this precaution the nurse prevents injury to the:
    ① Basilic plexus
    ② Brachial plexus
    ③ Celiac plexus
    ④ Solar plexus

675. Injury to the brain is particularly likely to cause death if it involves the:
① Medulla
② Midbrain
③ Pons
④ Thalamus

676. Mr. Brown's temperature, soon after admission to the hospital, registered 102.2° F (39° C), a fact suggesting injury of the:
① Hypothalamus
② Pallidum
③ Temporal lobe
④ Thalamus

677. After Mr. Brown recovers consciousness, he complains of hearing ringing noises, a fact suggesting injury of:
① Cranial nerve VI (abducent)
② Cranial nerve VIII (vestibulocochlear)
③ Frontal lobe
④ Occipital lobe

678. Mr. Brown has a grand mal seizure. The physician prescribes phenytoin (Dilantin) to control the seizures. The expected effect of this drug is to:
① Alter the permeability of the cell membrane to potassium
② Control nerve impulses originating in the motor cortex
③ Prevent depression of the central nervous system
④ Produce an antispasmodic action on the muscles

679. Mr. Brown's condition has stabilized and he is transferred out of the intensive care unit. The nurse should automatically place at the bedside:
① A sphygmomanometer
② Oxygen equipment
③ A padded tongue blade
④ A rubber or plastic airway

680. Mr. Brown questions the nurse regarding the scheduling of his medication. The nurse informs him that the medications:
① Can usually be stopped after a year's absence of seizures
② Need to be taken only in periods of emotional stress
③ Will probably have to be continued for life
④ Will prevent the occurrence of seizures

681. Mr. Brown has no paralysis after his accident. This suggests noninvolvement of the:
① Basal ganglia
② Parietal lobe
③ Precentral gyrus
④ Postcentral gyrus

Situation: Mrs. Crane, a 32-year-old woman who has intermittently been having painful, swollen knee and wrist joints during the past 3 months, is being admitted to the hospital for treatment of rheumatoid arthritis. Questions 682 through 685 refer to this situation.

682. The nurse would expect the physician to order the following diet for Mrs. Crane:
① High protein
② Salt free
③ General diet, supplemented with vitamins and iron
④ Bland diet

683. The medication the nurse would expect to be prescribed to relieve the pain in Mrs. Crane's knees would be:
① Codeine, 30 mg, q4h
② Aspirin, 0.6 g, q4h
③ Codeine, 30 mg, q4h prn
④ Nembutal, 90 mg, q4h

684. To prevent deformity of the knee joint, the nurse should:
① Immobilize the joint with pillows for a period of several weeks
② Discourage use of the knee joint
③ Encourage motion of the joint within limits of pain
④ Keep Mrs. Crane on a bed rest regimen

685. Mrs. Crane asks the nurse why the physician may inject hydrocortisone into the knee joint. The nurse explains that the most important reason for doing this is to:
① Prevent ankylosis of the joint
② Reduce inflammation
③ Provide psychotherapy
④ Relieve pain

Situation: Mr. Wilson has a herniated lumbar disc. Questions 686 through 690 refer to this situation.

686. Mr. Wilson generally experiences a sudden increase in pain when he:
① Sits on cold surfaces
② Lies prone with knees flexed
③ Sneezes
④ Stands for extended periods

687. Mr. Wilson is to undergo a myelogram before surgery. Postoperatively it would be unnecessary for the nurse to:
① Do a thorough neurologic evaluation
② Maintain him in a horizontal position
③ Encourage fluids to replace lost CSF
④ Apply cold compresses distal to the puncture

688. In caring for Mr. Wilson after the laminectomy, the nurse should give the lowest priority to:
① Keeping him flat in bed
② Turning him from side to side
③ Ambulating him with a back brace
④ Assessing him for symmetry of movement

689. The main postoperative complication that the nurse should observe for following the laminectomy is:
① Spasms of the bladder
② Pain referred to the flanks
③ Compression of the cord
④ Cerebral edema

690. In contrast to caring for a client with a lumbar laminectomy, when caring for a client with a cervical laminectomy the nurse:
① Should provide range-of-motion exercise early during the postoperative period
② Has the added responsibility of removing oral secretions
③ Should maintain the client's head in a flexed position
④ Must keep the client's head at a 45-degree angle from the spine

Situation: Mr. Fritz, a 32-year-old car salesman, suffered a spinal cord injury in an auto accident, resulting in paraplegia. Questions 691 through 697 refer to this situation.

691. Good nursing care of Mr. Fritz will provide that he be turned every 2 hours. This is necessary mainly to:
 ① Keep the client comfortable
 ② Prevent pressure sores
 ③ Improve circulation in the lower extremities
 ④ Prevent flexion contractures of all the extremities

692. The least effective method of preventing contractures of the joints of Mr. Fritz's lower extremities would be:
 ① Changing bed position q2h
 ② Maintaining proper bed positions
 ③ Passively moving the extremities through ROM several times daily
 ④ Providing the client with active exercise instructions

693. Mr. Fritz questions the need for a tilt table. The nurse explains that the tilt table is used to help:
 ① Prevent hypertension
 ② Encourage circulation to prevent pressure sores
 ③ Prevent loss of calcium from long bones
 ④ Encourage increased activity

694. Formation of urinary calculi is a complication that may be encountered by the client with paraplegia. A factor that contributes to this condition is:
 ① High fluid intake
 ② Increased intake of calcium
 ③ Inadequate kidney function
 ④ Increased loss of calcium from the skeletal system

695. Rehabilitation plans for Mr. Fritz:
 ① Should be considered and planned for early in his care
 ② Are not necessary, since he will return to his usual activities
 ③ Should be left up to the client and his family
 ④ Are not necessary, since he will not be able to work again

696. Since Mr. Fritz has paraplegia, the nurse recognizes that one major early problem will be:
 ① Use of mechanical aids for ambulation
 ② Client education
 ③ Quadriceps setting
 ④ Bladder control

697. The nurse may expect that Mr. Fritz will have some spasticity of the lower extremities. To prevent the development of contractures, careful consideration must be given to:
 ① Proper positioning
 ② Use of a tilt board
 ③ Active exercise
 ④ Deep massage

Situation: Mr. and Mrs. Lund, a retired couple who spent the winter in Florida, flew back to New York to see their newest grandson. On returning to their apartment after a family dinner, Mrs. Lund, age 72, tripped over a rug in the foyer. X-ray films at the hospital reveal a fracture of the acetabulum. Mrs. Lund's general state of health appears good except for the necessity to take enemas periodically. Questions 698 through 703 refer to this situation.

698. A fracture of the acetabulum most likely involves the part of the femur known as the:
 ① Head
 ② Shaft
 ③ Neck
 ④ Trochanteric region

699. Mrs. Lund expresses concern about the treatment she will need. The nurse should be aware that the treatment of choice in this instance will probably be:
 ① Insertion of a hip prosthesis with traction
 ② Hip pinning or nailing
 ③ Application of a spica cast
 ④ Skeletal traction

700. To prevent pulmonary and circulatory complications, the nurse should make sure that Mrs. Lund is:
 ① Turned from side to side q3h
 ② Ambulated as soon as the effects of anesthesia are gone
 ③ Turned on the unaffected side q2h
 ④ Permitted to be up in a chair as soon as the effects of anesthesia are gone

701. Mrs. Lund has an Austin-Moore prosthesis inserted. After surgery the nurse should avoid placing Mrs. Lund:
 ① On her affected side
 ② On her unaffected side
 ③ In a low semi-Fowler's position
 ④ In a supine position

702. Since Mrs. Lund is accustomed to taking enemas periodically to avoid constipation, the nurse should:
 ① Arrange to have enemas ordered
 ② Realize that enemas will be necessary because the normal conditioned reflex has been lost
 ③ Offer Mrs. Lund a large glass of prune juice in warm water each morning
 ④ Arrange to have laxatives ordered

703. Elderly people have a high incidence of hip fractures because of:
 ① Carelessness
 ② Fragility of bone
 ③ Rheumatoid diseases
 ④ Sedentary existence

Situation: Mrs. Bond, 35 years of age, has undergone a midthigh amputation following injury in an automobile accident. Questions 704 through 709 refer to this situation.

704. To promote early and efficient ambulation, the nurse should:
 ① Place pillows under the stump
 ② Encourage her to lie supine
 ③ Turn her to the prone position frequently
 ④ Keep backrest elevated

705. When Mrs. Bond is allowed to be up, the nurse should teach her to:
 ① Keep her hip in extension and adduction
 ② Keep her hip raised with stump elevated
 ③ Lift her shoulder and hip of affected side when taking a step
 ④ Walk with crutches until stump is completely healed

706. Before ambulation is started, in order to make walking with crutches easier the nurse should teach:
① Use of the trapeze to strengthen the biceps muscles
② Push-up exercises with sawed-off crutches to strengthen the triceps, finger flexors, wrist extensors, and elbow extensors
③ Isometric exercises of the hamstring muscles while sitting in a chair until circulatory status is stable
④ The importance of keeping limb in extension and abduction to prevent contractures

707. The crutch gait the nurse should teach the client wearing a prosthesis after a single leg amputation is the:
① Tripod crutch gait
② Four-point gait
③ Three-point gait
④ Swing-through crutch gait

708. In preparing Mrs. Bond for ambulation with crutches, the nurse should recognize she needs further teaching when she states, "I must practice:
① Standing and maintaining balance."
② Ambulating several hours a day."
③ Doing active exercises for muscle strengthening."
④ Sitting down and standing up."

709. Rehabilitation of Mrs. Bond should begin:
① Before the surgery
② During the convalescent phase
③ On discharge from the hospital
④ When she is ready for a prosthesis

Situation: Mr. Styles is brought to the ophthalmologist's office by his wife. He has minimum vision in his left eye and tells the nurse, "I'm sure it's a cataract; my brother just had cataract surgery." Questions 710 through 713 refer to this situation.

710. A cataract is:
① A thin film over the cornea
② A crystallinization of the pupil
③ An opacity of the lens
④ An increase in the density of the conjunctiva

711. After a client has cataract surgery, the nurse should:
① Encourage coughing and deep breathing
② Discourage vigorous brushing of teeth and hair
③ Keep the client in the supine position with sand bags on each side of the head
④ Encourage eye exercises to strengthen the ocular musculature

712. After examination the physician informs Mr. Styles that he has a detached retina. Retinal detachment is a:
① Separation between the photoreceptor and neural layers of the retina
② Separation between the sensory portion of the retina and the pigment layer
③ Consequence of optic-retinal atrophy
④ Separation of the choroid and optic chiasm

713. The goal of surgery for the treatment of a detached retina is to:
① Create a scar that aids in healing retinal holes
② Graft a healthy piece of retina in place
③ Promote growth of new retinal cells
④ Adhere the sclera to the choroid layer

Situation: Mrs. Johns tells the nurse preparing her for surgery that she is "terribly scared." The nurse recognizes that fear has stimulated Mrs. Johns autonomic nervous system. Questions 714 through 716 refer to this situation.

714. In thinking about autonomic activity, the nurse should be aware that a common misconception is that:
① Both sympathetic and parasympathetic impulses continually affect most visceral effectors
② Sympathetic impulses stimulate while parasympathetic impulses inhibit the functioning of any visceral effector
③ The autonomic nervous system is regulated by impulses from the hypothalamus and other parts of the brain
④ Visceral effectors (i.e., cardiac muscle, smooth muscle, glandular epithelial tissue) receive impulses only via autonomic neurons

715. In caring for Mrs. Johns, an indication of sympathetic control identifiable by the nurse would be:
① Constriction of pupils
② Skin pallor
③ Dry skin
④ Pulse rate of 60

716. An indication of parasympathetic dominance in Mrs. Johns would be:
① Excess epinephrine secretion
② Excess hydrochloric acid secretion
③ Constipation
④ Goose pimples

Situation: After an accident, Mrs. Jean Boyhout is admitted unconscious to the medical unit with internal bleeding and head injuries. The physician orders a type and cross match for 1000 ml of whole blood to be administered within the next 6 hours. Questions 717 through 721 refer to this situation.

717. Mr. Boyhout refuses to allow his wife to be transfused with the whole blood, since they are Jehovah's Witnesses. The nurse involved in this situation should:
① Gently explain to the husband why the transfusion is necessary, emphasizing the implications of not having the transfusion
② Institute the blood transfusion anyway, since the physician ordered it and the client's survival depends on volume replacement
③ Phone the physician for a special administrative order to give the blood under these circumstances
④ Have the husband sign a treatment refusal form and notify the physician so a court order can be obtained

718. Mrs. Boyhout remains unresponsive to sensory stimulation. The lobe of the cerebral cortex which registers general sensations such as heat, cold, pain, and touch is the:
① Frontal lobe
② Occipital lobe
③ Parietal lobe
④ Temporal lobe

719. The relay center for sensory impulses is the:
    ① Medulla oblongata
    ② Hypothalamus
    ③ Cerebellum
    ④ Thalamus

720. Internal organs, such as the bladder and the esophagus, are most directly under the control of the:
    ① Peripheral nervous system
    ② Central nervous system
    ③ Autonomic nervous system
    ④ Spinal cord

721. As Mrs. Boyhout regains consciousness, she is extremely confused. The nurse provides new information slowly and in small amounts because:
    ① Destruction of brain cells has occurred, interrupting mental activity
    ② Confusion or delirium can be a defense against further stress
    ③ A minimum of information should be given, since she is unaware of her surroundings
    ④ Teaching is based on information progressing from the simple to the complex

Situation: Mrs. Martin, age 68, is admitted with severe back pain. She has a history of osteoporosis. Questions 722 through 724 refer to this situation.

722. Osteoporosis may be caused by:
    ① Estrogen therapy
    ② Excess calcium intake
    ③ Hypoparathyroidism
    ④ Prolonged immobility

723. Because of her disease, Mrs. Martin is vulnerable to:
    ① Fatigue fractures
    ② Pathologic fractures
    ③ Compound fractures
    ④ Greenstick fractures

724. The nurse should encourage Mrs. Martin to increase her intake of:
    ① Enriched grains
    ② Large amounts of protein
    ③ Turnip greens
    ④ Soft drinks

Situation: Mrs. Zeno, a client with a history of myasthenia gravis, is admitted with respiratory distress. Questions 725 through 731 refer to this situation.

725. Respiratory complications are common for individuals with myasthenia gravis because of:
    ① Narrowed airways
    ② Ineffective coughing
    ③ Impaired immunity
    ④ Viscosity of secretions

726. In providing safe care for Mrs. Zeno it is most important for the nurse to check her bedside for the presence of:
    ① An intravenous setup
    ② A syringe and Tensilon (edrophonium HCl)
    ③ A tracheostomy set
    ④ A hypothermia blanket

727. Tensilon (edrophonium HCl) is used for the diagnosis of myasthenia gravis because this drug will cause a temporary:
    ① Increase in symptoms
    ② Drying of the mouth and throat
    ③ Increase in blood pressure
    ④ Increase in muscle strength

728. Neural impulses travel in one direction because:
    ① Polarization occurs laterally
    ② Axons secrete acetylcholine
    ③ Sodium pump does not work in reverse
    ④ Cholinesterase acts along the entire axon

729. The terminals of axons supplying skeletal muscle:
    ① Release acetylcholine
    ② Release ATP
    ③ Release cholinesterase
    ④ Release epinephrine

730. Mrs. Zeno has been receiving neostigmine (Prostigmin). This drug acts by:
    ① Stimulating the cerebral cortex
    ② Blocking cholinesterase action
    ③ Replacing deficient neurotransmitters
    ④ Accelerating transmission along neural sheaths

731. Mrs. Zeno's weakness continues despite treatment with neostigmine. Tensilon (edrophonium HCl) is ordered:
    ① To confirm the diagnosis of myasthenia
    ② Because of her resistance to neostigmine
    ③ For its synergistic effect
    ④ To rule out cholinergic crisis

732. Allopurinol is used to treat gout. The objective of therapy is to:
    ① Increase uric acid excretion
    ② Decrease uric acid production
    ③ Prevent crystallization of uric acid
    ④ Decrease synovial swelling

733. One drug that may be prescribed and that has long been known to be of value in the prevention and treatment of acute attacks of gout is:
    ① Hydrocortisone
    ② Colchicine
    ③ Phenylbutazone (Butazolidin)
    ④ Probenecid (Benemid)

734. A client with degenerative arthritis may require a total-hip replacement. This surgery is done:
    ① Using a "laminar airflow room"
    ② Using three separate stages
    ③ With the patient in lithotomy position
    ④ Early in the disease process

735. A sprain accompanied by edema is treated with the application of compresses. The appropriate temperature range for the compresses would be:
    ① 65° to 80° F (18° to 26.6° C)
    ② 80° to 93° F (26.6° to 34° C)
    ③ 93° to 98° F (34° to 36.6° C)
    ④ 98° to 105° F (36.6° to 40.5° C)

736. In preparing a teaching plan for a client with hypertrophic arthritis it would be inappropriate for the nurse to include a discussion of:
    ① Degenerative arthritis
    ② Nonankylosing arthritis
    ③ Heberden's nodes
    ④ Marie-Strümpell disease

737. The synovial fluid of the joints minimizes:
    ① Velocity of movements
    ② Friction in the joints
    ③ Efficiency
    ④ Work output

738. Mrs. Paul is hospitalized for an acute exacerbation of rheumatoid arthritis. In talking with the nurse, she states that she does not want cortisone even if it is prescribed by the physician. Later the nurse attempts to administer cortisone that has been ordered by the physician. When Mrs. Paul asks what the medication is, the nurse gives an evasive answer. The client takes the medication and later finds that she has been given cortisone. She states that she intends to sue. The decision in this suit would take into consideration the fact that:
    ① A physician's order takes precedence over a client's preference
    ② The client has insufficient knowledge to make such a decision
    ③ The nurse is required to answer the client truthfully
    ④ The nurse should have notified the physician

739. The type of membrane that lines the knee joint is called the:
    ① Serous
    ② Synovial
    ③ Mucous
    ④ Epithelial

740. Compact bone is stronger than cancellous bone because of its greater:
    ① Volume
    ② Size
    ③ Weight
    ④ Density

741. An overexercised muscle that has an insufficient oxygen supply may become sore from a buildup of:
    ① Butyric acid
    ② Lactic acid
    ③ Acetoacetic acid
    ④ Acetone

742. Electric stimulation by the use of a peripheral nerve implant or dorsal column stimulator is used in intractable pain. The nurse should explain that after surgery:
    ① The client should not take tub baths
    ② The device may interfere with the television remote control
    ③ Analgesics will no longer be necessary
    ④ The transmitter must be worn externally

743. A procedure done to relieve intractable pain in the upper torso is:
    ① Chondrectomy
    ② Cordotomy
    ③ Rhizotomy
    ④ Wolfgang's procedure

744. The vision cycle in the eye requires vitamin A. Here the vitamin functions as:
    ① A necessary component of rhodopsin (visual purple), which controls light-dark adaptations
    ② A part of the rods and cones that controls color blindness
    ③ The material in the cornea that prevents cataract formation
    ④ An integral part of the retina's pigment known as melanin

745. Vitamin A is a fat-soluble vitamin produced by humans and other animals from its precursor carotene-provitamin A. One of the main sources of this vitamin is:
    ① Skim milk
    ② Leafy greens
    ③ Oranges
    ④ Tomatoes

746. The preferred treatment for malignant melanoma of the eye is:
    ① Chemotherapy
    ② Radiation
    ③ Cryosurgery
    ④ Enucleation

747. The optic chiasm:
    ① Receives nerve impulses from the optic tracts
    ② Is the space posterior to the lens with the consistency of jelly
    ③ Is a crossing of some optic nerves in the cranial cavity
    ④ Is the cavity in which the eyeball is fixed

748. Stimulation of the vagus nerve results in:
    ① Tachycardia
    ② Dilation of the bronchioles
    ③ Slowing of the heart
    ④ Coronary artery vasodilation

749. A feeling of pleasantness or unpleasantness, varying in degree from mild to intense, occurs when sensory impulses reach the:
    ① Basal ganglia
    ② Cerebral cortex
    ③ Hypothalamus
    ④ Thalamus

750. An arterial anastomosis present at the base of the brain is the:
    ① Volar arch
    ② Brachiocephalic sinus
    ③ Circle of Willis
    ④ Brachial plexus

751. The most frequently occurring type of brain tumor is a:
    ① Pituitary adenoma
    ② Neurofibroma
    ③ Glioma
    ④ Meningioma

752. The part of the ear which contains the receptors for hearing is the:
    ① Cochlea
    ② Middle ear
    ③ Tympanic cavity
    ④ Utricle

753. The ear bones that transmit vibrations to the oval window of the cochlea are found in the:
    ① Outer ear
    ② Inner ear
    ③ Middle ear
    ④ Eustachian tube

754. Nerve deafness would most likely result from an injury or infection that damaged the:
① Cochlear nerve
② Vestibular nerve
③ Trigeminal nerve
④ Vagus nerve

755. The medulla has centers for:
① Control of sexual development
② Fat metabolism, temperature regulation, water balance
③ Voluntary movement, taste, skin sensations
④ Control of breathing, heartbeat, blood vessel diameter

756. Reflex control of respiration occurs in the:
① Medulla and pons
② Cerebral cortex
③ Hypothalamus
④ Cerebellum

757. A labyrinthectomy is frequently performed to treat Ménière's syndrome. This procedure results in:
① Absence of pain
② Permanent deafness
③ Anosmia
④ Reduction of tinnitus

758. Otosclerosis is the most common cause of conductive hearing loss. With this disorder:
① The client is usually unable to hear bass tones
② Air conduction is more effective than bone conduction
③ Hearing aids usually restore hearing
④ Stapedectomy is the procedure of choice

759. A client who complains of tinnitus is describing a symptom that is:
① Functional
② Prodromal
③ Objective
④ Subjective

The Integumentary System

Situation: Mr. Anthony has second- and third-degree burns and is to receive a skin graft over the third-degree burn of his arm. Questions 760 through 765 refer to this situation.

760. The graft is taken from his left buttock. This graft is referred to as:
① A homograft
② An autograft
③ A heterograft
④ An allograft

761. A pigskin graft is often applied to burned areas. This graft is known as:
① A homograft
② An allograft
③ A heterograft
④ An isograft

762. The laboratory test that will best reflect loss of fluid due to burns is the:
① Blood pH
② Sedimentation rate
③ Hematocrit
④ BUN

763. In a burned client the relationship between body surface area and fluid loss is:
① Directly proportionate
② Inversely proportionate
③ Equal
④ Unrelated

764. The medication that a burned client usually receives as soon after admission as possible is:
① Phytonadione (Aquamephyton)
② Gamma globulin
③ Tetanus toxoid
④ Isoproterenol (Isuprel)

765. Mr. Anthony is to have mafenide (Sulfamylon) cream applied to his burned areas. A serious side effect of Sulfamylon therapy is:
① Renal shutdown
② Hemolysis of RBCs
③ Metabolic acidosis
④ Curling's ulcer

Situation: Miss Renee, 32 years old, is admitted to the emergency room with second-degree burns over 42% of her body and face, which she received when her nightgown caught fire. A urinary catheter is inserted. Questions 766 through 771 refer to this situation.

766. Because of her burns, Miss Renee's condition would be considered:
① Good
② Fair
③ Poor
④ Critical

767. The problem of least importance during the first few hours after the injury is:
① Edema of the larynx and trachea
② Maintenance of blood volume
③ Rapid decrease in the leukocyte count
④ The occurrence of pain

768. In the immediate shock period after Miss Renee's injury, nutritional care is centered on replacement therapy by IV fluids. The nurse should question the physician's order if it is designed to provide:
① Plasma expanders such as dextran
② Electrolytes, sodium and chloride, by use of a saline solution such as lactated Ringer's solution
③ Potassium added to replace losses
④ Water (dextrose solution) to cover additional insensible losses

769. It can be anticipated that the physician will wish to prevent tetanus from developing. If it is impossible to determine whether Miss Renee has been immunized against tetanus, the preparation used to produce passive immunization for several weeks with minimal danger of allergic reactions is:
① Tetanus antitoxin
② Tetanus toxoid
③ Tetanus immune globulin
④ DPT vaccine

770. Sulfisoxazole (Gantrisin), which is often used to combat urinary tract infections, belongs to the group of drugs known as:
① Antiseptics
② Analgesics
③ Uricosurics
④ Sulfonamides

771. When the urinary catheter is removed, Miss Renee is unable to empty her bladder. A drug used to relieve urinary retention is:
① Bethanechol (Urecholine)
② Pilocarpine hydrochloride
③ Carbachol injection
④ Neosporin

Situation: Mrs. Johnson, an 84-year-old widow, is admitted with metastatic melanoma. Questions 772 through 776 refer to this situation.

772. The nurse assesses Mrs. Johnson for the presence of:
① Oily skin
② Lymphadenopathy
③ Nikolsky's sign
④ Erythema of the palms

773. The physician suspects Mrs. Johnson also has other primary cancerous lesions in her connective tissue. The nurse understands that these lesions are classified as:
① Osteoblastomas
② Collagenomas
③ Sarcomas
④ Carcinomas

774. Mrs. Johnson is now terminally ill and is in the hospice unit. The nurse is aware that characteristic behavior in the initial stage of coping with dying includes:
① Asking for additional medical consultations
② Ringing a call light as soon as the nurse has left the room
③ Criticism of medical care
④ Sleeping for long periods

775. The family is likely to require more understanding when Mrs. Johnson reaches the:
① Denial stage
② Anger stage
③ Depression stage
④ Acceptance stage

776. Mrs. Johnson reaches the stage of acceptance. The nurse can best help her during this stage by:
① Allowing unrestricted visiting
② Being around though not necessarily speaking
③ Explaining all that is being done
④ Allowing her to cry

777. Psoriasis is characterized by:
① Shiny, scaly lesions
② Pruritic lesions
③ Multiple petechiae
④ Erythematous macules

778. Treatment of psoriasis usually involves:
① Avoiding exposure to the sun
② Potassium permanganate baths
③ Topical application of steroids
④ Debridement of necrotic placques

779. When caring for a client with scabies, the nurse should be aware that scabies is:
① Highly contagious
② Caused by a fungus
③ Associated with other allergies
④ A chronic problem

780. Pemphigus vulgaris primarily affects the:
① Gastrointestinal system
② Reproductive system
③ Neuromuscular system
④ Integumentary system

781. The best first-aid treatment for acid burns on the skin is to flush them with water and then apply a solution of:
① Sodium hydroxide
② Sodium chloride
③ Sodium bicarbonate
④ Sodium sulfate

782. A good first-aid treatment for an alkali (base) burn is to flush it with water and then flood it with:
① A weak acid
② A weak base
③ A solution of salt
④ Alcohol

783. Systemic lupus erythematosus (SLE) is a collagen disease characterized by:
① A butterfly rash
② An inflammation of small arteries
③ Muscle mass degeneration
④ Firm skin fixed to tissue

784. Mrs. Laukhardt is diagnosed as having scleroderma. Although no cause has been determined for this disorder, it is thought to be a defect in:
① Amino acid metabolism
② Sebaceous gland formation
③ Autoimmunity
④ Ocular motility

785. Mrs. Laukhardt discusses her prognosis with the nurse. She states, "I'm sure I'll live to a ripe old age. It's not too serious." In responding, the nurse should bear in mind that 50% of the clients with this disease:
① Recover completely
② Die within 6 months to 1 year
③ Succumb within 3 years
④ Have extended remissions

786. Mrs. Joyce, an elderly woman, is admitted to the surgical unit from a nursing home for treatment of decubitus ulcers. She is obviously dehydrated and her skin is dry and scaly. On admission the nurse immediately introduces fluids, applies emollients to her skin, and changes the dressings on her decubitus ulcers. Legally:
① No treatment should have been instituted for Mrs. Joyce until a physician ordered it
② The nurse should have instituted a plan for active range of motion exercise to all joints
③ The nurse provided supportive nursing care for the well-being of Mrs. Joyce
④ Debridement of the decubiti should have been done by the nurse before the dressing was applied

Infectious Diseases

Situation: Mr. McGee, a 31-year-old private in the Marines recently returned from Southeast Asia after a 13-month tour of duty, complains of chills along with a high fever. On the basis of the history and physical examination, the physician believes the most likely diagnosis is malaria. Questions 787 through 796 refer to this situation.

787. The most important diagnostic test in malaria is:
① Smear of peripheral blood
② Blood leukocyte count
③ Erythrocyte sedimentation rate
④ Splenic puncture

788. The nurse is reviewing Mr. McGee's physical examination and laboratory test. An important finding in malaria is:
① Splenomegaly
② Leukocytosis
③ Elevated sedimentation rate
④ Erythrocytosis

789. Mr. McGee asks the nurse how he could have prevented the disease. The nurse should explain that prophylaxis for the control of malaria includes:
① Vaccination
② Client isolation
③ Prompt detection and effective treatment
④ Antibiotic therapy

790. Blackwater fever occurs in some clients with malaria; therefore, the nurse should observe Mr. McGee for:
① Diarrhea
② Coffee ground emesis
③ Low-grade fever
④ Dark red urine

791. A serious complication of acute malaria is:
① Anemia and cachexia
② Congested lungs
③ Changes in water and electrolyte balance
④ Impaired peristalsis

792. In caring for Mr. McGee, the nurse should know that:
① Peritoneal dialysis is usually indicated
② He should be awakened only for nourishment after a paroxysm
③ Attention should be focused on rest and nourishing food between paroxysms
④ Isolation is necessary to prevent cross infection

793. Because Mr. McGee has a chloroquine-resistant malaria, the physician orders 650 mg of quinine dihydrochloride to be given over an 8-hour period by IV drip in 1000 ml of normal saline. The IV equipment is calibrated at 20 drops per milliliter. To deliver the correct dosage, the solution must be set to flow at the rate of:
① 10 drops/min
② 21 drops/min
③ 34 drops/min
④ 42 drops/min

794. Whenever quinine is used, the nurse should be alert to symptoms of severe cinchonism, which include:
① Tinnitus, decreased auditory acuity, nausea
② Deafness, vertigo, and severe visual, GI, and central nervous system disturbances

③ Pruritus, urticaria, and difficulty in breathing
④ Leg cramps, fever, and swollen painful joints

795. After several days of IV therapy, the physician replaces the IV injection with quinine sulfate, 2 g per day in divided doses. The nurse should administer this medication after meals to:
① Delay its absorption
② Minimize gastric irritation
③ Decrease stimulation of appetite
④ Decrease its antiarrhythmic action

796. When teaching Mr. McGee about drug therapy against *Plasmodium falciparum,* the nurse should include the fact that:
① The infections can generally be eliminated
② Transmission by the *Anopheles* mosquito can occur
③ The infections are controlled
④ Immunity will prevent reinfection

Situation: Ms. Simone, a 34-year-old computer programmer, is admitted to the hospital with a wound that is swollen and painful. The diagnosis of tetanus is suspected. Questions 797 through 801 refer to the situation.

797. The nurse must observe Ms. Simone for a symptom of tetanus that could be life-threatening. The nurse should assess Ms. Simone for:
① Muscle rigidity
② Spastic voluntary muscle contractions
③ Restlessness and irritability
④ Respiratory tract spasms

798. Ms. Simone is started on tetracycline therapy. When giving oral tetracycline to Ms. Simone, the nurse should:
① Provide orange or other citrus fruit juice with the medication
② Offer antacids 30 minutes after administration if GI side effects occur
③ Provide medication an hour before or after milk products have been ingested
④ Administer medication with meals or a snack

799. The physician orders additional antibiotic therapy with ampicillin. After 3 days, Ms. Simone has an urticarial response. Diphenhydramine hydrochloride (Benadryl) is administered to:
① Destroy histamine in tissues and reverse the urticarial response
② Inhibit release of vasoactive substances and dilate tissue capillaries
③ Metabolize histamine and inhibit release of substances causing intense itching
④ Compete with histamine for receptors and interfere with vasodilation

800. Ms. Simone may also be given penicillinase (Neutrapen) to:
① Displace penicillin from receptor sites
② Counteract the effects of penicillin in tissues
③ Destroy the penicillin allergen
④ Maintain therapy with a nonallergenic form of penicillin

801. Ms. Simone asks the nurse about immunizations against tetanus. The nurse explains that the major benefit in using tetanus antitoxin is that it:
① Stimulates plasma cells directly
② Provides high titer of antibodies
③ Provides immediate active immunity
④ Stimulates long-lasting passive immunity

Situation: Mr. Banks, a 22-year-old door-to-door salesman, is bitten by an uncollared dog while attempting to sell his merchandise. Mr. Banks treats the leg bite at home and several days later is depressed and does not go to work. He loses his appetite and goes to the hospital for a diagnostic workup. Rabies is suspected. Questions 802 through 804 refer to this situation.

802. With a suspected diagnosis of rabies, the nurse would expect to find that Mr. Banks has:
① A dry mouth
② Cardiac arrhythmias
③ Hematuria
④ Diplopia

803. The diagnosis of rabies is confirmed and Mr. Banks is admitted to the hospital for treatment. A special need for this client is protection from:
① The sight of fluids
② Diarrhea
③ Urinary stasis
④ Memory loss

804. Considering Mr. Banks' developmental level, the nurse when planning teaching for his discharge should include the potential health problems common in his age group. This can be accomplished by making him aware of:
① Eye problems, such as glaucoma
② Cardiovascular diseases
③ Kidney dysfunction
④ Accidents and their prevention

---

805. Infection with Group A beta-hemolytic streptococci is associated with:
① Rheumatoid arthritis
② Infectious hepatitis
③ Spinal meningitis
④ Rheumatic fever

806. The common factor of puerperal sepsis, scarlet fever, otitis media, bacterial endocarditis, rheumatic fever, and glomerulonephritis is that all:
① Can be easily controlled through childhood vaccination
② Result from streptococcal infections that enter via the upper respiratory tract
③ Are noncontagious, self-limiting infections by spirilla
④ Are caused by parasitic bacteria that normally live outside the body

807. The darkening of tissue seen in the various forms of gangrene is due to the breakdown of hemoglobin with subsequent formation of:
① Ferrous sulfide
② Ferric chloride
③ Heme
④ Insoluble proteins

808. Antibodies are also produced by:
① Plasma cells
② Eosinophils
③ Lymphocytes
④ Erythrocytes

809. A disease produced when a *Clostridium* organism enters wounds and produces a toxin causing crepitus is:
① Tetanus
② Gas gangrene
③ Botulism
④ Anthrax

Fundamental Concepts

Situation: A small urban community in the western area of the country is flattened by a severe, wide-spread tornado. Questions 810 through 814 refer to this situation.

810. Immediately after the storm has passed, the rescue team with which the nurse is working is searching for injured people. The nurse finds a man lying next to a broken natural gas main. He is not breathing and is bleeding heavily from a wound on the foot. The nurse's first step would be to:
① Remove him from the immediate vicinity
② Apply surface pressure to the foot wound
③ Start rescue breathing immediately
④ Treat him for shock

811. The nurse finds a young boy under the wreckage of a frame house. He is conscious, breathing satisfactorily, and lying on his back. He complains of pain in his back and is unable to move his legs. The nurse should first:
① Gently raise him to a sitting position to see if the pain either diminishes or increases in intensity
② Leave him lying on his back, give him instructions not to move, and seek additional help
③ Roll him on his abdomen, place a pad under his head, and cover him
④ Gently lift him onto a flat piece of lumber and, using any available transportation, rush him to medical help

812. The nurse finds another injured person, obviously in shock. The nurse should keep him lying on his back and:
① Elevate the head higher than the rest of the body; give stimulant in small sips
② Surround the body with hot water bottles or chemical heating pads if available
③ After evaluation, allow him to walk around if injuries permit
④ Raise the legs higher than the rest of the body, prevent chilling, and give fluids if possible

813. When a disaster occurs, the nurse may have to treat the mass hysteria first. The person or persons to be cared for immediately would be those in:
① Depression
② Euphoria
③ Panic
④ Comatose state

814. In any disaster concerning a number of people, the function that contributes most to saving of lives is sorting, or triage. When determining priority of needs, the people who need immediate care are those with:
    ① Second-degree burns of 10% of the body
    ② Severe lacerations involving open fractures of major bones
    ③ Closed fractures of major bones
    ④ Significant penetrating or perforating abdominal wounds

Situation: The nurse at a first aid station at an ocean beach is called to assist with a near drowning. Questions 815 through 817 refer to this situation.

815. The nurse must establish and maintain an airway. One danger of near drowning that must be assessed for is:
    ① Hypervolemia
    ② Renal failure
    ③ Alkalosis
    ④ Pulmonary edema

816. The victim must be assessed for hypothermia. Hypothermia would be manifested by:
    ① A slowed pulse and lowered temperature
    ② An irregular pulse and stupor
    ③ An increased blood pressure and rapid respirations
    ④ A temperature below 84° F (28° C) and erythema

817. When transferred to the hospital, the victim should be instructed to expect:
    ① Core rewarming with heated oxygen
    ② Ambulation to increase metabolism
    ③ Gastric tube feedings to increase fluids
    ④ Frequent oral temperature assessment

---

818. A nursing diagnosis is a nurse's:
    ① Actual nursing intervention
    ② Proposed plan of care
    ③ Assessment of client data
    ④ Identification of the client's health problems

819. Where primary nursing is practiced, the nurse who plans for and delegates care with full authority to see that the plan is followed is the:
    ① Clinical specialist
    ② Head nurse
    ③ Nurse clinician
    ④ Primary nurse

820. An example of primary health care by the nurse would be:
    ① Correction of dietary deficiencies
    ② Assisting in immunization programs
    ③ Prevention of disabilities
    ④ Rehabilitation

821. An objective method of data collection includes:
    ① Direct observation of the client
    ② Speaking with the client's family
    ③ The client's description of the illness
    ④ Collection of specimens

822. The determining factor in the revision of a nursing care plan is the:
    ① Correctness of the original diagnosis
    ② Method for providing care
    ③ Time available for care
    ④ Effectiveness of implementation

823. Nursing process can be defined as the:
    ① Activities a nurse employs to identify a nursing problem
    ② Process the nurse uses to determine nursing goals
    ③ Steps the nurse employs in planning and giving nursing care
    ④ Implementation of nursing care by the nurse

824. To begin the nursing process, the nurse must first:
    ① State the client's nursing needs
    ② Identify goals for nursing care
    ③ Obtain information about the client
    ④ Evaluate the effectiveness of nursing actions

825. The effectiveness of nurse-client communication is validated by:
    ① Health team conferences
    ② Medical assessments
    ③ Client feedback
    ④ Client's physiologic adaptations

826. The most important aspect of hand washing is:
    ① Water
    ② Soap
    ③ Friction
    ④ Time

827. When the fluid in a bottle is allowed to flow into a person intravenously:
    ① Chemical energy is converted to kinetic energy
    ② Potential energy is converted to kinetic energy
    ③ Potential energy is converted to chemical energy
    ④ Kinetic energy is converted to potential energy

828. The primary reason for the ease of penetration of the needle through the tissue when administering an IM injection is:
    ① The force used by the nurse when inserting the needle
    ② The extremely high pressure developed at the tip of the needle due to its very small area
    ③ The softness of the tissue compared with the hardness of the needle
    ④ The long, slender shape of the needle

829. A client has a temperature of 99.8° F. This temperature can be converted to:
    ① 37.7° C
    ② 38.2° C
    ③ 37.0° C
    ④ 36.5° C

830. A client with pyrexia will probably demonstrate:
    ① Dyspnea
    ② Elevated blood pressure
    ③ Increased pulse rate
    ④ Precordial pain

831. The stage of sleep associated with psychologic rest is:
    ① Stage 1
    ② REM sleep
    ③ Stage 2
    ④ Stage 4

832. The absorption of fluids by gauze is best explained by the principle of:
    ① Diffusion
    ② Osmosis
    ③ Capillarity
    ④ Dialysis

833. The temperature range for a tepid application is:
① 80° to 93° F (26.6° to 34° C)
② 70° to 78° F (21° to 25.5° C)
③ 60° to 68° F (15.5° to 20° C)
④ 55° to 65° F (12.8° to 18° C)

834. Local hot and cold applications transfer temperature to and from the body by:
① Radiation
② Convection
③ Insulation
④ Conduction

835. Cold applications for short periods of time produce:
① Depression of vital signs
② Peripheral vasodilation
③ Decreased viscosity of blood
④ Local anesthesia

836. The best definition of a tort is:
① Doing something that a reasonable person under ordinary circumstances would not do
② The application of force to the person of another by a reasonable individual
③ An illegality committed by one person against the property or person of another
④ An illegality committed against the public and punishable by the law through the courts

837. Examples of intentional torts include:
① Malpractice and assault
② False imprisonment and battery
③ Negligence and invasion of privacy
④ Malpractice and negligence

838. Nurses are protected from all legal action when they:
① Report incidences of suspected child abuse to the appropriate authorities identified in legislation and policies
② Administer CPR measures on an unconscious child pulled from a swimming pool
③ Offer first aid at the scene of an automobile-bus accident
④ Offer health teaching regarding family planning

839. Regulating the practice of nursing has as its primary purpose the protection of:
① The public
② Practicing nurses
③ Professional standards
④ The employing agency

840. Mr. Manor, 21 years old, admits himself to the psychiatric unit for help. He develops severe pain in the right lower quadrant and is diagnosed as having acute appendicitis. In preparing Mr. Manor for an appendectomy the nurse should:
① Ask him to sign his own preoperative consent after he is informed of the procedure and required care
② Phone his next of kin to come in to sign his consent because he is on a psychiatric unit
③ Have the surgeon and the psychiatrist sign for the surgery, since it is an emergency procedure
④ Have two nurses witness the operative consent as the client signs it

CHAPTER 4

Psychiatric Nursing

Since nursing is concerned with the basic needs of people, the nurse must be able to understand and assist the individual, being constantly aware of the many factors that influence a person's behavioral response. Individuals are constantly interacting with both the internal and the external environments and at any given moment stand as a conglomerate of their own and their forebears' experiences. The individual is continuously faced with emotional stress from the moment of birth until the moment of death. How people adapt to this stress and the problems resulting from the adaptations are the focus of psychiatric nursing. Psychiatric nursing is therefore the care of clients with emotional problems. But the principles used in the care of psychiatric clients are applicable to all clients regardless of their diagnosis. Nursing, which is concerned with total care, must provide for the individual's physical (soma) as well as emotional (psyche) needs.

Background Information from the Behavioral Sciences
BASIC CONCEPTS FROM ANTHROPOLOGY
A. All people are influenced by the culture into which they are born
B. Cultural factors include race, nationality, and religion
C. Groups that share a common race, nationality, religion, or language are known as ethnic groups
D. Society as a whole frequently develops a fixed set of expected responses for certain ethnic groups
E. When each member of an ethnic group is expected to respond in a specific manner, the expected responses are called stereotypes
F. Cultural variability occurs in all stages of the life cycle: child rearing, marriage patterns, health maintenance, etc.

Cultural Influences
Race
A. Defined as a certain combination of physical traits that are transmitted by lineage or heredity
B. Physical traits of a race include skin color; texture and/ or color of hair; eye shapes and folds; shape of nose, lips, and cheekbones; contour of the head; and body build
C. Of all the factors involved in ethnic group membership, race, which is given a great deal of emphasis, appears to be a biologic phenomenon that seems to contribute few specifics to the cultural background

Nationality
A. Defined as original or acquired membership in a particular nation
B. The culture of nationalities is passed down through generations in the form of

1. Beliefs and superstitions
2. Foods and national dishes
3. Festivals and feast days
4. Language and the meanings of certain words
C. Nationality and the culture that it imparts frequently become even more important when a group of people immigrate to a new country where the members tend to join together to form a subculture of the new national culture
D. The subculture provides its members with a sense of security by furnishing a collective identity and maintaining the familiar

Religion
A. Defined as the quest for values of the ideal life usually embodied in a particular set of beliefs practiced individually or within an organized system
B. Religious beliefs in some form have existed in every group during every period of history
C. Organized religions have been instrumental in developing an ethical and moral system that has frequently been based on a society's needs
D. Most of the world's religions have developed many rituals as part of their worship, and these rituals form the basis of the religious culture that is passed down from generation to generation
E. In contrast to traditional religion there exist numerous religious cults; persons seeking a sense of belonging and purpose join a religious cult that gives them a group identity through communal living and rigorous rituals

Culture and Health
A. General influences
1. Cultural background influences the way in which people view both health and disease
2. The cultural influences seem to be derived from the areas of nationality and religion rather than race
B. Specific influences
1. National culture may influence an individual's
a. Response to illness
b. Response to pain and even the tolerance of pain
c. Need for superstitions and rituals
d. Acceptance of dietary change both in type or in consistency of food
e. Need for support and comfort from the family
f. Ability to communicate in understandable terms
g. Response to loss of independence
h. Feelings about loss of privacy and exposure of parts of the body
i. Feelings about loss of body parts
j. Need for specific rites and rituals associated with dying
2. Religious culture may influence an individual's
a. Views on conception, birth, and child care
b. Views about the meaning of pain and suffering
c. Feelings about the meaning of death
d. Desire for guidance from the clergy
e. Acceptance of certain treatments such as immunizations and blood transfusions
f. Concept of illness as a punishment

g. Dietary restrictions including the types of food and their preparation

h. Need for specific rites and rituals associated with dying

BASIC CONCEPTS FROM SOCIOLOGY

A. Every human society has institutions for the socialization of its members
   1. Process by which individuals are compelled or induced to conform to the customs of the group
      a. Group establishes rules and codes of conduct governing its members, and these become the norms, values, and mores of the group
      b. Role of members includes specified rights, duties, attitudes, and actions
   2. Controls established through a system of rewards and punishment
      a. Reward leads to acceptance as a member of the group
      b. Punishment for antisocial behavior leads to rejection and separation from the group
B. Development of society requires sanction of group members
   1. Growth takes place in social space
      a. Social boundaries separate one group from another
      b. Barriers to participation are established through mores and customs
   2. Leader's influence is always limited to conditions placed on it by the total group
   3. Behavioral roles are established by members of the group
C. A society is a reflection of all the functional relationships that occur between its individual members
   1. Products of group life are a major determinant in an individual's intellect, creativity, memory, thinking, and feeling
      a. Human beings have no memory, thought, or feeling that does not include society
      b. Intellect and creativity can be enhanced or hampered by society
   2. Members of a society have functional and rewarding social contact
      a. Members are accepted and approved and then participate in establishing rules, norms, and values
      b. The nonmembers have, at best, limited social contacts with the members; this causes a segmentation of relationships and provides few rewarding experiences for the nonmembers
D. Society or a group can change because of conflict among members
   1. This conflict is greatest when there is an absence of certain members, an introduction of new members, or a change in leadership
   2. Ensuing reorganization goes through three stages
      a. Tension: caused by conflict
      b. Integration: during which members learn about "the other's" problem
      c. Resolution: during which a reconstruction of the group's norms and values takes place
   3. Resolution of conflict and the restoring of equilibrium
      a. This takes place when people interact with one another and the group is dynamic
      b. Conflicts are not resolved when groups are rigid with fixed membership and ideas
E. Family is the primary group
   1. Helps society to establish and maintain its code of behavior
   2. Provides individual family members with
      a. Strong emotional ties
         (1) Members experience sensory stimuli through close contacts
         (2) Members learn to care about the emotional and physical well-being of each other
         (3) Members are responsive to one another's feelings, acts, and opinions
         (4) Members learn empathy by vicariously living the experiences of others
         (5) Members view selves through the eyes of others
      b. A feeling of security by meeting dependent needs
      c. A system of communication
         (1) Overt: words
         (2) Covert: body language
      d. Role identification and intimacy that helps them to internalize the acceptable behavioral patterns of the group
      e. A spirit of cooperation and competition through sibling interaction
   3. Changes that have influenced the family's ability to indoctrinate children with the norms of society
      a. The Industrial Revolution changed an agrarian society into an industrial one
         (1) Families became nuclear rather than extended
         (2) Families depended more on secondary groups for survival
         (3) New social groups were established to replace the extended family
         (4) Labor unions replaced patriarchal management
            (a) Laws enacted to protect the rights of children and other dependent people of society
            (b) Laws enacted to establish minimum wage and hourly benefits
         (5) Increased mobility of individuals reduced contact with family
      b. Altered male and female role patterns
         (1) Changing status of women
            (a) More women go outside the home to work
            (b) Women have an increased role in decision making and are better educated
         (2) Changing status of men
            (a) More men are willing to assume homemaking responsibilities
            (b) Men share decision making with women, thus decreasing dominance

(3) Increased partnership in home and financial management has resulted in less stereotyped sex roles

  c. Factors resulting in a reduction in the size of families

    (1) Increase in financial cost involved in raising and educating children

    (2) Emphasis on limited population growth

    (3) Wide dissemination of birth control information

    (4) Legalization of abortions

    (5) Persons choosing to marry in later adulthood

    (6) Couples deciding to delay the start of a family until later years

F. Peer groups help youth to establish norms of behavior and assist in the rites of passage from the family group to society

  1. Youth learns about society through contact with the peer group

  2. Youth develops further self-concept in contact with other youths

  3. Peer group interaction can produce change in its individual members

  4. Members have a strong loyalty to the peer group because of the reciprocal relationships and other rewards the group offers

  5. Peer group norms may conflict with family or society's norms

G. Group membership helps individuals achieve goals that are not attainable through individual effort

  1. Types of groups are task oriented, therapy, self-awareness, social

  2. Group functional roles include task roles, group building or maintenance roles, individual or self-serving roles

  3. Group content refers to the subject matter or task being worked on

  4. Group process refers to what is happening between and to group members while working; it deals with morale, feeling tones, influence, competition, conflict

H. Type of leadership in a group depends on the needs of the group members as well as the personality of the leader

  1. Authoritarian leader: rigid and uses leadership role as an instrument of power; the leader makes all the decisions, which are then handed down to the membership; little communication and interrelating between leader and group

  2. Democratic leader: fair and logical, uses the leadership role to stimulate others to achieve a collective goal; the leader encourages interrelating among members by relating to all members; weaknesses as well as strengths are accepted; the contributions of all members are fostered and utilized

  3. Emotional leader: reflects the feeling tones, norms, and values of the group

  4. Laissez-faire leader: passive and unproductive; usually assumes the role of a participant-observer and exerts little control or guidance over group behavior

5. Bureaucratic leader: rigid and assumes a role that is determined by formal criteria or rules that are inherent in the organization and frequently unrelated to the present group; the leader is not emotionally involved and avoids interrelating with the group members

6. Charismatic leader: can assume any of the above behaviors, since the group attributes supernatural power to this person or the office and frequently follows directions without question

I. Types of roles assumed by members of the group

  1. Harmonizer: brings other group members into accord while reconciling opposing positions

  2. Questioner: asks questions, seeks information, and gives constructive criticism to other group members

  3. Deserter: talks about irrelevant material; is indifferent and usually disruptive in some manner

  4. Tension reducer: introduces levity when it is needed and appropriate

  5. Encourager: contributes to the ego of others in the group; is a warm responsive member

  6. Monopolizer: attempts to control and assert authority over group; does not allow others to talk

  7. Clarifier: restates issues for clarification and then summarizes for rest of the group

  8. Opinion giver: uses own experience to back up opinion or belief

  9. Initiator: proposes ideas or topics for discussion and suggests possible solutions for group discussion

  10. Listener: shows interest in the group by expressions on face or by body language while making little or no comment

  11. Negativist: pessimistic, argumentative, and uncooperative

  12. Energizer: pushes the group into action

  13. Aggressor: hostile, aggressive; seeks attention; verbally attacks other group members

J. Community is a social organization that is considered the individual's secondary group

  1. Relationships among members are usually more impersonal

  2. Individuals participate in a more delimited manner or in a specific capacity

  3. The group frequently functions as a means to an end

    a. The group enables diversified groups to communicate

    b. The group helps other groups to identify community problems and possible solutions

  4. The secondary group is usually rather large and meets on an intermittent basis; contacts are usually maintained through correspondence

  5. Leaders of the community facilitate group interaction

    a. They have a knowledge of the community and its needs

    b. They have the skill to stimulate others to act

  6. Secondary groups help establish laws that are necessary to limit antisocial behavior

    a. Laws provide diversified groups with a common base of acceptable behavior

b. Some laws may favor and protect the vested interests of specific groups within the society

Sociology and Health

A. Role of society
1. Traditionally societies have placed great emphasis on caring for their members when they are ill
2. Recently society's role in health maintenance and the prevention of disease has been given an increased priority
3. Society's provision for health maintenance includes
   a. Protection of food, water, and drug supplies
   b. Establishment of public health agencies for the supervision, prevention, and control of disease and illness
   c. Development of public education programs
   d. Awarding scholarship grants for health education and research
   e. Development of unemployment insurance programs
   f. Establishment of workmen's compensation insurance
   g. Establishment of Social Security and Medicare programs
   h. Establishment of social welfare services and Medicaid programs
   i. Supervision of medical and hospital insurance programs
B. Health agency as a social institution has
1. A bureaucratic structure
2. Policies, rules, and regulations governing behavior of its members
3. An impersonal viewpoint
4. A status hierarchy
5. An increasingly specialized subculture
C. Hospital as a subculture of society
1. Employees develop both written and unwritten hospital policies that
   a. Set standards of acceptable behavior for both clients and staff
   b. Regulate the hospitalized client's contact with the primary group by limiting visitors
   c. Force both clients and staff to relate to the secondary group
   d. Punish unacceptable behavior by any members of the group, including the client
2. Folklores and folkways of the hospital serve to
   a. Maintain the mystique of medicine by fostering the use of a unique language and system of symbols
   b. Attach stigmas to various social illnesses such as AIDS and other sexually transmitted diseases, mental illness, drug addiction, and alcoholism, which are associated with certain patterns of living and acting that are not acceptable to the group
   c. Perpetuate the roles and values of the health team members and maintain the status quo
3. Hospital has several functions
   a. Primary: to help the client regain health and resume a role in society by providing services directed toward
      (1) Treatment of illness
      (2) Rehabilitation
      (3) Maintenance of health
      (4) Protecting the client's legal rights
   b. Secondary: to help society by providing services directed toward
      (1) Education of health professionals
      (2) The education of the general public
      (3) Research
D. Delivery of health services: responsibility of the community
1. Members of society become active participants in prevention of illness
2. Community health centers care for the ill in the home rather than in the hospital
3. Extended care facilities are established with more community and homelike atmosphere
4. Nonmedical community leaders take an active role in establishing health policy for society
5. Lay members of the community become involved with health agencies' policies and decisions
6. Health maintenance and treatment are no longer considered a privilege but the right of all members of society

BASIC CONCEPTS FROM NEUROPHYSIOLOGY
Neurophysical Theory of Behavior

A. Studies reveal that a malfunction of certain CNS neurons, which excrete substances known as neurotransmitters, appear to inhibit or trigger impulses in other neurons and may be responsible for distortions of behavior associated with psychiatric disorders
B. Neurotransmitters
1. Dopamine: an excess has been strongly linked with schizophrenia; a deficiency has been found in individuals with Parkinson's disease
2. Norepinephrine: an excess has been linked to manic behavior; a deficiency has been linked to depressed behavior
3. Serotonin: an excess has been found to result in hypersomnia (pathologically excessive sleep or drowsiness); a deficiency has been found to result in insomnia (abnormal wakefulness)

BASIC CONCEPTS FROM PSYCHOLOGY

A. Human beings must be able to perceive and interpret stimuli to interact with the environment
1. Perception and cognitive functioning are influenced by
   a. The nature of the stimuli
   b. Culture, beliefs, attitudes, and age
   c. Past experiences
   d. Present physical and emotional needs
2. Individual's personality development is influenced by the ability to perceive and interpret stimuli
   a. Through these processes the external world is internalized
   b. The external world may in turn be distorted by the individual's perceptions
B. Humans must communicate to be able to interact with the environment
1. Communication is a behavior that is learned through the process of acculturation
2. People must communicate with others to make needs known
   a. Infant uses the cry to bring attention to needs

b. Hearing is essential to the development of good speech, since one learns to form words by hearing the words of others

c. Written word usually replaces the spoken word when face-to-face encounters are impractical and supplements the spoken word when further clarification is necessary

3. Productive communication depends on the consensual validation of all involved

a. To understand the intent of the message, each person must be aware of the meaning of the spoken word as well as the inflections in the speaker's voice (verbal and nonverbal communication)

b. Validation can best be accomplished when participants are empathetic

c. Language and channels of communication must be adapted to the person and the purpose for which it is intended

d. Feedback is necessary to evaluate the effectiveness of the words and guide the communication

e. Satisfaction is enhanced for all involved when lines of communication are kept open

4. Barriers to effective communication include

a. Variations in culture, language, and education

b. Problems in hearing, speech, or comprehension: poor reception and perception

c. Refusal to listen to another point of view: inability to evaluate

d. Use of selective inattention, which may cause an interruption or distortion of the message

5. Nonverbal behavior communicates the inner feelings of the individual performing the behavior

a. Facial expression, posture, and body movement may express the anxiety, pain, tension, fear, happiness, joy, or satisfaction the individual is experiencing

b. Nonverbal communication may transmit a different message than the individual's verbal communication (covert vs. overt messages)

c. Confusion arises when there is a difference in the verbal and nonverbal message received

C. Psychologic experiences provide the energy that is transformed into behavior

1. Anxiety frequently provides the push that moves people to action because it

a. Develops when two goals or needs are in conflict

b. Is a state of apprehension or tension aroused by impulses from within

c. Prepares one for action or completely overwhelms and inhibits action

2. Anxiety develops in stages that progress from increased alertness to panic

3. The sympathetic nervous system prepares the body's physiologic defense for fight or flight by stimulating the adrenal medulla to secrete epinephrine and norepinephrine

a. The heartbeat is accelerated to pump more blood to the muscles

b. The peripheral blood vessels constrict to provide more blood to the vital organs

c. The bronchioles dilate, and breathing becomes rapid and deep to supply more oxygen to the cells

d. The pupils dilate to provide increased vision

e. The liver releases glucose for quick energy

f. The prothrombin time is shortened to protect the body from loss of blood in the event of injury

4. Selye's general adaptation syndrome (GAS) is the body's physiologic adaptation to stress (anxiety)

a. The adrenal cortex secretes cortisone during the emergency stage

b. When stress continues, the increased secretion of cortisone causes the body to go through a resistive stage

c. If the process continues, the last stage is exhaustion and death

5. Defense mechanisms serve to protect the personality by controlling anxiety and reducing emotional pressures

Development of the Personality
Definition

A. Sum of all traits that differentiate one individual from another

B. Total behavior pattern of an individual through which the inner interests are expressed

C. The individual's unique and distinctive way of behaving and interacting with others

D. Constellation of defense mechanisms for dealing with inner and outer pressures

E. A functional role within a family system

Factors Involved in Personality Development

A. Behavior is a learned response that develops as a result of past experiences

B. To protect the individual's emotional well-being, these experiences are organized in the psyche on three different levels

1. Conscious: composed of past experiences, easily recalled, that create little if any emotional discomfort and tend to be somewhat pleasant

2. Subconscious: composed of material that has been deliberately pushed out of conscious but can be recalled with some effort

3. Unconscious: contains the largest body of material, greatly influences behavior

a. This material cannot be deliberately brought back into awareness, since it is usually unacceptable and painful to the individual

b. If recalled, it is usually disguised or distorted, as in dreams; however, it is still capable of producing a good deal of anxiety

C. According to Freud the personality consists of three parts: the id, ego, and superego

1. Id contains the instincts, impulses, and urges; is totally self-centered and unconscious

2. Ego is the conscious self, the "I" that deals with reality; the part of the personality that is shown to the environment

3. Superego controls, inhibits, and regulates impulses and instincts whose uncontrolled expression would endanger the emotional well-being of the individual and the stability of the society

Critical Periods in the Formation of the Personality

A. Personality of an individual develops in overlapping stages that shade and merge together
   1. Certain goals must be accomplished during each stage in the development from infancy to maturity
   2. If these goals are not accomplished at specific periods, the basic structure of the personality will be weakened
   3. Factors in each stage persist as a permanent part of the personality
   4. Each stage has particular frustrations and major traumas that must be overcome
   5. Successful resolution of the conflicts associated with each stage is essential to development
   6. Unresolved conflicts remain in the unconscious and may, at times, result in maladaptive behavior
B. Tasks related to personality development during infancy
   1. Freud: oral stage—infant obtains gratification by taking everything in; begins to develop self-concept from the responses of others
   2. Erikson: trust versus mistrust—trust develops from the inner feeling of self-worth that is transmitted through maternal care; child learns to depend on the satisfaction that is derived from this care, and when the need is met, trust develops
   3. Sullivan: need for security—infant learns to rely on others to gratify needs and satisfy wishes; develops a sense of basic trust, security, and self-worth when this occurs
   4. Piaget: sensorimotor stage—infant develops physically with a gradual increase in the ability to think and use language; progresses from simple reflex responses through repetitive behaviors to deliberate and imaginative activity
C. Tasks related to personality development during early childhood
   1. Freud: anal stage—struggle of giving of self and breaking the symbiotic ties to mother; as the ties are broken, the child learns independence
   2. Erikson: autonomy versus shame and doubt—the struggle of holding on to or letting go; an internal struggle for self-identity; love versus hate
   3. Sullivan: child learns to communicate needs through the use of words and the acceptance of delayed gratification and interference with wish fulfillment
   4. Piaget: preoperational thought stage—child learns to imitate and play; begins to use symbols and language although interpretation is literal
D. Tasks related to personality development during preschool period
   1. Freud: oedipal stage—love for and desire to possess parent of the opposite sex creates fear and guilt feelings; desires are repressed and role identification with parent of the same sex occurs
   2. Erikson: initiative versus guilt—stage of intensive activity, play, and consuming fantasies where child interjects parents' social consciousness

3. Sullivan: development of body image and self-perception—organizes and uses experiences in terms of approval and disapproval received; begins using selective inattention and disassociates those experiences which cause physical or emotional discomfort and pain
   4. Piaget: preoperational thought stage continues—child begins understanding relationships and develops basic conceptual thought and intuitive reasoning
E. Tasks related to personality development during school age or preadolescence
   1. Freud: latency stage—period of low sexual activity; identifies with peer groups
   2. Erikson: industry versus inferiority—the child learns how to make things with others and strives to achieve success
   3. Sullivan: the period of learning to form satisfying relationships with peers—uses competition, compromise, and cooperation; the preadolescent learns to relate to peers of the same sex
   4. Piaget: concrete operational thought stage—thinking is more socialized and logical with increased intellectual and conceptual development; begins problem solving by use of inductive reasoning and logical thought
F. Tasks related to personality development during adolescence
   1. Freud: genital stage—sexual activity increases; sexual identity is strengthened or attacked
   2. Erikson: identity versus identity diffusion—childhood identifications are integrated with the basic drives, native endowments, and opportunities offered in social roles
   3. Sullivan: learns independence and how to establish satisfactory relationships with members of the opposite sex
   4. Piaget: formal operational stage—develops true abstract thought by application of logical tests; achieves conceptual independence and problem solving ability
G. Tasks related to personality development during young adulthood
   1. Erikson: intimacy versus isolation—moves from the relative security of self-identity to the relative insecurity involved in establishing intimacy with another
   2. Sullivan: becomes economically, intellectually, and emotionally self-sufficient
H. Tasks related to personality development during later adulthood
   1. Erikson: generativity versus self-absorption—the mature person becomes interested in establishing and guiding the next generation
   2. Sullivan: learns to be interdependent and assumes responsibility for others
I. Tasks related to personality development during senescence
   1. Erikson: adapts to triumphs and disappointments with a certain ego integrity
   2. Sullivan: develops an acceptance of responsibility for what life is and was and of its place in the flow of history

Influence of Basic Needs on the Development of Personality

A. Humanity has certain basic needs that must be satisfied
1. Need to communicate
   a. Through communication, humans maintain contact with reality
      (1) The individual needs to validate findings with others to correctly interpret reality
      (2) Validation is enhanced when communication conveys an understanding of feelings
   b. Through communication, the individual develops a concept of self in relation to others
2. Need for security
   a. To feel secure as an assurance of survival is fundamental
   b. Fear emerges when survival is threatened
   c. Initially the infant's security is related to the satisfaction of physical needs
   d. Security is enhanced when the same individual meets the infant's physical needs in a consistent manner
   e. The infant must also perceive love to feel secure
   f. Security is derived from the individual's perception of self in relation to others
   g. How the individual handles these perceptions influences personality development
3. Need to move from dependence to independence
   a. The infant is dependent on the parents but through learning acquires faculties for independence
   b. There is no real security or deep assurance of survival in being dependent on others, since uncertainties develop if one's security is totally derived from this source
   c. The infant must feel love and security before reaching out to struggle with the problems in the environment
   d. When the need for love and security is met, the child is sustained in the failures and hurts associated with learning and independence
   e. Denial of the opportunity to learn or frustration in the drive for independence will produce emotional problems
4. Need to develop a self-concept
   a. Self-concept begins to develop early in infancy
   b. Determination of the self-concept develops primarily through interaction with significant persons in the environment
   c. An integral part of the self-concept is the body image
   d. First and most deeply learned perception of body image develops from the attitudes of significant others, since children view themselves as others view them
   e. Concept of the self is root of security and future developmental needs
   f. Communication enhances the development of self
   g. A person's self-concept is the basis for emotional stability or instability; a secure person has strength and capacity for independence and becomes less anxious when circumstances require the help of others
5. Need to find relief from organic discomfort
   a. Through experience, one learns the most satisfying ways of relieving discomfort
   b. Adjustment to illness depends on how the individual adjusts to life
B. Needs of a specific individual at a given time will vary according to internal and external environmental factors.
C. To attain psychologic equilibrium and achieve need satisfaction, the individual attempts to maintain a feeling of safety and comfort in adapting to life's situations; this is often achieved by maintaining a feeling of worth and a feeling of being needed by others

Anxiety and Behavior

A. Anxiety
1. Is a state of apprehension, tension, or uneasiness
2. Is an internal phenomenon aroused by impulses
3. Occurs when the ego is threatened
4. Frequently stems from an anticipation of danger
5. May arise from known, unknown, or unrecognized sources
B. Levels of anxiety
1. Alertness level: automatic response of the central nervous system that
   a. Prepares the body for danger by regulating internal processes
   b. Concentrates all energies for internal activity
2. Apprehension level: response to anticipation of short-term danger that
   a. Prepares the individual for efficient performance
   b. Occurs when facing new situations
   c. Creates some conscious awareness of discomfort
3. Free-floating level: response to generalized anxiety that
   a. Creates a feeling of impending doom
   b. Produces an acute feeling of discomfort
4. Panic level: total response to anxiety characterized by uncontrolled, unrealistic behavior that
   a. Lessens perception of the environment to protect the ego from awareness
   b. Increases the danger to the entire system
C. Behavioral defenses against anxiety
1. Conscious: these are the first-line defenses against anxiety; used by all people in times of stress; comprise the individual's deliberate effort to maintain control, reduce tension, and limit anxiety (individual may be aware of behavior but is not always aware of underlying reason); the individual
   a. Removes self from the source of anxiety
   b. Escapes through bodily satisfactions
   c. Focuses psychic energy on other, more pleasant, activities
   d. Uses substitute gratifications
   e. Consciously avoids painful subjects
   f. Gives socially acceptable reasons for behavior
   g. Releases tensions by acting out impulsively
2. Unconscious: these include the second-, third-, and fourth-line defenses against anxiety; may be used by all people in extremely stressful situations; how-

ever, if used consistently, indicate that the individual is emotionally ill

   a. Second-line defenses are the personality traits developed to handle interpersonal relationships and protect the ego; these defenses include

     (1) Exaggerated dependency and immaturity

     (2) Passive submission

     (3) Domination of others

     (4) Aggression toward others

     (5) Withdrawal from others

     (6) Compulsive ambition

     (7) Perfectionism and grandiosity

   b. Third-line defenses are the neurotic traits developed to handle interpersonal relationships and protect the ego; these defenses include

     (1) Repudiation and opposition of inner drives by the use of reaction formation

     (2) Avoidance of emotional or feeling level by placing complete emphasis on intellectual reasoning

     (3) Inhibition of affective, autonomic, and visceral functions to deaden actual awareness of repressed impulses

     (4) Displacement of impulses to an external object, which is then feared and avoided

     (5) Use of compulsive rituals to magically neutralize inner impulses

   c. Fourth-line defenses are the psychotic traits developed to handle interpersonal relationships and protect the ego; these defenses include

     (1) Regression to dependency level of development frequently accompanied by childish attitudes and behavior

     (2) Denial and withdrawal from others and reality

     (3) Internalization of hostility

     (4) Excited, uncontrolled acting out

  3. As anxiety and the threat to the ego are increased or decreased, shifts in the lines of defense will occur; the individual's behavior is altered by these shifts

D. Major sources of anxiety

  1. Threat to one's biologic integrity; interference with one's basic physiologic needs

  2. Threat to one's self system: self-esteem, self-worth, self-respect

Personality Defenses
Defense Mechanisms Provide Initial Protection for the Personality

A. Although all individuals may, in times of severe emotional stress, use many of the behaviors listed, it is the repetitive use of these behaviors in most situations that is indicative of problems

B. Identifiable patterns of response begin to form when individuals respond to most situations they encounter with the same type of behavior

C. Commonly used normal defense mechanisms that help an individual to deal with reality are

  1. Identification: the individual internalizes the characteristics of an idealized person

  2. Substitution: the individual replaces one goal for another

  3. Compensation: the individual makes up for a perceived lack in one area by emphasizing capabilities in another

  4. Sublimation: a socially acceptable behavior is substituted for an unacceptable instinct; this mechanism is used when the expression of these instincts would prove a threat to the self

  5. Compromise: reciprocal give-and-take necessary in many relationships to salvage some part of the situation or the goal

  6. Rationalization: the individual makes acceptable excuses for behavior and feelings; attempts to explain behavior by logical reasoning

D. In addition to the normal defenses, all individuals may use compensatory-type defenses in times of stress; these, when used in moderation, are adaptive; if used to excess, they frequently create greater emotional problems

  1. As the use of these compensatory defenses increases and encompasses more of the individual's life, contact with reality is interrupted and distortions begin

  2. These patterns of behavior are considered deviations and are usually looked on as symptoms of emotional problems

   a. Conversion: emotional conflict is unconsciously changed into a physical symptom that can be expressed openly and without anxiety

   b. Denial: emotional conflict is blocked from the conscious mind and the individual refuses to recognize its existence

   c. Displacement: emotions related to an emotionally charged situation or object are shifted to a relatively safe substitute situation or object

   d. Fantasy: conscious distortion of unconscious wishes and needs to obtain gratification and satisfaction

   e. Projection: unconscious denial of unacceptable feelings and emotions in oneself while attributing them to others

   f. Reaction formation: the individual unconsciously reverses unacceptable feelings and behaves in the exact opposite manner

   g. Regression: return to an earlier stage of behavior when stress creates problems at the present stage

   h. Repression: involuntary exclusion from consciousness of those ideas, feelings, and situations which are creating conflict and causing discomfort

   i. Suppression: voluntary exclusion from consciousness of those ideas, feelings, and situations which are creating conflict and causing discomfort

   j. Transference: positive or negative feelings and emotions that were previously present toward important figures are applied and attributed to another person in the present

k. Intellectualization: use of thinking, ideas, or intellect to avoid emotions
l. Introjection: complete acceptance of another's opinions and values as one's own

Motivation, Learning, and Behavior

A. All behavior is motivated
1. Motive always implies some purpose
2. Social motives are often changed through learning
3. Symbolic rewards are the major factors in learning
4. Social approval is an important form of symbolic reward
B. Behavior and emotions
1. Emotions act as motives for behavior, since they often involve a reaction to some external situation
2. Behavior is always accompanied and often controlled by the emotions
3. Emotions may facilitate or hinder the learning process
4. Emotions exert a strong influence on the thinking process
C. Automatic behavior
1. Is the predetermined or repetitive type behavior that has been used successfully in prior situations
2. Requires little effort or thought
3. Is adapted to definite situations and can be difficult to alter if the situation changes
4. Is integrated with cognition in the functioning of a mature and independent adult
D. Life is a continually changing process, and when these changes occur in areas of significance they often produce rather distinct emotional responses; these changes include
1. Resistance to change: the individual hesitates to accept or adapt to the change and may attempt to deny its occurrence or reject its outcome
2. Regression: the individual returns to an earlier type of behavior that, at the time, provided some satisfaction and gratification and now provides an escape from the unacceptable or anxiety-producing situation
3. Acceptance and progression: the individual adapts to the change and expends energy on outside objects rather than self-centered aims

Deviate Patterns of Behavior
Withdrawn Behavior

A. Definition: pathologic retreat from, or an avoidance of; people and the world of reality
B. Developmental factors
1. Unhappy childhood caused by conflict, tension, and anxiety in the home
2. Inconsistent relationships with parents
a. Lack of firm standards for reward or punishment
b. Variations between verbal and nonverbal communications
3. Failure to develop a sense of security
4. Failure to develop positive self-image
5. Interpersonal relationships create a continuous source of anxiety

6. Chronic anxiety results in loss of interest in interpersonal relationships and reality testing
7. Extreme sensitivity, narcissim, and introversion develop
C. Compensatory mechanisms used to reduce and avoid stress include
1. Fixation
2. Rigidity and compulsiveness
3. Reaction formation
4. Sublimation
5. Rationalization
6. Regression
D. Effects of compensatory mechanisms on behavior
1. Isolation and failure to test reality result in greater distortions of reality situations
2. Behavior can progress until loss of contact with reality develops and individual retreats into the condition usually identified as schizophrenia

Projective Behavior

A. Definition: pathologic denial of one's own feelings, faults, failures, and emotions while continually attributing them to others
B. Developmental factors
1. Parents set extremely high demands and continually raise expected standards of performance
2. Expectations of failure are fostered, creating feelings of inadequacy and feelings of inferiority
3. Childhood experiences continue to reinforce these feelings and chronic insecurity, suspiciousness, and extreme sensitivity develop
4. Feelings of hostility develop and cannot be expressed
5. Inability to establish interpersonal relationships with others interferes with reality testing
6. The individual develops a rigid, structured, narcissistic personality
7. Competitive society fosters and supports projective patterns of behavior
C. Compensatory mechanisms used to reduce and avoid stress include
1. Displacement
2. Projection
3. Rigidity
4. Denial
5. Rationalization
6. Delusions
7. Ideas of reference
D. Effects of compensatory mechanisms on behavior
1. The individual is unable to tolerate suspense, prolonged anxiety, or tension
2. Unacceptable impulses and wishes are denied and faults and failures are disclaimed for self and attributed to others
3. Delusional ideas develop and begin to dominate behavior
4. Ideas of reference result in continual misinterpretation of events
5. Delusions become more systematized and spread out

6. Behavior can progress until loss of contact with reality is complete and the individual retreats into the condition usually identified as paranoid type schizophrenia or paranoid states

Aggressive Behavior

A. Definition: pathologic anger and hostility that are turned outward onto others or inward on oneself
B. Developmental factors
   1. Security is chronically threatened, resulting in a continual struggle to maintain it
   2. Strong need for approval
   3. Failure to develop self-concept and self-esteem
   4. Chronic anxiety and tension, which are often increased by the real or imagined loss of a love object
   5. Demands and responsibilities are high
C. Compensatory mechanisms used to reduce and avoid stress include
   1. Displacement
   2. Rigidity
   3. Denial
   4. Rationalization
   5. Repression
   6. Hostility that can be directed on
      a. Self
      b. Environment
D. Effects of compensatory mechanisms on behavior
   1. Need for approval results in compliance to demands
   2. Necessary compliance creates resentment
   3. Hostility develops and fosters feeling of guilt
   4. Self-doubt increases anxiety and tension
   5. Increased anxiety and tension reduce interpersonal relationships and reality testing
   6. Behavior can progress until there is a complete loss of contact with reality and the individual retreats into the condition usually identified as a mood disorder

Neurotic Behavior

Includes anxiety reactions, conversion reactions, phobic reactions, and obsessive-compulsive reactions
A. Definition: maladjustive type of response, characterized by many fears, anxieties, and/or physical symptoms
B. Developmental factors
   1. Usually lack a stable family life and effective guidance
   2. Frequently overprotected and fail to acquire the necessary skills to cope with problems
   3. Experience chronic insecurity, anxiety, and tension
   4. Goals are set for them by the parents, and acceptance depends on achieving the goals
   5. Constant struggle to gain reassurance and security
   6. Gains satisfaction from behavior and substitutes this satisfaction for the satisfaction desired but not obtained through interpersonal relations
C. Compensatory mechanisms used to reduce anxiety and avoid stress include
   1. Displacement
   2. Rationalization
   3. Regression
   4. Rigidity and compulsiveness
   5. Conversion
   6. Denial

D. Effects of compensatory mechanisms on behavior
   1. Behavior is purposeful and is unconsciously resorted to when the person feels threatened
   2. Continued use of behavior can
      a. Create new problems for the individual
      b. Be out of proportion to the degree of stress, impair social effectiveness, and dominate the individual's total life
   3. When impairment of functioning occurs, the individual is usually considered to be deviating from the normal and to have an anxiety disorder

Socially Aggressive Behavior

A. Definition: maladjustive response resulting from a defect in the development of the personality that is characterized by peculiar actions or misbehavior
B. Developmental factors
   1. Approval and disapproval do not appear sufficiently strong in childhood to influence the behavior along accepted patterns
   2. Long history of maladjustment that creates more problems as child matures and standards for acceptable behavior are increased
   3. The individual may show a history of severe emotional trauma in early life that interferes with emotional development
   4. Parents frequently provide a cold, emotionally sterile environment
C. Compensatory mechanisms used to reduce anxiety and avoid stress include
   1. Displacement
   2. Repression
   3. Denial
   4. Regression
   5. Hostility
   6. Rejection
D. Effects of compensatory mechanisms on behavior; the individual
   1. Appears competent but is usually unreliable and lacks a sense of responsibility
   2. Has the potential to succeed but shows a history of repeated failure
   3. Lacks perseverance, honesty, and sincerity
   4. Is completely egocentric and incapable of emotional investment in others
   5. Experiences no remorse or shame
   6. Is explosive under pressure
   7. Is unable to tolerate criticism
   8. Fails to profit from past experiences and cares little about the consequences for present acts
   9. Has impaired judgment, which usually creates problems and brings the individual into conflict with society; usually classified as personality disturbances

Addictive Behavior

A. Definition: repeated or chronic use of alcohol or drugs with a resulting dependency on these substances
B. Developmental factors
   1. Feelings of loneliness and isolation develop
   2. Chronic anxiety, fears, and low tension tolerance develop as a result of early relationships
   3. Feelings of inadequacy in interpersonal relationships serve to increase anxiety

4. Inability to delay satisfaction
5. Struggle for independence yet unconscious desire to be dependent
6. Impulsiveness and resentment of responsibility
7. Peer pressure and drug availability
8. Sexual conflict
9. Family factors
C. Compensatory mechanisms used to reduce anxiety and avoid stress include
   1. Denial
   2. Regression
   3. Rationalization
   4. Addiction
   5. Displacement
   6. Fantasy
   7. Repression
   8. Intellectualization
D. Effects of compensatory mechanisms on behavior
   1. Drug or alcohol reduces inhibitory self-control
   2. Drug or alcohol allows for expression of inner feelings but increases the guilt and requires more of the substance to relieve the guilt.
   3. Alcohol and drugs decrease feelings of inferiority and reduce anxiety
   4. Alcohol and drugs increase social isolation and cause deterioration of personal habits
   5. The individual becomes increasingly less efficient and devotes less energy to goals and ambitions
   6. Dependency and tolerance develop and the substances are needed in increasing amounts to achieve the same dulling of reality
   7. Securing the alcohol or drug becomes the main objective in life, and functioning is totally impaired; these individuals are then classified as drug addicts or alcoholics

Self-Destructive Behavior

A. Definition: Chronically indulging in self-destructive behavior by noncompliance with medical regimens; habitually abusing food, drugs, alcohol, or cigarettes, or engaging in high-risk activities
B. Developmental factors:
   1. Failure to develop a sense of security and/or self-worth
   2. Superficial interpersonal relationships
   3. Inconsistent relationship with parents
      a. Lack of firm standards for reward or punishment
      b. Variations between verbal and nonverbal communications
   4. Lack of faith in the future
   5. Anxiety results in difficulty in changing goals and expectations
   6. Sense of failure or shame when goals are not attained
   7. Sense of isolation
C. Compensatory mechanisms used to reduce and avoid stress include
   1. Rigidity
   2. Rationalization
   3. Withdrawal
   4. Denial
   5. Fantasy

D. Effects of compensatory mechanisms on behavior
   1. Greater risk of self-destructive behavior
   2. Greater risk of suicide
      a. Talking, threatening, or planning suicide in either very vague or specific terms throughout planning
      b. Making a suicide attempt in an acute crisis state by seriously and deliberately executing a plan
      c. The suicide is completed, but there is difficulty in determining whether the act was accidental or deliberate (e.g., autoeroticism practiced by adolescents; reckless driving)
      d. Copycat suicide: suicidal acts carried out by adolescents knowing or reading about similar acts

Psychologic Factors Affecting Physical Condition

A. Physical illnesses where psychogenic factors are the predominant causative agents
B. Anxiety stimulates the autonomic nervous system, and the nervous and endocrine impulses appear to center on one particular organ, creating actual physical illness and changes in the tissue structure
C. Reason a certain organ is involved with one client and a different organ with another is still undetermined
   1. Pathology: premorbid personality appears to be one of unexpressed aggression resulting from the unresolved struggle between dependent need and independent striving; may be familial
   2. Symptoms
      a. Skin
         (1) In neurodermatitis, dermatitis factitia, pruritus, and trichotillomania, psychic factors appear to dominate
         (2) There appears to be a relationship between endocrine imbalance and disturbances in the autonomic regulation of skin physiology
         (3) Stress seems to lead to rash, itching, and discomfort
      b. Musculoskeletal
         (1) Anxiety and fear often create a tightening of muscles
         (2) This becomes an aggravating factor in arthritis, backache, tension headache, or any other musculoskeletal disorder in which increased tension and spasm are involved
      c. Respiratory
         (1) Hyperventilation syndrome
            (a) Panting occurs with tension and excitement and this forced respiration can produce biochemical changes in the blood
            (b) These changes can alter the cerebral circulation and cause a reduction in consciousness and syncope
         (2) Bronchial asthma
            (a) Stress and tension appear to create increased secretions and changes in the bronchi
            (b) Individuals with asthma tend to exhibit a strong desire for protection and dependency yet fear rejection or engulfment

(c) Wheeze associated with asthma is considered by some to be a suppressed cry for this protection

d. Cardiovascular
   (1) Essential hypertension
      (a) Anxiety and other stresses are believed to play a role in releasing a pressor from the kidneys, which causes chronic vasoconstriction of the vessels
      (b) All other primary causes for hypertension must be ruled out before this cause can be diagnosed
      (c) Individuals with hypertension have difficulty handling hostile feelings, are less assertive, and have more obsessive-compulsive traits than nonhypertensive people
      (d) Hypertension may be considered a state of chronically unexpressed rage that arises from conflicts between passive/dependent longings and the struggle for independence
   (2) Coronary occlusion and angina
      (a) Coronary attacks frequently occur following periods of fatigue and anxiety
      (b) These individuals place a high value on work and success; they become depressed when inactive
e. Hemolymphatic
   (1) Certain blood dyscrasias and responses can be linked to emotional stress
   (2) In some individuals the neutrophil count drops, the clotting time is decreased, both blood viscosity and erythrocyte sedimentation rate rise
   (3) Nature of this response to stress is still controversial
f. Gastrointestinal
   (1) Peptic ulcer
      (a) Anxiety and other stress appear to create a condition of hyperactivity, hypersecretion, hyperacidity, and engorgement of the mucosa
      (b) Related to stresses in life, particularly those concerned with conflicts between passivity and aggression
      (c) Use reaction formation to cover the strong, somewhat irrational need to achieve security from others
   (2) Ulcerative colitis
      (a) Parasympathetic stimulation of the lower bowel produces an enzyme that interferes with the protective coating of the bowel
      (b) May occur as a reaction to a variety of stresses but most often in situations that demand accomplishment and arouse fear of not succeeding
      (c) Many clients are immature and have not gained any feelings of independence

g. Genitourinary
   (1) Disturbances in genital and urinary problems may occur under stress
   (2) Enuresis, amenorrhea, frigidity, and impotence appear to be related to psychologic factors
   (3) Depression and feelings of helplessness may be related to urinary retention
   (4) Fear may be related to urgency and frequency
h. Endocrine
   (1) Eating patterns and dependency on food for satisfaction and reduction of stress appear related to both diabetes mellitus and obesity
   (2) Feelings of insecurity and an unusual sense of responsibility appear associated with onset of hyperthyroidism
i. Organs of special sense: some evidence that certain neurologic disturbances, such as atypical facial neuralgia, are related to emotional conflict
3. Therapy: must be directed toward both the physical and emotional problems
4. Nursing care
   a. Reduce emotional stimulation when possible
   b. Explain all procedures carefully and allow client time for questions
   c. Provide the client with talking time
   d. Avoid material that appears to stimulate conflict for the client
   e. Accept the client's behavior and encourage expression of feelings
   f. Remember that the client is really physically ill and the symptoms have a physiologic basis

Nursing in Psychiatry
BASIC PRINCIPLES OF PSYCHIATRIC NURSING

A. These principles
   1. Are by necessity general in nature
   2. Form the guidelines for the emotional care of all clients
B. In caring for clients, the nurse should attempt to
   1. Accept and respect people as individuals regardless of their behavior
   2. Limit or reject the individual's inappropriate behavior without rejecting the individual
   3. Recognize that all behavior has meaning and is meeting the needs of the performer regardless of how distorted or meaningless it appears to others
   4. Accept the dependency needs of individuals while supporting and encouraging moves toward independence
   5. Help individuals set appropriate limits for themselves or set limits for them when they are unable to do so
   6. Encourage individuals to express their feelings in an atmosphere free of reprisal or judgment
   7. Recognize that individuals need to use their defenses until other defenses can be substituted
   8. Recognize how feelings affect behavior and influence relationships

9. Recognize that individuals frequently respond to the behavioral expectations of others: family, peers, authority (staff)
10. Recognize that all individuals have a potential for movement toward higher levels of emotional health

THERAPEUTIC NURSING RELATIONSHIPS

A. Phases
   1. Orientation or introductory: the nurse establishes a trust relationship which the client tests by discussing only what he or she wishes to discuss; clients are never pushed to discuss areas of concern that are upsetting to them
   2. Working: the nurse and the client discuss areas of concern and the client is helped to plan, implement, and evaluate a course of action
   3. Termination: end of the therapeutic relationship between the nurse and the client; the time parameters should be set early in the relationship with meetings spaced further and further apart near the end
B. Themes of communication: recurring thoughts and ideas that give insight into what an individual is feeling and tie the communication together
   1. Content: conversation may appear superficial but careful attention to the underlying theme helps the nurse identify problem areas while providing insight into the client's self-concept
   2. Mood: emotion or affect that the client communicates to the nurse; includes personal appearance, facial expressions, and gestures that reflect the client's mood and feelings
   3. Interaction: how the client reacts or interacts with the nurse; includes how the client relates and what role he or she assumes when communicating with the nurse and others
C. Fundamental requirements of a therapeutic relationship
   1. Ability to communicate therapeutically requires a basic understanding and use of interviewing techniques in developing a trusting relationship through
      a. Open-ended rather than probing questions
      b. Reflection of words and feelings and paraphrasing
      c. Acceptance of the client's behavior
      d. Nonjudgmental objective attitude
      e. Focusing on the emotional needs of the client
      f. Having a therapeutic goal for the interview
   2. Recognition that an individual has potential for growth
      a. Individuals need to learn about their own behavior in relation to others
      b. Exchanging experiences with others provides the reassurance that reactions are valid and feelings shared
      c. Participating with groups increases knowledge of interpersonal relationships and helps individuals to identify their strengths and resources
      d. The identification of the individual's strengths and resources helps to convey the expectation of growth

3. Recognition that an individual needs to be accepted
   a. Acceptance is an active process designed to convey respect for another through empathetic understanding
   b. Acceptance of others implies and requires acceptance of self
   c. To be nonjudgmental, one must become aware of one's own attitudes and feelings and their affect on perception
   d. Acceptance requires that individuals be permitted and even encouraged to express their feelings and attitudes even though they may be divergent from the general viewpoint
      (1) Individuals should be encouraged to express both positive and negative feelings
      (2) This encouragement must occur on both the verbal and nonverbal level
   e. Acceptance means showing interest in another person; interest requires
      (1) Face-to-face contact and really listening to what the other person has to say
      (2) Developing an awareness of the other person's likes and dislikes
      (3) Attempting to understand another's point of view
      (4) Using nonverbal as well as verbal expressions of acceptance
   f. Acceptance requires the development of interpersonal techniques that encourage others to express problems; the listener's
      (1) Reflection of feelings, attitudes, and words help the speaker to identify feelings
      (2) Open-ended questions permit the speaker to focus on problems
      (3) Paraphrasing assists the speaker in clarifying statements
      (4) Use of silence provides both the listener and the speaker with the necessary time for thinking over what is being discussed
   g. Acceptance requires the recognition of factors that block communication, including
      (1) Any overt or covert response that conveys a judgmental or superior attitude
      (2) Direct questions that convey an invasive or probing attitude
      (3) Ridicule that conveys a hostile attitude
      (4) Talking about one's own problems and not listening, which conveys a self-serving attitude and loss of interest in the speaker
D. Recognition of behavioral changes that result from physical illness
   1. Anxiety, fear, and depression occur whenever there is a health problem
      a. Body image and feelings of being in control of one's body have their basis in the early developmental period
      b. Anxiety develops whenever a real or imagined threat to the body image occurs
   2. Signs of the anxiety, fear, and depression associated with illness are variable and include
      a. Indifference to symptoms: usually related to failure to accept the occurrence of a health problem

b. Denial of reality: usually related to attempts to maintain stability and integrity of the personality

c. Reaction formation: usually related to attempts to block the reality from consciousness and acting as if nothing is wrong

d. Failure to keep appointments and follow physician's or nurse's directions: usually related to fear of finding additional problems or admitting there is something wrong

e. Overconcern with body functions and symptoms: usually related to fear of death

f. Asking many questions and offering many complaints: usually related to attempts at keeping a staff member by the bedside because of fears associated with illness; fear of abandonment

g. Opportunity to ventilate feelings

3. Emotional needs of the ill person include
   a. Security of continuous relationships with friends and members of their families
   b. Some way of achieving the feeling of self-worth and self-esteem
   c. Assistance in accepting the dependent role of the client
   d. Assistance in resolving conflicts while maintaining security
   e. Assistance in refocusing inner resources
   f. Contact with the reality of the external world

4. To help the individual maintain the self-concept during illness, the nurse must understand the normal emotional stages of illness
   a. Denial: the individual cannot believe it is happening
   b. Anger: something has happened that one cannot control
   c. Bargaining: promising to be a better person if something occurs
   d. Depression: one grieves for loss or expected loss
   e. Acceptance of the illness and learning how to adapt: this stage can only be reached when the individual has resolved the conflicts that develop during the earlier stages

5. Common reactions occur to the change in body image associated with many health problems
   a. Attitudes toward one's body and self-concept greatly influence response
   b. Fear is a universal response; individual may focus on fear of
      (1) Pain
      (2) Incapacitation
      (3) Disfigurement
      (4) Altered self-concept
      (5) Rejection of loved ones
      (6) Death
   c. Questioning is a universal response; the individual may focus on
      (1) This can't be happening to me
      (2) Is this really happening to me?
      (3) What did I do to deserve this?
      (4) Why am I being punished?

d. Grief and mourning are universal responses; the individual may focus on
   (1) What was in the past
   (2) What could have been for the future
   (3) Loss of missed opportunities
   (4) A magnified view of the loss
   (5) Avoiding interpersonal contacts

6. Caring for the dying client involves caring for the body, the mind, and the spirit
   a. Demands an understanding and acceptance of the nurse's own feelings, beliefs, and fears about death
   b. The last stages of life should be viewed as a positive rather than negative achievement

Pharmacology Related to Emotional Disorders
MINOR TRANQUILIZERS
Description

A. Used to produce sedation and relieve anxiety without producing sleep

B. Act by dose-related CNS depression with inhibition of the limbic and reticular activating systems of the brain; many also exert skeletal muscle relaxant and anticonvulsant effects

C. Minor tranquilizers are available in oral and parenteral (IM, IV) preparations

D. Used when the individual has difficulty in coping with environmental stresses and accomplishing daily activities

Types

A. chlordiazepoxide hydrochloride (Librium)
B. clorazepate dipotassium (Tranxene)
C. diazepam (Valium)
D. hydroxyzine hydrochloride, hydroxyzine pamoate (Atarax, Vistaril)
E. oxazepam (Serax)
F. alprazolam (Xanax)
G. meprobamate (Miltown)

Precautions

A. Drug interactions: drugs potentiate depressant effects of alcohol or sedatives

B. Adverse effects: drowsiness, hypotention, muscle relaxation, decreased ability to concentrate occur frequently in initial days of therapy; hypersensitivity reactions

Nursing Care

A. Utilize safety precautions for hospitalized clients upon initiating therapy (supervise ambulation)

B. Assess for signs of dependence

C. Monitor blood work during long-term therapy

D. Instruct client to
   a. Avoid engaging in hazardous activity
   b. Avoid concurrent use of alcohol
   c. Avoid administration with other CNS depressants

E. Administer controlled substances according to appropriate schedule restrictions

F. Evaluate client's response to medication and understanding of teaching

MAJOR TRANQUILIZERS
Description

A. Used to alter the symptoms of individuals experiencing detachment from reality and having the potential for manifesting destructive behavior
B. Act by blocking dopamine receptors in the CNS and sympathetic nervous system activity; some also exert antiemetic, anticholinergic, and antihistaminic effects
C. Major tranquilizers are available in oral and parenteral (IM, IV) preparations
D. Used when the individual is incapable of coping with environmental stresses and accomplishing daily activities
E. Major tranquilizers control behavior when the client's uncontrolled actions are destructive to self, others, or the environment

Types

A. Phenothiazine derivatives
  1. chlorpromazine hydrochloride (Thorazine)
  2. fluphenazine hydrochloride (Prolixin)
  3. perphenazine (Trilafon)
  4. prochlorperazine (Compazine)
  5. promazine hydrochloride (Sparine)
  6. thioridazine hydrochloride (Mellaril)
  7. trifluoperazine (Stelazine)
  8. triflupromazine hydrochloride (Vesprin)
  9. fluphenazine decanoate injection (Prolixin Deconate): maintenance dose effective in controlling symptoms for 4 weeks or longer
B. Butyrophenones
  1. droperidol (Inapsine)
  2. haloperidol (Haldol)
C. Dihydroindolone: molidone hydrochloride (Moban)
D. Thioxanthenes
  1. chlorprothixene (Taractan)
  2. thiothixene (Navane)

Precautions

A. Drug interactions: potentiate the action of alcohol, barbiturates, antihypertensives, and anticholinergics; concomitant use should be avoided when possible; antipsychotic medications should be temporarily discontinued when spinal or epidural anesthesia is necessary
B. Adverse effects of major tranquilizers: agranulocytosis (manifested by cold or sore throat), jaundice, signs of extrapyramidal tract irritation, drowsiness (highest incidence in initial days of therapy), orthostatic hypotension, constipation, urinary retention, anorexia, hypersensitivity reactions (tissue fluid accumulation, photoallergic reaction, impotence, cessation of menses or ovulation), cardiac toxicity
  1. Extrapyramidal symptoms
    a. Acute dystonic reaction: occurs early in treatment, sometimes after a single dose of tranquilizer; involves bizarre and severe muscle contractions
    b. Pseudoparkinsonism: resembles true parkinsonism (tremor, masklike facies, drooling, restlessness)
    c. Akinesia: fatigue, weakness of arms and legs

    d. Akathisia: motor restlessness
    e. Tardive dyskinesia: most severe extrapyramidal effect characterized by involuntary movements of face, jaw, and tongue resulting in bizarre grimacing, lip smacking, protrusion of tongue, jerking of the head and neck, extension and flexion of fingers, and clonic motion of the spine; occurs after prolonged use of antipsychotic drugs; antiparkinsonian drugs ineffective and condition is usually irreversible; all medication is usually stopped to see if syndrome will spontaneously disappear
  2. Antiparkinsonian drugs: block the extrapyramidal symptoms
    a. benztropine (Cogentin)
    b. biperiden (Akineton)
    c. diphenhydramine (Benadryl)
    d. trihexyphenidyl (Artane)

Nursing Care

A. Monitor for signs of hepatic toxicity (e.g., jaundice)
B. Monitor for signs of infection (e.g., sore throat)
C. Monitor blood pressure in standing and supine positions
D. Offer sugar-free chewing gum or hard candy to increase salivation
E. Assist with ambulation as necessary; keep siderails up when nonambulatory
F. Assess for extrapyramidal symptoms (antiparkinsonism agent may be prescribed to decrease symptoms)
G. Monitor blood work during long-term therapy
H. Instruct client to
  1. Avoid administration with other CNS depressants, including concurrent use of alcohol
  2. Avoid engaging in potentially hazardous activities
  3. Avoid exposure to direct sunlight; wear protective clothing
  4. Recognize extrapyramidal symptoms and report their occurrence to the physician immediately
  5. Avoid changing positions rapidly
  6. Notify physician if sore throat, fever, or weakness occurs; avoid crowded, potentially infectious places
I. Evaluate client's response to medication and understanding of teaching

ANTIDEPRESSANTS
Description

A. Used to improve the general behavior and mood of clients experiencing depressive episodes
B. Antidepressant drugs increase the level of norepinephrine at subcortical neuroeffector sites
C. Available in oral and parenteral (IM) preparations
D. Norepinephrine blockers provide elevated levels of the neurohormone by preventing reuptake and storage at the axon (tricyclic compounds)
E. Monoamine oxidase inhibitors (MAOIs) elevate norepinephrine levels in brain tissues by interfering with the enzyme MAO; act as psychic energizers
F. fluoxetine hydrochloride promotes the uptake of serotonin in the CNS

Types

A. Norepinephrine blockers
1. amitriptyline hydrochloride (Elavil)
2. desipramine hydrochloride (Norpramin, Pertofrane)
3. doxepin hydrochloride (Adapin, Sinequan)
4. imipramine hydrochloride (Presamine, Tofranil)
5. nortriptyline hydrochloride (Aventyl)
6. protriptyline hydrochloride (Pamelor, Vivactil)
B. Monoamine oxidase inhibitors (MAOIs)
1. isocarboxazid (Marplan)
2. phenelzine sulfate (Nardil)
3. tranylcypromine sulfate (Parnate)
C. fluoxetine hydrochloride (Prozac)

Precautions

A. Norepinephrine blockers
1. Drug interactions: potentiate effects of anticholinergic drugs and CNS depressants (e.g., alcohol and sedatives)
2. Adverse effects: orthostatic hypotension, skin rash, drowsiness, dry mouth, blurred vision, constipation, urine retention, tachycardia, CNS stimulation in elderly clients (excitement, restlessness, incoordination, fine tremor), nightmares, delusions, disorientation, insomnia
B. Monoamine oxidase inhibitors (MAOIs)
1. Drug interactions: MAOIs potentiate the effects of alcohol, barbiturates, anesthetic agents (cocaine), antihistamines, narcotics, corticoids, anticholinergics, and sympathomimetic drugs
2. Drug-food interactions: hypertensive crisis with vascular rupture, occipital headache, palpitation, stiffness of neck muscles, emesis, sweating, photophobia, and cardiac arrhythmias may occur when neurohormonal levels are elevated by ingestion of foods with high tyramine content (pickled herring, beer, wine, chicken livers, aged or natural cheese, chocolate)
3. Adverse effects: CNS stimulation (headache, restlessness, insomnia), peripheral edema, orthostatic hypotension, dry mouth, constipation, urine retention, transient impotence, anorexia, nausea
C. Fluoxetine hydrochloride
1. Drug interactions: may interact with Tryptophan, diazepam, warfarin, and digitoxin; should be discontinued for 2 weeks prior to administration of MAOIs
2. Adverse effects: insomnia, headache, flu-like syndrome, dry mouth, and sexual dysfunction

Nursing Care

A. Assess for effectiveness of drug action
B. Maintain suicide precautions, especially as depression begins to lift; carefully monitor blood sugar in diabetics
C. Instruct client to
1. Change positions slowly
2. Avoid engaging in hazardous activities
3. Utilize sugar-free chewing gum or hard candy to stimulate salivation
4. Check all OTC preparations with physician before use

5. Expect therapeutic effect to be delayed; may take 3 to 4 weeks with tricyclics; 2 weeks with Prozac; 1 to 4 weeks with MAOIs
D. MAOIs
1. Maintain dietary restrictions; avoid foods containing tyramine (aged cheeses, beer, chianti wine, yogurt, soy sauce, chocolate)
2. Monitor client for occurrence of hypertensive crisis (severe headache, palpitations)
E. Avoid concurrent administration of adrenergic drugs
F. Evaluate client's response to medication and understanding of teaching

LITHIUM
Description

A. Used to control the manic episode of mood disorders
B. Acts by reducing adrenergic neurotransmitter levels in cerebral tissue through alteration of sodium transport
C. Lithium is available in oral capsules and tablets, both regular and sustained release forms, and liquid preparations
D. Improves productivity by decreasing psychomotor activity or response to environmental stimuli
E. Norepinephrine uptake accelerator which alters sodium transport in nerve and muscle cells and affects a shift in intraneural metabolism of norepinephrine

Types

lithium carbonate (Eskalith, Lithane, Lithonate)

Precautions

A. Drug interactions: diuretics increase the reabsorption of lithium resulting in possible toxic effects; haloperidol and thioridazine can result in encephalopathic syndrome; sodium bicarbonate or sodium chloride increase the excretion of lithium
B. Drug-food interaction: restriction of sodium intake increases drug substitution for sodium ions, which causes signs of hyponatremia (nausea, vomiting, diarrhea, muscle fasciculations, stupor, convulsions); therefore salt intake must be maintained
C. Adverse effects: excess voiding and extreme thirst caused by drug suppression of antidiuretic hormone (ADH) function, which causes dehydration; slurred speech, disorientation, confusion, cogwheel rigidity, ataxia, renal failure, respiratory depression, and coma are toxic side effects; toxic effects can easily occur because the difference between the therapeutic level and toxic level is slight

Nursing Care

A. Recognize that therapeutic effects will be delayed for several weeks
B. Recognize that dehydration and hyponatremia predispose the client to lithium toxicity
C. Assess therapeutic blood levels (0.6-1.2 mEq/L) during course of therapy
D. Avoid concurrent administration of adrenergic drugs
E. Maintain normal sodium intake during course of therapy
F. Encourage increased fluid intake

G. Supervise ambulation if necessary

H. Administer with meals to reduce GI irritation

I. Teach the client that the nausea, polyuria, and thirst that occurs initially will subside after several days

J. Teach client and family to observe for signs of toxicity such as diarrhea, vomiting, drowsiness, muscular weakness, and ataxia

K. Evaluate client's response to medication and understanding of teaching

DRUGS THAT PRODUCE SEDATION AND SLEEP
Description

A. Sedatives and hypnotics can be used in addition to tranquilizers for psychiatric and other clients

B. Central nervous system depressants have antianxiety effects in low dosages, produce sleep in high dosages, and general anesthetic-like states in very high dosages

C. All hypnotic drugs probably alter either the character or the duration of REM sleep

Types with Related Precautions

A. Trichloroacetic acid: produces natural sleep
   1. Drugs
      a. chloral betaine (Beta-Chlor)
      b. chloral hydrate (Felsules, Lorinal, Noctec, Somnos)
      c. petrichloral (Periclor)
   2. Adverse effects: gastric irritation causing diarrhea
   3. Drug interactions: potentiates the effects of alcohol taken concurrently causing sudden loss of consciousness
   4. Considerations during therapy: drug metabolites cause false positive reaction for glycosuria when Benedict's reagent is used for testing

B. Paraldehyde: used primarily to diminish hyperactivity in alcoholics or to control convulsions; has a pungent odor and taste, and elimination from the lungs results in an environmental odor

C. Phenothiazine derivatives: act like antihistamines; used for sleep induction in anxious clients
   1. Drugs
      a. methotrimeprazine hydrochloride (Levoprome)
      b. promazine hydrochloride (Sparine)
      c. propiomazine hydrochloride (Largon)
   2. Adverse effects: hypotension, dizziness, dry mouth, cardiac palpitations, pseudoparkinsonism symptoms, cholestatic jaundice, agranulocytosis

D. Barbiturate sedatives: most frequently used hypnotics
   1. High lipoid tissue affinity: rapid response, short acting
      a. hexobarbital (Sombucaps, Sombulex)
      b. pentobarbital sodium (Nembutal)
      c. secobarbital sodium (Seconal)
   2. Moderate lipoid tissue affinity: moderately slow response, intermediate acting
      a. amobarbital (Amytal)
      b. aprobarbital (Alurate)
      c. butabarbital sodium (Bubartal Sodium, Butisol Sodium)
      d. probarbital calcium (Ipral)
      e. talbutal (Lotusate)

   3. Low lipoid tissue affinity: slow response
      a. barbital (Neuronidia)
      b. phenobarbital (Luminal)
   4. Adverse effects: morning drowsiness, hypersensitivity reactions (photosensitivity, dermatologic reactions), respiratory depression, and hypotension (most frequent with parenteral use)
   5. Fatalities from overdosage: depend on degree of lipoid tissue affinity
      a. High lipotropic group: rapid respiratory depression, marked hypotension after ingestion of excess
      b. Moderate lipotropic group: protracted period of sedation, but allows time-lapse for resuscitation or reconsideration
      c. Low lipotropic group: excretion concurrent with slow action, least popular for self-induced overdosage
   6. Drug interaction: lowers blood levels of orally administered griseofulvin and decreases the therapeutic effect; increases activity of hepatic microsomal enzymes; the accelerated metabolism of oral anticoagulants lowers their hypoprothrombinemic effect

E. Other sedatives and hypnotics and their adverse effects
   1. ethchlorvynol (Placidyl): morning drowsiness, blurred vision, transient hypotension
   2. ethinamate (Valmid): morning drowsiness
   3. flurazepam hydrochloride (Dalmane): dizziness, tachycardia, GI disturbances
   4. methaqualone (Quaalude, Sopor): morning drowsiness, GI disturbances
   5. methyprylon (Noludar): morning drowsiness, GI disturbances
   6. sodium bromide (primarily for daytime sedation): gastric irritation, generalized rash, tremors of the hands, tremulousness of the lips and tongue, impaired mental processes, auditory and visual hallucinations, coma with long-term use
   7. glutethimide (Doriden)
      a. Morning drowsiness, transient hypotension, and infrequently produces pharyngeal and laryngeal reflex depression
      b. Acts synergistically with oral anticoagulants to decrease their effectiveness

F. Excess ingestion
   1. Any of the sedative-hypnotics may cause unconsciousness, coma, death
   2. Addiction to these drugs alone or in combination has increased
   3. Removal of drug from the stomach by aspiration, resuscitative measures (assisted ventilation, cardiac massage), hemodialysis of diffusible drug, vasopressor administration to counteract vascular collapse, and correction of acidosis
   4. Follow-up supervision to avoid repetition of the problem

G. Drugs are habit forming; withdrawal after long-term use many precipitate severe symptoms: anxiety, tremor, insomnia, confusion, perceptual distortions, agitation, delirium, GI disturbances, orthostatic hypotension, convulsions leading to cardiovascular collapse and death

Nursing Care

See Nursing care under Minor tranquilizers

Classification of Mental Disorders*

A. Disorders usually first evident in infancy, childhood, or adolescence
  1. Mental retardation
  2. Pervasive developmental disorders
  3. Disruptive behavior disorders
  4. Anxiety disorders of childhood and adolescence
  5. Eating disorders
  6. Gender identity disorders
  7. Tic disorders
  8. Elimination disorders
  9. Speech disorders
B. Organic mental syndromes and disorders
  1. Organic mental syndromes
    a. Delirium
    b. Dementia
  2. Organic mental disorders (dementias arising in the sensium and presensium)
    a. Primary degenerative dementia, senile onset
    b. Primary degenerative dementia, presenile onset
  3. Psychoactive substance-induced organic mental disorders
C. Psychoactive substance use disorders
  1. Alcohol abuse
  2. Drug dependence
D. Schizophrenia
E. Paranoid disorder
F. Mood disorders
  1. Major mood disorders
    a. Bipolar disorder
    b. Major depression
  2. Other mood disorders
G. Anxiety disorders
  1. Phobic disorders
  2. Anxiety states
  3. Obsessive compulsive disorder
  4. Post-traumatic stress disorder
H. Somatoform disorders
I. Dissociative disorders
J. Sexual disorders
K. Adjustment disorders
L. Personality disorders

Disorders Usually First Evident in Infancy, Childhood, or Adolescence
NURSING PROCESS FOR CLIENTS WITH DISORDERS USUALLY FIRST EVIDENT IN INFANCY, CHILDHOOD, OR ADOLESCENCE
Probable Nursing Diagnoses Based on Assessment

A. Impaired verbal communication related to
  1. Cerebral deficits
  2. Psychologic barriers

B. Ineffective family coping: disabling, related to
  1. Unresolved emotions
  2. Prolonged denial of problem
  3. Ambivalent family relationships
  4. Inadequate resources
  5. Abusive or destructive behavior
C. Altered family processes related to
  1. Disturbed family interactions
  2. Disturbed behavior of infant, child, or adolescent
  3. Failure of infant, child, or adolescent to meet role expectations
D. Ineffective individual coping related to
  1. Inadequate support system
  2. Personal vulnerability
  3. Inability to meet basic needs
  4. Inability to meet role expectations
  5. Poorly developed or inappropriate use of defense mechanisms
E. Impaired home maintenance management related to
  1. Inadequate support system
  2. Difficulty in maintaining child or adolescent in the home because of threats to safety
  3. Lack of or failure to use community resources
  4. Disturbed or destructive behavior of child or adolescent
F. Potential for injury related to
  1. Sensory deficits
  2. Altered judgment
G. Altered nutrition: less or more than body requirements related to
  1. Disturbed body image
  2. Dysfunctional emotional conditioning in relationship to food
H. Feeding, bathing/hygiene, dressing/grooming, toileting self-care deficit related to
  1. Perceptual or cognitive impairment
  2. Emotional dysfunctioning
I. Sensory/perceptual alterations (visual, auditory, kinesthetic, gustatory, tactile, olfactory) related to
  1. Perceptual or cognitive impairment
  2. Emotional dysfunction
  3. Misinterpretation of stimuli
  4. Inability to evaluate reality
J. Sleep pattern disturbance related to emotional dysfunctioning
K. Altered thought processes related to
  1. Inability to evaluate reality
  2. Disturbed interpretation of environment
  3. Disturbed mental activities
  4. Altered sensory perception, reception, and transmission
L. Violence, potential for: self-directed or directed at others, related to
  1. Feelings of suspicion or distrust of others
  2. Inability to discharge emotions verbally
  3. Misinterpretation of stimuli
M. Chronic low self-esteem related to
  1. Perceptual or cognitive impairment
  2. Emotional dysfunctioning
  3. Disturbed relationships
  4. Frequent lack of success

---

*Adapted from Diagnostic and statistical manual of mental disorders, ed. 3, Revised, Washington, D.C., 1987, American Psychiatric Association.

N. Body image disturbance related to
1. Inability to evaluate reality
2. Perceptual or cognitive impairment
O. Personal identity disturbance related to
1. Inability to establish self boundaries
2. Inability to interpret reality
3. Failure to develop meaningful relationships
4. Nonacceptance of gender
P. Anxiety related to
1. Frequent lack of success
2. Inability to meet expectations of others
3. Failure to develop meaningful relationships

Nursing Care for Clients with Disorders Usually First Evident in Infancy, Childhood, Or Adolescence

A. Recognize that all children, especially these children, require
1. Protection from danger
2. Love and acceptance
3. Basic physiological needs to be met
4. Meaningful relationships
5. An opportunity to explore the environment
B. Direct care toward helping the child grow up emotionally by
1. Establishing a favorable environment in which the child can gain or regain a favorable equilibrium
2. Establishing a constructive relationship
3. Helping the child to see self as a worthwhile person
4. Recognizing that the behavior has meaning for the child
5. Being as realistic and as truthful as possible in dealing with the child
6. Attempting to establish trust
7. Setting limits that are as realistic as possible but as firm as necessary
8. Pointing out reality, but accepting the child's views of it while pointing it out
9. Being consistent both in approach and in rules and regulations
10. Making all explanations as clear as possible
11. Supporting and encouraging the child's moves toward independence but allowing dependency when necessary
C. Evaluate client's response and revise plan as necessary

MENTAL RETARDATION

Mental retardation is covered in Pediatric Nursing

PERVASIVE DEVELOPMENTAL DISORDER— AUTISTIC DISORDER

A. Many theories as to cause are being studied; however, no definitive cause has been established
B. Failure to develop satisfactory relationships with significant adults, regardless of the cause, appears to be an underlying problem
C. Symptoms
1. An alienation or withdrawal from reality
2. A severe disturbance in the child's feeling of self-identity
3. Inability to differentiate between self and environment

4. Confusion in self-boundaries frequently characterized by speaking of self only in the third person
5. A defect in ego formation or an inadequately functioning ego system
6. A conflict between self and reality
7. Defect in the adaptive, inhibitory, and steering mechanisms of the personality
8. Interference with intellect may be so profound, child appears to be mentally retarded
9. Lack of meaningful relationships with outside world
10. Use of autistic fantasy resulting in communication defects
11. Turning to inanimate objects and self-centered activity for security
12. Symptoms associated with severe autism include
a. Profound apathy
b. Looseness of association
c. Autistic thinking
d. Ambivalence
e. Absence of communication skills
f. Poor grasp of reality
g. Bizarre, unpredictable, uncontrolled behavior
h. Inability to relate to others
i. Total interference with intellectual functioning
D. Therapy
1. Psychotherapy directed toward the developmental level of the child: play, group, or individual therapy
2. Medications: tranquilizers and amphetamines provide some reduction of symptoms
3. Removal from the home situation may be necessary, although day school situations frequently provide enough relief so that hospitalization can be avoided
E. Nursing care
1. For general nursing care see Nursing care at the beginning of this classification
2. Accept child's need to push away but continue to make physical contact on a regular basis
3. Provide a consistent routine for activities of daily living
4. Maintain a consistent familiar environment
5. Use picture and letter boards to assist in communication
6. Set consistent and firm limits for behavior
7. Prevent acts of self-distructive behavior
8. Evaluate client's response and revise plan as necessary

DISRUPTIVE BEHAVIOR DISORDERS
Attention-deficit Hyperactivity Disorder

A. Diagnosis difficult, since the pathology must be separated from normal disturbances that occur during this period of life
B. Evident before 7 years of age; lasting at least 6 months
C. Symptoms
1. Inappropriately inattentive
2. Excessive impulsiveness
3. Short attention span
4. Squirming and fidgeting
5. Hyperactivity may or may not be present
D. Therapy
1. Psychological counseling
2. Antianxiety medications

E. Nursing care
 1. For general nursing care see Nursing care at the beginning of this classification
 2. Plan activities that provide a balance between expenditure of energy and quiet time
 3. Set realistic, attainable goals
 4. Structure situations to provide less stimulation (play with only one other child rather than group)
 5. Provide firm and consistent discipline; ignore temper tantrums
 6. Provide exercises in perceptual-motor coordination and balance
 7. Structure learning experience to utilize the child's ability
 8. Provide opportunities so the child can experience success and satisfaction
 9. Administer drugs such as methylphenidate (Ritalin) or dextroamphetamine sulfate
 10. Evaluate client's response and revise plan as necessary

Conduct Disorders

A. The child may be socialized (evidence of social attachment) or undersocialized (little evidence of social attachment)
B. The child may be aggressive or nonaggressive
C. Symptoms
 1. Behavior is destructive to the child's own general aims
 2. Behavior is repeated despite rational arguments to the contrary and despite punishment
 3. Behavior leads to getting caught and punished
 4. Behavior includes stealing, truancy, running away, excessive rebelliousness, and physical cruelty to others and animals
 5. Conduct involves the discharge of affects stemming from unconscious conflicts
D. Therapy
 1. Psychological counseling
 2. Milieu therapy
E. Nursing care
 1. For general nursing care see Nursing care at the beginning of this classification
 2. Set a firm system of rewards and punishments within set limits
 3. Do not permit manipulation
 4. Evaluate client's response and revise plan as necessary

ANXIETY DISORDERS OF CHILDHOOD AND ADOLESCENCE

A. Separation anxiety disorder
 1. Excessive anxiety centered on harm befalling self, family, or those to whom child has attachment
 2. Equally common in males and females
 3. Symptoms
  a. Problems with sleeping unless near the person to whom child has attachment
  b. Refusal to attend school in order to remain near the person to whom child has attachment
  c. Physical complaints of headache and stomachaches when threat of separation is anticipated

B. Avoidant disorder of childhood and adolescense
 1. Limited social functioning and avoidance of new relationships for 6 months or longer
 2. More common in females than males
 3. Symptoms
  a. Avoidance of contact with unfamiliar people
  b. Social involvement limited to family members or people who are familiar to the child
  c. Excessive shyness and timidity when confronted with strangers
C. Overanxious disorder
 1. Excessive and unrealistic anxiety and worry
 2. Equally common in males and females
 3. Symptoms
  a. Worry about future events as well as appropriateness of past or future performance
  b. Physical complaints of headache, nausea, or shortness of breath
  c. Difficulty falling asleep at night
  d. Tense or nervous appearance and behavior
D. Therapy
 1. Psychotherapy: in children, usually in the form of play therapy
 2. Medications: amphetamines and mild tranquilizers are quite effective with children
E. Nursing care
 1. For general nursing care see Nursing care at the beginning of this classification
 2. Provide consistent caregivers
 3. Introduce child to new situations gradually; permit child to bring a familiar comforting toy
 4. Allow parent to stay with child as long as possible
 5. Evaluate client's response and revise plan as necessary

EATING DISORDERS
Anorexia Nervosa

A. Most common in adolescent through 30-year-old population
B. More common in females
C. Avoidance of food may result from excessive concern with obesity
D. Apparent failure to separate from mother and become autonomous
E. Usually triggered by an adolescent crisis
F. Symptoms
 1. Weigh less than 85% of expected weight
 2. Distorted self-image: appear fat to themselves even when emaciated
 3. Intense fear of becoming fat
 4. May have history of compulsive traits
 5. Usually very manipulative
 6. Usually high achievers academically
 7. Frequent discord in family relationships, especially with mother
 8. Often interested in food and cooking in general
 9. Cessation of menses in females
 10. Inability to sustain self-starvation may result in bulimic episodes: binging of food followed by self-induced vomiting
 11. Fatigue or hyperactivity
 12. Feeling of fullness after small intake

13. Nausea
14. Constipation
15. Emaciation
16. Hypotension
17. Low blood glucose
18. Anemia
19. Low BMR

G. Therapy
1. Unified team approach
2. Behavior modification techniques which focus on client's responsibility for weight gain
3. Time limit on meals
4. Use of nasogastric tube if weight loss is so great or fluid and electrolyte imbalance is so severe that it causes a threat to life
5. Psychotherapy focusing on self-image
6. Group therapy
7. Family therapy with all members of family involved
8. Gradually increase caloric and protein intake

H. Nursing care
1. For general nursing care see Nursing care at the beginning of this classification
2. Develop a therapeutic environment and offer emotional support; develop a trusting relationship
3. Briefly discuss dietary modification with the individual in a nonthreatening manner; encourage diet high in nutrient-dense foods; do not focus on eating or weight loss
4. Evaluate client's response and revise plan as necessary

Bulimia Nervosa

A. Most common in adolescent through 30-year-old population
B. More common in females
C. Obesity is frequently found in parents or siblings
D. Predisposition to depression
E. Discord in family relationships
F. Obsession with food results from a morbid fear of obesity and the pathologic need to binge
G. Symptoms
1. Compulsive eating binges characterized by rapid consumption of excessive amounts of high caloric foods in brief periods followed by induced purging (vomiting, enemas, laxatives, or diuretics)
2. Periods of severe dieting or fasting between binges
3. Sporadic vigorous exercising between binges
4. Weight may be within normal range with frequent fluctuations, above or below normal range due to alternating binges and fasts
5. Awareness that the eating pattern is abnormal along with a fear of not being able to stop voluntarily
6. Depression and self-deprecating thoughts follow binges
7. Impulsive
8. Extroverted
9. Possible intermittent substance abuse
10. Very concerned with body image and appearance
11. Repeated attempts to control or lose weight
H. Therapy
See Therapy under Anorexia nervosa

I. Nursing care
1. See Nursing care under Anorexia nervosa
2. Keep client under close observation to prevent purging
3. Evaluate client's response and revise plan as necessary

Obesity Related to Compulsive Overeating

A. Excessive weight gain that occurs when intake of calories exceeds expenditure of energy over time
B. Compulsive intake of food without the purging associated with bulimia nervosa
C. Although binges may occur, overeating is usually fairly constant over time
D. Overeating seems to be related to
1. View of food in a context other than satiation of hunger
2. Use of food as a panacea or reward
3. Social and emotional stresses
4. Although calorie intake is excessive there appears to be some relationship to lack of exercise, genetic predisposition, or metabolic imbalances
5. Problem usually starts in childhood where eating patterns are established
E. Overeating can result in multiple biochemical disturbances including increased insulin resistance, glucose intolerance, changes in fatty acid metabolism, and alterations in other hormonal and enzymatic processes resulting in disturbed cell physiology
F. Symptoms
1. Continued ingestion of food after hunger is satiated
2. Lack of control over eating
3. Frequent attempts at weight loss; history of trying multiple diets
4. Low self-esteem related to feelings of lack of willpower or weakness
5. Weight gain that exceeds 15% of ideal weight on the standard height-weight table
6. Skinfold thickness greater than 26 mm measured on triceps, or suprailiac, with skinfold calipers
G. Therapy
1. Balanced calorie-restricted diet that is followed for a more long-term effect; 1 or 2 pound per week loss yields optimal results
2. Behavior modification program
a. Food diary (self-monitoring)
b. Control speed of eating; food should be chewed for preset length of time
c. Reinforce compliance (system of rewards should be established for changes in eating patterns or reduction of pounds)
3. Support groups
4. Psychotherapy
5. Hypnotherapy
H. Nursing care
1. For general nursing care see Nursing care at the beginning of this classification
2. Provide emotional support by assisting the client to separate eating behavior from evaluation of self as good or bad
3. Praise client for progress but expect and accept lapses

4. Encourage client to plan special treats in the diet
5. Help client uncover new outlets for emotional expression other than food
6. Help client set realistic, attainable short-term goals
7. Evaluate client's response and revise plan as necessary

GENDER IDENTITY DISORDERS

Persistent discomfort with one's assigned gender and a feeling that it is inappropriate or inaccurate

A. Prepubescent gender identity disorder
   1. Has intense discomfort with own gender and desires to be the opposite sex or believes that he or she is the opposite sex
   2. Rejects anatomical structures associated with own gender
   3. Cross-dresses and participates in activities associated with opposite sex
   4. Has not reached puberty
B. Transsexualism
   1. Has intense desire to exchange own sexual characteristics for those of the opposite sex
   2. Complains of discomfort wearing clothing of assigned sexual role
   3. Has anxiety and depression related to conformity with assigned sexual role
   4. Has reached puberty
   5. Can be asexual, homosexual, or heterosexual
C. Nontranssexual type
   1. Has no intense desire to acquire sexual characteristics of opposite sex, yet a persistent feeling of discomfort with one's assigned gender
   2. Cross-dressing is practiced but without the purpose of sexual excitement
   3. Anxiety and depression are usually decreased when the person is cross-dressing
   4. Has reached puberty
   5. Can be asexual, homosexual, or heterosexual
D. Therapy
   1. Individual or group psychotherapy
   2. Antianxiety medication if necessary
E. Nursing care
   1. For general nursing care see Nursing care at the beginning of this classification
   2. Accept and understand client's discomfort with gender
   3. Accept own feelings about client's cross-dressing
   4. Encourage client to become involved with support groups
   5. Be aware that if discomfort or depression is severe, self-mutilation or suicide are possibilities
   6. Evaluate client's response and revise plan as necessary

TIC DISORDERS

A. Classified as gross motor movement disorders
   1. Transient tic disorder
   2. Chronic motor tic disorder
   3. Tourette's syndrome
   4. It is not known if these three tic disorders are separate and distinct disorders or one disorder exhibiting progressively severe symptoms

B. Symptoms
   1. Involuntary, uncontrolled, multiple, rapid movements of muscles such as eye blinking, twitching, and head shaking that occur in bouts throughout the day
   2. Involuntary production of sounds such as throat clearing, grunting, barking, or socially unacceptable words
   3. Can often be controlled for short duration; not present during sleep; increased during times of stress
   4. Starts in early childhood
   5. More common in boys than girls
C. Therapy
   1. Treat any precipitating factor such as head injury, psychoactive substance intoxication, or infection
   2. Supportive individual or group counseling
   3. Medications such as sedatives or Dilantin may be prescribed although they are not shown to be effective with these disorders
D. Nursing care
   1. For general nursing care see Nursing care at the beginning of this classification
   2. Accept behavior recognizing that it is often uncontrollable
   3. Support client's attempts to control tic
   4. Note precipitating factors, if present, and frequency and duration of stereotyped movements

ELIMINATION DISORDERS

A. Classification
   1. Functional encopresis: involuntary or intentional defecation in inappropriate places, including clothing, after the age of 4
   2. Functional enuresis: involuntary or intentional micturition in inappropriate places, including clothing, after the age of 4
B. Symptoms
   1. These disorders are more common in boys than girls
   2. No identifiable physical problems are present
   3. Can occur before toilet training has been accomplished (primary) or after a period of controlled continence (secondary)
   4. Nocturnal bedwetting is most frequent; child may or may not be aware of voiding or recall a dream about the act of urinating
   5. Academic difficulties
   6. Loss of self-esteem
   7. Rejection by peers
   8. Severe anxiety
C. Therapy
   1. Rule out structural or organic causes
   2. Psychotherapy
   3. Medications such as antidepressants (Elavil) have been found to be effective with some clients
D. Nursing care
   1. For general nursing care see Nursing care at the beginning of this classification
   2. Change linen and clothing in a nonjudgmental manner to avoid further embarrassment for the client

3. Recognize and accept that the act is not motivated by hostility
4. Evaluate client's response and revise plan as necessary

SPEECH DISORDERS

A. Classification
   1. Cluttering: abnormally rapid, erratic, dysrhythmic speech patterns that make communication very difficult to follow
   2. Stuttering: frequent repitition of sounds or syllables impairing speech fluency although child has normal laryngeal skills; usually occurring at the beginning of a word or phrase
B. Symptoms
   1. Presence of faulty speech patterns that are persistent and increased by stress
   2. Anxiety
   3. Avoidance of social situations
   4. Loss of self-esteem
C. Therapy
   1. Speech therapy
   2. Counseling to reduce anxiety
D. Nursing care
   1. For general nursing care see Nursing care at the beginning of this classification
   2. Encourage client to adhere to speech therapy routine
   3. Allow individual time to verbalize; do not complete word or speech for the individual
   4. Evaluate client's response and revise plan as necessary

Organic Mental Syndromes and Disorders

Associated with actual changes in the tissue of the brain

NURSING PROCESS FOR CLIENTS WITH ORGANIC MENTAL SYNDROMES AND DISORDERS
Probable Nursing Diagnoses Based on Assessment

A. Anxiety related to
   1. Recognized early memory loss
   2. Threat to self-concept
   3. Change in environment
   4. Motor and sensory loss
B. Impaired verbal communication related to
   1. Progressive cerebral impairment
   2. Progressive neurological losses
   3. Aphasia
   4. Apathy and/or withdrawal from others
C. Ineffective individual coping related to
   1. Change in usual communication patterns
   2. Inability to meet role expectations
   3. Inability to meet basic needs
   4. Alteration in social participation
   5. High incidence of accidents
D. Altered family processes related to
   1. Change of roles within the family
   2. Change in family member's ability to function

3. Difficulty in dealing with progressive degeneration of family member; resultant guilt from feelings of resentment
4. Institutionalization of family member
E. Potential for injury related to
   1. Cognitive deficits
   2. Psychomotor deficits
F. Sensory/perceptual alterations (visual, auditory, kinesthetic, gustatory, tactile, olfactory) related to
   1. Progressive cerebral impairment
   2. Progressive neurological losses
G. Feeding, bathing/hygiene, dressing/grooming, toileting self-care deficit related to
   1. Cognitive or sensory impairment
   2. Increasing inability to carry out activities of daily living
H. Altered thought processes related to
   1. Inability to transmit messages
   2. Destruction of cerebral tissue
I. Impaired home maintenance management related to
   1. Impaired mental status
   2. Progressive inability to carry out activities of daily living
   3. Difficulty in maintaining self or family in the home because of threats to safety
J. Altered nutrition: less than body requirements related to
   1. Confusion
   2. Depression
   3. Anorexia
K. Situational low self-esteem related to
   1. Inability to handle situation or events
   2. Difficulty making decisions
L. Potential for violence: self-directed or directed at others, related to
   1. Sensory perceptual alterations
   2. Toxic reactions in or progressive deterioration of cerebral tissue

Nursing Care for Clients with Organic Mental Syndromes and Disorders

A. Provide a safe environment; provide direct supervision as necessary
B. Continually orient the client to time, date, and place
C. Keep client involved in reality and in the home situation as long as possible
D. Allow client to assume as much responsibility for self-care as possible
E. Provide a quiet environment, reduce stimuli
F. Plan care so the staff approaches these clients when they appear receptive
G. Keep the schedule of activities flexible to make use of the client's lability of mood and easy distractability
H. Encourage adequate nutritional intake; monitor intake and output
I. Provide diversional activities including exercises that the client enjoys and can handle
J. Observe for changing physiological and neurologic symptoms
K. Support family caregivers; maintain nonjudgmental attitude

L. Help provide some relief from responsibility of total care; refer to community agencies that provide home care helpers or respite care if appropriate
M. Support the family's decision to place client in a nursing home
N. Evaluate client's response and revise plan as necessary

DELIRIUM

A. Syndromes from which the client usually recovers, since the situation is often reversible and temporary
B. Characteristics
   1. Infection
     a. Intracranial or nervous system (e.g., meningitis or encephalitis)
     b. Systemic or toxic (e.g., pneumonia or typhoid)
   2. Trauma to the head
   3. Circulatory disturbances resulting in impairment of blood flow to the brain
   4. Metabolic disorders: electrolyte imbalance (e.g., dehydration, diarrhea, vomiting)
C. Symptoms
   1. Delirium and its accompanying confusion, hallucinations, and delusions
   2. Disorientation and confusion as to time, place, identity
   3. Memory defects for both recent and remote events and facts
   4. Slurring of speech may occur along with an indistinct pronunciation or use of words
   5. Tremors, incoordination, imbalance, and incontinence may develop
D. Therapy
   1. Reduce causative agent such as fever or toxins
   2. Prevent further damage
   3. Provide diet high in calories, protein, and vitamins
   4. Provide mild sedative if necessary
E. Nursing care
   See Nursing care at the beginning of this classification

DEMENTIA

A. Syndromes from which the client does not recover, since the damage is irreversible and permanent; there may be some improvement with treatment of the underlying cause, but disturbances in memory and judgment will remain
B. Characteristics
   1. Prenatal injury or malformation (e.g., hydrocephalus, microcephalus, neurosyphilis)
   2. Infections such as general paresis
   3. Trauma in which a head injury results in permanent brain damage
   4. Circulatory disturbances causing anoxia and permanent brain damage (e.g., cerebral arteriosclerosis, CVA)
   5. Nutritional deprivation of brain cells (e.g., pellagra)
   6. Damage resulting from generalized diseases (e.g., multiple sclerosis, hepatolenticular disease, Huntington's chorea, Parkinson's disease)
   7. Damage resulting from pressure of brain tumors
C. Symptoms: same as those resulting from delirium

D. Therapy: same as those for delirium, with greater emphasis on preventing further damage
E. Nursing care
   See Nursing care at the beginning of this classification

DEMENTIAS ARISING IN THE SENIUM AND PRESENIUM

(Alzheimer's disease and dementia of the Alzheimer's type most common)
A. Primary degenerative dementia, senile onset: occurs after age 65
B. Primary degenerative dementia, presenile onset: occurs before age 65
C. Characteristics
   1. Atrophy of brain accompanied by widened cortical sulci and enlarged cerebral ventricles
   2. Microscopic brain changes include senile plaques and a granulovacuolar degeneration of neurons
   3. Believed to be related to the brain's inability to produce sufficient neurotransmitters which transmit messages through the brain
D. Symptoms
   1. See Dementia
   2. More common in females than males; effects between 2% and 4% of population over age 65 but can occur as early as 35; appears to be a familial or genetic predisposition
   3. Differs from normal changes associated with aging
   4. Dementia has an insidious onset with symptoms following a progressively downhill course; changes are unrelated to any other specific cause
   5. Progression moves from mild forgetfulness for recent events to mutism, inability to carry out any activities of daily living, and incontinence; degeneration usually ends in a vegetative state and coma; disease is 100% fatal and death usually occurs within 5 years; currently the fourth leading cause of death in the United States
E. Therapy
   1. Rule out causes such as fluid and electrolyte or vitamin deficiencies, excessive medication, exogenous poisons, or metabolic disorders
   2. Provide supportive care including good nutrition with supplemental vitamins
   3. Admit to a total care institution when necessary
F. Nursing care
   See Nursing care at the beginning of this classification

PSYCHOACTIVE SUBSTANCE-INDUCED ORGANIC MENTAL DISORDERS

A. Nervous system, particularly the CNS, directly affected by substances taken nonmedically (alcohol, opiates, barbituates, cocaine, etc.) to alter mood and behavior
B. Usually occurs in individuals with substance abuse disorders
C. Behavioral changes may be related to a vitamin deficiency, especially in long-term alcohol abuse such as Korsakoff's syndrome
D. Symptoms
   1. Specific neurological and psychological signs and maladaptive behavior such as euphoria; dysphoria;

apathy; and psychomotor agitation, excitement, or depression; hypervigilance; fighting or violent behavior

2. Symptoms of dementia or delirium may be present depending upon the substance used
3. Physical symptoms such as depressed respiration, cardiac irregularities, and gastrointestinal changes may occur
E. Therapy
   See Delirium
F. Nursing care
   See Nursing care at the beginning of this classification

Psychoactive Substance-Use Disorders
NURSING PROCESS FOR CLIENTS WITH PSYCHOACTIVE SUBSTANCE-USE DISORDERS
Probable Nursing Diagnoses Based on Assessment

A. Anxiety related to
   1. Threat to self-concept
   2. Inability to deal with responsibility
   3. Feelings of inadequacy
   4. Concern regarding continued source of abused substance
B. Impaired verbal communication related to
   1. Inability to verbalize feelings and thoughts
   2. Mental confusion or CNS depression because of substance use
C. Ineffective family coping: compromised, related to
   1. Individual's preoccupation with abused substance
   2. Anger, frustration, and exhaustion associated with client's negative response to attempts at assistance or support
D. Ineffective individual coping related to
   1. Inability to meet basic needs or role expectations
   2. Inability to tolerate frustration
   3. Inappropriate use of defense mechanisms
   4. Excessive use of an abusing substance
E. Defensive coping related to
   1. Denial of obvious problem
   2. Projection of blame/responsibility
   3. Rationalization of failures
   4. Lack of participation in treatment or therapy
F. Denial related to inability to admit impact of problem on pattern of life
G. Self-esteem disturbance related to
   1. Inability to meet role expectations
   2. Feelings of inadequacy and expectation of failure
   3. Inability to accept strengths
   4. Negative feelings about self
H. Altered health maintenance related to
   1. Unhealthy life-style because of substance abuse
   2. Inability to take responsibility for health needs
   3. Failure to recognize that a problem exists
I. Altered nutrition: less than body requirements, related to
   1. A lack of interest in food
   2. Satiety of hunger by use of "empty calories" in alcohol
   3. Chemical dependence

J. Potential for injury related to
   1. Altered cerebral or perceptual function
   2. Altered judgment
   3. Altered mobility
K. Noncompliance with abstinence and supportive therapy related to
   1. Inability to stop using substance because of dependence
   2. Refusal to alter life-style
L. Sensory-perceptual alterations (visual, kinesthetic, tactile) related to intake of mind-altering substances
M. Potential for violence: self-directed or directed at others, related to
   1. Intake of mind-altering substances
   2. Misinterpretation of stimuli
   3. Feelings of suspicion or distrust of others

Nursing Care for Clients with Psychoactive Substance-use Disorders

See Nursing care under Alcohol abuse and Drug dependence

ALCOHOL ABUSE

Alcohol intake that interferes with normal functioning or is necessary as a prerequisite to normal functioning
A. Characteristics: premorbid personality utilizes the compensatory mechanisms of the addictive pattern of behavior
B. Patterns of drinking and symptoms
   1. Intoxication: state in which coordination or speech is impaired and behavior is altered
   2. Episodic excessive drinking: becoming intoxicated as infrequently as four times a year; episodes may vary in length from hours to days or weeks
   3. Habitual excessive drinking: becoming intoxicated more than 12 times a year or being recognizably under the influence of alcohol more than once a week even though not considered intoxicated
   4. Alcohol addiction: direct or strong presumptive evidence of dependence on alcohol; demonstrated by withdrawal symptoms or by the inability to go for a day without drinking; when there is a history of heavy drinking for 3 or more months, the individual is considered addicted to alcohol
   5. Early symptoms of alcoholism: frequent drinking sprees, increased intake, drinking alone or in the early morning, occurrence of blackouts
C. Therapy
   1. Should be multifaceted social and medical; involves psychotherapy (group, family, and individual counseling), especially with Alcoholics Anonymous
   2. Negative conditioning with disulfiram (Antabuse) appears to help but never given without the client's full knowledge, understanding, and consent
   3. Clients can be assisted only when they admit they need help
   4. Physical needs must be cared for, since dietary needs have often been ignored for long periods
D. Nursing care
   1. Provide a well-controlled, alcohol-free environment
   2. Plan a full program of activities but with adequate rest periods

3. Meet the client's needs for a great deal of support without criticism or judgment
4. Avoid trying to talk the client out of the problem
5. Accept the smooth facade that the client may present while approaching the lonely and fearful individual behind it
6. Accept failures without judgment or punishment
7. Accept hostility without criticism or retaliation
8. Recognize ambivalence and limit the need for decision making
9. Maintain the client's interest in a therapy program
10. Evaluate client's response and revise plan as necessary

DRUG DEPENDENCE

Misuse of drugs, usually by self-administration, in such a way as to bring about physical, emotional, or behavioral changes

A. Characteristics: premorbid personality, utilizing compensatory mechanisms of the addictive pattern of behavior
B. Definitions
1. Addiction: habituation to and tolerance of drugs other than alcohol, tobacco, and ordinary caffeine-containing beverages; medically prescribed drugs are excluded if they are taken under medical direction; addiction can occur simultaneously to two or more drugs or to alcohol and drugs (polysubstance abuse); lately, combined addiction to a multiplicity of drugs has become more common
2. Habituation: may be both physical and psychologic dependency
3. Tolerance: physical dependency to a drug in which the presence of the drug in increasingly higher dosage is needed to achieve the same effect; tolerance can exceed the usual lethal limits of a drug
4. Potentiation: two or more substances interact in the body to produce an effect greater than the sum of the effects of each substance taken alone
5. Antagonism: two or more substances interact in the body to produce an effect less than the sum of the effects of each substance taken alone
6. Withdrawal: characteristic pattern of reactions and behavior which occur when the used substance is abruptly stopped or amount taken significantly reduced; withdrawal syndrome varies with the specific substance, the amount being used, the length of time the substance has been used, and the individual taking the substance
C. Symptoms
1. Needle marks on limbs along the path of a vein
2. Addicted individuals may tend to wear long-sleeved shirts, even in warm weather
3. Yawning, lacrimation, rhinorrhea, and perspiration appear 10 to 15 hours after the last opiate injection; unrealistic high; pronounced depression
4. Severe abdominal cramps if too much time has elapsed between injections
5. Physical examination may reveal an underweight, malnourished individual with multiple dental caries and depressed CNS functioning
6. Job or academic failure; marital conflicts; poor reality testing; personality change
7. History of violent acting out with total disregard for human life or suffering
8. History of stealing to support habit
9. Nasal discharge with possible distruction of nasal septum if cocaine snorting has been practiced
10. Inability to maintain activities of daily living or fulfill role obligations
11. Marked tolerance with a progressive need for higher doses to achieve desired effects
12. Marked letdown with progression to severe depression after cocaine use
13. Hallucinations, hypervigilance, and paranoid ideation with cocaine use
D. Therapy
1. Treatment for drug overdose
a. Narcotic antagonists
(1) Nalorphine (Nalline) a partial antagonist, or naloxone (Narcan) a pure antagonist, will improve respiratory rate although they may not affect level of consciousness
(2) Nalline will increase respiratory depression if barbiturates have also been used, so Narcan is the drug of choice when in doubt about the substance used
(3) These antagonists completely or partially reverse narcotic depression and may produce an acute abstinence (withdrawal) syndrome by blocking the euphoric and physiologic effects of the narcotic
b. Gastric lavage may be done if substance had been taken orally within the past several hours
2. Treatment for withdrawal symptoms
a. Antidepressants seem to block the "high" from stimulant abuse and diminish the craving for the substance
b. Clonidine (Catapres) suppresses narcotic withdrawal symptoms and decreases adrenergic excess while opiate receptors return to normal levels
(1) Heroin addicts who are first stabilized on methadone before detoxification do better than those who go directly from heroin to clonidine
(2) Clonidine should not be used in those addicted individuals who also abuse alcohol or those who have unstable psychiatric or cardiovascular conditions
c. Decreasing amounts of tranquilizers are often administered to reduce physiologic and psychologic discomfort of withdrawal
3. Methadone maintenance for opiate addiction: programs do not treat addiction but change the addiction from an illegal drug to a legal drug, which is administered under supervision; has proved successful only in individuals with long-standing addictions
4. High-calorie, high-protein, high-vitamin diet because of poor eating habits
5. Treatment in groups run by ex-addicts
6. Therapeutic community setting

7. Psychotherapy and family therapy on an outpatient basis
8. Vocational counseling

E. Nursing care
   1. Set firm controls and keep area drug free when the client is hospitalized
   2. Keep atmosphere pleasant and cheerful but not overly stimulating
   3. Contribute to the client's self-confidence, self-respect, and security in a realistic manner
   4. Walk the fine line between a relatively permissive and a firm attitude
   5. Expect and accept evasion, manipulative behavior, and negativism; but require the client to shoulder certain standards of responsibility
   6. Accept the client without approving the behavior
   7. Do not permit the client to become isolated
   8. Introduce the client to group activities as soon as possible
   9. Protect clients from themselves and others
   10. Evaluate client's response and revise plan as necessary

Schizophrenia
CHARACTERISTICS

A. Premorbid personality: individuals use the compensatory mechanisms of the withdrawn pattern of behavior; in addition, those individuals with paranoid schizophrenia use the compensatory mechanisms of the projective pattern of behavior
B. Severe emotional problems: although unrecognized, begin early in life; however, most commonly occurs between 18 to 34 years of age
C. Chronic insecurity and an almost total failure in interpersonal relationships
D. Etiology still unknown; however, some interesting findings in genetics, biochemistry, psychology, family therapy, and sociology present hope for a breakthrough
E. Regardless of the ultimate etiology, a disturbed relationship with the environment and the family is an almost universal characteristic
F. Course of the disease: either acute or chronic; although it can stop or retrogress at any point, the disorder does not appear to permit a full restoration of integrity of the personality

SYMPTOMS

A. Alterations in feeling, thinking, and relating to the external world
B. Association defects occur, and association links weaken; the individual appears incoherent, bizarre, and unpredictable
C. Distortions interfere with attention, perception, concentration, and memory
D. Affect and emotional expression are flattened
E. Ambivalence is common and frequently is so exaggerated that any action or decision becomes impossible
F. Detachment from reality results in autistic thinking and serves to further distort reality
G. Disturbance occurs in body image, since the undeveloped ego has few strengths and no boundaries; the individual frequently refers to self in the second or third person (e.g., Tom or he) instead of using the first person (e.g., I or me)
H. Secondary symptoms such as hallucinations, delusions, confusion, stupor, and catatonia may or may not be present

TYPES

Although historically much time and effort were directed toward identifying types of schizophrenia, it should be recognized that the classification is not static; there is a great deal of overlapping symptomatology; individuals diagnosed as being in one classification frequently are diagnosed at a later time in another classification

A. Catatonic type: picture of withdrawal and distortions in reality testing, accompanied by total ambivalence, which is frequently exhibited in rather unpredictable motor activity; the ambivalence can render movement and decision making impossible, since the individual is unable to decide how or where to move; may literally be frozen in position, akinetic (stuporous)—or forced into aimless hyperkinetic fugue (excited) movements
B. Disorganized type: picture of severe and pronounced mental incapacity; great mental and emotional deterioration occurs; behavior is retarded, with sexual preoccupations, emotional dulling, and infantile silliness; onset is usually between 12 and 25 years of age
C. Paranoid type: uses withdrawal compensatory mechanisms to distort reality and then develops a rather intricate delusional system by using the projective pattern of behavior; is secretive and suspicious; uses ideas of reference, finally develops delusions of grandeur
D. Undifferentiated type: demonstrates the primary thought, affect, and withdrawal defects of schizophrenia but cannot be classified under a specific type because of mixed symptoms
E. Residual type: continues to use many of the compensatory mechanisms common to this disorder in the absence of prominent delusions, hallucinations, incoherence, or grossly disorganized behavior

THERAPY

A. Psychotherapy (individual, family, and group counseling)
B. Motivational therapy
C. Occupational and vocational therapy
D. Day-care treatment programs in community settings
E. Pharmacologic approach: antipsychotic drugs (major tranquilizers)—control behavior when the client's uncontrolled actions are destructive to self, others, or the environment (see Pharmacology related to emotional disorders)

NURSING PROCESS FOR CLIENTS WITH SCHIZOPHRENIA
Probable Nursing Diagnoses Based on Assessment

A. Anxiety related to
   1. Disturbed thought processes
   2. Pervasive ambivalence
   3. Mistrust of others
   4. Difficulty in dealing with reality

B. Impaired verbal communication related to
1. Inappropriate use of words and unique patterns of speech
2. Anxiety
3. Disturbed and disruptive thought processes

C. Ineffective family coping: compromised or disabling, related to
1. Ambivalent family relationships
2. Abusive or destructive behavior
3. Inadequate resources

D. Ineffective individual coping related to
1. Inability to meet basic needs
2. Poorly developed or inappropriate use of defense mechanisms
3. Inability to meet role expectations

E. Potential for injury related to
1. Sensory or perceptual deficits
2. Cognitive or psychomotor deficits
3. Altered judgment

F. Feeding, bathing/hygiene, dressing/grooming, toileting self-care deficit related to
1. Perceptual or cognitive impairment
2. Emotional dysfunctioning
3. Increasing inability to carry out activities of daily living

G. Sleep pattern disturbance related to
1. Emotional dysfunctioning
2. A side effect of psychotrophic drugs

H. Altered thought processes related to
1. Inability to evaluate reality
2. Disturbed interpretation of environment
3. Disturbed mental activities
4. Altered sensory perception, reception, and transmission

I. Potential for violence: self-directed or directed at others, related to
1. Feelings of suspicion or distrust of others
2. Inability to discharge emotions verbally
3. Misinterpretation of stimuli
4. Disturbed thought processes

J. Personal identity disturbance related to
1. Altered thought processes
2. Detachment from reality
3. Lack of boundaries between self and environment

K. Decisional conflict (generalized) related to
1. Altered perceptions
2. Ambivalence

L. Impaired social interaction related to
1. Withdrawal
2. Delusions and hallucinations
3. Distrust of others

M. Sensory perceptual alterations (visual, auditory, kinesthetic, gustatory, tactile, olfactory) related to
1. Emotional misinterpretation of stimuli
2. Inability to test reality

Nursing Care for Clients with Schizophrenia

A. Observe for adverse drug reactions whenever large doses of the major tranquilizers are being administered

B. Encourage the client to follow a plan of organized activity and a prescribed drug regimen

C. Encourage the client to continue medications even after symptoms abate

D. Respect the client as a human being with both dignity and worth

E. Accept the client at his or her present level of functioning

F. Avoid trying to argue the client out of delusions or hallucinations

G. Accept that the client's hallucinations and delusions are real and frightening

H. Encourage the development of interpersonal relationships between the client and others

I. Point out reality to the client but do not impose staff's concept of reality

J. Protect client from injury because of poor judgment

K. Evaluate client's response and revise plan as necessary

Paranoid Disorder

Individuals who demonstrate the suspiciousness and delusions common to paranoid conditions but do not exhibit the thinking and behavioral disorganization or the personality disintegration found in the other psychoses

CHARACTERISTICS

A. Premorbid personality: uses the compensatory mechanisms of the projective pattern of behavior

B. Paranoid defenses considered by some to be a protective mechanism against unconscious homosexuality or overt hostility

C. Exact etiology unknown

SYMPTOMS

A. Exhibits a rather elaborate, highly organized paranoid delusional system while preserving other functions of the personality

B. Thinking is not interfered with

C. Personality function continues

D. Delusions are drawn from real life situations

E. Hallucinations are not prominent

F. Behavior is not bizarre

G. Predominent theme of delusions determines type of paranoia (e.g., grandiose, jealous, persecutory)

THERAPY

A. Chemotherapy with major tranquilizers considered most helpful (see Pharmacology related to emotional disorders)

B. Individual psychotherapy may provide some relief of symptoms

C. Paranoid clients are the most challenging to reach, since none of the present therapies appear to be helpful in breaking down the delusional system

NURSING PROCESS FOR CLIENTS WITH PARANOID DISORDER
Probable Nursing Diagnoses Based on Assessment

A. Anxiety related to
1. Disturbed thought processes about specific areas
2. Mistrust of others
3. Difficulty in dealing with certain aspects of reality
4. Threat to security

B. Ineffective individual coping related to poorly developed or inappropriate use of defense mechanisms
C. Self-esteem disturbance related to
    1. Perceptual or cognitive impairment
    2. Feelings of grandiosity
    3. Feelings of persecution
D. Altered thought processes related to misinterpretations of events
E. Potential for violence: directed at others, related to
    1. Feelings of suspicion or distrust of others
    2. Misinterpretation of stimuli

Nursing Care for Clients with Paranoid Disorder

A. Provide an environment with some intellectual challenge that does not threaten security
B. Avoid counteraggression and retaliation against the client
C. Accept and recognize the client's need for a superior attitude
D. Meet sarcasm and ridicule in a matter-of-fact manner
E. Guard the client's self-esteem from attack by other clients
F. Accept the client's misinterpretations of events
G. Point out reality but do not directly challenge the client's delusions
H. Evaluate client's response and revise plan as necessary

Other Psychotic Disorders
SCHIZOAFFECTIVE DISORDER

A. Does not meet the criteria for either schizophrenia or a mood disorder
B. Occurs in early adulthood
C. Demonstrates a mixture of symptoms from both schizophrenia and mood disorders
D. The thought processes and bizarre behavior appears schizophrenic, but there is usually marked elation or depression; often proves to be basically schizophrenic in nature
E. Therapy depends upon the symptoms exhibited
F. Nursing care depends upon the type of symptoms exhibited (see Nursing care under Schizophrenia and Mood disorders)

POSTPARTUM PSYCHOSES

A. Psychotic symptoms develop after the birth of a baby
B. No organic factor present to initiate or maintain disorder
C. Often thought to be basically schizophrenia
D. Symptoms
    1. Delusions and hallucinations
    2. Incoherency and loosening of associations
    3. Catatonic-type stupor or excitement
    4. Grossly disorganized behavior
E. Therapy depends upon the type of symptoms exhibited; major tranquillizers or antidepressant drugs may be used
F. Nursing care
    1. See Nursing care for schizophrenia
    2. See Nursing care for mood disorders
    3. Supervise mother when caring for infant; remove child from mother's care if necessary
    4. Evaluate client's response and revise plan as necessary

Mood Disorders

Characterized by a disturbance of mood, encompassing two emotional extremes; individual demonstrates the vehement energy of mania, the despair and lethargy of depression, or both

NURSING PROCESS FOR CLIENTS WITH MOOD DISORDERS
Probable Nursing Diagnoses Based on Assessment

A. Anxiety related to
    1. Disturbed thought processes
    2. Difficulty in dealing with reality
    3. Feelings of failure and unworthiness
B. Impaired verbal communication related to
    1. Pressured speech and psychomotor activity
    2. Lethargy and psychomotor depression
    3. Inability to verbalize feelings and thoughts
C. Ineffective individual coping related to
    1. Inadequate support system
    2. Inability to meet basic needs
    3. Inability to meet role expectations
    4. Overwhelming feeling of unworthiness
D. Dysfunctional grieving related to actual or perceived object loss
E. Potential for injury related to impaired judgment
F. Altered nutrition: less than body requirements, related to
    1. Hyperactivity and excessive expenditure of calories
    2. Inability to sit down long enough to eat
    3. Lack of interest in food
    4. Feelings of unworthiness
G. Feeding, bathing/hygiene, dressing/grooming self-care deficit related to
    1. Disinterest in activities of daily living
    2. Emotional dysfunctioning
H. Sleep pattern disturbance related to
    1. Emotional dysfunctioning
    2. A side effect of psychotrophic drugs
I. Social isolation related to
    1. Object loss
    2. Absence of support group
    3. Alterations in mental functioning
J. Altered thought processes related to
    1. Impaired judgment
    2. Impaired ability to make decisions
    3. Altered attention span
    4. Overinvolvement with or withdrawal from environment
K. Potential for violence: self-directed or directed toward others, related to
    1. Inability to discharge emotions verbally
    2. Disturbed thought processes
    3. Feelings of unworthiness
L. Self-esteem disturbance related to
    1. Disturbed sensory perceptions resulting in somatic delusions
    2. Emotional dysfunctioning
    3. Feelings of inadequacy
    4. Feelings of grandiosity

M. Altered role performance related to
1. Disturbed sensory perceptions resulting in somatic delusions
2. Emotional dysfunctioning
3. Feelings of inadequacy
4. Feelings of grandiosity
N. Altered sexuality patterns related to
1. Increased or decreased sex drive
2. Level of energy

Nursing Care for Clients with Mood Disorders
A. General care
1. Monitor intake and output
2. Keep the environment nonchallenging and non-stimulating
3. Avoid irritating routines as much as possible
4. Protect the client against suicide during the entire episode
5. Keep activities simple, uncomplicated, and repetitive in nature; they should be of short duration and should require little concentration
6. Observe for adverse effects of drugs; monitor lithium blood levels weekly; white cell count less often
7. Encourage the client to continue medications even after symptoms abate
8. Caution and teach the client regarding special dietary precautions with lithium and the MAO inhibitors
9. Evaluate client's response and revise plan as necessary

BIPOLAR DISORDER
Presence of one or more manic or hypomanic episodes in a client with a history of depressive episodes

Characteristics
A. Premorbid personality: uses the compensatory mechanisms associated with aggressive patterns of behavior
B. Generally occurs between 20 and 40 years of age, although it has been reported in clients over 50 years of age
C. Usually a response to a loss, change in life events, or role change
D. Biochemical changes in the body, specifically a disturbance in biogenic amines
E. Cyclic, periodic episodes of acute self-limiting mood swings; can be all manic, all depressed, or mixed manic and depressed
F. Resumption of customary activities between episodes
G. Obesity a frequent precursor of attack; onset can be slowed or modified by dieting

Depressive Episode
A. Symptoms
1. Triad of symptoms with lowering of the mood tone; dejection, slowing of thinking and speech, decrease in psychomotor activity
2. Insomnia: difficulty in falling asleep and staying asleep, tending to wake early
3. Decreased appetite
4. Feelings of guilt and worthlessness
5. Difficulty in performing daily tasks

6. Tearful with suicidal ruminations
7. Speaking slowly using monosyllabic words
8. Orientation and logic unaffected
9. Sex drive decreased
10. Constipation and urinary retention may occur
B. Therapy
1. Dexamethosone suppression test (DST): used to identify depressed clients who may be responsive to antidepressant drug therapy or electroconvulsant therapy (ECT)
2. Electroconvulsive therapy to reduce depression; succinylcholine chloride (Anectine), a depolarizing muscle relaxant causing paralysis, is used to reduce the intensity of muscle contractions during the convulsive stage; used most often for clients with recurrent depressions, delusions, suicidal ideation, and those who are resistant to drug therapy
3. High-protein, high-carbohydrate diet is provided for energy
4. Psychotherapy
5. Pharmacologic approach in depressive phase: antidepressant drugs that increase the level of norepinephrine at subcortical neuroeffector sites (see Pharmacology related to emotional disorders)
C. Nursing care
1. For general nursing care see Nursing care at the beginning of this classification
2. Accept client's inability to carry out daily routines
3. Set expectations that can be achieved by the client
4. Help client express hostility and accept client's responses without rejection
5. Provide realistic praise whenever possible
6. Involve client in simple repetitious tasks and activities
7. Accept client's feelings of worthlessness as real; client's feelings should be accepted but not denied, condoned, or approved
8. Protect client against suicidal acting out, especially when the depression begins to lift; suicide is a real and ever-present danger throughout the entire illness
9. Evaluate client's response and revise plan as necessary

Manic Episode
A. Symptoms
1. Begins suddenly with rapid acceleration of symptoms
2. Excessive involvement in pleasurable activities which may have painful consequences (e.g., spending spree, questionable schemes)
3. Marked impairment of occupational functioning, social activities, or relationships
4. Mood is elevated, expansive, or irritable
5. Psychomotor aggitation
6. Flight of ideas
7. Easy distractability
8. Difficulty sleeping; decreased need for sleep
9. Extremely active; always in a hurry
10. Humor good, although remarks can be caustic; euphoric

11. Monopolizing conversations; irritability only superficially covered
12. Orientation clear, but judgment poor
13. Always planning and scheming
14. Increased sex drive
15. Inflated self-esteem; grandiosity
16. Excessive spending of money

B. Therapy
1. High-protein, high-carbohydrate diet is provided for energy, especially in manic phase
2. Psychotherapy
3. Pharmacologic approach in manic phase: improves productivity by decreasing psychomotor activity or response to environmental stimuli (see Pharmacology related to emotional disorders)

C. Nursing care
1. For general nursing care see Nursing care at the beginning of this classification
2. Accept client even though objectionable behavior should be rejected
3. Permit expression of hostility and ambivalence without reinforcement of guilt feelings
4. Approach in a calm, collected manner and maintain self-control
5. Set limits for behavior
6. Communicate in a nonargumentative manner
7. Use client's easy distractibility to interrupt hyperactive behavior to avoid injury and exhaustion
8. Advise all care givers to approach client in a consistent manner
9. Evaluate client's response and revise plan as necessary

MAJOR DEPRESSION

A. Characteristics
1. Similar to bipolar disorder
2. No organic factors are present; psychosocial stresses play a role
3. Usually occurs in late twenties but may occur at any age, including infancy

B. Symptoms
1. Diminished interest or pleasure in all activities
2. Decreased appetite with weight loss
3. Psychomotor retardation
4. Anxiety and tearfulness
5. Insomnia or hypersomnia
6. Feelings of worthlessness
7. Inappropriate guilt
8. Interruption in thinking and concentration which may interfere with occupational and social functioning
9. Recurrent thoughts of death; suicidal ideation with or without a specific plan to carry it out

C. Therapy
Same as depressive episode of bipolar disorder

D. Nursing care
1. For general nursing care see Nursing care at the beginning of this classification
2. For specific nursing care see Nursing care for depressive episode of bipolar disorder

MAJOR DEPRESSION—MELANCHOLIC TYPE

A. Characteristics
1. Frequently there is a history of a previous major depressive episode
2. Depression is agitated rather than retarded
3. Depression occurs after 40 years of age and before 60 years of age
4. Precipitating factors such as the marriage of children, loss of a job, breakup of a marriage, or death of a partner frequently are identified
5. Depression often closely related to the menopause or climacteric; hormonal and endocrine changes are considered by many to play an important role although current thinking does not make a distinction between this depression and depressions occurring at other periods of life
6. Usually rigid, inflexible, overassertive, overly meticulous, and worrisome

B. Symptoms
1. Wakes early after having had trouble falling asleep
2. Feelings of unreality and sinfulness
3. Complains of somatic delusions
4. Extremely jumpy and agitated
5. Pacing and wringing of hands as well as other increased motor activity
6. Loss of interest or pleasure in usual activities
7. Inability to react to pleasurable stimuli
8. Triad of symptoms: delusions of sin and/or poverty, obsession with death, somatic delusions especially related to the GI tract

C. Therapy
Same as Depressive episode of bipolar disorder

D. Nursing care
1. For general nursing care see Nursing care at the beginning of this classification
2. For specific nursing care see Nursing care for depressive episode of bipolar disorder

OTHER MOOD DISORDERS
Cyclothymic Disorder

A. Symptoms include alternating mood swings between elation and sadness; apparently unrelated to external environment
B. The individual is usually warm and friendly; approaches life with an obvious enthusiasm
C. Mood swings do not demonstrate great emotional intensity
D. Therapy
1. Often unnecessary; if required, same as for depressive or manic episode of bipolar disorder
2. Medication often unnecessary; if required, same as for manic or depressive episode of bipolar disorder
E. Nursing care
See Nursing care at the beginning of this classification and Nursing care under Depressive and Manic episodes of bipolar disorder

Dysthymic Disorder (Depressive Neurosis)

A. Guilt and depression used unconsciously to relieve anxiety

B. Symptoms of depression, insomnia, anorexia, decreased sexual drive, weight loss, constipation, fatigue; closely resembles bipolar disorder but differs in depth and awareness of reality
C. Depression is real, and suicide can occur
D. Therapy
1. Often unnecessary; if required, same as for Depressive episode of bipolar disorder
2. Medication often unnecessary; if required, same as for Depressive episode of bipolar disorder
E. Nursing care
1. For general nursing care see Nursing care at the beginning of this classification
2. For specific nursing care see Nursing care under Depressive episode of bipolar disorder

Anxiety Disorders

Common responses to emotional problems that are rarely treated in psychiatric settings; disturbances in personality, but there is no great defect in reality testing or severe antisocial behavior

NURSING PROCESS FOR CLIENTS WITH ANXIETY DISORDERS
Probable Nursing Diagnoses Based on Assessment

A. Anxiety related to
1. Threat to security
2. Threat to self-concept
3. Feelings of inadequacy
4. Recall of traumatic experiences
B. Ineffective individual coping related to
1. Inability to meet role expectations
2. Inadequate support system
3. Difficulty in meeting basic needs
4. Pervasive anxiety and fear
C. Potential for injury related to
1. Flight from the stress-producing object or situation
2. Feelings of panic
3. Altered judgment
D. Chronic or situational low self-esteem related to
1. Feelings of inadequacy and hostility
2. Disturbed relationships
3. Pervasive anxiety
4. Inability to meet role expectations
E. Altered role performance related to
1. Feelings of inadequacy and hostility
2. Disturbed relationships
3. Pervasive anxiety
4. Inability to meet role expectations
F. Fear related to
1. Feelings of panic
2. Altered judgment
3. Pervasive anxiety
G. Impaired social interaction related to
1. Pervasive anxiety
2. Irrational fear
H. Decisional conflict related to pervasive anxiety
I. Powerlessness related to overwhelming, pervasive anxiety
J. Posttrauma response related to experiencing an event that is outside of usual human experience

K. Potential for violence: self-directed or directed toward others, related to
1. Altered judgment
2. Pervasive anxiety and fear

Nursing Care for Clients with Anxiety Disorders

A. Establish a trusting relationship
B. Accept symptoms as real to the individual
C. Attempt to limit the use of defenses, but do not stop them until the individual is ready to give them up
D. Encourage the individual to develop a balance between work and play so anxiety is lessened
E. Help the individual develop better ways of handling anxiety-producing situations through problem solving
F. Accept physical symptoms but do not emphasize or call attention to them
G. Reduce demands on the individual as much as possible
H. Recognize when anxiety is interrupting ability to think clearly
I. Intervene to protect client from acting out on impulses that may harm self or others
J. Evaluate client's response and revise plan as necessary

PANIC DISORDER

A. Characteristics
1. Uses the compensatory mechanisms of the psychoneurotic pattern of behavior
2. Development of the symptoms usually permits some measure of social adjustment
3. Commonly begins in early 20s as a result of environmental factors in childhood
4. Early life rigid and orderly
5. Pressures of decision making regarding life-style that occur in the early adult years seem to act as precipitating factors
6. Discrete periods of intense discomfort or fear
B. Symptoms
1. Feeling of suffocating
2. Shortness of breath
3. Hyperventilation
4. Fluttering in the stomach
5. Diaphoresis
6. Vertigo
7. Faintness
C. Therapy
1. Complete medical workup to reassure the individual and rule out medical problems
2. Psychotherapy, family therapy, group therapy
3. Sedatives and minor tranquilizers if necessary
4. Pharmacologic approach: antianxiety drugs (minor tranquilizers) used when the individual is incapable of coping with environmental stresses and accomplishing daily activities
D. Nursing care
1. For general nursing care see Nursing care at the beginning of this classification
2. Remain with client during an attack
3. Do not get caught up in client's panic; remain calm and in control of the situation
4. Evaluate client's response and revise plan as necessary

PHOBIC DISORDERS

A. Characteristics
1. Uses the compensatory mechanisms of the psycho-neurotic pattern of behavior
2. Development of the phobia usually permits some measure of social adjustment
3. Commonly begins in early 20s as a result of environmental factors in childhood
4. Early life rigid and orderly
5. Pressures of decision making regarding life-style that occur in the early adult years seem to act as precipitating factors
6. Anxiety unconsciously transferred to an inanimate object or situation, which then symbolically represents the conflict and can be avoided

B. Types of phobias
1. Agoraphobia: fear of being alone or in public places where help would not be immediately available if necessary; includes tunnels, bridges, crowds, buses, and trains
2. Social phobia: fear of public speaking or situations in which public scrutiny may occur
3. Simple phobia: fear of specific objects, animals, or situations

C. Symptoms
1. Anxiety appears when clients find themselves in places that threaten their sense of security
2. Attempts are made to avoid these distressing situations
3. Depending on the phobic object, the individual's life-style is often greatly limited
4. Fear of being trapped, embarrassed, or humiliated in social situations

D. Therapy
1. Same as Panic disorders
2. Behavior modification with exposure to phobic object or situation in controlled doses

E. Nursing care
1. For general nursing care see Nursing care at the beginning of this classification
2. Recognize client's feelings about phobic object or situation
3. Provide constant support if exposure to phobic object or situation cannot be avoided
4. Evaluate client's response and revise plan as necessary

OBSESSIVE-COMPULSIVE DISORDER

A. Characteristics
1. Uses the compensatory mechanisms of the psycho-neurotic pattern of behavior
2. Development of the ritual usually permits some measure of social adjustment
3. Commonly begins in early 20s as a result of environmental factors in childhood
4. Early life rigid and orderly
5. Pressures of decision making regarding life-style that occur in the early adult years seem to act as precipitating factors
6. Unconscious control of anxiety by the use of rituals and thoughts

B. Symptoms
1. Thoughts persist and become repetitive and obsessive
2. Thoughts may be turned into compulsions that are repetitive acts of irrational behavior which the individual is emotionally forced to carry out although they serve no rational purpose
3. Client is indecisive and demonstrates a striving for perfection and superiority
4. Intellectual and verbal defenses are used
5. Anxiety and depression may be present in various degrees, particularly if rituals are prevented

C. Therapy
1. Same as Panic disorders
2. Behavior modification to attempt to limit the length and/or frequency of the ritual

D. Nursing care
1. For general nursing care see Nursing care at the beginning of this classification
2. Allow the client to continue the ritual but attempt to limit the length and frequency of the ritual
3. Support clients in their attempt to reduce dependency on the ritual
4. Evaluate client's response and revise plan as necessary

POST-TRAUMATIC STRESS DISORDER

A. Characteristics
1. Follows a devastating event that is outside the range of usual human experience (e.g., rape, assault, military combat, hostage situations)
2. The traumatic event is persistently re-experienced as flashbacks, distressing dreams, sense of reliving the experience, or one is exposed to situations that foster recall of the event (including anniversaries)

B. Symptoms
1. Feeling of isolation
2. Difficulty sleeping
3. Violent outbursts of anger
4. Depression
5. Interrupted concentration
6. Hypervigilance

C. Therapy
1. Same as Panic disorders
2. Behavior modification to provide controlled exposure to recall of the event

D. Nursing care
1. For general nursing care see Nursing care in the beginning of this classification
2. Stay with client when memory of the event returns to the conscious level
3. Protect client from acting out violently with disregard for the safety of self or others
4. Evaluate client's response and revise plan as necessary

GENERALIZED ANXIETY DISORDER

A. Characteristics
1. Uses the compensatory mechanisms of the psycho-neurotic pattern of behavior
2. Development of the anxiety usually permits some measure of social adjustment

3. Commonly begins in early 20s as a result of environmental factors in childhood
4. Early life rigid and orderly
5. Pressures of decision making regarding life-style that occur in the early adult years seem to act as precipitating factors
6. Excessive anxiety and worry about at least two of life situations

B. Symptoms
1. Pervasive continuous feeling of free-floating anxiety, tension, and apprehension
2. Episodes of dyspnea, palpitations, irritability, dizziness, insomnia, fainting, weakness, chest pain, trembling, and headaches
3. Symptoms usually appear in relation to stress situations such as crowded rooms, public gatherings, pregnancy, military service
4. The client appears anxious; often mildly depressed

C. Therapy
Same as Panic disorder

D. Nursing care
1. For general nursing care see Nursing care at the beginning of this classification
2. See Nursing care for panic disorders

Somatoform Disorders
NURSING PROCESS FOR CLIENTS WITH SOMATOFORM DISORDERS
Probable Nursing Diagnoses Based on Assessment

A. Anxiety related to
1. Threat to security
2. Threat to self-concept
3. Inability to meet role expectations

B. Ineffective individual coping related to
1. Development of physical symptoms to escape stressful situations and control anxiety
2. Inability to verbalize feelings
3. Inability to accept that the symptoms lack a physiologic basis

C. Body image disturbance related to
1. Passive acceptance of disabling symptoms which would alter body image
2. Inability to meet idealized role expectations and performance

D. Altered role performance related to
1. Passive acceptance of disabling symptoms which would alter body image
2. Inability to meet idealized role expectations and performance
3. Preoccupation with physical symptoms

Nursing Care for Clients with Somatoform Disorders

A. Establish a trusting relationship
B. Accept symptoms as real to the individual
C. Attempt to limit the use of defenses, but do not stop them until the individual is ready to give them up
D. Encourage the individual to develop a balance between work and play so anxiety is lessened
E. Help the individual develop better ways of handling anxiety-producing situations through problem solving

F. Accept physical symptoms but do not emphasize or call attention to them
G. Reduce demands on the individual as much as possible
H. Evaluate client's response and revise plan as necessary

CONVERSION DISORDER
A. Characteristics
1. Anxiety unconsciously converted to physical symptoms that are not under voluntary control; these symptoms permit the individual to avoid some unacceptable activity
2. Development of symptoms usually permits some measure of social adjustment
3. Generally begins before 30 years of age
4. Early life often rigid and orderly; physical illness frequently used by the family as an excuse for problems
5. Pressures of decision making regarding life-style in the early adult years seem to be precipitating factors

B. Symptoms
1. History of lost motor or sensory function without any adequate physical cause (e.g., paralysis, blindness, deafness)
2. Noticeable lack of concern about the problem; this lack of concern has been labeled *la belle indifférence*
3. Impairment may vary over different episodes and does not follow anatomic structure; paralysis or numbness may circle the foot or arm instead of beginning at the joint and is known as stocking-and-glove anesthesia
4. The individual appears relieved by symptoms and demonstrates little anxiety when observed

C. Therapy
1. Complete medical workup to reassure the individual and rule out medical problems
2. Psychotherapy, family therapy, group therapy
3. Sedatives and minor tranquilizers if necessary
4. Pharmacologic approach: antianxiety drugs (minor tranquilizers) used when the individual is incapable of coping with environmental stresses and accomplishing daily activities

D. Nursing care
See Nursing care at the beginning of this classification

BODY DYSMORPHIC DISORDER
A. Characteristics
1. Preoccupation with imagined defect in a normal-appearing person (not of delusional intensity)
2. Generally begins in early adolescence and lasts several years
3. No predisposing factor in early life or family patterns has been identified
4. A minor defect is grossly exaggerated

B. Symptoms
1. History of multiple visits to plastic surgeons to correct imagined defects
2. Avoidance of social situations because of anxiety over minor defects
3. Often exhibits symptoms of depression or obsessive-compulsive personality traits

C. Therapy
   Same as Conversion disorder
D. Nursing care
   See Nursing care at the beginning of this classification

HYPOCHONDRIASIS (HYPOCHONDRIACAL NEUROSIS)

A. Characteristics
   1. Preoccupation with the belief that one has a serious illness because of how physical symptoms are interpreted
   2. A positive medical evaluation does not allay their fears
   3. Knowledge of symptoms associated with a given disease aids in the client's developing a similar set of symptoms, leading them to conclude that they have the disease
   4. Psychosocial stresses are believed to lead to development of this disorder
   5. Usually begins between 20 and 30 years of age
B. Symptoms
   1. Misinterpretation and exaggeration of physical symptoms
   2. Inability to accept reassurance even after exhaustive testing and therapy; leads to "doctor-shopping"
   3. History of repeated absences from work
   4. Adoption of sick role and invalid life-style
C. Therapy
   Same as Conversion disorder
D. Nursing care
   See Nursing care at the beginning of this classification

Sexual Disorders

Changing social and cultural mores have caused many of the sexual behaviors that were once considered deviations to be removed from the list of "abnormal practices." Today sexual activities are considered abnormal only if they are directed toward anything other than consenting adults or are performed under unusual circumstances.

NURSING PROCESS FOR CLIENTS WITH SEXUAL DISORDERS
Probable Nursing Diagnoses Based on Assessment

A. Anxiety related to
   1. Threat to security and fear of discovery
   2. Conflict between sexual desires and societal norms
B. Potential for injury related to
   1. Retaliation for sexual behavior
   2. Risks involved in masochistic gratification
C. Sexual dysfunction related to
   1. Actual or perceived sexual limitations
   2. Feelings of vulnerability
   3. Values conflict
   4. Inability to achieve sexual satisfaction without the use of paraphiliac behaviors
D. Potential for infection related to
   1. Frequent changes in sexual partners
   2. Sadistic or masochistic acts
E. Potential for violence: directed toward others, related to obtaining sexual gratification through sadism

Nursing Care for Clients with Sexual Disorders

A. Accept the individual as a person in emotional pain
B. Avoid punitive remarks or responses
C. Protect the individual from others
D. Set limits on the individual's sexual acting out
E. Provide diversional activities
F. Evaluate client's response and revise plan as necessary

PARAPHILIAS

A. Characteristics
   1. Sexual urges or fantasies that are directed toward nonhuman objects, the pain to self or partner, or children and other nonconsenting individuals
   2. Diagnosis is made when the individual has acted on urges or is extremely distressed by the urges
   3. Sexual arousal accompanies paraphilic fantasies or stimuli
   4. Person may or may not be able to function sexually without the paraphilic fantasy or stimuli
   5. May be symptomatic of other personality or psychiatric disorders or may occur as a behavior aberration or a disordered personality
B. Types and symptoms
   1. Fetishism: substitution of an inanimate object for the genitals
   2. Transvestism: wearing clothes of the opposite sex to achieve sexual pleasure
   3. Exhibitionism: sexual pleasure obtained by exposing the genitals
   4. Pedophilia: attraction to children as sex objects
   5. Voyeurism: sexual gratification obtained by watching the sexual play of others
   6. Sadism: sexual gratification obtained from cruelty to others; used as a substitute for or an accompaniment of the sex act
   7. Masochism: sexual gratification obtained from self-suffering; used as a substitute for or an accompaniment of the sex act
   8. Frotteurism: sexual pleasure obtained by touching or rubbing against a nonconsenting person; usually occurs in crowds or public transportation
C. Therapy
   1. Rather unsuccessful with these individuals unless they really want to change
   2. If change is desired, psychotherapy may be effective
D. Nursing care
   See Nursing care at the beginning of this classification

SEXUAL DYSFUNCTION

Inhibition or interference with the appetitive, excitement, orgasm, or resolution phases of the sexual response cycle which can be psychogenic alone or psychogenic and biogenic, lifelong or acquired, generalized or situational

Adjustment Disorders

Acute reactions to overwhelming environmental stress

CHARACTERISTICS

A. No apparent underlying mental disorder in these individuals, although present behavior may be extremely disturbed

B. The individual seems to have the capacity to adapt to the overwhelming stress when given the time to do so

C. Problems with distortions or interruptions in thinking process and decision making tend to resolve themselves

SYMPTOMS

A. Infancy: extremely upset; demonstrating grief when separated from the mother

B. Childhood: regression to an earlier level of development when a new sibling arrives; intense anxiety on entering school

C. Adolescence: struggle for independence; leads to hypersensitivity and frequent episodes of heightened anxiety

D. Adult life: heightened anxiety in response to the stresses associated with marriage, pregnancy, divorce, change of employment, purchase of a house, etc.

E. Later life: menopause and climacteric, plan for retirement, "loss" of children to marriage, and death of a mate all serve to produce extreme stress situations

THERAPY

Determine the underlying cause of the conflict and work toward resolution

NURSING PROCESS FOR CLIENTS WITH ADJUSTMENT DISORDERS
Probable Nursing Diagnoses Based on Assessment

A. Anxiety related to
1. Inability to handle overwhelming stress effectively
2. Threat to self-concept
3. Threat to security

B. Ineffective individual coping related to
1. Overwhelming environmental stress, which is usually resolved over time
2. Failure of support system
3. Developmental level

C. Chronic low self-esteem related to
1. Overwhelming stress
2. Inability to cope

D. Altered role performance related to
1. Overwhelming stress
2. Inability to cope

Nursing Care for Clients with Adjustment Disorders

A. Recognize and accept that a problem exists
B. Help the individual and/or parents identify the problem
C. Support and avoid humiliation of the individual
D. Provide emphatic understanding
E. Evaluate client's response and revise plan as necessary

Personality Disorders

Borderline states characterized by defects in the development of the personality or by pathologic trends in its structure

CHARACTERISTICS

A. Habitual attitudes and reaction patterns in human relationships develop early in life and form the character structure of the individual

B. In most instances these behaviors create little discomfort or stress

C. Personality disturbances are, in reality, the selection and utilization of specific defense mechanisms which are used so often that they form a life-long pattern of action that, although not normal, is neither neurotic nor psychotic

D. Premorbid personality of individuals demonstrating any of the 11 classified personality disturbances resembles the compensatory mechanisms associated with the pathologic counterpart

TYPES AND SYMPTOMS

A. Paranoid personality disorder
1. Frequent use of projective mechanisms
2. Suspiciousness, fear, irritability, and stubbornness
3. Reality testing not greatly impaired

B. Schizoid personality disorder
1. Avoidance of meaningful interpersonal relationships
2. Use of autistic thinking, emotional detachment, and daydreaming
3. Introverted since childhood but maintaining fair contact with reality

C. Schizotypal personality disorder
1. Unattached, withdrawn
2. Affectively and intellectually diminished
3. Frequently part of the vagabond or transient groups of society

D. Antisocial personality disorder
1. Chronic life-long disturbances that conflict with society's laws and customs
2. Unable to postpone gratification
3. Randomly act out their aggressive egocentric impulses on society
4. Do not profit from past experience or punishment; live only for the moment
5. Have the ability to ingratiate themselves but "do not wear well"
6. Are in contact with reality but do not seem to care about it

E. Borderline personality disorder
1. Unstable and intense interpersonal relationships
2. Impulsive unpredictable behavior which is potentially self-destructive
3. Marked mood shifts
4. Identity disturbance
5. Chronic feeling of emptyness

F. Histrionic personality disorder
1. Emotional instability and hyperexcitability
2. Extroverted and directed toward gaining attention
3. Vain and deliberately manipulative

G. Narcissistic personality disorder
1. Overblown sense of importance
2. Strong need for attention and admiration
3. Relationships marked by ambivalence
4. Preoccupation with appearance

H. Avoidant personality disorder
1. Social discomfort and timidity
2. Loner; unwilling to get involved with other people
3. Fear of negative evaluation from others

I. Dependent personality disorder
   1. Unable to make decisions
   2. Lack of self-confidence
   3. Dependent and submissive
   4. Induces others to assume responsibility
J. Obsessive-compulsive personality disorder
   1. Rigidity, overconscientiousness, inordinate capacity for work
   2. Driven by obsessive concerns
   3. Behavior contains many rituals
K. Passive-aggressive personality disorder
   1. Rather helpless and indecisive, demonstrating passive obstructionism while clinging and pouting
   2. Frequent outbursts and temper tantrums when frustrated
   3. Often creating problems for others

THERAPY

A. Individual, group, and family psychotherapy
B. Crisis intervention when necessary
C. Vocational and occupational therapy

NURSING PROCESS FOR CLIENTS WITH PERSONALITY DISORDERS
Probable Nursing Diagnoses Based on Assessment

A. Anxiety related to
   1. Threat to security
   2. Threat to self-concept
   3. Inability to meet role expectations
   4. Difficulty in interpersonal relationships
B. Ineffective family coping: compromised, related to
   1. Abusive or destructive behavior
   2. Ambivalent family relationships
   3. Denial that problem exists
C. Ineffective individual coping related to
   1. Inability to learn from experience
   2. Poorly developed or inappropriate use of defense mechanisms
   3. Inability to tolerate frustrations
   4. Inability to form meaningful relationships
D. Social isolation related to the absence of meaningful relationships
E. Potential for violence: directed toward others, related to poor impulse control

Nursing Care for Clients with Personality Disorders

A. Maintain consistency and concern
B. Accept the individual as is; do not retaliate if provoked
C. Protect the individual from others while protecting others from the individual
D. Place realistic limits on behavior; make known what those limits are
E. Evaluate client's response and revise plan as necessary

Community Mental Health Services
CONCEPTS

A. Purposes
   1. To provide prevention, treatment, and rehabilitation services for individuals with emotional problems; also support for families
   2. To maintain these individuals and families in the community

3. To provide hospital care within the community in those instances when the individual cannot be maintained on an outpatient basis
B. Types of settings in which services are provided
   1. Outpatient services
      a. Storefront clinics
      b. Walk-in clinics in hospitals
      c. Emergency rooms
      d. Crisis intervention centers, including hot-line phone centers
      e. Day-care centers
      f. Private offices
   2. Inpatient services
      a. Specialized psychiatric hospitals
      b. General hospital psychiatric units
   3. Aftercare services
      a. Foster homes
      b. Halfway houses
      c. Sheltered workshops
      d. Day-care centers
C. Types of services
   1. Observation and diagnosis
   2. Assessment of the client's needs
   3. Crisis intervention
   4. Provide direct care services to clients including
      a. Individual, family, and group therapy
      b. Medications
      c. Electroconvulsive therapy
      d. Occupational therapy
      e. Recreational therapy
   5. Provide a therapeutic milieu that
      a. Supports the individual during the period of crisis
      b. Helps the individual learn new ways of coping with problems
   6. Referral to proper community agencies for necessary services
   7. Provide an educational setting for various professional groups in mental health concepts
   8. Vocational counseling
   9. Health screening

NURSE'S ROLE

A. Case finding
B. Assessment of the individual's needs
C. Establishment of the therapeutic milieu
D. Consultation with other professionals (e.g., physicians, psychologists, social workers, school teachers, clergy)
E. Active participation with the health team, including the individual and family
F. Involvement in individual, family, and group therapy
G. Coordination of health services for the individual and family
H. Education of groups within the community

Emotional Problems Associated with the Aged
GENERAL CONCEPTS

Feelings of loss associated with aging produce some of the behaviors often exhibited by the elderly. These behaviors are, in reality, defense mechanisms utilized to reduce anxiety and maintain self-esteem.

A. Often withdrawal when there is a felt loss or an actual change in body image or loss of a significant other; the individual turns inward, becomes unresponsive to others and the environment

B. Aggressive behavior often develops in response to feelings of guilt and anger when the individual feels helpless to control the situation; aggression may be turned inward on the self, resulting in depression, or turned outward on the environment, resulting in overt anger or hostility

C. Pattern of projective behavior may result when the individual needs to protect the self from the anxiety that feelings of blame or guilt elicit; decreased sensory perceptions associated with aging often contribute to the individual's belief that others are talking about and plotting against him or her

NURSING CARE

A. Help the client meet physical needs
B. Allow client sufficient time to assume and accomplish responsibilities for self-care
C. Seek the client out for short frequent periods of contact
D. Allow and encourage expression of feelings
E. Help the client set realistic goals that can be achieved
F. Recognize accomplishments of the client
G. Provide aids that will allow the client to be more involved with the environment
H. Try to involve the client in activities and social interactions
I. Evaluate client's response and revise plan as necessary

Psychiatric Nursing Review Questions

1. Mental experiences operate on different levels of awareness. The level that best portrays one's attitudes, feelings, and desires is the:
   ① Foreconscious
   ② Preconscious
   ③ Conscious
   ④ Unconscious

2. The level of anxiety which best enhances an individual's power of perception is:
   ① Mild
   ② Moderate
   ③ Severe
   ④ Panic

3. Sublimation is a defense mechanism that helps the individual:
   ① Act out in reverse something already done or thought
   ② Channel unacceptable sexual desires into socially approved behavior
   ③ Return to an earlier, less mature stage of development
   ④ Exclude from the conscious things that are psychologically disturbing

4. An example of displacement is:
   ① Ignoring unpleasant aspects of reality
   ② Imaginative activity to escape reality
   ③ Pent-up emotions directed to other than the primary source
   ④ Resisting any demands made by others

5. Personality is unique for every individual because it is the result of the person's:
   ① Genetic background, placement in family, and autoimmunity
   ② Biologic constitution, psychologic development, and cultural setting
   ③ Childhood experiences, intellectual capacity, and socioeconomic status
   ④ Intellectual capacity, race, and socioeconomic status

6. In the process of development the individual strives to maintain, protect, and enhance the integrity of the ego. This is normally accomplished through the use of:
   ① Ritualistic behavior
   ② Withdrawal patterns
   ③ Defense mechanisms
   ④ Affective reactions

7. Another term for the superego is:
   ① Self
   ② Ideal self
   ③ Narcissism
   ④ Conscience

8. The relationship which is of extreme importance in the formation of the personality is the:
   ① Parent-child
   ② Sibling
   ③ Peer
   ④ Heterosexual

9. The part of the nervous system that is primarily affected during a "fight or flight" reaction is the:
   ① Central nervous system
   ② Peripheral nervous system
   ③ Parasympathetic nervous system
   ④ Sympathetic nervous system

10. The superego is that part of the self which says:
    ① I want what I want
    ② I can wait for what I want
    ③ I should not want that
    ④ I like what I want

11. Groups are important in the emotional development of the individual because groups:
    ① Go through the same developmental phases
    ② Always protect their members
    ③ Are easily identified by their members
    ④ Identify acceptable behavior for their members

12. The family is important in the emotional development of the individual because the family:
    ① Gives rewards and punishment
    ② Helps one to learn identity and roles
    ③ Provides support for the young
    ④ Reflects the mores of a larger society

13. Communication ties people to their:
    ① Physical surroundings
    ② Environmental surroundings
    ③ Social surroundings
    ④ Materialistic surroundings

14. The primary emergence of the personality is demonstrated around the age of:
    ① 6 months
    ② 9 months
    ③ 2 years
    ④ 6 years

15. Problems with dependence versus independence develop during the stage of growth and development known as:
    ① Infancy
    ② Toddler
    ③ Preschool
    ④ School age

16. Strict toilet training before a child is ready will cause problems in personality development because at this age a child is learning to:
    ① Identify own needs
    ② Satisfy parents' needs
    ③ Live up to society's expectations
    ④ Satisfy own needs

17. The basic emotional task for the toddler is:
    ① Trust
    ② Independence
    ③ Identification
    ④ Industry

18. The problem of separation anxiety initially occurs during the:
    ① Oral stage
    ② Anal stage
    ③ Phallic stage
    ④ Latency stage

19. For an emotional balance the individual always needs:
    ① Family, work, and play
    ② Biologic satisfaction and social acceptance
    ③ Individual recognition and group acceptance
    ④ Security and social recognition

20. A 5-year-old boy is constantly found slapping his little sister. This behavior is probably caused by:
    ① Sibling rivalry
    ② Unresolved oedipal conflicts
    ③ Negativistic id impulses
    ④ Overcompensation efforts of superego

21. Since people need some gratifying communication to learn, to grow, and to function in a group, all events that significantly curtail communication will eventually produce:
    ① Some degree of mental deficiency
    ② Severe disturbances
    ③ Further attempts to increase communication
    ④ Withdrawal

22. In applying mental health principles to the care of any person with children, the nurse should be aware that:
    ① Many parents experience feelings of resentment toward their children
    ② Every parent has inborn feelings of love and acceptance for children
    ③ It is pathologic to feel anger and resentment toward a child
    ④ It is easier to adjust to the first child than to later ones

23. Surgery should be delayed, if possible, because of the effects on personality development during the:
    ① Oral stage
    ② Anal stage
    ③ Oedipal stage
    ④ Latency stage

24. A person has a mature personality if the:
    ① Ego acts as a balance between the id and the superego pressures
    ② Ego responds to the demands of the superego
    ③ Ego responds to the demands of society
    ④ Superego has replaced and increased all the controls of the parents

25. Play for the preschool-age child is necessary for the emotional development of:
    ① Projection
    ② Competition
    ③ Introjection
    ④ Independence

26. During the oedipal stage of growth and development, the child:
    ① Loves the parent of the same sex and hates the parent of the opposite sex
    ② Loves the parent of the same sex and the parent of the opposite sex
    ③ Has ambivalence toward both parents
    ④ Loves the parent of the opposite sex and hates the parent of the same sex

27. The stage of growth and development basically concerned with role identification is the:
    ① Oral stage
    ② Oedipal stage
    ③ Latency stage
    ④ Genital stage

28. The main personality problem for clients who need props to blur reality is usually:
    ① Dependency
    ② Mistrust
    ③ Role blurring
    ④ Ego ideal

29. Many persons who are "well adjusted" in ordinary daily living become dependent and demanding when physically ill and hospitalized. This is probably an example of the mechanism of:
    ① Denial
    ② Compensation
    ③ Reaction formation
    ④ Regression

30. The defense mechanism in which emotional conflicts are expressed through motor, sensory, or somatic disability is identified as:
    ① Dissociation
    ② Psychosomatic
    ③ Compensation
    ④ Conversion

31. A college boy who is smaller than average and unable to participate in sports becomes the life of the party and a stylish dresser. This is an example of the mechanism of:
    ① Reaction formation
    ② Compensation
    ③ Sublimation
    ④ Introjection

32. A person, seeing a design on the wallpaper, perceives it as an animal. This is an example of:
    ① Delusion
    ② Hallucination
    ③ Illusion
    ④ Idea of reference

33. The ability to tolerate frustration is an example of one of the functions of the:
    1. Id
    2. Superego
    3. Ego
    4. Unconscious
34. An emotional experience in childhood becomes traumatic when:
    1. The ego is overwhelmed by anxiety it cannot handle
    2. The superego has not been internalized
    3. The child is unable to verbalize own feelings
    4. The parents are harsh and restrictive
35. Resolution of the oedipal complex takes place when the child overcomes the castration complex and:
    1. Rejects the parent of the same sex
    2. Identifies with the parent of the opposite sex
    3. Identifies with the parent of the same sex
    4. Introjects behaviors of both parents
36. A generally accepted concept of personality development is:
    1. The personality is capable of change and modification throughout life
    2. By the end of the first 6 years, the personality has reached its adult parameters
    3. The capacity for personality change decreases rapidly after adolescence
    4. The basic personality is rather firmly set by 2 years of age
37. The superego is that part of the psyche which:
    1. Is the source of creative energy
    2. Develops from internalizing the concepts of parents and significant others
    3. Contains the instinctual drives
    4. Operates on the pleasure principle and demands immediate gratification
38. Evidence of the existence of the unconscious is best demonstrated by:
    1. Déjà vu experiences
    2. Slips of the tongue
    3. The ease of recall
    4. Free-floating anxiety
39. The most common characteristic of emotionally disturbed children is that they:
    1. Respond to any stimulus
    2. Are totally involved with the environment
    3. Respond to little external stimulus
    4. Seem unresponsive to the environment
40. The nurse should observe the autistic child for signs of:
    1. Not wanting to eat
    2. Crying for attention
    3. Catatonic-like rigidity
    4. Enjoying being with people
41. Hyperkinesis in children is usually treated with:
    1. Chlorpromazine hydrochloride (Thorazine)
    2. Haloperidol (Haldol)
    3. Methylphenidate hydrochloride (Ritalin)
    4. Methocarbamol (Robaxin)
42. A person who deliberately pretends an illness is usually thought to be:
    1. Out of contact with reality
    2. Neurotic
    3. Malingering
    4. Using conversion defenses

43. Two 20-year-old female clients have become very much attached to one another and were recently found in bed together. They became angry and sarcastic when the nurse asked one of them to return to her own bed. The nurse can best handle this situation by:
    1. Asking the physician to transfer one of the clients to another unit
    2. Supervising them carefully and separating them when possible throughout the day and especially at night
    3. Restricting both their privileges for several days because their behavior is undesirable and immature
    4. Adopting a matter-of-fact, noncondemning attitude while setting limits on their behavior
44. A frequent finding in clients with paraphilic sexual disorders is that they usually have:
    1. An inadequate physical development of the sexual organs
    2. A deficiency of gonadal and pituitary hormones
    3. Other covert or overt emotional problems
    4. A poor adjustment due to association with society's fringe groups
45. Jim Howard, a 52-year-old man with a diagnosis of schizophrenia, is about to be discharged to a halfway house. This is the fifth admission in less than 1 year for Jim. He improves while in the hospital but after discharge he forgets to take his medication, is unable to function, and must be hospitalized again. A medication that could be given IM to Jim on an outpatient basis every 2 weeks would be:
    1. Stelazine
    2. Thorazine
    3. Prolixin decanoate
    4. Lithium carbonate
46. Projection, rationalization, denial, and distortion by hallucinations and delusions are examples of a disturbance in:
    1. Thought process
    2. Association
    3. Logic
    4. Reality testing
47. A client expresses the belief that the FBI is out to kill him. This is an example of:
    1. A hallucination
    2. A self-accusatory delusion
    3. A delusion of persecution
    4. An error in judgment
48. Mr. James is withdrawn and noncommunicative; to encourage him to talk, the best plan of nursing intervention would be to:
    1. Ask simple questions that require answers
    2. Focus on nonthreatening subjects
    3. Try to get him to discuss his feelings
    4. Sit and look through magazines with him
49. When caring for clients exhibiting withdrawn patterns of behavior, an important aspect of nursing care is to:
    1. Help the client understand that it is harmful to withdraw from situations
    2. Involve the client in activities throughout the day
    3. Help keep the client oriented to reality
    4. Encourage the client to discuss why he does not mix with other people

50. Observation is an important aspect of nursing care. It is especially important in the care of the withdrawn client because it:
    ① Helps in understanding the client's feelings
    ② Is useful in making a diagnosis
    ③ Indicates the degree of psychic depression
    ④ Tells the staff how ill the client is
51. The best approach in helping a very withdrawn client is to provide an environment with:
    ① A large variety of activities
    ② A specific routine
    ③ A trusting relationship
    ④ Group involvement
52. The most accurate definition of "depression," as used in psychiatry, is:
    ① A disturbance in mood as a reaction to the loss of a love object
    ② A total loss of control over emotional impulses
    ③ An inability to make decisions or function
    ④ A disturbance in mood as a result of frustration of instinctual strivings
53. Schizophrenia is considered a functional illness. This means that the:
    ① Genes of the child may carry the schizophrenic factor
    ② Brain itself undergoes actual physical change that produces the symptoms of schizophrenia
    ③ Brain itself undergoes no physical change, but the operation of the organ is disturbed, producing the symptoms of schizophrenia
    ④ Individual is predisposed to schizophrenia because of poor housing and living conditions during childhood
54. The affect most commonly found in the client with schizophrenia is one of:
    ① Happiness and elation
    ② Apathy and flatness
    ③ Sadness and depression
    ④ Anger and hostility
55. Mental illness is evidenced when an individual:
    ① Has difficulty relating to others
    ② Experiences frequent periods of high anxiety
    ③ Expresses little desire for work or social activities
    ④ Has difficulty completing activities
56. Carolyn Demarke has been a client on the psychiatric unit for several days. She arouses anxiety and frustration in the ward staff and manipulates so well that she intimidates any nurse who comes near her. One morning, Carolyn yells out at the nurse, "You've worked it so that I can't go out with the group today to bowl. You're as cunning as a fox—I hate you! Get out or I'll hit you." The best response by the nurse would be:
    ① "You are being rude and I don't like it. Your behavior is stopping me from wanting to stay with you."
    ② "Go ahead and hit me if you have a need to."
    ③ "Tell me what I did to hurt you."
    ④ "I don't really like to hear your threats and insults. Can you tell me why you feel this way?"
57. Functional mental illnesses are mainly the result of:
    ① Genetic endowment
    ② Social environment
    ③ Infection and inflammation
    ④ Deterioration of brain tissue
58. When there is nothing organically wrong with the organs of communication and yet the individual is unable to communicate, the condition is referred to as:
    ① Organic mental disorder
    ② Mental deficiency
    ③ Functional mental disorder
    ④ Chronic brain pathology
59. Mrs. Ray is hospitalized because of a severe depression. While at home she refused to eat, stayed in bed most of the time, and did not talk with family members. Finally, unable to cope with the problem, her husband took her to the hospital. Here the symptoms persist and she will not leave her room. The nurse caring for her attempts to talk to her, asking questions but receiving no answers. Finally, in exasperation, the nurse tells the client that if she does not respond she will be left alone. The nurse:
    ① Attempts to use reward and punishment to motivate the client
    ② Is really assaulting the client and should have refrained from this
    ③ Recognizes that the client has the right to make the decision
    ④ Should get her involved in group therapy rather than attempting one-to-one therapy
60. Mr. James, a client on the psychiatric unit, becomes upset in the day room. In attempting to deal with the situation the nurse should:
    ① Lead him from the room by taking him by his arm
    ② Allow him to act out until he tires
    ③ Give directions in a firm low-pitched voice
    ④ Instruct him to be quiet
61. While talking to another client Susan comes up and yells, "I hate you. You're talking about me again," and throws a glass of juice at the nurse. The best nursing approach would be to:
    ① Remove Susan to an isolation room because she needs to have limits placed on her behavior
    ② Understand her behavior; then say, "You hate me? Tell me about that."
    ③ Ignore both the behavior and Susan, clean up the juice, and talk to her when she is better
    ④ Verbalize feelings of annoyance as an example to Susan that it is more acceptable to verbalize feelings than to act out
62. The nurse recognizes that it would be unusual for an individual with an anxiety disorder to handle the anxiety by:
    ① Converting it into a physical symptom
    ② Acting it out with antisocial behavior
    ③ Displacing it onto less threatening objects
    ④ Regressing to earlier levels of adjustment
63. A phobic reaction will rarely occur unless the person:
    ① Thinks about the feared object
    ② Absolves the guilt of the feared object
    ③ Introjects the feared object into the body
    ④ Comes into contact with the feared object

64. School phobia is usually treated by:
    ① Calmly explaining why attendance at school is necessary
    ② Returning the child to school immediately
    ③ Allowing the parent to accompany child to classroom
    ④ Allowing the child to enter classroom before other children

65. The person with socially aggressive behavior needs an environment that:
    ① Allows freedom of expression
    ② Is mainly group oriented
    ③ Provides control by setting limits
    ④ Can be manipulated

66. The individual who demonstrates obsessive-compulsive behavior can best be treated by:
    ① Calling attention to the behavior
    ② Restricting the client's movements
    ③ Supporting but limiting the behavior
    ④ Keeping the client busy to distract him or her

67. Many people control anxiety by ritualistic behavior. When taking care of these individuals it is important for the nurse to:
    ① Allow them time to carry out the ritual
    ② Prevent them from carrying out the ritual
    ③ Explain the meaning of the ritual
    ④ Avoid mentioning the ritual

68. Sally, age 16, is admitted to the psychiatric service. She has lost 20 pounds in 6 weeks. She is very thin but excessively concerned about being overweight. Her daily intake is 10 cups of coffee. The most important initial nursing intervention would be to:
    ① Compliment her on her lovely figure
    ② Explain the value of good nutrition
    ③ Explore the reasons why she does not eat
    ④ Try to establish a relationship of trust

69. Shortly after admission, Sally falls to the floor and has tonic and clonic movements. She does not respond verbally but the nurse notes that she is still chewing gum. The nurse should:
    ① Remove the chewing gum
    ② Send another client for help
    ③ Report and record all observations
    ④ Insert a tongue blade between her teeth

70. A young handsome man with a diagnosis of antisocial personality disorder is being discharged from the hospital next week. He asks the nurse for her phone number so he can call her for a date. The nurse's best response would be:
    ① "No, you are a client and I am a nurse."
    ② "We are not permitted to date clients."
    ③ "I like you, but our relationship is professional."
    ④ "It is against my professional ethics to date clients."

71. The client with an antisocial personality disorder:
    ① Is generally unable to postpone gratification
    ② Suffers from a great deal of anxiety
    ③ Has a great sense of responsibility toward others
    ④ Rapidly learns by experience and punishment

72. A person with an antisocial personality disorder has difficulty relating to others because of never having learned to:
    ① Count on others
    ② Be dependent on others
    ③ Communicate with others socially
    ④ Empathize with others

73. When pouring liquid Thorazine, the nurse should:
    ① Keep it away from the face during inspiration
    ② Mix it with fruit juice immediately
    ③ Administer immediately after pouring
    ④ Avoid contact with skin

74. Mrs. Somers is an elderly client who has been taking chlorpromazine hydrochloride (Thorazine) for several months. After noticing that she sits rigidly in her chair, the nurse observes her closely for other evidence of adverse effects of the drug, including:
    ① Inability to concentrate, excess salivation
    ② Minimal use of nonverbal expression, rambling speech
    ③ Incoordinated movement of extremities, tremors
    ④ Reluctance to converse, nonverbal clues indicating fear

75. In assessing the client for adverse effects of chlorpromazine hydrochloride (Thorazine), the nurse would also:
    ① Examine her eyeballs and question her about the color of her stools
    ② Assess her appetite and weigh her weekly.
    ③ Take her blood pressure and ask if she has frequent headaches
    ④ Examine her skin and ask if she has numbness or coldness of her feet

76. A client receiving high-dosage chlorpromazine HCl (Thorazine) has developed tremors of the hands. The nurse should:
    ① Report the symptoms to the physician
    ② Withhold the medication
    ③ Tell the client it is transitory
    ④ Give the client finger exercises to perform

77. An extrapyramidal symptom that is a potentially irreversible side effect of chlorpromazine and other antipsychotic drugs is:
    ① Pseudoparkinsonism
    ② Torticollis
    ③ Tardive dyskinesia
    ④ Occulogyric crisis

78. Lithium carbonate is the drug of choice for:
    ① Acute agitation of schizophrenia
    ② Agitated phase of paranoid state
    ③ Modification of depressive phase of major depression
    ④ Control of manic episode of bipolar disorders

79. A common manageable side effect of the major tranquilizers is:
    ① Jaundice
    ② Unintentional tremors
    ③ Ptosis
    ④ Melanocytosis

80. When monoamine oxidase inhibitors (MAOIs) are prescribed, the client should be cautioned against:
    ① The use of medications with an elixir base
    ② Prolonged exposure to the sun
    ③ Ingesting wines and aged cheeses
    ④ Engaging in active physical exercise

81. Photosensitization is a side effect associated with the use of:
    ① Chlorpromazine hydrochloride (Thorazine)
    ② Thioridazine hydrochloride (Mellaril)
    ③ Methylphenidate hydrochloride (Ritalin)
    ④ Lithium carbonate (Lithane)

82. The major tranquilizers are the drugs of choice to relieve symptoms of:
    ① Narcotic withdrawal
    ② Depression
    ③ Hyperkinesis
    ④ Psychosis

83. Drugs such as trihexyphenidyl (Artane), biperiden (Akineton), and benztropine (Cogentin) are often prescribed in conjunction with:
    ① Major tranquilizers
    ② Minor tranquilizers
    ③ Barbiturates
    ④ Antidepressants

84. Many psychiatric clients are given the drugs Cogentin or Artane in conjunction with the phenothiazine derivatives to:
    ① Potentiate the effect of the drug
    ② Reduce postural hypotension
    ③ Combat extrapyramidal side effects
    ④ Modify depression that often accompanies schizophrenia

85. Mrs. Jane, a 45-year-old woman, is hospitalized because of chronic alcoholism. She is irritable with the nurses and seems only to wait for a friend who visits daily. After such visits Mrs. Jane seems happier and more relaxed. One day the nurse sees the visitor give her a package, which she puts away quickly. Later Mrs. Jane, obviously intoxicated, tells the staff that her friend has brought gin regularly. Mrs. Jane's husband is very upset and threatens to sue. The decision in this suit would take into consideration the fact that:
    ① Clients may have gifts brought to them without prior inspection
    ② Mrs. Jane's response to her friend's visit was a clue that the nurse missed
    ③ The nurse is responsible for observing the client's behavior
    ④ Psychotic clients need close supervision

86. Chronic alcoholic clients with Wernicke's encephalopathy associated with Korsakoff's syndrome are treated initially by:
    ① Oral administration of paraldehyde
    ② Judicious use of tranquilizers
    ③ Providing a high-protein diet
    ④ Intramuscular injections of thiamine

87. In thinking about alcohol and drug abuse the nurse should be aware that:
    ① Most polydrug abusers also abuse alcohol
    ② Most alcoholics become polydrug abusers
    ③ An unhappy childhood is a causative factor in addictions
    ④ Addictive individuals tend to use hostile abusive behavior

88. For most nurses the most difficult part of the nurse-client relationship is:
    ① Developing an awareness of self and the professional role in the relationship
    ② Being able to understand and accept the client's behavior
    ③ Accepting responsibility in identifying and evaluating the real needs of the client
    ④ Remaining therapeutic and professional at all times

89. The goal of the therapeutic psychiatric environment is to:
    ① Help the client become popular in a controlled setting
    ② Improve the client's ability to relate to others
    ③ Help the staff to help the client
    ④ Make the hospital atmosphere more home-like

90. During a group meeting a client, Mr. Thomas, tells everyone of his fear of his impending discharge from the hospital. It would be most appropriate for the group leader to respond:
    ① "Maybe you're not ready to be discharged yet, Mr. Thomas."
    ② "Maybe others in the group have similar feelings that they would share."
    ③ "You ought to be happy that you're leaving, Mr. Thomas."
    ④ "How many in the group feel that Mr. Thomas is ready to be discharged?"

91. The emotional leader of a group is one who:
    ① Reflects the feeling tone of the group
    ② Has an authoritarian role within the group
    ③ Designates the roles within the group
    ④ Selects those who are to be members of the group

92. Group therapy can best help those who:
    ① Are emotionally ill
    ② Are dependent on others
    ③ Feel they have a problem
    ④ Have no one to listen to them

93. The group setting is especially conducive to therapy, since it:
    ① Creates a new learning environment
    ② Fosters one-to-one relationships
    ③ Decreases the focus on the individual
    ④ Confronts individual members with their shortcomings

94. When providing group therapy, the nurse must focus on:
    ① Behavior of individual members
    ② Personal feelings affecting behavior
    ③ Jointly experienced stress
    ④ Confrontation between members

95. In helping to resolve a crisis situation it is most important for the nurse to:
    ① Meet all dependency needs
    ② Encourage socialization
    ③ Support ego strengths
    ④ Involve the person in a therapy group

96. The current trend in the treatment of the emotionally ill is to:
    ① Medicate during stressful periods
    ② Maintain them in the community
    ③ Encourage the assumption of responsibility
    ④ Provide occupational therapy

97. The referral of discharged psychiatric clients to a psychiatric day hospital facility in their own community is done primarily to assist them to:
    ① Maintain goals attained during hospitalization
    ② Increase social skills and awareness
    ③ Avoid direct confrontation with the community
    ④ Get out of the house for a few hours daily

Situation: Mrs. Avery, age 29, was a capable librarian before her marriage. However, she was always very sensitive, aloof, withdrawn, and lacking in the ability to feel warm toward others; she rarely joined any organizations and distrusted people in general. Shortly after the birth of her last child she was admitted to a psychiatric hospital for care. At this time she is convinced that the neighbors are accusing her of indiscretions and that they have her home "bugged" so that they may overhear any conversations taking place there. Since her admission she has remained aloof from the others, paces the floor, and believes that the hospital is a house of torture and the food poisoned. Questions 98 through 106 refer to this situation.

98. Mrs. Avery's prepsychotic personality might be described as:
   ① Suspicious and socially inadequate
   ② Rigid and controlling
   ③ Dependent and immature
   ④ Schizoid and introverted

99. Nursing interventions for Mrs. Avery should appropriately be directed toward:
   ① Convincing her that the hospital staff is trying to help
   ② Helping her enter into group recreational activities
   ③ Arranging the hospital environment so that her contact with other clients is limited
   ④ Helping her learn to trust the staff through selected experiences

100. Mrs. Avery frequently refuses to eat because she believes that the food is poisoned. One of the most appropriate ways in which the nurse might initially handle this situation is to:
   ① Simply state that the food is not poisoned
   ② Suggest that food be brought in from home
   ③ Taste the food in her presence
   ④ Tell her that she will have to be tube fed if she does not eat

101. After the initial intervention the nurse should pursue the matter of Mrs. Avery's belief by saying:
   ① "Why do you think the food is poisoned?"
   ② "You feel someone wants to poison you?"
   ③ "Your feeling is a symptom of your illness."
   ④ "You'll be safe with me. I won't let anyone poison you."

102. Mrs. Avery has refused to eat for 36 hours. She states that the voice of her dead father has commanded her to atone for her sins by fasting for 40 days. The initial intervention on the part of the nurse that might interrupt her delusional system is:
   ① Asking the physician to write an order for tube feeding
   ② Asking Mrs. Avery exactly what the voice said
   ③ Telling Mrs. Avery that she has nothing to atone for
   ④ Suggesting other means of atonement that may be less damaging

103. Mrs. Avery remains aloof from all other clients. The nurse with whom she has developed a friendly relationship may help her participate in some ward activity by:
   ① Inviting another client to take part in a joint activity with the nurse and Mrs. Avery
   ② Asking the physician to speak to Mrs. Avery about entering into ward activities

③ Finding solitary pursuits that Mrs. Avery can enjoy on the ward
④ Speaking to Mrs. Avery about the importance of entering into activities

104. Mrs. Avery has been assigned to a four-bed room. The night nurse reports that she has been awake for several nights. The cause of her sleeplessness may be related to:
   ① Fear of the other clients
   ② Worry about her family
   ③ Trying to work out her problems
   ④ Watching for an opportunity to escape

105. The nurse could most appropriately begin to help Mrs. Avery with her sleep problem by saying:
   ① "Don't worry, you'll sleep when you're tired."
   ② "I'm going to move you to a private room."
   ③ "I'll get you the sedative your doctor ordered."
   ④ "You seem unable to sleep at night."

106. While talking with the nurse about her problem of not being able to make friends with any of the other clients, Mrs. Avery begins to cry. At this time it would be most therapeutic for the nurse to:
   ① Suggest that they play a game of Scrabble
   ② Tell her that her crying isn't going to help
   ③ Sit quietly with her
   ④ Point out how she can change this

Situation: Mr. Frank, 21 years of age, is an only child who has never earned his own living and has always been pampered and coddled by his domineering mother and ignored by his quiet retiring father. When he started dating, his mother chose the girls he took out. Recently Mr. Frank married a woman several years older than he, even though his mother seriously disapproved of her. Despite this, he brought his wife to his home to live. Both the mother and the wife are unhappy with this arrangement. Mr. Frank had many guilt feelings about his marriage and soon began to complain of pain in his right arm, which progressed to the point of paralysis. After seeking help from competent orthopedic specialists, he was referred for psychiatric evaluation. Questions 107 through 109 refer to this situation.

107. Mr. Frank's symptoms may be an unconscious attempt to solve a conflict evolving from:
   ① Hostile feelings toward his home
   ② Ambivalent feelings toward his wife
   ③ Inadequate feelings in regard to assuming the role of husband
   ④ Needs to be a dependent child and an independent adult

108. In discussing Mr. Frank's prognosis with the staff the nurse informs them that:
   ① His symptoms of paralysis may spread to other parts of his body
   ② Continuous psychiatric treatment will be required to maintain him as a functioning individual
   ③ Recovery of the use of the arm can be expected, but under stress he may utilize similar symptoms
   ④ It is not possible to predict what the future for this client holds

109. In dealing with Mr. Frank, the nurse should realize that:
    ① This symptom is necessary for him to cope with his present situation.
    ② This symptom is an unconscious method of getting attention
    ③ He can get well if he is helped to focus on other things
    ④ His problem will be solved when he learns to deal with his mother and wife

Situation: Mrs. Sam, a 45-year-old homemaker, was recently admitted to the psychiatric hospital because of a history of hopelessness, anxiety, and suicide attempts. In the hospital she paces the halls, cries, and says that the terrible condition of the world is her fault. She believes that her insides are decayed, that her husband and children are dead, and that the food she eats is of no nutritional value to her. Mrs. Sam has three daughters, all of whom are away at college. Her life has always centered about her family and her meticulously kept home. She has never had any hobbies or outside interests, and her moral standards have been strict and unbending. Questions 110 through 115 refer to this situation.

110. Mrs. Sam's prepsychotic personality can best be described as:
    ① Withdrawn and seclusive, with an active fantasy life
    ② Rigid, narrow, overly conscientious
    ③ Suspicious, sensitive, aloof
    ④ Dependent, immature, insecure

111. One of the nurse's primary responsibilities in caring for Mrs. Sam is to:
    ① Help her realize that her children are not dead
    ② Protect her against her suicidal impulses
    ③ Reassure her that she is a good woman
    ④ Keep up her interest in the outside world

112. One of the nursing goals is to help Mrs. Sam pace the halls less frequently, since this wears her out physically. This can best be accomplished by:
    ① Supplying her with simple monotonous tasks
    ② Restraining her in a chair so she is unable to pace
    ③ Requesting a sedative order from her physician
    ④ Placing her in a single room so she can pace in a smaller area

113. In reassuring Mrs. Sam concerning the many fears that are upsetting to her, it would be helpful to say:
    ① "Your daughters and your husband love you very much."
    ② "You know that you are not a bad woman."
    ③ "Mrs. Sam, those ideas of yours are in your imagination."
    ④ "Those ideas are part of your illness and you will change as you improve."

114. The nurse continues to sit with Mrs. Sam, although there is little verbal communication. One day, Mrs. Sam asks her, "Do you think they'll ever let me out of here?" The nurse's best response is:
    ① "Why, do you think you are ready to leave?"
    ② "You have the feeling that you might not leave?"
    ③ "Everyone says you're doing just fine."
    ④ "Why don't you ask your doctor?"

115. Mrs. Sam confides to the nurse that she has been thinking about suicide. The nurse recognizes that Mrs. Sam:
    ① Feels safe with the nurse and can share her feelings with her
    ② Wishes to frighten the nurse
    ③ Is fearful of her own impulses and is seeking protection from them
    ④ Wants attention from the staff

Situation: Mrs. Jones, a 29-year-old woman, believes that doorknobs are contaminated and refuses to touch them, except with a paper tissue. Questions 116 through 118 refer to this situation.

116. In dealing with this behavior the nurse should:
    ① Encourage her to touch doorknobs by removing all available paper tissue until she learns to deal with the situation
    ② Explain to her that her idea about doorknobs is part of her illness and is not necessary
    ③ Encourage her to scrub the doorknobs with a strong antiseptic so she does not need to use tissues
    ④ Supply her with paper tissues to help her function until her anxiety is reduced

117. Symptoms such as using tissues to touch doorknobs develop because the client is:
    ① Consciously using this method of punishing herself
    ② Unconsciously controlling unacceptable impulses or feelings
    ③ Listening to voices that tell her the doorknobs are unclean
    ④ Fulfilling a need to punish others by carrying out an annoying procedure

118. Therapeutic treatment of Mrs. Jones should be directed toward helping her to:
    ① Forget her fears by administering antianxiety medications
    ② Understand her behavior is caused by unconscious impulses that she fears
    ③ Redirect her energy into activities to help others
    ④ Learn that her behavior is not serving a realistic purpose

Situation: Mrs. Smith has been admitted to a psychiatric hospital with the diagnosis of organic mental disorder. Questions 119 through 124 refer to this situation.

119. The nurse recognizes that it would be most unusual for Mrs. Smith to demonstrate:
    ① Resistance to change
    ② A tendency to dwell on the past and ignore the present
    ③ Preoccupation with personal appearance
    ④ An inability to concentrate on new activities or interests

120. An organic mental disorder is characterized by:
    ① Areas of brain destruction called senile plaques
    ② Periodic remissions and exacerbations
    ③ Aggressive acting out behavior
    ④ Hypoxia of selected areas of brain tissue

121. The approach that would be most helpful in meeting Mrs. Smith's needs is:

① Simplifying the environment as much as possible while eliminating need for choices
② Providing a nutritious diet high in carbohydrates and proteins
③ Developing a consistent nursing plan with fixed time schedules to provide for emotional and physical needs
④ Providing an opportunity for many alternative choices in the daily schedule to stimulate interest

122. In attempting to understand Mrs. Smith's behavior the nurse recognizes that Mrs. Smith is probably:
① Attempting to develop new defense mechanisms to meet her current life situation
② Not capable of using any defense mechanisms
③ Making exaggerated use of old familiar mechanisms
④ Using one method of defense for every situation

123. The nursing care plan for the client with organic brain deterioration should include:
① An extensive reeducation program
② Details for protective and supportive care
③ The introduction of new leisure time activities
④ Plans to involve the client in group therapy sessions

124. In planning care for Mrs. Smith the nurse should appropriately:
① Maintain the daily routine of living with which she is familiar
② Discuss current events to keep her in contact with reality
③ Teach her new social skills to encourage participation
④ Encourage her to talk of her youth and early experiences

Situation: Dr. Kay, a 45-year-old physician, is admitted to the psychiatric unit of a general hospital. He is restless, loud, aggressive, and resistive during the admission procedure. Questions 125 through 127 refer to this situation.

125. Dr. Kay shouts at the nurse who is trying to take his admission blood pressure, "I'm a physician. Do you think you're more qualified than I? I'll do it myself." The most therapeutic response by the nurse would be:
① "Right now, doctor, you're just another client."
② "If you'd rather, doctor. I'm sure you'll do it OK."
③ "I'm sorry but I can't allow that. I must take it."
④ "If you won't cooperate, I'll get the attendants in to hold you down."

126. After the admission examination a nurse is assigned to introduce Dr. Kay to the other clients. He tells her that he wishes to be introduced as Dr. Kay. The nurse's response should be:
① "I can't do that. It's better if they don't know you are a doctor."
② "That's fine, Dr. Kay; that's how I'll introduce you."
③ "All the clients here call one another by their first names."
④ "Why do you insist on being called Doctor?"

127. By the time Dr. Kay has been a client on the service for 3 days he has questioned everyone's authority, has advised other clients that their treatments are wrong, and has talked four other clients into forming their own therapy group. The staff's most appropriate response would be to:

① Ignore him and hope he will stop trying to disrupt the ward
② Understand that he is unable to control his actions and that limits must be set for him
③ Tell the other clients that he is just another client and they should not pay attention to him
④ Restrict his contact with other clients until he stops bothering everyone

Situation: The nurse is assigned to care for Mr. Bishop, a 39-year-old, hyperactive, elated client who exhibits flight of ideas. Questions 128 through 131 refer to this situation.

128. The nursing care plan for Mr. Bishop should appropriately include plans to:
① Encourage him to talk as much as needed
② Arouse and focus his interest in reality
③ Persuade him to complete any task that he begins
④ Provide constructive channels for redirecting his excess energy

129. In approaching Mr. Bishop during a period of great overactivity it is essential to:
① Use a firm, warm, consistent approach
② Anticipate and physically control his hyperactivity
③ Allow him to choose the activities in which he will participate
④ Let him know you will not tolerate destructive behavior

130. Mr. Bishop is not eating. The nurse recognizes that this may be because he:
① Feels that he does not deserve the food
② Believes that he does not need the food
③ Wishes to avoid the clients in the dining room
④ Is so busy that he does not take time to eat

131. The nurse can best respond to Mr. Bishop's eating problem by:
① Providing a tray for him in his room
② Assuring him that he is deserving of food
③ Ordering foods that he can hold in his hand to eat while moving around
④ Pointing out that the energy he is burning up must be replaced

Situation: Mrs. Lord, 23 years old, has been married 3 months. She was admitted to a psychiatric hospital after a month of unusual behavior that included eating and sleeping very little, talking or singing constantly, charging hundreds of dollars' worth of furniture to her father-in-law, and picking up dates on the street. In the hospital, Mrs. Lord monopolizes conversation, insists on unusual privileges, and frequently becomes demanding, bossy, and sarcastic. She has periods of great overactivity and sometimes is destructive. She frequently uses vulgar and profane language. Mrs. Lord was formerly witty, gay, and the "life of the party." Questions 132 through 137 refer to this situation.

132. The symptoms that Mrs. Lord exhibits are usually found in clients experiencing:
① Mood disorders
② Schizophrenic disorders
③ Personality disorders
④ Major depressions

133. When Mrs. Lord's language becomes vulgar and profane, the nurse should:
     ① State: "We don't like that kind of talk around here."
     ② State: "When you can talk in an acceptable way, we will talk to you."
     ③ Recognize it as part of her illness but set limits on it
     ④ Ignore it, since she is using it only to get attention

134. During Mrs. Lord's phase of extreme elation and hyperactivity the nursing staff should consider her nutritional needs by:
     ① Following her around the dining room with her tray
     ② Providing her with frequent high-calorie feedings that can be held in the hand
     ③ Accepting the fact that she will eat when she is hungry
     ④ Allowing her to prepare her own meals and eat when she pleases

135. Mrs. Lord's hyperactivity might be redirected therapeutically by:
     ① Giving her cleaning equipment and suggesting that she assist with the ward work
     ② Asking her to guide other clients as they clean their rooms
     ③ Suggesting that she initiate social activities on the ward for the client group
     ④ Giving her a pencil and paper and encouraging her to write

136. In helping Mrs. Lord with personal hygiene the nurse should:
     ① Keep makeup away from her because she will apply it too freely
     ② Suggest that she wear hospital clothing to avoid confrontations
     ③ Allow her to apply makeup in whatever manner she chooses
     ④ Encourage her to dress attractively and in her own clothing

137. Three new staff members are assigned to the unit on which Mrs. Lord is a client. During their orientation tour, Mrs. Lord greets them by saying, "Welcome to the funny farm. I'm Jo-Jo the head yo-yo." This comment might mean that she is:
     ① Looking for attention from the new staff
     ② Unable to distinguish fantasy from reality
     ③ Anxious over the arrival of the new staff members
     ④ Trying to fill her role as "life of the party"

Situation: Mr. Long, age 35, has been admitted to the mental health unit of a general hospital. Over the past month he has had difficulty in sleeping and has lost his appetite. Although very anxious and tense, he appears sad and has lost all initiative. He has difficulty in concentrating, and most of his thoughts center on his unworthiness and his failures. Questions 138 to 147 refer to this situation.

138. Mr. Long is being interviewed by the admitting nurse. The statement that would be the most appropriate at this time would be:
     ① "Tell me what has been bothering you."
     ② "Why do you feel so bad about yourself?"
     ③ "Tell me how you feel about yourself."
     ④ "What can we do to help you during your stay with us?"

139. Mr. Long's feelings of self-effacement are best observed by his:
     ① Quiet and monotonous voice
     ② Lack of initiative
     ③ Inappropriate gestures and affect
     ④ "Don't listen to me" attitude

140. The nurse needs to evaluate Mr. Long's potential for suicide. The approach that would best gain this information would be:
     ① Asking his family if he has ever attempted suicide
     ② Asking him if he has ever thought of suicide
     ③ Asking other clients about suicide while in a group
     ④ Asking him what his plans are for the future

141. The action by the nurse that would be most therapeutic when Mr. Long states, "I am no good. I'm better off dead." would be:
     ① Unobtrusively removing those articles which could be used in a suicide attempt
     ② Stating, "I think you are good; you should think of living."
     ③ Stating, "I will stay with you until you are less depressed."
     ④ Alerting the staff to provide 24-hour observation of the client

142. In making a nursing care plan for Mr. Long, the approach that would be most therapeutic would be:
     ① Allowing time for his slowness when planning activities
     ② Encouraging the client to perform menial tasks to meet the need for punishment
     ③ Helping Mr. Long focus on family strengths and support systems
     ④ Reassuring him that he is worthwhile and important

143. Mr. Long refuses to cooperate with the staff. All planned activities are rejected, since he is "just too tired." The nursing approach that best expresses an understanding of his needs is:
     ① Explaining why the activities are therapeutic for him
     ② Accepting his behavior calmly and, without excessive comment, setting firm limits
     ③ Helping him express his feelings of hostility toward the activities
     ④ Planning a rest period for him during activity time

144. The nurse understands that one of the most difficult tasks for Mr. Long is to express his:
     ① Feelings of low self-esteem
     ② Remorse and guilt
     ③ Anger toward others
     ④ Need for comforting

145. Mr. Long is to have electroconvulsive therapy (ECT). The nurse, when discussing this therapy, should tell him that:
     ① He will be put to sleep and will have no pain
     ② With new methods of administration, treatment is totally safe
     ③ It is better not to talk about it, but he can ask any question
     ④ He will have complete memory loss as a result of the treatment

146. The physician has ordered imipramine (Tofranil), 75 mg tid, for Mr. Long. An appropriate nursing action in giving this drug is:

① Warning him not to eat cheese, fermenting products, and chicken liver

② Avoiding administration of barbiturates or steroids with this drug

③ Having him checked for intraocular pressure and instruct him to watch for symptoms of glaucoma

④ Observing him for increased tolerance so that therapeutic dosage is maintained

147. Mr. Long is to be discharged from the hospital. The statement by the nurse that gives the most understanding at this time is:
    ① "I am going to miss you; we have become good friends."
    ② "Call the unit night or day if you have problems."
    ③ "This is my phone number; call me and let me know how you are doing."
    ④ "I know you are going to be all right when you go home."

Situation: Mr. James has been admitted to the psychiatric unit for psychologic testing. He is a 43-year-old well-dressed man whom the nurse finds sitting with his face in his hands. He is charged with molesting a 7-year-old child. Questions 148 and 149 refer to this situation.

148. When the nurse asks Mr. James to come to dinner, he refuses, stating "I don't want anyone to see me. Leave me alone." The nurse's best response would be:
    ① "Certainly, Mr. James. I respect your wishes."
    ② "It will be easier to face other people right away."
    ③ "Only the staff members know why you are here."
    ④ "You are the hardest judge you must face, Mr. James."

149. Mr. James looks intently at the nurse without saying anything else. The nurse could best respond by stating:
    ① "I'll be at the desk if you need me."
    ② "Pull yourself together, Mr. James. I'll walk you to dinner."
    ③ "Tell me what you are feeling now, Mr. James."
    ④ "It must be difficult to be on a psychiatric unit."

Situation: Mrs. Jordon is admitted with a severe anxiety disorder. She is crying, wringing her hands, and pacing. Questions 150 through 155 refer to this situation.

150. The first nursing intervention should be to:
    ① Ask her what is bothering her
    ② Tell her to sit down and try to relax
    ③ Stay physically close to her
    ④ Get her involved in a nonthreatening activity

151. Unsatisfied needs create anxiety that motivates an individual to action. This action is brought about mainly to:
    ① Relieve physical discomfort
    ② Reduce tension
    ③ Remove the problem
    ④ Deny the situation

152. The nurse should teach Mrs. Jordon's family that anxiety can be recognized as:
    ① Fears that are related to the total environment
    ② A behavior pattern observable in ourselves and others

③ A totally unique experience and feeling

④ Consciously motivated thoughts and wishes

153. The nurse can minimize Mrs. Jordon's psychologic stress by:
    ① Learning what is of particular importance to her
    ② Explaining in fine detail the procedures and therapies
    ③ Confidently advising her that the nurse is in charge of the situation
    ④ Avoiding the discussion of any areas that may be emotionally charged

154. Physiologically, the nurse would expect Mrs. Jordon's anxiety to be manifested by:
    ① Dilated pupils, dilated bronchioles, increased pulse rate, hyperglycemia, and peripheral vasoconstriction
    ② Constricted pupils, constricted bronchioles, increased pulse rate, hypoglycemia, and peripheral vasodilation
    ③ Dilated pupils, constricted bronchioles, decreased pulse rate, hypoglycemia, and peripheral vasoconstriction
    ④ Constricted pupils, dilated bronchioles, increased pulse rate, hyperglycemia, and peripheral vasodilation

155. The most appropriate way to decrease Mrs. Jordon's anxiety is by:
    ① Prolonged exposure to fearful situations
    ② Introducing an element of pleasure into fearful situations
    ③ Avoiding unpleasant objects and events
    ④ Acquiring skills with which to face emergencies

Situation: Mrs. Queen, 28 years old, is admitted to the hospital with a diagnosis of conversion disorder. Questions 156 through 159 refer to this situation.

156. Mrs. Queen states that she is unable to move her legs. The nurse would expect to observe that Mrs. Queen:
    ① Appears greatly depressed
    ② Exhibits free-floating anxiety
    ③ Appears calm and composed
    ④ Demonstrates anxiety when discussing symptoms

157. When caring for Mrs. Queen, a positive nursing intervention would be to:
    ① Encourage her to try to walk
    ② Avoid focusing on her physical symptoms
    ③ Tell her there is nothing wrong
    ④ Help her follow through with the physical therapy plan

158. In a client such as Mrs. Queen, anxiety is:
    ① Diffuse and free floating
    ② Localized and relieved by the symptom
    ③ Consciously felt by the client
    ④ Projected onto the environment

159. In planning nursing care for Mrs. Queen, the nurse recognizes that:
    ① It is best to ignore her complaints
    ② Her behavior indicates a lack of willpower
    ③ Her symptoms are evidence of a disturbed personality
    ④ If additional stress is added, she will become psychotic.

Situation: The staff and clients have just learned that, while on a weekend pass from the hospital, Sally Finn has committed suicide. A meeting is called to attempt to deal with the feelings this incident has aroused among staff and clients alike. The collective mood of the group is tense and restless. Questions 160 through 162 refer to this situation.

160. The nurse sitting beside Mrs. Smith observes that she is sobbing and rocking back and forth in a sitting position while she hugs her arms around herself and moans softly, "I'm next. Oh, my God, I'm next. They couldn't stop Sally and they can't protect me." The nurse could best respond by saying:
    ① "Sally was a lot sicker than you are, Mrs. Smith."
    ② "It's different, Mrs. Smith. Sally was home; you're here."
    ③ "You are afraid you will hurt yourself, Mrs. Smith?"
    ④ "Don't worry. All passes will be canceled for a while."

161. Jim May, a friend of Sally's, stands up and shouts, "Oh! I know what you're all thinking; you think that I should have known that she was going to kill herself. You think that I helped her plan this." The group leader's response should be:
    ① "Oh no, Jim, we all know you liked Sally."
    ② "You feel we're blaming you for Sally's death, Jim?"
    ③ "It'll help if you tell us the truth, Jim."
    ④ "Helping her plan her suicide would not be healthy."

162. During the group discussion it is learned that Sally had not shared her strong suicidal feelings and had successfully masked her depression. The group leader should be prepared primarily to deal with:
    ① The guilt that the group feels because it could not prevent Sally's suicide
    ② The fear and anxiety which some members of the group may have that their own suicidal urges may go unnoticed and unprotected
    ③ The guilt, fear, and anger of the staff, that they have failed to anticipate and prevent Sally's suicide
    ④ The lack of concern over Sally's suicide expressed by some of the group

Situation: Miss Hayes, 19 years of age, came to the psychiatric hospital from a girl's dormitory on a nearby college campus where she was a freshman. Throughout high school she had always been an excellent student who was interested in modern art, ballet, dancing, symphony concerts, and good literature. She played the violin very well. She had no close friends and was considered a loner. Her family states that she always has been sensitive and different from other girls. She was admitted to the psychiatric hospital when she refused to get out of bed and go to classes. Her personal appearance deteriorated steadily during the past month, and recently she did not bother to comb her hair or put on makeup. In the hospital she talks to unseen people, voids on the floor, sometimes masturbates openly, occasionally eats with her hands, and refuses to shower or wear her own clothes. Questions 163 through 171 refer to this situation.

163. The nurse's efforts should be directed toward helping Miss Hayes by:
    ① Providing frequent rest periods to avoid exhaustion
    ② Attempting to establish a meaningful relationship with her
    ③ Reducing environmental stimuli and maintaining dietary intake
    ④ Facilitating her social relationships with her peer group

164. The most appropriate way to begin to help Miss Hayes accept the realities of daily living would be to:
    ① Encourage her to join the other clients in group singing
    ② Assist her to care for her own personal hygiene
    ③ Encourage her to take up playing the violin again
    ④ Leave her alone when she is disinterested in the activities at hand

165. When Miss Hayes openly masturbates, the nurse should most appropriately:
    ① Restrain her hands
    ② Not react to the behavior
    ③ Put her in seclusion
    ④ State that such behavior is unacceptable

166. Miss Hayes starts to repeat phrases that others have just said. This type of speech is known as:
    ① Autism
    ② Echopraxia
    ③ Echolalia
    ④ Neologism

167. The nurse could best handle the problem of Miss Hayes voiding on the floor by:
    ① Making her mop the floor
    ② Restricting her fluids throughout the day
    ③ More frequent toileting with supervision
    ④ Withholding privileges each time she voids on the floor

168. When Miss Hayes eats with her hands, the nurse can handle this problem by:
    ① Placing the spoon in her hand and suggesting that she use it
    ② Commenting, "I thought college girls had better manners than that."
    ③ Removing the food and saying, "You can't have any more until you can use your spoon."
    ④ Saying in a joking way, "Well, fingers were made before forks."

169. While watching TV in the day room Miss Hayes suddenly screams, bursts into tears, and runs out of the room to the far end of the hallway. The most therapeutic action for the nurse to take would be to:
    ① Write up the incident on her chart while memory is fresh
    ② Ask another client what made Miss Hayes act as she did
    ③ Walk to the end of the hallway where Miss Hayes is standing
    ④ Accept the action as just being the impulsive behavior of a sick person

170. Miss Hayes feels that "a man on television" is responsible for her being sick. This is an example of:
    ① Autistic thinking
    ② Illusion
    ③ Hallucination
    ④ Delusion

171. Miss Hayes, who has been watching the nurse for a few days, suddenly walks up and shouts, "You think you're so damned perfect and good. I think you stink!" The most appropriate response for the nurse to make would be:
    ① "I can't be all that bad can I?"
    ② "You seem angry with me."
    ③ "Stink? I don't understand."
    ④ "Boy, you're in a bad mood."

Situation: Mrs. Ohream is a 46-year-old woman who was admitted to the psychiatric hospital because she drank poison and slashed her wrists. She cries a great deal, refuses food, and says that she is not fit to live. The physician has ordered electroconvulsive therapy (ECT) for her. Questions 172 through 176 refer to this situation.

172. Mrs. Ohream has just awakened from her first ECT treatment. The most appropriate nursing intervention would be to:
    ① Get Mrs. Ohream up and out of bed as soon as possible and back into her normal routine
    ② Orient Mrs. Ohream to time and place and tell her that she has just had a treatment
    ③ Arrange for the attendant to bring Mrs. Ohream a lunch tray
    ④ Take Mrs. Ohream's blood pressure and pulse rate every 15 minutes until she is fully awake

173. The factor that is most important in helping to evaluate the risk of suicide in a depressed client such as Mrs. Ohream is the:
    ① Length of time the depression has existed
    ② Impending anniversary of the loss of a loved one
    ③ Development of plans for discharge from hospital or program
    ④ Presence of multiple personal problems

174. A positive nursing action in caring for Mrs. Ohream is to:
    ① Allow her to make decisions for herself
    ② Provide her with frequent periods of thinking time
    ③ Hold her hand while sitting with her
    ④ Play a game of chess with her

175. The nurse is caring for Mrs. Ohream on a day when she seems more withdrawn and depressed. An appropriate nursing action would be to:
    ① Ask her if you may sit with her
    ② Tell her you will spend some time with her
    ③ Remain visible to her
    ④ Get her involved in group activities

176. Depressed clients such as Mrs. Ohream seem to do best in settings where they have:
    ① Many varied activities
    ② A great deal of stimuli
    ③ A simple daily schedule
    ④ To make only simple decisions

Situation: Mr. Daniels, 19 years old and a known heroin addict, is unconscious when admitted to the emergency room with the diagnosis of narcotic (heroin) overdose. Questions 177 through 179 refer to this situation.

177. The medication used to combat an overdose of narcotics is:
    ① amphetamine sulfate (Benzedrine)
    ② naloxone hydrochloride (Narcan)

③ dextroamphetamine (Dexedrine)
④ caffeine sodium benzoate

178. The planned effect of this drug is to:
    ① Stimulate cortical sites controlling consciousness and cardiovascular function
    ② Accelerate metabolism of heroin and stimulate respiratory centers
    ③ Compete with narcotics for receptors controlling respiration
    ④ Decrease analgesia and the comatose state induced by heroin

179. Within an hour Mr. Daniels is responding. Close observation of his status is indicated because:
    ① The combined action of naloxone hydrochloride and heroin causes cardiac depression
    ② Naloxone hydrochloride may cause neuropathy and convulsions
    ③ The narcotic effect may cause return of symptoms after the nalaxone chloride is metabolized
    ④ Hyperexcitability and amnesia may cause the client to thrash about and become abusive

Situation: James Cote is a narcotic addict who had surgery to repair a laceration of his heart caused by a bullet. Postoperatively he is receiving methadone hydrochloride orally. Questions 180 through 185 refer to this situation.

180. Methadone hydrochloride:
    ① Provides postoperative pain control without causing narcotic dependence
    ② Counteracts the depressive effects of long-term opiate usage on cardiac and thoracic muscles
    ③ Allows symptom-free termination of narcotic addiction
    ④ Converts narcotic use from an illicit to a legally controlled drug

181. Drug abuse is best defined as:
    ① A physiologic need for a drug
    ② A psychologic dependence on a drug
    ③ An excessive drug use inconsistent with acceptable medical practice
    ④ A compulsion to take a drug on either a continuous or periodic basis

182. Hard drugs easily cause dependence because of their ability to:
    ① Ease pain
    ② Clear sensorium
    ③ Blur reality
    ④ Decrease motor activity

183. How many hours after the last dose of methadone would the nurse expect Mr. Cote's withdrawal symptoms to reach a peak?
    ① 8 to 24
    ② 24 to 48
    ③ 48 to 72
    ④ 72 to 96

184. The nurse would expect Mr. Cote's basic personality to be marked by insecurity and:
    ① Infantile passion for self-gratification
    ② The need to delay gratification
    ③ The use of psychosomatic mechanisms
    ④ Weak id drives

185. When methadone hydrochloride dosage is lowered, Mr. Cote must be observed closely for evidence of:
     ① Agitation, attempts to escape from the hospital
     ② Piloerection, lack of interest in surroundings
     ③ Skin dryness, scratching under incisional dressing
     ④ Lethargy, refusal to participate in therapeutic exercise

Situation: Mr. Winford, a 42-year-old executive, is admitted for treatment of his alcoholism. Questions 186 through 191 refer to this situation.

186. Mr. Winford is suspicious of others and blames them for his difficulty. The nurse understands that he is using this behavior because he has problems:
     ① In identifying who bothers him
     ② With dependence and independence
     ③ In telling the truth
     ④ Meeting his ego ideal

187. Mr. Winford asks if the nurse can see the bugs that are crawling on his bed. The nurse's best reply would be:
     ① "I will get rid of them for you."
     ② "No, I don't see any bugs."
     ③ "I will stay with you until you are calmer."
     ④ "Those bugs are a part of your sickness."

188. Mr. Winford often makes up stories to fill in the blank spaces of his memory. This is known as:
     ① Denying
     ② Confabulating
     ③ Lying
     ④ Rationalizing

189. As Mr. Winford begins to feel better, he denies excessive use of alcohol. The nurse understands that denial is meeting Mr. Winford's need to:
     ① Make him look better in the eyes of others
     ② Live up to others' expectations
     ③ Make him seem more independent
     ④ Reduce his feelings of guilt

190. Mr. Winford asks if it is required that he attend Alcoholics Anonymous. The nurse's best reply would be:
     ① "No, it is best to wait until you feel you really need them."
     ② "Yes, because you will learn how to cope with your problem."
     ③ "Do you have feelings about going to these meetings?"
     ④ "You'll find you'll need their support."

191. Groups such as Alcoholics Anonymous help people like Mr. Winford because in a group the person learns that:
     ① He does not need a crutch
     ② His problems are not unique
     ③ His problems are caused by alcohol
     ④ People stand stronger together

Situation: Mr. Ray, a 32-year-old salesman, is attending his first meeting of Alcoholics Anonymous because he finally realized and admitted that he is an alcoholic. Questions 192 through 196 refer to this situation.

192. The most effective treatment of alcoholism is accomplished by:
     ① Admission to an alcoholic unit in a hospital
     ② Individual or group psychotherapy

③ The daily administration of disulfiram (Antabuse)
④ Active membership in Alcoholics Anonymous

193. Self-help groups such as Alcoholics Anonymous are successful because they meet the client's need to:
     ① Be trusted
     ② Grow
     ③ Be independent
     ④ Belong

194. Self-help groups assist their members to:
     ① Deal with present behavior and changes in behavior
     ② Identify with their peers
     ③ Set long-term goals
     ④ Identify the underlying cause of their behavior

195. For clients with alcoholism, the primary rehabilitator is the:
     ① Nurse
     ② Physician
     ③ Entire health team
     ④ Client

196. The most important factor in Mr. Ray's rehabilitation is:
     ① His emotional or motivational readiness
     ② The qualitative level of his physical state
     ③ His family's accepting attitude
     ④ The availability of community resources

Situation: Donald Raye, a 19-year-old college sophomore, has been admitted through the university health service. He had become increasingly withdrawn, unkempt, isolated, and depressed. The referring psychiatrist notes strong suicidal tendencies. A contributing factor appears to be an abrupt ending of a relationship with a 22-year-old senior. His grades have fallen to the extent that he is in danger of failing all his courses. Questions 197 through 200 refer to this situation.

197. Donald's prognosis for a reasonably rapid recovery is:
     ① Poor, since he has suicidal tendencies
     ② Bad, since he is failing in all sectors of his life
     ③ Fair, since he is intelligent enough to pull himself together
     ④ Good, since the onset is fairly sudden and no previous emotional problems existed

198. On the second day after his admission Donald asks the nurse why he is being observed around the clock and has his freedom of movement restricted. The nurse's most appropriate reply would be:
     ① "Your doctor has ordered it. He's the one you should ask."
     ② "Why do you think we are observing you?"
     ③ "We are concerned that you might try to harm yourself."
     ④ "What makes you think that, Donald?"

199. On the fourth day Donald tells the nurse, "Hey look! I was feeling pretty depressed for a while, but I'm certainly not going to kill myself." The nurse's best response to his communication would be:
     ① "Kill yourself? I don't understand."
     ② "We have to observe you until your doctor tells us to stop."
     ③ "Suppose we talk some more about this."
     ④ "You do seem to be feeling better."

200. With treatment Donald progresses satisfactorily and is to be discharged within a day or two. He appears to be responsible for his actions and the staff is pleased with his progress. The day before discharge the nurse leaves the door to the unit unlocked. On her return a few minutes later Donald is gone. He is found in a bathroom where he has hanged himself. In this situation:
   ① Determined clients almost always succeed at suicide, even with constant supervision
   ② The lifting of the depression demonstrated Donald's recovery, so supervision was unnecessary
   ③ Suicidal clients should be observed until all symptoms of depression have disappeared
   ④ Donald's actions should have been anticipated by the nurse

Situation: Mrs. Jameson has been hospitalized for a major depressive episode. For the past 5 days she has been receiving Parnate (tranylcypromine sulfate) 10 mg po bid. Questions 201 through 206 refer to this situation.

201. This morning Mrs. Jameson refused her medication stating. "It doesn't help, so what's the use of taking it." The response by the nurse that would best demonstrate an understanding of the action of this medication would be:
   ① "Sometimes it takes 2 to 3 weeks to see an improvement."
   ② "You should have felt a response by now. I'll notify your physician."
   ③ "It takes 6 to 8 weeks for this medication to have an effect."
   ④ "I'll talk to the physician about increasing the dosage, and that will help."

202. An important aspect of teaching for Mrs. Jameson regarding her understanding of her medication should be that:
   ① The therapeutic level of Parnate and the toxic level are very close
   ② Clients taking this type medication have special dietary restrictions
   ③ It is necessary to wear a hat outdoors and avoid the sun
   ④ Drowsiness is an expected side effect of this medication

203. An activity that would be most appropriate for Mrs. Jameson, during the early part of her hospitalization, would be a:
   ① Small dance-therapy group
   ② Card game with three other clients
   ③ Project involving drawing
   ④ Game of Trivial Pursuit

204. Mrs. Jameson has been having daily one-to-one therapy sessions with Ms. Morgan, her primary nurse. A long-term goal that Ms. Morgan and Mrs. Jameson have planned for might be that Mrs. Jameson will:
   ① Be able to develop new defense mechanisms
   ② Understand the unconscious source of her anger
   ③ Be able to talk about her depressed feelings
   ④ Be more realistic in accepting herself and others

205. As her depression begins to lift, Mrs. Jameson is asked to join a small discussion group that meets on the unit every evening. She tells the nurse that she does not want to join because she has nothing to talk about. The best response by the nurse would be:
   ① "Could you start off by talking about your children?"
   ② "A woman your age has a great deal to offer the group."
   ③ "Maybe tomorrow you will feel more like talking."
   ④ "You feel you will not be accepted by the group unless you have something to say?"

206. If Mrs. Jameson does not abide by her diet restrictions while on Parnate, it is most likely she will develop:
   ① A sudden severe hypotension
   ② Severe muscle spasms
   ③ An occipital headache
   ④ Generalized urticaria

Situation: Elsie Anglim, 38 years old, has been admitted for medical supervision of her withdrawal from seconal which she has depended on for sleep for many years. Questions 207 and 208 refer to this situation.

207. A standard regimen for her withdrawal process would be the administration of gradually decreased amounts of:
   ① Methadone
   ② Lithium
   ③ Thorazine
   ④ Phenobarbital

208. The nurse caring for Mrs. Anglim is aware that abrupt withdrawal from barbiturates could cause a person to experience:
   ① Convulsions
   ② Diarrhea
   ③ Urticaria
   ④ Ataxia

Situation: Maura Collins, a registered nurse on the psychiatric unit of a general hospital, has been asked to talk with a group of senior high school students and their parents on career advisement day. Questions 209 and 210 refer to this situation.

209. When Maura defines her role as a psychiatric nurse, the statement that would best describe the practice of psychiatric nursing would be:
   ① Assuring clients' legal and ethical rights by acting as a client advocate
   ② Focusing interpersonal skills on people with physical or emotional problems
   ③ Helping people with present or potential mental health problems
   ④ Acting in a therapeutic way with people diagnosed as having a mental disorder

210. When asked by one student to describe a mentally healthy individual, Ms. Collins defines such a person as one who:
   ① Has insight into his or her own problems
   ② Is able to meet his or her own basic needs
   ③ Is not exhibiting pathological symptoms
   ④ Is free from both physical and emotional problems

CHAPTER 5

Pediatric Nursing

Pediatric nursing encompasses the care of well and ill children, stressing preventive as well as restorative interventions. This section is divided into the descriptive age groups of childhood, that is, infancy, toddlerhood, preschool years, school-age years, and adolescence. Principles of growth and development, age-specific achievements, health maintenance objectives, and disease-related states are discussed for each age category. Such an organization attempts to present the nursing of children as one that incorporates their physical and psychologic needs toward optimum promotion of health.

Introduction
BASIC CONCEPTS

A. Children are individuals, not little adults, who must be seen as part of a family
B. Family-centered care is the objective in the care of children to provide total health maintenance
C. Children are influenced by genetic factors, home and environment, and parental attitudes
D. Chronologic and developmental ages of children are the most important contributing factors influencing their care
E. Prevention of illness and maintenance of health are the main thrusts in health care of children
F. Play is a natural medium for expression, communication, and growth in children

THE FAMILY
Structure of the Family

A. The basic unit of a society
B. Composition varies although one member is usually recognized as head
C. Usually share common goals and beliefs
D. Roles change within the group and reflect both the individual's and the group's needs
E. Status of members determined by position in family in conjunction with views of society

Functions of the Family

A. Reproduction: group developed to reproduce and rear members of a society
B. Maintenance to provide
   1. Clothing, housing, food, and medical care
   2. Social, psychologic, and emotional support for family members
   3. Protection, since immaturity of young children necessitates that care be given by adults
   4. Status: child is a member of a family that is also a part of the larger community

C. Socialization
   1. Child is "acculturated" by introduction to social situations and instruction in appropriate social behaviors
   2. Self-identity develops through relationships with other family members
   3. Child learns appropriate sex roles and responsibilities
D. Growth of individual members toward maturity and independence

HUMAN GROWTH AND DEVELOPMENT
Principles of Growth

A. Traditional definition of growth is limited to physical maturation
B. Integrated definition includes functional maturation
C. Growth is complex with all aspects closely related
D. Growth is measured both quantitatively and qualitatively over a period of time
E. Although the rate is not even, growth is a continuous and orderly process
   1. Infancy: most rapid period of growth
   2. Preschool to puberty: slow and uniform rate of growth
   3. Puberty: (growth spurt) second most rapid growth period
   4. After puberty: decline in growth rate till death
F. There are regular patterns in the direction of growth and development, such as the cephalocaudal law (from head to toe) and the proximodistal law (from center of body to periphery)
G. Different parts of the body grow at different rates
   1. Prenatally: head grows the fastest
   2. During the first year: elongation of trunk dominates
H. Both rate and pattern of growth can be modified, most obviously by nutrition
I. There are critical or sensitive periods in growth and development, such as brain growth during uterine life and infancy
J. Although there are specified sequences for achieving growth and development, each individual proceeds at own rate
K. Development is closely related to the maturation of the nervous system; as some primitive reflexes disappear, they are replaced by a voluntary activity such as grasp

Characteristics of Growth

A. Circulatory system
   1. Heart rate decreases with increasing age
      a. Infancy: 120 beats per minute
      b. One year: 80 to 120
      c. Childhood: 80 to 100
      d. Adolescence to adulthood: 70 to 90 (after maturity, women have slightly higher pulse rate than men)

2. Blood pressure increases with age
   a. Ranges from 40 to 70 mm Hg diastolic to 65 to 140 mm Hg systolic
   b. These levels increase about 2 to 3 mm Hg per year beginning at age 7 years
   c. Systolic pressure in adolescence: higher in males than in females
3. Hemoglobin
   a. Highest at birth, 17 g per 100 ml of blood; then decreases to 10 to 15 g per 100 ml by 1 year
   b. Fetal hemoglobin (60% to 90% of total hemoglobin) gradually decreases during the first year to less than 5%
   c. Gradual increase in hemoglobin level to 14.5 g per 100 ml between 1 and 12 years of age
   d. Level higher in males than in females

B. Respiratory system
1. Rate decreases with increase in age
   a. Infancy: 30 to 40 per minute
   b. Childhood: 20 to 24 per minute
   c. Adolescence and adulthood: 16 to 18 per minute
2. Vital capacity
   a. Gradual increase throughout childhood and adolescence, with a decrease in later life
   b. Capacity in males exceeds that in females
3. Basal metabolism
   a. Highest rate is found in the newborn
   b. Rate declines with increase in age, higher in males than in females

C. Urinary system
1. Premature and full-term newborns have some inability to concentrate urine
   a. Specific gravity (newborn): 1.001 to 1.020
   b. Specific gravity (others): 1.001 to 1.030
2. Glomerular filtration rate greatly increased by 6 months of age
3. Glomerular filtration rate reaches adult values between 1 and 2 years of age
4. Glomerular filtration rate gradually decreases after 20 years of age

D. Digestive system
1. Stomach size small at birth, rapidly increases during infancy and childhood
2. Peristaltic activity decreases with advancing age
3. Blood sugar levels gradually rise from 75 to 80 mg per 100 ml of blood in infancy to 95 to 100 mg during adolescence
4. Premature infants have lower blood sugar levels than do full-term infants
5. Enzymes are present at birth to digest proteins and a moderate amount of fat but only simple sugars (amylase is produced as starch is introduced)
6. Secretion of hydrochloric acid and salivary enzymes increases with age until adolescence; then decreases with advancing age

E. Nervous system
1. Brain reaches 90% of total size by 2 years of age
2. All brain cells are present by end of the first year, although their size and complexity will increase
3. Maturation of the brainstem and spinal cord follows cephalocaudal and proximodistal laws

F. Impact on medications
1. Pediatric dosages differ from adult medication dosages due to differences in physiology
   a. Immature liver function
   b. Immature kidney function
   c. Decreased gastric function
   d. Decreased plasma protein concentration
   e. Altered body composition
      (1) Decreased fat
      (2) Increased water
2. Calculate dosage based on body surface area (m^2) to ensure that the child receives the correct drug dosage within a safe therapeutic range
3. Dosage can also be calculated based on body weight, although it is not as accurate as surface area
4. Child must be closely monitored for signs and symptoms of toxicity

PLAY
Functions of Play
A. Educational
B. Recreational
C. Physical development
D. Social and emotional adjustment
   1. Learn moral values
   2. Develop the idea of sharing
E. Therapeutic

Types
A. Active, physical
   1. Push-and-pull toys
   2. Riding toys
   3. Sports and gym equipment
B. Manipulative, constructive, creative, or scientific
   1. Blocks
   2. Construction toys such as erector sets
   3. Drawing sets
   4. Microscope and chemistry sets
   5. Books
   6. Computer programs
C. Imitative, imaginative, and dramatic
   1. Dolls
   2. Dress-up costumes
   3. Puppets
D. Competitive and social
   1. Games
   2. Role playing

Criteria for Judging the Suitability of Toys
A. Safety
B. Compatibility
   1. Child's age
   2. Level of development
   3. Experience
C. Usefulness
   1. Challenge to development of the child
   2. Enhancing social and personality development
   3. Increasing motor and sensory skills
   4. Developing creativity
   5. Expressing emotions
   6. Achieving mastery
   7. Implementating therapeutic procedures

Criteria for Judging the Nonsuitability of Toys
A. Unsafe
B. Beyond the child's level of growth and development
C. Overstimulating; frustrating
D. Limited uses and transient value (see also play for each age group)
E. Foster isolation from peer group

The Infant
GROWTH AND DEVELOPMENT
Developmental Timetable
A. One month
  1. Physical
    a. Weight: gains about 150 to 210 g (5 to 7 oz) weekly during the first 6 months of life
    b. Height: grows about 2.5 cm (1 inch) a month for the first 6 months of life
    c. Head circumference: grows about 1.5 cm (⅗ inch) a month for the first 6 months of life
  2. Motor
    a. May lift the head temporarily, but generally the head must be supported
    b. Holds the head parallel with the body when placed prone
    c. Can turn the head from side to side when prone or supine
    d. Asymmetrical posture dominates, such as tonic neck reflex
    e. Primitive reflexes still present
  3. Sensory
    a. Follows a light to midline
    b. Eye movements coordinated most of the time
    c. Visual acuity 20/100 to 20/50
  4. Socialization and vocalization
    a. Watches face intently while being spoken to
    b. Utters small throaty sounds
B. Two to 3 months
  1. Physical: posterior fontanel closed
  2. Motor
    a. Holds the head erect for a short time and can raise chest supported on the forearms
    b. Bears some weight on legs when held in standing position
    c. Actively holds rattle but will not reach for it
    d. Grasp, tonic neck, and Moro reflexes are fading
    e. Step or dance reflex disappears
    f. Plays with fingers and hands
  3. Sensory
    a. Follows a light to the periphery
    b. Has binocular coordination (vertical and horizontal vision)
    c. Listens to sounds
  4. Socialization and vocalization
    a. Smiles in response to a person or object
    b. Laughs aloud and shows pleasure in making sounds
    c. Cries less
C. Four to 5 months
  1. Physical
    a. Birth weight doubles
    b. Drools because salivary glands are functioning but child does not have sufficient coordination to swallow saliva

  2. Motor
    a. Balances the head well in a sitting position
    b. Can sit when the back is supported; knees will be flexed and back rounded
    c. Symmetrical body position predominates
    d. Can sustain a portion of own weight when held in a standing position
    e. Reaches for and grasps an object with the whole hand
    f. Can carry hand or an object to the mouth at will
    g. Reaches for attractive objects but misjudges distances
    h. Can roll over from abdomen to back
    i. Lifts head and shoulders at a 90-degree angle when prone
    j. Primitive reflexes (e.g., grasp, tonic neck, and Moro) have disappeared
    k. Neurologic reflexes
      (1) Landau (6 to 8 months-12 to 24 months): when infant is suspended in a horizontal prone position, the head is raised, legs and spine are extended
      (2) Parachute (7 to 9 months, persists indefinitely): when the infant is suspended in a horizontal prone position and suddenly thrust forward, hands and fingers extend forward as if to protect from falling.
  3. Sensory
    a. Recognizes familiar objects and people
    b. Has coupled eye movements; accommodation is developing
  4. Socialization and vocalization
    a. Coos and gurgles when talked to
    b. Definitely enjoys social interaction with people
    c. Vocalizes displeasure when an object is taken away
D. Six to 7 months
  1. Physical
    a. Weight: gains about 90 to 150 g (3 to 5 oz) weekly during second 6 months of life
    b. Height: grows about 1.25 cm (½ inch) a month
    c. Head circumference: grows about 0.5 cm (⅕ inch) a month
    d. Teething may begin with eruption of two lower central incisors, followed by upper incisors
  2. Motor
    a. Can turn over equally well from stomach or back
    b. Sits fairly well unsupported, especially if placed in a forward-leaning position
    c. Hitches or moves backward when in a sitting position
    d. Can transfer a toy from one hand to the other
    e. Can approach a toy and grasp it with one hand
    f. Plays with feet and puts them in mouth
    g. When lying down, lifts head as if trying to sit up
    h. Transfers everything from hand to mouth
  3. Sensory
    a. Has taste preferences
    b. Will spit out disliked food
  4. Socialization and vocalization
    a. Begins to differentiate between strange and familiar faces and shows "stranger anxiety"
    b. Makes polysyllabic vowel sounds

    c. Vocalizes "m-m-m-m" when crying

    d. Cries easily on slightest provocation but laughs just as quickly

E. Eight to 9 months

  1. Motor

    a. Sits steadily alone

    b. Has good hand-to-mouth coordination

    c. Developing pincer grasp, with preference for use of one hand over the other

    d. Crawls, may go backward at first

    e. Can raise self to a sitting position but may require help to pull self to feet

  2. Sensory

    a. Depth perception is beginning to develop

    b. Displays interest in small objects

  3. Socialization and vocalization

    a. Shows anxiety with strangers by turning or pushing away and crying

    b. Definite social attachment is evident: stretches out arms to loved ones

    c. Is voluntarily separating self from mother by desire to act on own

    d. Reacts to adult anger: cries when scolded

    e. Has imitative and repetitive speech, using vowels and consonants such as "Dada"

    f. No true words as yet, but comprehends words such as "bye-bye"

    g. Responds to own name

F. Ten to 12 months

  1. Physical

    a. Weight: birth weight triples

    b. Height: birth length increases by 50%

    c. Head and chest circumferences are equal

    d. Upper and lower lateral incisors usually have erupted, for total of 6 to 8 teeth

  2. Motor

    a. Stands alone for short times

    b. Creeps (creeping is more advanced because the abdomen is supported off the floor)

    c. Walks with help: moves around by holding onto furniture

    d. Can sit down from a standing position without help

    e. Can eat from a spoon and a cup but needs help; prefers using fingers

    f. Can play pat-a-cake and peek-a-boo

    g. Can hold a crayon to make a mark on paper

    h. Helps in dressing, such as putting arm through sleeve

  3. Sensory

    a. Visual acuity 20/50 +

    b. Amblyopia may develop with lack of binocularity

    c. Discriminates simple geometric forms

  4. Socialization and vocalization

    a. Shows emotions such as jealousy, affection, anger

    b. Enjoys familiar surroundings and will explore away from mother

    c. Fearful in strange situation or with strangers; clings to mother

    d. May develop habit of "security" blanket

    e. Can say two words besides *Dada* or *Mama* with meaning

    f. Understands simple verbal requests, such as "Give it to me."

PLAY DURING INFANCY (SOLITARY PLAY)

A. Safety is chief determinant in choosing toys (aspirating small objects is one cause of accidental death)

B. Mostly used for physical development

C. Toys need to be simple because of short attention span

D. Visual and auditory stimulation is important

E. Suggested toys

  1. Rattles

  2. Soft stuffed toys

  3. Mobiles

  4. Push-pull toys

  5. Simple musical toys

  6. Strings of big beads and large snap toys

  7. Unbreakable mirrors

  8. Weighted or suction toy

  9. Squeeze toys

  10. Teething toys

  11. Books with textures

  12. Activity boxes

  13. Simple take-apart toys

  14. Nestled boxes and fitting forms

HEALTH PROMOTION DURING INFANCY
Developmental Milestones Associated with Feeding

A. At birth the full-term infant has sucking, rooting, and swallowing reflexes

B. Newborn feels hunger and indicates desire for food by crying

C. At 1 month the infant has strong extrusion reflex

D. By 5 to 6 months the infant can use fingers to eat zwieback or toast

E. By 6 to 7 months the infant is developmentally ready to chew solids

F. By 8 to 9 months the infant can hold a spoon and play with it during feeding

G. By 9 months the infant can hold own bottle

H. By 12 months the child usually can drink from a cup, although fluid may spill and bottle may be preferred at times

Infant Nutrition

A. Nutrition as it affects growth

  1. Birth weight usually doubled by 5 months of age and tripled by 1 year (small babies may gain more weight in a shorter period)

  2. Growth during the first year should be charted to observe for comparable gain in length, weight, and head circumference

  3. Generally, growth charts demonstrate the percentile of the child's growth rate (below the fifth and above the ninety-fifth percentile are considered abnormal)

  4. Percentiles of growth curves must be seen in relation to

    a. Deviation from a steady rate of growth

    b. Hereditary factors of parents (size and body shape)

    c. Comparison of height and weight

5. Satisfactory rate of growth judged by
   a. Weight and length (overweight and underweight constitute malnutrition)
   b. Muscular development
   c. Tissue tone and turgor
   d. General appearance and activity level
   e. Amount of crying and needed sleep
   f. Presence or absence of illness
   g. Mental status and behavior in relation to norms for the age
B. Proper feeding essential to growth and development
   1. General good nutrition that promotes growth but prevents overweight
   2. Prevention of nutritional deficiencies
   3. Prevention of GI disturbances, such as vomiting or constipation
   4. Establishment of good eating habits later in life
   5. Consistency of foods should progress from liquid to semisoft to soft to solids as the dentition and jaw develop

Guidelines for Infant Feeding

A. Breast milk is the most desirable complete diet for the first 6 months but requires supplements of fluoride (regardless of the fluoride content of the local water supply), iron by 6 months, and vitamin D if the mother's supply is deficient or the infant is not exposed to frequent sunlight
B. Iron-fortified commercial formula is an acceptable alternative to breast-feeding; requires fluoride supplements in areas where the fluoride content of drinking water is below 0.3 ppm (Table 5-1)
C. Breast milk or commercial formula is recommended for the first year, but after this age the infant can be given homogenized vitamin D–fortified whole milk; the use of milk with reduced fat content (skimmed or low-fat) is not recommended because increased quantities of solids would be required to supply the caloric needs, leading to overfeeding, and the high solute load would place excessive demands on the immature kidneys; in addition, essential fatty acids are missing
D. Solids can be introduced by about 6 months; the first food is often commercially prepared iron-fortified infant cereals; rice is usually introduced first because of its low allergenic potential; infant cereals should be continued until 18 months of age
E. With the exception of infant cereals, the order of introducing other foods is variable; recommended sequence is weekly introduction of other foods such as fruits and vegetables, and then meats
F. First solid foods are strained, puréed, or finely mashed
G. Finger foods such as toast, zwieback, raw fruit, or crisp-cooked vegetables are introduced at 6 to 7 months
H. Chopped table food or commercially prepared junior foods can be started by 9 to 12 months
I. Fruit juices should be offered from a cup as early as possible to reduce development of nursing bottle caries
J. Method
   1. Feed when the baby is hungry, after a few sucks of breast milk or formula
   2. Introduce one food at a time, usually at intervals of 4 to 7 days, to allow for identification of food allergies
   3. Begin spoon feeding by placing food on back of the tongue, because of the infant's natural tendency to thrust tongue forward
   4. Use a small spoon with straight handle; begin with 1 or 2 teaspoons of food; gradually increase to a couple of tablespoons per feeding
   5. As the amount of solid food increases, the quantity of milk needs to be decreased to approximately 900 ml (30 oz) daily to prevent overfeeding
   6. Never introduce foods by mixing them with the formula in the bottle
K. Weaning
   1. Giving up the bottle or breast for a cup is psychologically significant, since it requires the relinquishing of a major source of pleasure
   2. Usually, readiness develops during second half of the first year because of
      a. Pleasure from receiving food by a spoon
      b. Increasing desire for more freedom
      c. Acquiring more control over body and the environment
   3. Weaning should be gradual, replacing only one bottle at a time with a cup and finally ending with the nighttime bottle
   4. If breast-feeding must be terminated before 5 or 6 months of age, a bottle should be used to allow for the infant's continued sucking needs; after about 6 months wean directly to a cup
L. Diseases or conditions during infancy with possible diet modifications
   1. Diarrhea: decreased fat and carbohydrate
   2. Constipation: increased fluids, added prune juice or strained fruit, change in type of carbohydrate
   3. Celiac disease (malabsorption syndrome): results from gluten sensitivity; diet should be low in gluten, which is found in wheat, rye, barley, and oat grains, so these grains are eliminated and rice and corn are substituted
   4. Allergy: individual diet modification according to specific food sensitivity; e.g., if milk allergy exists, substitute forms of soybean or meat formula preparations are used
   5. Lactose intolerance: found in non-Caucasian races; lactose-free diet used with Nutramigen as a milk substitute
   6. See Inborn errors of metabolism for other disorders.

Table 5-1. Supplemental fluoride dosage schedule (mg/day*)

Age	Concentration of fluoride in drinking water (ppm)		
	<0.3	0.3 to 0.7	>.07
2 weeks to 2 years	0.25	0	0
2 to 3 years	0.50	0.25	0
3 to 16 years	1.00	0.50	0

From American Academy of Pediatrics, Committee on Nutrition: Fluoride supplementation, Pediatrics 77(5): 758-768, 1986.
*2.2 mg sodium fluoride contains 1 mg fluoride.

Immunizations (see Tables 5-2 and 5-3)

A. Specific characteristics of immunizations
1. Diphtheria toxoid: about 80% effective; febrile reaction more commonly seen in older children, so the adult-type Td (tetanus and diphtheria toxoid) given
2. Tetanus toxoid: nearly 100% effective; induces prolonged immunity
3. Pertussis vaccine (vaccine of whole organism): least effective of DTP; has the most side effects
   a. Started early since no passive immunity from mother exists, as with diphtheria and tetanus
   b. Not given after the child's seventh birthday because of more severe reactions
4. Td, after 6 years of age: given routinely every 10 years and at 5-year intervals in the event of a possibly contaminated wound
5. Measles vaccine (live attenuated vaccine): generally not given before 15 months of age because of the presence of natural immunity from mother; if given before 15 months of age, a second dose should be administered
6. Rubella given to children mainly to prevent occurrence of the disease in women during the first trimester of pregnancy
   a. Not given to any unimmunized pregnant woman or if pregnancy is suspected because of potential infection of the fetus
   b. Pregnancy must be prevented until 3 months after immunization to eliminate danger to the fetus

Table 5-2. Recommended schedule for active immunization of normal infants and children

Age	Immunization recommended
2 months	DTP,[a] TOPV[b]
4 months	DTP, TOPV
6 months	DTP[c]
1 year	Tuberculin tests[d]
15 months	Measles, rubella, mumps[e]
18 months	DTP, TOPV
24 months	HBPV[f]
4-6 years	DTP, TOPV
14-16 years	Td[g]—repeat every 10 years

Adapted from American Academy of Pediatrics: Report of the Committee on Infectious Diseases, Ill., ed. 20, 1986. Copyright American Academy of Pediatrics, 1986
(a) DTP—diphtheria and tetanus toxoids combined with pertussis vaccine.
(b) TOPV—trivalent oral poliovirus vaccine. This recommendation is suitable for breast-fed as well as bottle-fed infants.
(c) A third dose of TOPV is optional but may be given in area of high endemicity of poliomyelitis
(d) Frequency of tuberculin testing depends on risk of exposure of the child and on the prevalence of tuberculosis in the population group. The initial test should be at or preceding the measles vaccine.
(e) May be given at 15 months as measles-rubella or measles-mumps-rubella combined vaccines.
(f) HBPV Haemophilus influenza type B polysaccharide vaccine
(g) Td—combined tetanus and diphtheria toxoids (adult type) for those more than 6 years of age, in contrast to diphtheria and tetanus (DT) toxoids, which contain a larger amount of diphtheria antigen.

Table 5-3. Recommended immunization schedules for infants and children not initially immunized at usual recommended times in early infancy

Recommended time	Immunization(s)	Comments
Younger than 7 years old		
First visit	DTP, OPV, MMR	MMR if child ≥15 months old; tuberculin testing may be done
Interval after first visit		
1 mo	HBPV*	For children 24-60 months
2 mo	DTP, OPV	
4 mo	DTP (OPV)	OPV is optional (may be given in areas with increased risk of poliovirus exposure)
10-16 mo	DTP, OPV	OPV is not given if third dose was given earlier
4-6 yr (at or before school entry)	DTP, OPV	DTP is not necessary if the fourth dose was given after the fourth birthday; OPV is not necessary if recommended OPV dose at 10-16 months following first visit was given after the fourth birthday
Age 14-16 yr	Td	Repeat every 10 years throughout life
7 years old and older		
First visit	Td, OPV, MMR	
Interval after first visit		
2 mo	Td, OPV	
8-14 mo	Td, OPV	
Age 14-16 yr	Td	Repeat every 10 years throughout life

DTP, diphtheria and tetanus toxoids with pertussis vaccine; *HBPV, Haemophilus influenzae* type b polysaccharide vaccine; *MMR,* live measles, mumps, and rubella viruses in combined vaccine; *OPV,* oral poliovirus vaccine; *Td,* tetanus toxoid and diphtheria toxoid.
Haemophilus influenzae type b polysaccharide vaccine can be given, if necessary, simultaneously with DTP (at separate sites). The initial three doses of DTP can be given at 1- to 2-month intervals; so, for the child in whom immunization is initiated at 24 months old or older, one visit could be eliminated by giving DTP, OPV, MMR at the first visit; DTP and HBPV at the second visit (1 month later); and DTP and OPV at the third visit (2 months after the first visit). Subsequent DTP and OPV 10 to 16 months after the first visit are still indicated.
From American Academy of Pediatrics: Report of the Committee on Infectious Diseases, ed. 20, Elk Grove Village, Ill, 1986. Copyright American Academy of Pediatrics, 1986.

7. Haemophilus influenza type B (Hib) polysaccharide vaccine recommended for children 2 years and older; should only be used at 18 months if child is in high-risk category; e.g., child who attends day-care center, is asplenic, or has sickle cell anemia; DPT can be given at same visit, but different site should be used

B. General considerations for immunizations (see Table 5-4)
   1. Presence of maternal antibodies
   2. Administration of blood transfusion or immune serum globulin within 3 months
   3. High fever, serious illness (common cold is not a contraindication)
   4. Diseases in which immunity is impaired
   5. Immunosuppressive therapy
   6. Generalized malignancy such as leukemia
   7. Anaphylactic reaction to egg protein
   8. Neurologic problems such as convulsions during administration of pertussis vaccine
   9. Allergic reaction to a previously administered vaccine or a substance in the vaccine such as preservatives or neomycin

Injury Prevention

A. Accidents are one of the leading causes of death during infancy
   1. Mechanical suffocation causes most accidental deaths in children under 1 year of age
   2. Aspiration of small objects and ingestion of poisonous substances occurs most often during second half of the first year and into early childhood
   3. Trauma from rolling off a bed or falling down stairs can occur at any time

B. Teaching is an essential aspect
   1. Birth to 4 months
      a. Aspiration
         (1) Not as great a danger to this age group but should begin practicing safeguarding early (see under 4 to 7 months)
         (2) Inform parents of dangers from baby powder; encourage its proper use and storage
      b. Suffocation
         (1) Keep all plastic bags stored away from infant's reach; discard large plastic garment bags after tying in a knot
         (2) Do not cover mattress or pillows with plastic

Table 5-4. General considerations for immunizations

Immunization	Reaction	Nursing responsibilities*
Diphtheria	Fever usually within 24 to 48 hours Soreness, redness, and swelling at site of injection	Instructions for DTP: Advise parents of possible side effects May recommend prophylactic use of acetaminophen if fever occurred following previous DTP immunization
Tetanus	Same as for diphtheria but may include urticaria and malaise All may have delayed onset and last several days Lump at injection site may last for weeks, even months, but gradually disappears	Recommend use of antipyretics if fever occurs following present immunization Advise parents to notify physician *immediately* of any unusual side effects, such as those listed under pertussis
Pertussis	Same as for tetanus but may include loss of consciousness, convulsions, persistent screaming episodes, generalized and/or focal neurologic signs, fever of or above 104°F (40°C), systemic allergic reactions, thrombocytopenia, or hemolytic anemia	Before administering next dose of DTP, inquire about reactions, especially those listed under pertussis
Poliovirus (TOPV)	Essentially no side effects Vaccine-associated paralysis rarely occurs within 2 months of immunization	Assess presence of family members at risk from TOPV
Measles	Anorexia, malaise, rash, and fever may occur 7 to 10 days after immunization Rarely (estimated risk 1:1 million doses) encephalitis may occur	Advise parents of more common side effects and use of antipyretics for fever If a persistent high fever with other obvious signs of illness occurs, have them notify physician immediately
Mumps	Essentially no side effects other than a brief, mild fever	See general comment to parents
Rubella	Mild rash that lasts 1 or 2 days within a few days after immunization Arthralgia, arthritis, and/or paresthesia of the hands and fingers may occur about 2 weeks after vaccination and is more common in older children and adults	Advise parents of side effects, especially of time delay before joint swelling and pain Assure them that these symptoms will disappear May recommend use of mild analgesics for pain
Haemophilus influenza type B (Hib)	Low-grade fever, mild local reactions at injection site, rarely fever above 104°F (40°C)	Advise parents of possible mild side effects

*General comment to parents regarding each immunization: the benefit of being protected by the immunization is believed to greatly outweigh the risk from the disease.

(3) Use a firm mattress, no pillows, and loose blankets

(4) Make sure crib design follows federal regulations and mattress fits snugly

(5) Position crib away from other furniture

(6) Avoid sleeping in bed with infant

(7) Do not tie pacifier on string around infant's neck

(8) Remove bibs at bedtime

(9) Drowning: never leave infant alone in bath

c. Falls

(1) Always raise crib rails; tie rails to crib if malfunctioning

(2) Never leave infant on a raised, unguarded surface

(3) When in doubt where to place child, use the floor

(4) Restrain child in the infant seat and never leave unattended while the seat is resting on a raised surface

(5) Avoid using a high chair until child is old enough to sit well

d. Poisoning

Not as great a danger to this age group but should begin practicing safeguarding early (see 4 to 7 months)

e. Burns

(1) Check bath water and warmed formula and food

(2) Do not pour hot liquids when infant is close by, such as sitting on lap

(3) Beware of cigarette ashes that may fall on infant

(4) Do not leave infant in the sun for more than a few minutes, use hats and sunscreens

(5) Wash flame-retardant clothes according to label directions

(6) Use cool mist vaporizers

(7) Do not keep child in parked car

(8) Check surface heat of car restraint

f. Motor vehicles

(1) Transport infant (even newborn) in a specially constructed rear-facing car seat with shoulder and waist restraints

(2) Do not place infant on the seat or in your lap

(3) Do not place a carriage or stroller behind a parked car

g. Bodily damage

(1) Avoid sharp, jagged-edged objects

(2) Keep diaper pins closed and away from infant

2. Four to 7 months

a. Aspiration

(1) Keep buttons, beads, and other small objects out of infant's reach

(2) Use pacifier with one-piece construction and loop handle

(3) Keep floor free of any small objects

(4) Do not feed infant hard candy, nuts, food with pits or seeds, or whole hot dogs

(5) Inspect toys for removable parts

(6) Avoid balloons as playthings

b. Suffocation

May begin to teach swimming as part of water safety

c. Falls

(1) Restrain in high chair

(2) Keep crib rails raised to full height

d. Poisoning

(1) Make sure that paint for furniture or toys does not contain lead

(2) Place toxic substances on a high shelf and/or locked cabinet

(3) Hang plants or place on a high surface rather than on floor

(4) Avoid storing large quantities of cleaning fluids, paints, pesticides, and other toxic substances

(5) Discard used containers of poisonous substances

(6) Do not store toxic substances in food containers

(7) Know telephone number of local poison control center

e. Burns

(1) Keep faucets out of reach

(2) Place hot objects (cigarettes, candles, incense) on high surface

f. Motor vehicles

(See birth to 4 months)

g. Bodily damage

(1) Give toys that are smooth and rounded, preferably made of wood or plastic

(2) Avoid long, pointed objects as toys

3. Eight to 12 months

a. Aspiration

(see 4 to 7 months)

b. Suffocation

(1) Keep doors of ovens, dishwashers, refrigerators, and front-loading clothes washers and dryers closed at all times

(2) If storing an unused appliance, such as a refrigerator, remove the door

(3) Fence swimming pools; always supervise when near any source of water, such as cleaning buckets

(4) Keep bathroom doors closed

c. Falls

Fence stairways at top and bottom if child has access to either end

d. Poisoning

(1) Administer medications as a drug, not as a candy

(2) Do not administer adult medications unless prescribed by a physician

(3) Replace medications and poisons immediately after use; replace caps properly if a child protector cap is used

(4) Advise parents regarding proper use of syrup of ipecac

e. Burns

(1) Place guards in front of any heating appliance, fireplace, or furnace

(2) Keep electrical wires hidden or out of reach

(3) Place plastic guards over electrical outlets; place furniture in front of outlets

(4) Keep hanging tablecloths out of reach

(5) Do not allow infant to play with electrical appliance

f. Motor vehicles

(1) Do not use adult seat or shoulder belt without infant car seat

(2) Do not allow to crawl behind a parked car

(3) If infant plays in a yard have the yard fenced or use a playpen

g. Bodily damage

(1) Do not allow infant to use a fork for self-feeding

(2) Use plastic cups or dishes

(3) Check safety of toys and toybox

(4) Protect from animals, especially dogs

Nursing Responsibilities for Parental Guidance During the Infant's First Year

A. First 6 months

1. Understand each parent's adjustment to newborn, especially mother's postpartal emotional needs

2. Teach infant care and assist parents to understand infant's individual needs and temperament and that infant expresses wants through crying

3. Encourage parents to establish a schedule that meets their needs and their child's

4. Help parents understand infant's need for stimulation in environment

5. Support parent's pleasure in seeing child's growing friendliness and social response, especially smiling

6. Plan anticipatory guidance for safety

7. Stress need for immunization against disease

8. Prepare for introduction of solid foods

B. Second 6 months

1. Prepare parents for child's "stranger anxiety"

2. Encourage parents to allow child to cling to mother or father and avoid long separation from either

3. Guide parents concerning discipline because of infant's increasing mobility

4. Teach accident prevention because of child's advancing motor skills and curiosity

5. Encourage parents to leave child with suitable mother substitute to allow some free time

6. Discuss readiness for weaning

HEALTH PROBLEMS DURING INFANCY
Hospitalization During Infancy

A. Reactions to parental separation (begins later in infancy: see the toddler)

B. General problems in care of the infant

1. Small size

a. Body warmth and temperature control

b. Maintenance of fluids: prone to edema, dehydration, and electrolyte imbalance

(1) Infants have a higher percentage of extracellular fluid than do adults, which can be quickly excreted

(2) Infants' kidneys are unable to concentrate urine

2. Immature organ systems

a. Primary defense mechanisms just developing: loss of antibodies from fetal life increases the infant's susceptibility to infection

(1) Antibody levels lowest at 6 weeks to 2 months of age; then infants begin to develop their own system

(2) Problem subsides as infants grow older

b. Blood vessels still developing; increased fragility causes hemorrhage

c. Some essential enzymes (e.g., glucuronyl transferase, which is necessary for conjugation of bilirubin) still developing: more chance for jaundice and brain damage

NURSING PROCESS FOR INFANTS WITH HEALTH PROBLEMS
Probable Nursing Diagnoses Based on Assessment

A. Ineffective airway clearance related to

1. Accumulation of secretions

2. Immobility

3. Fatigue

B. Anxiety related to

1. Strange environment

2. Perception of impending event

3. Separation

4. Anticipated discomfort

5. Knowledge deficit

6. Discomfort

7. Difficulty breathing

8. Feelings of powerlessness

C. Pain related to

1. Disease process

2. Interventions

D. Ineffective family coping: compromised, related to

1. Situational crisis

2. Temporary family disorganization

E. Potential for aspiration related to

1. Disease process

2. Impaired swallowing

F. Altered family processes related to

1. Situational crisis

2. Knowledge deficit

3. Temporary family disorganization

4. Inadequate support systems

G. Diversional activity deficit related to lack of sensory stimulation

H. Fear related to

1. Separation from support systems

2. Uncertain prognosis

3. Perceived inability to control events

I. Potential fluid volume deficit related to

1. Inability to concentrate urine

2. Higher percentage extracellular to intracellular water

3. Inability to regulate input

J. Anticipatory parental grieving related to

1. Expected loss

2. Gravity of infant's physical status

K. Impaired home maintenance management related to

1. Inadequate support systems

2. Family member illness

3. Unfamiliarity with resources

L. Potential for injury related to
   1. Use of specific therapies and appliances
   2. Incapacity for self-protection
   3. Immobility
M. Altered parenting related to
   1. Separation
   2. Skill deficit
   3. Family stress
   4. Knowledge deficit
   5. Interrupted parent-infant bonding
N. Feeding, bathing/hygiene, dressing/grooming, and toileting self-care deficit related to developmental level
O. Sensory-perceptual alteration: tactile related to protective environment
P. Potential impaired skin integrity related to
   1. Immature structure and function
   2. Immobility
Q. Sleep pattern disturbance related to
   1. Excessive crying
   2. Frequent assessment
   3. Therapies
   4. Interventions
   5. Fear of child's prognosis
R. Spiritual distress (parental) related to
   1. Inadequate support systems
   2. Challenged belief and value system due to moral/ethical implications of therapy
S. Impaired breast-feeding related to
   1. Mother-infant separation
   2. Inability of infant to suck
T. Powerlessness related to health care environment
U. Knowledge deficit related to anxiety
V. Potential for infection related to
   1. Immature immune system
   2. Impaired skin integrity
   3. Presence of infective organisms

Probable Nursing Diagnoses for the Family of a Child with a Disability

A. Parental role conflict related to complex care of child
B. Family coping: potential for growth, related to child's disability and care
C. Anticipatory grieving related to
   1. Loss of ideal child
   2. Projected death of child
D. Decisional conflict related to
   1. Need for medical therapies
   2. Proposed care for child
E. Situational low self-esteem related to loss of image of ideal child
F. Fatigue related to care requirements of child with a disability
G. Spiritual distress related to decisions regarding "right to life" conflicts
H. Diversional activity deficit related to inadequate support systems to provide respite
I. Altered parenting related to
   1. Unrealistic expectations of child
   2. Knowledge deficit

Nursing Care for Infants with Health Problems

See specific diseases for nursing care

Nursing Care for the Family of a Child with a Disability

A. Recognize that parents will exhibit a variety of responses, such as grief and mourning, chronic grief, and excessive use of defense mechanisms
B. Understand the stages of chronic grief
   1. Shock and disbelief: parents tend to
      a. Learn about the deformity but deny the facts
      b. Feel inadequate and guilty
      c. Feel insecure in their ability to care for the child
      d. "Doctor shop" in hope of finding solutions
   2. Awareness of the handicap: parents tend to
      a. Feel guilty, angry, and depressed
      b. Envy well children: closely related to bitterness and anger
      c. Search for clues or reasons why this happened to them
      d. Reject and feel ambivalent toward the child
   3. Restitution or recovery phase: parents tend to
      a. See the child's disability in proper perspective
      b. Function more effectively and realistically
      c. Socially and emotionally accept the child
      d. Reintegrate family life without centering it around the handicapped child
C. Help parents gain awareness of the child's disability
   1. Learning cannot take place until awareness of the problem exists
   2. Help the parents develop an awareness through their own realization of the problem rather than identifying problem for them
   3. Help the parents see the problem by drawing attention to certain manifestations such as failure to walk or talk
D. Help the parents understand the child's potential ability and assist them in setting realistic goals
   1. Help them feel a sense of adequacy in parenting by emphasizing good care, identifying small steps in learning process of child, and acquainting them with parents of children with similar problems
   2. Teach them how to work with their handicapped child in simple childhood tasks of walking, talking, toileting, feeding, and dressing
   3. Teach them how to stimulate the child's learning of new skills
E. Encourage the parents to treat the child as normally as possible
   1. Encourage them to avoid overprotection and to use consistent, simple discipline
   2. Help them become aware of the effects of this child on siblings who may resent the excessive attention given to this child
F. Provide the family with an outlet for own emotional tensions and needs
   1. Acquaint them with organizations, especially parent groups, who have children with similar problems
   2. Be a listener, not a preacher
   3. Assist siblings who may fear the possibility of giving birth to children with similar problems
G. Teach parents the importance of follow-up, long-term, medical supervision
H. Evaluate clients' response and revise plan as necessary

CHROMOSOMAL ABERRATIONS
Nursing Process for Children with Chromosomal Abberations
Probable Nursing Diagnoses Based on Assessment

A. Ineffective airway clearance related to
   1. Nasal obstruction
   2. Excessive thick secretions
   3. Impaired musculature
B. Potential for aspiration related to
   1. Impaired swallowing
   2. Nasogastric tube feedings
   3. Impaired gag reflex
C. Constipation related to
   1. Impaired musculature
   2. Decreased activity
D. Bowel incontinence related to cognitive/perceptual impairment
E. Impaired verbal communication related to cognitive impairment
F. Diversional activity deficit related to cognitive or sensory impairment
G. Fear related to hospitalization
H. Knowledge deficit related to cognitive or sensory impairment
I. Altered nutrition: potential for more than body requirements related to immobility
J. Chronic low self-esteem related to
   1. Unrealistic self-expectations
   2. Sterility (Turner and Klinefelter syndromes)
   3. Lack of pubertal changes (Turner and Klinefelter syndromes)
K. Body image disturbance related to
   1. Unrealistic self-expectations
   2. Sterility (Turner and Klinefelter syndromes)
   3. Lack of pubertal changes (Turner and Klinefelter syndromes)
L. Potential impaired skin integrity related to
   1. Immobility
   2. Dermatological changes (Down's syndrome)
M. See Nursing diagnoses for infants with health problems and for the family of child with a disability

Nursing Care for Children with Chromosomal Aberrations

A. See Nursing care under each disorder
B. See Nursing care for the Family of a child with a disability

Down's Syndrome

A. Chromosomal causes
   1. Trisomy 21: associated with advanced parental age (40 to 44 years of age—1%; over 45 years of age—2%); can occur in all age groups
   2. Translocation 15/21: translocated chromosome transmitted most often by the mother who is a carrier; age not a factor
   3. Mosaicism: mixture of normal cells and cells that are trisomic for 21 (usually leads to a less severe phenotype)
B. Associated defects
   1. Small, rounded skull with a flat occiput
   2. Inner epicanthal folds and oblique palpebral fissures
   3. Speckling of the iris (Brushfield's spots)
   4. Small nose with a depressed bridge (saddle nose)
   5. Protruding, sometimes fissured, tongue
   6. Small, sometimes low-set, ears
   7. Short, thick neck
   8. Hypotonic musculature (protruding abdomen, umbilical hernia)
   9. Hyperflexible and lax joints
   10. Simian line (transverse crease on the palmar side of the hand)
   11. Broad, short, and stubby hands and feet
   12. Delayed or incomplete sexual development (men with Down's syndrome usually are infertile)
C. Nursing care
   1. Provide emotional support to parents
   2. Encourage genetic counseling appropriate for type of problem
   3. Assist parents in setting realistic expectations and goals for the child
   4. Prevent infection, especially respiratory
   5. Provide activity consistent with defects
   6. Provide physical supervision and habilitation
   7. Refer for careful testing of intellectual functioning for guidance to parents
   8. See Nursing care for the child with mental retardation
   9. See Nursing care for the family of a child with a disability
   10. Evaluate client's response and revise plan as necessary

Trisomy 18

A. Several physical anomalies of the head, ears, mandible, hands, feet, heart, and kidneys
B. Failure to thrive and short survival; if survive, severe mental retardation
C. Nursing care
   1. Refer parents for genetic counseling
   2. Because of short survival, prepare the parents for loss of their child
   3. See Nursing care for the family of a child with a disability
   4. Evaluate client's response and revise plan as necessary

Turner's Syndrome (Gonadal Dysgenesis)

A. Chromosome monosomy (XO karyotype) in females
B. Congenital malformations such as short stature, webbed neck, infantile genitalia, and developmental failure of secondary sexual characteristics at puberty
C. Usually normal intelligence; problems in directional sense and space-form recognition
D. Nursing care
   1. Provide for genetic counseling of parents
   2. Prepare child for lack of pubertal changes and need for hormonal replacement
   3. Counsel with emphasis on adoption rather than on the person's inability to conceive
   4. See Nursing care for the family of a child with a disability
   5. Evaluate client's response and revise plan as necessary

Klinefelter's Syndrome

A. Sex-chromosomal abnormality of XXY in males
B. Physical characteristics: tall, skinny, long legs and arms, small firm testes, gynecomastia, and poorly developed secondary sex characteristics at puberty
C. Behavioral disorders and mental defects often present
D. Nursing care
   1. Counsel with emphasis on positive aspects such as adoption or donor insemination
   2. Recognize that emotional problems may require lifelong counseling
   3. See Nursing care for the child with mental retardation
   4. See Nursing care for the family of a child with a disability
   5. Evaluate client's response and revise plan as necessary

GASTROINTESTINAL MALFORMATIONS (STRUCTURAL ANOMALIES PRESENT AT BIRTH)
Nursing Process for Children with Gastrointestinal Malformations
Probable Nursing Diagnoses Based on Assessment

A. Activity intolerance related to generalized weakness
B. Pain related to
   1. Bowel distention
   2. Alteration in bowel motility
C. Potential fluid volume deficit related to excessive losses
D. Potential for infection related to
   1. Presence of infectious organisms
   2. Damaged tissues
E. Impaired breast-feeding related to infant's inability to suck
F. Altered nutrition: potential for less than body requirements related to
   1. Difficulty of sucking
   2. Lack of appetite
G. Feeding, bathing/hygiene, dressing/grooming, toileting self-care deficit related to discomfort
H. Body image disturbance related to perception of physical defect or disease
I. Potential impaired skin integrity related to irritation from body secretions or excretions
J. See Nursing diagnoses for infants with health problems and for the family of child with a disability

Nursing Care for Children with Gastrointestinal Malformations

A. See Nursing care under each disorder
B. See Nursing care for the family of a child with a disability

Facial Malformations

A. Failure of union of embryonic structure of face
   1. Fusion of maxillary and premaxillary processes between 5 and 8 weeks of fetal life
   2. Palatal structures fuse between 9 and 12 weeks
B. Cause unknown; evidence of hereditary influence
   1. Incidence in general population is 1 in 800 births
   2. If one child is born with a cleft lip or palate but no history of the anomaly in family, the chance that it will occur in the next child is about 4%
   3. If a history of either anomaly exists in one parent, there is about a 4% chance that the first child will have the defect

Cleft Lip

A. Bilateral or unilateral; if unilateral, more common on the left side
B. More common in males
C. Can be of several degrees; complete cleft usually continuous with cleft palate
D. Treatment is surgical repair, usually done soon after birth because of psychologic difficulties of the parents associated with the visual effects of the defect and the child's inability to meet sucking needs
E. Main difficulty is feeding since the child cannot form a vacuum with the mouth to suck but may be able to breast-feed (sometimes the breast fills the cleft, making sucking easier)
F. Problem of swallowed air caused by mouth breathing results in
   1. Distended abdomen, pressure against the diaphragm
   2. Mucous membranes of the orpharynx become dried and cracked, leading to infection
G. Nursing care
   1. Preoperative nursing care
      a. Feed in an upright position
      b. Feed with a soft large-holed nipple or rubber-tipped syringe placed on the top and side of the tongue, toward back of the mouth
      c. Burp frequently because of swallowed air
      d. Teach parents to give water after each feeding to cleanse the infant's mouth
      e. Prevent infection from irritation of the lip
         (1) Restrain infant's arms, if needed
         (2) Provide a pacifier to increase sucking pleasure
   2. Postoperative nursing care
      a. Maintain a patent airway
         (1) Problem because of edema of the nose, tongue, and lips combined with the child's habit of breathing through the mouth
         (2) Proper equipment such as laryngoscope, endotracheal tube, and suction at or near the bedside
      b. Cleanse the suture line to prevent crust formation and eventual scarring
      c. Prevent crying, because of pressure on suture line (encourage the parent to stay with the infant)
      d. Place the child supine with arm or elbow restraints
         (1) Change position to the side or sitting up, to prevent hypostatic pneumonia
         (2) Remove restraints only when supervised
      e. Feed (same as before surgery)
      f. Support the parents by accepting and treating the child as normal
   3. See Nursing care for the family of a child with a disability
   4. Evaluate client's response and revise plan as necessary

Cleft Palate

A. More common in girls
B. May involve the soft or hard palate and may extend into the nose, forming an oronasal passageway
C. Age for repair is usually after the child has grown but before speech is well developed
D. Infection, especially aspiration pneumonia
E. Speech
  1. Palate is needed to trap air in the mouth
  2. Tonsils usually not removed because they provide an additional mechanism to trap air
  3. The child will need a speech appliance to help prevent guttural sounds if repair is delayed beyond speech development
F. Dental development
  1. Excessive dental caries
  2. Malocclusion from displacement of the maxillary arch
G. Hearing problems caused by recurrent otitis media (eustachian tube connects the nasopharynx and middle ear and easily transports foreign material to the ear)
H. Nursing care
  1. Preoperative nursing care: same as for cleft lip except
    a. Feed upright to prevent aspiration
    b. Feed by gavage if necessary
    c. Encourage early use of spoon and cup
    d. Teach parents the need for proper dental hygiene and regular dental supervision
  2. Postoperative nursing care: same as for cleft lip except
    a. In maintaining a patent airway, try to avoid use of suction that traumatizes the operative site
    b. Place the child in a prone Trendelenburg position to prevent aspiration and promote postural drainage
    c. Avoid trauma to suture line by instructing child not to rub tongue on roof of mouth
    d. Provide liquid diet; no milk, because of curd formation on suture line
    e. Avoid the use of straw or spoon
    f. Recognize the need for emotional support of the parents is greater, since recovery is longer and the prognosis uncertain
  3. See Nursing care for the family of a child with a disability
  4. Evaluate client's response and revise plan as necessary

Tracheoesophageal Anomalies

A. Absence of the esophagus
B. Atresia of the esophagus without a tracheal fistula
C. Tracheoesophageal fistula
D. The most common type of anomaly is proximal esophageal atresia combined with distal tracheoesophageal fistula
E. Signs and symptoms
  1. Excessive drooling
  2. Excessive mucus in nasopharynx causing cyanosis, which is easily reversed by suctioning
  3. Choking, sneezing, and coughing during feeding, with regurgitation of formula through the mouth and nose
  4. Inability to pass a catheter into the stomach
F. Treatment: surgical correction
G. Preoperative nursing care
  1. Keep NPO
  2. Maintain in upright position
  3. Suction oropharynx to remove accumulated secretions
  4. Observe for signs of respiratory distress
  5. Change position to prevent pneumonia
  6. Monitor intake and output
H. Postoperative nursing care
  1. Frequently suction mouth and pharynx
  2. Provide high humidity to liquefy thick secretions
  3. Stimulate crying and change of position to prevent pneumonia
  4. Perform proper care of chest tubes if used
  5. Maintain nutrition by oral, parenteral, or gastrostomy method
  6. Provide a pacifier if oral feedings are contraindicated
  7. Provide comfort and physical contact, because hospitalization is usually long
I. See Nursing care for the family of a child with a disability
J. Evaluate client's response and revise plan as necessary

Intestinal Obstruction

A. Congenital life-threatening obstruction of the intestine
B. Signs alerting the nurse to life-threatening obstruction
  1. Abdominal distention
  2. Absence of stools, especially meconium in the newborn (meconium ileus)
  3. Vomiting of bile-stained material; may be projectile
  4. Cyanosis and weak grunting respirations from abdominal distention, causing the diaphragm to compress the lungs
  5. Paroxysmal pain
  6. Weak, thready pulse
C. Preoperative nursing care
  1. Keep NPO
  2. Monitor intake and output
  3. Observe for signs of dehydration
  4. Maintain nasogastric suction
D. Treatment: immediate surgical correction
E. Postoperative nursing care: dependent on the type of surgery performed
  1. Keep operative sites clean and dry, especially after passage of stool
  2. Position the infant on side rather than abdomen to prevent pulling legs up under the chest
  3. Care of colostomy: prevent excoriation of the skin by frequent cleansing and use of a diaper held on by a belly binder
  4. Instruct the parents about colostomy care (include avoidance of tight diapers and clothes around the abdomen)
  5. See Nursing care for the family of a child with a disability
  6. Evaluate client's response and revise plan as necessary

Imperforate Anus

A. Most common intestinal anomaly
B. Failure of the membrane separating the rectum from the anus to absorb during eighth week of fetal life
C. Fistulas within the vagina, urinary tract, or scrotum are common
D. Symptoms
   1. Failure to pass meconium stool
   2. Inability to insert a catheter or small finger into the rectum
   3. Abdominal distention
E. Treatment: immediate surgical correction unless a fistula is present
F. Preoperative and postoperative nursing care: same as for intestinal obstruction

Pyloric Stenosis

A. Congenital hypertrophy of muscular tissue of the pyloric sphincter, usually asymptomatic until 2 to 4 weeks after birth
B. Clinical signs
   1. Vomiting, progressively projectile
   2. Non-bile-stained vomitus
   3. Constipation
   4. Dehydration and weight loss
   5. Distention of the epigastrium, visible peristalsis, and palpable olive-shaped mass in the right upper quadrant
C. Treatment generally surgical: the Fredet-Ramstedt procedure: longitudinal splitting of the hypertrophied muscle
D. Preoperative nursing care
   1. Keep NPO
   2. Monitor intake and output
   3. Monitor for signs of dehydration
E. Postoperative nursing care
   1. Same as for any abdominal surgery
   2. Teach parents the specific feeding method
      a. Give small frequent feedings and feed slowly
      b. Hold the baby in a high-Fowler's position during feeding and place on the right side after feeding with head of bed slightly elevated
      c. Bubble frequently during feeding and avoid unnecessary handling afterward
   3. See Nursing care for the family of a child with a disability
   4. Evaluate client's response and revise plan as necessary

Megacolon (Hirschsprung's Disease)

A. Absence of parasympathetic ganglion cells in a portion of the bowel, which causes enlargement of the bowel proximal to the defect
B. Symptoms may occur gradually
   1. Constipation, or passage of ribbon or pellet-like stool
   2. Intestinal obstruction
C. Treatment: surgical
   1. Removal of aganglionic portion of the bowel
   2. Colostomy if necessary

D. Nursing care
   1. Teach parents the correct procedure for enemas if indicated (point out danger of water intoxication)
   2. Use only isotonic solutions
   3. Prepare isotonic saline by using 1 tsp table salt to 500 ml (1 pint) of tapwater
   4. Use the following suggested amounts of fluid for enemas

Age	Amount (ml)
Infant	120 to 240
2 to 4 years	240 to 360
4 to 10 years	360 to 480
11 years	480 to 720

   5. Postoperative nursing care: dependent on the type of surgery performed
   6. See Nursing care for the family of a child with a disability
   7. Evaluate client's response and revise plan as necessary

RESPIRATORY MALFORMATIONS
Nursing Process for Children with Respiratory Malformations
Probable Nursing Diagnoses Based on Assessment

A. Potential activity intolerance related to
   1. Generalized weakness
   2. Hypoxia
B. Ineffective airway clearance related to
   1. Excess thick secretions
   2. Fatigue
   3. Position requirements
C. Potential for aspiration related to
   1. Presence of tracheostomy or endotracheal tube
   2. Depressed cough and gag reflexes
D. Diversional activity deficit related to environmental restrictions (bed rest, mist tent, ventilatory appliances)
E. Potential for infection related to
   1. Aspiration of foreign substances
   2. Excessive secretions
   3. Presence of infectious organisms
F. Altered nutrition: less than body requirements, related to lack of energy to suck and chew
G. Body image disturbance related to perceived effect of chronic illness
H. Sensory-perceptual alteration related to
   1. Hospital environment
   2. Isolation
   3. Mechanical appliances
I. Potential impaired skin integrity related to
   1. Excessive secretions on skin
   2. Irritation of appliances (tracheostomy tube)
J. Sleep pattern disturbance related to
   1. Position requirements
   2. Discomfort
K. See Nursing diagnoses for children with health problems (specific age group) and for the family of child with a disability

Nursing Care for Children with Respiratory Malformations

A. See Nursing care under each disorder
B. See Nursing care for the family of a child with a disability

Diaphragmatic Hernia

A. Protrusion of abdominal viscera through an opening into the thoracic cavity
B. Symptoms alerting the nurse
  1. Severe respiratory difficulty with cyanosis
  2. Relatively large chest, especially on the affected side
  3. Failure of affected side of the chest to expand during respiration, absence of breath sounds
  4. Relatively small abdomen
C. Treatment: immediate surgical repair
D. Nursing care
  1. Support parents due to critical nature of the condition
  2. Gastric suction to remove secretions and swallowed air from the stomach and intestine before and after surgery
  3. Preoperatively position the infant on affected side with the head elevated to allow full expansion of the unaffected side
  4. Postoperatively feed the infant by gavage to decrease chances of swallowing air

Congenital Laryngeal Stridor (Laryngomalacia)

A. A crowing sound during inspiration caused by different factors, most often related flabbiness of the epiglottis
B. May correct itself as the infant grows, or may necessitate tracheostomy to sustain life
C. Symptoms
  1. Difficulty feeding
  2. Stridor
  3. Difficulty breathing
D. Nursing care
  1. Feeding
    a. Feed infant slowly; stop frequently to allow breathing and then reoffer bottle or breast
    b. Position correctly at the breast or select proper bottle nipple hole size to regulate flow
    c. Help parent to learn correct feeding method
  2. Breathing
    a. Encourage parents to listen to sound of stridor to detect a change
    b. Protect from respiratory tract infection, which increases breathing difficulty
  3. See Nursing care for the family of a child with a disability
  4. Evaluate client's response and revise plan as necessary

Choanal Atresia

A. Embryonic membrane obstructing the posterior nares at junction with the nasopharynx
B. Bilateral obstruction
C. Symptoms
  1. Mouth breathing
  2. Dyspnea that is relieved by crying and aggravated by sucking
D. Treatment: surgery if breathing is severly impaired
E. Nursing care is the same as for laryngeal stridor

CARDIAC MALFORMATIONS

A. Normal circulatory changes that occur at or shortly after birth
  1. Pulmonary circulation rapidly increases
  2. Decreased oxygen concentration results in closure of the foramen ovale, ductus arteriosus, and ductus venosus
B. General signs and symptoms of congenital heart defects in children
  1. Dypsnea, especially on exertion
  2. Feeding difficulty and failure to thrive, often first signs discovered by the parent
  3. Stridor or choking spells
  4. Heart rate over 200, respiratory rate about 60 in the infant
  5. Recurrent respiratory tract infections
  6. In the older child, poor physical development, delayed milestones, and decreased exercise tolerance
  7. Cyanosis, squatting, and clubbing of fingers and toes
  8. Heart murmurs
  9. Excessive perspiration
C. Classification of cardiac lesions
  1. Acyanotic: shunt from left to right side of heart
    a. No abnormal communication between pulmonary and systemic circulation
    b. If a connection within the heart chambers exists, pressure forces blood from the arterial (left) to the venous (right) side of the heart, where it is reoxygenated
  2. Cyanotic: shunt from the right to left side of the heart
    a. Abnormal connection between the pulmonary and systemic circulations
    b. Venous or unoxygenated blood enters the systemic circulation
    c. Polycythemia (increase in the number of red blood cells) occurs as the body tries to compensate for inadequate supply of oxygen
    d. Squatting or knee-chest position is preferred because it decreases venous return by occluding the femoral veins, which have a very low oxygen content; consequently a smaller volume of this blood enters the right ventricle so that the blood shunted into the aorta has a higher oxygen content; it also increases systemic vascular resistance, which diverts right ventricular blood from the aorta into the pulmonary artery, increasing pulmonary blood flow; this increases the amount of oxygenated blood in the left side of the heart and eventually into systemic circulation
    e. Compensation and the nature of the defect cause clubbing of fingers and toes, retarded growth, and increased viscosity of blood; can lead to congestive heart failure

Types of Acyanotic Defects
Ventricular Septal Defect (VSD)

A. Abnormal opening between the two ventricles
B. Severity of the defect depends on size of the opening
C. High pressure in the right ventricle causes hypertrophy, with development of pulmonary hypertension
D. Low, harsh murmur heard throughout systole
E. Treatment procedure: closure of the opening in the septum

Atrial Septal Defect (ASD)

A. Types
1. Ostium secundum defect, in which the hole is in the center of the septum
2. Ostium primum defect, in which there is inadequate development of the endocardial cushions
3. Sinus venosus defect, in which the superior portion of the atrial septum fails to form near the junction of the atrial wall with the superior vena cava
B. Murmur heard high on the chest, with fixed splitting of the second heart sound
C. Treatment procedure: closure of the opening in the septum

Patent Ductus Arteriosus (PDA)

A. Failure of the fetal connection between the aorta and pulmonary artery to close
B. Blood shunted from the aorta back to the pulmonary artery; may progress to pulmonary hypertension and cardiomegaly
C. Machinery-type murmur heard throughout the heartbeat in the left second or third interspace
D. Treatment procedure: closure of the opening between the aorta and the pulmonary artery; in critically ill newborns, pharmacologic closure may be attempted with a prostaglandin inhibitor (e.g., indomethacin)

Coarctation of the Aorta

A. In utero, failure of aorta to develop completely; stricture usually occurs below level of the aortic arch
B. Increased systemic circulation above the stricture: bounding radial and carotid pulses, headache, dizziness, epistaxis
C. Decreased systemic circulation below the stricture: absent femoral pulses, cool lower extremities
D. Increased pressure in aorta above the defect causes left ventricular hypertrophy
E. Murmur may or may not be heard
F. Treatment procedure: resection of the defect and anastomosis of the ends of the aorta

Aortic Stenosis

A. Narrowing of the aortic valve
B. Causes increased workload on the left ventricle, and the lowered pressure in the aorta reduces coronary artery flow
C. Treatment procedures: division of the stenotic valves of the aorta

Pulmonary Stenosis

A. Narrowing of the pulmonary valve
B. Causes decreased blood flow to the lungs and increased pressure to the right ventricle
C. Treatment procedures: valvotomy or balloon angioplasty

Types of Cyanotic Defects
Tetralogy of Fallot

A. Four associated defects
1. Pulmonary valve stenosis
2. Ventricular septal defect, usually high on the septum
3. Overriding aorta, receiving blood from both ventricles, or an aorta arising from the right ventricle
4. Right ventricular hypertrophy
B. Palliative treatment procedures performed to increase pulmonary blood flow
1. Waterston-Cooley procedure: aorta to pulmonary artery anastomosis
2. Blalock-Taussig procedure: subclavian artery to pulmonary artery anastomosis
C. Complete repair: closure of the ventricular septal defect and resection of the infundibular stenosis, possibly with a pericardial patch to enlarge the right ventricular outflow tract

Transposition of the Great Vessels

A. Aorta arises from the right ventricle, and pulmonary artery arises from the left ventricle
B. Incompatible with life unless there is a communication between the two sides of the heart, such as an atrial septal defect, ventricular septal defect, or patent ductus arteriosus
C. Palliative treatment procedures performed to prevent pulmonary vascular resistance and congestive heart failure until the child is able to tolerate complete repair
1. Rashkind procedure: enlargement of an existing atrial septal defect by pulling a balloon through the defect (balloon septostomy) during a cardiac catheterization
2. Blalock-Tarrearg anastomosis creation of a systemic-pulmonary shunt if pulmonic stenosis is present
3. Pulmonary artery banding if a ventricular septal defect is present to decrease blood flow to the lungs and increase shunting of oxygenated blood intraventricularly to the aorta
4. Pharmacologic dilation of a patent ductus arteriosus with use of prostaglandins (e.g., Prostin VR)
5. Blalock-Hanlen operation: surgical creation of an atrial septal defect
D. Complete repair
1. Rastelli procedure: closure of VSD (directing left ventricular blood through VSD into aorta, pulmonic valve closed and conduit made from right ventricle to pulmonary artery) results in physiologic normal circulation but requires revision as child grows; procedure of choice for infants with transposition of the great vessels, VSD, and severe pulmonic stenosis
2. Mustard's or Senning's procedure: removing the entire atrial septum and creating a new atrial septum from existing pericardium or a prosthesis that tunnels or baffles blood for more effective oxygenation, with creation of two new functionally correct atrial chambers
3. Jatene operation: transposing the great vessels to their correct anatomic placement with reimplantation of the coronary arteries

Tricuspid Atresia

A. Absence of the tricuspid valve
B. Incompatible with life unless there is a communication between the right and left sides of the heart, such as atrial septal defect, ventricular septal defect, or patent ductus arteriosus

C. Palliative treatment procedures: same as for tetralogy of Fallot

D. Complete repair: Fontan procedure: conversion of the right atrium into an outlet for the pulmonary artery, which involves placing a tubular conduit with a valve between the two and closing the atrial septal defect; physiologically corrects tricuspid atresia by preventing any mixing of systemic blood in the left atrium and shunting the entire venous blood to the lungs for oxygenation

Truncus Arteriosus

A. Single great vessel arising from the base of the heart, serving as a pulmonary artery and aorta

B. Systolic murmur is heard, and a single semilunar valve produces a loud second heart sound that is not split

C. Palliative treatment: banding the pulmonary arteries as they arise from the truncus to decrease blood flow to lungs

D. Complete repair: Rastelli's operation: excising pulmonary arteries from aorta and attaching them to the right ventricle by means of a prosthetic valve conduit; septal defects also repaired

Treatment of Cardiac Malformations

A. Surgical intervention

B. Pharmacological approach: cardiac glycosides to increase the efficiency of heart action
  1. Positive inotropic effect is achieved by increasing the permeability of muscle membranes to the calcium and sodium ions required for contraction of muscle fibrils
     a. Forceful contraction during systole improves peripheral tissue perfusion
     b. Chamber emptying allows additional venous blood to enter the cardiac chambers during diastole
  2. Negative chronotropic effect is achieved through an action mediated by the vagus nerve that slows firing of the SA node and impulse transmission through the AV node (negative dromotropic action)
  3. Drug preparations have the same qualitative effect on heart action but differ in potency, rate of absorption, amount absorbed, onset of action, and speed of elimination
     a. digitalis: longer onset, peak action, and half-life
     b. digoxin (Lanoxin): rapid onset and peak action and short half-life; drug of choice in children, especially because the risk of toxicity is lessened by the shorter half-life
  4. Digitalization
     a. Provides an initial loading dose for acute effect on the enlarged heart
     b. After desired effect is achieved, the dosage is lowered to maintenance level, replacing the drug metabolized and excreted each day
  5. Adverse effects
     a. Most frequent: nausea, vomiting, headache, drowsiness, insomnia, vertigo, confusion; all attributable to drug action at CNS sites; oral forms also cause nausea and vomiting by irritation of the gastric mucosa

     b. Bradycardia attributable to drug-induced slowing of SA node firing
     c. Arrhythmias are first evidence of toxicity in one-third of clients; premature nodal or ventricular impulses; varying degrees of heart block caused by drug action that slows transmission of impulses through the AV node
     d. Xanthopsia (yellow vision) caused by drug effect on the visual cones
     e. Gynecomastia (mammary enlargement) in males resulting from the estrogenlike steroid portion of digitalis glycosides
  6. Considerations during therapy
     a. Premature contractions elevate the audible apical rate and mask the pacemaker conduction rate; apical pulse is taken before administration and drug is withheld when pulse rate drops to 110 to 90 in infants and below 70 in older children
     b. Immaturity of hepatic and renal systems in premature and newborn infants or depressed hepatic or renal function in children may result in cumulation
     c. Since potassium ions are required for interaction of digitalis glycosides with sodium-potassium dependent membranes, the lowering of serum levels of potassium ions may foster digitalis toxicity
     d. Since calcium ions act synergistically with digitalis on myocardial membranes, an elevation of serum calcium ion levels may increase sensitivity of cardiac muscle to digitalis action
  7. Drug interactions
     a. Phenobarbital, phenytoin, and phenylbutazone, by induction of hepatic microsomal enzymes, accelerate metabolism of digitalis glycosides; serum levels are lower when the drugs are used concomitantly
     b. Diuretics that cause hypokalemia may contribute to the incidence of serious arrhythmias when administered concurrently with digitalis glycosides; supplemental potassium may be used for replacement of losses, or potassium-sparing diuretics may be prescribed to prevent potassium ion losses

Nursing Process for Children with Cardiac Malformations
Probable Nursing Diagnoses Based on Assessment

A. Potential activity intolerance related to imbalance between oxygen supply and demand

B. Ineffective airway clearance related to fatigue

C. Diversional activity deficit related to activity intolerance

D. Fatigue related to excessive energy requirements of cardiac work

E. Potential fluid volume deficit related to
  1. Inadequate intake
  2. Fluid loss

F. Impaired physical mobility related to activity intolerance

G. Altered nutrition: less than body requirements related to inadequate intake

H. Feeding, bathing/hygiene, dressing/grooming, toileting self-care deficit related to activity intolerance
I. Body image disturbance related to perceived body imperfection
J. Sensory-perceptual alteration: visual, auditory, related to hospital environment
K. Social isolation related to physical limitations
L. See Nursing diagnoses for infants with health problems and for the family of child with a disability

Nursing Care for Children with Cardiac Malformations

A. Correctly calculate the dosage of digoxin; usually prescribed in micrograms (1000 μg = 1 mg)
B. Take the apical pulse prior to administering the drug
C. Observe for signs of digitalis toxicity
D. Teach the parents home administration of digoxin
   1. Give digoxin at regular intervals, usually every 12 hours, such as 8 AM and 8 PM
   2. Plan the times so that the drug is given 1 hour before or 2 hours after feedings
   3. Use a calendar to mark off each dose that is given or post a reminder, such as a sign on the refrigerator
   4. Have the prescription refilled before the medication is completely used
   5. Administer the drug carefully by slowly squirting it in the side and back of the mouth
   6. Do not mix it with other foods or fluids, since refusal to consume these results in inaccurate intake of the drug
   7. If the child has teeth, give water after administering the drug; whenever possible, brush the teeth to prevent tooth decay from the sweetened liquid
   8. If a dose is missed and more than 6 hours has elapsed, withhold the dose and give the next dose at the regular time; if less than 6 hours has elapsed, give the missed dose
   9. If the child vomits within 15 minutes of receiving the digoxin, repeat the dose once; if more than 15 minutes has elapsed, do not give a second dose
   10. If more than two consecutive doses have been missed, notify the physician
   11. Do not increase or double the dose for missed doses
   12. If the child becomes ill, notify the physician immediately
   13. Keep digoxin in a safe place, preferably a locked cabinet
   14. In case of accidental overdose of digoxin, call the nearest poison control center immediately
E. Help the parents cope with symptoms of the disease
   1. During dyspneic/cyanotic spell, place the child in a side-lying knee-chest position, with the head and chest elevated
   2. Keep the child warm; encourage rest and sleep
   3. Decrease the child's anxiety by remaining calm
   4. Feed the child slowly; allow frequent burping
   5. Administer small, frequent meals
   6. Introduce solids and spoon feeding early
   7. Encourage the anorexic child to eat
   8. Encourage parents to include others in the child's care to prevent their own exhaustion

F. Foster growth-promoting family relationships
   1. Encourage family members to discuss their feelings about each other and the child's defect
   2. Maintain expectations from all siblings as equally as possible
   3. Provide consistent discipline, especially from infancy, to prevent behavioral problems
   4. Encourage acceptable pursuits for the child
   5. Discuss school entry with the teacher and school nurse
   6. Guide parents to the eventual hazards of fostering overdependency
   7. Help the parents feel adequate in their maternal-paternal roles by emphasizing growth and developmental progress of the child
   8. Help the parents foster the child's development by stimulating the child to age-appropriate goals consistent with his or her activity tolerance
   9. Provide social experiences for the child
G. Preoperative assessment areas necessary for planning postoperative care
   1. Keep a sleep record so care can be organized around the child's usual rest pattern
   2. Avoid constipation and straining after surgery
      a. Assess the child's elimination pattern
      b. Know words the child uses
      c. Have the child practice using a bedpan
   3. Record the level of activity and list favorite toys or games that require gradually increased exertion
   4. Determine the child's fluid preferences for postoperative maintenance
   5. When recording vital signs, always indicate the child's activity at the time of measurement
   6. Observe the child's verbal and nonverbal responses to pain
H. Prepare the child physically and emotionally for surgery
   1. Main assessment factor in preparation of the child is the developmental and chronologic age
      a. Explanation of the heart differs according to age of the child
      b. Children 4 to 6 years of age know that the heart is in the chest, describe it as valentine shaped, and characterize its function by the sound of "tick tock"
      c. Children 7 to 10 years of age do not see the heart as valentine shaped, know it has veins, have an idea of its function (e.g., "It makes you live"), but do not understand the concept of pumping
      d. Children over 10 years of age have a concept of veins, valves, circulation, and why death occurs when the heart stops
   2. Preparation is based on the principle that fear of the unknown increases anxiety
   3. The same nurse should participate in preoperative and postoperative preparation as a source of support for the child and parents
   4. Nurse must know what equipment is usual after open or closed heart surgery
   5. Let the child play with equipment such as stethoscope, blood pressure machine, oxygen mask, suction, and syringes

6. For the young child, especially the preschooler, use dolls and puppets to describe procedures
7. Preparation for cardiac catheterization prior to surgery is essential as well
8. For the young child, talk about the size of the bandage; for the older child, discuss the actual incision
9. Familiarize the child with the postoperative environment such as recovery room and intensive care unit, stressing the strange noises there (e.g., the monitors)
10. Have the child practice coughing, using blow bottles, and breathing on the IPPB machine
11. Explain to the child why coughing and moving are necessary even though they may be uncomfortable
12. Explain to the child what tubes may be used and what they will look like
13. For more specific discussion of the aforementioned, see specific age groups under Pediatric Nursing

I. Specifics of postoperative care are similar to those for any major surgery
J. Help the child and family adjust to correction of the cardiac defect
1. Improved physical status is often difficult for the child who has become accustomed to the sick role and its secondary gains
2. Improved physical status of the child is also difficult for the parents, since it reduces child's dependency
3. The child may have difficulty learning to relate to peers and siblings on a competitive basis
4. The child can no longer use the disability as a crutch for educational and social shortcomings
5. Parental expectations must be adjusted to accommodate the child's new physical vigor and search for independence
K. See Nursing care for the family of a child with a disability
L. Evaluate client's response and revise plan as necessary

NEUROLOGICAL MALFORMATIONS
Nursing Process for Children with Neurological Malformations
Probable Nursing Diagnoses Based on Assessment

A. Ineffective airway clearance related to excessive secretions
B. Potential for aspiration related to
1. Disease process
2. Impaired swallowing
C. Constipation related to immobility
D. Pain related to positioning
E. Diversional activity deficit related to
1. Immobility
2. Difficulty coordinating movements
3. Muscular weakness
F. Altered parenting related to
1. Sick child
2. Physical limitations
G. Potential for injury related to
1. Impaired coordination
2. Immobility
3. Environmental hazards

H. Altered nutrition: potential for more than body requirements, related to immobility
I. Feeding, bathing/hygiene, dressing/grooming, toileting self-care deficit related to
1. Developmental level
2. Muscular weakness
3. Immobility
J. Social isolation related to
1. Impaired mobility
2. Disturbance in self-concept
K. Sensory-perceptual alterations: visual, auditory, related to environmental factors
L. Impaired skin integrity related to
1. Immobility
2. Secretions or excretions on the skin
M. Social isolation related to
1. Impaired mobility
2. Self-concept disturbance
N. See Nursing diagnoses for infants with health problems and for the family of child with a disability

Nursing Care for Children with Neurological Malformations

A. See Nursing care under each disorder
B. See Nursing care for the family of a child with a disability

Spina Bifida

A. Malformation of the spine in which the posterior portion of the laminae of the vertebrae fails to close; most common site is the lumbosacral area
1. Spina bifida occulta: defect only of the vertebrae; spinal cord and meninges are intact
2. Meningocele: meninges protrude through the vertebral defect
3. Meningomyelocele: meninges and spinal cord protrude through the defect; most serious type
B. Associated defects include weakness or paralysis below the defect, bowel and bladder dysfunction, clubfeet, dislocated hip, and hydrocephalus
C. Arnold-Chiari syndrome: defect of the occipito-cervical region with swelling and displacement of medulla into the spinal cord
D. Surgical repair of the sac to maintain neurological function and prevent infection
E. Nursing care
1. Protect against infection because breakdown of the sac leaves the spinal cord open to the environment
   a. Area must be kept clean, especially from urine and feces
   b. Diaper is not used, but sterile gauze with antibiotic solution may be placed over the sac
   c. Avoid pressure on sac
2. Maintain function through proper position: place in prone position, hips slightly flexed and abducted, feet hanging free of mattress, and a slight Trendelenburg slope to reduce spinal fluid pressure
3. Because of restriction in position, feed child in prone position; establish eye contact and encourage parents to visit and feed the child

4. Foster elimination in the infant with a neurogenic bladder:
   a. Use the Credé method or slight pressure against the abdomen for complete emptying of the bladder
   b. While the infant is prone, apply pressure to the abdomen above symphysis pubis with sides of the fingers and counterpressure with thumbs against the buttocks
5. Postoperative nursing care
   a. Measure head size to determine whether hydrocephalus is occurring
   b. Monitor for signs of increased intracranial pressure
6. Care is same as for cardiac surgery, with emphasis on development of the child's abilities
7. See Nursing care for the family of a child with a disability
8. Evaluate client's response and revise plan as necessary

Hydrocephalus

A. Abnormal accumulation of cerebrospinal fluid within the ventricular system
   1. Noncommunicating: obstruction within the ventricles such as congenital malformation, neoplasm, or hematoma
   2. Communicating: inadequate absorption of cerebrospinal fluid resulting from infection, trauma, or obstruction by thick arachnoid membrane or meninges
B. Symptoms
   1. Increasing head size in the infant because of open sutures and bulging fontanels
   2. Prominent scalp veins and taut shiny skin
   3. "Sunset" eyes (sclera visible above iris), bulging eyes, and papilledema of retina
   4. Head lag, especially important after 4 to 6 months
   5. Increased intracranial pressure: projectile vomiting not associated with feeding, irritability, anorexia, high shrill cry, convulsions
   6. Damage to the brain because increased pressure decreases blood flow to the cells, causing necrosis
C. Treatment
   1. Removal of the obstruction
   2. Mechanical shunting of fluid to another area of the body
      a. Ventricular peritoneal shunt: catheter passed subcutaneously to the peritoneal cavity
      b. Ventricular atrial shunt: catheter passed from a lateral ventricle to the internal jugular vein to the right atrium of the heart
D. Nursing care
   1. Prevent breakdown of scalp, infection, and damage to spinal cord
      a. Place the infant in a Fowler's position to facilitate draining of fluid; postoperative positioning should be flat with no pressure on the shunted side
      b. When holding the child, support the neck and head
      c. Observe shunt site (abdominal site in peritoneal procedure) for infection

2. Monitor for increasing intracranial pressure
   a. Carefully observe neurologic signs
   b. Measure head circumference
   c. Use minimal sedatives or analgesics, which can mask symptoms
   d. Check the valve frequently for patency
3. Promote adequate nutrition
   a. Monitor for vomiting, irritability, lethargy, and anorexia because these will decrease the intake of nutrients
   b. Perform all care before feeding to prevent vomiting; hold infant if possible
   c. Observe for signs of dehydration
4. Keep eyes moist and free of irritation if eyelids incompletely cover corneas
5. Postoperative nursing care: similar to that for cardiac surgery except
   a. Place the child on bed rest after surgery, with minimal handling to prevent damage to shunt
   b. Support parents
      (1) Continued shunt revisions are usually necessary as growth occurs
      (2) Usually very concerned about retardation
   c. Observe for brain damage by recording milestones during infancy
   d. Teach parents
      (1) Pumping of the shunt
      (2) Signs of increasing intracranial pressure
      (3) Evidence of dehydration
6. See Nursing care for the family of a child with a disability
7. Evaluate client's response and revise plan as necessary

GENITOURINARY MALFORMATIONS
Nursing Process for Children with Genitourinary Malformations
Probable Nursing Diagnoses Based on Assessment

A. Pain related to
   1. Response to deformity
   2. Postoperative response
B. Fluid volume excess related to intake greater than output
C. Potential for infection related to residual urine
D. Body image disturbance related to perception of physical defect
E. Potential impaired skin integrity related to
   1. Presence of incontinent urine
   2. Irritation to edematous tissues
   3. Presence of artificial drainage system or appliance
F. Social isolation related to
   1. Frequent hospitalization
   2. Body image disturbance
G. See Nursing diagnoses for infants with health problems and for the family of child with a disability

Nursing Care for Children with Genitourinary Malformations

A. See Nursing care under each disorder
B. See Nursing care for the family of a child with a disability

Exstrophy of the Bladder

A. Entire lower urinary tract, from bladder to external urethral meatus, is outside the abdominal cavity
B. May be accompanied by defects such as inguinal hernia, epispadias, undescended testes, or short penis in boys and a cleft clitoris or absent vagina in girls
C. Treatment
   1. Plastic surgery
   2. Closure of the bladder within 48 hours if possible; final repair attempted before school age
   3. Ileal conduit (also called ureteroileal cutaneous ureterostomy): a small section of the ileum or colon is resected, and the remaining bowel is reanastomosed; one end of the resected bowel is sutured closed and the other end is attached to a small opening in the lower abdomen, forming a stoma; the distal ends of the ureters are severed from the bladder and attached to the ileum, which acts like a bladder, although there is no voluntary control in the regulation of voiding; the child wears an ileostomy appliance over the stoma, which collects the continuously flowing urine; in a young child diapers serve the same purpose as the collecting appliance
   4. Cutaneous ureterostomy: the ureters are attached directly to the abdominal wall, usually at a site proximal to the level of the kidneys; two collecting appliances are worn over the bilateral openings
D. Nursing care
   1. Help the parents to accept the disorder and the long term sequelae
   2. Scrupulously clean the area around bladder and apply sterile petrolatum gauze
   3. Use loose clothing to avoid pressure over the area
   4. Change clothing frequently because of odor
   5. Care for the urine-collecting appliance; change frequently
   6. See Nursing care for the family of a child with a disability
   7. Evaluate client's response and revise plan as necessary

Displaced Urethral Opening

A. Hypospadias
   1. In boys the urethra opens on the lower surface of the penis from just behind the glans to the perineum (placement varies)
   2. In girls the urethra opens into the vagina
B. Epispadias
   1. Occurs only in boys
   2. Urethra opens on dorsal surface of the penis; often associated with exstrophy of the bladder
C. Defect can be a sign of ambiguous genitalia
D. Procreation may be interfered with in severe cases
E. Increased risk of urinary tract infection
F. Treatment: surgical repair of the defect; repair may be in several stages
G. Nursing care
   1. Provide the parents with an explicit explanation of child's future functioning

   2. Prepare child for surgery; the boy needs help in coping with anatomical difference from peers and the adjustments to voiding in the sitting position
   3. See Nursing care for the family of a child with a disability
   4. Evaluate client's response and revise plan as necessary

SKELETAL MALFORMATIONS
Nursing Process for Children with Skeletal Malformations
Probable Nursing Diagnoses Based on Assessment

A. Constipation related to immobility
B. Pain related to position
C. Diversional activity deficit related to
   1. Immobility
   2. Corrective devices
D. Potential for injury related to
   1. Knowledge deficit
   2. Use of corrective devices
E. Altered nutrition: more than body requirements related to immobility
F. Feeding, bathing/hygiene, dressing/grooming, toileting self-care deficit related to
   1. Immobility
   2. Discomfort
G. Body image disturbance related to
   1. Perception of disability
   2. Corrective devices
H. Potential impaired skin integrity related to
   1. Immobility
   2. Use of corrective devices
I. Social isolation related to
   1. Impaired mobility
   2. Self-concept disturbance
J. See Nursing diagnoses for infants with health problems and for the family of child with a disability

Nursing Care for Children with Skeletal Malformations

A. See Nursing care under each disorder
B. See Nursing care for the family of a child with a disability

Club Foot

A. Foot has been twisted out of position in utero
B. Most common type: talipes equinovarus: foot is fixed in plantar flexion (downward) and deviated medially (inward)
C. Treatment is most successful when started early in infancy, since delay causes muscles and bones of legs to develop abnormally, with shortening of tendons
D. Nonsurgical treatment: gentle repeated manipulation of the foot or forcible correction under anesthesia and application of a wedge cast
E. Surgical treatment: Done if nonsurgical treatment not effective
   1. Tight ligaments released
   2. Tendons lengthened or transplanted
F. Follow-up care of the client
   1. Extended medical supervision is required, since there is a tendency for this deformity to recur (considered cured when the child is able to wear normal shoes and walk properly)

2. Care emphasizes muscle reeducation (by manipulation) and proper walking
3. Heels and soles of braces or shoes prescribed following correction must be kept in repair
4. Corrective shoes may have sole and heel lifts on lateral border to maintain proper position

G. Nursing care
   1. Observe toes for signs of circulatory impairment; make sure toes are visible at the end of the cast
   2. Watch for signs of weakness and wear of the cast, especially if the child is allowed to walk on it
   3. Teach parents all the necessary care and emphasize the need for follow-up which may be prolonged
   4. For other areas of cast care, see Treatment of a dislocated hip
   5. See Nursing care for the family of a child with a disability
   6. Evaluate client's response and revise plan as necessary

Congenital Hip Dysplasia

A. Head of the femur does not lie deep enough within the acetabulum and slips out on movement (may be caused by lack of embryonic development of the joint or position in utero)
B. Symptoms
   1. Limitation in abduction of leg on the affected side
   2. Asymmetry of gluteal, popliteal, and thigh folds
   3. Audible click when abducting and externally rotating the hip on the affected side: Ortolani's sign
   4. Apparent shortening of the femur: Galeazzi's sign
   5. Waddling gait and lordosis when the child begins to walk
C. Treatment
   1. Directed toward enlarging and deepening the acetabulum by placing the head of the femur within the acetabulum and applying constant pressure
   2. Proper positioning: legs slightly flexed and abducted
      a. Pavlik harness
      b. Frejka pillow: a pillow splint that maintains abduction of the legs
      c. Bryant's traction
      d. Spica cast; from the waist to below the knees
      e. Brace
   3. Surgical intervention such as open reduction with casting
D. Nursing care when a spica cast is applied (see Fractures in Medical-Surgical Nursing for care of client with cast)
   1. Respiratory problems: hypostatic pneumonia
      a. Change position frequently from back to stomach
      b. Teach parents postural drainage and exercises for child such as blowing bubbles to increase lung expansion
      c. Encourage parents to seek immediate medical care if the child develops congestion or cough
   2. Infection and excoriation of skin
      a. Observe for circulation of toes, pedal pulses, and blanching
      b. Do not let the child put small toys or food inside cast

   c. Use gauze strips inside cast as a scratcher
   d. Alert parents to signs of infection, such as odor
   e. Protect cast edges with adhesive tape or waterproof material, especially around perineum
   f. Use diapers and plastic lining to minimize soiling of cast by feces and urine
   3. Constipation from immobility
      a. Teach parents to observe for straining on defecation and constipation
      b. Increase fluids and fiber to prevent constipation
   4. Nutrition
      a. Provide small, frequent meals because of inflexibility of cast around waist (a window may be made over the abdominal area to allow for expansion with meals)
      b. Adjust calorie intake, since less energy expenditure can lead to obesity
   5. Transportation and positioning
      a. Use wagon or stroller with back flat
      b. Protect child from falling when positioned
      c. Never pick up child by the bar between the legs of the cast (use two people to provide adequate body support if necessary)
   6. Meet emotional needs
      a. Use touch as much as possible; small children can be picked up and cuddled
      b. Stimulate and provide for play activities appropriate to age
   7. Provide parents with help and support
      a. Give written instructions
      b. Schedule routine home visits with telephone counseling available
      c. Stress need for follow-up care since treatment may be prolonged
      d. Prepare parents for the possible use of an abduction brace after the cast is removed
   8. See Nursing care for the family of a child with a disability
   9. Evaluate client's response and revise plan as necessary

Developmental Anomalies of the Extremities

A. Polydactyly: extra digits
B. Syndactyly: partial or complete fusion of two or more digits
C. Amelia: absence of a limb
D. Treatment: if possible, early correction and preparation for use of a prosthesis
E. Nursing care
   1. Recognize own reaction to the deformity
   2. Accept the parents' reactions of guilt, anger, and hopelessness
   3. Assist the parents in setting realistic goals for the child
   4. Prepare the parents to answer the child's questions about the deformity and what it will mean in the future
   5. See Nursing care for the family of a child with a disability
   6. Evaluate client's response and revise plan as necessary

INBORN ERRORS OF METABOLISM
Nursing Process for Children with Inborn Errors of Metabolism
Probable Nursing Diagnoses Based on Assessment

A. Altered growth and development related to changes in metabolism

B. Altered nutrition: less than body requirements, related to restrictive diet

C. Feeding, bathing/hygiene, dressing/grooming, toileting self-care deficit related to uncompensated cognitive perceptual impairment

D. Body image disturbance related to dietary restrictions

E. Knowledge deficit related to special dietary needs

F. See nursing diagnoses for infants with health problems and for the family of child with a disability

Nursing Care for Children with Inborn Errors of Metabolism

A. See Nursing care under each disorder

B. See Nursing care for the family of a child with a disability

Phenylketonuria (PKU)

A. Lack of the enzyme phenylalanine hydroxylase, which changes phenylalanine (essential amino acid) into tyrosine

B. Transmitted by autosomal recessive gene

C. Symptoms
1. Mental retardation from damage to the nervous system by buildup of phenylalanine
   a. Often noticed by 4 months of age
   b. IQ is usually below 50 and most frequently under 20
2. Strong musty odor in urine from phenylacetic acid
3. Absence of tyrosine reduces the production of melanin and results in blond hair and blue eyes
4. Fair skin is susceptible to eczema

D. Treatment
1. Early detection: test for PKU at birth
   a. Guthrie blood test: effective in newborns; testing can be done during first 48 hours of life; if testing is done during initial 24 hours, it should be repeated by the third week of life
   b. Ferric chloride urine test: effective only when infant is over 2 weeks of age, when brain damage may have occurred
2. Dietary: low-phenylalanine: use Lofenalac PKU 1, or Phenylfree as a milk substitute and restrict foods to those low in this amino acid (usually continued until the child is 6 to 8 years of age)
3. Treat eczema (see Nursing care for eczema)

E. Nursing care
1. Help parents to understand the disease and the role of diet
2. Refer parents for genetic counseling
3. See Nursing care for the family of a child with a disability
4. Evaluate client's response and revise plan as necessary

Galactosemia

A. Missing enzyme that converts galactose to glucose

B. Transmitted by autosomal recessive gene

C. Treatment
1. Early detection: test for galactosemia at birth; Beutler test (method similar to Guthrie test for PKU) mandatory in many states
2. Dietary reduction of lactose: use a soy-base formula as a milk substitute and restrict foods to those low in lactose (usually continued until the child is 7 to 8 years of age) followed by a relaxed modification throughout life

D. Nursing care similar to that for phenylketonuria

Congenital Hypothyroidism

A. Failure of embryonic development of the thyroid gland or inborn enzyme defect in the formation of thyroxine

B. Symptoms
1. Prolonged physiologic jaundice, feeding difficulties, inactivity (excessive sleeping, little crying), anemia, problems resulting from hypotonic abdominal muscles (constipation, protruding abdomen, and umbilical hernia)
2. Appears at 3 to 6 months of age in formula-fed babies; may be delayed in breast-fed babies
3. Impaired development of nervous system leads to mental retardation; level depends on degree of hypothyroidism and interval before therapy is begun
4. Decreased growth and decreased metabolic rate resulting in increased weight
5. Characteristic infant facies: short forehead; wide puffy eyes; wrinkled eyelids; broad, short, upturned nose; large protruding tongue; hair is dry, brittle, and lusterless with low hairline
6. Skin is mottled due to decreased heart rate and circulation
7. Skin is yellowish from carotenemia due to decreased conversion of carotene to vitamin A

C. Detection: neonatal screening for thyroxine (T_4) and thyroid-stimulating hormone (TSH)

D. Treatment: indefinite replacement therapy with thyroid hormone; if therapy begun prior to 3 months of age, chances for normal growth and normal IQ increased

E. Nursing care
1. Instruct parents regarding administration of thyroid replacement and signs of overdose (rapid pulse, dyspnea, insomnia, irritability, sweating, fever, and weight loss)
2. Teach parents to take pulse
3. See Nursing care for the family of a child with a disability
4. Evaluate client's response and revise plan as necessary

NONCONGENITAL HEALTH PROBLEMS IN INFANCY
Intussusception

A. Telescoping of one portion of the intestine into another; occurs most frequently at the ileocecal valve

B. Symptoms
1. Healthy, well-nourished infant who wakes up with severe paroxysmal abdominal pain, evidenced by kicking and drawing legs up to the abdomen

2. One or two normal stools, then bloody mucous stool ("currant jelly" stool)
3. Palpation of sausage-shaped mass
4. Other signs of intestinal obstruction usually present
C. Treatment
  1. Medical: reduction by hydrostatic pressure (barium enema)
  2. Surgical reduction; sometimes with intestinal resection
D. Nursing diagnoses based on assessment for children with intussusception
  1. Anxiety related to separation from significant others
  2. Pain related to surgical procedure
  3. Potential for infection related to surgical incision
  4. Feeding, bathing/hygiene, dressing/grooming, toileting self-care deficit related to
    a. Age
    b. Pain
  5. Altered nutrition: less than body requirements related to
    a. Decreased intake
    b. Increased peristalsis
  6. Potential fluid volume deficit related to
    a. Decreased intake
    b. Diarrhea
  7. See Nursing diagnoses for infants with health problems and for the family of child with a disability
E. Nursing care
  1. Same as for any abdominal surgery
  2. Make provisions for frequent parental visits since the problem usually occurs when the child is 6 to 8 months of age and separation anxiety is acute
  3. See Nursing care for the family of a child with a disability
  4. Evaluate client's response and revise plan as necessary

Failure to Thrive (FTT)

A. The term used to describe infants and children whose weight and sometimes height fall below the fifth percentile for their age
B. There are two distinct categories of FTT
  1. Organic: result of a physical cause, such as congenital heart defects, neurologic lesions, microcephaly, chronic urinary tract infection, gastroesophageal reflux, renal insufficiency, malabsorption syndrome, endocrine dysfunction, or cystic fibrosis
  2. Nonorganic: caused by psychosocial factors, problem being between the child and the primary care giver, usually the mother; in this situation the lack of physical growth is secondary to the lack of emotional and sensory stimulation (other terms include maternal deprivation, environmental deprivation, and deprivation dwarfism)
    a. Characteristics of nonorganic FTT children
      (1) Growth failure: below the fifth percentile in height and weight
      (2) Developmental retardation: social, motor, adaptive, language
      (3) Apathy
      (4) Poor hygiene
      (5) Withdrawing behavior

      (6) Feeding or eating disorders, such as vomiting, anorexia, voracious appetite, pica, rumination
      (7) No fear of strangers (at the age when stranger anxiety is normal)
      (8) Avoidance of eye-to-eye contact
      (9) Wide-eyed gaze and continual scan of the environment ("radar gaze")
      (10) Stiff and unyielding or flaccid and unresponsive
      (11) Minimal smiling
    b. Characteristics of the parent providing care
      (1) Difficulty perceiving and assessing the infant's needs
      (2) Frustrated and angered at the infant's dissatisfied response
      (3) Frequently under stress and in crisis, with emotional, social, and financial problems
      (4) Often with marital disturbances (e.g., absent spouse or one who gives little emotional support)
      (5) Tending to lead lonely, solitary lives with few outside interests or friends
      (6) Experienced poor parenting as a child
C. Nursing diagnoses based on assessment for children with FTT
  1. Diversional activity deficit related to developmental deprivation
  2. Potential for fluid volume deficit related to
    a. Knowledge deficit
    b. Inadequate support systems
  3. Impaired home maintenance management related to
    a. Knowledge deficit
    b. Inadequate support systems
  4. Potential for infection related to nutritional deficit
  5. Knowledge deficit related to parenting skills
  6. Altered growth and development related to
    a. Emotional environment
    b. Health problems
    c. Nutritional deficit
  7. Parental role conflict related to
    a. Knowledge deficit
    b. Lack of role model
  8. Altered parenting related to disturbed parent-child relationship
  9. Potential impaired skin integrity related to malnutrition
  10. See Nursing diagnoses for infants with health problems and for the family of child with a disability
D. Nursing care
  1. Provide a consistent care giver who can begin to satisfy routine needs
  2. Provide optimum nutrients
    a. Make feeding a priority goal
    b. Keep an accurate record of intake to determine daily calories
    c. Weigh daily and record to ascertain weight gain
  3. Introduce a positive feeding environment
    a. Assign one nurse for feeding
    b. Maintain a calm, even temperament; be persistent

c. Provide a quiet, unstimulating environment

d. Hold the young child for feeding

e. Maintain eye-to-eye contact with the child

f. Talk to the child by giving appropriate directions and praise for eating

g. Follow the child's rhythm of feeding

h. Establish a structured routine and follow it consistently

4. Increase stimulation, appropriate to the child's present developmental level

5. Provide the parent an opportunity to talk

6. When necessary, relieve the parent of child-rearing responsibilities until able and ready emotionally to support the child

7. Demonstrate proper infant care by example, not lecturing (allow the parent to proceed at own pace)

8. Supply the parent with emotional support without fostering dependency

9. Promote the parent's self-respect and confidence by praising achievements with child

10. Evaluate client's response and revise plan as necessary

Sudden Infant Death Syndrome: SIDS (Crib Death)

A. A definite syndrome with unknown cause

B. No. 1 cause of death in infants between 1 week and 1 year of age; incidence of 2 in every 1000 live births

C. Peak age of occurrence: healthy infant 2 to 4 months of age—90% occur by 6 months

D. Higher incidence in
1. Males
2. Premature infants
3. Multiple births
4. Newborns with low Apgar scores
5. Infants with CNS disturbances

E. Feeding habits not significant; breast-feeding does not prevent SIDS

F. May be a greater incidence in siblings of SIDS children

G. Nursing diagnoses based on assessment for the family who experiences SIDS
1. Family coping: potential for growth, related to successfully coping with loss
2. Ineffective family coping: disabling, related to situational crisis
3. Altered family processes related to disruption of life-style
4. Fear related to loss of child
5. Dysfunctional grieving related to loss of child
6. Potential altered parenting related to grief
7. See Nursing diagnoses for the family of a child with a disability

H. Nursing care to assist parents
1. Know signs of SIDS to distinguish it from child neglect or abuse; do or say nothing that instills guilt in the parents
2. Reassure the parents that they could not have prevented the death or predicted its occurrence
3. Reinforce that an autopsy should be done on every child to confirm diagnosis
4. Visit the parents at home to discuss the cause of death and help them with their guilt and grief

5. Refer the parents to a national SIDS parent group

6. Evaluate clients' response and revise plan as necessary

Diarrhea

A. Frequent watery stools due to increased peristalsis resulting from a variety of causes, local or systemic

B. Symptoms
1. Frequent watery stools
2. Loss of fluids and electrolytes
3. If fluid loss is severe
   a. Weight loss greater than 10% (severe dehydration)
   b. Poor skin turgor and dry mucous membranes
   c. Depressed fontanels and sunken eyeballs
   d. Decreased urine output, increased specific gravity, and increased hematocrit
   e. Irritability, stupor, convulsions from loss of intracellular water and decreased plasma volume
   f. Metabolic acidosis which decreases available bicarbonate

C. Treatment
1. In severe diarrhea correct fluid and electrolyte imbalance
2. Identify the causative agent and institute proper therapy (antibiotics are used if a bacterial agent is present)

D. Nursing diagnoses based on assessment for children with diarrhea
1. Diarrhea related to intestinal irritation that increases peristalsis
2. Potential fluid volume deficit related to excessive fluid losses
3. Potential for infection related to damaged tissue
4. Altered nutrition: less than body requirements, related to increased peristalsis with decreased absorption
5. Potential impaired skin integrity related to excretions on the skin
6. See Nursing diagnoses for infants with health problems and for the family of child with a disability

E. Nursing care
1. Isolate the infant until stool culture results are reported as negative
2. Explain to the parents why antibiotics and an increase in food are ineffective in treating viral diarrhea
3. Teach parents progressive increase in diet: alterations in diet may control mild diarrhea
   a. Clear fluids to decrease inflammation of the intestinal mucosa
   b. If tolerated, half-strength formula
   c. Regular diet of bland foods
4. Evaluate client's response and revise plan as necessary

Vomiting

A. Ejection of stomach contents associated with many conditions such as poor feeding technique, relaxation or constriction of the cardiac sphincter, or local or systemic infections

B. Symptoms
  1. One or more episodes of regurgitation or emesis
  2. If vomiting is severe
    a. Dehydration
    b. Tetany and convulsions in severe alkalosis resulting from hypokalemia and hypocalcemia
    c. Metabolic alkalosis from loss of hydrogen ion
C. Treatment: care directed toward correction of the underlying problem
D. Nursing diagnoses based on assessment for children with vomiting
  See Nursing diagnoses for infants with health problems, for the family of child with a disability, and for children with diarrhea
E. Nursing care
  1. Maintain in prone position with body inclined at 30° at all times
  2. Do not disturb infant after feeding
  3. If associated with gastroesophageal reflux or cardiac sphincter problems
    a. Thicken the consistency of foods given
    b. Provide small volume feedings every 2 to 3 hours
  4. Evaluate client's response and revise plan as necessary

Colic

A. Paroxysmal intestinal cramps
B. May be caused by cow's milk sensitivity, but often no cause is found
C. May be associated with excessive swallowing of air, size of nipple opening or shape of nipple, too rapid feeding or over-feeding, and tenseness or anxiety in the mother
D. Symptoms
  1. Pulling up of arms and legs
  2. Red-faced crying over long periods of time
  3. Presence of excessive gas
E. Treatment: directed toward correction of the underlying cause when identified
F. Nursing diagnoses based on assessment for children with colic and their parents
  1. Pain related to abdominal cramping
  2. Altered sleep patterns related to pain
  3. Knowledge deficit related to infant feeding practices
  4. Diversional activity deficit related to limited energy resources
  5. Altered sleep patterns related to interrupted sleep from infant crying
  6. Ineffective family coping: compromised, related to alterations in family life-style and relationships related to infant's discomfort
  7. See Nursing diagnoses for infants with health problems, for the family of child with a disability, and for the child with diarrhea
G. Nursing care
  1. Watch the parent feed the infant before attempting to counsel
  2. Teach the parent to bubble the infant frequently and to position on the abdomen after feeding
  3. Encourage the mother to take time away from the infant

  4. Reassure mother that the condition is not life-threatening, the infant will gain weight, and the condition will eventually subside
  5. Evaluate client's response and revise plan as necessary

Constipation

A. Hard, dry stools which are hard to pass or are infrequent
B. Usually a result of diet, although may have a psychologic component
C. Treatment
  1. Dietary: increased fiber and fluid
  2. If mineral oil is used, it should not be given with foods, since it decreases the absorption of nutrients
  3. Enemas should be avoided; bowel retraining should be instituted
D. Nursing diagnoses based on assessment for children with constipation
  1. Altered nutrition: less than body requirements, related to inadequate intake of fiber
  2. Potential fluid volume deficit related to inadequate intake
  3. Pain related to
    a. Bowel distention
    b. Alteration in bowel motility
  4. See Nursing diagnoses for infants with health problems and for the family of child with a disability
E. Nursing care
  1. Teach parents to provide foods with fiber and avoid those that bind
  2. Teach parents to increase amount of fluid given to infant
  3. Place infant in knee-chest position if abdominal distention or cramping is present
  4. Cuddle infant to provide comfort as necessary
  5. Evaluate client's response and revise plan as necessary

Respiratory Tract Infections

A. Frequent cause of morbidity
B. Acute infection may be bacterial or viral (see Review of microbiology in Medical-surgical nursing)
  1. Acute nasopharyngitis (common cold)
  2. Pneumonia
  3. Bronchitis
  4. Tonsillitis
  5. Epiglottitis
  6. Croup
  7. Acute laryngotracheobronchitis
C. Probable nursing diagnoses for children with respiratory disorders
  1. Activity intolerance related to
    a. Altered breathing pattern
    b. Fatigue
  2. Ineffective airway clearance related to
    a. Excessively thick secretions
    b. Fatigue
    c. Positioning difficulties
  3. Pain, related to positioning difficulties
  4. Diversional activity deficit related to
    a. Environmental restrictions
    b. Fatigue

5. Potential for infection related to
    a. Aspiration of foreign substances
    b. Presence of secretions
    c. Positioning difficulties
6. Potential impairment of skin integrity related to secretions/excretions on skin
7. Potential fluid volume deficit related to fluid losses
8. Altered Nutrition: less than body requirements, related to inability to eat (fatigue, difficulty breathing)
9. Sleep pattern disturbance related to
    a. Difficulty breathing
    b. Sensory overload
    c. Discomfort
10. See nursing diagnoses for infants with health problems and for the family of child with a disability
D. Nursing care
    1. Increase fluid intake
        a. Prevents dehydration from fever and perspiration
        b. Loosens thickened secretions
    2. Increase humidity and coolness
        a. Liquifies secretions
        b. Decreases the febrile state and inflammation of the mucous membrane
        c. Causes vasoconstriction and bronchiolar dilation
    3. Promote nasal and pulmonary drainage
        a. Clean the nares with a bulb syringe
        b. Suction the oronasal pharynx
        c. Perform postural drainage, clapping, and vibrating
    4. Provide rest by decreasing stimulation
    5. Increase oxygen
    6. Never use tongue blade to visualize posterior pharynx in children with epiglottitis
    7. If a tracheotomy is necessary see Medical-surgical nursing for nursing care of clients with a tracheotomy
    8. Evaluate client's response and revise plan as necessary

Otitis Media

A. Acute: infection of the middle ear; causative organism usually *Haemophilus influenzae, Staphylococcus* organism, or *Streptococcus* organism
B. Symptoms of acute otitis media
    1. Pain: infant frets and rubs ear or rolls head from side to side
    2. Drum bulging, red, may rupture; no light reflex
C. Serous: accumulation of uninfected serous or mucoid matter in the middle ear; cause unknown
D. Symptoms of serous otitis media
    1. No pain or fever, but "fullness" in the ear
    2. Drum appears gray, bulging
    3. Possible loss of hearing from scarring of the drum
E. Treatment
    1. Antibiotics
    2. Surgery including myringotomy or insertion of tympanotomy tubes
F. Nursing diagnoses based on assessment for children with otitis media
    1. Pain related to infectious process
    2. Sensory-perceptual alterations (auditory) related to recurrent otitis media

3. See Nursing diagnoses for infants with health problems and for the family of child with a disability
G. Nursing care
    1. Teach parents proper administration of antibiotics; stress importance of full course of therapy
    2. Teach parent proper instillation of ear drops
        a. If the child is under 3 years of age, pull the auricle down and back
        b. For an older child, pull the auricle up and back
    3. Minimize recurrence
        a. Eliminate environmental allergies
        b. Feed in upright position
    4. Encourage medical follow-up to check for complications such as chronic hearing loss, mastoiditis, or possible meningitis
    5. Evaluate client's response and revise plan as necessary

Meningitis

A. Causative agent may be viral or bacterial, such as *Haemophilus influenzae, Neisseria meningitidis,* or *Streptococcus pneumoniae*
B. Symptoms (more severe in bacterial infections)
    1. Opisthotonos: rigidity and hyperextension of the neck
    2. Headache
    3. Irritability and high-pitched cry
    4. Signs of increased intracranial pressure
    5. Fever, nausea, and vomiting
C. Treatment: massive doses of intravenous antibiotics
D. Nursing diagnoses based on assessment for children with meningitis
    1. Ineffective airway clearance related to level of consciousness
    2. Potential for aspiration related to
        a. Impaired swallowing
        b. Decreased level of consciousness
    3. Potential fluid volume deficit related to
        a. Excess losses
        b. Inability to manage own intake
    4. Altered nutrition: less than body requirements, related to inability to tolerate food
    5. Feeding, bathing/hygiene, dressing/grooming, toileting self-care deficit related to neuromuscular impairment
    6. Sensory-perceptual alteration related to environmental factors
    7. See Nursing diagnoses for infants with health problems and for the family of child with a disability
E. Nursing care
    1. Provide for rest
    2. Decrease stimuli from the environment (control light and noise)
    3. Position on the side with head gently supported in extension
    4. Institute respiratory isolation
    5. Decrease fluids because of meningeal edema
        a. Record carefully intake and output
        b. Monitor IV fluid
    6. Provide emotional support for the parents, since the child usually becomes ill very suddenly

7. Administer antibiotic therapy as prescribed
8. Evaluate client's response and revise plan as necessary

Febrile Convulsions

A. Caused by elevation of temperature
B. Usually occur in children between 6 months and 3 years of age
C. Treatment
   1. Treat the underlying cause
   2. Reduce the fever
D. Nursing diagnoses based on assessment for children with febrile convulsions
   1. Potential ineffective airway clearance related to decreased level of consciousness
   2. Potential for aspiration related to seizures
   3. Potential for injury related to environmental hazards
   4. See Nursing diagnoses for infants with health problems and for the family of a child with a disability
E. Nursing care
   1. Reduce fever with antipyretic drugs
   2. General seizure precautions
      a. Protect the child from injury; do not restrain; pad crib rails; do not use tongue blade
      b. Place in side-lying position to prevent aspiration
      c. Record the time of seizure, duration, and body parts involved
      d. Suction the nasopharynx and administer oxygen after the seizure as required
      e. Observe the degree of consciousness and behavior after the seizure
      f. Provide rest after the seizure
   3. For further discussion of convulsive disorders, see Medical-Surgical Nursing
   4. Evaluate client's response and revise plan as necessary

Eczema

A. Atopic manifestation of a specific allergen that may have an emotional component
B. Most common during first 2 years of life
C. Symptoms
   1. Erythema and edema from dilation of capillaries
   2. Papules, vesicles, and crusts
   3. Itching that may precipitate infection from scratching
   4. Periods of remission and exacerbation
   5. Seen mostly on cheeks, scalp, neck, and flexor surfaces of arms and legs
D. Treatment
   1. Identify allergen
   2. Local or systemic antipruritics
E. Nursing diagnoses based on assessment for children with eczema
   1. Pain, related to
      a. Tissue damage
      b. Therapies
      c. Position requirements
   2. Potential for infection related to
      a. Denuded skin
      b. Presence of infective organisms

3. Sleep pattern disturbance related to
   a. Physical discomfort
   b. Schedule of therapies
4. See Nursing diagnoses for infants with health problems and for the family of child with a disability
F. Nursing care
   1. Support the parents because this long-term problem is often discouraging, since the infant is difficult to comfort
   2. Restrain hands to keep the infant from scratching when unsupervised, but provide supervised unrestrained play periods
   3. Pick up frequently since the infant is irritable, fretful, and anorectic
   4. Avoid using wool clothing or blankets or any furry toys
   5. Provide the parent with a list of foods permitted and omitted on an elimination or restricted diet
   6. Instruct the parent how to apply topical ointments prescribed
   7. Evaluate client's response and revise plan as necessary

EMOTIONAL DISORDERS

For common emotional disorders of infancy see Disorders usually first evident in infancy, childhood, or adolescence in Psychiatric Nursing

The Toddler
GROWTH AND DEVELOPMENT
Developmental Timetable

A. Fifteen months
   1. Motor
      a. Walks well alone by 14 months, with a wide-based gait
      b. Creeps upstairs
      c. Builds tower of two blocks
      d. Drinks from a cup and can use a spoon
      e. Enjoys throwing objects and picking them up
   2. Vocalization and socialization
      a. Can use four to six words including name
      b. Has learned "no", which may be said while doing a requested demand
B. Eighteen months
   1. Physical
      a. Growth has decreased and appetite lessened— "physiologic anorexia"
      b. Anterior fontanel is usually closed
      c. Abdomen protrudes, larger than chest circumference
   2. Motor
      a. Runs clumsily
      b. Climbs stairs or up on furniture
      c. Scribbles vigorously, attempting a straight line
      d. Drinks well from a cup, manages a spoon well
      e. Builds tower of three to four cubes
   3. Vocalization and socialization
      a. Says 10 or more words
      b. Has new awareness of strangers
      c. Begins to have temper tantrums
      d. Very ritualistic, has favorite toy or blanket, thumb-sucking may be at peak

C. Two years
   1. Physical
      a. Weight—about 11 to 12 kg (26 to 28 pounds)
      b. Height—about 80 to 82 cm (32 to 33 inches)
      c. Teeth—16 temporary
   2. Motor
      a. Gross motor skills quite refined
      b. Can walk up and down stairs, both feet on one step at a time, holding onto rail
      c. Builds tower of six to seven cubes or will make cubes into a train
      d. May be ready for daytime bladder and bowel control
   3. Sensory
      a. Accommodation well developed
      b. Visual acuity 20/40
   4. Vocalization and socialization
      a. Vocabulary of about 300 words
      b. Uses short two-to-three-word phrases, also pronouns
      c. Obeys simple commands
      d. Still very ritualistic, especially at bedtime
      e. Can help undress self and pull on simple clothes
      f. Shows signs of increasing autonomy and individuality
      g. Does not share possessions, everything "mine"
D. Thirty months
   1. Physical
      a. Full set of 20 temporary teeth
      b. Decreased need for naps
   2. Motor
      a. Walks on tiptoe
      b. Stands on one foot momentarily
      c. Builds tower of eight blocks
      d. Copies horizontal or vertical line
   3. Vocalization and socialization
      a. Beginning to see self as a separate individual from reflected appraisal of significant others
      b. Still sees other children as "objects"
      c. Increasingly independent, ritualistic, and negativistic

Major Learning Events

A. Toilet training: most important task of the toddler
   1. Physical maturation must be reached before training is possible
      a. Sphincter control adequate when the child can walk
      b. Able to retain urine for at least 2 hours
      c. Usual age for bowel training: 24 to 30 months
      d. Daytime bowel and bladder control: during second year
      e. Night control: by 3 to 4 years of age
   2. Psychologic readiness
      a. Aware of the act of elimination
      b. Able to inform the parent of the need to urinate or defecate
      c. Desire to please the parent
   3. Process of training
      a. Usually begin with bowel, then bladder
      b. Accidents and regressions frequently occur

   4. Parental response
      a. Choose a specific word for the act
      b. Have a specific time and place
      c. Do not punish for accidents
B. Need for independence without overprotection; the parents should
   1. Be consistent: set realistic limits
   2. Reinforce desired behavior
   3. Be constructive, geared to teach self-control
   4. Punish immediately after a wrongdoing
   5. Punish appropriately

PLAY (PARALLEL PLAY)

A. The child plays alongside other children but not with them
B. Mostly free and spontaneous, no rules or regulations
C. Attention span is still very short, and change of toys occurs at frequent intervals
D. Safety is important; there is danger of
   1. Breaking a toy through exploration and ingesting small pieces
   2. Ingesting lead from lead-based paint on toys
   3. Being burned by potentially flammable toys
E. Imitation and make-believe play begins by end of the second year
F. Suggested toys
   1. Play furniture, dishes, cooking utensils
   2. Play telephone
   3. Puzzles with a few large pieces
   4. Pedal-propelled toys, such as tricycle
   5. Straddle toys and rocking horse
   6. Clay, sandbox toys, crayons, finger paints
   7. Pounding toys, blocks
   8. Push-pull toys

HEALTH PROMOTION DURING CHILDHOOD
Childhood Nutrition

A. Nutritional objectives
   1. Provide adequate nutrient intake to meet continuing growth and development needs
   2. Provide a basis for support of psychosocial development in relation to food patterns, eating behavior and attitudes
   3. Provide sufficient calories for increasing physical activities and energy needs
B. Diet: calorie and nutrient requirements increase with age
   1. Increased variety in types and textures of foods
   2. Increased involvement in the feeding process, stimulation of curiosity about food environment, language learning
   3. Consideration for the child's appetite, choices, motor skills
C. Possible nutritional problem areas
   1. Anemia: increase foods containing iron (e.g., enriched cereals, meat, egg, green vegetables)
   2. Obesity or underweight: increase or decrease calories; maintain core foods
   3. Low intake of calcium, iron, vitamins A and C: usually caused by dietary fads
   4. Often omitting breakfast

5. Influence of commercialism on selection of foods and emphasis on fast foods, "empty-calorie" snacks, and high-carbohydrate convenience foods

Injury Prevention

A. Leading cause of death in children over 1 year of age
B. Children under 5 years of age account for over half of all accidental deaths during childhood
C. More than half of accidental child deaths are related to automobiles and fire
D. Accidents can be viewed in terms of the child's growth and development, especially curiosity about the environment
   1. Motor vehicle
      a. Walking or running, especially after objects thrown into the street
      b. Poor perception of speed, lack of experience to foresee danger
      c. Child often unseen because of small size; can be run over by a car backing out of the driveway, or when playing in leaves or snow
      d. Failure to restrain in a car (sitting in a person's lap, improper use of seat belts rather than appropriate car restraint)
   2. Burns
      a. Investigating: pulls a pot off the stove, plays with matches, inserts an object into wall socket
      b. Climbing: reaches the stove, oven, ironing board and iron, cigarettes on the table
   3. Poisons
      a. Learning new tastes and textures, puts everything into mouth
      b. Developing fine motor skills: able to open bottles, cabinets, jars
      c. Climbing to previously unreachable shelves and cabinets
   4. Drowning
      a. Child and parents do not recognize the danger of water
      b. Child is unaware of inability to breathe under water
   5. Aspirating small objects and putting foreign bodies in ear or nose
      a. Puts everything in mouth
      b. Very interested in body and newly found openings
   6. Fractures
      a. Climbing, running, and jumping
      b. Still developing sense of balance
E. Prevention, through parent education and child protection, is the goal

HEALTH PROBLEMS OF THE TODDLER
Hospitalization of the Toddler

A. Toddler experiences basic fear of loss of love, fear of unknown, fear of punishment
B. Immobilization and isolation represent additional crises to the toddler
C. Stages of separation anxiety: the specific response of toddler
   1. Protest
      a. Prolonged loud crying, consoled by no one but the parent or usual care giver
      b. Continually asks to go home
      c. Rejection of the nurse or any other stranger
   2. Despair
      a. Alteration in sleep pattern
      b. Decreased appetite and weight loss
      c. Diminished interest in environment and play
      d. Relative immobility and listlessness
      e. No facial expression or smile
      f. Unresponsive to stimuli
   3. Detachment or denial
      a. Cheerful undiscriminating friendliness
      b. Lack of preference for parents

NURSING PROCESS FOR TODDLERS WITH HEALTH PROBLEMS
Probable Nursing Diagnoses Based on Assessment

A. Anxiety related to
   1. Strange environment
   2. Perception of impending event (specify)
   3. Separation
   4. Anticipated discomfort
   5. Knowledge deficit
   6. Discomfort
   7. Difficulty breathing
   8. Feelings of powerlessness
B. Pain related to
   1. Disease process
   2. Interventions
C. Family coping: potential for growth, related to successful parenting
D. Ineffective family coping: compromised, related to situational crisis
E. Ineffective individual coping related to situational crisis
F. Altered family process related to
   1. Situational crisis
   2. Knowledge deficit
   3. Temporary family disorganization
   4. Inadequate support systems
G. Diversional activity deficit related to
   1. Lack of sensory stimulation
   2. Frequent or prolonged hospitalization
H. Fear related to
   1. Separation from support systems
   2. Uncertain prognosis
I. Anticipatory grieving (parental) related to
   1. Expected loss (specify)
   2. Gravity of child's physical status
J. Impaired home maintenance management related to
   1. Knowledge deficit
   2. Inadequate support system
K. Potential for aspiration related to
   1. Impaired swallowing
   2. Disease process
L. Potential for injury related to
   1. Use of specific therapies and appliances
   2. Incapacity for self-protection
   3. Immobility
M. Parental role conflict related to
   1. Illness of child
   2. Inability to care for child

N. Potential altered parenting related to
1. Separation
2. Skill deficit
3. Family stress
O. Feeding, bathing/hygiene, dressing/grooming, toileting self-care deficit related to developmental level
P. Sensory-perceptual alteration (tactile) related to protected environment
Q. Potential impaired skin integrity related to
1. Immature structure and function
2. Immobility
R. Sleep pattern disturbance related to
1. Excessive crying
2. Frequent assessment
3. Therapies
S. Spiritual distress (parental) related to
1. Inadequate support systems
2. Decisions regarding "right to life" conflicts
T. See Nursing diagnoses for the family of child with a disability

Nursing Care for Toddlers with Health Problems

A. Prevent separation anxiety
1. Encourage the parent to stay with the child in hospital or to visit as frequently as possible
2. Provide a consistent care giver
3. Provide individual attention, physical touch, sensory stimulation, and affection
4. Prepare the parent for the child's reaction to separation
5. Involve the parent in the child's care as much as possible
6. If the parent is unable to visit, establish phone contact
7. Establish routine similar to the child's home routine
8. Provide the child with favorite items from home, for example, a blanket, a toy, a bottle, or a pacifier
9. Maintain the child's familiarity with home by talking about the parents, having the child listen to a tape recording of family members' voices, and showing photographs of family members
10. When family members leave, stay with child for comfort and to reassure parents
11. Associate the parents' visits with familiar events, such as "Mommy is coming after lunch"
12. Encourage the parents to visit at frequent intervals for shorter times, rather than one long visit
B. Prepare parents and the child for hospitalization
1. Give primary consideration to maintaining the parent-child relationship by limiting separation
2. Based on assessment, establish routines and rituals that the child is accustomed to in the areas of
a. Toilet training
b. Feeding
c. Bathing
d. Sleep patterns
e. Recreational activities
3. Prepare the parent for regression of the child to previous modes of behavior and loss of newly learned skills

4. Avoid teaching the child new skills during hospitalization
5. Allow the child's release of tension, especially aggression, through play (banging a drum, knocking blocks over, scribbling on paper)
6. Recognize that only minimal advance preparation of the child for hospitalization is possible, since cognitive ability to grasp verbal explanation is limited
C. See Nursing care for specific diseases
D. Evaluate client's response and revise plan as necessary

ACQUIRED IMMUNE DEFICIENCY SYNDROME (AIDS)

See Medical-Surgical Nursing for additional information
A. Results from infection with the human immunodeficiency virus (HIV) acquired through
1. Sexual contact with infected partner
2. Parenteral exposure to infected blood
3. Perinatal exposure to infected mother
4. Breast feeding a possible source of exposure
B. Symptoms
1. Failure to thrive
2. Interstitial pneumonitis
3. Hepatosplenomegaly
4. Diffuse lymphadenopathy
5. Protracted diarrhea
6. Low birth weight
7. Eczema
8. Recurrent otitis media
9. Developmental failure
C. Therapy
1. Nutritional support
2. Treatment and prophylaxis of HIV infection
3. Treatment of lymphocytic interstitial pneumonia
4. Intravenous gamma globulin
5. Treatment of tumors, end organ failure, and chronic pain
D. Nursing diagnoses based on assessment for children with AIDS
1. Anticipatory grieving related to the perceived loss of child
2. Diversional activity deficit related to restricted environment
3. Alteration in family process related to situational crisis
4. Potential for infection related to altered body defenses
5. See Nursing diagnoses for the toddler with health problems and for the family of a child with a disability
E. Nursing care
1. Prevent transmission of virus
a. Blood and body secretion precautions
b. Education of child and parent about modes of transmission
2. Support child and family
3. Monitor child for signs and symptoms of sepsis and other complications
4. See Nursing care for the family of a child with a disability
5. Evaluate client's response and revise plan as necessary

BURNS

See Medical-Surgical Nursing

A. Treatment
   1. Stop the burning process
      a. Remove from source of danger
      b. Remove smoldering clothes
      c. For superficial burns, immerse the affected area in cool water
   2. Administer prompt first aid
      a. Maintain a patent airway
      b. For first-degree burns, cleanse the area, apply sterile dressing soaked in sterile saline if possible
      c. Do not apply creams, butter, or any household remedies
      d. Do not give oral fluids for severe burns (more than 10% of body)
   3. Transport the client to a proper care facility
      a. Children are hospitalized with burns of 5% to 12% of body surface or more
      b. Child's large body surface in proportion to weight results in greater potential for fluid loss
      c. Shock: primary cause of death in first 24 to 48 hours
      d. Infection: primary cause of death after initial period
   4. Treat fluid and electrolyte loss
      a. Greatest in first 24 to 48 hours because of tissue damage
      b. Immediate replacement of both fluids and electrolytes is essential
      c. Determination of hematocrit, hemoglobin, and chemistries should be done daily to provide a guide for replacement
B. Nursing diagnoses based on assessment for children with burns
   1. Constipation related to
      a. Less than adequate intake
      b. Immobility
   2. Pain related to
      a. Wound care
      b. Trauma to skin
   3. Altered family processes related to situational crisis (child with a serious injury)
   4. Fluid volume deficit related to active loss through skin
   5. Potential for injury related to
      a. Tissue damage
      b. Presence of infective agents
      c. Smoke inhalation
      d. Metabolic derangements
   6. Impaired physical mobility related to
      a. Pain
      b. Impaired joint movement
   7. Altered nutrition: less than body requirements, related to
      a. Increased catabolism
      b. Loss of appetite
   8. Feeding, bathing/hygiene, dressing/grooming, toileting self-care deficit related to
      a. Variable disability
      b. Immobility
   9. Body image disturbance related to
      a. Perception of appearance
      b. Mobility
   10. Actual or potential impaired skin integrity related to
      a. Thermal injury
      b. Immobility
   11. See Nursing diagnoses for the toddler with health problems and for the family of a child with a disability
C. Nursing care
   1. Monitor fluids and electrolytes
      a. Administer prescribed fluids accurately, both time and volume
      b. Accurate measurement of intake and output is critical (daily weights, diaper count and weight)
   2. Maintain isolation
      a. The child has feelings of guilt and punishment
      b. Children under 5 years of age rarely understand the reason for isolation
      c. Furthers separation between parents and the child
      d. Encourage the child to express feelings
   3. Compensate for touch deprivation
      a. Touch, a child's main means of comfort and security, is now painful
      b. Pleasurable touch must be reestablished (apply lotion to unaffected areas)
      c. Maximize the use of other senses to promote security and comfort
   4. Provide for adequate nutrition
      a. High in protein, vitamins, and calories
      b. The child is frequently anorectic because of discomfort, isolation, emotional depression
      c. Provide the child food preferences when feasible; do not force eating or use it as a weapon; encourage parent participation
      d. Alter the diet as needs change, especially when high-calorie foods are no longer needed and can cause obesity
   5. Prevent contractures
      a. Make moving a game; use play that utilizes the affected part, such as throwing a ball for arm movement
      b. Provide for proper body alignment; place the child so attention is focused on an object that will keep the body in specific position
      c. Do passive exercises during bath or whirlpool
      d. Give analgesics before exercise
   6. Meet child's emotional needs
      a. Allow the child to play with gown, mask, gloves, and bandages so that they are less strange
      b. Prepare the child for baths and whirlpool treatments which can be frightening and painful
      c. Allow child to reenact treatments and care on a doll to work through feelings
      d. Help child deal with changes in body
         (1) For the younger child, more of a concern to parents (whose reactions are communicated to the child)
         (2) For the older child, especially the adolescent, body damage is of great concern

(3) Emphasize what can be done to improve looks (plastic surgery, wigs, appropriate clothing, makeup)

7. Help limit pain
   a. Assess extent of pain by observing behavior of the young child, as well as verbal complaints
   b. Distinguish pain from fear of dark, being left alone, or being in strange surroundings
   c. Administer analgesics prior to procedures; often narcotics may be required
8. See Nursing care for the family of a child with a disability
9. See Nursing care for the toddler with health problems
10. Evaluate client's response and revise plan as necessary

D. Nurse's role in prevention of burn injuries
   1. Educate children regarding fire safety
      a. Tell the child to leave the house as soon as smoke is smelled or flames are seen, without stopping to retrieve a pet or toy
      b. Involve all members of the family in fire drills
      c. Demonstrate "stop, drop, and roll" rather than running if clothes are on fire
   2. Educate parents especially in regard to the child's growth and development and specific dangers at each age level
   3. Help parents prevent fires in the home
      a. Teach cautious use of heaters, barbecue, and fireplace; place shield in front of heating unit
      b. Supervise children at all times
      c. Maintain integrity of the electrical system
      d. Regulate water heater to safe level
      e. Use and maintain smoke detectors
      f. Maintain escape route
   4. Evaluate parents' and child's understanding of teaching

POISONING
Nursing Process for Children with Poisoning
Nursing Diagnoses Based on Assessment

A. Altered family processes related to
   1. Guilt
   2. Sudden hospitalization
   3. Emergency aspect of illness
B. Fear related to
   1. Sudden onset of problem
   2. Potential life-threatening nature of incident
C. Potential for poisoning related to
   1. Immature judgment of child
   2. Presence of toxic substance
D. Potential for aspiration related to
   1. Induced vomiting
   2. Decreased level of consciousness
E. Knowledge deficit related to child safety precautions
F. See Nursing diagnoses for the toddler with health problems and the family of a child with a disability

Nursing Care for Children with Poisoning

A. Terminate the exposure
   1. Empty the mouth of pills, plant parts, or other material

2. Thoroughly flush eyes and/or skin with tap water if they were involved
3. If gasoline was spilled, remove contaminated clothing
4. Bring the victim into fresh air if an inhalation poisoning
5. Give water to dilute ingested poison

B. Identify that a poisoning has occurred
   1. Call the local poison control center, emergency facility, or physician for immediate advice regarding treatment
   2. Save all evidence of poison (container, vomitus, urine, etc.)

C. Do not induce vomiting
   1. If the person is comatose, in severe shock, convulsing or has lost the gag reflex; these conditions can increase the risk of aspiration
   2. If the poison is a low-viscosity hydrocarbon; once aspirated, it can cause a severe chemical pneumonitis
   3. If the poison is a strong corrosive (acid or alkali); emesis of the corrosive redamages the mucosa of the esophagus and pharynx

D. Remove the poison
   1. Dilute with water
   2. Induce vomiting except as contraindicated by administering ipecac syrup (for 1- to 2-year-olds 15 ml with 1 to 2 glasses of water) if vomiting has not occurred; repeat once in 20 minutes
   3. Administer activated charcoal only *after* inducing vomiting
   4. Prepare appropriate equipment for potential medical use, such as gastric lavage

E. Whether vomiting is spontaneous or induced, prevent aspiration
   1. Keep the child's head lower than the chest
   2. When alert, place the head between the legs
   3. When unconscious, position on the side

F. Observe for latent symptoms and complications of poisoning
   1. Monitor vital signs
   2. Treat as appropriate (e.g., institute seizure precautions, keep warm and position correctly in case of shock, reduce temperature if hyperpyrexic)

G. Support the child and parent
   1. Keep calm and quiet
   2. Do not admonish or accuse the child or parent of wrongdoing

H. See specific Nursing care under specific type of poisoning

I. See Nursing care for the toddler with health problems

J. Evaluate client's response and revise plan as necessary

K. Nurse's role in prevention of poisoning
   1. Assess possible contributing factors in the occurrence of an accident, such as discipline, parent-child relationship, developmental ability, environmental factors, and behavior problems
   2. Institute anticipatory guidance for possible future accidents based on the child's age and maturational level

3. Refer to a visiting nurse agency for evaluation of the home environment and the need for safety measures
4. Provide assistance with environmental manipulation when necessary
5. Educate the parents regarding safe storage of all substances
6. Teach children the hazards of ingesting nonfood items without supervision
7. Caution against keeping large amounts of drugs on hand, especially children's varieties
8. Discourage transferring drugs to containers without safety caps
9. Discuss problems of discipline and children's non-compliance
10. Evaluate parents' understanding and revise plan as necessary

Salicylate Poisoning

A. One of the most common drugs taken by children
B. Toxic dose: 4 to 7 gr per kilogram of body weight or 7 adult aspirins (28 baby aspirin) for a 9-kg (20-lb) child
C. Symptoms of mild salicylate toxicity (numbers 6 to 8 are of little value in small children)
   1. Sweating
   2. Nausea
   3. Vomiting
   4. Diarrhea
   5. Delirium
   6. Ringing in the ears
   7. Dizziness
   8. Disturbances of hearing and vision
D. Symptoms of salicylate poisoning
   1. Hyperventilation: confusion, coma
   2. Metabolic acidosis: anorexia, sweating, increased temperature
   3. Bleeding, especially if chronic ingestion
E. Treatment
   1. Induce vomiting, gastric lavage, activated charcoal, saline cathartics
   2. IV fluids
   3. Vitamin K if bleeding
   4. Peritoneal dialysis in severe cases
F. Nursing care
   1. Identify the salicylate overdose
   2. Assist with removal of the drug and other therapies
      a. Administer ipecac syrup
      b. Assist with gastric lavage if appropriate
      c. Administer activated charcoal after ipecac syrup
      d. Administer a saline cathartic
      e. Assist with peritoneal dialysis, hemodialysis, or exchange transfusion if necessary
      f. Administer intravenous fluids as prescribed
      g. Assess blood gases and serum electrolyte concentration frequently
      h. Administer sodium bicarbonate, electrolytes, and vitamin K as indicated
      i. Measure intake and output
      j. Check urine specific gravity
      k. Place on a cooling blanket
      l. Observe vital signs frequently
      m. Obtain serial blood and urine specimens
      n. Assess the level of unconsciousness and other neurologic signs
      o. Administer anticonvulsants
      p. Insert nasogastric tube to detect gastric bleeding
      q. Assess stools for occult blood (guaiac test)
   3. Support the child and parents
      a. Explain procedures and tests according to developmental level of the child
      b. Allow for expression of feelings
      c. Provide comfort measures
      d. Encourage parents to visit
      e. Allow expression of feelings regarding circumstances related to the poisoning
      f. Provide reassurance as appropriate
      g. Keep parents informed of the child's progress
   4. See Nursing care for children with poisoning
   5. Evaluate client's response and revise plan as necessary

Acetaminophen Poisoning

A. Symptoms of overdose
   1. Profuse diaphoresis
   2. Nausea and vomiting
   3. Skin eruptions
   4. Weakness
   5. Cyanosis
   6. Slow, weak pulse
   7. Depressed respirations
   8. Decreased urine output
   9. Hypothermia
   10. Circulatory collapse
   11. Coma
   12. Liver failure
B. Treatment
   1. Induce vomiting with ipecac syrup, lavage
   2. Administer IV fluid
   3. Administer an antidote (acetylcysteine)
C. Nursing care: essentially the same as those discussed under salicylate poisoning
   1. Monitor the electrocardiograph
   2. Measure intake and output
   3. Measure and record the vital signs frequently
   4. Obtain blood for hepatic and renal function tests
   5. Support the child and family
   6. See Nursing care for children with poisoning
   7. Evaluate client's response and revise plan as necessary

Petroleum Distillates

(Kerosene, turpentine, gasoline, lighter fluid, furniture polish, metal polish, benzene, naphtha, some insecticides, cleaning fluid)
A. Symptoms of toxicity
   1. Gagging, choking, and coughing
   2. Nausea
   3. Vomiting
   4. Alterations in sensorium, such as lethargy
   5. Weakness
   6. Respiratory symptoms of pulmonary involvement
      a. Tachypnea
      b. Cyanosis
      c. Substernal retractions
      d. Grunting

B. Vomiting is not induced: aspiration is a particular danger because of the risk of a chemical pneumonia
C. Nursing care
   1. Identify ingestion of distillates
   2. Prevent further irritation
      a. Avoid causing emesis
      b. Implement gastric lavage or emesis *only* as indicated
   3. Support the child and family
   4. See Nursing care for children with poisoning
   5. Evaluate client's response and revise plan as necessary

Corrosive Chemicals

(Oven and drain cleaners, electric dishwasher granules, strong detergents)
A. Symptoms of toxicity
   1. Severe burning pain in the mouth, throat, and stomach
   2. White, swollen mucous membrane, edema of the lips, tongue, and pharynx (respiratory obstruction)
   3. Violent vomiting; hemoptysis, hematemesis
   4. Signs of shock
   5. Anxiety and agitation
B. Never induce vomiting, since regurgitation of the substance will cause further damage to the mucous membranes
C. Nursing care
   1. Identify ingestion
   2. Maintain a patent airway
      a. Examine the pharynx for burns
      b. Observe for respiratory difficulty
      c. Provide an airway if necessary; have emergency equipment available
      d. Administer steroids if prescribed
   3. Prevent further irritation
      a. Avoid causing emesis
      b. Dilute with water if advised
      c. Give nothing by mouth except as ordered and tolerated
   4. Provide comfort and support to the child and family
      a. Administer analgesics as needed
      b. Remain with the child
      c. Keep parents informed of the child's progress
   5. See Nursing care for children with poisoning
   6. Evaluate client's response and revise plan as necessary

Lead Poisoning (Plumbism)

A. Most common between 9 months and 3 years of age, usually from eating lead chips from peeling paint or sucking on objects painted with lead-based paint
B. Characteristics of the child and parents
   1. High level of oral activity in the child (e.g., use of pacifier, thumb-sucking)
   2. Oral gratification used as method of relieving anxiety in the child
   3. Parents, regardless of income, education, or age
      a. Use few resources to stimulate child
      b. Provide less adequate child care
      c. Are less affectionate
      d. Are immature

C. Symptoms of chronic ingestion
   1. Loss of weight, anorexia
   2. Abdominal pain, vomiting
   3. Constipation
   4. Anemia, pallor, listlessness, fatigue
   5. Lead line on teeth; density of long bones
   6. Behavior changes (impulsiveness, irritability, hyperactivity, or lethargy)
   7. Headache, insomnia, joint pains
   8. Brain damage, convulsions, death
   9. Increased blood lead level
      a. Normal: below 40 μg per 100 ml of blood
      b. Borderline: below 60 μg per 100 ml of blood
      c. Treatment begun at 60 μg or higher
      d. Convulsions and irreversible brain damage: about 80 μg
D. Treatment
   1. Objective: reduce concentration of lead in the blood and soft tissue by promoting its excretion and deposition in bones
      a. Calcium disodium edetate (Calcium Disodium Versenate)
         (1) Urine lead content monitored; peak excretion in 24 to 48 hours
         (2) Adverse effects: acute tubular necrosis, malaise, fatigue, numbness of extremities, GI disturbances, fever, pain in muscles and joints
      b. Dimercaprol (BAL)
         (1) Generally used in conjunction with calcium disodium edetate
         (2) Adverse effects: local pain at the site of injection; may cause persistent fever in children receiving therapy; rise in blood pressure accompanied by tachycardia after injection
      c. Vitamin D, calcium, and phosphorus
   2. Prevention of further ingestion
E. Nursing care
   1. Prevent lead poisoning through education, proper housing, supervision of children
   2. Screen children at risk by recognizing signs, especially behavior changes
   3. Plan for rotation of injection sites and preparation of the child
   4. Observe carefully
   5. Plan discharge and follow-up care of the child
   6. Teach parents to prevent further ingestion
   7. See Nursing care for children with poisoning
   8. Evaluate client's response and revise plan as necessary

FRACTURES

See Medical-Surgical Nursing for additional information on fractures
A. Greenstick fractures: incomplete break and bending of a long bone, occurring in young children because the bones are soft and not fully mineralized
B. Treatment of fractures: splint, traction, or cast
   1. Bryant's traction: for fractured femur
      a. Generally used for children under 2 years of age

b. Legs are suspended vertically with buttocks slightly off bed and upper body maintaining countertraction

2. Spica cast may be used for child of any age

C. Nursing diagnoses for children with fractures
   1. Pain related to
      a. Fracture
      b. Cast
   2. Diversional activity deficit related to immobility
   3. Fear related to perception of cast removal
   4. Potential for injury related to
      a. Edema
      b. Immobility
      c. Presence of traction
      d. Limited respiratory excursion (spica cast)
   5. Impaired physical mobility related to
      a. Musculoskeletal injury
      b. Use of immobilizing devices
   6. Altered Nutrition: more than body requirements, related to immobility
   7. Altered family processes related to
      a. Situational crisis
      b. Injured child
   8. Feeding, bathing/hygiene, dressing/grooming, toileting self-care deficit related to musculoskeletal impairment
   9. Potential impaired skin integrity related to
      a. Immobility
      b. Presence of cast
   10. See nursing diagnoses for the toddler with health problems

D. Nursing care
   1. The child must be kept flat on back
   2. Restraining jacket may be necessary to prevent moving
   3. Provide activity to keep child occupied and entertained
   4. See Nursing care for the toddler with health problems
   5. Evaluate client's response and revise plan as necessary

ASPIRATION OF FOREIGN OBJECTS

A. Symptoms of complete obstruction
   1. Substernal retractions
   2. Inability to cough or speak
   3. Increased pulse and respiratory rate
   4. Cyanosis

B. Treatment
   1. If incomplete obstruction, do not intervene; allow child to continue coughing until object is dislodged
   2. Immediate first aid if object is completely obstructing the trachea
      a. Try to pull the object out if possible without forcing it further down
      b. Turn the small child upside down (head lower than chest) and deliver four quick sharp back blows with the heel of the hand; turn the child over and deliver four quick chest thrusts using the technique for CPR

c. Abdominal thrust for children 1 year and older (Heimlich maneuver): grasp the victim from behind around the upper abdomen and squeeze, forcing the diaphragm up

3. Medical removal by bronchoscopy

4. Surgical relief by a tracheotomy below level of the object

C. Nursing diagnoses based on assessment for children who have aspirated a foreign object
   1. Anxiety related to
      a. Parents' perceived threat to life of child
      b. Child's inability to breathe
   2. Potential for suffocation related to knowledge deficit of risk factors
   3. Ineffective airway clearance related to obstruction
   4. See Nursing diagnoses for the toddler with health problems

D. Nursing care
   1. Keep small objects such as balloons, buttons, and batteries out of the child's reach
   2. Inspect larger toys for removable objects
   3. Teach the child not to run or laugh with food or fluid in the mouth
   4. Avoid giving young children foods easily aspirated, such as nuts or hotdogs
   5. Teach the child to chew food well before swallowing
   6. See Nursing care for the toddler with a health problem
   7. Evaluate client's response and revise plan as necessary

CHILD ABUSE

A. Refers to both physical and sexual abuse and emotional neglect

B. Majority of abused children are under 4 years of age

C. About 70% to 80% of abuse is by parents

D. Characteristics of abusing parents
   1. Their own childhood included abuse
   2. Have incorrect concept of what a small child is and can do
   3. Plagued by a low self-esteem and lack of identity
   4. Tend to be young, immature, and dependent
   5. Frequently expect the child to provide them with nurturing and love
   6. Tend to be depressed, lonely people, yearning for love and understanding
   7. Have no outside resources for emotional support or relief from responsibility, especially in time of crisis; thus they take out their frustration on the child

E. Nursing diagnoses based on assessment for abused children and abusing parents
   1. Potential for trauma related to
      a. Characteristics of child
      b. Characteristics of care giver
      c. Environmental characteristics
   2. Potential for violence: directed at others, related to
      a. Inability to control impulses, especially anger
      b. Chronic low self-esteem
      c. Their own parental role models

3. Chronic low self-esteem related to
   a. The self-degrading concepts developed as children
   b. Inability to control impulses, especially anger
   c. Lack of a support system
4. Ineffective individual coping related to
   a. Inability to respond to environmental pressure
   b. Lack of respite from parenting responsibilities
   c. Inability to use problem-solving techniques
5. Ineffective family coping: disabling, related to
   a. Ambivalent family relationships
   b. Use of physical force to control family members (actual or threatened)
   c. Feelings of powerlessness related to abusing family member
   d. Use of mind-altering substances such as alcohol or drugs
6. Social isolation related to a lack of personal and nurturing relationships
7. Pain related to physical or emotional abuse
8. Hopelessness related to inability to deal with or escape abusing individual
9. Altered growth and development related to
   a. Physical abuse
   b. Lack of nurturing
   c. Neglect
   d. Environmental deficiencies
10. For additional nursing diagnoses see specific injuries child has sustained

F. Nursing care
1. Be alert for clues that indicate child abuse or neglect
   a. The child has many unexplained injuries, scars, bruises
   b. Parents offer inconsistent stories explaining child's injuries when questioned
   c. Emotional response of parents is inconsistent with the degree of the child's injury
   d. Parents may resist or fail to be present for questioning
   e. The child exhibits physical signs of neglect: malnourished, dehydrated, unkempt
   f. The child cringes when physically approached and appears unduly afraid
   g. The child responds in a manner that indicates avoiding punishment rather than gaining reward
   h. The child has excessive interest in sexual matters
   i. The child has a sexually transmitted disease
2. Be aware of child abuse laws
3. Recognize that the main objective must be to protect the child from further abuse
4. Focus on helping parents with their own dependency needs
   a. Group therapy
   b. Home visiting
   c. Foster grandparents
5. Help parents learn to control frustration through other outlets
6. Educate parents about the child's normal needs and development, new modes of discipline, and realistic expectations

7. Provide emotional support and therapy for the child since abused children frequently grow up to be abusing parents
8. Evaluate client's response and revise plan as necessary

MENTAL RETARDATION

A. Usually defined as low IQ (70 or below); about 3% of the population
B. Retardation can be further classified by the use of the following intelligence test scores (these numbers are approximate and should not be used in a fixed manner for diagnosis)
1. Normal: 90 to 110 IQ
2. Borderline: 71 to 89 IQ
3. Mild: 50/55 to 70 IQ
   a. Educable: can achieve a mental age of 8 to 12 years
   b. Can learn to read, write, do arithmetic, achieve a vocational skill, and function in society
4. Moderate: 35/40 to 50/55 IQ
   a. Trainable: can achieve a mental age of 3 to 7 years
   b. Can learn the activities of daily living, social skills; can be trained to work in a sheltered workshop
5. Severe: below 20/25 to 35/40 IQ
   a. Barely trainable: can achieve a mental age of 0 to 2 years
   b. Totally dependent on others and in need of custodial care
6. Profound: below 20/25 IQ
   a. May attain mental age of young infant
   b. Requires total care

C. Causes
1. Prenatal: heredity, PKU, Down's syndrome, severe malnutrition (relationship is under study), rubella, other infections, maternal drug use (including alcohol)
2. Natal: kernicterus (high bilirubin level), intracranial hemorrhage, anoxia, physical injury
3. Postnatal: lead poisoning, meningitis, encephalitis, neoplasms, recurrent convulsions
4. Metabolic: imbalance in essential nutrients, metabolic or endocrine disorders such as PKU or hypothyroidism

D. Characteristics of mentally retarded children
1. Delayed milestones
   a. Infant fails to suck
   b. Head lag after 4 to 6 months of age
   c. Slow in learning self-help; slow to respond to new stimuli
   d. Slow or absent speech development
2. Mental abilities are concrete: abstract ability is limited
3. Lack power of self-appraisal
4. Do not learn from errors
5. Cannot carry out complex instructions
6. Do not relate with peers: more secure with adults
7. Comforted by physical touch
8. Learn rote responses and socially acceptable behavior

9. May repeat words (echolalia)
10. Short attention span, but usually attracted to music

E. Conditions that may lead to a false diagnosis of mental retardation
  1. Emotional disturbance, such as autism or maternal deprivation
  2. Sensory problems, such as deafness or blindness
  3. Cerebral dysfunctions, such as cerebral palsy, learning disorders, hyperkinesia, epilepsy

F. Nursing diagnoses based on assessment for children with mental retardation
  1. Altered family processes related to a child with a disability
  2. Potential for injury related to knowledge deficit
  3. Feeding, bathing/hygiene, dressing/grooming, toileting self-care deficit related to developmental delay
  4. Altered growth and development related to maturational lag
  5. Impaired verbal communication related to retarded developmental level
  6. Impaired social interaction related to
    a. Communication difficulties
    b. Knowledge deficit
    c. Developmental lag
  7. Sensory-perceptual alterations (visual, auditory, kinesthetic, gustatory, tactile, olfactory) related to developmental delay
  8. See Nursing diagnoses for the toddler with health problems and for the family of child with a disability

G. Nursing care
  1. Always deal with the child's developmental not chronologic age
    a. Educate the parent regarding developmental age
    b. When the child is nearing adolescence, sexual feelings accompany maturation and need to be explained according to the child's mental capacity
  2. Set realistic goals; teach by simple steps for habit formation rather than for understanding or transference of learning
    a. Break the process of skills learning down into simple steps that can be easily achieved
    b. Ensure each step is learned completely before teaching the child the next step
    c. Recognize that behavior modification is a very effective method of teaching these children
    d. Praise for accomplishments to develop the child's self-esteem
    e. Keep discipline simple, geared toward learning acceptable behavior rather than developing judgment
    f. Recognize that routines are the foundation of the child's life-style; hospitalization should be based on the child's normal schedule
    g. See Nursing care for the family of a child with a disability
    h. Evaluate client's response and revise plan as necessary

CEREBRAL PALSY

A. Neuromuscular disability or difficulty in controlling voluntary muscles (caused by damage to some portion of the brain, with associated sensory, intellectual, emotional, or convulsive disorders)

B. Characteristics of cerebral palsy
  1. Affects young children, usually becoming evident before 3 years of age
  2. Nonprogressive, but persists throughout life
  3. Some motor dysfunction always present
  4. Mental deficiency may or may not be present

C. Major causes
  1. Anoxia of the brain caused by a variety of insults at or near the time of birth
  2. Congenital or neonatal infection of the central nervous system

D. Types: classified according to predominant clinical manifestation
  1. Spastic (65%): hyperactivity of muscle stretch reflex, which becomes worse with rapid passive motion
  2. Dyskinetic: major manifestation is athetosis; slow, wormlike, involuntary purposeless movement
  3. Ataxic failure of muscle coordination
  4. Tremor: a rhythmic purposeless movement that becomes worse with excitement or intentional movement
  5. Flaccid: decreased muscle tension
  6. Rigid: persistent stiffness of the muscles on movement, which becomes less severe with rapid passive motion

E. Symptoms
  1. Difficulty in feeding, especially sucking and swallowing
  2. Asymmetry in motion or contour of body
  3. Delayed motor development and speech
  4. Excessive or feeble cry
  5. Any of the muscular abnormalities listed under types

F. Nursing diagnoses based on assessment for children with cerebral palsy
  1. Activity intolerance related to
    a. Decreased energy and fatigue
    b. Perceptual/cognitive impairment
  2. Impaired verbal communication related to neuromuscular impairment
  3. Altered family processes related to the birth of a child with a disability
  4. Potential for trauma related to neuromuscular impairment
  5. Impaired physical mobility related to neuromuscular impairment
  6. Feeding, bathing/hygiene, dressing/grooming, toileting self-care deficit related to impaired neuromuscular development
  7. Sensory-perceptual alterations (visual, auditory, kinesthetic, tactile) related to neurologic deficit
  8. Altered growth and development related to physical disability
  9. Altered nutrition: less than body requirements, related to greater than normal energy expenditure

10. Body image disturbance related to
    a. Physical disability
    b. Appearance
11. See Nursing diagnoses for the toddler with health problems and for the family of child with a disability
G. Nursing care
    1. Feeding
       a. Recognize drooling results from difficulty in swallowing
       b. Use a spoon and blunt fork, with plate attached to the table, for easier self-feeding
       c. Provide child with increased calories because of excessive energy expenditure, increased protein for muscle activity, and increased vitamins (especially B_6) for amino acid metabolism
    2. Relaxation
       a. Provide rest periods in an area with few stimuli
       b. Set limits and control activity level
    3. Safety
       a. Protect from accidents resulting from poor balance and lack of muscle control
       b. Provide helmet for protection against head injuries
       c. Always restrain in chair, bed, etc.
    4. Play
       a. Keep safety as main objective
       b. Do not overstimulate; should have educational value, appropriate to child's developmental level and ability
    5. Elimination
       a. Recognize difficulty in toilet training is because of poor muscle control
       b. Provide special bowel and bladder training
    6. Speech
       a. Recognize poor coordination of lips, tongue, cheeks, larynx, and poor control of diaphragm make formation of words difficult
       b. Refer for speech therapy
    7. Breathing
       a. Recognize poor control of the intercostal muscles and diaphragm causes the child to be prone to respiratory tract infection
       b. Protect the child from exposure to infection as much as possible; be alert for symptoms of aspiration pneumonia
    8. Dental problems
       a. Recognize problems in muscular control affect development and alignment of teeth
       b. Explain that frequent dental caries occur and there is a great need for dental supervision and care
       c. Teach the parent to brush the child's teeth if muscular dysfunction present
    9. Vision
       a. Recognize common ocular problems such as strabismus and refractive errors may be related to poor muscular control
       b. Look for such disorders to prevent further problems such as amblyopia
   10. Hearing
       a. Recognize hearing problems may be present depending on the basic cause of the brain damage
       b. Encourage parents to have child's hearing checked periodically
   11. See Nursing care for the family of a child with a disability
   12. See Nursing care for the toddler with health problems
   13. Evaluate client's response and revise plan as necessary

HEARING DISORDERS

A. Types
    1. Conductive: loss from damage to middle ear
       a. Accounts for about 80% of reduced hearing
       b. Conductive loss of 30 dB or more may require a hearing aid
    2. Sensorineural: damage to inner ear structures of the auditory nerve
       a. Distortion in clarity of words
       b. Problem in discrimination of sounds
    3. Mixed conductive-sensorineural
    4. Central auditory
       a. Not explained by other three causes
       b. The child hears but does not understand
B. Causes
    1. Maternal factors: rubella, syphilis
    2. Perinatal: anoxia, kernicterus, prematurity, excessive noise
    3. Postnatal: mumps, otitis media, head trauma, drugs such as streptomycin
C. Developmental and behavioral manifestations of hearing loss
    1. Lack of the Moro reflex in response to a sharp clap
    2. Failure to respond to loud noise
    3. Failure to locate a source of sound at 61 to 95 cm (2 to 3 feet) after 6 months of age
    4. Absence of babble by 7 months of age
    5. Inability to understand words or phrases by 12 months of age
    6. Use of gestures rather than verbalization to establish wants
    7. History of frequent respiratory tract infections and otitis media
D. Nursing diagnoses based on assessment for children with hearing disorders
    1. Altered family processes related to
       a. Situational crisis
       b. Difficulty in communication
    2. Potential for injury related to cognitive-perceptual impairment
    3. Impaired verbal communication related to loss of hearing before speech is established
    4. Social isolation related to difficulty with communication
    5. Sensory-perceptual alteration (auditory) related to hearing impairment
    6. See Nursing diagnoses for the toddler with health problems and for the family of child with a disability

E. Nursing care
1. Observe for manifestations beginning at birth
2. Face the child to facilitate lipreading
3. Do not walk back and forth while talking
4. Have a good light on speaker's face
5. Be level with the child's face and speak toward the good ear
6. Always enunciate and articulate carefully
7. Do not talk too loudly, especially if the loss is sensorineural
8. Use facial expressions, since verbal intonations are not communicated
9. Encourage active play to build self-confidence
10. See Nursing care for the family of a child with a disability
11. See Nursing care for the toddler with health problems
12. Evaluate client's response and revise plan as necessary

VISUAL DISORDERS

A. Functional definition of blindness: visual loss of acuity to read print, must use braille, may have light perception
B. Strabismus: imbalance of the extraocular muscles causing a physiologic incoordination of the eye
1. A cause of blindness: amblyopia develops in the weak eye from disuse
2. Must be corrected before 4 years of age to prevent blindness
3. Treatment
a. To force the weak eye to fixate: patch the good eye and exercise the weak eye
b. Surgery to lengthen or shorten the extraocular muscles
C. Causes other than strabismus
1. Maternal: albinism, congenital cataracts, rubella, galactosemia
2. Perinatal: retrolental fibroplasia
3. Postnatal: trauma, diabetes, syphilis, tumor
D. Developmental and behavioral manifestations indicating a reduction in vision
1. Delayed motor development
2. Rocking for sensory stimulation
3. Squinting, rubbing eyes
4. Sitting close to television, holding book close to face
5. Clumsiness, bumping into objects
E. Nursing diagnoses based on assessment for children with visual disorders
1. Altered family processes related to situational crisis
2. Potential for injury related to cognitive-perceptual impairment
3. Sensory-perceptual alteration (visual) related to visual impairment
4. See nursing diagnoses for the toddler with health problems and for the family of child with a disability
F. Nursing care
1. Be aware of early signs of visual problems
2. Explain and encourage parents to follow treatments for strabismus and other conditions

3. Always talk so the child can hear clearly
4. Use noise so the child can locate your position
5. Help the child learn through other senses, especially touch through play activities
6. Facilitate eating
a. Arrange food on the plate at clock hours and teach the child its location
b. Provide finger foods when possible
c. Provide a light spoon and deep bowl so the child can feel weight of food on spoon
7. See Nursing care for the family of a child with a disability
8. See Nursing care for the toddler with health problems
9. Evaluate client's response and revise plan as necessary

PINWORMS

A. Most common intestinal parasite in United States
B. Children reinfest themselves by fingers to anus to mouth route
C. Can also be infested by breathing air-borne ova
D. Symptoms
1. Severe pruritus of the anal area
2. Vaginitis
3. Irritability and insomnia
4. Poor appetite and weight loss
5. Eosinophilia
E. Diagnosis: cellophane tape test to isolate eggs from the anal area (must be done in morning before the first BM)
F. Treatment: anthelmintics
1. Mebendazole (Vermox)
a. Selectively and irreversibly inhibits uptake of glucose and other nutrients of pinworms
b. Adverse effects: occasional, transient abdominal pain and diarrhea
2. Piperazine citrate (Antepar)
a. Paralyzes musculature of pinworms and roundworms by curarelike action
b. Within 3 days pinworms are passed active and alive; roundworms paralyzed and alive
3. Pyrantel pamoate (Antiminth)
a. Blocks neuromuscular transmission in roundworms, hookworms, pinworms
b. Adverse effects: anorexia, nausea, vomiting, diarrhea, abdominal cramps, headache, dizziness, drowsiness, rash
4. Pyrvinium pamoate (Povan)
a. Inhibits respiratory enzymes and anaerobic metabolism to inactivate pinworms, threadworms
b. Adverse effects: nausea, vomiting, abdominal cramps; cyanine dye origin of the drug colors stool, emesis, and most materials bright red or orange
G. Nursing diagnoses based on assessment for children with pinworms
1. Potential impaired skin integrity related to irritation of perianal area
2. See Nursing diagnoses of the toddler with health problems

H. Nursing care
   1. Prevent reinfestation
     a. Do not allow the child to scratch the anus; child may need to wear mittens
     b. Keep fingernails short
     c. Place a tight diaper or underpants on child
     d. Wash anal area thoroughly at least once a day
     e. Change child's clothes daily; wash in hot water
     f. Air out bedroom, dust and vacuum house thoroughly
   2. Teach parent about administration of medication
     a. Overdose will not produce a quicker recovery
     b. Stools may turn bright red from medication
   3. See Nursing care for the toddler with health problems
   4. Evaluate client's response and revise plan as necessary

LYME DISEASE

A. Caused by spirochete transmitted by ticks
B. Three stages of infection
   1. Tick bite at time of innoculation
   2. Development of erythematous papule that enlarges radially, resulting in a large circumferential ring with a raised edematous doughnut-like border
   3. Systemic involvement of neurologic, cardiac, and musculoskeletal systems which appears several weeks after the cutaneous phase is completed
C. Symptoms
   Symptoms depend upon which organ system is involved after the initial cutaneous phase
D. Treatment
   1. Antibiotics used for treatment in the second phase will prevent most disease progression
   2. Neurologic symptoms are treated with oral prednisone or antibiotics when present less than 24 hours
   3. Cardiac symptoms are treated with daily prednisone and aspirin
   4. Musculoskeletal pain treated with aspirin and prednisone
E. Nursing diagnoses based on assessment for the child with Lyme disease
   1. Pain related to disease process
   2. Fear related to uncertain prognosis
   3. See Nursing diagnoses for the toddler with health problems
F. Nursing care
   1. Teach parents to examine children for ticks
   2. Support child and family
   3. For further information see Lyme disease in Medical-Surgical Nursing
   4. See Nursing care for the toddler with health problems
   5. Evaluate client's response and revise plan as necessary

ANEMIA

A. Most prevalent nutritional disorder among children in the United States; caused by lack of adequate sources of dietary iron
   1. Infant usually has iron reserve for 6 months
   2. Premature infant lacks reserve
   3. Children receiving only milk have no source of iron

B. Insidious onset: usually diagnosed because of an infection or chronic GI problems
C. Symptoms
   1. Pallor, weakness
   2. Slow motor development
   3. Poor muscle tone
   4. Hemoglobin level below the normal for age (general rule: below 11 g)
D. Treatment
   1. Food sources rich in iron
   2. Iron replacement
     a. Oral iron sources
       (1) Drug: ferrous sulfate—most absorbable form of iron
       (2) Adverse effects: nausea, vomiting; fatalities in children who ingest enteric-coated tablets, thinking they are candy
       (3) Drug interactions: ferrous sulfate binds tetracycline and decreases absorption; magnesium trisilicate decreases absorption of iron preparations
     b. Parenteral iron sources
       (1) Drug: iron-dextran injection (Imferon)
       (2) Adverse effects: tissue staining (use Z tract for injection), fever, lymphadenopathy, nausea, vomiting, arthralgia, urticaria, severe peripheral vascular failure, anaphylaxis, secondary hematochromatosis
E. Nursing diagnoses based on assessment for children with anemia
   1. Activity intolerance related to generalized weakness
   2. Altered family processes related to situational crisis
   3. Potential for infection and trauma related to lowered body defenses
   4. Fatigue related to decreased oxygen-carrying capacity of blood
   5. Altered nutrition: less than body requirements, related to knowledge deficit of appropriate foods
   6. See Nursing diagnoses for the toddler with health problems
F. Nursing care
   1. Prevent development of anemia
     a. Teach pregnant women the importance of their iron intake
     b. Encourage feeding of iron-fortified infant formula or breast feeding
     c. Encourage feeding iron-fortified infant cereal
     d. Introduce foods high in iron
   2. Provide for good nutrition and proper administration of supplemental iron
     a. Vitamin C aids absorption
     b. Hydrochloric acid aids absorption
     c. Oxalates, phosphate, and caffeine decrease absorption
     d. Use a straw since some liquid preparations stain teeth
     e. Discolors stools; may cause gastric irritation or constipation
   3. See Nursing care for the toddler with health problems
   4. Evaluate client's response and revise plan as necessary

CELIAC DISEASE

A. Chronic intestinal malabsorption and inability to digest gluten, a protein found mostly in wheat, rye, oats, and barley
B. Usually begins in infancy or toddler stage, but later in breast-fed infants
C. Symptoms
   1. Progressive malnutrition: secondary deficiencies: anemia, rickets
      a. Stunted growth
      b. Wasting of extremities
      c. Distended abdomen
   2. Steatorrhea: fatty, foul, frothy, bulky stools
   3. Celiac crisis: severe episode of dehydration and acidosis from diarrhea
D. Treatment: dietary
   1. Low in glutens; no wheat, rye, oats, or barley
   2. High in calories and protein
   3. Low fat
   4. Small, frequent feedings; adequate fluids
   5. Vitamin supplements, all in water-miscible form
   6. Supplemental iron
E. Nursing diagnoses based on assessment for children with celiac disease
   1. Diarrhea related to intestinal malabsorption
   2. Altered family processes related to situational crisis (child with a chronic illness)
   3. Potential for injury related to
      a. Sensitivity to gluten
      b. Knowledge deficit (diet and food composition)
   4. Alteration in nutrition: less than body requirements, related to impaired intestinal absorption
   5. See Nursing diagnoses for the toddler with health problems and for the family of a child with a disability
F. Nursing care
   1. Protect the child from infection
   2. Teach parents dietary restrictions
   3. Explain need for frequent follow-up supervision, home visits
   4. See Nursing care for the family of a child with a disability
   5. See Nursing care for the toddler with health problems
   6. Evaluate client's response and revise plan as necessary

CYSTIC FIBROSIS

A. Autosomal recessive disorder affecting the exocrine glands
B. Pathology: defect is in overproduction of mucus or an absence of normal mucus-removing mechanism
   1. Pancreas: becomes fibrotic, with a decreased production of pancreatic enzymes (late complication — diabetes)
      a. Lipase: causes steatorrhea (fatty, foul, bulky stools)
      b. Trypsin: causes increased nitrogen in stool
      c. Amylase: inability to break down polysaccharides
   2. Rectal prolapse
   3. Sweat glands: high electrolyte content of sodium and chloride (3 to 5 times higher than normal); chloride levels above 60 mEq/L are diagnostic
   4. Respiratory system: increased viscous mucus in the trachea, bronchi, and bronchioles resulting in
      a. Obstruction, interfering with expiration (emphysema)
      b. Infection
   5. Liver: possible cirrhosis from biliary obstruction, malnutrition, or infection; portal hypertension leads to esophageal varices
   6. Sexual organs: infertility possible
C. Symptoms
   1. Based on pathophysiology listed in B.
   2. Similar to celiac disease
   3. Some early manifestations during infancy
      a. Meconium ileus at birth (about 15%)
      b. Failure to regain normal 10% weight loss at birth
      c. Presence of cough or wheezing during first 6 months of age
   4. Because of respiratory involvement, there may be clubbing of fingers, barrel-shaped chest, cyanosis, distended neck veins
   5. Cardiac enlargement, particularly right ventricular hypertrophy (cor pulmonale)
D. Nursing diagnoses based on assessment for children with cystic fibrosis
   1. Activity intolerance related to
      a. Imbalance between oxygen supply and demand
      b. Ineffective airway clearance
   2. Ineffective airway clearance related to secretion of thick, tenacious mucus
   3. Ineffective breathing pattern related to tracheobronchial obstruction
   4. Altered family processes related to situational crisis (child with a chronic illness)
   5. Anticipatory grieving related to perceived potential loss of child
   6. Potential for injury related to impaired body defenses
   7. Altered nutrition: less than body requirements, related to inability to digest nutrients
   8. Body image disturbance related to perception of being different
   9. Sleep pattern disturbance related to
      a. Frequent coughing
      b. Ineffective breathing
   10. Social isolation related to
      a. Hospitalization
      b. Confinement to home
      c. Fatigue
   11. See Nursing diagnoses for the toddler with health problems and for the family of child with a disability
E. Nursing care
   1. Prevent respiratory tract infections
      a. Postural drainage, percussion, vibrating
      b. Aerosal therapy
      c. Use of expectorants and antibiotics
      d. Avoid antitussives and antihistamines

2. Promote optimal nutrition
   a. Replacement of pancreatic enzymes, given with cold food in middle of meal
   b. Replacement of fat-soluble vitamins in water-miscible form
   c. High-protein diet of easily digested food, normal fat, high calories
3. Promote mobility and activity
   a. Encourage activity and regular exercise
   b. Help the child regulate activity to own tolerance
4. Promote a positive body image
   a. Help child deal with barrel-shaped chest, poor weight gain, thin extremities, bluish coloring, smell of stools, poor posture
   b. Encourage good hygiene and select clothes that compensate for protuberant abdomen and emaciated extremities
5. Provide for emotional support and counseling for child and family
   a. Long-term problem causing financial and emotional stresses
   b. Illness can become a major controlling factor in the family
      (1) The child begins to recognize that wheezing brings attention and uses this knowledge
      (2) Parents can deal with such behavior by recognizing false attacks and using consistent discipline
   c. Encourage the family to join the Cystic Fibrosis Foundation
   d. Refer family for genetic counseling
6. See Nursing care for the family of a child with a disability
7. See Nursing care for the toddler with health problems
8. Evaluate client's response and revise plan as necessary

SICKLE CELL ANEMIA

A. Autosomal disorder affecting hemoglobin
B. Defective hemoglobin causes red blood cells to become sickle shaped and clump together under reduced oxygen tension
C. Symptoms of sickle cell crises
   1. Vaso-occlusive crisis: most common and only painful type
      a. Results from sickled cells obstructing blood vessels causing occlusion, ischemia, and potential necrosis
      b. Symptoms include: fever, acute abdominal pain (visceral hypoxia), hand-foot syndrome, and arthralgia without an exacerbation of anemia
   2. Splenic sequestration crisis
      a. Results from the spleen pooling large quantities of blood, which causes a precipitous drop in blood pressure and ultimately shock
      b. Acute episode occurs most commonly in children between 8 months and 5 years of age; can result in death from anemia and cardiovascular collapse
      c. Chronic manifestation is termed functional asplenia

3. Aplastic crisis: diminished red blood cell production
   a. May be triggered by a viral or other infection
   b. Profound anemia results due to rapid destruction of red blood cells combined with a decreased production
4. Hyperhemolytic crisis: increased rate of red blood cell destruction
   a. Characterized by anemia, jaundice, and reticulcytosis
   b. Rare complication which frequently suggests a coexisting abnormality such as glucose-6-phosphate dehydrogenase deficiency
D. Nursing diagnoses based on assessment for children with sickle cell anemia
   1. Activity intolerance related to generalized weakness
   2. Pain related to tissue ischemia
   3. Altered family processes related to situational crisis (child with a chronic health problem)
   4. Fear related to
      a. Unfamiliar environment
      b. Separation from support system
   5. Potential fluid volume deficit related to
      a. Sickling phenomena
      b. Pain
      c. Immobility
   6. Potential for infection and trauma related to
      a. Weakened bones
      b. Anemia
      c. Dehydration
   7. Body image disturbance related to
      a. Retarded growth and maturation
      b. Limited activity tolerance
      c. Chronic illness
   8. Altered tissue perfusion (cardiovascular) related to decreased oxygen tension
   9. See Nursing diagnoses for the toddler with health problems and for the family of a child with a disability
E. Nursing care
   1. Prevent crisis
      a. Avoid infection, dehydration, and other conditions causing strain on body, which precipitates a crisis; prophylactic use of pneumococcal, meningococcal, and H. flu vaccines
      b. Avoid hypoxia: treat respiratory tract infections immediately
      c. Avoid dehydration
         (1) May cause a rapid thrombus formation
         (2) Daily fluid intake should be calculated according to body weight (130 to 200 ml per kilogram [2 to 3 oz per pound])
         (3) During crisis, fluid needs to be increased, especially if the child is febrile
   2. During crisis provide for
      a. Adequate hydration (may need IV therapy)
      b. Proper positioning, careful handling
      c. Exercise as tolerated (immobility promotes thrombus formation and respiratory problems)
      d. Adequate ventilation
      e. Control of pain; use narcotics; schedule to prevent pain
      f. Blood transfusions for severe anemia

3. Provide for genetic counseling
   a. Disorder mostly of blacks; can be found in Mediterranean people
   b. Parents need to know the risk of having other children with the trait or disease
   c. If both parents are carriers, each pregnancy has 25% chance of producing a child with the disease
   d. Screen young children for the disorder, since clinical manifestations usually do not appear before 6 months of age
4. See Nursing care for the family of a child with a disability
5. See Nursing care for the toddler with health problems
6. Evaluate client's response and revise plan as necessary

β-THALASSEMIA (COOLEY'S ANEMIA)

A. Autosomal disorder with varied expressivity
B. Basic defect seems to be a deficiency in the synthesis of β-chain polypeptides, which results in a decreased rate of production of the globin molecule
C. Symptoms
   1. Severe anemia
   2. Unexplained fever
   3. Poor feeding
   4. Markedly enlarged spleen
   5. Enlarged abdomen, reflecting significant hepatomegaly
   6. Impaired physical growth
   7. Exercise intolerance
   8. Headache
   9. Listlessness
   10. Anorexia
   11. Bone changes: seen later in untreated cases
       a. Enlarged head
       b. Prominent frontal and parietal bone bosses
       c. Prominent malar eminences
       d. Depressed bridge of the nose
       e. Oblique appearance of the eyes
       f. Enlarged maxilla with upward protrusion of the lip and upper central incisors
D. Treatment
   1. Use of blood transfusions to maintain adequate hemoglobin levels
   2. Transfusions greatly increase the risk of hemosiderosis (excessive iron storage in various tissues of the body, especially the spleen, liver, lymph glands, heart, and pancreas) and hemochromatosis (excessive iron storage with resultant cellular damage)
   3. Iron-chelating agents such as deferoxamine (Desferal) are given to reduce iron storage
E. Nursing diagnoses based on assessment for children with β-thalassemia
   1. Activity intolerance related to generalized weakness
   2. Altered family processes related to situational crisis (child with a disability/serious illness)
   3. Fear related to
      a. Unfamiliar environment
      b. Separation from support system

4. Anticipatory grieving related to perceived potential loss of child
5. Potential for infection and trauma related to
   a. Weakened bones
   b. Anemia
6. Body image disturbance related to
   a. Retarded growth and maturation
   b. Limited activity tolerance
   c. Chronic illness
7. See Nursing diagnoses for the toddler with health problems and for the family of child with a disability
F. Nursing care
   1. Be alert for signs and symptoms in older infants or young children of Mediterranean descent (Italian, Greek, Syrian)
   2. Prevent infection
      a. Avoid contact with persons who have infections
      b. Administer prophylactic antibiotics
   3. Prevent complications
      a. Carry out careful observation during transfusion
      b. Administer chelating agents as ordered
      c. Administer folic acid
      d. Avoid activities that increase risk of fractures
      e. Observe for signs of cholecystitis in the adolescent
   4. Assist the child in coping with the disorder and its effects
      a. Explore the child's feelings about being different from other children
      b. Emphasize the child's abilities and focus on realistic endeavors
      c. Encourage quiet activities, creative efforts, and "thinking" games
      d. Emphasize good hygiene and grooming
      e. Encourage interaction with peers
      f. Help plan therapies and medical care so they do not interfere with the child's regular activities and social interaction
      g. Assist the child with vocational planning
      h. Introduce the child to other children who have adjusted well to this or a similar disorder
   5. Support the parents
      a. Explore feelings of guilt regarding the hereditary nature of the disease
      b. Emphasize the need for the child to lead as normal a life as possible
      c. Help the family deal with the potentially fatal nature of the disease
   6. Prevent the occurrence of β-thalassemia
      a. Refer for genetic counseling
      b. Reinforce and clarify counseling information
   7. See Nursing care for the family of a child with a disability
   8. See Nursing care for the toddler with health problems
   9. Evaluate client's response and revise plan as necessary

EMOTIONAL DISORDERS

For common emotional disorders of the toddler see Disorders usually first evident in infancy, childhood, or adolescence in Psychiatric Nursing

The Preschool-Age Child
GROWTH AND DEVELOPMENT
Developmental Timetable

A. Three years
  1. Physical
     a. Usual weight gain 1.8 to 2.7 kg (4 to 6 pounds)
     b. Usual height gain 7.5 cm (3 inches)
  2. Motor
     a. Jumps off bottom step
     b. Rides a tricycle using pedals
     c. Walks upstairs alternating feet
     d. Builds tower of 9 or 10 cubes
     e. Constructs three-block bridge
     f. Can unbutton front or side button
     g. Usually toilet trained at night
  3. Sensory: visual acuity 20/30
  4. Vocalization and socialization
     a. Vocabulary of about 900 words; uses 3- to 4-word sentences
     b. May have normal hesitation in speech pattern
     c. Uses plurals
     d. Begins to understand ideas of sharing and taking turns
  5. Mental abilities
     a. Beginning understanding of the past, present, future, or any aspect of time
     b. Stage of magical thinking
B. Four years
  1. Physical
     a. Height and weight increases are similar to previous year
     b. Length at birth is doubled
  2. Motor
     a. Skips and hops on one foot
     b. Walks up and down stairs like an adult
     c. Can button buttons and lace shoes
     d. Throws ball overhand
     e. Uses scissors to cut outline
  3. Vocalization and socialization
     a. Vocabulary of 1,500 words or more
     b. May have an imaginary companion
     c. Tends to be selfish and impatient, but takes pride in accomplishments
     d. Exaggerates, boasts, and tattles on others
  4. Mental abilities
     a. Unable to conserve matter
     b. Can repeat four numbers and is learning number concept
     c. Knows which is the longer of two lines
     d. Has poor space perception
C. Five years
  1. Physical: height and weight increases are similar to previous year
  2. Motor
     a. Gross motor abilities well developed
     b. Can balance on one foot for about 10 seconds
     c. Can jump rope, skip, and roller skate
     d. Can draw a picture of a person
     e. Prints first name and other words as learned
     f. Dresses and washes self
     g. May be able to tie shoelaces
  3. Sensory
     a. Minimal potential for amblyopia to develop
     b. Color recognition is well established
  4. Vocalization and socialization
     a. Vocabulary of about 2,100 words
     b. Talks constantly
     c. Asks meaning of new words
     d. Generally cooperative and sympathetic toward others
     e. Basic personality structure is well established
  5. Mental abilities (Piaget's phase of intuitive thought)
     a. Beginning understanding of time in terms of days as part of a week
     b. Beginning understanding of conservation of numbers
     c. Has not mastered the concept that parts equal a whole regardless of their appearance

PLAY (COOPERATIVE PLAY)

A. Loosely organized group play where membership changes readily and rules are absent
B. Through play, the child deals with reality, learns control of feelings, and expresses emotions more through words than through actions
C. Play is still physically oriented but is also imitative and imaginary
D. Increasing sharing and cooperation among preschool children, especially 5-year-olds
E. Suggested toys (same principles as discussed before)
  1. Puppets
  2. Additional dress-up clothes, dolls, house, furniture, small trucks, animals, etc.
  3. Painting sets, coloring books, paste, and cut-out sets
  4. Illustrated books
  5. Puzzles with large pieces and more shapes
  6. Tricycle, swing, slide, and other playground equipment

HEALTH PROBLEMS OF THE PRESCHOOLER
Hospitalization of the Preschooler

A. Reaction of the child
  1. Fears about body image are now greater than fear of separation
  2. The fears include
     a. Intrusive experiences: needles, thermometer, otoscope
     b. Punishment and rejection
     c. Pain
     d. Castration and mutilation
B. If possible parents can be helped to prepare the child beforehand, since increased cognitive and verbal ability makes explanations possible

NURSING PROCESS FOR THE PRESCHOOLER WITH HEALTH PROBLEMS
Probable Nursing Diagnoses Based on Assessment

A. Anxiety related to
  1. Strange environment
  2. Perception of impending event
  3. Anticipated discomfort
  4. Knowledge deficit

5. Discomfort
6. Difficulty breathing
7. Feelings of powerlessness
B. Pain, related to
1. Disease process
2. Interventions
C. Family coping: potential for growth related to successful parenting
D. Ineffective family coping: compromised related to situational crises
E. Ineffective individual coping related to situational crises
F. Diversional activity deficit related to
1. Lack of sensory stimulation
2. Frequent or prolonged hospitaliza tion
G. Altered family processes related to
1. Situational crisis
2. Knowledge deficit
3. Temporary family disorganization
4. Inadequate support system
H. Fear related to
1. Separation from support systems
2. Uncertain prognosis
3. Potential change in body
I. Parental role conflict related to
1. Sick child
2. Inability to care for child
J. Anticipatory grieving (parental) related to
1. Expected loss
2. Gravity of child's physical status
K. Impaired home maintenance management related to
1. Knowledge deficit
2. Inadequate support systems
L. Feeding, bathing/hygiene, dressing/grooming, toileting self-care deficit related to
1. Fatigue
2. Pain
3. Developmental level
4. Limitations of treatment modalities
M. Potential for injury related to
1. Use of specific therapies and appliances
2. Incapacity for self-protection
3. Immobility
N. Potential altered parenting related to
1. Separation
2. Skill deficit
3. Family stress
O. Sensory-perceptual alterations (tactile) related to protected environment
P. Potential impaired skin integrity related to immobility
Q. Sleep pattern disturbance related to
1. Excessive crying
2. Frequent assessment
3. Therapies
R. Spiritual distress (parental) related to
1. Inadequate support systems
2. Decisions regarding "right to life" conflicts
S. See Nursing diagnoses for the family of child with a disability

Nursing Care for Preschoolers with Health Problems

A. Begin preparing for hospitalization a few days before but not too early because of the child's poor concept of time
B. Clarify cause and effect because of the child's phenomenalistic thinking (in the child's mind, proximity of two events relates them to each other)
C. Explain routines of hospital admission but not all procedures at one time, since this would be overwhelming
D. Recognize play is an excellent medium for preparation (use dolls, puppets, make-believe equipment, dress-up doctor and nurse clothes)
E. Provide time for play as an outlet for fear, anger, and hostility, as well as a temporary escape from reality
F. Keep verbal explanation as simple as possible and always honest
G. Add details about procedures, drugs, surgery, and the like as the child's cognitive level and personal experiences increase
H. See nursing care under each disorder

CANCER

Leading cause of death related to illness in children; second only to accidents

Leukemia

A. The most common type of childhood cancer; prognosis is improving
B. Peak incidence: 2 to 6 years of age
C. Malignant neoplasm of blood-forming organs
D. In children, overproduction of immature leukocytes: blast-cell or stem-cell leukemia
1. Lymphocytic: about 85% of cases; better prognosis than for myelogenous
2. Myelogenous: about 10%; poorer prognosis
E. Symptoms: caused by overproduction of immature nonfunctional cells
1. Anemia: pallor, weakness, irritability
2. Infection: fever
3. Tendency toward bleeding: petechiae and bleeding into joints
4. Pain in joints caused by seepage of serous fluid
5. Tendency toward easy fracture of bones
6. Enlargement of spleen, liver, lymph glands
7. Abdominal pain and anorexia resulting in weight loss
8. Necrosis and bleeding of gums and other mucous membranes
9. Later symptoms: CNS involvement and frank hemorrhage
F. Treatment objectives
1. Induce remission by chemotherapy (see Pharmacology related to neoplastic disorders)
   a. Prednisone: steroid
   b. Vincristine: plant alkaloid
   c. Methotrexate: folic acid antagonist
   d. L-asparaginase: enzyme
   e. 6-mercaptopurine: purine antagonist
   f. Cyclophosphamide: alkylating agent
   g. Doxorubicin hydrochloride: cytotoxic antibiotic
2. Prevent CNS involvement by use of irradiation and intrathecal methotrexate, because leukemic cells invade the brain but most antileukemic drugs do not pass the blood-brain barrier
3. Transfusions to replace and provide needed blood factors such as red blood cells, platelets, and white cells

G. Nursing diagnoses based on assessment for children with cancer
1. Activity intolerance related to
   a. Anemia
   b. Reduced energy and fatigue
2. Constipation related to
   a. Medications
   b. Pain on defecation
3. Pain related to physiologic effect of neoplasia and treatment
4. Altered family processes related to situational crisis (child with life-threatening disease)
5. Anticipatory grieving related to perceived potential loss of child
6. Potential for infection related to
   a. Decreased immune response
   b. Use of chemotherapy
7. Potential for injury (including hemorrhage) related to
   a. Decreased strength and endurance
   b. Pain and discomfort
   c. Decreased platelets
8. Impaired physical mobility related to
   a. Decreased strength and endurance
   b. Pain and discomfort
   c. Neuromuscular impairment
9. Altered nutrition: less than body requirements related to loss of appetite
10. Body image disturbance related to
    a. Loss of hair
    b. Moon face
    c. Debilitation
11. Potential impaired skin integrity related to
    a. Immobility
    b. Administration of antimetabolites
    c. Disease process
12. See Nursing diagnoses for the preschooler with health problems and for the family of a child with a disability
H. Nursing care
1. Encourage adjustment to chronic illness; stress need for normal life-style
2. Deal with the child's idea of death: discussion should be appropriate to level of understanding
   a. Preschooler: concept that death is reversible; greatest fear is separation
   b. Child 6 to 9 years of age: concept that death is personified; a person actually comes and removes the child
   c. Child over 9 years of age: adult concept of death as irreversible and inevitable
3. Be alert for and attempt to support the child experiencing side effects of drugs
   a. Cytoxan: severe nausea, vomiting, cystitis, and alopecia
   b. Vincristine: constipation, alopecia, neurotoxicity
   c. Methotrexate: oral and rectal ulcers
4. Prevent infection by hand washing; avoid contact with people who have active infections, and crowded places
5. Handle the child carefully because of pain and hemorrhage; use analgesics for pain

6. Provide gentle oral hygiene; soft, bland foods; increased liquids
7. Provide for frequent rest periods, quiet play
8. See Nursing care for the family of a child with a disability
9. See Nursing care for the preschooler with health problems
10. Evaluate client's response and revise plan as necessary

Wilms' Tumor (Nephroblastoma)

A. Most frequent intraabdominal childhood tumor
B. Estimated occurrence 1 in 10,000 live births
C. Slightly higher prevalence in males
D. Peak incidence at 3 years of age
E. Increased occurrence in siblings and identical twins
F. Symptoms
1. Swelling or nontender mass in abdomen; confined to one side of midline
2. Symptoms associated with compression of neighboring organs or metastasis (lungs: cough, dyspnea, shortness of breath)
3. Hematuria occurs in less than 25%
4. Anemia possible secondary to hematuria
5. Hypertension
G. Treatment
1. Surgery: should be scheduled soon after confirmation of renal mass
   a. Tumor, kidney, and associated adrenal gland removed; precautions taken not to rupture the capsule of the tumor
   b. Contralateral kidney inspected
   c. Regional lymph nodes and organs inspected and biopsied; when indicated, they are removed
   d. When bilateral kidney involvement, partial nephrectomy is done on the less affected side
2. Radiation therapy: indicated for all children except those in stage I with favorable histology
3. Chemotherapy
   a. Indicated for all stages
   b. Drugs used include actinomycin D, vincristine, adriamycin
   c. Treatment continued for 6 to 15 months
4. Prognosis
   a. Stage I and II with localized tumor: 90% cure with multimodal therapy
   b. When metastasis present: 50% survival
H. Nursing diagnoses based on assessment for children with Wilms' tumor
1. Anxiety related to
   a. Fear of the unknown
   b. Strange environment
2. Altered family processes related to situational crisis (child with a serious illness)
3. Potential for infection related to
   a. Lowered body defenses
   b. Abdominal surgery
4. Potential for injury related to
   a. Presence of tumor cells
   b. Abdominal surgery
5. Altered nutrition: less than body requirements, related to loss of appetite

6. See Nursing diagnoses for the preschooler with health problems and for children with leukemia

I. Nursing care
1. Preoperative
   a. Handle and bathe carefully to prevent trauma to the abdomen, which may result in rupture of the tumor capsule
   b. Place sign over bed: "Do not palpate abdomen"
   c. Prepare parents and child for large size of incision and drainage
   d. Monitor blood pressure
   e. Begin teaching family about chemotherapy and radiation therapy
2. Postoperative
   a. Monitor BP carefully
   b. Monitor intake and output to assess function of remaining kidney
   c. Encourage child to turn, cough, and deep breathe to prevent pulmonary complications
   d. Teach parents to identify untoward reactions from chemotherapy and radiation therapy
3. See Nursing care for the family of a child with a disability
4. See Nursing care for the preschooler with health problems
5. See Nursing care for the child with leukemia
6. Evaluate client's response and revise plan as necessary

NEPHROSIS (MINIMAL CHANGE NEPHROTIC SYNDROME)

A. Pathology: abnormal, increased permeability of the glomerular basement membrane to plasma albumin
B. Cause unknown: theories include
   1. Hypersensitivity
   2. Antigen-antibody response (rationale for the use of glucocorticoids and other immunosuppressive drugs)
C. Peak incidence: 2 to 7 years of age
D. Symptoms
   1. Generalized dependent edema, especially genital, periorbital, and abdominal (ascites)
   2. Proteinuria
   3. Hypoproteinemia: poor general health, loss of appetite
   4. Hyperlipemia
   5. May also see symptoms usually associated with nephritis
      a. Hematuria
      b. Hypertension
E. Nursing diagnoses based on assessment for children with nephrosis
   1. Potential activity intolerance
      a. Bed rest
      b. Fatigue
   2. Diversional activity deficit related to
      a. Activity intolerance
      b. Hospitalization
   3. Altered family processes related to situational crisis (child with a serious illness)
   4. Potential fluid volume deficit related to protein and fluid loss

5. Potential for infection related to
   a. Presence of infective organisms
   b. Lowered body defenses
6. Altered nutrition: less than body requirements related to loss of appetite
7. Body image disturbance related to change in appearance
8. Potential impaired skin integrity related to
   a. Edema
   b. Lowered body defenses
9. See Nursing diagnoses for the preschooler with health problems and for the family of a child with a disability

F. Nursing care
1. Infection: both disease state and drug therapy increase susceptibility
   a. Protect the child from others who are ill
   b. Teach parents the signs of impending infection and encourage them to seek medical care
2. Malnutrition caused by loss of protein and poor appetite
   a. Provide regular diet; discourage the use of salt and salty foods
   b. Encourage the child to select foods from high-protein choices
   c. Restrict fluids if ordered
3. Respiratory difficulty caused by ascites
   a. Place in a Fowler's position to decrease pressure against the diaphragm
   b. Monitor vital signs
4. Discomfort caused by edema, pressure areas
   a. Provide some relief by positioning and giving skin care
   b. Support the genitalia if edematous
5. Change in body image caused by edema and steroids
   a. Recognize that this becomes a greater problem as the child gets older
   b. Emphasize clothes, hairdo, etc. that make the child attractive
   c. Stress that "diets" will not help weight loss
6. Behavioral changes such as irritability and depression
   a. Help parents understand that mood swings are influenced by physical condition
   b. Encourage the child to participate in own care
   c. Encourage diversionary activities that provide satisfaction
7. See Nursing care for the family of a child with a disability
8. See Nursing care for the preschooler with health problems
9. Evaluate client's response and revise plan as necessary

URINARY TRACT INFECTION

A. Very common in females because of anatomy of the lower urinary tract: urethra is short and meatus is close to the anus
B. Symptoms
   See Cystitis in Medical-Surgical Nursing

C. Nursing diagnoses based on assessment for children with urinary tract infections
 1. Altered patterns of urinary elimination related to infectious process
 2. Potential for infection related to
  a. Presence of infective organisms
  b. Chemical characteristics of the genitourinary tract
 3. See Nursing diagnoses for the preschooler with health problems
D. Nursing care (teach prevention)
 1. Cleanse genitalia (front to back)
 2. Void when necessary as opposed to holding urine in bladder
 3. Increase fluids, particularly those that acidify urine
 4. Identify asymptomatic infections
 5. See Nursing care for the family of a child with a disability, if a chronic problem
 6. See Nursing care for the preschooler with health problems
 7. Evaluate client's response and revise plan as necessary

ALLERGY

A. Altered tissue response to a substance that has been inhaled or ingested or that has contacted the skin
B. Most common types in children
 1. Eczema
 2. Asthma
C. General considerations
 1. Family history can be a significant factor
 2. Comprehensive study of the child and environment essential
  a. Prepare the child for skin tests
  b. Study the environment in terms of emotional stresses as well as physical allergens
 3. Teach the parents to eliminate allergenic substances and to administer drugs properly

Eczema

See Eczema under Infant with health problems

Asthma

A. Pathology
 1. Spasms of bronchi and bronchioles
 2. Edema of mucous membranes
 3. Increased secretions
 4. Respiratory acidosis from buildup of carbon dioxide
B. Symptoms
 1. Wheezing, especially on expiration
 2. Labored breathing, cough, increased secretions
 3. Flaring nares, distended neck veins
C. Treatment for respiratory allergies
 1. Bronchodilators
  a. Theophyllines
   (1) Drugs
    (a) Aminophylline
    (b) Theophylline
   (2) Actions
    (a) Act directly on the bronchial smooth muscle to decrease spasm, relax smooth muscle of the vasculature

 (b) Direct stimulatory effect on the myocardium increases cardiac output, which improves blood flow to kidneys
 (c) Direct action on the renal tubules provides diuretic effect by increasing excretion of sodium and chloride ions
   (3) Adverse effects: oral forms cause gastric irritation
  b. Epinephrine hydrochloride: drug of choice in respiratory emergency, such as status asthmaticus
   (1) Actions
    (a) Effect is on the beta-adrenergic receptors in the bronchi; relaxes smooth muscle and increases respiratory volume
    (b) Inhalants cause vasoconstriction, which reduces congestion or edema
   (2) Adverse effects: cardiac palpitation; overuse of inhalants may cause "congestive rebound"
  c. Isoproterenol hydrochloride (Isuprel hydrochloride, Proternol)
   (1) Action: similar to that of theophyllines
   (2) Adverse effects: action at cardiovascular beta receptors causes tachycardia, peripheral blood vessel dilation (hypotension)
  d. Metaproterenol (Alupent, Metaprel)
  e. Terbutaline (Bricanyl): little effect on cardiac tissue
  f. Cromolyn sodium (Aarane, Intal): acts primarily by preventing release of mediators of type I allergic reactions (histamine, slow-reacting substance of anaphylaxis) from sensitized mast cells; prophylactic use by inhaling capsule contents lessens bronchoconstriction
  g. Adverse effects common to bronchodilator group: anxiety, nervousness, tremors, nausea, vomiting, headache, dizziness
 2. Expectorants: increase the production of thinner, less viscid secretions that protect bronchial tissues
  a. Drugs
   (1) Calcium iodide
   (2) Glyceryl guaiacolate (Robitussin)
   (3) Iodinated glycerol (Organidin)
   (4) Potassium iodide (Enkide)
  b. Act to raise the osmolality of bronchial glandular secretions, causing fluids to move to dilute the secretions
  c. Adverse effects: nausea, skin eruptions; long-term use of iodides may cause iodism (inflammation of respiratory tract tissues, skin eruptions, accumulation of fluid in nasal passages, lungs, eyelids)
 3. Corticosteroids
  a. Antiinflammatory effect diminishes the inflammatory component of asthma and reduces airway obstruction
  b. Used in status asthmaticus; however, less often for long-term control because of side effects
D. Nursing diagnoses based on assessment for children with asthma
 1. Activity intolerance related to imbalance between oxygen supply and demand

2. Ineffective airway clearance related to
   a. Hyperventilation
   b. Fatigue
3. Ineffective breathing pattern related to
   a. Bronchiolar edema
   b. Increased mucus secretions
   c. Bronchiolar constriction
4. Diversional activity deficit related to
   a. Frequent hospitalization
   b. Allergen-free environment
5. Altered family processes related to situational crisis (illness of child)
6. Fear related to
   a. Hospitalization
   b. Difficult breathing
7. Potential fluid volume deficit related to
   a. Difficulty swallowing
   b. Increased loss through respiratory tract
8. Potential for suffocation related to interaction between individual and environmental allergen
9. Body image disturbance related to perception of physiologic changes
10. Sleep pattern disturbance related to
    a. Illness
    b. Separation
11. Social isolation related to
    a. Hospitalization
    b. Confinement to home
12. See Nursing diagnoses for the preschooler with health problems and for the family of a child with a disability

E. Nursing care
1. Recognize that cumulation of drug can occur unless dosage is regulated
2. Administer parenteral drugs slowly over a 4- to 5-minute period to avoid peripheral vasodilation (hypotension, facial flushing), cerebral vascular constriction (headache, dizziness), cardiac palpitation, and precordial pain
3. Teach parents how to give antispasmodic drugs and bronchodilators and why they must be given even if child does not have an attack
4. Teach parents postural drainage, need for increased fluids, and the use of a cool mist humidifier to provide high humidity in home to promote good respiratory hygiene
5. Improve ventilating capacity
   a. Position in a high-Fowler's, leaning slightly forward
   b. Teach breathing exercises and controlled breathing
6. Teach parents that a controlled environment can limit attacks
   a. Keep environment as allergen free as possible
   b. Avoid exertion, exposure to cold air, and people with infections
   c. Avoid as much as possible emotional factors that precipitate attacks
7. See Nursing care for the family of a child with a disability
8. See Nursing care for the preschooler with health problems
9. Evaluate client's response and revise plan as necessary

MUCOCUTANEOUS LYMPH NODE SYNDROME (KAWASAKI DISEASE)

A. Acute febrile illness of unknown etiology; the principal area of involvement is the cardiovascular system, with extensive perivasculitis of arterioles, venules, and capillaries, including the coronary arteries; panvasculitis and perivasculitis of the main coronary arteries may result in stenosis or obstruction with aneurysm formation, pericarditis, interstitial myocarditis and endocarditis, and phlebitis of the larger veins
B. Symptoms
1. Fever for 5 or more days
2. Bilateral congestion of the ocular conjunctiva without exudation
3. Changes of the mucous membranes of the oral cavity, such as erythema, dryness, and fissuring of the lips, oropharyngeal reddening, or "strawberry tongue"
4. Changes in the extremities, such as peripheral edema, peripheral erythema and desquamation of the palms and soles, particularly periungual peeling
5. Polymorphous rash, primarily of the trunk
6. Cervical lymphadenopathy
7. Other signs, including diarrhea, photophobia, tympanitis, and arthralgia and arthritis, especially involving the larger joints such as elbows, wrists, knees, and ankles
C. Treatment: primarily supportive and directed toward controlling fever, preventing dehydration, and minimizing possible cardiac complications
1. Large doses of aspirin
2. Intravenous gamma globulin
3. Monitoring the cardiac status
D. Nursing diagnoses for children with Kawasaki disease
1. Anxiety related to concern for child's prognosis
2. Potential impaired skin integrity related to
   a. Edema
   b. Desquamation
3. Pain related to disease process
4. See Nursing diagnoses for the preschooler with health problems and for the family of a child with a disability
E. Nursing care
1. Administer aspirin to control fever; assess for early signs of toxicity
2. Provide optimal nutrition
3. Administer analgesics for joint pain if needed in addition to aspirin
4. Monitor for any signs of heart disease, especially arrhythmias
5. See Nursing care for the family of a child with a disability
6. See Nursing care for the preschooler with health problems
7. Evaluate client's response and revise plan as necessary

TONSILLECTOMY AND ADENOIDECTOMY

Not done routinely, since lymphoid tissue helps prevent invasion of organisms
A. Indications for surgical removal
1. Recurrent tonsillitis or otitis media
2. Enlargement that interferes with breathing or swallowing

B. Contraindications for removal
1. Occasional infections that clear up rapidly
2. Cleft palate, hemophilia, or debilitating disease such as leukemia
C. Complications after surgery
1. Hemorrhage: first 24 hours
   a. Frequent swallowing, bright red blood in the vomitus
   b. Restlessness
   c. Increased pulse rate, pallor
2. Hemorrhage from sloughing of tissue: 5 to 10 days postoperative
D. Nursing diagnoses based on assessment for children undergoing a tonsillectomy and adenoidectomy
1. Ineffective airway clearance related to discomfort when swallowing and coughing
2. Pain related to surgical incision
3. Altered family processes related to situational crisis
4. Fear related to
   a. Discomfort
   b. Unfamiliar surroundings
   c. Separation from support people
5. Potential fluid volume deficit related to
   a. NPO prior to surgery
   b. Reluctance to swallow
6. Knowledge deficit related to unfamiliar routine and environment
7. Potential altered nutrition: less than body requirements, related to difficulty when swallowing
8. See Nursing diagnoses for the preschooler with health problems
E. Nursing care
1. Keep the child on the abdomen or side with head turned to the side
2. After surgery give child cool liquids, not red in color and not thick or mucus-producing
3. Ask the child to talk; provide assurance that it is possible
4. Apply ice collar to decrease edema
5. Administer analgesics as necessary for comfort
6. See Nursing care for the preschooler with health problems
7. Evaluate client's response and revise plan as necessary

EMOTIONAL DISORDERS

For common emotional disorders of the preschooler see Disorders usually first evident in infancy, childhood, or adolescence in Psychiatric Nursing

The School-Age Child
GROWTH AND DEVELOPMENT
Developmental Timetable

A. Physical growth
1. Permanent dentition, beginning with 6-year molars and central incisors at 7 or 8 years of age
2. Tends to look lanky because bone development precedes muscular development
   a. Six years: height and weight gain slower, 5 cm (2 inches) and 2 to 3 kg (4½ to 6½ pounds)
   b. Seven years: continues to grow, 5 cm (2 inches) and 2.5 kg (5½ pounds) a year

   c. Eight to 9 years: continues to grow, 5 cm (2 inches) and 3 kg (6½ pounds) a year
   d. Ten to 12 years: slow growth in height compared to rapid weight gain, 6.25 cm (2½ inches) and 4.5 kg (10 pounds) a year; pubescent changes may begin to appear, especially in females
B. Motor
1. Refinement of coordination, balance, and control is ocurring
2. Motor development necessary for competitive activity becomes important
C. Sensory: visual acuity of 20/20
D. Mental abilities
1. Readiness for learning, especially in perceptual organization: names months of year, knows right from left, can tell time, can follow several directions at once
2. Acquires use of reason and understanding of rules
3. Trial-and-error problem solving becomes more conceptual rather than action oriented
4. Reasoning ability allows greater understanding and use of language
5. Concrete operations (Piaget): knows that quantity remains the same even though appearance differs

PLAY
Play Activities Vary with Age

A. Number of play activities decreases while the amount of time spent in one particular activity increases
B. Likes games with rules because of increased mental abilities
C. Likes games of athletic competition because of increased motor ability
D. Should learn how to work as well as play, with a beginning appreciation for economics and finances
E. In beginning of school years, boys and girls play together but gradually separate into sex-oriented type of activities
F. Suggested play for 6-to-9-year-olds
1. More housekeeping toys that work, doll accessories, paper doll sets, simple sewing machine, and needlework
2. Simple work and number games (i.e., calling for increased skills)
3. Physically active games such as hopscotch, jump rope, climbing trees
4. Collections and hobbies such as stamp collecting and building simple models
5. Bicycle riding
G. Suggested play for 9-to-12-year-olds
1. Handicrafts of all kinds
2. Model kits, collections, hobbies
3. Archery, dart games, chess, jigsaw puzzles
4. Sculpturing materials such as pottery clay
5. Science toys, magic sets

HEALTH PROBLEMS OF THE SCHOOL-AGE CHILD
Hospitalization of the School-Age Child

A. Reactions of the school-age child
1. Usually handles separation well but prefers parents to be near

2. Fears the unknown, especially when dependency or loss of control is expected; fears bodily harm, especially disfigurement
3. Possesses realistic concept of death by 9 to 10 years of age
4. Self-image about reaction to pain is important; may use avoidance to deal with physical discomfort
5. Wants to know scientific rationale for treatments and procedures

B. If possible parents can be helped to prepare the child beforehand, since increased cognitive and verbal ability makes explanations possible

NURSING PROCESS FOR THE SCHOOL-AGE CHILD WITH HEALTH PROBLEMS
Probable Nursing Diagnoses Based on Assessment

A. Anxiety related to
1. Strange environment
2. Perception of impending event
3. Anticipated discomfort
4. Knowledge deficit
5. Discomfort
6. Difficulty breathing
7. Feelings of powerlessness

B. Pain related to
1. Disease process
2. Interventions

C. Family coping: potential for growth related to successful parenting

D. Ineffective family coping: compromised related to situational crises

E. Ineffective individual coping related to situational crises

F. Diversional activity deficit related to
1. Lack of sensory stimulation
2. Frequent or prolonged hospitalization

G. Altered family processes related to
1. Situational crisis
2. Knowledge deficit
3. Temporary family disorganization
4. Inadequate support system

H. Fear related to
1. Separation from support systems
2. Uncertain prognosis
3. Potential change in body

I. Parental role conflict related to
1. Sick child
2. Inability to care for child

J. Anticipatory grieving (parental) related to
1. Expected loss
2. Gravity of child's physical status

K. Impaired home maintenance management related to
1. Knowledge deficit
2. Inadequate support systems

L. Feeding, bathing/hygiene, dressing/grooming, toileting self-care deficit related to
1. Fatigue
2. Pain
3. Developmental level
4. Limitations of treatment modalities

M. Potential for injury related to
1. Use of specific therapies and appliances
2. Incapacity for self-protection
3. Immobility

N. Potential altered parenting related to
1. Separation
2. Skill deficit
3. Family stress

O. Sensory-perceptual alterations (tactile) related to protected environment

P. Potential impaired skin integrity related to immobility

Q. Sleep pattern disturbance related to
1. Excessive crying
2. Frequent assessment
3. Therapies

R. Spiritual distress (parental) related to
1. Inadequate support systems
2. Decisions regarding "right to life" conflicts

S. See Nursing diagnoses for the family of child with a disability

Nursing Care for the School-Age Child with Health Problems

A. Begin preparing child for hospitalization before admission if possible

B. Explain diagnostic modalities and treatments at level of child's understanding

C. Involve child and parents in planning care

D. Provide time for play as an outlet for fear, anger, and hostility, as well as a temporary escape from reality

E. Keep verbal explanation as simple as possible and always honest

F. Add details about procedures, drugs, surgery, and the like as the child's cognitive level and personal experiences increase

G. Encourage and allow child to express feelings, emotions, and fears

H. Provide for tutoring if absence from school is prolonged

I. Encourage visits from siblings and peers and the formation of new peer relationships

J. Recognize that although play is diversional, this age group enjoys games with challenge and skill

K. Allow dependency but foster independence as much as possible

L. See Nursing care under each disorder

DIABETES MELLITUS

A. Peak incidence in the school-age group
1. Around 6 years of age
2. Around 12 years of age

B. Differences in diabetes in children and adults
1. Onset
   a. Rapid in children
   b. Insidious in adults
2. Obesity
   a. Not a factor in children
   b. Predisposing factor in adults
3. Dietary treatment
   a. Rarely adequate for children
   b. May be beneficial for some adults

4. Oral hypoglycemics
   a. Contraindicated for children
   b. May be beneficial for some adults
5. Insulin
   a. Almost universally necessary in children
   b. May be beneficial for some adults
6. Hypoglycemia and ketoacidosis
   a. Quite frequent in children
   b. More uncommon in adults
7. Degenerative vascular changes
   a. Develop after adolescence in children
   b. May be present at the time of diagnosis in adults

C. Symptoms: juvenile onset diabetes is always type I insulin-dependent diabetes mellitus (IDDM); not the same disease process as type II non-insulin-dependent diabetes mellitus (NIDDM)
1. Onset: rapid, obvious
2. Child usually thin, underweight
3. Increased thirst, fluid intake, appetite, and urinary output
4. Hyperglycemia: ketoacidosis or diabetic coma
   a. Causes
      (1) Decreased insulin
      (2) Emotional stress
      (3) Fever
      (4) Infection
      (5) Increased food intake
   b. Symptoms
      (1) Weakness, drowsiness
      (2) Lack of appetite, thirst
      (3) Abdominal and/or generalized pain
      (4) Acetone breath
      (5) Late signs: Kussmaul breathing (deep, rapid respirations), cherry red lips, loss of consciousness, death
5. Hypoglycemia: insulin therapy related
   a. Causes
      (1) Overdose of insulin
      (2) Decreased food intake
      (3) Excessive physical exercise: increases muscle activity and movement of glucose into muscle cells
   b. Symptoms
      (1) Sweating, flushing, pallor
      (2) Numbness, trembling, chilliness
      (3) Unsteadiness, nervousness, irritability
      (4) Hunger
      (5) Hallucinations
      (6) Late signs: convulsions, coma, death

D. Treatment
1. Control calorie, carbohydrate, fat, and protein intake
2. Insulin (see Pharmacology related to the endocrine system)
3. Exercise
4. Hyperglycemia: hospitalization with administration of fluids and insulin
5. Hypoglycemia: immediate supply of readily available glucose followed by a complex carbohydrate or protein

E. Nursing diagnoses based on assessment for children with diabetes mellitus
1. Diversional activity deficit related to hospitalization
2. Altered family processes related to situational crisis (child with a chronic illness)
3. Potential fluid volume deficit related to increased urine output
4. Potential for injury related to
   a. Dehydration
   b. Frequent injections
   c. Disease process
5. Body image disturbance related to perceived body changes (insulin dependence)
6. Self-esteem disturbance related to
   a. Need to restrict diet
   b. Need for insulin injections
   c. Feeling of being different from peers
7. Altered nutrition: less than body requirements, related to altered ability/inability to utilize nutrients
8. Potential for infection related to disease process
9. Knowledge deficit (diabetic management) related to newly diagnosed diabetes
10. Powerlessness related to diagnosis of chronic illness
11. See Nursing diagnoses for the school-age child with health problems and for the family of child with a disability

F. Nursing care: main objective is control of diabetes and education of child and family
1. Explain the differences between childhood and adult-onset diabetes to parents, who may think the child is faking because their own illness does not cause serious problems
2. Teach factors that affect insulin requirements and signs of insulin overdose and diabetic coma
   a. Give family a written list explaining symptoms
   b. Emphasize that skim milk can be given if insulin reaction is suspected but that insulin should *not be* increased if diabetic coma is developing
   c. Emphasize the need for close medical supervision
3. Teach need for prevention of infection
   a. Good skin care, frequent baths
   b. Properly fitting shoes
   c. Prompt treatment of any small cut
   d. Protection from undue exposure to illness
4. Encourage well-balanced diet, with fairly equal quantities of food eaten frequently and regularly, usually unrestricted within reason
5. Help plan exercise and adjust food and insulin to meet child's requirements
6. Teach child how to do blood glucose and urine testing to increase independence
7. Teach child how to administer insulin (by injection or pump)
   a. The child should be taught as early as motor and mental ability allows, usually by 7 or 9 years of age
   b. Explanations should be simple; diagrams for rotating sites should be used
   c. Periodic observation by an adult should be routine to discover faulty or careless technique

8. See Nursing care for the family of a child with a disability
9. See Nursing care of the school-age child with health problems
10. Evaluate client's response and revise plan as necessary

HEMOPHILIA

A. Defects in clotting mechanism of blood: two most common deficiencies
   1. Factor VIII, classic hemophilia
   2. Factor IX, Christmas disease
B. Hereditary influence: X-linked gene, classically occurring in males
C. Symptoms
   1. Prolonged bleeding from any wound
   2. Bleeding into the joints (hemarthrosis), resulting in pain, deformity, and retarded growth
   3. Anemia
   4. Intracranial hemorrhage
D. Treatment
   1. Control of bleeding
   2. Prevention of bleeding with use of factor replacement
      a. Drugs that replace deficient coagulation factors
         (1) Antihemophilic factor
            (a) Obtained from human sources
            (b) Provides concentrated factor VIII
         (2) Antihemophilic plasma
         (3) Factor IX complex contains factors II, VII, IX, X (concentrated)
      b. Adjunctive measures
         (1) Episilon-aminocaproic acid (Amicar): inhibits the enzyme that destroys formed fibrin and increases fibrinogen activity in clot formation
         (2) Fibrinogen: maintains plasma fibrinogen levels required for clotting materials
         (3) Thrombin: supplies physiologic levels of natural material at superficial bleeding sites to control bleeding
E. Nursing diagnoses based on assessment for children with hemophilia
   1. Diversional activity deficit related to activity limitations
   2. Altered family processes related to situational crisis (child with a chronic illness)
   3. Potential for injury (hemorrhage) related to disease process
   4. Knowledge deficit related to
      a. Disease process
      b. Home management
      c. Activity limitations
   5. Body image disturbance related to
      a. Perception of self as different
      b. Inability to participate in selected activities
   6. See Nursing diagnoses for the school-age child with health problems and for the family of child with a disability

F. Nursing care: objective now is to strive for home care, with self-administration of coagulation factors such as factor VIII
   1. Instruct the child and parents in the treatment of bleeding, especially of joints
      a. Immobilization of the area
      b. Compression of the area
      c. Elevation of the body part
      d. Application of cool compresses
   2. Provide for appropriate activity that lessens the chance of trauma, which is often difficult since boys are so physically active
   3. Select safe toys and inform parents to safe-proof house to minimize injuries; secure throw rugs
   4. Avoid use of aspirin or ibuprofen
   5. Control joint pain so the child uses extremities to prevent muscle atrophy
   6. Provide counseling, since disease is genetic and parents need assistance
   7. Encourage parents to treat the child as normally as possible, avoiding overprotection or overpermissiveness
   8. See Nursing care for the family of a child with a disability
   9. See Nursing care of the school-age child with health problems
   10. Evaluate client's response and revise plan as necessary

RHEUMATIC FEVER

A. Collagen disease: characterized by damage to connective tissue and usually blood vessels
B. Cause unknown: frequently follows infection with group A beta-hemolytic streptococci
C. Symptoms
   1. Heart: mitral and aortic stenosis may occur
   2. Joints: edema, inflammations and effusion especially in knees, elbows, hips, shoulders, and wrists
   3. Skin: erythematous macule with a clear center and wavy demarcated border usually on trunk and proximal extremities
   4. Neurologic: chorea
   5. Low-grade fever, epistaxis, abdominal pain, arthralgia, weakness, fatigue, pallor, anorexia, and weight loss
D. Treatment: antibiotics to eradicate organism and prevent recurrence
E. Nursing diagnoses based on assessment for children with rheumatic fever
   1. Potential for injury related to autoimmune response
   2. Decreased cardiac output related to disease process
   3. Altered nutrition: less than body requirements related to
      a. Anorexia
      b. Fatigue
   4. Potential for impaired skin integrity related to disease process
   5. Impaired physical mobility related to joint pain
   6. Pain related to inflammation of joints
   7. Fatigue related to decreased cardiac output
   8. Activity intolerance related to decreased cardiac output

9. Diversional activity deficit related to long-term illness
10. Altered growth and development related to disease process
11. Body image disturbance related to disease process
12. See Nursing diagnoses for the school-age child with health problems and for the family of child with a disability

F. Nursing care
1. Encourage bed rest to reduce work load of the heart
2. Encourage child to do schoolwork and keep up with class
3. Stimulate the development of quiet hobbies and collections
4. Gradually increase activities over a period of weeks to months
5. Handle painful joints carefully
6. Maintain proper body alignment to prevent deformities
7. Monitor need for pain medication and administer when necessary
8. Encourage an increased intake of nutritious fluids
9. Provide small, frequent, nutritious meals
10. Prevent invalidism by emphasizing abilities rather than limitations
11. Maintain child's status in home and school by keeping channels of communication open during illness
12. Help parents with home problems that may have served as predisposing factors
13. See Nursing care for the family of a child with a disability
14. See Nursing care of the school-age child with health problems
15. Evaluate client's response and revise plan as necessary

JUVENILE RHEUMATOID ARTHRITIS

A. Collagen disease, cause unknown, may occur in response to stress
B. Two peak ages of onset 2 to 5 and 9 to 11 years of age
C. Symptoms
1. Joint enlargement
   a. Stiffness, pain, and limited motion, especially in morning on awakening
   b. Spindle-fingers: thick proximal joint with slender tip
2. Low-grade fever
3. Erythematous rash on the trunk and extremities
4. Weight loss, fatigue, weakness
5. Tachycardia
6. Enlargement of the spleen, liver, and lymph nodes
D. Treatment
1. Salicylates: used in large doses for antiinflammatory properties
   a. Adverse effects: gastric irritation, salicylism with long-term use (visual disturbances, tinnitus, dizziness, mental confusion, diaphoresis, nausea, vomiting, intense thirst)
   b. Drug interactions
      (1) Salicylates have an intrinsic hypoglycemic effect and require a decrease in the dosage of

oral hypoglycemics for diabetics (they displace sulfonylurea hypoglycemics from protein-binding sites, which causes a greater hypoglycemic effect)
      (2) Salicylates decrease absorption of indomethacin from the intestinal tract and lower its effective circulating level
      (3) Salicylates antagonize the effect of sulfinpyrazone and probenecid in reducing serum uric acid levels by inhibiting tubular excretion of uric acid
      (4) Salicylates have a hypoprothrombinemic action and potentiate the effect of oral anticoagulants primarily by inhibiting platelet aggregation
2. Other nonsteroidal antiinflammatory drugs
3. Steroids
4. Physical therapy
E. Nursing diagnoses based on assessment for children with juvenile rheumatoid arthritis
1. Impaired physical mobility related to pain
2. Pain related to musculoskeletal impairment
3. Diversional activity deficit related to
   a. Pain
   b. Decreased mobility
4. Altered family processes related to situational crisis (child with a chronic illness)
5. Potential for injury related to
   a. Impaired mobility
   b. Musculoskeletal impairment
6. Altered nutrition: potential for more than body requirements, related to decreased mobility
7. Feeding, bathing/hygiene, dressing/grooming, toileting self-care deficit related to
   a. Pain
   b. Musculoskeletal impairment
8. Body image disturbance related to
   a. Perception of self as different
   b. Inability to participate in selected activities
9. See Nursing diagnoses for the school-age child with health problems and for the family of child with a disability
F. Nursing care
1. Emphasize that medication must be taken regularly, even in periods of remission, to decrease inflammation and pain
2. Promote proper body alignment and provide passive range of motion
3. Encourage a warm bath in the morning to decrease stiffness and increase mobility
4. Encourage exercises such as swimming
5. Encourage parents to accept the child's illness but to limit the use of the disease to foster dependency or control relationships
6. Teach the family why aspirin is given in large dosages and why other medications are not used
7. Encourage use of enteric-coated aspirin if there is GI irritability
8. Observe for signs of aspirin toxicity as demonstrated by tinnitus, vertigo, nausea, vomiting, sweating, and other signs of salicylate poisoning

9. See Nursing care for the family of a child with a disability
10. See Nursing care of the school-age child with health problems
11. Evaluate client's response and revise plan as necessary

SKIN INFECTIONS
Nursing Process for Children with Skin Infections
Nursing Diagnoses Based on Assessment

A. Pain related to skin lesions
B. Altered family processes related to situational crisis (child with a skin disorder)
C. Infection related to impairment of skin integrity
D. Body image disturbance related to perceived appearance
E. Impaired skin integrity related to
   1. Somatic factors
   2. Environmental agents
F. Potential impaired skin integrity related to
   1. Mechanical trauma
   2. Depressed defense mechanisms
G. Sleep pattern disturbance related to discomfort from skin lesions
H. Social isolation related to self-concept disturbance
I. See Nursing diagnoses for the school-age child with health problems

Nursing Care for Children with Skin Infections

A. Keep nails short to prevent injury from scratching
B. Administer medications to limit pruritus
C. Encourage daily bathing with tepid water; dry thoroughly
D. Prevent spread of infection to other members of the family
   1. Prevent direct contact between children
   2. Keep oozing lesions covered
   3. Prevent athlete's foot; do not walk barefooted, dry feet carefully, wear lightweight shoes to decrease heat, disinfect shoes and socks
E. Teach proper hair care
F. Encourage frequent bathing and change of clothes
G. Encourage completion of the full regimen of antimicrobial medication
H. Avoid use of strong alkalis such as bleach in clothes washing
I. Keep area clean and dry, rinse wastes from skin
J. Expose area to light and air
K. Apply bland ointment at night
L. Encourage screening in schools to identify the source of infection
M. See Nursing care of the school-age child with health problems
N. Evaluate client's response and revise plan as necessary

Pediculosis (lice)

A. May infest the hair on the head, body, pubic area
B. Nits (grayish white oval eggs) attach to hair
C. Severe itching may lead to secondary infection
D. Treatment: special shampoo, use of a fine-toothed comb to remove nits

Scabies

A. Produced by itch mite
B. Female burrows under the skin to lay eggs (usually in folds of skin)
C. Intensely pruritic: scratching can lead to secondary infection with the development of papules and vesicles
D. Treatment: all members of the family must be treated, since it is highly contagious
   1. Must wear clean clothes
   2. Must wash with sulfur or other special soap

Ringworm (fungal disease)

A. Scalp (tinea capitis)
   1. Reddened, oval or round areas of alopecia
   2. Treated topically or orally with an antifungal drug such as griseofulvin
   3. Head should be covered to prevent spread of infection
B. Feet (athlete's foot, tinea pedis)
   1. Scaly fissures between toes, vesicles on sides of feet, pruritus
   2. Particularly common in summer; contracted in swimming areas and gymnasium locker rooms
C. Treatment: griseofulvin, micronized (Fulvicin-U/F, Grifulvin V, Grisactin)
   1. Acts as an analog of purine and is incorporated into new epithelial cells during synthesis of nucleic acids
   2. Adverse effects: peripheral neuritis, vertigo, fever, dryness of mouth, arthralgia, mild transient urticaria, nausea, diarrhea, headache (may disappear as therapy continues), drowsiness, fatigue

Intertrigo

A. Excoriation of any adjacent body surfaces
B. Caused by moisture and chafing

Impetigo

A. Bacterial infection of skin by streptococci or staphylococci
B. Highly contagious; other areas of body frequently become infected
C. Treatment: antibiotics systemically and locally; isolate child; keep from scratching other areas of the body

REYE'S SYNDROME

A. Acute encephalopathy with fatty degeneration of the liver
B. Cause unknown although there appears to be a relationship with antecedent viral infection and administration of aspirin
C. Symptoms: prodromal symptoms include malaise, cough, rhinorrhea, or sore throat, followed by worsening cerebral signs as seen in the clinical stages:
   1. Stage I: Vomiting, lethargy, drowsiness
   2. Stage II: Disorientation, delirium, aggressiveness and combativeness, central neurologic hyperventilation (or sometimes shallow breathing), hyperactive reflexes, and stupor
   3. Stage III: Obtundence, coma, hyperventilation, cerebral decortication

4. Stage IV: Deepening coma, decerebrate rigidity, loss of ocular reflexes, large fixed pupils, divergent eye movements
5. Stage V: Seizures, loss of deep tendon reflexes, flaccidity, respiratory arrest

D. Treatment: determined by the clinical stage of the disease
  1. Stage I treatment is primarily supportive and directed toward restoring blood sugar levels, controlling cerebral edema, correcting acid-base imbalances, and eliminating factors known to increase intracranial pressure
  2. Stages II through V require invasive support, intracranial pressure monitoring and tracheal intubation with controlled ventilation; a radical approach is curarization and sedation

E. Nursing diagnoses based on assessment for children with Reye's syndrome
  1. Fear (parental) related to sudden critical nature of illness
  2. Potential for aspiration related to
    a. Vomiting
    b. Decreased level of consciousness
  3. Potential for injury related to
    a. Disorientation
    b. Delirium
    c. Impaired coagulation
  4. Potential fluid volume deficit related to intractable vomiting
  5. Sensory/perceptual alteration (all) related to cerebral edema
  6. Altered breathing pattern related to increased intracranial pressure
  7. Altered family processes related to situational crisis (acute illness of child)
  8. Parental role conflict related to sudden illness of child
  9. See Nursing diagnoses for the school-age child with health problems

F. Nursing care
  1. Assess vital signs and neurologic status continuously
  2. Assist with numerous invasive procedures
  3. Explain all therapies to the child (if alert) and parents
  4. Monitor intake and output and invasive equipment (intracranial line, central venous pressure)
  5. Keep parents informed of child's progress
  6. Include parents in child's care whenever possible
  7. Support the family, who will be frightened by the sudden and critical nature of the illness
  8. Foster dissemination of information concerning the role of aspirin in relation to viral disease and the development of Reye's syndrome
  9. See Nursing care of the school-age child with health problems
  10. Evaluate client's response and revise plan as necessary

LEGG-CALVÉ-PERTHES DISEASE (COXA PLANA)

A. A disturbance of circulation to the femoral capital epiphysis producing an ischemic aseptic necrosis of the femoral head, epiphysis, and acetabulum

B. Cause unknown
C. Symptoms
  1. Persistent pain in the affected hip(s)
  2. Limitation of movement in the affected hip(s)
  3. Limp
D. Treatment
  1. Aim is to keep the head of the femur in the acetabulum and maintain a full range of motion
  2. Conservative therapy must be continued for 2 to 4 years, whereas surgical correction returns the child to normal activities in 3 to 4 months
  3. Use of non-weight-bearing devices such as an abduction brace, leg casts, or a leather harness sling that prevents weight bearing on the affected limb
  4. Use of abduction-ambulation braces or casts after a period of bed rest and traction
  5. Surgical reconstructive and containment procedures

E. Nursing diagnoses based on assessment for children with Legg-Calvé-Perthes disease
  1. Potential for injury related to
    a. Musculoskeletal impairment
    b. Unaccustomed use of appliance
  2. Impaired physical mobility related to
    a. Pain
    b. Use of non-weight-bearing devices
  3. Body image disturbance related to
    a. Perception of self as different
    b. Inability to participate in selected activities
  4. Diversional activity deficit related to impaired mobility
  5. Altered family processes related to situational crisis (child with a temporary but extensive disability)
  6. See Nursing diagnoses for the school-age child with health problems and for the family of child with a disability

F. Nursing care
  1. Instruct the child and parents regarding what constitutes non-weight-bearing (e.g., no standing or kneeling on the affected leg)
  2. Educate the child and parents regarding correct use of appliances
  3. Assist the child and family in selecting activities according to the child's age, interests, and physical limitations
    a. Quiet games
    b. Hobbies such as collections, model building, crafts, indoor gardening
  4. Encourage peer interaction
  5. Involve the child in planning activities and therapy
  6. Help the child determine alternatives to weight-bearing activity (e.g., scorekeeping, sideline "coach")
  7. Help the child devise explanations for appliances and the inability to participate actively with peers
  8. See Nursing care for the family of a child with a disability
  9. See Nursing care of the school-age child with health problems
  10. Evaluate client's response and revise plan as necessary

EMOTIONAL DISORDERS

For common emotional disorders of the school-age child see Disorders usually first evident in infancy, childhood, or adolescence in Psychiatric Nursing

The Adolescent
GROWTH AND DEVELOPMENT
Developmental Timetable

A. Physical growth: includes the physical changes associated with puberty such as secondary sexual characteristics
B. Pubertal growth spurt
   1. Females between 10 and 14
      a. Weight gain 7 to 25 kg (15 to 55 pounds), mean 17.5 kg (38 pounds)
      b. Approximately 95% of mature height achieved by the onset of menarche or skeletal age of 13 years; height gain 5 to 25 cm (2 to 10 inches), mean 20.5 cm (8¼ inches)
   2. Males between 12 and 16 years
      a. Weight gain 7 to 30 kg (15 to 65 pounds), mean 23.7 kg (52 pounds)
      b. Approximately 95% of mature height achieved by skeletal age of 15 years; height gain 10 to 30 cm (4 to 12 inches), mean 27.5 cm (11 inches)
C. Mental abilities
   1. Abstract thinking
      a. New level of social communication and understanding
         (1) Can comprehend satire and double meanings
         (2) Can say one thing and mean another
      b. Can conceptualize thought; more interested in exploring ideas than facts
      c. Can appreciate scientific thinking, problem solve, and theoretically explore alternatives
   2. Perception
      a. Can appreciate nonrepresentational art
      b. Can understand that the whole is more than the sum of its parts
   3. Learning
      a. Much longer span of attention
      b. Learns through inference, intuition, and surmise, rather than repetition and imitation
      c. Enjoys regressing in terms of language development by using jargon to suit changing moods
D. Social patterns
   1. Peer group identity
      a. One of the strongest motivating forces of behavior
      b. Extremely important to be part of the group and like everyone else in every way
      c. Clique formation; usually based on common denominators such as race, social class, ethnic group, or special interests
   2. Interpersonal relationships
      a. Major goal is learning to form a close intimate relationship with the opposite sex
      b. Adolescents may develop crushes and worship many idols
      c. Time of sexual exploration and questioning of one's sexual role
   3. Independence
      a. By 15 or 16 years of age, adolescents feel they should be treated as adults
      b. Ambivalence: adolescent wants freedom but is not happy about corresponding responsibilities and frequently yearns for more care-free days of childhood
      c. Parental ambivalence and discipline problems are common as parents try to allow for increasing independence but continue to offer constructive guidance and enforce discipline

HEALTH PROMOTION DURING ADOLESCENCE
Adolescent Nutrition

A. Nutritional objectives
   1. Provide optimum nutritional support for demands of rapid growth and high energy expenditure
   2. Support development of good eating habits through variety of foods, regular pattern, good quality snacks (high in protein, low in refined carbohydrate, primarily sugar)
B. Nutrient needs increased in all respects, so adequate intake of all nutrients should form basis of diet
C. Possible nutritional problems
   1. Low intakes of calcium, vitamin A and C, iron in girls
   2. Anemia: increase foods containing iron
   3. Obesity or underweight: decrease or increase calories as needed
   4. Nutritional deficiencies related to
      a. Psychologic factors: food aversions, emotional problems
      b. Fear of overweight: crash diets, mainly in girls; cultural pressure
      c. Fad diets: caused by misinformation; need for sound counseling
      d. Poor choice of snack foods: usually high in sugar; use more fruit and protein forms
      e. Irregular eating pattern
   5. Additional stress of pregnancy: need high protein and calorie intake
D. Nutrition education may be made through association with teenagers' concerns about physical appearance, figure control, complexion, physical fitness, athletic ability

Injury Prevention

A. Appropriate education regarding sexual maturity, reproduction, and sexual behavior
B. Driver education
C. Education regarding use and abuse of drugs, especially alcohol
D. Education on health hazards associated with smoking

HEALTH PROBLEMS OF THE ADOLESCENT
Hospitalization of the Adolescent

A. Reaction of the adolescent
   1. Increased need for privacy, sense of control, and independence
   2. Increased concern for mutilation, disfigurement, and loss of function; needs to be like peers; body image important

3. Concerned about separation from peers and possible loss of status in group
B. Parents and medical/nursing team can help prepare the adolescent for hospitalization by providing full explanations and answering questions completely and honestly

NURSING PROCESS FOR ADOLESCENTS WITH HEALTH PROBLEMS
Probable Nursing Diagnoses Based on Assessment

A. Anxiety related to
   1. Strange environment
   2. Perception of impending event (specify)
   3. Separation from family/peer group
   4. Anticipated discomfort
   5. Knowledge deficit
   6. Feelings of powerlessness
B. Pain related to
   1. Disease process
   2. Interventions
C. Potential for aspiration related to
   1. Disease process
   2. Impaired swallowing
D. Family coping: potential for growth related to
   1. Successful parenting
   2. Resolution of situational crisis
E. Ineffective family coping: compromised related to situational crisis
F. Ineffective individual coping related to situational crisis
G. Parental role conflict related to
   1. Ill child
   2. Inability to care for child
H. Diversional activity deficit related to
   1. Frequent or prolonged hospitalization
   2. Separation from peer group
I. Altered family processes related to
   1. Situational crisis
   2. Knowledge deficit
   3. Temporary family disorganization
   4. Inadequate support system
J. Fear related to
   1. Separation from support system
   2. Uncertain prognosis
   3. Body image disturbance
K. Anticipatory grieving related to expected loss of life or limb or severity of illness
L. Impaired home maintenance management related to
   1. Knowledge deficit
   2. Inadequate support system
M. Potential for injury related to
   1. Use of specific therapies and appliances
   2. Incapacity for self-protection
   3. Immobility
N. Knowledge deficit related to new medical regimen
O. Potential noncompliance with therapy and health teaching related to
   1. Perceived invulnerability
   2. Denial of illness
   3. Desire not to be different from peers
P. Potential altered parenting related to
   1. Separation
   2. Skill deficit
   3. Family stress

Q. Body image disturbance related to
   1. Change in body characteristics
   2. Perceived developmental imperfections
R. Potential impaired skin integrity related to radiotherapy
S. Sleep pattern disturbance related to
   1. Frequent assessment
   2. Therapies
T. Spiritual distress related to
   1. Inadequate support system
   2. Decisions regarding "right to life" conflicts
U. See Nursing diagnoses for the family of a child with a disability

Nursing Care for Adolescents with Health Problems

A. Involve the adolescent in planning care
B. Answer questions honestly and directly
C. Be as open as possible concerning feelings, care, and prognosis
D. Foster independence as much as possible
E. Provide for contact with peers
F. Encourage compliance with health program
G. Arrange for continuity in school work
H. Recognize that problems of adolescence are magnified by an illness during this period of development
I. Encourage involvement of positive support systems
J. Accept the adolescent's self-appraisal but point out reality
K. Encourage use of clothing or makeup to minimize perceived shortcomings
L. See Nursing care under specific diseases in Pediatric Nursing, Medical-Surgical Nursing, Maternity Nursing, and Psychiatric Nursing
M. See Nursing care for the family of a child with a disability

COMMON PROBLEMS OF THE ADOLESCENT

A. Accidents: leading cause of death, with motor vehicle accidents causing the most fatalities
B. Homicide and suicide: next two causes of death among this age group
C. Drug abuse
D. Delinquency
E. Alcoholism
F. Pregnancy
G. Obesity
H. Acne
I. Anorexia nervosa and bulimia
J. Orthopetic problems
K. Cancer

SCOLIOSIS

A. Lateral curvature of the spine usually associated with a rotary deformity that eventually causes cosmetic and physiologic alterations in the spine, chest, and pelvis
B. Nonstructural scoliosis: curve is flexible and corrects by bending
C. Structural scoliosis: curve fails to straighten on side-bending; characterized by changes in the spine and its supporting structures

D. Cause in 70% of cases is "idiopathic"; probably transmitted as an autosomal dominant trait with incomplete penetrance
E. Symptoms
1. Prominence of one hip
2. Deformity of the rib cage
3. Prominence of one scapula
4. Difference in shoulder or scapular height
5. Curve in the vertebral spinous process alignment
6. Breasts appear unequal in size
7. Other clues
   a. Clothes do not fit right
   b. Skirt hems are uneven
F. Screening for scoliosis
1. Have the child stand erect, clothed only in underpants (and bra if older girl) and observe from behind; note asymmetry of the shoulders and hips
2. Have the child bend forward so the back is parallel with the floor; observe from the side, noting asymmetry or prominence of the rib
3. Diagnosis: confirmed by x-ray examination
G. Treatment: depending on severity of the curvature
1. Exercise can be used in nonstructural scoliosis
2. Mild to moderate curvature
   a. Milwaukee brace, an individually adapted steel and leather brace that extends from a chin cup and neck pads to the pelvis, where lumbar pads rest on the hips
      (1) Worn 23 hours a day
      (2) The child is gradually weaned from the brace over a 1- to 2-year period
      (3) Brace then worn only at night until the spine is mature
   b. Electrical stimulation to the convex side of the curvature may prevent progression of the scoliosis
3. More severe curves usually require surgery: techniques consist of spinal realignment and straightening by way of external or internal fixation and instrumentation combined with bony fusion (arthrodesis) of the realigned spine
   a. Harrington rods
   b. Lugue segmental instrumentation
   c. Dwyer instrumentation
4. Most severe scoliotic curvatures require traction devices and exercises for a time before spinal fusion to provide partial correction and more flexibility
H. Nursing diagnoses based on assessment for the adolescent with scoliosis
1. Altered family processes related to situational crisis (child with a structural defect)
2. Potential for injury related to use of supportive devices
3. Knowledge deficit related to disorder
4. Body image disturbance related to
   a. Perceived alteration in body structure
   b. Altered appearance when using supportive devices
5. Potential impaired skin integrity related to
   a. Presence of brace
   b. Use of electrical stimulation

6. Chronic low self-esteem related to perceived difference from peers
7. Impaired physical mobility related to use of supportive devices
8. Altered growth and development related to disease process
9. Pain related to medical/surgical therapies
10. See Nursing diagnoses for the adolescent with health problems and for the family of a child with a disability
I. Nursing care
1. Check spinal alignment as part of child assessment
2. Reinforce and clarify explanations provided by the orthopedist in regard to
   a. Appliance
   b. Plan of care
   c. Activities allowed or restricted
   d. Child's and parents' responsibilities in therapy
3. Examine skin surfaces in contact with the brace or electrical stimulator for signs of irritation; implement corrective action to treat or prevent skin breakdown
4. Help in selection of the appropriate wearing apparel to wear over the brace to minimize altered appearance and footwear to maintain proper balance
5. Prepare for surgery if required
6. See Nursing care for the family of a child with a disability
7. See Nursing care for the adolescent with health problems
8. Evaluate client's response and revise plan as necessary

BONE TUMORS

A. Osteogenic sarcoma
1. Most frequent bone tumor in children
2. Primary tumor site: diaphysis (shaft) of a long bone, especially the femur
3. Arises from osteoid tissue
B. Ewing's sarcoma
1. Most frequent sites: shaft of the long and trunk bones, especially the femur, tibia, fibula, humerus, ulna, vertebra, scapula, ribs, pelvic bones, and skull
2. Arises from medullary tissue (marrow)
C. Symptoms
1. Localized pain in the affected site
2. Limp
3. Voluntary curtailment of activity
4. Inability to hold heavy objects
5. Weight loss
6. Frequent infections
D. Diagnosis
1. X-ray examination
2. Computerized tomography (bone)
3. Bone scan
4. Bone marrow aspiration
5. Surgical biopsy (Ewing's sarcoma)
E. Treatment
1. Osteogenic sarcoma: amputation of the affected bone followed by high-dose methotrexate or pre-

operative and postoperative use of chemotherapy with en bloc resection of the primary tumor followed by a prosthetic replacement
   2. Ewing's sarcoma: intensive irradiation of the involved bone and chemotherapy
F. Nursing diagnoses based on assessment for the adolescent with a bone tumor
   1. Altered family processes related to
      a. Hospitalization
      b. Child with a life-threatening disease
   2. Fear related to knowledge deficit (surgical/medical care)
   3. Anticipatory grieving (parental) related to perceived loss of child
   4. Anticipatory grieving (adolescent) related to possible loss of limb
   5. Potential for injury related to tumor growth
   6. Impaired physical mobility related to amputated extremity
   7. Body image disturbance related to altered physical appearance following amputation and other therapies
   8. Potential impaired skin integrity related to radiation therapy and use of prosthesis
   9. Potential for infection related to surgery and other medical therapies
   10. Pain related to
      a. Disease process
      b. Medical therapies
   11. Decisional conflict related to variety of treatment modalities
   12. Ineffective individual coping related to medical/surgical interventions
   13. See Nursing diagnoses for the adolescent with health problems, for children with cancer, and for child with a disability
G. Nursing care
   1. Prepare the child and family for surgery
      a. Employ straightforward honesty
      b. Avoid disguising the diagnosis with terms such as "infection"
      c. Emphasize lack of alternatives if amputation is planned
      d. Answer questions regarding information presented by the surgeon and clarify any misconceptions
      e. Avoid overwhelming the child or parents with too much information
   2. Prepare the child and family for radiotherapy (Ewing's sarcoma)
      a. Explain the procedure
      b. Remain with the child during the procedure
      c. Explain the undesirable side effects of radiotherapy
      d. Suggest and/or implement measures to reduce the physical effects of radiotherapy, such as selecting loose-fitting clothing over the irradiated areas to decrease additional irritation, protection of the area from sunlight and sudden changes in temperature (avoid ice packs, heating pads)

   3. Prepare the child and family for chemotherapy
      a. Impress on the child the importance of therapy
      b. Explain the probable side effects of antimetabolites (e.g., nausea, hair loss)
   4. Assist the child in adjusting to his or her disability
      a. Assist the child in becoming adept at using the appliances
      b. Help the child select clothing to camouflage the prosthesis
      c. Encourage good hygiene, grooming, and sex-appropriate items to enhance appearance such as wig (for hair loss from antimetabolites), makeup, attractive (sex-appropriate) clothing
      d. Allow the child time and opportunity to go through the grief process
      e. Allow for expression of feelings regarding the loss and the undesirable effects of chemotherapy
      f. Help the child cope with the side effects of chemotherapy and irradiation
      g. Allow dependance but encourage independence
   5. Support the child and family
      a. Allow for expression of feelings
      b. Clarify misconceptions and provide technical information as needed
      c. Impress upon both child and family the need for continuing normal activities, interactions, and behaviors
   6. See Nursing care for the family of a child with a disability
   7. See Nursing care for the adolescent with health problems
   8. Evaluate client's response and revise plan as necessary

EMOTIONAL DISORDERS

For common emotional disorders of the adolescent see Disorders first evident in infancy, childhood, or adolescence in Psychiatric Nursing

OTHER HEALTH PROBLEMS

Many problems of adolescence are similar to those of adults; see specific areas in Maternity Nursing and Medical-Surgical Nursing for further discussion

Pediatric Nursing Review Questions

1. Play during infancy is:
   ① Initiated by the child
   ② A way of teaching how to share
   ③ More important than in later years
   ④ Mostly used for physical development
2. The primary task to be accomplished between 12 and 15 months of age is to learn to:
   ① Use a spoon
   ② Climb stairs
   ③ Walk
   ④ Say simple words

3. Preschool children role play. This is an important part of socialization, since it:
   ① Encourages expression
   ② Helps children think about careers
   ③ Teaches children about stereotypes
   ④ Provides guidelines for adult behavior

4. Learning processes associated with a particular stage of development often are referred to as "developmental tasks." A characteristic of developmental tasks is that:
   ① There is no uniform time for learning a task
   ② Tasks are learned at the same age in children
   ③ Tasks occur with predictable rhythm
   ④ Most development tasks are learned by school age

5. Parents can predispose their children to problems with nutrition by using food in early childhood as a means of:
   ① Socializing
   ② Reward and punishment
   ③ Acculturation
   ④ Teaching discipline

6. The major influence on eating habits of the *early* schoolage child is the:
   ① Example of parents at mealtime
   ② Food preferences of the peer group
   ③ Availability of food selections
   ④ Smell and appearance of food

7. Selection of drugs of choice for the treatment of pneumonia depends primarily on:
   ① Selectivity of the organism
   ② Tolerance of the client
   ③ Preference of the physician
   ④ Sensitivity of the organism

8. Mrs. Legere and her son Johnny are seen at the clinic. They both have severe upper respiratory tract infections, and the physician plans to prescribe tetracycline (Achromycin). The nurse reminds him that Johnny is 6 years old and that Mrs. Legere is in her eighteenth week of pregnancy. The data are important because the drug may cause:
   ① Persistent vomiting when given to small children and pregnant women
   ② Tooth enamel defects in children under 8 years of age and in the maturing fetus
   ③ Lower red blood cell production at times in their development when anemia is a common problem
   ④ Changes in the bone structure of young children and pregnant women

9. A viral infection characterized by red blotchy rash and Koplik's spots in the mouth is:
   ① Rubeola
   ② Rubella
   ③ Chickpox
   ④ Mumps

10. Under certain circumstances the virus that causes chickenpox can also cause:
    ① Athlete's foot
    ② Infectious hepatitis
    ③ Herpes zoster
    ④ German measles

11. Using live virus vaccines against measles is contraindicated in children receiving corticosteroids or antineoplastic or irradiation therapy because these children may:
    ① Have had the disease or have been immunized previously
    ② Be unlikely to need this protection during their shortened life span
    ③ Be allergic to rabbit serum, which is used as a basis for these vaccines
    ④ Be susceptible to infection because of their depressed immune response

12. An injection consisting of bacterial cells that have been modified is:
    ① A vaccine
    ② An antitoxin
    ③ A toxoid
    ④ A toxin

13. A child comes to the hospital after exposure to diphtheria and is given antitoxin. This type of immunity is known as:
    ① Active natural immunity
    ② Active artificial immunity
    ③ Passive natural immunity
    ④ Passive artificial immunity

14. Immunity by antibody formation during the course of a disease is:
    ① Active natural immunity
    ② Active artificial immunity
    ③ Passive natural immunity
    ④ Passive artificial immunity

15. A viral disease that begins with respiratory inflammation and skin rash and may result in grave complications is:
    ① Rubeola
    ② Rubella
    ③ Yellow fever
    ④ Chickenpox

16. Mary has received her primary immunizations, so her mother asks the nurse which ones she should receive prior to starting kindergarten. The nurse suggests the following booster doses:
    ① DTP, OPV
    ② Measles, DTP
    ③ OPV, rubella
    ④ DTP, tuberculin test

17. Occasionally infants are born without an immune system. They can live normally with no apparent problems during their first months after birth because:
    ① Limited antibodies are produced by the fetal thymus during the eighth and ninth months of gestation
    ② Antibodies are passively received from the mother through the placenta and milk
    ③ Limited antibodies are produced by the infant's colonic bacteria
    ④ Exposure to pathogens during this time can be limited

18. James, a 2-year-old child, is admitted to the hospital with a diagnosis of pneumonia. He is given antibiotics, forced fluids, and oxygen. James' temperature continues to rise until it reaches 103° F (39.4° C). The nurse calls the physician at the mother's request, but the physician sees no cause for alarm or change in treatment, even though James has a history of convulsions during previous periods of high fever. Although the nurse is concerned, she takes no further action. Later James has a convulsion that results in neurologic impairment of the left arm and leg. Legally:
    ① The nurse's actions did not derive from observations, client's history, or scientific fact
    ② The physician's decision takes precedence over the nurse's concern
    ③ High temperatures are common in children, and this situation presented little cause for undue concern
    ④ The physician is totally responsible for the client's health history and treatment regimen

19. Four-year-old Bobby has a seizure disorder and has been taking phenytoin (Dilantin) for 3 years. An important nursing measure for Bobby would be to:
    ① Offer the urinal frequently
    ② Administer scrupulous oral hygiene
    ③ Check for pupillary reaction
    ④ Observe for flushing of the face

20. When teaching parents at the school about communicable diseases, the nurse reminds them that these diseases are serious, and that encephalitis can be a complication of:
    ① Chickenpox
    ② Pertussis
    ③ Poliomyelitis
    ④ Scarlet fever

21. A viral disease caused by one of the smallest human viruses that infect the motor cells of the anterior horn of the spinal cord is:
    ① Rubeola
    ② Rubella
    ③ Poliomyelitis
    ④ Chickenpox

22. A *Streptococcus* infection characterized by swollen joints, fever, and the possibility of endocarditis and death is:
    ① Whooping cough
    ② Measles
    ③ Tetanus
    ④ Rheumatic fever

23. A skin infection that can be a sequela of a staphylococcal infection or glomerulonephritis is:
    ① Herpes simplex
    ② Scabies
    ③ Intertrigo
    ④ Impetigo

24. A small toddler is admitted to the hospital because of sudden hoarseness and an insistence on continuous and somewhat unintelligible speech. In talking with the mother, the nurse will be particularly concerned about:
    ① Acute respiratory tract infection
    ② Undetected laryngeal abnormality
    ③ Respiratory tract obstruction due to a foreign body
    ④ Retropharyngeal abscess

25. An infection caused by the yeast *Candida albicans* often occurring in infants and debilitated individuals is:
    ① Typhoid fever
    ② Thrush
    ③ Malta fever
    ④ Dysentery

26. A mother talks to the nurse about her sick infant and she is disturbed because she did not realize the baby was ill. A major indication of illness in an infant is:
    ① Longer periods of sleep
    ② Grunting and rapid respirations
    ③ Profuse perspiration
    ④ Desire for increased fluids during the feedings

27. Among the last signs of heart failure in the infant and child is:
    ① Rapid respiratory rate in the supine position
    ② Orthopnea
    ③ Tachypnea
    ④ Peripheral edema

28. A newborn of a few hours appears to be less cyanotic when he cries. The nurse should observe for:
    ① Twitching of the body resulting from neural damage
    ② Unequality of chest expansion associated with atelectasis
    ③ Alterations in heart rate associated with an atrioventricular septal defect
    ④ Sternal retractions of respiratory distress syndrome

29. A mother brings her week-old newborn to the clinic because he continually regurgitates. Chalasia is suspected. The nurse instructs the mother to:
    ① Keep the infant prone following feedings
    ② Not permit the infant to cry for prolonged periods
    ③ Keep the infant in a semisitting position, particularly after feedings
    ④ Administer a minimumn of 8 oz of formula at each feeding

30. The best legal definition of assault is:
    ① The application of force to another person without lawful justification
    ② Threats to do bodily harm to the person of another person
    ③ A legal wrong committed by one person against the property of another
    ④ A legal wrong committed against the public and punishable by law through the state and courts

31. In legal terminology, the term battery means:
    ① Doing something that a reasonable person with the same education or preparation would not do
    ② A legal wrong committed by one person against the property of another
    ③ The application of force to the person of another person without lawful justification
    ④ Maligning the character of an individual while threatening to do bodily harm

32. Dietary treatment of PKU includes a:
    ① Low-phenylalanine diet
    ② Phenylalanine-free diet
    ③ Dietary supplement for phenylalanine
    ④ Protein-free diet

33. Alan, age 3 months, has been diagnosed as having cretinism. If care is not instituted until after early infancy, he will probably:
    ① Have myxedema
    ② Be somewhat mentally retarded
    ③ Have abnormal deep tendon reflexes
    ④ Have thyrotoxicosis

34. Three-month-old Lisa is diagnosed as having cretinism. She is to receive thyroxine sodium, 0.35 mg, qd po. The medication is available in elixir form, 0.25 mg/ml. The nurse should administer:
    ① 0.8 ml
    ② 1.4 ml
    ③ 0.6 ml
    ④ 1.0 ml

35. Three-year-old Karen Allen may have celiac disease. One symptom common in children with celiac disease is stools that are:
    ① Large, frothy, dark green
    ② Small, pale, mucoid
    ③ Large, pale, foul smelling
    ④ Moderate, green, foul smelling

36. Mrs. Joyce asks the nurse how to tell the difference between measles (rubeola) and German measles (rubella). The nurse tells Mrs. Joyce that with rubeola the child has:
    ① A high fever and Koplik's spots
    ② Symptoms similar to a cold, followed by a rash
    ③ Nausea, vomiting, and abdominal cramps
    ④ A rash on the trunk with pruritus

37. The physician orders a tap water enema for 6-month-old Bart. The nurse considers that a tap water enema could:
    ① Cause a fluid and electrolyte imbalance
    ② Increase his fear of intrusive procedures
    ③ Result in shock from a sudden drop in temperature
    ④ Result in loss of necessary nutrients

38. Chickenpox can sometimes be fatal to children who are receiving:
    ① Antibiotics
    ② Steroids
    ③ Anticonvulsants
    ④ Insulin

39. The nurse explains to the parent group that the most important complication of mumps in postpubertal males is:
    ① Decrease in libido
    ② Hypopituitarism
    ③ Sterility
    ④ A decrease in androgens

40. Paula, a 3-year-old with eczema of the face and arms, has not heeded the nurse's warnings to "stop scratching—or else!" The nurse finds Paula scratching so intensely that her arms are bleeding. With great flurry, the nurse ties Paula's arms to the crib sides saying, "I'm going to teach you one way or another." In this situation, the nurse:
    ① Had to protect Paula's skin and acted as any reasonably prudent nurse would do
    ② Tried to explain to Paula and rightly expected her to understand and cooperate

③ Has used actions that can be interpreted as assault and battery
④ Has merely done her job with considerable accountability

41. Nancy, age 8, is receiving tetracycline (Achromycin). Her fever is down and secretions have lessened; but she is eating poorly, is withdrawn, lethargic, and irritable, and sobs readily. The nurse should promptly discuss the problem with the physician because:
    ① She needs a higher food intake to fight the infection
    ② Anemia is a frequent occurrence after infection and treatment with antibiotics
    ③ Concurrent bladder infection may be present as an extension of her gram-negative infection
    ④ Generalized physical symptoms and behavior problems may precede drug-induced liver damage

42. Fourteen-year-old Evelyn is severely hurt while on a skateboard and develops muscle contractures in all her limbs. She refuses to move, so the nurse should encourage her by:
    ① Explaining that some pain is inevitable
    ② Allowing friends to visit every day
    ③ Permitting her to make decisions regarding her care
    ④ Setting strict limits to increase her security

43. Nine-year-old Harold has a fractured femur and a full leg cast has just been applied. Which of the following observations made by the nurse should be reported to the physician immediately?
    ① Pedal pulse of 90
    ② Cast still damp and warm after 4 hours
    ③ Inability to move the toes
    ④ Increased urinary output

44. Two-year-old Jimmy swallowed kerosene from a soda bottle stored in the garage. Immediate treatment for ingestion of petroleum distillates is to have the child swallow:
    ① Milk of magnesia
    ② Strong tea
    ③ Weak salt solution
    ④ Mineral oil

45. A toddler has swallowed a liquid drain cleaner containing lye. The immediate intervention is to administer:
    ① Syrup of ipecac
    ② Two ounces of milk
    ③ Dilute vinegar solution
    ④ Sodium bicarbonate and water

46. Susan is found by her mother playing with an open bottle of diuretic tablets. The physician tells Susan's mother to give syrup of ipecac to Susan. The effect of the drug will be enhanced by:
    ① Resting until vomiting occurs
    ② Drinking 2 to 3 glasses of water
    ③ Actively playing until vomiting occurs
    ④ Stimulating the gag reflex

47. The primary reason for using prednisone in the treatment of acute leukemia in children is that it is able to:
    ① Suppress mitosis in lymphocytes
    ② Reduce irradiation edema
    ③ Decrease inflammation
    ④ Increase appetite and sense of well-being

48. A combination of drugs, which includes vincristine (Oncovin) and prednisone, is prescribed for a child with leukemia. Because of their toxicity the nurse should expect:
    1. Neurologic symptoms
    2. Irreversible alopecia
    3. Anemia and fever
    4. Gastrointestinal symptoms
49. Which of the following responses is unusual in infants subjected to prolonged hospitalization?
    1. Lack or slowness of weight gain
    2. Looking at ceiling lights rather than at persons caring for them
    3. Limited emotional response to stimuli
    4. Excessive crying and clinging when approached
50. A characteristic of infants and young children who have experienced maternal deprivation is:
    1. Extreme activity
    2. Proneness to illness
    3. Responsiveness to stimuli
    4. Tendency toward overeating
51. Naomi, 9 years old, is about to have surgery. The physician orders meperidine (Demerol), 20 mg, IM preoperatively. The container reads "50 mg/ml." The nurse should administer:
    1. 0.6 ml
    2. 0.4 ml
    3. 0.8 ml
    4. 1.0 ml
52. An infant scheduled for surgery is diagnosed as having a diaphragmatic hernia. Measures that the nurse would expect to be employed at this time include:
    1. Positive pressure oxygen by mask
    2. Positive pressure oxygen by endotracheal tube
    3. Increased oxygen concentration by any method
    4. Humidity of 40%
53. It is expected that, after some surgical intervention for atelectasis, lung expansion will recur within:
    1. 1 hour
    2. 48 to 72 hours
    3. 4 hours
    4. 12 to 48 hours
54. Dina, 18 months old, is to receive 5% dextrose and Ringer's lactate, 1000 ml IV, in 24 hours. The drop factor of the minidropper is 60 drops/ml. The nurse should regulate the IV to run at:
    1. 34 drops per minute
    2. 38 drops per minute
    3. 42 drops per minute
    4. 21 drops per minute
55. When picked up by either the mother or the nurse, an 8-month-old infant screams. The scream seems to be that of pain. At his clinic visit the nurse will note and talk particularly to the mother about:
    1. The infant's food and specific vitamins given to him, including vitamins C and D
    2. Accidents and injuries and the importance of their prevention
    3. Any other behavior of the infant that may have been noticed by the mother
    4. Limiting the play time and activities that this infant has with other children in the family

56. Eleven-year-old Harry has gained weight. His mother is concerned that Harry, who loves sports, may become obese. The nurse:
    1. Urges a decreased caloric intake
    2. Explains this is normal for a preadolescent
    3. Advises an increase in activity
    4. Discusses the relationship of genetics and weight gain
57. Exposure to hepatitis B may be expected to occur in hospitals because of:
    1. Needle sticks and mucous membrane exposure
    2. Careless handling of excreta by staff
    3. Newer treatments for hemophilia A
    4. Increasing use of ventilating systems
58. Elouise, 8 months old, has a gastrostomy tube and is given 240 ml of tube feeding q4h. One of the primary nursing responsibilities at the time of the feeding is to:
    1. Elevate the tube 30 cm (12 inches) above the mattress
    2. Give 10 ml of normal saline before and after feeding
    3. Position on the right side after feeding
    4. Open the tube 1 hour before feeding
59. Prior to administering a gastrostomy tube feeding to an infant, the nurse should:
    1. Slowly instill 5 ml of water
    2. Aspirate the tube
    3. Provide the baby with a pacifier
    4. Place in a semi-Fowler's position
60. Sal has been admitted to the hospital for surgery to correct his congenital megacolon. Enemas are ordered preoperatively to cleanse the bowel. The nurse should use:
    1. Soap suds
    2. Hypertonic phosphate
    3. Isotonic saline
    4. Tap water
61. If monocular strabismus is not corrected early enough:
    1. Vision in both eyes will be diminished
    2. Peripheral vision will disappear
    3. Dyslexia will develop
    4. Amblyopia develops in the weak eye

Situation: Mr. Crew, a nursing student, is doing therapeutic play with the children in the playroom of the well-baby clinic. To understand how to plan for children of various ages, he needs to have knowledge of their developmental norms. Questions 62 through 65 refer to this situation.

62. Mr. Crew observes that 2-year-old Mark:
    1. Builds houses with blocks
    2. Is very possessive of toys
    3. Attempts to stay within the lines when coloring
    4. Amuses himself with a picture book for 15 minutes
63. Mr. Crew observes 4-year-old Colin having difficulty playing with the other children. He understands that it is normal for Colin to:
    1. Exaggerate and boast to impress others
    2. Have fierce temper tantrums and negativism
    3. Engage in parallel or solitary play
    4. Be almost totally dependent on parents

64. Fifteen-month-old Nadia is playing in the playpen. Mr. Crew observes her activities and realizes that her physical tasks are within the norms when she is able to:
    ① Build a tower of six blocks
    ② Stand in the playpen holding onto the sides
    ③ Throw all the toys out of the playpen
    ④ Walk across the playpen with ease

65. Mr. Crew would encourage two 6-year-old boys in the playroom to play with:
    ① A board game
    ② An erector set
    ③ Checkers
    ④ Clay

Situation: Mr. and Mrs. Bee were emotionally upset when their baby girl Sue was born with a cleft palate and double cleft lip. Questions 66 through 70 refer to this situation.

66. To give the most support to the parents, the nurse should:
    ① Discourage them from talking about the baby
    ② Encourage them to express their worries and fears
    ③ Tell them not to worry because the defect can be repaired
    ④ Show them postoperative photographs of babies who had similar defects

67. The most critical factor in the immediate care of Sue after repair of the lip is:
    ① Maintenance of a patent airway
    ② Administration of drugs to reduce oral secretions
    ③ Administration of parenteral fluids
    ④ Prevention of vomiting

68. Additional nursing care for Sue after the surgical lip repair would include:
    ① Placing the infant in a semisitting position
    ② Keeping the infant from crying
    ③ Spoon feeding for the first 2 days after surgery
    ④ Keeping the baby NPO

69. At 2 years of age Sue returned for palate surgery. The most important factor in preparing her for this experience is:
    ① Her previous hospital visits
    ② Gratification of all her wishes
    ③ Never leaving her with strangers
    ④ Assurance of affection and security

70. A toothbrush would not be used on Sue immediately after palate surgery because:
    ① The suture line might be injured
    ② She was not accustomed to a brush at home
    ③ She probably has no teeth
    ④ It might be frightening to her

Situation: David, age 1 year, weighs 12.6 kg (28 pounds) but is pale and lethargic. His hemoglobin level is 5 g and he has an enlarged heart. When taking a nursing history from his mother, the nurse learns that he refuses food so she gives him a quart of milk per day from a bottle. Questions 71 through 77 refer to this situation.

71. The nurse suggests that his mother:
    ① Put a large hole in the nipple and put baby food in with his milk
    ② Take him to the metabolic clinic for a checkup
    ③ Immediately begin the weaning process
    ④ Give him finger foods such as raisins and chopped meat

72. David should have been started on solid foods by at least 5 or 6 months of age because:
    ① His fetal reserve of iron was depleted
    ② It would have taught him how to chew
    ③ His bone marrow activity had slacked off at this time
    ④ It would have helped control his weight

73. The most prevalent nutritional disorder among children in the United States is iron deficiency anemia. A major reason for this in young children is:
    ① Overfeeding of milk
    ② Lack of adequate iron reserves from the mother
    ③ Blood disorders
    ④ Introduction of solid foods too early for proper absorption

74. Anemia, a nutritional problem encountered in children and adults, involves several different nutrients. The nutrients include proteins, iron, vitamin B_{12} and:
    ① Carbohydrates
    ② Thiamine
    ③ Calcium
    ④ Folic acid

75. The food that the nurse would emphasize to David's mother as a source of iron to be included in his diet daily is:
    ① Orange juice
    ② Lamb
    ③ Mineral-fortified cereal
    ④ Milk

76. David's mother also states that he has eight teeth and asks when she should take him to the dentist. For dental prophylaxis, the nurse encourages her to take him:
    ① The next time another family member goes to the dentist
    ② Before starting school
    ③ Between 2 and 3 years of age
    ④ When he begins to lose his deciduous teeth

77. The nurse's background knowledge of the basic nutrients that act as partners in building red blood cells will form the basis for a teaching plan. These nutrient partners of iron are:
    ① Calcium and vitamins
    ② Carbohydrates and thiamine
    ③ Proteins and ascorbic acid
    ④ Vitamin D and riboflavin

Situation: Four-year-old Ann weighs 18 kg (40 pounds) and is in a private pediatric room on "gown, glove, and linen precautions." She was admitted for weight loss, anorexia, vaginitis, and insomnia. A diagnosis of pinworm infestation was made. Questions 78 through 82 refer to this situation.

78. The most effective time for the nurse to collect a cellophane tape test for pinworms is:
    ① At bedtime before bathing
    ② Just following a BM
    ③ Immediately after meals
    ④ Early morning before arising

79. Pinworms cause a number of symptoms besides anal itching. A rare sequela of pinworm infestation that the nurse should observe for is:
   ① Pneumonitis
   ② Stomatitis
   ③ Hepatitis
   ④ Appendicitis

80. Pyrvinium pamoate (Povan) is an effective single-dose drug to eliminate pinworms. How many milligrams will Ann receive if 5 mg per kilogram of body weight are ordered?
   ① 90 mg
   ② 18 mg
   ③ 40 mg
   ④ 200 mg

81. After administering pyrvinium pamoate (Povan) to Ann, it is important to alert the staff that a normal side effect of this drug is that it colors the stool or vomitus:
   ① Dark brown
   ② Light green
   ③ Bright red
   ④ Gentian blue

82. The nurse's decision to alert the staff is based on the knowledge that:
   ① Irritation by pinworms in the rectum may cause ulceration and bleeding
   ② The cyanine dye origin of the drug colors the stool
   ③ The stool contains hemoglobinlike metabolic products of disintegrating pinworms
   ④ The drug is irritating to the intestinal mucosa and may cause transient bleeding

Situation: Seven-year-old Johnny has been admitted for a tonsillectomy. Questions 83 through 85 refer to this situation.

83. An essential nursing action preoperatively is to:
   ① Encourage parent to stay until Johnny goes to the operating room
   ② Provide him with his favorite toy
   ③ Observe his ASO titer
   ④ Check for loose teeth and report to physician

84. The nurse suspects hemorrhage postoperatively when Johnny:
   ① Snores noisily
   ② Becomes pale
   ③ Complains of thirst
   ④ Swallows frequently

85. Johnny is complaining of pain in his throat. Which of the following medications for pain would be best for him at this time?
   ① Aspirin, 300 mg
   ② Tylenol, 300 mg
   ③ Phenobarbital, 15 mg
   ④ Demerol, 50 mg

Situation: Two-day-old Edward has a meningomyelocele. He is scheduled for surgery. Questions 86 through 88 refer to this situation.

86. Prior to the surgical correction, a primary nursing goal in caring for a child with a meningomyelocele is to:
   ① Observe for bowel and bladder dysfunction
   ② Prevent infection
   ③ Prevent skin breakdown
   ④ Observe for increasing paralysis

87. After closure of Edward's meningomyelocele, it is essential that his nursing care include:
   ① Decrease of environmental stimuli
   ② Strict limitation of leg movement
   ③ Measurement of head circumference daily
   ④ Observation of serous drainage from the nares

88. To meet a major developmental need of Edward's the nurse should:
   ① Provide a soft cuddly toy
   ② Give him a pacifier
   ③ Warm his formula before feeding
   ④ Put a mobile over his crib

Situation: Eight-year-old John Kee is being discharged following treatment for sickle cell crisis. He is allowed to return to school and resume normal activities. Questions 89 through 93 refer to this situation.

89. The nurse explains to Mrs. Kee that a very important aspect of care for John at home should include:
   ① At least 14 hours sleep per day
   ② Rigorous exercise and play
   ③ Ingestion of large quantities of liquids
   ④ High-calorie diet

90. Infants with sickle cell anemia may not be diagnosed as having this disorder because of:
   ① The presence of fetal hemoglobin during the first year of life
   ② Compensation of increased hematocrit and hemoglobin if well fed
   ③ Absence of respiratory disorders
   ④ General good health and an excellent growth curve

91. The sickling process of the red blood cell occurs in conditions of:
   ① Hemodilution
   ② Hypoxia
   ③ Thrombocytopenia
   ④ Hypocalcemia

92. To prevent thrombus formation in capillaries, as well as other problems from stasis and clotting of blood in the sickling process, the main nursing intervention is:
   ① Administration of oxygen
   ② Increasing fluids by mouth and a humidifier
   ③ Complete bed rest
   ④ Use of heparin or other anticoagulants

93. Common nursing care that helps prevent both sickle cell crisis and celiac crisis is:
   ① Limitation of activity
   ② Protection from infection
   ③ High-iron, low-fat, high-protein diet
   ④ Careful observation of all vital signs

Situation: Johnny Smith, 12 months of age, is brought to the pediatric health clinic for a regular physical assessment. Questions 94 through 98 refer to this situation.

94. In reviewing his immunizations for the past 10 months the nurse would expect him to have been immunized against:
   ① Measles, rubella, polio, tuberculosis, and pertussis
   ② Polio, pertussis, tetanus, and diphtheria
   ③ Measles, mumps, rubella, and tuberculosis
   ④ Pertussis, tetanus, polio, and measles

95. Mrs. Smith asks the nurse how the DTP injection works. The nurse, in formulating a response, recalls that in active immunity:
    ① Blood antigens are aided by phagocytes in defending the body against pathogens
    ② Protein antigens are formed in the blood to fight invading antibodies
    ③ Protein substances are formed by the body to destroy or neutralize antigens
    ④ Lipid agents are formed by the body against antigens
96. The measles immunization is usually routinely given after 15 months of age because of the:
    ① Increased hazard of side effects in infants
    ② Presence of maternal antibodies during the first year
    ③ Interference it causes with effectiveness of pertussis, diphtheria, and tetanus immunizations
    ④ Rare incidence of measles infection prior to 12 months of age
97. Infants receive immunizations made up of attenuated viruses. This means that these immunizations:
    ① Contain passive antibodies
    ② Contain active antibodies
    ③ Cause the development of passive antibodies
    ④ Cause the development of active antibodies
98. In terms of preventive teaching for a 1-year-old, the nurse would speak to Mrs. Smith about:
    ① Adequate nutrition
    ② Accidents
    ③ Sexual development
    ④ Toilet training

Situation: Nancy Hand, a 5-year-old only child, is admitted to the hospital with pneumonia. She requires bed rest, a soft diet, liberal fluid intake, and ampicillin, 250 mg, po qid. She is restless and fretful and tells the nurse she feels sick. Questions 99 through 104 refer to this situation.

99. The immediate priority in Nancy's nursing care is:
    ① Nutrition
    ② Rest
    ③ Exercise
    ④ Elimination
100. Nursing care likely to be most effective in alleviating Nancy's fretfulness is:
    ① Giving her a jigsaw puzzle
    ② Putting her in a room by herself
    ③ Letting her play with a doll
    ④ Reading a story to her
101. The best choice of between-meal nourishment for Nancy is:
    ① Fresh fruit
    ② Hard candy
    ③ Skim milk
    ④ Creamed soup
102. When the nurse brings her dinner tray Nancy says, "I'm too sick to feed myself." The nurse should respond:
    ① "Try to eat as much as you can."
    ② "Be a big girl and don't act like a baby."
    ③ "Let it go until you feel better."
    ④ "Wait 5 minutes and I will help you."

103. Nancy's statement is most likely indicative of:
    ① Immaturity
    ② Loneliness
    ③ Regression
    ④ Temper tantrum
104. Nancy is apathetic about eating. Nursing care directed toward supporting her nutrition should include:
    ① Providing diversional activity at mealtime
    ② Eliminating all between-meal nourishment
    ③ Asking her parents to visit at mealtime
    ④ Giving her only the foods she likes best

Situation: Mrs. Bronson is informed that her infant daughter has phenylketonuria (PKU). Questions 105 through 108 refer to this situation.

105. Which of the following statements is true concerning PKU?
    ① PKU is transmitted by an autosomal dominant gene
    ② The infant is tested for PKU immediately after delivery
    ③ If PKU is untreated, mental retardation occurs
    ④ Treatment for PKU includes life-long diet therapy
106. A test that was done on Baby Bronson in the nursery to detect PKU is:
    ① Guthrie blood test
    ② Ferric chloride urine test
    ③ Phenistix test
    ④ Clinitest serum phosphopyruvic acid
107. When teaching Mr. and Mrs. Bronson about their daughter's disorder, the nurse should state that:
    ① Phenylalanine is not necessary for growth
    ② Other amino acids can be increased to substitute for phenylalanine
    ③ A low-phenylalanine diet is required
    ④ Phenylalanine can be administered to correct the deficiency
108. In terms of dietary counseling, the parents need much help and support in adhering to specific regimens. A frequent question asked by parents is, "How long will my child have to be on this diet?" An appropriate response by the nurse is:
    ① "Unfortunately, this is a life-long problem and dietary management must always be maintained."
    ② "Usually, if the child does well for 1 year, she then can gradually begin eating regular foods."
    ③ "As of now, research shows that a child needs to be on this diet until she is about 6 to 8 years of age. Then she can gradually begin to eat other foods."
    ④ "No one knows, but why don't you discuss it with your doctor."

Situation: Mrs. Simmons brings 3-year-old Sam to the emergency room, indicating he has had a fever for several days, has held his neck rigid, and is now vomiting. While being examined he has a convulsion and is admitted to the pediatric unit. Questions 109 through 114 refer to this situation.

109. While instituting nursing measures to reduce Sam's fever, the nurse recognizes that an important consideration is to:
    ① Monitor vital signs every 10 minutes
    ② Force oral fluids
    ③ Measure output every hour
    ④ Limit exposure to prevent shivering

110. One morning, while Sam is in his crib, the nurse notes his jaws are clamped and he is having a seizure. The most important nursing responsibility at this time is to:
    ① Insert a padded tongue blade
    ② Start oxygen at 10 L by mask
    ③ Protect Sam from harm from the environment
    ④ Restrain Sam to prevent injury to soft tissue
111. Febrile convulsions are common in children and:
    ① Usually occur after the first year of life
    ② The cause is usually readily identified
    ③ May occur in minor illnesses
    ④ Occur more frequently in females than males
112. The physician orders acetaminophen 150 mg, po, q4h, prn for fever above 101° F (38° C). The nurse has on hand a bottle labeled "1 tablet equals 80 mg." The nurse should administer:
    ① ½ tablet
    ② 1 tablet
    ③ 1½ tablets
    ④ 2 tablets
113. Sam is diagnosed as having meningococcal meningitis. The nurse observes Sam for the:
    ① Identifying purpuric skin rash
    ② Continual tremors of the extremities
    ③ Low-grade nature of the fever
    ④ Palatal paralysis and glossitis
114. The most serious complication of meningitis in young children is:
    ① Hydrocephalus
    ② Blindness
    ③ Peripheral circulatory collapse
    ④ Epilepsy

Situation: Three-month-old Matt Quincy is admitted to the hospital with bile-stained vomitus and abdominal distention. Questions 115 through 118 refer to this situation.

115. The nurse should also observe for:
    ① Constant severe pain and absence of stools
    ② Bounding pulse and hypotonicity
    ③ Paroxysmal pain and grunting respirations
    ④ High-pitched cry and weak thready pulse
116. Prior to surgery for the intestinal obstruction, Matt is kept NPO and has a Levin tube in place. To calm Matt and also to meet his developmental needs best, the nurse should:
    ① Allow him to suck on a pacifier
    ② Hang a brightly colored mobile in his crib
    ③ Place him on his abdomen and permit him to crawl
    ④ Allow him to hold his favorite toy
117. Matt develops diarrhea postoperatively and is given IV fluids. The rate of flow must be observed often by the nurse to:
    ① Avoid IV infiltration
    ② Prevent increased output
    ③ Prevent cardiac embarrassment
    ④ Replace all fluids lost
118. When Mrs. Quincy returns to the surgical clinic for follow-up care, the nurse includes the following preventive suggestion in her teaching:
    ① Remove all tiny objects from the floor
    ② Keep crib rails up to the highest position
    ③ Cover electric outlets with safety plugs
    ④ Remove poisonous substances from low areas

Situation: Five-year-old Sam has been hospitalized with acute glomerulonephritis. Questions 119 through 122 refer to this situation.

119. The nurse observes Sam primarily for:
    ① Polyuria, high fever
    ② Dehydration, hematuria
    ③ Hypertension, circumocular edema
    ④ Oliguria, hypotension
120. When planning nursing care for Sam, the nurse realizes that he needs help in understanding his restrictions, one of which is:
    ① Bed rest for at least 4 weeks
    ② A bland diet high in protein
    ③ Daily doses of IM penicillin
    ④ Isolation from other children with infections
121. The average 5-year-old is incapable of:
    ① Making decisions
    ② Tying his shoelaces
    ③ Abstract thought
    ④ Hand-eye coordination
122. Sam loves to ride his bike, and his parents are very concerned about his activity when he returns home. The nurse bases the answer to them on the fact that after the urinary findings are nearly normal:
    ① He must remain in bed for 2 weeks
    ② Activity does not affect the course of the disease
    ③ He must not play active games
    ④ Activity must be limited for 1 month

Situation: Sue Green, a 2-year-old girl, is admitted to the pediatric unit with respiratory wheezing, dyspnea, and cyanosis. One of the tentative diagnoses is cystic fibrosis. Questions 123 through 129 refer to this situation.

123. Cystic fibrosis can predispose Sue to bronchitis mainly because:
    ① Tenacious secretions obstruct the bronchioles and respiratory tract and provide a favorable medium for growth of bacteria
    ② Increased salt content in saliva can irritate and necrose mucous membranes in nasopharynx
    ③ Neuromuscular irritability causes spasm and constriction of the bronchi
    ④ The associated heart defects of cystic fibrosis cause congestive heart failure and respiratory depression
124. The problem of cystic fibrosis is sometimes first noted by the nurse in the newborn nursery because of the infant's:
    ① Increased heart rate
    ② Abdominal distention
    ③ Excessive crying
    ④ Sternal retractions
125. Sue is small and underdeveloped for her age primarily because she:
    ① Ingested little food for several months because of poor appetite
    ② Was unable to absorb nutrients because of a lack of pancreatic enzymes

③ Secreted less than normal amounts of pituitary growth hormone

④ Developed muscular and bony atrophy from lack of motor activity

126. When caring for the child with cystic fibrosis the nurse should:
① Perform postural drainage
② Encourage active exercise
③ Prevent coughing
④ Provide small frequent feedings

127. The foul-smelling, frothy characteristic of the stool in cystic fibrosis results from the presence of large amounts of:
① Sodium and chloride
② Semidigested carbohydrates
③ Undigested fat
④ Lipase, trypsin, and amylase

128. Medications that will problably be used for Sue in her therapeutic regimen include:
① A steroid and an antimetabolite
② Antibiotics, a multivitamin preparation, and cough drops
③ Pancreatic enzymes and antibiotics
④ Aerosol mists, decongestants, and fat-soluble vitamins

129. In cystic fibrosis, frequent stools and tenacious mucus often produce:
① Intussusception
② Anal fissures
③ Meconium ileus
④ Rectal prolapse

Situation: Two-year-old Mike Cox is admitted to the hospital for the second surgical repair of his clubfoot. Mrs. Cox cannot stay overnight with her son, since visiting hours are restricted. On the morning after admission, Mike is standing in his crib crying. He refuses to be comforted and calls for his mother. Questions 130 through 133 refer to this situation.

130. The nurse approaches Mike to bathe him and he screams louder. This behavior is recognized as the stage of protest, and the nurse:
① Picks him up and walks with him around the room
② Sits by his crib and bathes him later when his anxiety decreases
③ Decides he really does not need a bath when he is this upset
④ Fills the basin with water and proceeds to bathe him

131. On the third postoperative day Mike begins to regress and lies quietly in his crib with his blanket. The nurse recognizes that Mike is in the stage of:
① Denial
② Mistrust
③ Rejection
④ Despair

132. During his second week of hospitalization, Mike smiles easily, goes to all the nurses happily, and does not express a great deal of interest in his mother when she visits. After leaving Mike's room, Mrs. Cox tells the nurse she is pleased that Mike is adjusting well but expresses some concern about his reactions to her. Before responding to Mrs. Cox, the nurse should understand Mike's behavior and realize that he:
① Is repressing his feelings for his mother
② Has established a routine and feels safe
③ Feels better physically so his behavior has improved
④ Has given up fighting and accepts the separation

133. The nurse explains the meaning of Mike's behavior to Mrs. Cox and tells her that after he goes home she should expect that:
① Mike will miss the nurses and hospital routine
② It will be easier for Mike to adjust to his home situation
③ Mike will continue his happy, normal behavior
④ It will take some time before the mother-child relationship is reestablished

Situation: Sara, 12 years old, was diagnosed at the orthopedic clinic as having idiopathic scoliosis. Proper exercising and avoidance of fatigue are essential components of Sara's care. Questions 134 through 136 refer to this situation.

134. Early in Sara's treatment the nurse can suggest which of the following sports as therapeutic?
① Bowling
② Swimming
③ Badminton
④ Golf

135. To assist her curvature correction, Sara is fitted with a Milwaukee brace. The nurse explains to Sara and her parents that the length of time the brace must be worn varies but it is usually worn until:
① Cessation of bone growth at the time of physical maturity
② The curvature of the spine is completely straightened
③ Pain on prolonged standing diminishes
④ The iliac crests are at equal levels

136. One of the earliest signs of sexual maturity in a young girl such as Sara is:
① Interest in the opposite sex
② Attention to grooming
③ An increase in the size of the breasts
④ The appearance of axillary and pubic hair

Situation: At 2 weeks of age Baby Williams begins to vomit after his feedings and is admitted to the hospital for observation with a tentative diagnosis of pyloric stenosis. Questions 137 through 141 refer to this situation.

137. The nurse should carefully observe him for:
① Signs of dehydration
② Coughing and gagging after feeding
③ Quality of cry
④ Quality of stool

138. When vomiting is uncontrolled in an infant, the nurse should observe for signs of:
① Tetany
② Alkalosis
③ Acidosis
④ Hyperactivity

139. The maintenance of fluid and electrolyte balance is more critical in children than in adults because:
    ① Renal function is immature in children below the age of 4
    ② Cellular metabolism is less stable than in adults
    ③ The proportion of water in the body is less than in adults
    ④ The daily fluid requirement per unit of body weight is greater than in adults

140. What is the most critical factor confronting the nurse in the administration of IV fluids to a small, dehydrated infant?
    ① Maintenance of the prescribed rate of flow
    ② Maintenance of the fluid at body temperature
    ③ Calculation of the total necessary intake
    ④ Assurance of sterility

141. Surgery is performed and Baby Williams' condition is stable. The nurse caring for him notices that his postoperative orders are similar to those for other infants having undergone such surgery and include:
    ① Withholding all feedings for the first 24 hours
    ② Additional glucose feedings after the first 24 hours
    ③ Thickened formula 24 hours after surgery
    ④ Diluted formula feeding 24 hours after surgery

Situation: Karen Vale, a 5-year-old girl, is admitted to the hospital 1 week before surgery for tetralogy of Fallot. Questions 142 through 146 refer to this situation.

142. The defects associated with this heart anomaly include:
    ① Right ventricular hypertrophy, atrial and ventricular defects, and mitral valve stenosis
    ② Right ventricular hypertrophy, ventricular septal defect, stenosis of pulmonary artery, and overriding aorta
    ③ Origin of the aorta from the right ventricle and of the pulmonary artery from the left ventricle
    ④ Abnormal connection between the pulmonary artery and the aorta, right ventricular hypertrophy, and atrial septal defects

143. A common finding in most children with cardiac anomalies is:
    ① Mental retardation
    ② Cyanosis and clubbing of fingertips
    ③ A family history of cardiac anomalies
    ④ Delayed physical growth

144. Karen is to receive digoxin (Lanoxin) elixir, 0.010 mg, po. Based on developmental norms for a 5-year-old, the nurse would withhold the medication and notify the physician if the apical rate is below:
    ① 60 beats per minute
    ② 80 beats per minute
    ③ 90 beats per minute
    ④ 100 beats per minute

145. Karen's laboratory analysis indicates a high red blood cell count. This polycythemia can best be understood as a compensatory mechanism for:
    ① Cardiomegaly
    ② Low iron level
    ③ Low BP
    ④ Tissue oxygen need

146. Karen undergoes heart surgery to repair the anomaly. Postoperatively it is essential that the nurse prevent:
    ① Constipation
    ② Unnecessary movement
    ③ Crying
    ④ Coughing

Situation: Johnny, a 15-year-old, is taken to the emergency room of the local hospital because he stepped on a nail. Questions 147 and 148 refer to this situation.

147. The puncture wound is cleansed and a sterile dressing applied. While doing these tasks, the nurse asks the mother if Johnny has been immunized against tetanus. The reply is affirmative. Penicillin is administered, and Johnny is sent home with instructions to return if there is any change in the wound area. A few days later, Johnny is admitted to the hospital with a diagnosis of tetanus. Legally:
    ① The possibility of tetanus could not have been foreseen, since he had been immunized
    ② The nurse's judgment was adequate in view of the client's symptoms
    ③ Assessment by the nurse was incomplete and the treatment was inadequate
    ④ Hospital protocol should govern treatment in emergency room care

148. After Johnny's admission, one of the most important aspects of nursing care should be directed toward:
    ① Maintaining body alignment
    ② Encouraging high intake of fluid
    ③ Carefully monitoring urinary output
    ④ Decreasing external stimuli

Situation: Three-day-old Patty is diagnosed as having congenital hip dysplasia. Questions 149 through 151 refer to this situation.

149. An early sign able to be observed by the nurse in the newborn nursery is:
    ① Limitation in adduction of the leg
    ② Shortening of the leg on the unaffected side
    ③ Depressed dance reflex
    ④ Asymmetry of the gluteal folds

150. At 3 months of age Patty has a spica cast applied from below the axilla to below the knee. To prevent a serious complication that often occurs in infants in a spica cast, the nurse teaches Patty's parents to:
    ① Seek immediate medical care if Patty develops a cough
    ② Limit movement to prevent cast damage
    ③ Change Patty's diapers frequently
    ④ Feed Patty a low-calorie diet

151. When elevating Patty's head, the nurse is aware that it is important to:
    ① Limit this position to 1 hour at a maximum
    ② Raise the entire mattress and spring at the head of the bed
    ③ Use at least two pillows under her shoulders
    ④ Place folded diapers at the edge of the cast

Situation: Working on a cardiac care unit, the nurse will care for many children with a variety of congenital anomalies. Questions 152 through 155 refer to this situation.

152. Meg, 2 years old, has a cyanotic congenital heart disease. The nurse would expect to observe:
① Edema in the extremities
② An elevated hematocrit
③ Absence of pedal pulses
④ Orthopnea

153. Baby boy Vics has been found to have a patent ductus arteriosus, which is:
① A narrowing of the pulmonary artery
② An abnormal opening between the right and left ventricles
③ A connection between the pulmonary artery and the aorta
④ An enlarged aorta and pulmonary artery

154. The nurse is caring for a child with an acyanotic heart disease. A major common symptom of acyanotic heart disease is:
① Polycythemia
② Clubbing of fingers and toes
③ Severe retarded growth
④ The presence of an audible heart murmur

155. Alma has coarctation of the aorta. When taking her vital signs, the nurse can expect to observe:
① Weak, thready radial pulses
② Higher BP in upper extremities
③ Bounding femoral pulses
④ Notching of the clavicle

Situation: Ten-year-old Jim Smith is admitted to the emergency room after a car accident. However, normal measures to stop his bleeding are unsuccessful, and, on further study, Jim is found to have a mild case of classic hemophilia. Mr. and Mrs. Smith are very concerned about this and wonder how it happened. Questions 156 through 158 refer to this situation.

156. In discussing hemophilia with Mr. and Mrs. Smith the nurse should explain that:
① Hemophilia is an X-linked disorder in which the mother is usually the carrier of the illness but is not affected by it
② Hemophilia is an autosomal dominant disorder in which the woman carries the trait
③ Hemophilia follows regular laws of Mendelian inherited disorders such as sickle cell anemia
④ This disorder can be carried by either male or female but occurs in the sex opposite that of the carrier

157. Jim's parents are very worried about their other children, two girls and another boy, and want to know what the chances are concerning their having the disorder or being a carrier. An appropriate answer to this question would be that:
① All the girls will be normal and the other son a carrier
② Each son has a 50% chance of being a victim and each daughter a 50% chance of being a carrier

③ All the girls will be carriers and one half the boys will be victims
④ Each son has a 50% chance of being either a victim or carrier, and the girls will all be carriers

158. The most common site of internal bleeding in hemophiliacs is the:
① Cerebrum
② Ends of the long bones
③ Intestines
④ Joints

Situation: Eight-year-old Cara has juvenile rheumatoid arthritis. Drug therapy includes the administration of sodium salicylate, 10 gr, 4 times daily. Questions 159 through 161 refer to this situation.

159. During the salicylate therapy the nurse should observe Cara for:
① Nausea, dizziness, edema, headache
② Gastric distress, nausea, vomiting, tinnitus
③ Constipation, deafness, nausea, headache
④ Diarrhea, gastric distress, edema of the face

160. Sodium salicylate is classified as an:
① Antibiotic and antipyretic
② Analgesic and antipyretic
③ Analgesic and sedative
④ Antipyretic and hypnotic

161. While Cara is in bed convalescing, she becomes very bored and irritable. The nurse plans activities that a school-age child would like and suggests she:
① Play chess
② Start a collection
③ Watch game shows on TV
④ Do arithmetic puzzles

Situation: Nellie, a newborn, is admitted to the pediatric unit with the diagnosis of choanal atresia. Questions 162 through 164 refer to this situation.

162. Choanal atresia is an anomaly located in the:
① Nasopharynx
② Intestinal tract
③ Pharynx and larynx
④ Anal area

163. While feeding Nellie, the nurse notices that she:
① Lacks a swallow reflex
② Chokes on her feeding
③ Does not appear to be hungry
④ Takes only about half of her feeding

164. When reviewing the data recorded on Nellie's chart, the information that might indicate to the nurse that the baby requires special attention would be:
① Birth weight of 3500 g
② 20 ml of milky-colored fluid aspirated from stomach
③ The infant has a positive Babinski reflex
④ The Apgar score at birth was 3

Situation: Three-year-old Roger is admitted to the pediatric unit with a diagnosis of nephrosis. Questions 165 through 168 refer to this situation.

165. The most important nursing intervention for Roger is:
① Encouraging fluids
② Regulating his diet
③ Maintaining bed rest
④ Preventing infection

166. As Roger gets older and has repeated attacks of nephrosis, it is most important for the nurse to help him develop:
    ① Fine muscle coordination
    ② Acceptance of possible sterility
    ③ A positive body image
    ④ The ability to test his own urine

167. During his nap, Roger wets the bed. The best approach by the nurse would be to:
    ① Change his clothes and make no issue of it
    ② Explain that big boys should try to call the nurse
    ③ Tell him to help with remaking the bed
    ④ Change his bed, putting a rubber sheet on it

168. When providing nursing care to a preschool-age child, the nurse should remember that his greatest fear is of:
    ① Isolation
    ② Intrusive procedures
    ③ Death
    ④ Pain

Situation: Mary is hospitalized with a severe asthma attack. Questions 169 through 172 refer to this situation.

169. The acid-base imbalance complicating this condition is:
    ① Respiratory alkalosis caused by the accelerated respirations and loss of carbon dioxide
    ② Respiratory acidosis caused by the impaired respirations and increased formation of carbonic acid
    ③ Metabolic acidosis caused by excessive production of acid metabolites
    ④ Metabolic acidosis caused by the kidneys' inability to help compensate for the increased carbonic acid formed

170. Mary is in a Croupette and is given prednisone, 15 mg, po bid. The nurse should:
    ① Check her eosinophil count daily
    ② Prevent exposure to infection
    ③ Keep Mary NPO except for medications
    ④ Have her rest as much as possible

171. Mary has IV therapy of 5% dextrose in 0.5 normal saline started. Aminophylline is to be given IV for 20 minutes every 8 hours. Before administering the drug, the nurse should:
    ① Check her temperature
    ② Monitor BP
    ③ Administer oxygen
    ④ Take her pulse

172. When Mary's parents take her home, they should be taught to increase her fluid intake and to have her:
    ① Avoid exertion and exposure to cold
    ② Stay in the house for at least 2 weeks
    ③ Increase her calorie intake
    ④ Avoid foods high in fat

Situation: Two-month-old Paul Carr is brought to the clinic, and a diagnosis of colic is made. Mrs. Carr appears exhausted. Questions 173 through 176 refer to this situation.

173. The nurse realizes that Mrs. Carr needs help coping with Paul and suggests that she:
    ① Provide Paul with warm sweetened tea when he begins to cry
    ② Arrange for some time away from Paul each day to rest

③ Sit comfortably in a quiet darkened room to hold Paul when he cries
    ④ Give Paul a warm bath to calm him down

174. The behavior of an infant with colic is usually suggestive of:
    ① Inadequate peristalsis resulting in constipation
    ② A protective mechanism designed to rid the GI tract of foreign proteins
    ③ Paroxysmal abdominal pain due to excessive gas
    ④ An allergic response to certain proteins in milk

175. Paul returns with his mother for his 6-month check-up. When teaching Mrs. Carr how to prevent accidents when caring for her 6-month-old, the nurse should emphasize that this age child can usually:
    ① Sit up
    ② Stand while holding onto furniture
    ③ Roll over
    ④ Crawl lengthy distances

176. When Mrs. Carr returns with Paul for his 9-month check-up, she expresses concern about his development. The baby no longer has the same strong grasp that he had shortly after birth, nor does he have a similar response to startle that he had at an early age. The nurse should discuss with Mrs. Carr that:
    ① Neurologic examination is desirable
    ② Failure of these responses may be related to mental retardation
    ③ These responses are usually replaced by voluntary activity at 5 to 6 months of age
    ④ The infant needs additional sensory stimulation to aid in the return of these responses

Situation: Loren, age 14, is admitted to the hospital and is scheduled to undergo orthopedic surgery the following day. Questions 177 through 180 refer to this situation.

177. At the conclusion of visiting hours, Loren's mother hands the nurse a bottle of capsules and says, "These are for Loren's allergy. Will you be sure she takes one about 9 o'clock?" The nurse might best respond:
    ① "One capsule at 9 PM? Of course, I will give it to her."
    ② "Did you ask the doctor if she should have this tonight?"
    ③ "I am certain the doctor knows about Loren's allergy."
    ④ "We will ask Loren's doctor to write an order so we can give this medication to her."

178. In relation to obtaining an informed consent, the nurse should remember that the adolescent:
    ① Does not have the legal capacity to give consent
    ② Is not able to make an acceptable or intelligent choice
    ③ Is able to give voluntary consent when parents are not available
    ④ Will most likely be unable to choose between alternatives when asked to consent

179. Postoperatively, Loren complains of pain and is given 15 mg of codeine sulfate as ordered q3 to 4h prn. Two hours after she is given this medication she complains of severe pain. The nurse should:
    ① Administer another dose of codeine within 30 minutes, since it is a relatively safe drug
    ② Tell Loren she cannot have additional medication for 1 more hour

③ Report that Loren has an apparent idiosyncrasy to codeine

④ Request that the physician evaluate Loren's need for additional medication

180. About 8 hours later, Loren complains of itching. A drug that can be ordered to relieve this symptom is:
① Chlorpheniramine (Chlor-Trimeton)
② Nitrofurazone (Furacin)
③ Salicylanilide (Salinidol)
④ Hyaluronidase (Alidase)

Situation: Two-year-old Sue McMichael fractures her femur and is placed in Bryant's traction. Questions 181 through 184 refer to this situation.

181. While caring for Sue, the nurse should know that Bryant's traction:
① Helps by allowing the child to turn side to side
② Is skin traction to the affected leg
③ Is skin traction and elevates the hips slightly from the bed
④ Is attached to a pin placed in the affected femur

182. Sue becomes constipated and the physician orders an isotonic enema. The nurse is aware that the maximum amount of fluid to be given a small child without a physician's specific order is:
① 100 to 150 ml
② 155 to 250 ml
③ 255 to 350 ml
④ 355 to 500 ml

183. One evening Sue screams and cries frequently, particularly after her mother's visit. Her loud crying disturbs others on the unit, and the nurse finds it impossible to quiet her. She is in a four-bed room, adjacent to which is a storeroom large enough to hold a crib. When her crying is particularly loud and prolonged, the nurse puts her crib in the storeroom and closes the door. She is left there until her crying ceases, a matter of 30 or 45 minutes. Legally:
① The other children had to be considered, so Sue needed to be removed
② Sue needed to have limits set to control her crying
③ Sue had a right to remain in the room with the other children
④ Keeping the child by herself for more than 30 minutes was too long

184. Several days later, Mrs. McMichael asks the nurse what to do when Sue has her temper tantrums. The nurse suggests that Mrs. McMichael allow Sue another way of expressing her anger, such as the use of:
① A ball and bat
② A pounding board
③ Clay or Play-Doh
④ A punching bag

Situation: Karina, 7 years old, is to have an expioratory laparotomy and possible appendectomy. Questions 185 through 188 refer to this situation.

185. The physician orders atropine, gr 1/300, IM preoperatively. The vial reads "atropine 0.4 mg/ml." The nurse should administer:

① 0.5 ml
② 1 ml
③ 0.25 ml
④ 0.75 ml

186. Postoperatively, to help relieve Karina's anxiety, the nurse should:
① Tell her a story about a girl with similar surgery
② Allow her time to talk about her feelings
③ Provide her with bandage, tape, scissors, and a doll
④ Ask her mother to room with her for a few days

187. Karina begins thumb-sucking after her surgery. This was not Karina's behavior preoperatively. The nurse should:
① Report this behavior to the physician
② Distract her by playing checkers
③ Accept the thumb-sucking
④ Tell her thumb-sucking causes buck teeth

188. Karina develops a urinary tract infection. The physician orders a sulfonamide preparation. A major nursing responsibility when administering this drug is to:
① Weigh the child daily
② Administer the drug at the prescribed times
③ Give milk with the medication
④ Monitor the temperature frequently

Situation: Mr. Gioni, the father of three young children, is diagnosed as having tuberculosis. Questions 189 through 191 refer to this situation.

189. Members of the family who have a positive reaction to the tuberculin test are candidates for treatment with:
① Old tuberculin
② BCG vaccine
③ INH and PAS
④ Purified protein derivative of tuberculin

190. If a person has been exposed to tuberculosis but shows no signs or symptoms except a positive tuberculin test, prophylactic drug therapy is usually continued after the last exposure for a period of:
① 3 weeks
② 6 months
③ 1 year
④ 5 years

191. Children in the family who have been exposed to but show no evidence of tuberculosis:
① Can be considered to be immune
② Should be treated with INH and PAS
③ Are usually given massive doses of penicillin
④ Are given X-ray examinations every 6 months

Situation: The nurse in the outpatient pediatric clinic is talking to a group of parents whose children have been diagnosed as having attention deficit disorder. Questions 192 and 193 refer to this situation.

192. One of the major behavioral characteristics of children with attention deficit disorders is their:
① Inability to use abstract thought
② Overreaction to stimuli
③ Continued use of rituals
④ Retarded speech development

193. In helping the parents to cope with their children's behavior, the nurse suggests that one of their best approaches would be to:
    ① Write a list of expectations to avoid confusion
    ② Be consistent and firm about established rules
    ③ Avoid asking specific questions
    ④ Allow the child to set up his or her own routines

Situation: Brian Smith, age 4, is admitted to the pediatric unit exhibiting pallor, fever, and extensive bruising over the body. Laboratory reports indicate a massive proliferation of lymphoblasts. A bone marrow aspiration confirms a diagnosis of acute lymphocytic leukemia. Questions 194 through 199 refer to this situation.

194. In examining Brian's labwork the nurse notes that he is neutropenic. This alteration is a result of:
    ① Increased internal bleeding
    ② Overwhelming infection
    ③ Increased immature cell growth
    ④ Decreased intake of iron rich nutrients

195. Brian is placed on bed rest. While assisting with his morning care, the nurse notes bloody expectorant after he has brushed his teeth. The nurse should first:
    ① Tell Brian to be more careful when brushing his teeth
    ② Record and report the incident but do not alarm Brian
    ③ Secure a smaller toothbrush for his use
    ④ Rinse his mouth with half-strength hydrogen peroxide

196. Brian is started on chemotherapy, including prednisone. A side effect of prednisone that Brian may exhibit is:
    ① Alopecia
    ② Anorexia
    ③ Mood changes
    ④ Weight loss

197. Methotrexate is part of Brian's therapy. This chemotherapeutic agent accomplishes its action by:
    ① Competing for essential structural components, thus inhibiting white blood cell production
    ② Intervening in mitosis, thus inhibiting the growth of the malignant cells
    ③ Acting as an antibiotic to control the spread of infected white blood cells
    ④ Depressing bone marrow function, thus decreasing white blood cell production

198. Brian is to receive a blood transfusion. If an allergic reaction to the blood occurs, the nurse's first intervention should be to:
    ① Relieve the symptoms with an ordered antihistamine
    ② Call the physician immediately
    ③ Slow the flow rate of the transfusion
    ④ Stop the blood immediately and flush the tubing

199. As a preschooler, Brian's response to hospitalization is influenced by his:
    ① Fear of separation
    ② Belief in death's finality
    ③ Belief in the supernatural
    ④ Fear of bodily harm

Situation: Baby boy Harrison was born at 8:05 AM following an uneventful labor and delivery. His mother and father spent time with him in the delivery and recovery room and then he was taken to the nursery by his father and the nurse. Gestational age assessment placed him at 39 weeks. Questions 200 through 203 refer to this situation.

200. As part of the initial assessment the nurse counts baby Harrison's cord vessels. In a normal infant there are:
    ① Two vessels: one vein and one artery
    ② Three vessels: one vein and two arteries
    ③ Three vessels: two veins and one artery
    ④ Four vessels: two veins and two arteries

201. In performing gestational age scoring, the nurse should recognize as characteristic of a preterm infant the presence of:
    ① Plantar creases covering the entire sole
    ② Testes both descended with rugae covering scrotum
    ③ Square window sign (wrist forms 90° angle)
    ④ Ears contain cartilage with the pinna firm

202. Mrs. Harrison asks the nurse how frequently she should burp her infant when bottle feeding. Recognizing that baby Harrison has a strong sucking reflex and no physical abnormalities, the nurse should answer:
    ① "You should burp him at the end of the feeding only. Otherwise he could become confused at having his feeding stopped."
    ② "Burp him periodically; usually in the middle and at the end of a feeding. If he's been crying, you can burp him before starting."
    ③ "With new infants we recommend burping every 5 to 10 minutes. That gets him used to a routine and lets you see how much he's taking."
    ④ "Burp the baby five to six times during each feeding for the first month."

203. The nurse tells Mrs. Harrison that the best way to position her newborn son during the first week or two of life is to lay him:
    ① On his back with his head flat
    ② On his back with his head slightly elevated
    ③ On his stomach with his head slightly elevated
    ④ On either side with the head flat

Situation: Eight-year-old Jennifer Herron is admitted to the hospital with deep, rapid respirations; flushed, dry cheeks; nausea; and increased thirst. Her history reveals she has had type I diabetes mellitus for 2 years. Questions 204 and 205 refer to this situation.

204. In reviewing the pathophysiology of her illness with Jennifer, the nurse's plan should take into consideration that:
    ① Jennifer will respond favorably to opportunities to participate in her care
    ② Jennifer is in the abstract level of cognition
    ③ Peer influence will decrease in importance to her
    ④ Her current developmental task involves achieving a sense of identity

205. Jennifer receives a combination of NPH and regular insulin at 7 AM. The nurse should be aware that Jennifer's response prior to lunch at noon will be controlled by:
    ① The NPH rather than the regular insulin
    ② Equal effects of regular and NPH insulin
    ③ Decreasing effects of regular and increasing effects of NPH insulin
    ④ Increasing effects of regular and NPH insulin

CHAPTER 6

Maternity Nursing

This section, maternity nursing, covers reproductive problems and emphasizes the pubertal changes of adolescence; the normal processes of conception, embryologic development, pregnancy, labor, delivery, and postpartum developments; and family planning. In addition, the newborn and the mother are discussed in relation to prematurity, birth injuries, and complications of labor and delivery. Current topics such as abortion, infant narcotic addiction, sexually transmitted diseases, and sterility are included.

Childbirth is a family experience. Humanity's basic needs for survival are centered in the family because without continuous love, physical contact, food, and stimulation of the senses, the infant would never survive. As each new member becomes a part of the family unit, interactions with the environment and other human beings become a part of early physical and emotional development. What is learned is determined by the kinds of stimulation received from the interactions occurring within the family. It is through this reciprocal give-and-take between the newborn and the family that each person becomes an individual, unique self.

Although childbearing patterns differ the world over, there are constants. In order of priority, they are: immediate physical contact between the infant and the parents; ability of the parents to give the infant love, food, and protection from the environment; the biologic need in men and women to reproduce; and the maturation and growth process that occurs in males and females in their changing roles as parents.

The unique and changing responsibilities in the life-cycle event of parenthood can be a real crisis. The changes occurring in society, whether social, economic, technical, or political, directly affect the patterns of childbearing and childrearing. Parenthood today is given serious thought, since it concerns both the family and society with the emphasis on quality rather than quantity.

Reproductive Readiness
PUBERTY

A period during which the organs of reproduction mature and are prepared for their reproductive function
A. Physical and physiologic changes
   1. In males
      a. Occur between 10 and 14 years of age; less dramatic than in female
      b. Heralded by deepening of voice and growth of body hair on the face, axillae, and genitalia
      c. Second year after onset: increased activity of sweat glands, spermatogenesis occurs with periodic erections and emissions of mature sperm
      d. Dramatic body growth spurt
      e. Ejaculation is beginning of fertility and end of puberty
   2. In females
      a. Occur between 9 and 13 years of age
      b. Sudden enlargement of the breasts, growth of body hair on the axillae and genitalia; changes in size and vascularity of internal reproductive organs
      c. Heralded by first menstrual flow, called *menarche;* unlike the male's first ejaculation, many first menstrual cycles are anovulatory (infertile)
      d. Dramatic body growth more evident than in male
B. Psychologic changes
   1. Age differences in maturation
   2. Heterosexual interests: girls earlier than boys, girls interested in older boys
   3. Emancipation struggles with parents: independence versus dependence
   4. Need for belonging to a peer group
C. Menstrual cycle
   1. Rhythmic reproductive cycle in females extending from the onset of a period of uterine bleeding to the onset of the next period of bleeding; mean cycle length is 28 days; normal range is 20 to 45 days per cycle
   2. During each cycle several (about 20) follicles commence maturation, but usually only one reaches full maturity and ruptures its contained ovum (and some surrounding granulosa cells) into the abdominal cavity
   3. The rhythmic menstrual cycles begin at puberty and cease at menopause
   4. Menstrual cycle divided into three stages based on endometrial histologic makeup and may be correlated with concentration fluctuations in hypothalamic, hypophyseal, and ovarian hormones (which cause the endometrial and other reproductive tract histologic changes)
      a. First stage—menstruation or menses: lasts 4 to 6 days; characterized by endometrial hemorrhage with the discharge exiting through the vagina; estrogen and progesterone blood levels are relatively low; the FSH level is elevated and, combined with a steady low level of LH secretion, initiates ovarian estrogen secretion, leading to the second stage
      b. Second stage—follicular or proliferative: lasts 8 to 10 days culminating in ovulation; endometrium repairs and proliferates in preparation for possible implantation, and a single ovarian follicle approaches full maturation as the concentration of estradiol (the principal estrogenic hormone) in the blood rises; estradiol exerts a negative feedback on FSH secretion and a positive feedback on LH secretion (the latter hormone induces ovulation); estradiol's feedback effects are exerted on the hypothalamic secretion of FSH-RH and LH-RH (which control the hypophyseal secretion of FSH and LH)
      c. Third stage—luteal or secretory: final stage is 9 to 13 days and begins after ovulation; LH pro-

motes formation of a temporary endocrine gland, the corpus luteum, from the ruptured follicle; granulosa and theca interna cells of follicle enlarge, divide into and occupy the cavity (antrum) of the follicle, and secrete progesterone and estrogen; progesterone stimulates the already proliferated endometrium to become glandular with a high glycogen-secreting potential (uterus now prepared for implantation); if fertilization does not occur, the corpus luteum functions for 7 to 8 days after ovulation and then involutes, becoming nonfunctional (corpus albicans) 10 to 12 days after ovulation; progesterone and estrogen blood levels drop, the negative feedback effect of estradiol on FSH is released, and the first stage begins again

PREGNANCY CYCLE
Prenatal Period (Antepartal Period)
Formation of Gametes

A. The egg and spermatozoon each have one set of chromosomes (23); this is in contrast to other cells of the body, which have two sets, or 46 chromosomes (23 pairs)
B. The production of ova (eggs) and spermatozoa (sperm) requires a special type of nuclear division (meiosis) in which the chromosome number is reduced from two sets (46 chromosomes) to one set (23 chromosomes)

Fertilization

A. Spermatozoa are deposited in the vagina
B. Fertilization usually occurs in the uterine tube when the egg is about one third the way down the tube; usually this is about 24 hours after ovulation
C. Sperm must be in the genital tract 4 to 6 hours before they are able to fertilize an egg; during this period the enzyme hyaluronidase is activated; this enzyme is able to dissolve the cement substance (hyaluronic acid) which holds together the cells that surround the ovum
D. Male nucleus enters the cytoplasm of the egg and several events follow:
   1. Fertilization membrane forms around the egg to prevent the entrance of other sperm
   2. Sperm tail is lost and the male nucleus (male pronucleus) moves toward the female nucleus (female pronucleus)
E. Fertilization proper occurs when the male pronucleus unites with the female pronucleus; thus the chromosome number is restored to two sets (46 chromosomes)

Cleavage

A. In a short time after fertilization the zygote undergoes rapid division to produce a mass of cells (morula) that descends in the uterine tube
B. As it descends, it also divides to form a hollow ball referred to as the blastocyst

Implantation

A. The blastocyst implants in the uterine wall
   1. The blastocyst is differentiated into an inner cell mass, a blastocoele (internal cavity)

   2. An outer covering of cells, the trophectoderm, becomes the trophoderm and will form the fetal portion of the placenta, the vehicle for exchange of nutrients and wastes
   3. Implantation occurs 7 to 8 days after fertilization generally in upper fundal portion
   4. Increased maternal hormonal action is necessary for continued implantation of fetus in the uterus
B. Placentation and umbilical cord development
   1. Placenta
      a. Organ of dual origin (maternal and embryonic portions) serving interchange of food and wastes between mother and embryo (or fetus) during pregnancy
      b. Formed from villous portion of chorion (chorion frondosum) and the portion of the uterine endometrium (called the decidua during pregnancy) directly underlying the implanted embryo (decidua basalis): chorionic villi project into placental sinuses (in decidua basalis) filled with maternal blood
      c. Functions as the fetal digestive tract and also as fetal lungs, kidneys, and as a major endocrine gland (producing estrogens, progesterone, ACTH, growth hormone, and gonadotropic hormones HCG and HPL) (see Endocrine system in Medical-Surgical Nursing)
      d. Serves as a protective barrier against harmful effects of some drugs and microorganisms
   2. Umbilical cord
      a. Inserted close to the central portion of the placenta and attached to fetus
      b. Has one vein (which transports nourishment) and two arteries (which transport wastes) between the mother and baby
      c. Wharton's jelly, a protective covering, surrounds the entire cord

Embryonic Period

A. First 2 months, after this period it is called a fetus
B. The inner cell mass differentiates into germ layers
   1. Ectoderm: outer layer of skin and mouth cavity and nervous tissue
   2. Mesoderm: connective tissue, including blood and muscle tissue
   3. Endoderm: linings of the alimentary tract, respiratory system, and several glands
C. About the twelfth day after fertilization a fetal membrane, the amnion, forms around the embryo; another membrane, the yolk sac, develops beneath the embryo
   1. Amnion is fluid filled (amniotic fluid) and serves as a fetal shock absorber
   2. Yolk sac serves as an initial embryonic source of erythrocytes
D. Later an allantois develops that will supply the placental blood vessels
E. A chorion surrounds the embryo; this will eventually form the major part of the placenta; fingerlike projections of the chorion called chorionic villi grow into the endometrium; chorionic villi project into placental blood sinuses; the combination of chorionic villi, placental blood sinuses, and placental blood constitutes the placenta

F. Fetal development—differentiation of cells occurs
   1. 14 days: heart begins to beat; brain, early spinal cord, and muscle segments present
   2. 26 days: tiny buds for arms appear
   3. 28 days: tiny buds for legs appear
   4. 30 days: embryo ¼ to ½ inch (0.6 to 1.2 cm) in length, definite form, beginning of umbilical cord is visible
   5. 31 days: arm buds develop into hands, arms, and shoulders
   6. 33 days: finger outlines present
   7. 46 to 48 days: cartilage in upper arms replaced by first bone cells, amniotic fluid surrounds the fetus (amniotic fluid is a protective cushion, equalizes pressures, maintains temperature, and facilitates the baby's movements for adequate growth and development; first 8 weeks is period of rapid growth and development)
   8. 3 months (12 weeks): fetus moves body parts, swallows, practices inhaling and exhaling, weighs 28 g (1 oz); fetal heart audible with Doptone
   9. Any interference with maternal physiology may cause irreparable damage to fetus; no drugs should be taken during this period if possible
   10. 4 to 5 months (16 to 20 weeks): fetal movements felt by mother (known as quickening), weighs 170 g (6 oz), is 20 to 25 cm (8 to 10 inches) in length
   11. 5 to 6 months (20 to 24 weeks): hair growth on head, eyelashes and brow, skeleton hardens, eyelids closed, weighs 0.45 kg (1 lb), is 30.5 cm (12 inches) in length, fetal heart audible with fetoscope
   12. 6 to 7 months (24 to 28 weeks): eyelids open, amniotic fluid increases to 1 quart with a daily exchange of 6 gallons, weighs 0.5 kg (1¼ lb)
   13. 7 to 8 months (28 to 32 weeks): many fat deposits, weighs 0.45 to 0.7 kg (1 to 1½ lb)
   14. 8 to 9 months (32 to 36 weeks): stores protein for extrauterine life, gains 1.8 kg (4 lb)

G. Fetal circulation: contains mixed blood; less than maximal O_2 concentration; only exception is in the umbilical vessel upon its immediate entrance into liver
   1. Foramen ovale is an opening between the right and left atria during fetal life, bypassing fetal lungs
   2. Ductus arteriosus is a connection between pulmonary trunk and aorta, also bypassing fetal lungs
   3. Ductus venosus is a connection between umbilical vein and ascending vena cava, bypassing fetal liver

Chromosomes

A. Humans have 23 pairs of homologous chromosomes
B. In males the sex chromosomes (the X and Y) are not equal in size
C. Homologous chromosomes carry sets of matching genes (alleles) in which one may be dominant and the other recessive, or they may have blending expressions

Sex Determination in Humans

A. Genetic females have two sets of autosomes (nonsex chromosomes) and two X chromosomes, whereas genetic males have two sets of autosomes and one X chromosome and one Y chromosome

B. All eggs produced by females have one set of autosomes and one X chromosome; spermatozoa produced by a male have a set of autosomes and either an X or a Y chromosome
C. If an X-bearing spermatozoon fertilizes an egg, a female will result; if a Y-bearing spermatozoon fertilizes an egg, a male will result

Genes

A. Sex-linked genes: genes carried on the X chromosome are called sex-linked genes and are always expressed in the male, even though they may be recessive; examples of such genes cause hemophilia and color blindness
B. Multiple genes: many different genes may combine to produce cumulative effects, such as the degree of pigmentation or height
C. Multiple alleles: an example of human traits controlled by multiple alleles are the genes controlling normal blood types; the genes for type O are dominated by the genes for type A or type B; the genes for A and B are both expressed

Genes	Blood type
OO	O
AO	A
AA	A
BO	B
BB	B
AB	AB

D. Following are some other obvious human traits controlled by genes

Dominant	Recessive
Brown eyes	Blue eyes
Normal blood clotting	Hemophilia (sex-linked)
Normal color vision	Color blind (sex-linked)
Normal pigmentation	Albinism
Rh positive (multiple alleles)	Rh negative
Normal red blood cell development	Sickle cell trait

Chromosomal Alterations

A. In rare cases additional sex chromosomes may appear and produce abnormal individuals
   1. X chromosome and no Y chromosome: Turner's syndrome
   2. Two or more X chromosomes and a Y chromosome: Klinefelter's syndrome
B. Translocation of chromosome: a cytogenetic abnormality such as trisomy 21 (Down's syndrome)
C. Mutations
   1. Changes in the DNA are mutations; there may also be chromosomal changes
   2. The frequency of mutations may be increased by certain agents such as ultraviolet radiation, x-ray films, radioactive radiation, and certain chemical substances

Physical and Physiologic Changes in Mother During Pregnancy

Pregnancy is a normal physiologic process that affects all body systems and results in both objective and subjective changes; it is a stressful time requiring many adaptations and may lead to minor discomforts

A. Endocrine
1. During pregnancy the chorion of the placenta secretes a hormone, chorionic gonadotropin (HCG), that maintains the corpus luteum; the continuation of progesterone and estrogen secretion from the corpus luteum maintains the pregnancy during the early weeks of development; presence of hormone is an indicator of pregnancy
2. Chorionic gonadotropin reaches a peak in the third month and then drops
3. Estrogen and progesterone increase and continue to be secreted from the placenta during the last 6 months of pregnancy; progesterone acts to inhibit uterine contractions, which might occur due to uterine stretching as the fetus grows; increase in these hormones leads to sodium and water retention and muscle relaxation, which leads to fatigue
4. Thyroid activity is increased
5. Chorionic somatomammotrophin increased; a diabetogenic hormone which decreases maternal use of glucose, leaving it available for fetal use
6. Estriol levels increased; used as indicator of fetal well-being
7. In the last month uterine contents shift downward so that the fetus is in contact with the cervix; this contact may induce oxytocin secretion by the posterior pituitary
8. The secretion of oxytocin, which stimulates uterine contractions, coupled with the drop in progesterone brings about labor; uterine contractions increase in frequency and intensity, culminating in fetal expulsion (birth)

B. Reproductive
1. Amenorrhea occurs, since the corpus luteum persists and ovulation is inhibited by the high levels of circulating estrogen and progesterone
2. Breast changes such as fullness, tingling, soreness, darkening of the areolae and nipples occur along with an increase in hormonal levels
3. Leukorrhea is increased as hormonal levels rise, and the increased acidity is a protection from bacterial invasion
4. Changes in the uterus are circulatory, hormonal, and related to fetal growth
   a. Softening of the cervix: Goodell's sign
   b. Softening of the lower uterine segment: Hegar's sign
   c. Purplish hue to the vaginal mucosa: Chadwick's sign
   d. Uterus enlarges in size but not weight
   e. Changes in position of the uterus: first trimester uterus is in pelvic cavity, second and third trimester uterus is in abdominal cavity before lightening occurs

C. Gastrointestinal
1. Reduction in hydrochloric acid secretion which interferes with gastric motility, causing nausea and vomiting (morning sickness) and pyrosis (heartburn)

2. Elevated estrogen levels cause excessive salivation
3. Hyperemia and softening of gums with accompanying hyperacidity of oral secretions results in nonspecific gingivitis
4. Decreased emptying time of gallbladder may precipitate development of gallstones
5. Food cravings may occur; only significant if substance craved is unusual (pica), e.g., clay, starch, dirt
6. Constipation is secondary to hypoperistalsis, lack of fluids, poor dietary habits, pressure of the enlarged uterus on internal organs, effects of progesterone on muscle, and hemorrhoids

D. Excretory
1. Proximity of the uterus and bladder in early and late pregnancy causes urinary frequency
2. Bladder tone is reduced by effects of hormones on smooth muscle
3. Bladder capacity up to 1500 ml in second trimester
4. Increased urinary output results in lowered specific gravity
5. Increased excretion of sugar caused by lowered renal threshold
6. Pressure of enlarging uterus causes dilation of right ureter and kidney

E. Circulatory
1. Physiologic anemia occurs as a result of increased blood volume with no proportional increase in red blood cells
2. Cardiac output increases 25% to 50% during pregnancy, peaking at 7 or 8 months
3. Heart rate increases 10 beats per minute in the latter half of pregnancy: approximately 14,000 extra beats in 24 hours
4. Palpitations occur in early months from sympathetic nervous stimulation and in later months from increased thoracic pressure because of enlarged uterus
5. BP may drop slightly in second trimester
6. Supine hypotension syndrome: in supine position weight of enlarged uterus obstructs vena cava, which decreases blood return to heart; decreased cardiac output ensues with hypotension, lightheadedness, faintness, and palpitations
7. White blood cells, fibrinogen, and other clotting factors increase
8. Varicose veins of legs, vulva, and perianal area may occur
9. Edema of extremities common in the last 6 weeks of pregnancy because of stasis of blood

F. Respiratory
1. At 36 to 38 weeks, pressure of the enlarged uterus on diaphragm and lungs may cause dyspnea that subsides when lightening occurs
2. Oxygen consumption is increased by about 15% between the sixteenth and fortieth weeks, although there may be only a slight increase in vital capacity during pregnancy
3. Hyperventilation occurs due to mother's need to blow-off increased CO_2 transferred to her from fetus
4. Nasal congestion occurs as a response to increased estrogen levels

G. Integumentary
1. Excretion of wastes through the skin causes diaphoresis
2. Skin changes: darkening of the areolae, darkening patches on the face (chloasma), linea alba becomes nigra on the abdomen, related to increased estrogen; striae on the abdomen and legs caused by skin stretching as pregnancy advances; erythematous changes on the palms and face in some women

H. Skeletal
1. Softening of all ligaments and joints, especially symphysis and sacroiliac joint, caused by increased hormonal action of estrogens and relaxin
2. Leg cramps may occur from an imbalance of the calcium/phosphorus ratio in the body and from pressure of the gravid uterus on nerves supplying lower extremities

I. Emotional
1. Acceptance of biologic fact of pregnancy; usually occurs during first trimester
2. Acceptance of growing fetus as distinct from self; usually occurs during second trimester
3. Preparation for birth and relinquishing of child; usually occurs during third trimester
4. Ambivalence about child and parenting
5. Mood swings
6. Increase or decrease in sexual desire
7. Anxiety related to delivery and adult responsibilities

J. Affirmation and confirmation of pregnancy
1. Presumptive signs: mostly subjective; may be indicative of other illnesses
   a. Amenorrhea
   b. Fatigue
   c. Nausea and vomiting
   d. Breast changes
   e. Urinary frequency
   f. Darkening of pigmentation on face, breasts, and stomach
   g. Quickening: feeling of movement about 15 to 20 weeks
2. Probable signs: objective but still not definite confirmations of pregnancy
   a. Uterine changes
      (1) Chadwick's sign
      (2) Hegar's sign
      (3) Goodell's sign
      (4) Enlargement of the uterus
   b. Fetal outline
   c. Pregnancy tests: urine and blood of pregnant woman used to detect HCG (human chorionic gonadotropin)
   d. Ballottment
   e. Braxton Hicks contractions
3. Positive signs: confirm pregnancy
   a. Fetal heart beat
   b. Fetal outline and movement as felt by examiner
   c. Ultrasonography revealing movement of fetal heart
   d. Roentgenography of fetal skeleton (rarely used since x-ray may be damaging to fetus)

4. Estimating date of confinement (EDC) or estimating date of delivery (EDD) and duration of pregnancy
   a. Naegele's rule: count back 3 months from the first day of the last menstrual period and add 7 days (9 calendar months, 270 days or 10 lunar months, 280 days)
   b. Fundal height
   c. Ultrasonography: establishes fetal age from head measurements (term pregnancy: biparietal diameter is 9.8 cm or more); test is done when woman has full bladder (must be instructed to increase fluids before test)

K. Nutritional needs during pregnancy
1. Consideration of preconceptional nutritional status; age and parity of mother, biologic interactions between mother, fetus, and placenta; and individual needs such as in times of stress
2. Weight gain should be evaluated with regard to the quality of gain (Is weight gain caused by edema or fat deposition?)
3. Severe caloric restriction during pregnancy is contraindicated, since it is a potential hazard to the mother and fetus
4. Weight reduction should never be started as a regimen during pregnancy
5. Restriction of sodium and administration of diuretics are potentially dangerous to the mother and fetus during pregnancy
6. Nausea and vomiting: limited fluids with meals, small frequent feedings, restricted fat, high carbohydrate
7. Constipation: increased fluids and residue or fiber; appropriate activity level
8. Consideration of the demands of pregnancy related to growth and development of the fetus during the various trimesters; provide adequate nutrition to meet increased maternal and fetal nutrient demands
   a. Increased calories to meet increased basal metabolic needs and spare protein for growth, to promote weight gain to support pregnancy (average 11.4 kg, or 25 lb, but is individual according to need), and for lactation
   b. Increased protein to provide for growth demands
   c. Increased vitamins, especially folic acid supplement to prevent anemia
   d. Increased minerals with supplement of iron to prevent anemia
   e. Iodized salt to provide needed sodium and iodine
9. Lactating mother needs additional caloric requirements
10. Dietary assessment and counseling should be an integral part of prenatal care for every pregnant woman
11. Changes in dietary regimen should consider cultural, economic, and psychologic implications of food habits
12. Food guide may be based on basic four groups with
    a. Increased protein foods: 1 qt milk, two eggs, two servings of meat, added cheese

b. Additional servings from each of the remaining food groups: grains, vegetables, fruits
c. Additional calories, protein, and fluids during lactation
13. Adolescent nutritional needs
  a. Weight gain for normal pregnancy and expected weight gain for growth are added together
  b. Higher protein intake for young pregnant female
  c. Iron needs higher to support enlarging muscle mass and increasing blood volume
  d. Calcium intake increased by 400 mg
L. Medical supervision during pregnancy
1. History, including medical, surgical, gynecologic and obstetric data; family history of hereditary and transmittable diseases such as diabetes, tuberculosis, heart disease
2. Physical examination of the skin, thyroid, teeth, lungs, heart, and breasts, abdominal palpation, auscultation, height of fundus, vaginal examination, and pelvic evaluation (prior to last 4 weeks of pregnancy)
3. Cervical and vaginal smears for monilia, trichomonas, herpes, and chlamydia; Papanicolaou test for cancer
4. Blood pressure; weight; and urinalysis for acetone, albumin, and sugar done at all visits
5. Blood specimens taken for typing, cross-matching, Rh factor, serologic test for syphilis (repeated at 32 weeks), and rubella titer
6. Screening tests
  a. Alpha-fetoprotein (AFP) testing for neural tube defects
  b. Tine testing for tuberculosis
  c. Tay-Sachs screening, particularly for Jewish women
  d. Sickle cell screening, particularly for black women

Nursing Process During the Prenatal Period
Probable Nursing Diagnosis Based on Assessment

A. Fear related to diagnosis of pregnancy, lack of knowledge about body changes, and/or impending parenthood
B. Constipation related to less frequent bowel movements associated with slowed peristalsis and pressure from gravid uterus
C. Decreased cardiac output related to pressure on vena cava by gravid uterus when in supine position
D. Family coping: potential for growth related to acceptance of pregnancy and fulfillment of parental tasks
E. Potential fluid volume deficit related to increasing demands of pregnancy
F. Potential for trauma related to altered balance associated with increased weight of uterus and change in center of gravity
G. Knowledge deficit related to new experience of pregnancy
H. Altered nutrition: less than body requirements related to increased needs of pregnancy or nausea and vomiting
I. Potential disturbance in self-esteem related to altered appearance and ambivalence about pregnancy

J. Potential disturbance in body image related to actual appearance and other physical changes of pregnancy
K. Sexual dysfunction related to altered body contour
L. Altered patterns of urinary elimination related to pressure of gravid uterus

Nursing Care During the Prenatal Period

A. Assist the parents in understanding the anatomy and physiology of pregnancy, labor, and delivery
B. Teach mother to monitor for
1. Visual disturbances
2. Edema of face, fingers, or feet
3. Persistent severe headaches
4. Convulsions
5. Epigastric pain
6. Persistent severe vomiting
7. Any vaginal discharge, including blood
8. Signs of infection
9. Burning on urination
10. Abdominal pain
11. Absence of or decrease in fetal movements after initial presence
C. Teach mother about physiologic changes and related discomforts that occur during pregnancy (nausea, vomiting, backaches, varicosities, hemorrhoids, constipation, leg pain, etc.)
D. Respond to questions about bathing, douching, work, sex, exercise, etc.
E. Help the parents discuss and explore feelings related to childbearing and childrearing in attempting to alleviate fears
F. Prepare the mother for the physical work of labor through the use of muscle and breathing exercises for the various phases of labor
G. Identify parents' situational support systems
H. Prepare the father for a coaching and supporting role during pregnancy, labor, and delivery
I. Introduce families to health facilities available for continued health care of the family
J. Discuss various childbirth preparation techniques such as Lamaze, Reade, and Bradley
K. Teach the mother to avoid over-the-counter or prescription drugs without checking with the physician since many drugs considered harmless may be teratogenic to the developing fetus
L. Evaluate client's response and revise plan as necessary

Intrapartal Period (Period of Birth)

A. Labor: physiologic and mechanical process in which the baby, placenta, and fetal membranes are propelled through the pelvis and expelled from the birth canal
B. Anatomy of the bony pelvis
1. Parts: ischium, ilium, sacrum, coccyx
2. Joints: sacroiliacs, sacrococcygeal, symphysis pubis (all soften during pregnancy)
3. Divisions: false pelvis supports the enlarged uterus in the abdominal cavity; true pelvis is the bony inner pelvis through which the baby must pass
4. Diameters: at inlet: true conjugate (anteroposterior diameter), transverse (widest diameter at inlet), right and left oblique diameters; at outlet: conjugate diagonal (anteroposterior is widest diameter), transverse (one ischial tuberosity to the other)

5. Classification of pelvis: gynecoid (normal female pelvis), android (male pelvis), anthropoid, and platypelloid
6. Normal female pelvis has an ample pubic arch, curved sacrum, curved side walls, blunt ischial spines, and a movable coccyx

C. Attitude: relationship of fetal parts to each other
D. Lie: relationship of the long axis of the infant to the long axis of the mother
E. Presentation: baby's body part that engages in the true pelvis
1. Cephalic (head): vertex, brow, or face
2. Breech: frank, complete, single, or double footling
3. Shoulder: cannot be delivered vaginally
F. Position: relationship of presenting parts to four quadrants of the mother's pelvis (the letters L and R are used for left or right; A and P for anterior or posterior; O for occiput; M for mentum or face; S for sacrum)
1. Vertex: occiput, LOA, LOP, ROA, ROP
2. Face: chin (mentum), LMA, LMP, RMA, RMP
3. Breech: sacrum, LSA, LSP, RSA, RSP
G. Station: relationship of presenting part to the false and true pelves
1. Floating: presenting part movable above the true pelvic inlet
2. Engaged: suboccipitobregmatic diameter fixed into the pelvic inlet
3. Station O: presenting part at level of the ischial spines: levels below spines +1, +2, +3; levels above spines −1, −2, −3
H. Signs and symptoms prior to labor
1. Physiologic
   a. Lightening: baby drops down into the true pelvis
   b. Braxton Hicks contractions: painless tryout contractions in preparation for true labor
   c. Increased vaginal secretions
   d. Softening of cervix
   e. Rupture of membranes (ROM); for confirmation fluid can be tested with nitrazine paper
   f. Bloody show; softening and effacement of cervix causes mucus plug to be expelled; this is accompanied by small blood loss
2. Psychologic: mother shows signs of nesting (increased activity) due to sudden rise in energy level
I. Signs and symptoms of true labor
1. Uterine contractions that increase in frequency, strength, and duration and do not disappear when lying down or walking around
2. Effacement and progressive dilation of the cervix
J. Mechanisms of labor: rotation of vertex presentation through the true pelvis
1. Engagement, descent with flexion: at onset of labor, head descends and chin flexes on the chest
2. Internal rotation: as labor contractions and uterine forces move the baby downward, the head internally rotates to pass through the ischial spines
3. Extension: occiput emerges under the symphysis pubis and the head is delivered by extension
4. External rotation: to allow for rotation of the shoulders to an anteroposterior position
5. Expulsion: rest of baby is delivered

K. Stages of labor and maternal changes
1. First stage: from the onset of true labor to complete effacement and dilation of the cervix
   a. Latent phase: mild, short contractions, cervix dilated 0 to 3 cm; mother excited and happy that labor has started, some apprehension; follows directions readily
   b. Active phase: moderate to strong contractions 5 minutes apart, cervix dilates from 4 to 7 cm, bloody show, membranes may rupture, breathing techniques help in relaxing, medication may be necessary for discomfort, supportive measures (e.g., encouragement, praise, reassurance, keeping the mother informed of progress, providing rest between contractions, presence of a supporting person) by the husband or nurse help; has difficulty in following directions
   c. Transition phase: strong contractions 1 to 2 minutes apart (lasting 45 to 60 seconds or more with little rest in between); cervix dilates from 7 to 10 cm with a bloody show; mother becomes irritable, restless, agitated, highly emotional, belches, has leg tremors, perspires, pale white ring around mouth (circumoral pallor), flushed face, sudden nausea, and vomiting; feels need to have a BM due to pressure on anus; unable to communicate or follow directions
2. Second stage: beginning with full dilation of the cervix and ending with birth of the baby; perineum bulges, pushing with contractions, grunting sounds, behavior changes from great irritability to great involvement and work, sleep and relaxation occur between contractions, leg cramps are common
3. Third stage: following birth of the baby through expulsion of the placenta; placental separation (5 to 30 minutes) after delivery heralded by globular formation of uterus, lengthening of umbilical cord, and gush of blood; may have alteration in perineal structure either from episiotomy (prophylactic incision into perineum to allow for delivery of head) or laceration (may be 1°, 2°, 3°, or 4°) from rapid expulsion of presenting part
4. Fourth stage: following expulsion of placenta to 3 to 4 hours after delivery; fundus firm in the midline and at or slightly above the umbilicus; scant, bloody vaginal discharge (lochia rubra); fatigue, thirst, chills, nausea; excitement and intermittent dozing
L. Oxytocics
1. Description
   a. Drugs that stimulate the uterus to contract
   b. Used in the pregnant female to initiate labor
   c. Used to augment contractions that have already begun
   d. Capable of inducing contraction of the lacteal glands which aids in letdown reflex for nursing
   e. Exerts vasopressor and antidiuretic effects
   f. Used to control postpartum uterine atony
   g. Oxytocics are available in parenteral (IM, IV) and nasal preparations
2. Examples
   a. ergonovine maleate (Ergotrate)
   b. methylergonovine maleate (Methergine)
   c. oxytocin (Pitocin)

3. Major side effects
   a. Maternal
      (1) Hypertension (contracture of smooth muscles of blood vessels)
      (2) Tachycardia
      (3) Arrhythmias
      (4) Uterine rupture (excessive contraction)
      (5) Water intoxication (antidiuretic effect)
      (6) Convulsions (water intoxication)
      (7) Coma (water intoxication)
   b. Fetal
      (1) Anoxia, asphyxia
      (2) Arrhythmias (PVCs, bradycardia)
      (3) Hyperbilirubinemia
4. Nursing care
   a. Never leave client unattended
   b. Have O_2 and emergency resuscitative equipment available
   c. Utilize infusion-control device for IV administration
   d. Discontinue if prolonged uterine contractions occur
   e. Monitor uterine contractions
   f. Assess BP and pulse every 15 minutes
   g. Fetal monitoring is essential
   h. Instruct client on nasal administration technique
   i. Evaluate client's response to medication and understanding of teaching

M. Maternal analgesia and anesthesia
   1. Analgesia
      Meperidine hydrochloride (Demerol) most commonly-used narcotic analgesic given during active labor; may be given IM or IV; appears in fetus 1 to 2 minutes after administration
   2. Regional analgesia and anesthesia
      a. Epidural
      b. Spinal
      c. Pudendal
      d. Local infiltration; most frequently used
   3. Nursing care
      a. Observe mother and newborn for respiratory depression if narcotic analgesic is given; monitor mother for hypotension
      b. After epidural
         (1) Monitor for hypotension
         (2) If hypotension occurs, position client on left side, increase IV infusion, and administer oxygen
      c. Evaluate client's response to medication and understanding of teaching

Nursing Process During the Intrapartal Period
Probable Nursing Diagnoses Based on Assessment

A. Mother
   1. Fear related to lack of knowledge and unfamiliarity with labor process
   2. Potential ineffective individual coping related to exhaustion
   3. Potential disturbance in self-esteem related to inability to live up to behavioral expectations (self or others)
   4. Pain related to labor process and episiotomy
   5. Impaired gas exchange related to hyperventilation
   6. Impaired physical mobility related to need for fetal monitoring, bed rest, or positioning
   7. Altered patterns of urinary elimination related to pressure of enlarged uterus, analgesia or anesthesia, and trauma of labor and delivery
   8. Potential for injury related to lack of control, especially during transition phase, position during delivery, and administration of anesthesia
   9. Altered cardiopulmonary tissue perfusion associated with hypovolemia related to uterine relaxation following birth and/or cervical lacerations
B. Baby
   1. Decreased cardiac output related to prolonged contractions, short umbilical cord, head compression, pressure on umbilical cord, or uteroplacental insufficiency
   2. Ineffective airway clearance related to excessive mucus, aspiration of meconium, or inability to clear airway
   3. Potential for injury related to trauma of birth or maternal infection
   4. Ineffective thermoregulation related to immature heat regulation, inability to shiver, and lack of brown fat

Nursing Care During the Intrapartal Period

A. First stage
   1. Admit mother and labor coach
      a. Orient to unit
      b. Obtain history
         (1) Parity and gravidity
         (2) EDC/EDD
         (3) Onset of contractions
         (4) Status of membranes
         (5) Time and contents of last meal
         (6) Allergies
         (7) Intent to breast or bottle feed
      c. Obtain vital signs
      d. Perform Leopold's maneuvers
      e. Time and assess contractions
      f. Assist with vaginal examination
      g. Do perineal prep and give enema if ordered
      h. Test urine for protein and glucose
      i. Collect blood for CBC and cross-match
      j. Give emotional support to mother and labor coach
   2. Maintain asepsis
   3. Monitor frequency, duration, and strength of contractions
      a. Palpate fundus
      b. Interpret data on maternal uterine monitor
      c. Prolonged contractions of 90 seconds or more may occur with administration of oxytocin (Pitocin); discontinue drug
   4. Monitor fetal heart rate (FHR)
      a. Fetoscope
      b. Internal or external fetal monitor
   5. Interpret data of fetal monitoring
      a. Baseline FHR: normal heart rate between uterine contractions is 120 to 160 beats per minute

b. Tachycardia: heart rate above 160 beats per minute lasting over 10 minutes
   (1) Transient tachycardia may occur with fetal activity; may be due to maternal fever or dehydration and drugs such as atropine, Vistaril, or ritodrine
   (2) Nursing intervention includes reducing maternal fever, increasing fluids, and monitoring for amnionitis
c. Bradycardia: heart rate below 120 beats per minute lasting longer than 10 minutes
   (1) May be due to fetal hypoxia; anesthetics used for epidural, spinal, caudal, and pudendal blocks; maternal hypotension; prolonged umbilical cord compression
   (2) Nursing intervention includes repositioning mother on side assessing for prolapsed cord, positioning to relieve pressure on cord, elevating lower extremities
d. Variability: normal irregularity of cardiac rhythm (balance between sympathetic and parasympathetic divisions of autonomic nervous system); manifested by cyclic fluctuations and beat-to-beat changes of heart rate; usually transient; often occurs with fetal tachycardia
   (1) Absence of these fluctuations is indicative of fetal CNS depression
   (2) Associated with drugs such as narcotics and barbiturates, fetal hypoxia, acidosis, and immaturity of fetus
   (3) Nursing intervention includes administration of oxygen, repositioning of mother on left side
e. Decelerations: periodic decrease in FHR
   (1) Early decelerations
      (a) FHR decreases but not below 100 beats per minute
      (b) Occur early in contraction phase, before peak
      (c) Indicate head compression
      (d) No nursing intervention needed
   (2) Late decelerations
      (a) FHR rarely decreases below 100 beats per minute but, if severe, may decrease to 60 beats per minute
      (b) Begin as contraction peaks with lowest rate after peak of contraction
      (c) Long recovery time; FHR may not return to normal until well after contraction ends
      (d) Often associated with loss of variability; may be accompanied by bradycardia or tachycardia
      (e) Indicative of uteroplacental insufficiency caused by uterine tetany from oxytocin administration; maternal supine hypotension; regional anesthesia; hypertensive disorders; diabetes mellitus; and other chronic disorders
      (f) Ominous if persistent or associated with decreased variability

      (g) Nursing intervention includes discontinuing oxytocin if being administered, positioning mother on left side, administering oxygen by mask at 8 to 10 L/minute, increasing rate of intravenous fluids, assisting with fetal blood sampling; preparing for delivery if there is no improvement
6. Prevent supine hypotension by positioning mother on left side to keep gravid uterus from compressing vena cava
7. Assist the mother with breathing techniques throughout labor by teaching and encouraging appropriate breathing patterns in varying phases of labor and rebreathing techniques to correct and prevent hyperventilation
8. Utilize measures to promote comfort and rest by providing warmth, administering analgesics and tranquilizers as ordered, except in late phase of labor (less than 2 hours before birth) to prevent fetal depression; encourage use of relaxation techniques and positions learned in childbirth classes; support and encourage mother and coach; carefully monitor BP during administration of regional anesthetic
9. Observe perineum for bloody show and appearance of amniotic fluid (indicates ruptured membranes); note
   a. Amount
   b. Color; if greenish, check for breech position and obtain fetal heart
   c. Odor; if foul may indicate amnionitis
   d. FHR following amniotomy to artificially rupture membranes (AROM)
10. Assess body fluids, bladder, and bowel function
11. Monitor for
   a. Prolonged strong contractions; may indicate tetanic uterus
   b. Taut boardlike abdomen; may indicate abruptio placenta
   c. Increase in pulse and temperature; may indicate infection
   d. Hypertension; may indicate preeclampsia
   e. Hypotension; may occur following epidural or spinal anesthesia; turn client on side
   f. Vaginal bleeding; may indicate placenta previa
   g. Meconium-stained amniotic fluid; may indicate breech position or fetal distress
   h. Abnormal variations in FHR patterns; may indicate fetal distress
12. Evaluate client's response and revise plan as necessary
B. Second stage
   1. Assist mother with pushing
   2. Transfer to delivery room or prepare birthing bed
   3. Monitor FHR
   4. Prepare mother for delivery
   5. Evaluate client's response and revise plan as necessary
C. Third stage
   1. Care of baby
      a. Clear airway of mucus
      b. Observe frequently

c. Use Apgar scoring to determine respiratory effort
d. Maintain body heat
e. Assess the newborn for visible anomalies
f. Place in parent's arms or view
g. Instill silver nitrate or other medication into each eye after bonding to prevent ophthalmia neonatorum
h. Identify the mother and baby prior to leaving delivery room by use of prints and application of bands
2. Record delivery and accompanying events
3. Evaluate baby's response and revise plan as necessary
D. Fourth stage
1. Palpate the fundus frequently for firmness and height in relation to umbilicus; if relaxed and dextroverted, check for bladder fullness
2. Check for bladder distention; determine voiding pattern
3. Check the perineum for vaginal and suture line bleeding; count vaginal pads; assess for concurrent uterine relaxation; massage uterus
4. Monitor temperature, BP, and pulse; report fluctuations
5. Administer oxytocic medication as ordered; after delivery an oxytocic may be administered rapidly to enhance uterine contractions
6. Check episiotomy or laceration site for hematoma, bleeding, or edema; apply icebag to perineum immediately after delivery to reduce edema
7. Keep warm; chills are common after delivery
8. Provide fluid and food as tolerated
9. Evaluate client's response and revise plan as necessary

Postpartal Period

A. Puerperium: 6-week period following delivery in which the reproductive organs undergo physical and physiologic changes, a process called *involution*; because of the many physiologic and psychologic stresses of the postpartum period, there is a trend to increase this period to 3 months following delivery and call it the fourth trimester of pregnancy
B. Systemic changes during the peurperium
1. Reproductive system
a. Uterus: intermittent contractions bring about involution, after-contractions may cause discomfort necessitating analgesics; oxytocin release during breastfeeding speeds up involution
b. Lochia: vaginal flow following delivery, changes from rubra to serosa, then becomes alba (uterine lining regenerates with new epithelium in 2 or 3 days)
c. Vagina practically returns to its prepregnant state through a healing of soft tissue and cicatrization
d. Abdominal wall soft and flabby but eventually regains tone
e. Breasts
(1) As placenta is delivered, there is activation of luteinizing hormone in the anterior pituitary: secretion of prolactin also stimulates milk production

(2) Posterior pituitary secretes pitocin, an oxytocic that initiates the letdown reflex with milk ejection as the baby suckles
(3) Breast engorgement occurs on the second or third day because of vasodilation prior to lactation
2. Digestive system
a. Added proteins and calories to replenish those lost with the process of involution
b. Lactating mother needs added calories and fluids
c. Roughage and exercise relieve constipation and distention
3. Circulatory system
a. Blood volume usually back to normal by the third week after delivery
b. Blood fibrinogen levels increase during the first week
c. Increase in leukocytes; may go as high as 30,000/ μL, especially if labor was lengthy
d. Drop in hemoglobin and red blood count on the fourth postpartal day
4. Excretory system
a. Increased urinary output, second to fifth postpartal day
b. Bladder tone altered during pregnancy: retention with overflow may occur
c. Activation of lactogenic hormone may result in lactose in the urine
d. Excretion of nitrogen as involution occurs
5. Integumentary system: profuse diaphoresis as wastes are being excreted

Nursing Process During the Postpartal Period
Probable Nursing Diagnosis Based on Assessment

A. Impaired skin integrity related to episiotomy or laceration
B. Potential for infection related to inadequate perineal care
C. Constipation related to pain upon defecation and decreased peristalsis
D. Altered patterns of urinary elimination related to effects of anesthesia and edema of perineal area
E. Pain related to episiotomy, perineal edema, breast engorgement, or hemorrhoids
F. Sleep pattern disturbance related to discomfort, parenting activities, and anxiety
G. Anxiety related to insecurities about parental role and parenting activities
H. Knowledge deficit about parenting activities related to lack of experience
I. Potential altered parenting related to lack of support from significant others, interruption in bonding process, lack of knowledge, or unrealistic expectations for self, infant, or partner
J. Altered nutrition: less than body requirements related to increased need for protein for tissue repair and lactation
K. Impaired breastfeeding related to improper positioning, inverted nipples, or absence of infant sucking

Nursing Care During the Postpartal Period

A. Use aseptic techniques in giving perineal care; teach mother self-care

B. Inspect the breasts for tissue and nipple breakdown, palpate to rule out growths (teach breast self-examination for continued health), support breasts with well-fitted brassiere

C. Teach the importance of hand washing in caring for self and baby (important for personnel to avoid cross contamination)

D. Observe vital signs: a temperature of 100.4° F (38° C) or above for two consecutive days (excluding first 24 hours after delivery) considered sign of beginning puerperal infection; bradycardia is a normal phenomenon following delivery

E. Palpate the fundus for firmness and descent below the umbilical level (involution normally follows a one-finger breadth descent daily, by the fifth or sixth day fundus cannot be felt); a fundus that is boggy indicates poor contractile power of uterus and results in bleeding

F. Administer oxytocic medication as ordered to promote involution
   1. Ergonovine maleate (Ergotrate)
   2. Methylergonovine maleate (Methergine)
   3. Maintains the uterus in a slightly contracted state that controls bleeding from intrauterine sites and maintains tone, rate, and amplitude of rhythmic contractions required for involution of the uterus

G. Check lochia for color, amount, odor (foul odor indicates beginning infection); observe suture line for redness, ecchymosis, edema, or gapping

H. Assess for afterpains; more common in multiparas; treat as ordered

I. Promote bladder and bowel function

J. Encourage Kegel exercises to strengthen pubococcygeal muscles

K. Provide diet high in proteins and calories to restore body tissues

L. Ambulate early to prevent blood stasis

M. Monitor laboratory reports for Hgb, Hct, and WBC

N. Observe for postpartal blues, which may be caused by a drop in hormonal levels on the fourth or fifth day

O. Meet the mother's needs to enable her to meet the baby's needs

P. Assist the mother with self-care and care of the baby as needed

Q. Provide for group discussion on breast-feeding, infant care, etc.; encourage mother

R. Discuss resumption of intercourse and family planning; include information about when to expect menses

S. If Rh negative mother, assess need for administration of RhoGAM

T. Give rubella vaccine if indicated

U. Evaluate client's response and revise plan as necessary

The Newborn
ASSESSMENT OF FAMILY HISTORY

A. Chronic illness in the mother's or father's family

B. Previous medical-surgical illnesses of the mother and father

C. Age and present health status of the mother and father

D. History of previous pregnancies

E. Prenatal history
   1. Medical supervision during pregnancy
   2. Nutrition during pregnancy
   3. Course of pregnancy: illnesses, medications taken, or treatments required
   4. Duration of gestation
   5. Course and amount of sedation and anesthesia required
   6. Type of delivery and significant events during the immediate period after delivery
   7. Immediate response of newborn (Apgar score at 1 and 5 minutes following birth)

PROBABLE NURSING DIAGNOSES BASED ON ASSESSMENT OF THE NEWBORN

A. Ineffective airway clearance related to mucus obstruction

B. Potential for aspiration related to presence of meconium in amniotic fluid

C. Altered nutrition: less than body requirements, related to limited fluid intake or poor sucking ability

D. Pain related to circumcision and heel sticks for glucose, hematocrit, and PKU

E. Ineffective thermoregulation related to immaturity of nervous system

DETERMINANTS OF NURSING CARE TO FOSTER PARENT-CHILD RELATIONSHIPS

A. Concepts basic to parent-infant relationships
   1. Early and frequent parent-infant contact is essential for survival (bonding)
   2. Parenting abilities can be fostered and developed
   3. Biologic changes that occur at puberty and during pregnancy influence the development of nurturance
   4. Interaction between mother and child begins from the moment of conception and can be shared with the father
   5. Love for the infant grows as the parents interact and care for the infant
   6. As the parent gives to the infant and the infant receives, the parent in turn receives satisfaction from parenting tasks
   7. Any disturbance in the give-and-take cycle sets up frustrations in both the parent and the infant
   8. Parental behavior is learned and frequent parent-infant contact enhances development of parenting abilities

B. Infant's basic needs
   1. Physiological—food, clothing, bathing, and protection from environment
   2. Emotional—security, comfort, fondling, caressing, rocking, being spoken to, and contact with one person on a consistent basis

C. Mothering and fathering are
   1. Based on a biologic inborn desire to reproduce
   2. Role concepts that begin with own childhood experiences
   3. Primitive emotional relationships
   4. Maturing processes
   5. Conceptualizations of the physiologic and psychologic processes following infant's birth

6. Fostered by the parent-infant interaction that constantly reinforces gratification as needs are met and security develops
7. Abilities that are learned rather than innate

D. Parent-child relationships are affected by
1. Readiness for pregnancy
   a. Planned or unplanned
   b. Health status prior to pregnancy
   c. Financial status
   d. Determinants such as age, cultural backgrounds, number in family unit
   e. Political forces
2. Nature of the pregnancy
   a. Health status during pregnancy
   b. Preparation for parenthood
   c. Support from family members and members of the health team
3. Character of the labor and delivery
   a. Length and pattern of labor
   b. Type and amount of analgesia received
   c. Support from family and health team
   d. Anesthesia during delivery
   e. Type of delivery

E. Bonding
1. Significant phases
   a. Taking-in phase: mother's needs have to be met before she can meet the baby's; behavior: talks about self rather than the baby, doesn't seem too interested in the baby, doesn't touch the infant, cries easily
   b. Transition phase: characterized by the mother's starting to take hold, looking at and reaching for the baby, touching with fingertips, talking about the baby, etc.
   c. Taking-hold phase: kisses, embraces, gives care to infant, eye contact, uses whole hand to make contact, calls the baby by name, etc.
2. Nursing care to promote bonding
   a. Allow the parents to touch, fondle, and hold infant
   b. Give the mother ample time to inspect and begin to identify with baby
   c. Encourage give-and-take between parents and infant: rooming-in arrangement
   d. Support these beginning relationships
   e. Identify beginning of disturbed relationships
   f. Evaluate parent's and baby's response and revise plan as necessary

DETERMINANTS OF NURSING CARE TO FOSTER ADAPTATION TO EXTRAUTERINE LIFE

A. Immediate needs at the time of delivery
1. Aspiration of mucus to provide an open airway
2. Evaluation by use of Apgar score 1 and 5 minutes following birth (Table 6-1)
3. Maintenance of body temperature to prevent acidosis
4. Constant observation of physical condition
5. Eye care: prophylactic instillation of silver nitrate or other medication in each eye to prevent ophthalmia neonatorum

B. Appraisal of the newborn after delivery
1. Skin
   a. Body is normally pink with slight cyanosis of hands and feet for 24 hours (jaundice is abnormal during the first 24 to 48 hours of life)
   b. Check for abrasions, rashes, crackling, and elasticity, which indicates the status of tissue hydration; at times, milia (white pinpoint spots over the nose caused by retained sebaceous secretions), birthmarks, forceps marks, ecchymosis, or papules are present
2. Respirations are abdominal and irregular, with a rate of 30 to 50 per minute (retractions: depression of the sternum—are abnormal)
3. Head and sensory organs
   a. Head and chest circumference nearly equal to the crown-rump length; chest slightly smaller than head
   b. Symmetry of face: as the baby cries, sides of the face move equally
   c. Check the head for molding, abrasions, or skin breakdowns; observe for caput succedaneum: edema of soft tissue of the scalp; cephalhematoma: edema of the scalp caused by effusion of blood between the bone and periosteum; extend the head fully in all directions for adequacy in range of motion
   d. Observe the eyes for discharge or irritation; check the pupils for reaction to light, equality of eye movements (normally there is some ocular incoordination); check the sclerae for clarity, jaundice, or hemorrhage
   e. Nose: observe for patency of both nostrils
   f. Mouth: observe the gums and hard and soft palates for any openings; mucosa of the mouth normally clear (white patches that bleed on rubbing indicate thrush, a monilial infection)

Table 6-1. Apgar score chart*

Adaptation	0	1	2
Heart rate	Absent	Slow, below 100	Over 100
Respiratory effort	Absent	Weak cry	Strong cry
Muscle tone	Limp	Some flexion of extremities	Active motion
Reflex irritability	No response	Grimace	Cry
Color	Cyanotic, pale	Body pink, extremities cyanotic	Completely pink

*Scores: 7 to 10, good condition; 3 to 6, moderately depressed; 0 to 2, severely depressed.

g. Ears: auricles open; vernix covers tympanic membrane, making otoscopic examination useless (ring bell close to ear—baby should stir); both eyes should be same level as ears; upper earlobes normally curved (flatness indicative of kidney anomaly)

4. Chest and abdomen
   a. Chest auscultation: only respiratory sounds should be audible (noisy crackling sounds abnormal); heart rate: regular 120 to 160 per minute (rubbing or unusual sounds abnormal)
   b. Abdomen
      (1) Listen to bowel sounds over the abdomen
      (2) Palpate the spleen with fingertips under the left costal margin: tip should be palpable
      (3) Palpate liver on the right side: normally 1 cm below the costal margin
      (4) Observe umbilical cord for redness, odor, or discharge
      (5) Palpate the femoral pulses gently at inner aspect of the groin: indicate intact circulation to extremities

5. Genitalia
   a. Boys
      (1) Palpate the scrotum for testes: at times undescended at birth, which is normal (must descend by puberty or sperm will be destroyed by high temperature within the abdominal cavity)
      (2) Enlargement of scrotum: indicates hydrocele (diagnosis affirmed by transparent appearance of the scrotum when a flashlight is held close to the scrotal sac)
      (3) Observe tip of the penis for the urinary meatus: epispadias, meatus on upper surface of the penis; hypospadias, meatus on lower surface
   b. Girls: observe the genitalia for labia and vaginal opening; edema of labia and bloody mucoid discharge normal, resulting from transfer of maternal hormones

6. Extremities
   a. Hands and arms: thumbs clenched in fist
      (1) Check for number and variation of fingers
      (2) Check the clavicle and scapulae while putting arm through normal range of motion; clicking or resistance indicates dislocation or fracture
      (3) Palpate for fractures; crepitation is indicative
   b. Feet and legs
      (1) Check toes, pattern and number
      (2) Adduct and abduct feet through range of motion; there should be no resistance or tightness
      (3) Flex both legs onto the lower abdomen; there should be no resistance or tightness
      (4) Place both feet on a flat surface and bend the knees; knees should be at the same height (when unequal, known as Allis' sign, indicates hip dislocation)

7. Back: turn the baby on the abdomen, run a finger along the vertebral column; any separations or swellings indicative of spina bifida
8. Anus: patency confirmed with passage of meconium; inability to insert a rectal thermometer may be indicative of imperforate anus
9. Neuromuscular development: check reflexes
   a. Rooting: touch the baby's cheek; baby should search for finger
   b. Sucking: place an object close to the baby's mouth; baby should make an attempt to suck
   c. Grasp: place fingers in palm of the baby's hand and encircle palm with your hand; lift the infant off a firm surface, baby will grasp; infant's head will lag as baby is raised
   d. Babinski: run thumb up middle undersurface of infant's foot; toes will separate and flare out
   e. Plantar: run thumb up the lateral undersurface of infant's foot; toes will curl downward
   f. Moro: make a loud, sharp noise close to the baby; will result in the baby's bringing both arms and legs close to the body as if in an embrace (disappears by 4 months of age)
   g. Crawl: when the baby is on a firm surface and turned on its abdomen, crawling movements will follow
   h. Step or dance: while the infant is supported under both arms, stepping movements will occur when feet are placed on a firm surface

C. Changes in the newborn during the first week of life
   1. Circulatory
      a. Tying of cord at birth brings changes in fetal circulation: closure of the foramen ovale and ductus arteriosus and obliteration of the umbilical arteries produce an adultlike circulation within 1 hour after birth
      b. Heart rate regular; 120 to 180, but variable depending on the infant's activity; soft heart murmur common for first month of life
      c. Clotting mechanism poor because of low prothrombin concentration; vitamin K by injection is necessary
      d. Liver immature (although large): cannot destroy excessive red cells in the newborn, resulting in physiologic jaundice by third day
      e. Hemoglobin level high: 14 to 20 g/100 ml of blood
      f. White blood count high: 6,000 to 22,000
   2. Respiratory: respirations diaphragmatic, irregular, abdominal; 30 to 50 per minute, quiet with periods of apnea
   3. Excretory
      a. Kidneys immature: newborn should void during first 24 hours (2 weeks of age voids 20 times daily), albumin and urates (brick red staining on diaper) common during first week because of dehydration
      b. Stools: first stool, black-green and tenacious, called *meconium;* by third day, becomes mixed with light yellow, called *transitional*

4. Integumentary
   a. Lanugo: fine downy hair growth over the entire body
   b. Milia: small, whitish, pinpoint spots over the nose caused by retained sebaceous secretions
   c. Monogolian spots: blue-black discolorations on back, buttocks, and sacral region that disappear by first year
5. Digestive
   a. Has stores of nutrients from intrauterine existence; therefore needs very little nourishment first few days
   b. Roots and sucks when anything is brought to mouth
   c. Digests simple carbohydrates, fats, and proteins readily
   d. Cardiac sphincter of stomach not well developed, therefore regurgitates if stomach is over-full
   e. Needs to be bubbled frequently to get rid of air bubbles in stomach
6. Endocrine
   a. Metabolic: all newborns normally lose 10% of their body weight by first week of life
   b. PKU testing done 48 hours after ingestion of nutrients; infants with absence of phenylalanine will need special diet to prevent retardation
   c. Hormonal: enlargement of breasts in boys (gynecomastia) and girls is normal as a result of hormones transmitted to baby by mother
7. Neural
   a. CNS and brain not well developed: infant needs constant supply of oxygen
   b. Breathing, sucking, and crying are early neural activities necessary for the infant's survival

D. Needs of newborn
   1. Air for survival
      a. Suctioning of mucus as needed to maintain an open airway
      b. Positioning: side lying to facilitate drainage of mucus
      c. Observing any signs of air hunger (e.g., cyanosis, flaring of the nostrils, noisy respirations, sternal retractions) would warrant aspiration and administration of oxygen by inhalation
   2. Warmth, comfort, and protection from the environment
      a. Keep in a heated crib until body temperature is stabilized to prevent chilling; baby is unable to shiver and must break down brown fat to produce energy for warmth; premature or skinny infants can be compromised by chilling because they have a paucity of brown fat available for breakdown
      b. Clothing should be loose, soft
      c. Crib should be firm and provide protection
      d. Skin should be kept clean and dry to maintain integrity
   3. Human contact: body contact with another human is paramount for the newborn's survival; ministrations in giving care should be carried out with pur-

pose and awareness of the importance of these early beginning relationships (talking, rocking, singing are an essential part of body contact with a newborn)
   4. Food
      a. Initial weight loss of 10% of birth weight is normal and usually regained by tenth day of life
      b. Infant feeding usually delayed immediately after birth because of
         (1) General weakness and danger of aspiration
         (2) Reduced calorie requirement because of inactivity and low heat production of infant
      c. Phenylalanine cannot be detected until 24 hours after first feeding; tested 48 hours after first feeding
      d. Newborn needs to ingest simple proteins, carbohydrates, fats, vitamins, and minerals for continued cell growth
      e. Fluid (130 to 200 ml per kilogram or 2 to 3 oz fluid per pound of body weight)
      f. Calories (110 to 130 calories per kilogram or 50 to 60 calories per pound of body weight)
      g. Protein (2.2 to 2.0 g per kilogram of body weight from birth to 6 months of age; 1.8 g per kilogram of body weight from 6 to 12 months of age)
   5. Sleep: since sleep lowers body metabolism, it helps restore energy and assimilate nutriments for growth

BREAST-FEEDING
Determinants

A. Advantages
   1. Psychologic value of closeness and satisfaction in beginning mother-child relationship
   2. Optimum nutritional value for infant
   3. Economical and readily accessible
   4. Greater immunity to infection
   5. Infant is less likely to be allergic to mother's milk
   6. Develops facial muscles, jaw, and nasal passages of infant, since stronger sucking is necessary
   7. Assists in involution of uterus
   8. Reduces chances of infection because of maternal antibodies present in colostrum and milk
B. Prerequisites
   1. Psychologic readiness of mother is a major factor in successful breast-feeding
   2. Adequate diet must be available prenatally and postnatally to ensure high-quality milk
   3. Suitable rest, exercise, and freedom from tension for mother will provide increased satisfaction for both her and the infant
   4. Infant's sucking at the breast stimulates the maternal posterior pituitary to produce pitocin whose properties in the blood system constrict the lactiferous sinuses to move the milk down through the nipple ducts: known as the letdown reflex; a poor sucking reflex of the child will inhibit the letdown of milk; sucking also stimulates prolactin secretion
   5. Absence of emotional stress in the mother, since anxiety inhibits the letdown reflex

Nursing Care Related to Breast-Feeding

A. Teach feeding schedule
   1. Self-demand schedule is desirable
   2. Length of feeding time is usually 20 minutes with greatest quantity of milk consumed in first 5 to 10 minutes
B. Teach feeding techniques
   1. Mother and infant in comfortable position, such as semireclining or in rocking chair
   2. Entire body of infant should be turned towards mother's breast
   3. Initiate feeding by stimulating rooting reflex and direct nipple straight into baby's mouth (stroking cheek toward breast, being careful not to stroke other cheek, since this will confuse infant)
   4. Burp or bubble baby during and after feeding to allow for escape of air by
      a. Placing baby over shoulder
      b. Sitting baby on lap, flexed forward
      c. Rubbing or patting back (avoid jarring baby)
   5. Breast milk intake similar to formula intake
      a. 130 to 200 ml of milk per kilogram (2 to 3 oz of milk per pound) of body weight
      b. From one-sixth to one-seventh of baby's weight per day
   6. After lactation has been established, occasional bottle-feeding can be substituted
   7. Length of time for continuing breast-feeding is variable (may be discontinued when teeth erupt, since this can be uncomfortable for mother)
C. Teach care of breasts
   1. Cleanse with plain water once daily (soap or alcohol can cause irritation and dryness)
   2. Support breasts day and night with properly fitting brassiere
   3. Nursing pads should be placed inside bra cup to absorb any milk leaking between feedings
   4. Plastic bra liners should be avoided because they increase heat and perspiration and decrease air circulation necessary for drying of the nipple area

Contraindications

A. In mother
   1. Active tuberculosis
   2. Acute contagious disease
   3. Chronic disease such as cancer, advanced nephritis, cardiac disease
   4. Extensive surgery
   5. Narcotic addiction
B. In infant: cleft lip or palate or any other condition that interferes or prevents grasp of the nipple is the only real contraindication
C. Many drugs excreted in breast milk have harmful effects on the developing infant; these drugs must be avoided, or if they must be taken by the mother, breast-feeding is contraindicated; these drugs include:
   Analgesics and nonsteroidal antiinflammatory analgesics (NSAIA)
   Antibiotics (except cephalosporins, Mycostatin, oxacillin)
   Anticoagulants (except heparin)
   Anticonvulsants and sedatives
   Antihistamines
   Antineoplastic agents
   Autonomic drugs (except neostigmine, propantheline bromide)
   Cardiovascular drugs
   Diagnostic materials
   Diuretics (except furosemide)
   Heavy metals
   Hormones and contraceptives (except liothyronine sodium, medroxyprogesterone acetate)
   Narcotics
   Psychotropic agents
   Thyroid and antithyroid agents

BOTTLE-FEEDING
Determinants

A. Advantages
   1. Provides an alternative to breast-feeding
   2. Less restrictive than breast-feeding; may meet needs of working mothers
   3. Allows a more accurate assessment of intake
   4. May be indicated in the presence of a congenital anomaly such as cleft palate
   5. May be necessary for infants who require special formulas due to allergies or inborn errors of metabolism
B. Factors affecting success
   1. Pasteurization of milk
   2. Tuberculin testing of cows
   3. Sanitation in milk handling
   4. Adequate refrigeration and storage
   5. Preparation under clean conditions and sterilization to prevent contamination
   6. Formula designed to match nutrient ratio of breast milk composition: water dilution to reduce protein and mineral concentration; added carbohydrate to increase energy value
C. Types of formulas
   1. Fresh whole or skimmed milk
   2. Evaporated milk
   3. Dried milks (whole or skimmed)
   4. Commercial formulas

Nursing Care Related to Bottle-Feeding

A. Teach preparation of formula
   1. Calculation of formula to yield 110 to 130 calories and 130 to 200 ml of fluid per kilogram of body weight
   2. Proper preparation of formula by terminal heat method and feeding utensils (full 25 minutes of boiling)
   3. Proper refrigeration of formula
   4. Warming of formula before feeding by immersing bottle into warm water until approximately equal to body temperature (keep level of water in warmer below cap)
B. Teach feeding techniques
   1. Always hold infant during feeding to provide warm body contact (bottle propping may contribute to aspiration of formula)
   2. Hold bottle so nipple is always filled with milk to prevent excessive air ingestion

3. Adjust size of nipple hole to needs of baby (a premature infant needs a larger hole that requires less sucking)
4. After feeding and burping infant, place child on abdomen or side to aid digestion and prevent aspiration
5. Feeding should be offered on demand to meet the infant's needs

COMPARISON OF BREAST MILK AND COW'S MILK

	Breast milk	Cow's milk (whole)
Water	88%	88%
Protein	1.0% to 1.5%	3.5% to 4.0%
Sugar (lactose)	6.5% to 7.5%	4.5% to 5.0%
Fat	3.5% to 4.0%	3.5% to 5.0%
Minerals	0.15% to 0.25%	0.7% to 0.75%
Calories (per fluid ounce)	20	20

SELF-REGULATION SCHEDULE

A. Each infant born with different degree of maturity and rhythm of needs
B. Superior to rigid schedule, but should be modified to meet needs of infant and parents
C. Usually fed every 4 hours, with a nighttime feeding for first month, although schedule and amount are highly variable
D. Feeding behavior and degree of satisfaction reflect psychologic development of child
E. Close mother-infant relationship in feeding process meets basic need of trust (Erikson's stage of trust)

Deviations from the Normal Maternity Cycle in the Mother
COMPLICATIONS OF PREGNANCY
Pregnancy-induced Hypertension (PIH): Preeclampsia and Eclampsia (Formerly Referred to as Toxemia of Pregnancy)

A. Characterized by a triad of symptoms: edema, hypertension, and proteinuria occurring after the twentieth to twenty-fourth week of gestation and disappearing 6 weeks after delivery
B. Occurs in primiparas below 17 years of age and above 35 years of age, multiple pregnancies, women with chronic hypertension, diabetes mellitus, or severe nutritional deficiencies
C. Symptoms of pregnancy-induced hypertension
   1. Preeclampsia
      a. Mild: systolic pressure increased 30 mm/Hg or more above normal; diastolic pressure increased 15 mm/Hg or more above normal; proteinuria 1+; edema manifested by excessive weekly weight gain
      b. Severe: BP is 160/110 or above on two readings taken 6 hours apart after bed rest; proteinuria 3+ to 4+; extensive edema (puffiness of hands and face)
   2. Eclampsia: convulsions and/or coma associated with hypertension, proteinuria, and edema

D. Guidelines for prevention of pregnancy-induced hypertension
   1. Sound nutrition counseling during pregnancy and lactation: vitamins and minerals should complement a nutritious, protein-rich diet
   2. An additional 30 to 60 mg of supplemental iron daily in the second and third trimester (continue for 2 to 3 months postpartally in breast-feeding mother)
   3. Caloric intake should be increased 10% during pregnancy; severe calorie restriction is harmful during pregnancy
   4. Restriction of sodium is harmful during pregnancy and can result in electrolyte imbalance and elimination of essential nutritional components; may contribute to reduced circulatory volume
   5. Diuretics are contraindicated during pregnancy, since they cause hypovolemia and deplete essential nutrients for mother and fetus

Nursing Process for Clients with Pregnancy-induced Hypertension
Probable Nursing Diagnoses Based on Assessment

A. Fluid volume excess related to decreased urine output
B. Potential for injury related to sedation and possible convulsions
C. Anxiety related to course of pregnancy and possible death of fetus
D. Disturbance in body image related to massive edema and possible convulsions

Treatment and Nursing Care for Clients with Pregnancy-induced Hypertension

A. Treatment and nursing care for clients with preeclampsia
   1. High-protein diet
   2. Ambulatory care: frequent visits to obstetrician
   3. Instructions to report headaches, dizziness, blurring of vision, and scotoma
   4. Sedatives to ensure rest and sleep
   5. Blood chemistry: rise in hematocrit, uric acid, blood urea nitrogen, and decrease in CO_2 combining power indicate worsening of preeclampsia
   6. Qualitative urinalysis: increase in albumin output and/or decrease in urinary output indicates worsening of preeclampsia
   7. Administration of albumin concentrate increases renal flow by correcting the hypovolemia
   8. Conserve energy to decrease metabolic rate
   9. Assess anxieties and concerns
   10. Monitor to protect mother and fetus (includes respiratory rate, pulse, FHR, weight, intake and output, BP)
   11. Nonstress test (see Assessment techniques for high-risk pregnancy)
   12. Evaluate client's response and revise plan as necessary
B. Treatment and nursing care for clients with severe preeclampsia or impending eclampsia
   1. Hospitalization and complete bed rest
   2. Check vital signs, FHR, irritability, restlessness, signs of labor

3. When the client is receiving magnesium sulfate therapy, check frequently for depression of patellar reflexes and respirations (these side effects can be treated with the administration of calcium gluconate to the mother and levallorphan [Lorfan] to the newborn if respiratory depression occurs); magnesium sulfate also causes dizziness, diaphoresis, flushing, a feeling of warmth, and vomiting

4. Emergency equipment for possible convulsion, equipment to maintain an open airway, suction and oxygen, sedatives such as morphine sulfate and sodium luminal, tracheotomy set readily available on unit

5. Insertion of a Foley catheter ensures accurate measurement of urinary output

6. Limitation of visitors and reduction of environmental stimuli

7. Daily blood chemistry testing

8. Once symptoms are under control, labor may be induced or emergency cesarean delivery performed

9. Continue monitoring for 48 hours after delivery

10. Avoid all ergot products because of their hypertensive effects

11. Evaluate client's response and revise plan as necessary

Bleeding During the Maternity Cycle

Bleeding is an abnormal sign indicating a possible interruption of pregnancy

Nursing Process for Clients Experiencing Bleeding During the Maternity Cycle
Probable Nursing Diagnoses Based on Assessment

A. Anxiety related to unknown course of pregnancy and threat to life of mother or fetus

B. Anticipatory grieving related to outcome of pregnancy, threat of termination of childbearing ability, and loss of body part (uterus, ovary, fallopian tube)

C. Fluid volume deficit related to bleeding

D. Altered cardiopulmonary tissue perfusion related to hemorrhage

E. Situational low self-esteem related to feeling of guilt about failure to carry pregnancy to term

Nursing Care for Clients Experiencing Bleeding During the Maternity Cycle

A. Institute measures to alleviate fear and anxiety; assist with grieving process

B. Point out physiological reality, but encourage client to work through feelings of guilt

C. Encourage participation with thanatology services and bereavement groups when appropriate

D. Monitor amount and type of bleeding
   1. Save and count number of pads
   2. Distinguish between dark clotted blood and frank bleeding, which is bright red

E. Monitor vital signs; assess for hypovolemia and shock

F. Monitor laboratory work; prepare for administration of blood

G. Observe for signs of labor and imminent delivery

H. Monitor fetal heart if pregnancy is beyond twentieth week

I. Administer oxygen in late trimester bleeding

J. Maintain fluid and electrolyte balance

K. Provide double set-up (vaginal and cesarean) when vaginal examination is performed in suspected placenta previa

L. Administer RhoGAM to Rh negative client after abortion or delivery

M. Educate about necessity for follow-up care

N. Evaluate client's response and revise plan as necessary

First Trimester Bleeding

A. Abortion (see also induced abortion)
   1. Interruption of pregnancy in which there is complete expulsion or partial expulsion (incomplete) of the products of conception
   2. May be sudden, spontaneous, or induced by some external mechanical force
   3. Treatment consists of bed rest, immediate blood count, blood typing, Rh incompatibility, and cross-matching with availability of blood
   4. Vital signs and observing for signs of labor will indicate course of abortion and treatment
   5. Complete abortion: 24 to 48 hours observation for bleeding is imperative
   6. Incomplete abortion: dilation and curettage performed to empty the uterus of retained products of conception; same observation as with complete abortion
   7. Probable nursing diagnoses based on assessment
      a. Anxiety related to impending loss of pregnancy
      b. Anticipatory grieving related to loss of expected baby
      c. Pain related to uterine contractions
      d. Situational low self-esteem related to inability to carry pregnancy to term

B. Ectopic pregnancy
   1. Pregnancy in which implantation occurs outside the uterus (most frequent site is middle portion of fallopian tube, other sites are abdomen, ovaries, or cervix)
   2. Early signs and symptoms are usually concealed
   3. Pattern in tubal pregnancy is usually one in which spotting may occur after one or two missed menstrual periods, sharp lower right or left abdominal pain radiating to shoulder develops, concealed bleeding from site of rupture leads to sudden shock
   4. Treatment is immediate blood replacement and surgical removal of ruptured fallopian tube
   5. Probable nursing diagnoses based on assessment
      a. Pain related to tubal rupture
      b. Anticipatory grieving related to loss of expected baby
      c. Fear related to potential disturbance in future childbearing ability

Midtrimester Bleeding

A. Hydatidiform mole
   1. An abnormal pregnancy in which there is a benign growth of the chorion
   2. Spontaneous expulsion usually occurs between the sixteenth and eighteenth weeks of pregnancy
   3. Symptoms of PIH are common

4. Diagnosis: suspected when uterus is excessively large for period of gestation and fetal parts are not palpable
5. Treatment: if spontaneous evacuation does not occur, evacuation by delicate curettage or hysterotomy is performed
6. Dangers include uterine perforation, hemorrhage, and infection
7. Continued follow-up of serum gonadotropin levels is imperative for 1 year to rule out metastasis from chorionic carcinoma (increased gonadotropin levels warrant immediate hysterectomy)
8. Preventing a new pregnancy is essential for 1 year
9. Probable nursing diagnoses based on assessment
   a. Disturbance in self-esteem and/or body image related to carrying an abnormal pregnancy
   b. Fear related to development of cancer
   c. Ineffective coping related to uncertainty of continuing pregnancy associated with frequent human chorionic gonadotropin (HCG) level monitoring
B. Incompetent cervix
   1. Expulsion of products of conception due to cervical effacement and dilation in early midtrimester
   2. May result from forceful dilation and currettage, difficult delivery, or congenitally short cervix
   3. Painless contractions leading to delivery of dead or nonviable fetus
   4. Treatment includes cerclage procedure during fourteenth to sixteenth week of gestation; suture or ribbon placed beneath cervical mucosa to close cervix
   5. Probable nursing diagnoses based on assessment
      a. Situational low self-esteem related to inability to complete pregnancy
      b. Anticipatory grieving related to loss of expected baby
      c. Disturbance in body image related to feelings of failure and feelings of guilt associated with inability to complete pregnancy

Third Trimester Bleeding

A. Placenta previa
   1. Implantation of the embryo in the lower uterine segment
   2. Three types: marginal (placental edge is close to internal os), partial (placenta partially covers internal os), and complete (placenta completely covers internal os)
   3. Painless bleeding in the latter part of pregnancy is only symptom
   4. Treatment is to control bleeding: cesarean delivery may be performed
B. Abruptio placentae
   1. Premature separation of a normally implanted placenta
   2. Symptoms: with partially detached placenta there is external vaginal bleeding; with totally detached placenta, there is concealed bleeding, excruciating abdominal pain, and a boardlike abdominal wall
   3. Common in individuals with PIH, essential hypertension, and an abnormally short umbilical cord

4. Treatment
   a. Replacement of blood loss
   b. With fetal distress: emergency cesarean delivery
   c. Without fetal distress and in the presence of some cervical effacement and dilation: induction of labor may be attempted
C. Probable nursing diagnoses based on assessment
   1. Fear related to severe pain (abruptio placentae), frank bleeding (placenta previa), and possible death of fetus
   2. Pain related to pressure of trapped blood
   3. Anxiety related to unknown course of pregnancy and possibility of cesarean delivery
   4. Altered cardiopulmonary tissue perfusion in both mother and fetus related to hemmorhage and interruption of placental oxygen supply
   5. Sleep pattern disturbance related to frequent examinations

Postpartal Bleeding

A. Bleeding in excess of 500 ml within the first 24 hours following delivery
B. Frequent causes are uterine atony, vaginal and cervical lacerations, and retained placental fragments (bleeding occurring after 24 hours is usually caused by retained placental fragments)
C. Treatment for atony: massage fundal portion of uterus, administer oxytocics, and, with severe blood loss, blood replacement
D. Bleeding caused by retained placental fragments necessitates manual removal
E. Vaginal and cervical lacerations require surgical repair
F. Disseminated intravascular coagulopathy (DIC)
   1. Pathologic form of clotting
   2. Profuse uncontrollable bleeding from uterus; oozing of blood from episiotomy, laceration, or IV site
   3. Fragmental or distorted RBCs; decreased coagulation factors
   4. May occur from sepsis or shock
   5. Treatment includes cryoprecipitate, fresh frozen plasma
G. Probable nursing diagnoses based on assessment
   1. Fear related to uncontrollable bleeding and possible death
   2. Altered parenting related to interruption in bonding process
   3. Alterred cardiopulmonary tissue perfusion relative to hemorrhage resulting from uterine relaxation following birth and/or cervical laceration
   4. Altered cerebral or peripheral tissue perfusion related to pathologic clotting
   5. Fluid volume deficit related to hemorrhage

DEVIATIONS FROM THE NORMAL LABOR AND DELIVERY PROCESS
Nursing Diagnoses for Clients with Deviations from the Normal Labor and Delivery Process

A. See Nursing diagnoses under the specific deviations
B. See Nursing diagnoses during the intrapartal period and related nursing diagnoses for clients with reproductive disturbances

Induction of Labor

A. Elective induction: initiation of labor contractions by
   1. Pharmacologic means
      a. Administration of oxytocin (Pitocin) by infusion pump
      b. Vaginal insertion of prostaglandins
   2. Mechanical means
      a. Artificial rupture of membranes (amniotomy)
      b. Insertion of laminaria
      c. Breast stimulation
   3. May be done for medical or obstetric reasons; medical: diabetes, pyelonephritis; obstetric: PIH, Rh incompatibility, polyhydramnios, abruptio placentae, premature rupture of membranes at term without onset of labor
B. Augmentation of labor: assisting client when labor process is not progressing normally (prolonged labor) by pharmacologic or mechanical means
C. Induction or augmentation of labor is not done with cephalopelvic disproportion or malpresentation of fetus

Nursing Process During Induction of Labor
Probable Nursing Diagnoses Based on Assessment

A. Potential for trauma related to possibility of sustained contractions associated with administration of oxytocin, fetal cord prolapse following amniotomy, and mechanical method of induction
B. Potential for infection related to ruptured membranes and introduction of foreign bodies into vagina and uterus
C. Pain related to use of oxytocics
D. Anxiety related to uncertainty of the labor and delivery process

Nursing Care of Clients During Induction of Labor

A. Prepare mother and labor coach for induction
   1. Explain all procedures
   2. Obtain informed consent whenever necessary
B. Remain with mother and partner at all times
C. Obtain and record baseline information such as maternal vital signs, FHR, contractions for later comparison; continue to monitor all vital indices
D. Monitor Pitocin IV rate
   1. Increase drip rate until 2- to 3-minute contractions occur
   2. Discontinue Pitocin drip if
      a. A sustained uterine contraction occurs
      b. Fetal accelerations/decelerations persist
      c. Urinary flow decreases to 30 ml per hour; related to water intoxication
      d. Signs of placenta previa or abruptio placentae appear
E. Assist with artificial rupture of membranes (amniotomy)
   1. Maintain asepsis
   2. Immediately after rupture, monitor FHR
   3. Record time of rupture; prolonged membrane rupture may predispose client to sepsis
F. Maintain hydration
G. Provide for blood typing, Rh compatibility, crossmatching, and availability of blood
H. Have oxygen, suction, and resuscitation equipment readily available
I. Prepare for emergency cesarean delivery if necessary
J. Evaluate client's response and revise plan as necessary

Preterm or Premature Labor

A. Begins after twenty-eighth week but before thirty-seventh week gestation
B. Treatment
   1. Bed rest; left lateral position
   2. Tocolytic therapy (directed toward postponing labor)
      a. Terbutaline sulfate (Brethine)
      b. Ritodrine hydrochloride (Yutopar); administered intravenously first and then orally; used most often
      c. Magnesium sulfate

Nursing Process During Preterm or Premature Labor
Probable Nursing Diagnoses Based on Assessment

A. Anxiety related to uncertainty of the labor and delivery process and safety of the baby
B. Actual or potential altered parenting related to the physical condition of the baby
C. Parental role conflict related to need for specialized care and continued hospitalization of the newborn
D. Situational low self-esteem related to failure to carry pregnancy to full term

Nursing Care of Clients During Preterm or Premature Labor

A. Monitor vital signs, fetal heart rate, contractions, and progression of labor
B. Provide emotional support: reduce anxiety and prepare for possible loss of baby
C. Provide special care related to the administration of tocolytic medications
   1. Obtain baseline blood data and ECG readings
   2. Monitor vital signs; tachycardia and hypotension can occur
   3. Maintain hydration but monitor for pulmonary edema
   4. Monitor for signs of hypokalemia
   5. Monitor blood glucose levels
   6. Monitor intake and output
   7. Monitor neurological reflexes
D. Prepare for premature birth if labor continues
E. Evaluate client's response and revise plan as necessary

Postterm or Postdate Labor

A. Extends 2 weeks or 14 days past expected due date
   1. Poses no physiological risk for mother
   2. Decreased blood, oxygen, and nutrition to fetus because of placental change (decreased growth)
B. Induction of labor

Difficult Labor (Dystocia)

A. Mechanical
   1. Caused by contracted pelvis, obstruction in pelvis, malpresentation or position of fetus
   2. Treatment for mechanical dystocia is cesarean delivery

B. Functional
   1. Caused by faulty uterine contractions
   2. Treatment for functional dystocia: oxytocics to stimulate labor or cesarean delivery; deciding factors are length of labor, condition of mother and fetus, amount of cervical effacement and dilation, presentation, position, and station of presenting part

Nursing Process During Dystocia
Probable Nursing Diagnoses Based on Assessment

A. Pain related to prolonged unproductive contractions, administration of oxytocics, and cesarean delivery if necessary
B. Fatigue related to prolonged difficult labor
C. Anxiety related to the uncertainty of labor process
D. Potential for trauma related to failure of cervix to dilate adequately and/or mechanical problems

Nursing Care for Clients with Dystocia

A. Relieve back pain, caused by prolonged posterior pressure from fetus, by applying sacral pressure during contraction
B. Observe for signs of maternal exhaustion such as elevation of body temperature, fruity odor to breath, diminished urinary output with positive acetone reaction
C. Observe for signs of fetal distress
D. Have oxygen, suction, and resuscitation equipment readily available
E. Constantly monitor contractions, FHR, and vital signs when client is receiving oxytocic stimulation
F. Provide emotional support; keep client and family informed about progress
G. Evaluate client's response and revise plan as necessary

Precipitate Delivery

A. Rapid labor and delivery of less than 2-hour duration
B. Hazards to mother are perineal laceration and postpartum hemorrhage
C. Hazards to baby are anoxia and intracranial hemorrhage

Nursing Process During Precipitate Delivery
Probable Nursing Diagnoses Based on Assessment

A. Potential for maternal injury related to rapid expulsion of fetus resulting in lacerations and hemorrhage
B. Potential for fetal trauma related to cranial battering during rapid delivery

Nursing Care for Clients with Precipitate Labor

A. Remain with mother
B. Move to delivery room if possible or prepare for delivery in bed
C. Evaluate client's response and revise plan as necessary

Breech Delivery

Position of the baby in which the buttocks alone or the buttocks and feet descend through the birth canal first

Nursing Process During Breech Delivery
Nursing Diagnoses Based on Assessment

A. Pain related to prolonged posterior pressure from fetus
B. Potential for injury to baby related to possible prolapse of cord

Nursing Care of Clients with a Breech Delivery

A. Monitor the FHR in upper quadrants
B. Watch for prolapsed cord; if it occurs:
   1. Place the client in a knee-chest or Trendelenburg position to keep presenting part away from the cord
   2. Cover the cord with moist, sterile dressing to keep it from drying
C. Observation of frank meconium results from contraction of the uterus on lower colon of the fetus; not significant in breech delivery
D. Add Piper forceps to the delivery table if vaginal delivery is done
E. Prepare client for cesarean delivery; usually done in primigravidas
F. Evaluate client's response and revise plan as necessary

Cesarean Delivery

A. Delivery of baby via transabdominal incision
B. Indicated in cephalopelvic disproportion, dystocia, placenta previa and abruptio placentae, postmaturity, growths within the birth canal, diabetes, PIH, Rh incompatibility, malpresentation, fetal distress

Nursing Process During Cesarean Delivery
Nursing Diagnoses Based on Assessment

A. Pain related to incision and/or flatus associated with decreased peristalsis
B. Potential for infection related to surgical incision
C. Potential for trauma related to pelvic surgery
D. Situational low self-esteem related to inability to deliver vaginally

Nursing Care for Client with a Cesarean Delivery

A. Assist with bonding; offer emotional support; encourage touching; include father in process
B. Encourage early ambulation to prevent blood stasis
C. Check vital signs, fundus, and abdominal incision
D. Encourage eating of solids to promote peristalsis (prevents distention)
E. Record intake and output
F. Give analgesics as ordered
G. Promote lung aeration
H. Maintain fluid and electrolyte balance
I. Monitor urinary output
J. Evaluate client's response and revise plan as necessary

Childbirth Injuries

Injuries sustained by the mother as a result of pregnancy

Nursing Process Associated with Childbirth Injuries
Probable Nursing Diagnoses Based on Type of Injury and Assessment

A. Pain related to trauma to the perineum and/or displacement of reproductive organs
B. Potential for trauma related to a tear or rupture of an organ of reproduction
C. Stress incontinence (urinary or bowel) related to trauma associated with childbirth
D. Situational low self-esteem related to altered body function or loss of child-bearing ability

Nursing Care of Clients With Childbirth Injuries

See specific injury for related nursing care

Type of Childbirth Injury

A. Episiotomy: incision into the perineum to facilitate delivery and prevent lacerations and overstretching of the pelvic floor
  1. Routine procedure: closed surgically
  2. Nursing care
     a. Apply cold to limit edema
     b. Keep area clean and dry
     c. Administer analgesics as ordered for comfort
     d. Apply heat and local spray medications
     e. Teach perineal exercise
     f. Evaluate client's response to procedure
B. Lacerations are tears of the perineum or vulva resulting from a difficult or precipitate delivery: characterized as first, second, third, or fourth degree depending on the amount of involvement
  1. Treatment: surgical repair
  2. Nursing care: same as above; however, healing is slower following repair of a laceration
C. Relaxations of the vaginal outlet: an overstretching of the perineal supporting tissues resulting from childbirth (see Cystocele and rectocele in Medical-Surgical Nursing)
  1. Cystocele: a herniation of anterior vaginal wall with the descent and protrusion of the bladder
  2. Rectocele: a herniation of the pararectal fascia into the vagina
     a. Signs and symptoms: backache, feeling of heaviness and bearing down in the lower abdomen, urinary stress incontinence, (cystocele), and constipation (rectocele)
     b. Treatment: Kegel's exercises for stress incontinence (after childbearing period is completed, vaginoplasty is done)
     c. Nursing care with vaginoplasty consists of keeping perineal area clean and dry with insertion of Foley catheter or suprapubic catheter, warm sitz baths once healing has begun, analgesics for discomfort, antibiotics to prevent infection, high-protein diet to promote tissue repair; ambulation may be delayed to promote healing but leg motion and deep breathing are essential
D. Uterine prolapse: condition in which the uterus is found in a position lower than normal resulting from stretching and tearing of tissues during childbirth (see Prolapsed uterus in Medical-Surgical Nursing)
  1. Signs and symptoms: bearing-down sensation and a feeling of a dropping of the pelvic organs, leukorrhea with marked congestion of cervix or lacerations of exposed vaginal walls, frequency with retention, and eventually cystitis
  2. Treatment: dependent on age, desire for more children, and severity of symptoms; pessaries may be used as temporary measure; surgical intervention is usually a vaginal hysterectomy
E. Displacement of uterus: results from lesions of the pelvic organs or stretching and relaxation of the ligaments supporting the uterus (may be congenital or result from the trauma of childbirth)
  1. Signs and symptoms: backache, excessive bleeding during menstruation, sense of pressure or fullness

  2. Treatment: insertion of a pessary to relieve symptoms; severe symptoms warrant surgical intervention
F. Rupture of the uterus: usually occurs after the fetus reaches a viable size
  1. Causes: perforation during attempted abortion, rupture of a previous uterine scar, spontaneous rupture of an intact uterus with the abdominal overdistention that can occur with abruptio placentae, and/or labor induction
  2. Treatment: relieve symptoms of shock from hemorrhage and surgical intervention (the extent of surgical intervention depends on degree of rupture; usually hysterectomy)
  3. Nursing care for clients following hysterectomy
     a. Maintain patency of urinary catheter
     b. Assess urinary output while catheter is in place and after it is removed
     c. Monitor fluid and electrolyte balance
     d. Encourage coughing and deep breathing at frequent intervals
     e. Assess for gas pains and administer Harris flush, if ordered
     f. Institute measures, such as frequent ambulation and elevation of extremities when in a chair, to prevent thrombophlebitis
     g. Provide emotional support; encourage and provide for ventilation of feelings
     h. Provide postoperative teaching
        (1) Explain need to avoid driving for 3 to 6 weeks
        (2) Explain need to avoid sexual intercourse, dancing, jogging, and heavy lifting for 6 to 8 weeks
        (3) Emphasize importance of follow-up supervision
     i. Evaluate client's response and revise plan as necessary

Health Problems That Create a Risk During Pregnancy
ASSESSMENT TECHNIQUES FOR HIGH-RISK PREGNANCY

A. AFP—(alpha-fetoprotein) enzyme blood test: elevated levels may identify the pregnant woman carrying a baby with neural tube defects (spina bifida and anencephaly); may also indicate twins; if the AFP is elevated for two samples, it is followed by ultrasonography and amniocentesis for further confirmation; done at 14 to 16 weeks gestation
B. Ultrasonography: high-frequency sound wave testing; discerns placental location and gestational age by measurement of biparietal diameters
Nursing care: the client is encouraged to drink and refrain from voiding before the test to improve visualization
C. Chorionic villi sampling (CVS): supplies same data as amniocentesis but can be done earlier, and quicker results can be obtained
  1. Aspiration of villi done during the eighth to twelfth week of pregnancy
  2. Nursing care
     a. Obtain informed consent

b. Instruct client to drink water so that bladder is full
c. Place client in lithotomy position
d. After test monitor for uterine contractions, vaginal discharge, and teach client to observe for signs of infection

D. Amniocentesis: aspiration of amniotic fluid used to detect sex, chromosomal or biochemical defects, fetal age, L/S ratio (2/1 ratio indicates lung maturity), and increased bilirubin level associated with Rh disease
   1. Test done after sonogram; usually after 15 to 18 weeks of gestation
   2. Nursing care
      a. Obtain informed consent
      b. Explain procedure and expectations of client
      c. Have client empty bladder
      d. After test monitor for uterine contractions, vaginal discharge; teach client to observe for signs of infection and to remain on bed rest for 24 hours

E. Serum estriol levels: confirms healthy fetal-placental functioning; done particularly for clients with diabetes mellitus
   1. Results: falling levels at term may be indicative of impending fetal stress; two or more tests necessary to make diagnosis
   2. Nursing care: encourage the mother to return for testing; evaluate client's response to procedure

F. Nonstress test: to observe for accelerations of FHR in response to fetal movement
   1. Classification of results
      a. Reactive: two or more accelerations of FHR of 15 beats per minute lasting 15 seconds throughout any fetal movement; no intervention necessary
      b. Nonreactive: no FHR acceleration or accelerations less than 15 seconds; further monitoring necessary with use of the oxytocin challenge test
      c. Unsatisfactory: recording uninterpretable; test should be repeated in 24 hours
   2. Nursing care: observation of the fetal monitor; explanation of test to decrease the mother's anxiety; evaluate client's response to procedure

G. Oxytocin challenge test (OCT): to demonstrate whether a healthy fetus can withstand a decreased oxygen supply during the stress of a contraction produced by exogenous oxytocin (Pitocin); if late decelerations appear, the fetus may be compromised due to uteroplacental insufficiency
   1. Classification of results
      a. Negative: no late decelerations with a minimum of three contractions in 10 minutes; indicates that the fetus has good chance of surviving labor
      b. Positive: persistent and late decelerations occurring with more than half the contractions; indicates the need for considering premature intervention
      c. Suspicious: late decelerations occurring in less than half of uterine contractions; test should be repeated in 24 hours
   2. Nursing care: conscientious monitoring of the mother after the test to observe for possible initiation of labor; evaluate client's response to procedure

H. Biophysical profile (BPP): assesses breathing movements, body movements, tone, amniotic fluid volume, and FHR reactivity; a score of 2 is assigned to each finding, with a score of 8 to 10 indicating a healthy fetus
   1. Used for fetus that may have intrauterine compromise
   2. Nursing care: provide emotional support
   3. Evaluate client's response to procedure

I. Maternal assessment of fetal activity: need to contact physician or nurse midwife when there are fewer than 10 fetal movements in a 12-hour period, fewer than 3 fetal movements in an 8-hour period, or no fetal movements in the morning
   1. Used to determine vitality of fetus
   2. Nursing care: teach client how to record and report movements

J. Fetal scalp pH sampling: may be done during labor when fetal heart patterns begin to indicate distress; capillary blood samples are taken from the fetal scalp in utero
   1. Results: if acidosis present, immediate delivery of infant is indicated
   2. Nursing care: cleanse the vaginal area to avoid contamination when the test is done

HEART DISEASE

A. Origin: 90% rheumatic (incidence expected to decrease as incidence of rheumatic fever decreases); 10% congenital lesions or syphilis

B. Normal hemodynamics of pregnancy that adversely affect the client with heart disease
   1. Oxygen consumption increased 10% to 20%; related to needs of growing fetus
   2. Plasma level and blood volume increase and RBCs remain same (physiologic anemia)

C. Functional or therapeutic classification of heart disease during pregnancy
   1. Class I: no limitation of physical activity; no symptoms of cardiac insufficiency
   2. Class II: slight limitation of physical activity; may experience excessive fatigue, palpitation, or dyspnea in last trimester
   3. Class III: moderate to marked limitation of physical activity; bed rest indicated during most of pregnancy
   4. Class IV: marked limitation of physical activity; pregnancy should be avoided; indication for termination of pregnancy

Nursing Process for Pregnant Clients with Heart Disease
Probable Nursing Diagnoses Based on Assessment

A. Activity intolerance related to increased cardiac workload

B. Anxiety related to unknown course of pregnancy, possible loss of fetus, and inability to perform role responsibilities

C. Fear related to possible death

D. Fluid volume excess related to fluid shifts resulting from a decrease in intraabdominal pressure following delivery and/or a decrease in vascular space resulting from cessation of need for fetal circulation and uterine blood flow following delivery

Nursing Care for Pregnant Clients with Heart Disease

A. Prenatal period
1. Teach importance of rest and avoidance of stress
2. Instruct regarding use of elastic stockings
3. Teach importance of continued medical supervision by cardiologist
4. Teach appropriate dietary intake
   a. Adequate calories to ensure appropriate weight gain
   b. Limited, not restricted, salt intake
5. Administer medications as ordered; digitalis preparations, iron preparations, and prophylactic antibiotics (penicillin)

B. Intrapartal period
1. Encourage mother to remain in semi-Fowler's or left lateral position
2. Provide continuous cardiac monitoring
3. Provide electronic fetal monitoring
4. Assist mother to cope with discomfort; minimal analgesia and anesthesia is used
5. Assist with forceps delivery in second stage of labor to avoid work of pushing

C. Postpartal period: most critical time due to increased circulating blood volume after delivery of placenta
1. Institute early ambulation schedule; apply elastic stockings
2. Monitor for signs of congestive heart failure, such as respiratory distress and tachycardia
3. Refer to various agencies for family aid, if necessary, on discharge
4. Monitor heart rate; accelerated heart rate of mother in latter half of pregnancy puts extra workload on her heart
5. Provide for adequate rest; the increase in oxygen consumption with contractions during labor makes length of labor a significant factor
6. Keep under close supervision; the sudden tachycardia during delivery or the sudden bradycardia and the normal increase in cardiac output following delivery may cause cardiac arrest

DIABETES MELLITUS

A. Normal physiology of pregnancy that affects pregnant woman with diabetes
1. Vomiting during pregnancy, especially in first trimester, decreases carbohydrate intake with resulting acidosis
2. Increased activity of anterior pituitary decreases the tolerance for sugar
3. Elevated basal metabolic rate and decrease in carbon dioxide combining power increase tendency toward acidosis
4. Normal lowered renal threshold for glucose can result in glucosuria that might confuse diabetic picture
5. Muscular activity during labor depletes glycogen; therefore carbohydrate intake must be increased
6. During puerperium, hypoglycemia is common as involution and lactation occur

B. Hazards of diabetes during pregnancy
1. Often there is a history of repeated stillbirths and fetal deaths

2. Babies are excessively large, weighing over 4000 g
3. Neonatal deaths occur as a result of hypoxia, hypoglycemia, congenital anomalies, and premature labor
4. Toxemia and hydramnios are common
5. Insulin therapy instituted; oral hypoglycemics contraindicated
6. Frequent hospitalization may be necessary during prenatal period
7. Cesarean delivery usually indicated

Nursing Process for Pregnant Clients with Diabetes Mellitus
Probable Nursing Diagnoses Based on Assessment

A. Altered nutrition: less than body requirements related to fetal growth and increased maternal metabolism
B. Fluid volume deficit related to osmotic diuresis
C. Potential trauma related to large size of infant
D. Potential for infection related to increased susceptibility
E. Knowledge deficit related to newly diagnosed diabetes mellitus or management of previously diagnosed diabetes mellitus during pregnancy

Nursing Care for Pregnant Clients with Diabetes Mellitus

A. Encourage early medical and prenatal supervision
B. Encourage adherence to dietary regimen
C. Teach signs and symptoms of hyperglycemia (acidosis) and hypoglycemia (insulin reaction)
D. Teach hygiene and avoidance of stress
E. Teach urine testing and fingerstick procedures
F. Teach insulin administration
G. Reinforce need for various tests for fetal well-being, such as ultrasound, stress and nonstress tests, amniocentesis for L/S ratios and estriol levels
H. Prepare client for induction of labor or cesarean delivery if indicated
I. Continue monitoring for fluid and electrolyte balance and ketoacidosis during intrapartal and postpartal periods
J. Evaluate client's response and revise plan as necessary

Nursing Care for Infant of Diabetic Mother

A. Admit infant to neonatal intensive care unit
B. Keep the infant warm because of poor temperature control mechanisms
C. Observe respiration (stomach aspiration imperative at time of delivery, since hydramnios inflates stomach, which pushes up and interferes with diaphragm)
D. Observe for signs of hypoglycemia and hypocalcemia such as lethargy, poor sucking reflex, cyanosis, or muscular twitching; lowered blood glucose to 30 to 45 mg/dl
E. Provide glucose water feeding to prevent acidosis (with poor sucking reflex, glucose should be given parenterally)
F. Observe for congenital anomalies; there is an increased incidence in babies of diabetic mothers
G. Promote early mother-child interaction
H. Evaluate infant's response and revise plan as necessary

Deviations from the Normal Maternity Cycle in the Newborn
PRETERM (PREMATURE) OR LOW-BIRTH-WEIGHT INFANT

A. Prevention
1. Education of teenagers (prior to planning a family) in nutrition and general hygiene
2. Education of teenagers to the hazards of drug use and smoking
3. Adequate and early prenatal health supervision
4. Provisions for adequate housing and financial aid to persons of lower socioeconomic means
5. Adequate community agencies to facilitate available services to persons in need
6. Higher prematurity rates and low-birth-weight babies are frequently associated with malnutrition and underweight in the mother

B. Definitions
1. Classification of newborn infants is now made on the basis of gestational age as well as birth weight
2. An infant born at term (37 weeks or over) is called full size; an infant born before term (36 weeks or less) is called premature or preterm
3. A low-birth-weight infant is one who weighs 2500 g (5½ pounds) or less
4. Full-term infant may be of low birth weight; premature infant need not be

C. Management of the low-birth-weight infant immediately after delivery
1. Aspiration of mucus to maintain an open airway is vital
2. Absence of respirations necessitates direct laryngoscopy, tracheal aspiration, intubation, and mouth-to-tube insufflation
3. Maintenance of body temperature is difficult because of heat loss by skin evaporation; heated Isolette is needed
4. Aspiration of stomach contents at birth facilitates respirations and is often indicated for the low-birth-weight infant
5. Infant should be moved to the nursery in the heated unit with oxygen and resuscitation equipment available

D. Characteristics of preterm infant
1. Preterm infant has less subcutaneous fat, therefore the skin is wrinkled, blood vessels and bony structures are visible, lanugo present on face, eyebrows are absent, and ears are poorly supported by cartilage
2. Circumference of the head of the preterm infant is quite large in comparison with the chest; the fontanels are small and bones are soft
3. Skin color changes when preterm infant is moved; upper half of the body pale and lower half red, known as harlequin color change
4. Preterm infant's posture is one of complete relaxation with marked flexion and abduction of the thighs; random movements are common with slightest stimulus
5. Heat regulation poorly developed in the preterm infant because of poor development of CNS; heat loss caused by large skin surface area; poorly developed respiratory center with diminished oxygen consumption causing asphyxia; weak heart action, therefore slower circulation and poor oxygenation; insufficient heat production caused by inadequate metabolism
6. Respirations are not efficient in the preterm infant because of muscular weakness of lungs and rib cage; retraction at xiphoid is evidence of air hunger; infant should be stimulated if apnea occurs
7. Greater tendency toward capillary fragility and intracranial hemorrhage in the preterm infant; red and white blood cell counts are low with resulting anemia during first few months of life
8. Nutrition is difficult to maintain in the preterm infant because of weak sucking and swallowing reflexes, small capacity of stomach, low gastric acidity, and slow emptying time of the stomach; the usual caloric intake of 110 to 130 calories per kilogram (50 to 60 calories per pound) of body weight may need to be increased to 200 to 220 calories per kilogram (100 calories per pound) for adequate growth and development

Nursing Process for Preterm or Low-Birth-Weight Infants
Probable Nursing Diagnoses Based on Assessment

A. Impaired gas exchange related to interference with respiratory stimulation, lung immaturity, or airway obstruction
B. Ineffective breathing pattern related to lung immaturity, anoxia or hypoxia, damage to the cerebral respiratory center, or cerebral immaturity
C. Ineffective airway clearance related to weakness of respiratory musculature
D. Potential for aspiration related to weak or absent gag reflex and/or administration of tube feedings
E. Hypothermia related to decreased subcutaneous fat deposits, immature thermoregulation center, inadequate shiver response, large body surface area in relation to body weight, and/or lack of flexion of extremities toward the body
F. Altered nutrition: less than body requirements related to lack of energy to suck, and/or weak or absent gag and/or sucking reflex
G. Activity intolerance related to impaired oxygenation and reduced energy reserves
H. Potential for infection related to immature/impaired immune response, stasis of respiratory secretions, and/or aspiration

Nursing Care for Preterm or Low-Birth-Weight Infants

A. Maintain airway; check respirator function if employed; position to promote ventilation; suction when necessary; maintain temperature of environment
B. Observe for changes in respirations, color, and vital signs
C. Check efficacy of Isolette: maintain heat, humidity, and oxygen concentration; monitor oxygen carefully to prevent retrolental fibroplasia
D. Maintain aseptic technique to prevent infection
E. Adhere to the techniques of gavage feeding for safety of infant

F. Determine blood gases frequently to prevent acidosis
G. Institute phototherapy should hyperbilirubinemia occur
H. Support parents by letting them verbalize and ask questions to relieve anxiety
I. Provide flexible and liberal visiting hours for parents as soon as possible
J. Allow parents to do as much as possible for the infant after appropriate teaching
K. Arrange follow-up before and after discharge by a visiting nurse
L. Evaluate infant's response and revise plan as necessary

NEONATAL RESPIRATORY DISTRESS
Nursing Process for Infants with Neonatal Respiratory Distress
Probable Nursing Diagnoses Based on Assessment

See the probable nursing diagnoses under Nursing process for preterm or low-birth-weight infants

Nursing Care for Infants with Neonatal Respiratory Distress

In addition to the nursing care listed under the specific disorder, see the Nursing care under Nursing process for preterm or low-birth-weight infants

A. Asphyxia neonatorum occurs when respirations are not well established within 60 seconds after birth as a result of anoxia, cerebral damage, or narcosis
  1. Prevention: early prenatal care, prenatal education, early management of deviations from the normal pregnancy, adequate medical management during labor and delivery
  2. Signs and symptoms: asphyxia livida: persistent generalized cyanosis, good muscle tone; asphyxia pallida: marked pallor, poor muscle tone
  3. Nursing care
    a. Resuscitate immediately
    b. Keep infant under close observation for first 24 hours
    c. Keep equipment for intubation and oxygen administration readily available
    d. Evaluate infant's response and revise plan as necessary
B. Atelectasis: incomplete expansion of the lung or a partial or total collapse of the lung following initial expansion; common in prematurity, oversedation, damage to the respiratory center, or results from inhalation of mucus or amniotic fluid
  1. Signs and symptoms: cyanosis, rapid irregular respirations, flaring of nostrils, intercostal or suprasternal retraction, grunting on expiration
  2. Nursing care
    a. Maintain an open airway
    b. Administer oxygen with high humidity
    c. Stimulate respirations by frequently changing infant's position
    d. Administer antibiotics as ordered to prevent infection
    e. Evaluate infant's response and revise plan as necessary
C. Respiratory distress syndrome (hyaline membrane disease): condition in which a deficiency in surface-active (detergentlike) lipoproteins results in inadequate lung

inflation and ventilation; common following cesarean delivery and in low-birth-weight infants
  1. Symptoms: cyanosis, dyspnea, and sternal retraction
  2. Nursing care
    a. Admit to neonatal intensive care unit
    b. Keep the airway patent
    c. Keep the infant in an Isolette with oxygen and high humidity
    d. Administer antibiotics as ordered
    e. Maintain function of mechanical ventilation if employed
    f. Evaluate infant's response and revise plan if necessary

BIRTH INJURIES
Cranial Birth Injuries

A. Caput succedaneum: edema with extravasation of serum into scalp tissues caused by molding during the birth process
B. Cephalhematoma: edema of the scalp with effusion of blood between the bone and periosteum
C. Intracranial hemorrhage: bleeding into cerebellum, pons, and medulla oblongata caused by a tearing of the tentorium cerebelli; occurs following prolonged labor, difficult forceps delivery, precipitate delivery, version or breech extraction; symptoms—abnormal respirations; cyanosis; sharp, shrill, or weak cry; flaccidity or spasticity; restlessness; wakefulness; convulsions; poor sucking reflex

Nursing Process for Infants with Cranial Birth Injuries
Probable Nursing Diagnoses Based on Assessment

A. Trauma related to birth process
B. Altered cerebral tissue perfusion related to intracranial hemorrhage
C. See related nursing diagnoses under Nursing process for preterm or low-birth-weight infants

Nursing Care for Infants with Cranial Birth Injuries

A. No treatment is necessary for caput succedaneum since it subsides in a few days
B. No treatment of cephalhematoma is necessary since reabsorption usually occurs in a few days
C. Intracranial hemorrhage
  1. Keep infant in Isolette with oxygen
  2. Place infant in high Fowler's position
  3. Administer vitamins C and K as ordered to control and prevent further hemorrhage
  4. Institute ordered gavage feedings when sucking reflex is impaired
  5. Support parents because of guarded prognosis
  6. Evaluate infant's and parents' responses and revise plan as necessary

Neuromusculoskeletal Birth Injuries

A. Facial paralysis: asymmetry of face caused by damage to facial nerves from a difficult forceps delivery
B. Erb-Duchenne paralysis (brachial palsy): caused by a difficult forceps or breech extraction delivery; treatment depends on severity of paralysis

C. Dislocations and fractures are diagnosed by crepitation, immobility, and variations in range of motion; treatment depends on the site of fracture

Nursing Process for Infants with Neuromusculoskeletal Birth Injuries
Probable Nursing Diagnoses Based on Assessment

A. Trauma related to birth process
B. Impaired physical mobility related to injured nerves, muscles, or bones, prescribed restrictions, and/or pain
C. Pain related to injury
D. Potential impaired skin integrity related to impaired mobility and/or use of immobilizing devices
E. Potential for disuse syndrome related to injury

Nursing Care for Infants with Neuromusculoskeletal Birth Injuries

A. No treatment is necessary for facial paralysis since it usually is temporary and disappears in a few days
B. Erb-Duchenne paralysis
   1. Massage and exercise arm as ordered to prevent contractures
   2. Place in "traffic cop" position
   3. Apply ordered splints and braces which are used when paralysis is severe
C. Dislocations and fractures
   1. Apply swaddling, splints, slings, or casts as ordered
   2. Position as ordered
D. Reassure parents and teach necessary care and positioning
E. Refer to public health agency to ensure continuity of care
F. Refer to other community agencies as necessary
G. Evaluate infant's and parents' responses and revise plan as necessary

CONGENITAL ABNORMALITIES

Defects present at birth are structural or metabolic (birth injuries are not included); may be genetically determined or a result of environmental interference during intrauterine life (see Pediatric Nursing for congenital abnormalities)

HEMOLYTIC DISEASE

Hemolytic disease, and ABO or Rh incompatibility with destruction of red cells and resulting anemia; caused by a transfer of incompatible blood from the fetal to the maternal circulation, with antibody formation in the mother; the antibodies are then transferred through the placental barrier to the fetus, with a resulting agglutination and destruction of red cells (erythroblastosis fetalis)

A. Symptoms: jaundice within the first 24 hours of birth, anemia, enlargement of the liver and spleen, lethargy, poor feeding pattern, vomiting, tremors and convulsions indicative of kernicterus (signs of kernicterus are absence of Moro reflex, severe lethargy, apnea, high-pitched cry, and assuming an opisthotonos position)
B. Treatment: during pregnancy amniotic fluid determinations are done by chemical and spectrophotometric analysis; elevated readings warrant either intrauterine transfusion or induction of labor depending on the weeks of gestation; following delivery exchange transfusion is done on the infant to decrease the antibody level and increase red blood cells and hemoglobin levels

C. Prevention: RhoGAM, a preparation of Rh_o (D antigen) immune globulin is now given intramuscularly to the mother 72 hours after delivery or after abortion to prevent erythroblastosis fetalis in future pregnancies; mother must be negative for Rh antibodies to receive RhoGAM

INFECTIONS
Nursing Process for Infants with Infections
Probable Nursing Diagnoses Based on Assessment

A. Infection related to transmission during gestation, passage through infected birth canal, and/or cross contamination by care giver
B. Potential fluid volume deficit related to diarrhea
C. Potential altered body temperature related to microbial toxins and/or immature thermoregulatory center
D. Decreased cardiac output related to congenital anomaly
E. Diarrhea related to bacterial infection
F. Altered nutrition: less than body requirements, related to impaired sucking reflex, oral discomfort, diarrhea, and/or increased basal metabolic rate
G. Altered growth and development: actual or potential, related to microbial invasion of cardiac and/or cerebral tissue

Nursing Care for Infants with Infections

A. Collect specimens to identify causative organism
B. Institute isolation precautions
C. Employ strict medical asepsis with meticulous hand washing
D. Use disposable feeding equipment or sterilize as necessary
E. Teach mother to wash hands before and after handling or caring for baby
F. Teach mother how to cleanse breasts or feeding equipment
G. Teach mother how to administer or apply prescribed medications
H. For specific nursing care see disease entity
I. Evaluate infant's response and mother's understanding and revise plan as necessary

Specific Perinatal Infections

A. Thrush: mouth infection caused by *Candida albicans;* it may be transmitted as the baby passes through the mother's vaginal canal, by unclean feeding utensils, or improper hand washing techniques by staff or mother
   1. Symptoms are white patches on tongue, palate, and inner cheek surfaces that bleed on examination, and difficulty with sucking
   2. Nursing care
      a. Administer oral nystatin (Mycostatin)
      b. Apply 1% gentian violet to oral cavity
B. Impetigo: skin infection caused by *Staphylococcus* or *Streptococcus* organisms
   1. Symptoms are vesicles or pustules on the skin
   2. Nursing care
      a. Bathe daily with pHisoHex
      b. Break pustules with alcohol wipe
      c. Apply gentian violet, neomycin, or bacitracin locally
      d. Administer systemic antibiotics as ordered

C. Ophthalmia neonatorum: eye infection caused by the *Neisseria gonorrhoeae* transmitted from the genital tract during delivery or by infected hands of personnel; prophylactic eye care is administered to all infants at birth
  1. Symptoms include purulent conjunctivitis if prophylactic treatment is not used; permanent eye damage results if infection is untreated
  2. Nursing care
     a. Instill silver nitrate or prescribed ophthalmic antibiotic after providing an opportunity for initial bonding
     b. Treat infection with prescribed antibiotic
D. Epidemic diarrhea: gastrointestinal infection caused by *Escherichia coli* organism in stool
  1. Symptoms include forceful, watery, yellow-green stool, dry skin, rapid weight loss, and acidosis
  2. Nursing care
     a. Administer prescribed antibiotics
     b. Monitor fluid balance
     c. Administer intravenous fluids as ordered
E. Syphilis: a congenital systemic infection caused by *Treponema pallidum*
  1. Transmission
     a. Prenatal syphilis transmitted to fetus by the mother
     b. Incidence of fetal infection varies with stage of the disease in the mother at the time of pregnancy
     c. Fetus seldom infected prior to fourth month of pregnancy; Langhan's cells in chorion are protective barrier
     d. Prior to the fourth month of pregnancy, fetus not infected; after fourth month, the longer the infection goes untreated the greater the damage to the fetus; pregnant women treated immediately with penicillin
  2. Symptoms include maculopapular lesions of the palms of the hands and soles of the feet, restlessness, rhinitis, hoarse cry, enlargement of the spleen and palpable lymph nodes, enlarged ends of long bones on x-ray examination
  3. Nursing care
     a. Administer penicillin as ordered
     b. Teach importance of continued medical supervision and follow-up care
F. *Chlamydia* infection: a sexually-transmitted disease caused by *Chlamydia trachomatis,* which is transferred to the infant during passage through the birth canal
  1. Symptoms associated with inclusion neonatal conjunctivitis, trachoma, or pneumonia
  2. Nursing care
     a. Administer tetracycline or doxycycline to infant as ordered
     b. Administer erythromycin to pregnant woman as ordered to prevent transmission to infant during delivery
G. Acquired Immune Deficiency Syndrome (AIDS): generalized invasion of T-cells by the human immunodeficiency virus (HIV) rendering the infant unable to protect self from secondary infections; transmitted by mother who is HIV-positive
  1. Symptoms are usually not present at birth; infant screened for HIV infection when either parent is

HIV-positive or at high risk for AIDS; as child ages the presence of frequent and debilitating infections occurs
  2. Nursing care
     a. Obtain blood specimen for HIV testing
     b. Institute and teach parents blood and body fluid precautions
     c. Inform mother that the virus may be transmitted via breast milk and that infant should be bottle fed
     d. Stress the importance of continued medical supervision
H. Sepsis: bacterial infection precipitated by infected amniotic fluid or break in aseptic technique
  1. Symptoms include poor feeding, high temperature, lethargy, increasing irritability, vomiting, pallor, anemia, and increased number of stools
  2. Nursing care
     a. Administer IV antibiotic therapy as ordered
     b. Monitor intravenous fluid administration
     c. Administer oxygen as ordered
I. Necrotizing enterocolitis (NEC): necrotic lesions in intestines resulting from ischemia in area
  1. Occurs several weeks after birth; more common in preterm infant
  2. Symptoms include poor feeding, vomiting, loss of weight, GI bleeding, abdominal distention, disappearance of bowel sounds; severely compromises infant
  3. Nursing care
     a. Maintain NPO
     b. Administer IV therapy as ordered
     c. Maintain nasogastric decompression
     d. Monitor fluid and electrolyte balance
     e. Provide ileostomy or colostomy care if surgery has been performed
J. TORCH: acronym for the following infections
  1. T—Toxoplasmosis *(Toxoplasma gondii):* can be acquired by eating raw undercooked meat or contacting cat litter; organism crosses the placenta; severity of infection related to gestational age; can cause hydrocephalus, intracranial calcifications, or chorioretinitis in the infant
  2. O—Others (syphilis *[Treponema pallidum],* gonorrhea *[Neisseria gonorrhoeae]);* see syphilis (E)
  3. R—Rubella (rubella virus): greatest risk to the fetus when maternal infection occurs in first 12 weeks of gestation; baby may be born with encephalitis, ocular abnormalities, cardiac maldevelopment, and other defects; these infants may have active viral infection and should be isolated until pharyngeal mucus and urine are free of virus; for mothers who have not had rubella or who are serologically negative, rubella vaccine should be given in the immediate postdelivery period
  4. C—Cytomegalic inclusion disease (cytomegalovirus): pregnant woman usually asymptomatic; this sexually transmitted infection may cause hemolytic anemia, hydrocephalus, microcephalus, intrauterine growth retardation, or neonatal death

5. H—Herpes genitalis (herpesvirus): contracted by the mother during sexual relations; characterized by periods of exacerbations and remissions; first attack most severe; during active stage the infant must be delivered by cesarean delivery; if delivered vaginally, neonatal infection can be disseminated and result in death; surviving infants suffer central nervous system involvement

6. Care is directed toward prevention and early treatment in the pregnant woman to eliminate or reduce risk to the fetus

DRUG DEPENDENCE

A. Definition: infant born with physiologic dependence on drugs as a result of maternal drug use and/or abuse
B. Source: many preparations including
    1. Alcohol
    2. Morphine derivatives
    3. Synthetic opiates
    4. Methadone
    5. Cocaine
C. Perinatal mortality: 6 to 8 times higher than in normal control group
D. Alcohol abuse in the mother can result in fetal alcohol syndrome producing congenital defects and retardation
E. Withdrawal symptoms: appear soon after birth, depending on the length of maternal addiction, amount of drug taken, and time taken prior to birth
    1. Jittery
    2. Hyperactive
    3. Shrill and persistent cry
    4. Frequent yawning and sneezing
    5. Tendon reflexes increased
    6. Moro reflex decreased
    7. If untreated, may develop fever, vomiting, diarrhea, dehydration, apnea, convulsions; death may result

Nursing Process for Infants with Drug Dependence
Probable Nursing Diagnoses Based on Assessment

A. Pain related to withdrawal
B. Altered nutrition: less than body requirements, related to hyperactivity or lethargy and/or depressed sucking reflex
C. Sleep pattern disturbance related to withdrawal and/or use of sedatives
D. Potential ineffective breathing pattern related to mother's use of narcotic close to the time of delivery
E. Altered growth and development related to addiction to narcotics, congenital anomalies, and/or mental retardation associated with fetal alcohol syndrome

Nursing Care for Infants with Drug Dependence

A. Monitor infant's neuromuscular status
B. Monitor vital signs; support respiratory functioning
C. Administer supportive care to prevent injury
D. Administer sedatives or narcotics as ordered
E. Keep environmental stimuli to a minimum
F. Promote mother-infant bonding when possible; provide a constant care giver
G. Hold and cuddle frequently but provide for periods of uninterrupted rest

H. Use soft nipple to reduce sucking effort; administer supplemental methods of nutritional support as ordered
I. Encourage continued medical supervision
J. Refer to appropriate community service agencies for family support and supervision
K. Evaluate infant's and parents' responses and revise plan as necessary

Infertility and Sterility
DEFINITIONS

A. Sterility: presence of an absolute factor that makes a person unable to produce offspring
B. Infertility: inability on the part of a couple to reproduce after consistent attempts for a 1-year period

MALE INFERTILITY AND STERILITY

A. Coital difficulties: chordee (painful downward curving erection) or marked obesity
B. Spermatozoal abnormalities: small ejaculatory volume, low sperm count, increased viscosity, reduced mobility of spermatozoa, and/or more than 30% abnormal sperm forms
C. Testicular abnormalities: agenesis or degenesis of testes, cryptorchidism, poor maturation of the spermatozoa, physical injury due to trauma, irradiation, or increased temperature for prolonged periods
D. Abnormalities of the penis or urethra: hypospadias or urethral stricture
E. Prostate and seminal vesicle abnormalities: chronic prostatitis or seminal vesiculitis
F. Abnormalities of the epididymis and vas deferens: inflammation or closure
G. Severe nutritional deficiencies
H. Emotional factors

FEMALE INFERTILITY AND STERILITY

A. Endocrine disorders: pituitary, thyroid, or adrenal
B. Vaginal disorders: absence or stenosis of vagina, imperforate hymen, vaginitis, chronic infections
C. Cervical abnormalities: cervical obstruction by cervical polyps or tumors
D. Uterine abnormalities: hypoplasia, uterine neoplasms
E. Tubal disorders: obstruction (generally result of infection), perisalpingeal adhesions
F. Ovarian abnormalities: congenital abnormalities such as ovarian dysgenesis or agenesis, infections, tumors
G. Emotional problems: severe psychoneurosis or psychosis may cause anovulatory cycles
H. Coital factors: feminine hygiene preparations (including douches) that decrease vaginal pH may inactivate or destroy spermatozoa
I. Chronic disease states
J. Immunologic reactions to sperm
K. Nutritional factors such as a seriously faulty diet; anorexia nervosa

DIAGNOSTIC MEASURES

A. Male: history, physical examination, semen analysis
B. Female: history, physical examination, CBC, sedimentation rate, serologic tests, urinalysis, serum protein-bound iodine, x-ray films of the chest, basal metabolic rate determination, Sims or Huhner tests, endometrial biopsy, tubal insufflation, hysterosalpingography, culdoscopy

TREATMENT

Depends on causative factor

DRUGS THAT AFFECT GONADAL FUNCTION AND FERTILITY

A. Androgens are used to replace deficient hormones in males after puberty and before the climacteric to improve development of secondary sex characteristics or as single-incident therapy controlling lactogenic activity in the nonnursing mother
   1. Drugs
      a. fluoxymesterone (Halotestin, Ora-Testryl, Ultandren)
      b. methyltestosterone (Metandren, Neo-Hombreol-M, Oreton-M)
      c. testosterone (Androlan, Andronaq, Hormale Aqueous, Malogen, Neo-Hombreol-F, Oreton, Sterotate)
      d. testosterone cypionate (Depo-Testosterone, Durandro, Malogen CYP, T-Ionate-P.A.)
      e. testosterone enanthate (Delatestryl, Malogen LA, Repo-Test, Testate, Testostroval-P.A.)
      f. testosterone propionate (Hormale Oil, Neo-Hombreol, Oreton Propionate, Testonate)
   2. Adverse effects: adolescent males may have premature epiphyseal closure (decreased skeletal development, height stops increasing)
B. Estrogens primarily used to replace deficient hormones to control hormonal balance in menopausal or postmenopausal women or to maintain menses and fertility in females during reproductive years
   1. Drugs
      a. chlorotrianisene (Tace)
      b. conjugated estrogens (Conestron, Conjutab, Equgen, Menotabs, Premarin, Theogen)
      c. dienestrol (DV, Synestrol)
      d. esterified estrogens (Amnestrogen, Estrifol, Evex, Femogen, Glyestrin, Menest, SK-Estrogens, Trocosone, Zeste)
      e. estradiol (Aquadiol, Progynon)
      f. estrone (Estrusol, Menformon [A], Theelin, Wynestron)
      g. ethinyl estradiol (Estinyl, Feminone, Lynoral, Palonyl)
      h. hexestrol
      i. methallenestril (Vallestril)
      j. promethestrol dipropionate (Meprane Dipropionate)
   2. Adverse effects: anorexia, nausea, vomiting, tissue fluid accumulation
C. Conception enhancers
   1. Menotropins (Pergonal) stimulate growth and maturation of ovarian follicles in women with deficient ovum production by creating an effect on ovarian follicles comparable to that of natural FSH and LH
   2. Chorionic gonadotropin (A.P.L., Almetropin, Antuitrin-S, Chorex, Chorigon, Follutein, Glucotropin-Forte, Khorion, Libigen, Luton, Pregnyl, Riogon, Stemultrolin)
      a. Administered concurrently to support LH effect on ovulation when follicle maturation has occurred
      b. Adverse effects: 20% of clients have multiple births
   3. Clomiphene citrate (Clomid)
      a. Used during the fifth to the tenth day of the menstrual cycle to stimulate release of FSH and LH in anovulatory women
      b. Adverse effects: multiple births, visual changes, dizziness, light-headedness

NURSING PROCESS FOR CLIENTS EXPERIENCING INFERTILITY AND STERILITY
Probable Nursing Diagnoses Based on Assessment

A. Situational low self-esteem related to inability to reproduce
B. Health seeking behaviors to obtain help related to reproduction
C. Altered role performance related to inability to become a parent
D. Altered family processes related to inability to achieve a pregnancy
E. Sexual dysfunction related to physiological or emotional problems preventing pregnancy
F. Potential impaired adjustment related to inability to achieve desired goals
G. Anxiety related to inability to achieve a pregnancy and outcome of testing

Nursing Care for Clients Experiencing Infertility and Sterility

A. Apply principles of human relations and psychology
B. Listen to and discuss couple's particular problems, giving necessary support
C. Explain diagnostic procedures to alleviate anxiety and fear
D. Explain and discuss various treatment modalities
E. Encourage compliance with selected treatment modality; teach the reasons for the interventions
F. Listen to goals but point out reality
G. Help couples to support one another by
   1. Encouraging frank discussion of feelings
   2. Avoiding blaming behaviors
   3. Adjusting to altered roles
H. Accept and work with couple's realistic frustrations and disappointments
I. Evaluate clients' responses and revise plan as necessary

Family Planning
GOALS

A. Maintain optimum emotional and physical health of the family
B. Involve both partners in planning family size
C. Inform the couple of available methods of birth control and give them the freedom of choice

CONTRACEPTIVE METHODS

A. Oral contraceptives
   1. Description
      a. Used to prevent conception
         (1) Act by
            (a) Inhibiting ovulation causing a thickening of cervical mucus to inhibit sperm travel
            (b) Causing atrophic changes in the endometrium to prevent implantation

(2) Available in progestin mini pills or estrogen-progestin combination products

2. Examples
   a. Progestin products
      (1) Micronor
      (2) Ovrette
   b. Estrogen-progestin products
      (1) Demulen
      (2) Enovid
      (3) Norestrin
      (4) Ortho-novum
      (5) Ovral

3. Major side effects
   a. Thrombophlebitis; increased clot formation
   b. Hypertension due to fluid retention
   c. Libido changes related to hormonal effect
   d. Hyperglycemia related to decreased CHO tolerance
   e. CNS disturbances
   f. Breakthrough bleeding related to estrogen effect
   g. Breast tenderness due to fluid retention

4. Nursing care
   a. Obtain client health history for problems, which may contraindicate drug use; e.g., history of hypertension, thrombophlebitis, breast malignancy, CVA, breast-feeding mothers
   b. Assist client in choosing the best method of birth control by providing an accepting atmosphere
   c. Instruct client to
      (1) Keep scheduled appointments with gynecologist
      (2) Report occurrence of any side effects to physician
      (3) Use an additional method of birth control when beginning and ending therapy
   d. Review specific medication administration schedule with client and review procedure to follow if doses are missed

B. Intrauterine devices (IUD): mechanical devices inserted into isthmus of uterus; prevent pregnancy by increasing tubal motility so that ovum gets to uterus before lining is optimum for implantation; not as effective as oral contraceptives, since pregnancy may occur with device in place; may cause increased menstrual bleeding

C. Diaphragms: mechanical devices that fit over cervix and prevent sperm from entering cervical os; use with spermicide

D. Vaginal sponge: plastic sponge impregnated with spermicide; affords 48-hour protection

E. Condoms: rubber sheaths that cover penis and prevent semen from entering cervical os

F. Creams, jellies, foam tablets, and vaginal suppositories: spermicidal (generally low pH) preparations inserted into vaginal canal by applicator immediately prior to coitus (used in conjunction with the diaphragm and condom for added protection)

G. Coitus interruptus: withdrawal of the penis during sexual intercourse prior to ejaculation; least effective method

H. Gossypol: male contraceptive pill that inhibits spermatogenesis

I. Rhythm: the plotting of the basal body temperature to determine fertile period, with abstinence from coitus during that time

J. Surgical sterilization
   1. Bilateral vasectomy: small incision made into the scrotum and the vas deferens is ligated producing sterilization in the male by preventing ejaculation of sperm; usually performed on an outpatient basis
   2. Tubal ligation: interruption in the continuity of fallopian tubes by surgical transection, electric cautery, or compression with soft clamp preventing impregnation of ovum by sperm; accomplished by laparotomy, laparoscopy, or culdoscopy; usually requires short hospitalization

NURSING PROCESS FOR CLIENTS CONCERNED WITH FAMILY PLANNING
Probable Nursing Diagnoses Based on Assessment

A. Health seeking behaviors related to desire to control future pregnancies

B. Potential for injury related to physiological changes associated with oral contraceptives, and/or use of contraceptive devices

C. Potential for infection related to contraceptive devices

D. Decisional conflict related to lack of relevent information, uncertainty about alternative contraceptive methods, lack of experience with contraceptives, and/or challenge to a personal value

E. Fear related to failure of contraceptive method resulting in pregnancy

F. Anxiety related to potential irreversibility of some methods

Nursing Care for Clients Concerned with Family Planning

A. Explain and discuss various contraceptive modalities

B. Encourage compliance with selected regimen; teach and explain the steps in correct contraceptive use

C. Help couples to expand their knowledge about human sexuality

D. Support couples in their choice of contraceptive method; remain nonjudgmental

E. Teach couples electing surgical sterilization that in the female sterility is immediately achieved, while in the male sterility is not achieved until semen is sperm free (may take up to 6 weeks)

F. Encourage periodic physical examination for all women using oral or contraceptive devices; should include pelvic examination, Pap smear, and mammography

G. Evaluate clients' responses and understanding and revise plan as necessary

Abortion
METHODS OF INDUCED ABORTION

A. Menstrual extraction or minisuction: vacuum of uterine contents with a 50 ml syringe; done 5 to 7 weeks after last menstrual period

B. Vacuum aspiration: done under local paracervical, epidural, or general anesthesia in the first 12 weeks of pregnancy; the cervix is dilated and the products of conception are suctioned by a small hollow tube; the uterus is then curettaged to remove all fetal tissue

C. Dilation and curettage: performed during the first 12 to 14 weeks of pregnancy under local paracervical or general anesthesia; the cervix is dilated and uterus is curettaged

D. Saline injection: labor is induced when a pregnancy is 14 to 24 weeks in duration by injecting a sterile saline solution into the uterus by amniocentesis; labor usually begins within 20 to 36 hours after instillation of saline; produces a macerated fetus
E. Prostaglandins
1. Action: used during second trimester to trigger vasoconstriction and uterine contractions that interfere with endocrine function of placenta
2. Adverse effects: nausea, vomiting, diarrhea, pain at extrauterine sites, allergic reactions (not administered to clients with history of asthma)
F. Hysterotomy: performed after 16 weeks of pregnancy by surgically removing the fetus and placenta abdominally

NURSING PROCESS FOR CLIENTS HAVING AN ABORTION
Probable Nursing Diagnoses Based on Assessment

A. Situational low self-esteem related to possible feelings of frustration, fear, anger, or guilt
B. Decisional conflict related to termination of pregnancy and the diversity of options available
C. Knowledge deficit related to self-care after the abortion and/or alternate methods of contraception
D. Pain related to induced labor
E. Potential for injury related to mechanical termination of pregnancy
F. Potential for infection related to introduction of foreign objects or substances into the body

Nursing Care for Clients Having an Abortion

A. Be aware of own feelings about abortion (essential if the nurse is to intervene therapeutically with women having abortions)
B. Encourage the client's expression of frustration, fear, anger, or guilt
C. Be objective and support the client's decision about abortion
D. Make certain that a complete history and physical examination, complete laboratory workup, pelvic examination and Pap test, and a pregnancy test are done prior to induced abortion
E. Counsel in contraceptive methods if requested
F. Administer RhoGAM when client's blood is negative for antibodies
G. Evaluate client's response and revise plan as necessary

Menopause

A period in a woman's life when there is gradual cessation of ovarian function and menstrual cycles
A. Physiologic changes
1. Ovaries lose their ability to respond to gonadotropic hormones
2. Dramatic decrease in levels of circulating estrogens and progesterone because ovaries have atrophied
3. Increased FSH gonadotropin level in the blood, since production is no longer inhibited (negative feedback) by the ovaries; false-positive pregnancy test may occur

B. Symptoms
1. Somatic: atrophic changes in reproductive organs resulting in dyspareunia, weight gain, facial hair growth, cardiac palpitations, hot flashes, profuse diaphoresis, constipation, pruritus, faintness; long range changes may include osteoporosis
2. Psychic: headache, irritability, anxiety over loss of reproductive function, sexual feelings, and feelings of womanliness
C. Treatment
1. Support system to deal with stress
2. For dyspareunia: vaginal estrogen creams
3. Tranquilizers and phenobarbital if necessary
4. Hormone replacement therapy (HRT): although still controversial is now being used more frequently; small doses of conjugated estrogen with progestin is thought to reduce the risk of cancer that is present with the use of estrogen alone and prevent osteoporosis

NURSING PROCESS FOR CLIENTS DURING MENOPAUSE
Probable Nursing Diagnoses Based on Assessment

A. Potential for altered body temperature related to hormonal changes
B. Potential for ineffective individual coping related to hormonal changes
C. Potential disturbance in self-esteem, body image, or personal identity related to cessation of reproductive cycle
D. Potential altered role performance related to emotional perception of the aging process
E. Knowledge deficit related to lack of knowledge about the physiological changes associated with menopause

Nursing Care for Clients During Menopause

A. Teach the woman about the changes that may occur with menopause
B. Encourage the woman to ventilate her feelings
C. Explain the physiological basis for many of the temporary alterations associated with menopause
D. Refer for medical supervision if menopausal symptoms persist or interfere with functioning
E. Evaluate client's response and revise plan as necessary

Maternity Nursing Review Questions

1. The outermost membrane that helps form the placenta is the:
   ① Amnion
   ② Yolk sac
   ③ Chorion
   ④ Allantois
2. Progesterone is secreted in relatively large quantities by the:
   ① Corpus luteum
   ② Adrenal cortex
   ③ Endometrium
   ④ Pituitary gland

3. The developing cells are called a fetus from the:
   1. End of the second week to the onset of labor
   2. Implantation of the fertilized ovum
   3. Time the fetal heart is heard
   4. Eighth week to the time of birth

4. The ischial spines are designated as an important landmark in labor and delivery because the distance between the spines is:
   1. A measurement of the floor of the pelvis
   2. A measurement of the inlet of the birth canal
   3. The widest measurement of the pelvis
   4. The narrowest diameter of the pelvis

5. True labor can be differentiated from false labor in that in true labor contractions will:
   1. Occur immediately after membrane rupture
   2. Bring about progressive cervical dilation
   3. Be less uncomfortable if client is in side-lying position
   4. Stop when the client is encouraged to walk around

6. During pregnancy the volume of tidal air increases because there is:
   1. Increased expansion of the lower ribs
   2. A relative increase in the height of the rib cage
   3. Upward displacement of the diaphragm
   4. An increase in total blood volume

7. The uterus rises out of the pelvis and becomes an abdominal organ at about the:
   1. Eighth week of pregnancy
   2. Eighteenth week of pregnancy
   3. Tenth week of pregnancy
   4. Twelfth week of pregnancy

8. Most spontaneous abortions are caused by:
   1. Physical trauma
   2. Germ plasma defects
   3. Unresolved stress
   4. Congenital defects

9. In the dilation and suction evacuation method of elective abortion, laminarias are used in the dilation stage of the procedure because:
   1. They are stronger in action than instruments
   2. Dilation occurs within 2 hours
   3. Less anesthesia is necessary with this method
   4. They are hygroscopic and expand

10. The inner membrane that provides a fluid medium for the embryo is the:
    1. Amnion
    2. Yolk sac
    3. Chorion
    4. Funis

11. First fetal movements felt by the mother are known as:
    1. Ballottement
    2. Engagement
    3. Lightening
    4. Quickening

12. In prenatal development, growth is most rapid in the:
    1. Implantation period
    2. First trimester
    3. Second trimester
    4. Third trimester

13. The chief function of progesterone is the:
    1. Establishment of secondary male sex characteristics
    2. Stimulation of follicles for ovulation to occur
    3. Development of female reproductive organs
    4. Preparation of the uterus to receive a fertilized ovum

14. The practice of separating parents and child immediately after birth and limiting their time with the newborn in the first few days would appear to contradict studies based on:
    1. Rooming in
    2. Bonding
    3. Taking-in behaviors
    4. Taking-hold behaviors

15. Research indicates:
    1. Ambivalence and anxiety about mothering are common
    2. A rejected pregnancy will result in a rejected infant
    3. A good mother experiences neither ambivalence nor anxiety about mothering
    4. Maternal love is fully developed within the first week after birth

16. More than half the neonatal deaths in the United States are caused by:
    1. Atelectasis
    2. Prematurity
    3. Respiratory distress syndrome
    4. Congenital heart disease

17. The presence of multiple gestation should be detected as early as possible and the pregnancy managed with high risk in mind because:
    1. Perinatal mortality is two to three times greater than in single births
    2. Maternal mortality is much higher during the prenatal period in multiple gestation
    3. The mother needs time to adjust psychologically and physiologically after delivery
    4. Postpartum hemorrhage is an expected complication

18. During the process of gametogenesis, the male and female sex cells divide and then contain:
    1. A diploid number of chromosomes in their nuclei
    2. A haploid number of chromosomes in their nuclei
    3. Twenty-two pairs of autosomes in their nuclei
    4. Forty-six pairs of chromosomes in their nuclei

19. The placenta does not produce:
    1. Chorionic gonadotropin
    2. Follicle-stimulating hormone
    3. Progesterone precursor substances
    4. Somatotropin

20. After the first 3 months of pregnancy the chief source of estrogen and progesterone is the:
    1. Anterior hypophysis
    2. Placenta
    3. Adrenal cortex
    4. Corpus luteum

21. In fetal blood vessels the oxygen content is highest in the:
    1. Umbilical artery
    2. Ductus arteriosus
    3. Ductus venosus
    4. Pulmonary artery

22. The blood vessels in the umbilical cord consist of:
    ① Two arteries and one vein
    ② Two arteries and two veins
    ③ One artery and two veins
    ④ One artery and one vein
23. When assessing the significance of estriol studies in an antenatal client, the nurse should understand that:
    ① Elevations in estriol levels indicate fetal postmaturity
    ② Estriol is the hormone used in pregnancy tests
    ③ The fetus contributes precursors to the synthesis of estriol
    ④ Elevations in estriol levels indicate fetal demise
24. Physiologic anemia during pregnancy is a result of:
    ① Increased blood volume of the mother
    ② Decreased dietary intake of iron
    ③ Decreased erythropoiesis after first trimester
    ④ Increased detoxification demands on the mother's liver
25. The fetus is most likely to be damaged by the pregnant woman's ingestion of drugs during the:
    ① First trimester
    ② Second trimester
    ③ Third trimester
    ④ Entire pregnancy
26. The most common type of ectopic pregnancy is tubal. Within a few weeks after conception the tube may rupture suddenly, causing:
    ① Sudden knifelike, lower-quadrant abdominal pain
    ② Continuous dull, lower-quadrant abdominal pain
    ③ Painless vaginal bleeding
    ④ Intermittent abdominal contractions
27. In caring for a client with a tentative diagnosis of hydatidiform mole the nurse should be alert for:
    ① Painless heavy vaginal bleeding
    ② Unusually rapid uterine enlargement
    ③ Hypotension
    ④ Decreased FHR
28. The pituitary hormone that stimulates the secretion of milk from the mammary glands is:
    ① Prolactin
    ② Oxytocin
    ③ Progesterone
    ④ Estrogen
29. Breast-feeding is always contraindicated with:
    ① Pregnancy
    ② Herpes genitalis
    ③ Inverted nipples
    ④ Mastitis
30. Postpartal hemorrhage is usually not associated with:
    ① Delivery of twins or hydramnios
    ② Retained placenta
    ③ Toxemia of pregnancy
    ④ Overdistended bladder
31. Mrs. Pattern is admitted to the emergency room with vaginal bleeding. When taking a history, the nurse learns that the client has had five missed periods. Later the nurse reads the chart, which states, "stillborn delivered at 8 PM. . . ." The nurse understands this to mean that the products of conception:
    ① Were completely expelled
    ② Were previable

③ Weighed over 600 g
④ Measured 13.4 cm in length
32. A decision to withhold "extraordinary care" for a newborn with severe abnormalities is actually:
    ① The same as pediatric euthanasia
    ② A decision to let the newborn die
    ③ Presuming that the newborn has no rights
    ④ Unethical and illegal medical and nursing practice
33. The earliest clinical sign in idiopathic respiratory distress syndrome in the newborn is usually:
    ① Sternal and subcostal retractions
    ② Cyanosis
    ③ Rapid respiration
    ④ Grunting
34. Abruptio placentae is most likely to occur in a woman with:
    ① Toxemia
    ② Cardiac disease
    ③ Hyperthyroidism
    ④ Cephalopelvic disproportion
35. A predisposing factor in determining whether a woman will have a postpartum hemorrhage is the knowledge that:
    ① Her uterus is overdistended
    ② She has had more than five pregnancies
    ③ The duration of her labor was very short
    ④ She is over 40 years of age
36. The birth hazard unassociated with breech delivery is:
    ① Intracranial hemorrhage
    ② Cephalhematoma
    ③ Compression of cord
    ④ Separation of placenta prior to delivery of head
37. The care of a client with placenta previa includes:
    ① Limited ambulation until the bleeding stops
    ② Observation and recording of the bleeding
    ③ Vital signs at least once per shift
    ④ A tap water enema before delivery
38. The nurse would suspect an ectopic pregnancy if the client complained of:
    ① Lower abdominal cramping present over a long period of time
    ② Sharp lower right or left abdominal pain radiating to the shoulder
    ③ Leukorrhea and dysuria a few days after the first missed period
    ④ An adherent painful ovarian mass
39. The most effective position for a woman in labor when the nurse notes a prolapsed cord is:
    ① Sims
    ② Fowler's
    ③ Trendelenburg
    ④ Lithotomy
40. The two most important predisposing causes of puerperal infection are:
    ① Hemorrhage and trauma during labor
    ② Toxemia and retention of placenta
    ③ Malnutrition and anemia during pregnancy
    ④ Organisms present in the birth canal and trauma during labor

41. The most common symptom of congenital rubella syndrome that follows infection in the mother during the first trimester is:
    ① Hydrocephalus
    ② Phocomelia
    ③ Cardiac anomaly
    ④ Otosclerosis
42. Closure of the foramen ovale after birth is caused by:
    ① A decrease in the aortic blood flow
    ② An increase in the pulmonary blood flow
    ③ A decrease in pressure in the left atrium
    ④ An increase in the pressure in the right atrium
43. After birth, in a normal neonate, the ductus arteriosus becomes the:
    ① Ligamentum teres
    ② Venous ligament
    ③ Ligamentum arteriosum
    ④ Superior vesical artery
44. An infant's intestines are sterile at birth, therefore lacking the bacteria necessary for the synthesis of:
    ① Prothrombin
    ② Bile salts
    ③ Intrinsic factor
    ④ Bilirubin
45. Immunity transferred to the fetus from an immune mother through the placenta is:
    ① Active natural immunity
    ② Active artificial immunity
    ③ Passive natural immunity
    ④ Passive artificial immunity
46. The finding which would probably necessitate intense follow-up care of a newborn would be:
    ① An initial Apgar score of 5
    ② A birth weight of 3500 g
    ③ The aspiration of 20 ml of milky-colored fluid from newborn's stomach
    ④ An umbilical cord that contained only two vessels
47. The nurse encourages continued medical supervision for the pregnant woman with pyelitis because:
    ① Antibiotic therapy is given until the urine is sterile
    ② Toxemia frequently occurs following pyelitis
    ③ Pelvic inflammatory disease occurs with untreated pyelitis
    ④ A low-protein diet is given until pregnancy is terminated
48. A nurse tells a pregnant woman not to wear tight clothing around her abdomen because of possible damage to the fetus. The principle responsible for the potential damage is:
    ① Pascal's
    ② Archimedes'
    ③ Newton's
    ④ Einstein's
49. During pregnancy, the uterine musculature hypertrophies and is greatly stretched as the fetus grows. This stretching:
    ① By itself inhibits uterine contraction until oxytocin stimulates the birth process
    ② Is prevented from stimulating uterine contraction by high levels of estrogen during late pregnancy
    ③ Inhibits uterine contraction along with the combined inhibitory effects of estrogen and progesterone
    ④ Would ordinarily stimulate uterine contraction but is prevented by high levels of progesterone during pregnancy
50. During pregnancy a polypeptide similar to the adrenal steroids is responsible for:
    ① Symptoms of morning sickness
    ② Urinary frequency
    ③ Linea nigra and chloasma
    ④ Softening of the cervix
51. A normal woman who had a hemophilic father is mated to a man with normal blood clotting. Genetically it can be predicted that:
    ① All children will be hemophiliacs
    ② Half the male children will be hemophiliacs
    ③ All male children will be hemophiliacs
    ④ Female children will be unaffected
52. If anemia is present with a hemoglobin level of 8 g or lower, a mother with cardiac disease probably will go into:
    ① Cardiac failure
    ② Heart block
    ③ Atrial fibrillation
    ④ Cardiac compensation
53. The most frequent side effect associated with the use of IUDs is:
    ① Rupture of the uterus
    ② Excessive menstrual flow
    ③ Expulsion of the IUD
    ④ Ectopic pregnancy
54. Oral contraceptives during menopause:
    ① Prolong menses
    ② Intensify menopausal symptoms
    ③ Cause menorrhagia
    ④ Have no effect on menopause
55. An abandoned infant has been brought to the hospital. Ophthalmia neonatorum is diagnosed. The nurse can estimate the infant's age at:
    ① One day
    ② Less than 24 hours
    ③ About 3 to 4 days
    ④ Two days
56. If a woman with an untreated chlamydial infection is allowed to deliver vaginally, the infant is in danger of being born with:
    ① Ophthalmia neonatorum
    ② Congenital syphilis
    ③ Thrush
    ④ Pneumonia
57. The care of a newborn infant of a mother with untreated syphilis during the second trimester would be:
    ① Having the baby immediately screened for syphilis
    ② Assessing for a cleft palate
    ③ Observing for maculopapular lesions of the soles
    ④ Eliciting hypotonicity of skeletal muscles
58. Mrs. Peters enters the hospital for exploratory abdominal surgery. She is 3 months pregnant and has been informed that there are many dangers involved. The nurse has her sign a consent form for an exploratory laparotomy. Cancer of the uterus is discovered

and a hysterectomy is performed. On returning from surgery Mrs. Peters is informed that her uterus was removed. She sues the hospital, the surgeon, and the nurse. The decision in this case will be based on the fact that:
① The client received inadequate information to give consent
② The surgeon has the legal right to do what was deemed necessary in surgery
③ General consent forms signed on admission are sufficient
④ Consent for exploratory surgery implies permission for removing organs if this is justified

59. The operative procedure which would result in surgical menopause would be a:
① Bilateral oophorectomy
② Partial hysterectomy
③ Bilateral salpingectomy
④ Tubal ligation

60. Hot flashes are caused by:
① Overstimulation of the adrenal medulla
② Accumulation of acetylcholine
③ Cessation of pituitary gonadotropins
④ Hormonal stimulation of the sympathetic system

61. Menopause is the cessation of menstrual function. One of the reasons given is:
① An increase in the secretion of progesterone from the follicles in the ovary
② A decrease in the production of prostaglandins
③ The inability of the ovary to respond to gonadotropic hormones
④ A decrease in gonadotropin in the blood

62. Ovulation occurs when the:
① Blood level of LH is high
② Endometrial wall is sloughed off
③ Progesterone level is high
④ Oxytocin level is high

63. High concentration of estrogens in the blood:
① Causes ovulation
② Inhibits anterior pituitary secretions of FSH
③ Is one of the causes of osteoporosis
④ Stimulates lactation

Situation: Mrs. Greene, a 22-year-old primigravida, is attending prenatal clinic. She has missed two menstrual periods. She relates that the first day of her last menstrual period was July 22. Questions 64 through 69 refer to this situation.

64. Mrs. Greene's estimated date of delivery would be:
① May 5
② April 29
③ April 15
④ May 14

65. As Mrs. Greene is being prepared for the pelvic examination, she complains of feeling very tired and sick to her stomach, especially in the morning. The best response for the nurse to make is:
① "This is common during the early part of pregnancy. There is no need to worry."
② "This is a common occurrence during the early part of pregnancy; let's discuss some ways to deal with it."
③ "These are common occurrences during pregnancy with all the body changes; can you tell me how you feel in the morning?"
④ "Perhaps you might ask the doctor when he arrives."

66. Mrs. Greene works as a secretary in a large office. Her job has implications for her plan of care during pregnancy. The nurse would most likely recommend that Mrs. Greene:
① Ask for a break in the morning and afternoon so she can elevate her legs
② Inform her employer that she cannot work beyond the second trimester
③ Ask for a break in morning and afternoon for added nourishment
④ Try to walk about every few hours of her work day

67. The physician performs a pelvic examination and discovers that Mrs. Greene has a normal female pelvis, with the sacrum:
① Well hollowed, coccyx movable, spines not prominent, pubic arch wide
② Flat, coccyx movable, spines prominent, pubic arch wide
③ Deeply hollowed, coccyx immovable, pubic arch narrow, spines not prominent
④ Flat, coccyx movable, spines prominent, pubic arch narrow

68. Mrs. Greene is concerned because she has read that nutrition during pregnancy is important for proper growth and development of the baby. She wants to know something about the foods she should eat. The nurse should:
① Give her a list of foods so she can better plan her meals
② Assess what she eats by taking a diet history
③ Emphasize the importance of limiting salt and highly seasoned foods
④ Instruct her to continue eating a normal diet

69. Mrs. Greene states, "I'm worried about gaining too much weight because I've heard it's bad for me." The nurse should respond:
① "Yes, weight gain causes complications during pregnancy."
② "Don't worry about gaining weight. We are more concerned if you don't gain enough weight to ensure proper growth of your baby."
③ "The pattern of your weight gain will be of more importance than the total amount."
④ "If you gain over 15 pounds, you'll have to follow a low-calorie diet."

Situation: Mrs. Bey is 20 weeks pregnant and requests an abortion. Questions 70 through 73 refer to this situation.

70. During the salinization method of elective abortion, the nurse should be alert for side effects such as:
① Oliguria
② Thirst
③ Bradycardia
④ Edema

71. After the salinization procedure the client should be told that labor will probably begin within:
    1. Two hours after the procedure
    2. Several minutes following the procedure
    3. Eight hours after the procedure
    4. Twenty-four to 72 hours after the procedure

72. When Mrs. Bey returns to the clinic, she asks about an IUD for birth control. The nurse explains that the IUD is used to provide contraception by:
    1. Blocking the cervical os
    2. Increasing the mobility of the uterus
    3. Setting up a nonspecific inflammatory cell reaction
    4. Preventing the sperm from reaching the fallopian tube

73. The nurse should explain that a very common problem that has been associated with IUDs when they are used is:
    1. Development of vaginal infections
    2. Discomfort associated with coitus
    3. Spontaneous expulsion of the device
    4. Perforation of the uterus

Situation: Mrs. Johnson is in her first trimester and comes to the prenatal clinic. She has a cold and appears to be farther into her pregnancy than the history indicates. Questions 74 through 79 refer to this situation.

74. Mrs. Johnson asks if it is all right to take aspirin. The best advice the nurse can give to a pregnant woman in her first trimester is to:
    1. Avoid all drugs, including aspirin, and refrain from smoking and ingesting alcohol
    2. Take only prescription drugs, especially in the second and third trimesters
    3. Cut down on drugs, alcohol, and cigarettes
    4. Avoid smoking and all drugs except aspirin when needed, and limit alcohol to no more than 1 oz daily

75. Mrs. Johnson delivers twins during the seventh month, and they are diagnosed as having hyaline membrane disease. The principle underlying the respiratory distress of these infants is:
    1. Surface tension
    2. Pascal's principle
    3. Second law of thermodynamics
    4. Archimedes' principle

76. When caring for Mrs. Johnson's twins, the nurse should keep:
    1. Them prone to prevent aspiration
    2. Them in a high-humidity environment
    3. Oxygen concentration low to prevent eye damage
    4. Caloric intake low to decrease metabolic rate

77. While considering nursing measures to foster parent-child relationships, the nurse should be aware that the most important factor at this time is the:
    1. Duration and difficulty of labor
    2. Anesthesia during labor
    3. Health status during pregnancy
    4. Physical condition of the twins

78. Mrs. Johnson might experience postpartal hemorrhage for all the following reasons. However, the most common one is:
    1. Retained secundines
    2. Lacerations of the cervix
    3. Atony of the uterus
    4. Secondary infections

79. Overstretching of perineal supporting tissues as a result of childbirth can bring about a rectocele. The most common symptom is:
    1. Urinary stress incontinence
    2. Crampy abdominal pain
    3. A bearing-down sensation
    4. Recurrent urinary tract infections

Situation: Mrs. Unger delivers a baby spontaneously. Questions 80 through 85 refer to this situation.

80. The primary critical observation for Apgar scoring is the:
    1. Respiratory rate
    2. Heart rate
    3. Presence of meconium
    4. Evaluation of Moro reflex

81. Within 3 minutes after birth the normal heart rate of the infant may range between:
    1. 100 and 180
    2. 130 and 170
    3. 120 and 160
    4. 100 and 130

82. Within this same period the normal respiratory rate may be as high as:
    1. 100
    2. 80
    3. 60
    4. 50

83. The nurse may best obtain a Moro reflex by:
    1. Creating a loud noise suddenly
    2. Changing the infant's equilibrium
    3. Stimulating the infant's feet
    4. Grasping the infant's hand

84. The Moro reflex response is marked by:
    1. Extension of arms
    2. Extension of the legs and fanning of the toes
    3. Adduction of arms
    4. Abduction and then adduction of the arms

85. Asymmetric Moro reflexes are frequently associated with:
    1. Cerebral or cerebellar injuries
    2. Cranial nerve damage
    3. Brachial plexus, clavicle, or humerus injuries
    4. Down's syndrome

Situation: Mrs. Cohen, a 26-year-old primigravida, comes to the prenatal clinic during the first trimester. She states she weighed 47.6 kg (105 lb) before her pregnancy and currently weighs 49.4 kg (109 lb). Questions 86 through 90 refer to this situation.

86. Mrs. Cohen is concerned about regaining her figure after delivery and wishes to diet during pregnancy. The nurse should advise Mrs. Cohen that:
    1. Dieting is recommended to make delivery easier since she is so small
    2. Inadequate food intake during pregnancy can cause low-birth-weight infants
    3. Dieting is recommended to lessen the incidence of stillbirth
    4. Inadequate food intake during pregnancy can cause toxemia

87. The nurse should provide dietary teaching for Mrs. Cohen because:
    ① Pregnant women must adhere to a specific pregnancy diet
    ② Different sources of essential nutrients are favored by different cultural groups
    ③ Most weight gain during pregnancy is fluid retention
    ④ Dietary allowances should not increase during pregnancy

88. During the seventh month of pregnancy Mrs. Cohen exhibits dependent edema. The nurse explains the treatment for fluid retention during pregnancy, which is:
    ① Adequate fluid and a low-salt diet
    ② Adequate fluid and elevation of the lower extremities
    ③ A low-salt diet and elevation of the lower extremities
    ④ Judicious use of diuretics and elevations of the lower extremities

89. Mrs. Cohen develops painless vaginal bleeding during the last trimester. The nurse realizes that this may be caused by:
    ① Abruptio placentae
    ② Frequent intercourse
    ③ Placenta previa
    ④ Excessive alcohol ingestion

90. The best intervention to delay delivery of clients with vaginal bleeding in the last trimester is:
    ① Bed rest
    ② Oxygen by mask
    ③ Ultrasound test
    ④ Nonstress testing

Situation: Mrs. Elliot, 12 weeks pregnant, visits the obstetric clinic complaining of severe nausea and vomiting. Questions 91 through 97 refer to this situation.

91. The nurse suspects that Mrs. Elliot has hyperemesis gravidarum and knows that this is frequently associated with:
    ① High levels of chorionic gonadotropin
    ② Slowed secretion of free hydrochloric acid
    ③ A GI history of cholecystitis
    ④ Excessive amniotic fluid

92. On her next visit Mrs. Elliot is vastly improved and asks the nurse if she can continue to have sexual relations. The nurse's response is based on the knowledge that coitus during pregnancy would be contraindicated only in the presence of:
    ① Leukorrhea
    ② Gestation of 30 weeks or more
    ③ Premature rupture of membranes
    ④ Increased FHR

93. In the forty-first week of gestation, Mrs. Elliot has a bloody show but contractions have not begun. The head is at station +1. An acceptable method to induce labor at this time is:
    ① IM injection of oxytocin
    ② Artificial rupture of membranes
    ③ Administration of prostaglandins
    ④ A tap water enema

94. Mrs. Elliot has a bloody show and crampy abdominal pain. The nursing intervention at this time is:
    ① Typing and cross matching the client's blood for a possible transfusion
    ② Providing the client with comfort measures used for women in labor
    ③ Teaching the client how to avoid straining
    ④ Reviewing Lamaze breathing techniques with the client

95. During the postpartum period it is important that Mrs. Elliot voids regularly. Retention of fluid in the bladder is unrelated to the development of:
    ① Bladder atony
    ② Infection of the bladder
    ③ Diaphoresis following delivery
    ④ Postpartum bleeding

96. When Mrs. Elliot's male infant has been in the nursery for about 18 hours, the nurse caring for him notes that his breathing is below 35 per minute. No other changes are noted and, since the infant is apparently well, no record or report is made. Several hours later the infant experiences severe respiratory distress and emergency care is necessary. Legal responsibility in this instance would have to take into consideration that:
    ① A reading outside normal parameters is significant and should have been reported
    ② Respirations in the newborn are irregular and a drop is rarely important
    ③ Most infants experience slow respirations during the first 24 hours
    ④ The respiratory tract is underdeveloped in newborns and respiratory rate is not significant

97. During the taking-hold phase, the nurse would expect Mrs. Elliot to:
    ① Be concerned with her own needs
    ② Touch the baby with her fingertips
    ③ Call the baby by name
    ④ Talk about the baby

Situation: Mrs. Portridge has been married for 6 years and has been unable to become pregnant. Mr. and Mrs. Portridge have decided to discuss this problem with a physician, who suggests that some studies be done. Questions 98 through 101 refer to this situation.

98. A test commonly used to determine the number, motility, and activity of sperm is the:
    ① Rubin test
    ② Huhner test
    ③ Papanicolaou test
    ④ Friedman test

99. In the female, evaluation of all the pelvic organs of reproduction is accomplished by:
    ① Cystoscopy
    ② Biopsy
    ③ Culdoscopy
    ④ Hysterosalpingogram

100. After ovulation has occurred, the ovum is believed to remain viable for:
    ① 1 to 6 hours
    ② 12 to 18 hours
    ③ 24 to 36 hours
    ④ 48 to 72 hours

101. A factor in sterility may be related to the pH of the vaginal canal. A frequent medication that is ordered to alter the vaginal pH is:
    ① Sulfur insufflations
    ② Sodium bicarbonate douches
    ③ Lactic acid douches
    ④ Estrogen therapy

Situation: Mrs. Winder, age 24, complains of menstrual irregularity and infertility. Questions 102 through 104 refer to this situation.

102. A drug the physician might prescribe to treat both of Mrs. Winder's complaints is:
    ① Methallenestril (Vallestril)
    ② Ergonovine (Ergotrate)
    ③ Norethynodrel with mestranol (Enovid)
    ④ Relaxin (Releasin)

103. Eventually Mrs. Winder becomes pregnant. She is hospitalized when her membranes rupture during the thirty-eighth week of pregnancy. If the obstetrician decides to induce labor, the drug that will probably be used is:
    ① Ergonovine maleate
    ② Progesterone
    ③ Oxytocin (Pitocin)
    ④ Lututrin (Lutrexin)

104. During the period of induction, Mrs. Winder should be observed carefully for signs of:
    ① Uterine tetany
    ② Severe pain
    ③ Prolapse of the umbilical cord
    ④ Hypoglycemia

Situation: Mrs. King is a primigravida at term and is admitted to the labor room. She has attended education for childbirth classes together with her husband. When Mrs. King is admitted, she is experiencing contractions every 5 to 8 minutes, which last approximately 30 seconds. She also has a slight bloody discharge. The physician's examination reveals that the cervix is about 3 cm dilated and almost fully effaced. The vertex is presenting at a +1 station, with the occiput toward the left side of the symphysis pubis. Mrs. King is quite cheerful and at ease. Questions 105 through 111 refer to this situation.

105. Mrs. King asks the nurse if it is all right for her to get up and walk around. Based on observations of Mrs. King's contractions and knowledge of the physiology and mechanism of labor, the nurse could best respond:
    ① "Please stay in bed; walking may interfere with proper uterine contractions."
    ② "I can't make a decision on that, you will have to ask the doctor."
    ③ "You will have to stay in bed; otherwise your contractions cannot be timed and no one can listen to the fetal heart."
    ④ "It is quite all right for you to be up and about as long as you feel comfortable and your membranes are intact."

106. Mrs. King's contractions gradually increase in strength and become more frequent and last longer. Her membranes rupture. The first action for the nurse to take is to:
    ① Monitor the FHR
    ② Call the physician
    ③ Time the contractions
    ④ Check BP and pulse

107. The nurse observes the amniotic fluid and decides that it appears normal, since it is:
    ① Clear and dark amber colored
    ② Milky, greenish-yellow, containing shreds of mucus
    ③ Clear, almost colorless, containing little white specks
    ④ Cloudy, greenish-yellow, containing little white specks

108. An examination reveals that Mrs. King is 6 to 7 cm dilated and that the vertex is low in the midpelvis. To alleviate discomfort during contractions, the nurse should instruct Mr. King to encourage his wife to:
    ① Pant
    ② Abdominal breathe
    ③ Pelvic rock
    ④ Athletic chest breathe

109. Mrs. King becomes very tense with contractions and quite irritable. She frequently states "I cannot stand this a minute longer." This kind of behavior is indicative of the fact that she:
    ① Is entering the transition phase of labor
    ② Needs immediate administration of an analgesic or anesthetic
    ③ Is developing some abnormality in terms of uterine contractions
    ④ Has been very poorly prepared for labor in the parents' classes

110. Mr. King is becoming very tense at this time. He asks, "Do you think it is best for me to leave, since I don't seem to do my wife much good?" The most appropriate response by the nurse would be:
    ① "If you feel that way, you'd best go out and sit in the father's waiting room for a while because you may transmit your anxiety to your wife."
    ② "I know this is hard for you. Why don't you go have a cup of coffee and relax and come back later if you feel like it?"
    ③ "This is the time your wife needs you. Don't run out on her now."
    ④ "This is hard for you. Let me try to help you coach her during this difficult phase."

111. Mrs. King is now fully dilated, totally effaced, and the head is at +2. During each contraction the nurse should encourage her to:
    ① Relax by closing her eyes
    ② Push with lips closed
    ③ Pant to prevent cervical edema
    ④ Blow so as not to grunt

Situation: Mrs. Kelly is a 27-year-old gravida 1 para 0 with a childhood history of rheumatic fever. She has been admitted to the hospital at 35 weeks' gestation because of shortness of breath. Questions 112 through 119 refer to this situation.

112. Normal hemodynamics of pregnancy that affect the pregnant cardiac client include the:
    ① Decrease in the number of red blood cells
    ② Rise in cardiac output after the thirty-fourth week
    ③ Gradually increasing size of the uterus
    ④ Cardiac acceleration in the last half of pregnancy

113. Shortly after admission, Mrs. Kelly goes into labor. To prevent cardiac decompensation during labor the nurse should:
    ① Position Mrs. Kelly on her side with shoulders elevated
    ② Maintain an IV infusion of potassium chloride
    ③ Administer sodium IV infusion
    ④ Administer oxytocin to strengthen contractions

114. Nursing care of a women in premature labor includes:
    ① Reassuring her that the situation is under control
    ② Explaining why pain medication is kept at a minimum
    ③ Encouraging her not to bear down
    ④ Keeping her npo to prevent abdominal distention

115. During the postpartal period it is not uncommon for the new mother to have an increased cardiac output with tachycardia. The nurse should observe the client carefully for signs of:
    ① Irregular pulse
    ② Respiratory distress
    ③ Increased vaginal bleeding
    ④ Hypovolemic shock

116. Mrs. Kelly's infant weighs 2062 g (4 lb, 9 oz) with an Apgar of 8/9. On admission to the nursery it would be unnecessary for the nurse to:
    ① Evaluate the newborn's status
    ② Support body temperature
    ③ Administer oxygen
    ④ Record vital signs

117. The nurse must continuously monitor baby Kelly, since the most common complication in the preterm infant is:
    ① Brain damage
    ② Respiratory distress
    ③ Aspiration of mucus
    ④ Hemorrhage

118. The nurse must monitor baby Kelly's temperature and provide appropriate nursing care because the premature baby:
    ① Is unable to break down glycogen to glucose
    ② Has a limited ability to use shivering to produce heat
    ③ Has a limited supply of brown fat available to provide heat
    ④ Has an underdeveloped pituitary system to control internal heat

119. When meeting baby Kelly's hydration needs, the nurse must consider the fact that urinary function in the premature baby:
    ① Is the same as in a full-term newborn
    ② Causes the loss of large amounts of urine
    ③ Maintains stability of acid-base and electrolyte balance
    ④ Tends to overconcentrate the urine

Situation: Mrs. Kim, a 22-year-old primigravida at term, is brought to the hospital by her husband. They have attended preparation for childbirth classes and plan to be together during labor. On admission Mrs. Kim is having 3- to 5-minute contractions, she has a bloody show, and her membranes are intact. On vaginal examination the cervix is fully effaced and 6 cm dilated, the vertex presenting at a +1 station. Vital signs are temperature 37° C (98.6° F), pulse rate 76, respirations 20, FHR 140 L.L.Q., BP 118/74. Mr. Kim is coaching and supporting his wife well, and Mrs. Kim appears to be quite relaxed. Questions 120 through 125 refer to this situation.

120. According to these data, Mrs. Kim is in:
    ① Early phase of labor
    ② Midphase of labor
    ③ Transition phase of labor
    ④ Accelerated phase of labor

121. Station +1 indicates that the presenting part is:
    ① Slightly below the ischial spines
    ② Slightly above the ischial spines
    ③ High in the false pelvis
    ④ On the perineum

122. Mrs. Kim is uncomfortable and asks for medication. Demerol, 50 mg, and Phenergan, 50 mg, are ordered to be administered intramuscularly. This medication would:
    ① Induce sleep until the time of delivery
    ② Increase her pain threshold, resulting in relaxation
    ③ Act as an amnesic drug
    ④ Act as a preliminary to anesthesia

123. A few hours later Mrs. Kim becomes very restless, her face is flushed, and she is irritable, perspiring profusely, and feels she is going to vomit. These symptoms are indicative of:
    ① Second stage
    ② Late stage
    ③ Transition stage
    ④ Third stage

124. After delivery when inspecting her newborn baby girl, Mrs. Kim notices a discharge from the nipples of both breasts. The nurse should explain that this is evidence of:
    ① Monilia contracted during birth
    ② Congenital hormonal imbalance
    ③ An infection contracted in utero
    ④ The influence of the mother's hormones

125. During the postpartum period the nurse examines Mrs. Kim and identifies the presence of lochia serosa and a fundus four finger breadths below the umbilicus. This indicates that the time elapsed is:
    ① 1 to 3 days postpartum
    ② 4 to 5 days postpartum
    ③ 6 to 7 days postpartum
    ④ 8 to 9 days postpartum

Situation: Mrs. Rowan is admitted to the high-risk obstetric unit with preeclampsia. Questions 126 through 132 refer to this situation.

126. Mrs. Rowan is receiving magnesium sulfate. The nurse must be alert for the first sign of excessive blood magnesium levels, which is:
    ① Development of cardiac arrhythmia
    ② Disappearance of the knee-jerk reflex
    ③ Increase in respiratory rate
    ④ Disturbance in sensorium

127. In caring for Mrs. Rowan the nurse should:
    ① Encourage her to drink clear fluids
    ② Protect her against extraneous stimuli
    ③ Isolate her in a dark room
    ④ Maintain her in a supine position

128. The first assessable objective sign of a convulsion in a client with preeclampsia is frequently:
    ① Rolling of the eyes to one side with a fixed stare
    ② Spots or flashes of light before the eyes
    ③ Persistent headache and blurred vision
    ④ Epigastric pain, nausea, and vomiting

129. Mrs. Rowan has a convulsion. Following the convulsion she has an elevated temperature of 39° C (102° F). The nurse realizes that this may be caused by:
    ① Development of a systemic infection
    ② Dehydration caused by rapid fluid loss
    ③ Disturbance of the cerebral thermal center
    ④ Excessive muscular activity

130. Mrs. Rowan is afraid of having another convulsion and asks when the likelihood of convulsions will end. The nurse replies that the danger of a convulsion in a woman with eclampsia ends:
    ① After labor begins
    ② After delivery occurs
    ③ 24 hours postpartum
    ④ 48 hours postpartum

131. Mrs. Rowan's labor is long and the baby is delivered in the breech position. Since Erb-Duchenne paralysis may be seen as the result of a difficult forceps or breech delivery, the nurse should assess the neonate for:
    ① A flaccid arm with the elbow extended
    ② A negative Moro reflex on the unaffected side
    ③ Loss of grasp reflex on the affected side
    ④ Inability to turn the head to the affected side

132. If Erb-Duchenne paralysis occurred, nursing care of the infant would include:
    ① Constant immobilization of the affected arm
    ② Immediate active ROM exercises to the affected arm
    ③ Teaching the parents to manipulate the muscle
    ④ Daily measurement of girth and length of the affected arm

Situation: Mrs. Jackson, 2½ months pregnant, comes to the prenatal clinic for the first time. Questions 133 through 137 refer to this situation.

133. Mrs. Jackson asks the clinic nurse how smoking will affect the baby. The nurse's answer reflects the following knowledge:
    ① Fetal and maternal circulation are separated by the placental barrier
    ② The placenta is permeable to specific substances
    ③ Smoking relieves tension and the fetus responds accordingly
    ④ Vasoconstriction will affect both fetal and maternal blood vessels

134. Mrs. Jackson is concerned about the mask of pregnancy, her "dark nipples," and the "dark line" from her navel to her pubis. The nurse explains that these adaptations are caused by hyperactivity of the:
    ① Adrenal gland
    ② Thyroid gland
    ③ Ovaries
    ④ Pituitary gland

135. Mrs. Jackson complains of morning sickness. The nurse realizes that a predisposing factor which causes morning sickness during the first trimester of pregnancy is the adaptation to increased levels of:
    ① Estrogen
    ② Progesterone
    ③ Luteinizing hormone
    ④ Chorionic gonadotropin

136. The nurse can help Mrs. Jackson overcome morning sickness by suggesting she:
    ① Eat nothing until the nausea subsides
    ② Take an antacid before bedtime
    ③ Request her physician to prescribe an antiemetic
    ④ Eat dry toast before arising

137. Mrs. Jackson delivers a healthy baby boy. Two days postpartum, after receiving a phone call from her babysitter informing her that her 2-year-old has been very upset since her admission to the hospital and is not eating, Mrs. Jackson elects to sign her baby and herself out of the hospital. Staff members have been unable to contact her physician. Mrs. Jackson arrives at the nursery ready to leave and asks that her infant be given to her to dress and take home. Appropriate nursing action would be:
    ① Explain to Mrs. Jackson that her infant must remain in hospital until signed out by the physician and that she must leave the baby in the nursery
    ② Allow Mrs. Jackson time with the baby to cuddle him before she leaves, but emphasize that the baby is a minor and legally must remain until orders are received
    ③ Tell Mrs. Jackson that under the circumstances hospital policy prevents the staff from releasing the infant into her care, but she will be informed when he is discharged
    ④ Give the baby to Mrs. Jackson to take home, making sure that she receives information regarding care and feeding of a 2-day-old infant and any potential problems which may develop

Situation: Mr. and Mrs. Singer are Rh-incompatible partners. As the pregnancy progresses, the maternal serum antibody titer continues to rise. An amniocentesis is scheduled for the twenty-eighth week of pregnancy. Questions 138 through 141 refer to this situation.

138. A common method of locating the precise position of a fetus prior to an amniocentesis is:
    ① X-ray examination
    ② Fetoscopy
    ③ Fluoroscopy
    ④ Sonography

139. The results of the amniocentesis indicate that the fetus is only mildly affected but does, in fact, have Down's syndrome. Mr. and Mrs. Singer elect to have the pregnancy terminated. The nurse giving postoperative care to a client who has had her pregnancy surgically terminated by hysterotomy should be aware that:
    ① The client is emotionally unstable at this time.
    ② The client needs to express her feeling of guilt, anger, and frustration
    ③ Contraceptive counseling should be deferred to a later time
    ④ The risk of postoperative infection is high

140. After the hysterotomy, Rh_oD (RhoGAM) is administered intramuscularly to:
    ① Prevent antibody formation in the mother
    ② Expand the antibody pool of the mother
    ③ Accelerate the mother's production of immune bodies
    ④ Suppress the activity of Rh-negative antibodies

141. It is important for the nurse to support the decisions made by the parents of a fetus with a birth defect, since:
    ① The nurse's support will relieve the pressure associated with decision making
    ② Supporting them will eliminate feelings of guilt
    ③ The parents are legally responsible for the decision
    ④ It is essential for maintenance of family equilibrium

Situation: Mrs. Dowle delivers a 2811.6 g (6 lb, 3 oz) baby girl. Questions 142 through 144 refer to this situation.

142. While holding her baby, Mrs. Dowle calls the nurse and says, "My baby is sick; she sneezes a lot and look how she breathes. Her breathing is so rapid and shallow and not regular. My neighbor's baby had to return to the hospital after she was home a week because she had pneumonia. I hope this does not happen to my baby." The best action for the nurse to take is to:
    ① Pick up the baby and tell the mother that the nurses will watch her closely
    ② Look the baby over and tell the mother that the baby is fine, there is nothing wrong with her
    ③ Look the baby over and explain to the mother that sneezing is normal and helps the baby to get rid of mucus and that a baby normally has rapid, shallow, irregular respirations
    ④ Look the baby over, take her to the nursery immediately, and return to the mother to tell her that the physician has been called, since the baby is obviously in respiratory distress

143. The nurse's response is based on the knowledge that a normal infant's respirations are:
    ① Regular, initiated by the chest wall, 40 to 60 per minute, shallow
    ② Irregular, abdominal, 40 to 50 per minute, shallow
    ③ Regular, abdominal, 40 to 50 per minute, deep
    ④ Irregular, initiated by chest wall, 30 to 60 per minute, deep

144. Mrs. Dowle, who has three children under 5 years of age at home, comments to the nursery nurse that she cannot hold the baby for feedings once she gets home. She has just too much to do, and anyhow it spoils the baby. The best response for the nurse to make is:
    ① "That's entirely up to you, you have to do what works for you."
    ② "Holding the baby when feeding is important for her development."
    ③ "It is most unsafe to prop a bottle. The baby could aspirate the fluid."
    ④ "You seem concerned about time. Let's talk about it."

Situation: Mrs. Ballen is admitted to the obstetric unit in labor with contractions about 15 minutes apart. Her cervix is moderately effaced and 4 cm dilated. Questions 145 through 150 refer to this situation.

145. During labor the nurse must be aware that an early deceleration (Type I dip) is evidenced by a FHR of:
    ① 140 to 160 beats per minute early in the contraction
    ② 120 to 140 beats per minute early in the contraction
    ③ 100 to 119 beats per minute early in the contraction
    ④ 80 to 100 beats per minute early in the contraction

146. Mrs. Ballen's labor progresses uneventfully and she enters the transitional stage. When Mrs. Ballen is positioned on the delivery table, both legs should be placed simultaneously in the stirrups to prevent:
    ① Excessive pull on the fascia
    ② Pressure on the perineum
    ③ Trauma to the uterine ligaments
    ④ Venous stasis in the legs

147. During each contraction the FHR persistently drops from 140 to 110 per minute, but recovers at end of contraction. The nurse should:
    ① Continue to monitor the FHR during contractions
    ② Notify the physician and prepare for immediate delivery
    ③ Decrease the drip rate of oxytocin to slow contractions
    ④ Change mother's position from back to side or side to side

148. Mrs. Ballen has decided to breast feed her infant. When teaching breast feeding the nurse should recognize Mrs. Ballen needs further instructions when she states, "I will:
    ① Try to empty the breast at each feeding."
    ② Use an alternate breast at each feeding."
    ③ Wash breasts with soap and water before feeding."
    ④ Wash breasts with water before each feeding."

149. Mrs. Ballen complains of frequent leg cramps. The nurse should suspect:
    ① Hypercalcemia and tell her to increase her activity
    ② Hypokalemia and tell her to increase her intake of green, leafy vegetables
    ③ Hyperkalemia and tell her to see a physician immediately
    ④ Hypocalcemia and tell her to increase her intake of milk

150. Mrs. Ballen asks about the difference between cow's milk and the milk from her breasts. The nurse should respond that cow's milk differs from human milk in that it contains:
    ① More protein, more calcium, and less carbohydrate
    ② Less protein, less calcium, and more carbohydrate
    ③ Less protein, more calcium, and more carbohydrate
    ④ More protein, less calcium, and less carbohydrate

Situation: Baby Reisler is delivered at 29 weeks' gestation. He weighs 1619 g (3 lb, 9 oz). Questions 151 through 154 refer to this situation.

151. Baby Reisler is considered to be in critical condition. According to his size and length of gestation, he would be classified as:
    ① Preterm
    ② Immature
    ③ Nonviable
    ④ Low-birth-weight infant

152. Baby Reisler is being fed by gavage. This type of feeding is indicated for such infants because:
    ① The feeding can be given quickly, so handling is minimized
    ② Vomiting is prevented
    ③ It conserves the baby's strength and does not depend on the swallowing reflex
    ④ The amount of food given can be more accurately regulated

153. Baby Reisler is placed in an incubator to maintain his body temperature at a constant level, since the heat regulation mechanism in these infants is one of the least developed functions. This is related to the fact that:
    ① The surface area in these babies is smaller than in normal newborns
    ② These babies lack subcutaneous fat, which would furnish some insulation
    ③ These babies perspire a great deal, thus losing heat almost constantly
    ④ These babies have a limited ability to produce antibodies against infections

154. In caring for these infants, the precautions that should be taken against retrolental fibroplasia include:
    ① Keeping oxygen at less than 40% concentration and discontinuing it as soon as feasible
    ② Carefully controlling temperature and humidity
    ③ Maintaining a high concentration of oxygen (above 75%) together with high humidity
    ④ Using phototherapy to prevent jaundice and retinopathy

Situation: After a long and difficult delivery, Baby John is admitted to the newborn nursery. Questions 155 through 159 refer to this situation.

155. An Apgar score of 4 would most likely indicate that his:
    ① Body is pink but his extremities blue
    ② Heart rate is over 100
    ③ Muscle tone is flaccid
    ④ Respirations are 35

156. Baby John has muscle twitchings, convulsions, cyanosis, abnormal respirations, and a short shrill cry. The nurse should suspect that he has:
    ① Tetany
    ② Intracranial hemorrhage
    ③ Spina bifida
    ④ Hyperkalemia

157. When observing Baby John for signs of pathologic jaundice, the nurse should be alert for:
    ① The appearance of jaundice during the first 24 hours
    ② Jaundice developing between 24 and 72 hours
    ③ Neurologic signs during the first 24 hours
    ④ Muscular irritability at birth

158. The nurse observes Baby John lying in a supine position with his head turned to the side, his legs and arms extended on the same side and flexed on the opposite side. This is:
    ① The Landau reflex
    ② The tonic neck reflex
    ③ The Moro reflex
    ④ An abnormal reflex

159. Experience has shown that parents are better able to cope with the birth of an abnormal child if informed:
    ① After the first 48 hours, when the mother's strength has returned
    ② When bringing the baby to the mother for the first time
    ③ After the birth, while the mother is still in the delivery room
    ④ When the parents ask if something is wrong with their baby

Situation: Mr. and Mrs. Light want to practice the rhythm method of contraception but do not understand how it works. Questions 160 through 163 refer to this situation.

160. The nurse's explanation is based on ovulation occurring:
    ① Seven days after the completion of the menstrual period
    ② Fourteen days after the completion of the menstrual period
    ③ Seven days before the end of the menstrual cycle
    ④ Fourteen days prior to the onset of menstruation

161. The time of ovulation can be determined by taking the basal temperature. During ovulation the basal temperature:
    ① Drops markedly
    ② Drops slightly and then rises
    ③ Rises markedly and remains high
    ④ Rises suddenly and then falls

162. The nurse explains that the efficiency of rhythm is dependent on the basal body temperature. A factor that will alter its effectiveness is:
    ① Frequency of intercourse
    ② Age of those involved
    ③ Presence of stress
    ④ Length of abstinence

163. Mrs. Light has missed two periods. When she comes to the prenatal clinic, she complains of vaginal bleeding and one-sided pain. The nurse suspects that Mrs. Light has:
    ① An incomplete abortion
    ② An ectopic pregnancy
    ③ Abruptio placentae
    ④ A rupture of the graafian follicle

Situation: Mr. and Mrs. Quinn have been married almost 7 years when the physician confirms that Mrs. Quinn is 8 to 10 weeks pregnant. Mr. and Mrs. Quinn are overjoyed. About 10 days after her visit to the physician, at the time of her normal menstrual period, Mrs. Quinn starts to stain but denies pain. The physician tells her to go to bed immediately and remain on complete bed rest for at least 72 hours. Since Mr. Quinn cannot stay at home and Mrs. Quinn has no one else to care for her, she is admitted to the hospital. Questions 164 through 167 refer to this situation.

164. Mrs. Quinn is admitted with a diagnosis of:
    ① Threatened abortion
    ② Inevitable abortion
    ③ Ectopic pregnancy
    ④ Missed abortion

165. After a few hours Mrs. Quinn begins to experience bearing-down sensations and suddenly expels the products of conception in bed. To give safe nursing care, the nurse should first:
    ① Take her immediately to the delivery room
    ② Check the fundus for firmness
    ③ Give her the sedation ordered
    ④ Immediately notify the physician

166. After delivery the nurse should observe Mrs. Quinn for:
    ① Dehydration and hemorrhage
    ② Hemorrhage and infection
    ③ Subinvolution and dehydration
    ④ Signs of toxemia

167. When Mrs. Quinn returns to her room, both she and her husband are visibly upset. The nurse notices that Mr. Quinn has tears in his eyes and that Mrs. Quinn has her face turned to the wall and is sobbing quietly. The best approach for the nurse to take is to go over to Mrs. Quinn and say:
    ① "I know how you feel, but you should not be so upset now, it will make it more difficult for you to get well quickly."
    ② "I can understand that you are upset, but be glad it happened early in your pregnancy and not after you carried the baby for the full time."
    ③ "I know that you are upset now, but hopefully you will become pregnant again very soon."
    ④ "I see that both of you are very upset. I brought you a cup of coffee and will be here if you want to talk."

Situation: Mr. and Mrs. James are attending the infertility clinic. Questions 168 through 173 refer to this situation.

168. In dealing with a couple who have been identified as having an infertility problem, the nurse should know that:
    ① One partner has a problem that makes them unable to have children
    ② The couple has been unable to have a child after trying for a year
    ③ Infertility is usually psychologic in origin
    ④ Infertility and sterility are essentially the same problem

169. A diagnostic test used to evaluate fertility is the post-coital test. It is best timed:
    ① Immediately after menses
    ② Within 1 to 2 days of presumed ovulation
    ③ One week after ovulation
    ④ Just prior to the next menstrual period

170. A tubal insufflation test is done to determine whether there is a tubal obstruction. Infertility caused by a defect in the tube is usually related to a:
    ① Past infection
    ② Fibroid tumor
    ③ Congenital anomaly
    ④ Previous injury to a tube

171. Mrs. James returns to the clinic because she has missed her menstrual period and thinks she is pregnant. The laboratory tests for pregnancy are based on the presence of:
    ① Isoimmune bodies
    ② Chorionic gonadotropin
    ③ Estrogen
    ④ Progesterone

172. In assessing Mrs. James' physical condition the nurse is aware of the fact that a normal adaptation of pregnancy is an increased blood supply to the pelvic region. The resulting bluish purple discoloration of the vaginal mucosa and cervix is known as:
    ① Hegar's sign
    ② Ladin's sign
    ③ Goodell's sign
    ④ Chadwick's sign

173. Mrs. James is concerned about gaining weight during pregnancy. The nurse explains that the largest part of weight gain during pregnancy is due to:
    ① Metabolic alterations
    ② Fluid retention
    ③ Increased blood volume
    ④ The fetus

Situation: Mrs. Page has been in labor for 18 hours and is exhausted. A cesarean delivery is being considered. Questions 174 through 178 refer to this situation.

174. The most common indication for cesarean delivery is:
    ① Cephalopelvic disproportion
    ② Primary uterine inertia
    ③ Placenta previa
    ④ Vaginal atony

175. The physician reviews Mrs. Page's pelvic measurements. The anteroposterior diameter of the birth canal is one of the important measurements of the pelvis and is known as the:
    ① Diagonal conjugate
    ② Transverse conjugate
    ③ Conjugate vera
    ④ Transverse diameter

176. To determine if there is cephalopelvic disproportion the physician will order:
    1. Pelvimetry
    2. X-ray examination
    3. Amniocentesis
    4. Fetal scalp pH

177. Mrs. Page eventually delivers her baby vaginally. The newborn has asymmetric gluteal folds, and the nurse suspects:
    1. A dislocated hip
    2. Peripheral nervous system damage
    3. An inguinal hernia
    4. CNS damage

178. Mrs. Page asks the nurse why sugar is added to the baby's formula. The nurse's response would depend on the following understanding:
    1. Cow's milk contains fewer calories than breast milk
    2. Sugar in cow's milk is not assimilated well
    3. Diluted cow's milk provides less sugar than the baby needs
    4. Sugar in cow's milk is a disaccharide

Situation: Mrs. Allen is 2 weeks past her expected date of delivery. The physician has decided to perform an oxytocin challenge test (OCT), in which IV oxytocin solution is administered and the FHR and uterine contractions are recorded. Questions 179 through 184 refer to this situation.

179. Which of the following would be an indication for the OCT?
    1. Previous abruptio placentae
    2. Placenta previa
    3. Premature onset of labor
    4. Pregnancy of more than 40 weeks

180. Contraindications to an OCT would include:
    1. Prematurity
    2. Drug addiction
    3. Hypertension
    4. Uterine activity

181. Mrs. Allen responds well to the OCT and labor is induced. Several hours later Mrs. Allen is complaining of pain and asks for medication. A medication given to a woman in labor that might cause respiratory depression of the newborn is:
    1. Meperidine (Demerol)
    2. Scopolamine
    3. Promazine (Sparine)
    4. Promethazine (Phenergan)

182. Mrs. Allen delivers a 4260 g (9 lb, 6 oz) baby. In assessing the newborn, the nurse observes an unequal Moro reflex on one side and a flaccid arm in adduction. The nurse suspects:
    1. Brachial palsy
    2. Supratentorial tear
    3. Fracture of the clavical
    4. Crigler/Najjar syndrome

183. The evening after delivery, the nurse encourages Mrs. Allen to ambulate in order to:
    1. Increase the tone of the bladder
    2. Promote respiration
    3. Increase peripheral vasomotor activity
    4. Maintain tone of abdominal muscles

184. In caring for the family on a postpartum unit, the nurse must be aware that all the tasks, responsibilities, and attitudes which make up child care can be called mothering and that either parent can exhibit motherliness. A person is able to perform "mothering" because of:
    1. An inborn ability based on instinct
    2. Positive childhood roles and concepts
    3. A good education in growth and development
    4. A marriage with flexible roles

Situation: Mrs. Evans, a diabetic, suspects that she is pregnant because she is experiencing breast changes, has missed two periods, and has some early morning nausea and excessive fatigue. Despite the nausea and fatigue, her urine tests are consistently negative for sugar. Mrs. Evans seeks the advice of an obstetrician, who confirms the diagnosis of pregnancy. Mrs. Evans is taking 30 units of NPH insulin daily at this time. Questions 185 through 189 refer to this situation.

185. A diabetic mother's metabolism is significantly altered during pregnancy as a result of:
    1. The increased effect of insulin during pregnancy
    2. The effect of hormones produced in pregnancy on carbohydrate and lipid metabolism
    3. An increase in the glucose tolerance level of the blood
    4. The lower renal threshold for glucose

186. Regulation of usual insulin coverage in a pregnant diabetic woman is difficult, since:
    1. Sugar can normally be found in the urine of a pregnant woman
    2. Sugar is metabolized more rapidly during pregnancy
    3. The basal metabolic rate is altered during pregnancy
    4. Insulin is absorbed more rapidly because of increased blood volume

187. Mrs. Evans is referred to the clinic nutritionist for nutritional assessment and counseling. The dietary program worked out for her would be:
    1. A low-carbohydrate, low-calorie diet to stay within her present insulin coverage and avoid hyperglycemia
    2. A diet high in protein of good biologic value and decreased calories
    3. Adequate balance of carbohydrate and fat to meet energy demands and prevent ketosis
    4. Insulin adjusted as needed to balance increased dietary needs

188. When Mrs. Evans' newborn is admitted to the newborn nursery, the nurse should be aware that babies of diabetic mothers show symptoms of tremors, apnea, cyanosis, and poor sucking reflex because of:
    1. Congenital depression of the islets of Langerhans
    2. Hypoglycemia
    3. CNS edema
    4. Hyperglycemia

189. Mrs. Evans' baby weighs 4600.8 g (10 lb, 2 oz), and she expresses concern about its size. The nurse's reply should be based upon the knowledge that babies of diabetic mothers are larger than other babies because of:

① Increased somatotropin and lowered glucose utilization
② Increased somatotropin and increased glucose utilization
③ Decreased somatotropin and decreased glucose utilization
④ Decreased somatotropin and increased glucose utilization

Situation: Mrs. Sawyer suspects she is pregnant when she attends the prenatal clinic for the first time. This is her first pregnancy and she is unsure whether the pregnancy should be terminated, since she and her husband depend on her salary. Questions 190 through 195 refer to this situation.

190. Pregnancy and birth are called crises because:
① They are periods of change and adjustment to change
② There are hormonal and physiologic changes in the mother
③ There are mood changes during pregnancy
④ Narcissism in the mother affects the husband-wife relationship

191. The nurse should intervene to alleviate crisis by:
① Involving the mother in preparation classes
② Helping the mother express her feelings
③ Understanding the family interaction
④ Involving the father in preparation classes

192. The nurse suggests a pregnancy test. This is possible because in early pregnancy the urine contains:
① Prolactin
② Chorionic gonadotropin
③ Estrogen
④ Luteinizing hormone

193. At the time of her second visit to the prenatal clinic Mrs. Sawyer requests information about abortion. She is 8 weeks pregnant at this time. The nurse expresses the opinion that abortion is immoral and that many women have permanent guilt feelings after an abortion. Mrs. Sawyer leaves the clinic in a very disturbed state. Legally the:
① Nurse had a right to state feelings as long as they were identified as the nurse's own
② Client had a right to correct, unbiased information
③ Physician should have been called in, since the nurse cannot talk about it
④ Nurse's statements need not be based on scientific knowledge

194. Mrs. Sawyer returns to the clinic after deciding to continue with the pregnancy. She complains of nausea and urinary frequency. She states that she feels punished for her thoughts about abortion. The nurse explains that urinary frequency often occurs because the capacity of the bladder is diminished during pregnancy by:
① Atony of the detrusor muscle
② Compression by the ascending uterus
③ Constriction of the ureteral entrance at the trigone
④ Compromise of the autonomic reflexes

195. The nurse also informs her that morning sickness is not punishment but is associated with pregnancy and usually ends by the end of the:

① Second month
② Third month
③ Fifth month
④ Fourth month

Situation: Mrs. Pitis, a 28-year-old primipara, was admitted 8 hours ago, 2 cm dilated in active labor. She is now 3 or 4 cm dilated and the vertex is floating. Questions 196 through 203 refer to this situation.

196. One of the most common causes of hypotonic uterine dystocia is:
① Toxemia
② Maternal anemia
③ Pelvic contracture
④ Twin gestation

197. Nursing care would include a careful assessment for signs of maternal exhaustion such as:
① Circumoral cyanosis
② Lowered body temperature
③ Fruity odor to breath
④ Skeletal muscle irritability

198. When caring for Mrs. Pitis, who is having a prolonged labor, the nurse must be aware that the client is very concerned when her labor deviates from what she sees as the norm. A response conveying acceptance of the client's expressions of frustration and hostility would be:
① "Would you like to talk about what's bothering you?"
② "All women get weary and frustrated during labor."
③ "I'll rub your back; tell me if it helps."
④ "I'll leave so you can talk to your husband."

199. Because secondary uterine inertia has developed in Mrs. Pitis, the physician has ordered oxytocin to stimulate contractions. The most important aspect of nursing care at this time is:
① Monitoring the FHR
② Checking perineum for bulging
③ Timing and recording length of contractions
④ Preparing for an emergency cesarean delivery

200. After a trial labor with oxytocin and x-ray pelvimetry, the physician advises Mrs. Pitis that a cesarean delivery is necessary. In addition to the routine care given postpartum clients during the first 24 hours, the nurse should:
① Check the fundus gently but firmly
② Check vital signs for evidence of shock
③ Maintain IV infusion of oxytocin
④ Encourage early ambulation

201. Two-day-old Andrew Pitis, who weighs 2722 g (6 lb), is fed Enfamil every 4 hours. Newborns need about 73 ml (2 to 3 oz) of fluid per pound of body weight each day. Based on this information, the nurse knows at each feeding to give Andrew at least:
① 2 to 3 oz
② 1 to 2 oz
③ 3 to 4 oz
④ 4 to 5 oz

202. Andrew has begun to eat greedily and finishes the entire bottle of formula. Afterward he regurgitates and his mother is concerned. The nurse explains to the mother that this is normal and due to:
    ① An underdeveloped cardiac sphincter
    ② A spasm at the pyloric valve
    ③ Intake of air while sucking
    ④ His position after feeding

203. Andrew has just been circumcised. The most essential nursing action the first day is to observe for:
    ① Infection
    ② Decreased urinary output
    ③ Shrill, piercing cry
    ④ Hemorrhage

Situation: Baby Terrence, a full-term male child, is delivered by cesarean delivery from a mother who is a known drug user. He is admitted to the newborn nursery. Questions 204 and 205 refer to this situation.

204. About 4 days after delivery the nurse notes that Baby Terrence has a purulent discharge from his eyes. The nurse suspects that he has:
    ① Developed a reaction to the AgNo₃ drops
    ② Signs of acquired immune deficiency syndrome (AIDS)
    ③ Contracted ophthalmia neonatorum
    ④ Symptoms of *Chlamydia trachomatis* infection

205. If an infant develops purulent conjunctivitis on the fourth day, the nurse should first:
    ① Secure an order for allergy testing of the infant
    ② Observe the infant for signs of pneumonia
    ③ Bathe the infant's eyes with tepid boric acid solution
    ④ Teach the mother about hand washing

Situation: Helen Reading is a Class 1 cardiac client with a history of rheumatic fever. She is admitted to the labor room in active labor. Questions 206 through 208 refer to this situation.

206. Proper positioning for Mrs. Reading is:
    ① Semi-Fowler's; supine
    ② Lying on right side; head elevated 30°
    ③ Left lateral; semi-Fowler's
    ④ Supine; high-Fowler's

207. A specific nursing intervention during labor for a client with cardiac problems is:
    ① Auscultating for rales q 30 minutes
    ② Turning from side to side q 15 minutes
    ③ Monitoring BP every hour
    ④ Encouraging frequent voiding

208. In view of Mrs. Reading's past medical history, the nurse anticipates that after delivery Mrs. Reading will be prophylactically placed on:
    ① Digitalis
    ② Lasix
    ③ Ampicillin
    ④ Heparin

Situation: Mrs. Tracey, 6-months pregnant, is admitted with complaints of painful urination, flank tenderness, and hematuria. Questions 209 and 210 refer to this situation.

209. A diagnosis of pyelonephritis is made. An important nursing intervention for Mrs. Tracey during this attack is:
    ① Limiting fluid intake
    ② Observing for signs of premature labor
    ③ Examining the urine for albumin
    ④ Maintaining her on a low-salt diet

210. Mrs. Tracey is to receive antibiotic therapy. The nurse should recognize that the safest antibiotic for administration during pregnancy would be:
    ① Nitrofurantoin
    ② Gantrisin
    ③ Tetracycline
    ④ Ampicillin

Comprehensive Tests

The following two comprehensive examinations have been developed to simulate the NCLEX examination. In order for you to achieve maximum learning from this experience we have divided each Comprehensive Test into four sections. You should allow 90 minutes (1½ hours) for each part and complete each part at one sitting. This will reflect one of the four testing sessions of the present NCLEX.

In Comprehensive Test 1 we recommend that you review the answers and rationales for each part as you complete it. In Comprehensive Test 2 we recommend that you plan two separate 1½ hour sessions daily for 2 consecutive days and wait until you have completed all four parts before checking the answers and rationales. We have made these recommendations so that Test 1 continues and reinforces your immediate learning and Test 2, while reinforcing learning, better reflects the actual situation you will experience when taking the NCLEX.

To help you analyze your mistakes on the comprehensive examinations and to provide a data base for making future study plans, two types of worksheets have been included. One is designed to aid you in identifying and recording errors in the way you process information. The other is to help you identify and record gaps in knowledge. Follow directions that appear on each worksheet. Use a separate set of worksheets for each part of both examinations. Use Worksheet 1 to identify the frequency with which you made particular errors. As you review material in class notes or this review book, pay special attention to correcting your most common problems. Use Worksheet 2 to identify the topics you want to review. It might be helpful to set priorities; review the most difficult topics first so that you will have time to review them more than once. These worksheets can be used to focus your future study.

The comprehensive test questions, like those in the comprehensive licensing examinations, are classified by level of difficulty and by five categories: (1) phases of the nursing process, (2) cognitive level, (3) clinical area, (4) client needs, and (5) category of concern. Full descriptions of these categories and their subclassifications are presented in Chapter 1, pp. 1-2. The letters following the rationales for the correct answers indicate the applicable categories. A key to these letters is given at the beginning of the Answers and Rationales for Comprehensive Tests, p. 633.

COMPREHENSIVE TEST 1: PART 1

To simulate the National Council Licensure Examination, this test should be completed within 1½ hours.

Situation: Mrs. Kraft, a 45-year-old woman, is a severe diabetic who is admitted to the hospital for a midthigh amputation of her right leg because of a gangrenous leg ulcer. She also has a history of chronic angle closure glaucoma and has been using pilocarpine 2% eyedrops four times a day for the past year.

1. The chief aim of treatment in chronic glaucoma is:
   ① Controlling intraocular pressure
   ② Dilating the pupil to allow for an increase in visual field
   ③ Resting the eye to reduce pressure
   ④ Preventing secondary infections that can add to the visual problem

2. Mrs. Kraft seems able to accept the amputation but appears to have difficulty dealing with the glaucoma. The nurse arranges to spend more time with her, since the nurse realizes the client with glaucoma needs assistance in learning to accept the disease because:
   ① There is usually restriction in the use of both eyes
   ② Lost vision cannot be restored
   ③ Total blindness is inevitable
   ④ Surgery will only temporarily help the problem

3. The ocular symptom that the nurse should expect Mrs. Kraft to exhibit is:
   ① A complete loss of central vision
   ② Attacks of acute pain
   ③ Impairment of peripheral vision
   ④ Constant blurred vision

4. Before the amputation, the anesthesiologist prescribes meperidine (Demerol), 50 mg, and atropine, 0.4 mg, for Mrs. Kraft. The nurse should:
   ① Withhold the atropine, since it is contraindicated
   ② Give the medication as ordered
   ③ Administer the pilocarpine before the atropine
   ④ Ask the anesthesiologist to verify the order

5. Postoperatively, to prevent contractures of the hip, the nurse should:
   ① Place pillows under the stump
   ② Encourage Mrs. Kraft to lie in the prone position several times daily
   ③ Remove pillows from under the stump and elevate the head of the bed
   ④ Encourage Mrs. Kraft to sit in a chair as much as possible

6. To promote early and efficient ambulation when Mrs. Kraft is allowed out of bed, the nurse should encourage her to:
   ① Keep hip in extension and abduction
   ② Keep hip in extension and adduction
   ③ Keep hip in flexion and adduction
   ④ Keep right shoulder raised when swinging stump

7. Stump shrinkage is an important step in the healing process. There are two factors that contribute to stump shrinkage: one is atrophy of the muscles, and the other is:
   ① Postoperative edema
   ② Development of skin turgor
   ③ Reduction of subcutaneous fat
   ④ Loss of tissue and bone during operation

8. In helping Mrs. Kraft prepare her stump for a prosthesis, the nurse should encourage her to:
   ① Abduct the stump when ambulating
   ② Hang the stump off the bed frequently
   ③ Soak the stump in warm water twice a day
   ④ Periodically press the end of the stump against a pillow

9. When preparing Mrs. Kraft for dinner, it is the nurse's responsibility to:
   ① Remove the pillow under the stump and raise the head of the bed
   ② Check Mrs. Kraft's urine for sugar and acetone
   ③ Get Mrs. Kraft out of bed and into a chair
   ④ Make sure that Mrs. Kraft uses salt substitutes

10. In planning for discharge with Mrs. Kraft, the nurse discusses stump care. Because of her glaucoma, Mrs. Kraft should:
    ① Use mydriatrics regularly
    ② Restrict fluid intake
    ③ Avoid bright lights or darkness
    ④ Avoid bending exercises

Situation: Ten-year-old Marc has rheumatoid arthritis. His joints are enlarged, and he has a low-grade fever with an erythematous rash on his trunk.

11. When planning nursing care for Marc, the nurse should know that he will most often have pain and limited movement of his joints:
    ① When the latex fixation test is positive
    ② When the room is cool
    ③ In the morning on awakening
    ④ After assistive exercise

12. A major difference between juvenile rheumatoid arthritis and the polyarthritis of rheumatic fever is that with rheumatoid arthritis there may be:
    ① Some permanent cardiac damage
    ② An exacerbation during the winter months
    ③ Some residual joint deformity
    ④ A link with the *Streptococcus* organism

13. In a client receiving prolonged aspirin therapy, the nurse should be alert for symptoms of:
    ① Urinary calculi
    ② Prolonged clotting time
    ③ Atrophy of the liver
    ④ Premature erythrocyte destruction

14. When 10-year-old Marc is able to move to a two-bed room, the best suited roommate would be:
    ① An 11-year-old boy with an appendectomy
    ② A 10-year-old girl with a fractured femur
    ③ A 9-year-old boy with asthma
    ④ A 12-year-old girl with colitis

Situation: Mr. Ray is admitted to the surgical unit with a diagnosis of cancer of the colon. His physician plans to do a colon resection with a permanent colostomy. During the 3 days prior to surgery, Mr. Ray is very cooperative in all preoperative procedures, responds pleasantly when approached by the nurses, and does not question staff about what is being done to him.

15. From his behavior, the nurse recognizes that Mr. Ray most likely:
    ① Is totally denying his illness
    ② Has been fully informed by his physician about what to expect
    ③ Is not verbalizing his feelings about what will happen to him
    ④ Feels reassured by his frequent contacts with the nurses

16. The night before Mr. Ray's surgery the nurse notices that each time rounds are made he is awake, despite adequate sedation. He has no requests but invites the nurse to have a cigarette with him. Based on an understanding of Mr. Ray's behavior, the nurse's response should be to:
    ① Send in a nurse's aide to keep him company while he smokes
    ② Point out to him that nurses cannot smoke in clients' rooms
    ③ Light his cigarette and tell him to call again if he still can't sleep
    ④ Light his cigarette and indicate that his inability to sleep has been noticed

17. After surgery the most effective way of helping Mr. Ray accept his colostomy would be to:
    ① Give him literature containing factual data about colostomies
    ② Point out to him the number of important people who have had colostomies
    ③ Begin to teach him self-care of his colostomy immediately
    ④ Contact a member of Colostomies, Inc. to speak with him

18. Mr. Ray's postoperative diet order reads "diet as tolerated". Principles that should guide food choices include:
    ① A low-residue diet should be followed indefinitely to avoid overstimulating the intestine
    ② A return to a regular diet as soon as possible gives psychologic support and more rapid physical rehabilitation
    ③ Many foods will cause all individuals with a colostomy the same discomfort
    ④ More rigid dietary rules limiting food choices are needed to provide security

19. During a colostomy irrigation, if Mr. Ray complains of abdominal cramps, the nurse should:
    ① Raise the irrigating can so the irrigation can be completed quickly
    ② Reassure him and continue the irrigation
    ③ Pinch the tubing so that less fluid enters the colon
    ④ Clamp the tubing and allow Mr. Ray to rest

20. Mr. Ray's colostomy is located on the left side of the abdomen. The type of stool the nurse would expect Mr. Ray to expel would be:
    ① Moist, formed
    ② Pencil shaped
    ③ Liquid
    ④ Mucus coated

21. During the rehabilitation period, when discussing with Mr. Ray the regaining of some measure of bowel control, the nurse should emphasize:
    ① Having a set time each day for his colostomy irrigation
    ② The importance of a soft low-residue diet
    ③ The importance of managing his fluid intake
    ④ The necessity for a high-protein diet

Situation: Johnny has been attending a day care center for autistic children.

22. Autism can usually be diagnosed when the child is about:
    ① 6 months of age
    ② 1 to 3 months of age
    ③ 2 years of age
    ④ 6 years of age
23. In planning activities for Johnny the nurse must remember that autistic children respond best to:
    ① Loud cheerful music
    ② Their own self-stimulating acts
    ③ Individuals in small groups
    ④ Large group activity
24. Since autistic children withdraw into their own world, relationships are difficult to establish. The nurse may be able to reach Johnny by:
    ① Body contact, such as cuddling
    ② Encouraging his participation in group activities
    ③ Imitating and participating in his activities
    ④ Providing a quiet, safe place for rocking
25. The nurse would expect Johnny to demonstrate:
    ① Sad, blank facial expressions
    ② Flapping of hands and rocking
    ③ Inappropriate smiling with flat emotions
    ④ Lack of response to any stimulus
26. When using play as therapy with Johnny the nurse should:
    ① Play music and dance with Johnny
    ② Provide mechanical and inanimate objects for play
    ③ Talk with Johnny while touching his hands
    ④ Provide brightly colored toys and blocks that he can handle
27. Given a choice, the autistic child would usually enjoy playing with a:
    ① Cuddly toy
    ② Large red block
    ③ Small yellow block
    ④ Playground merry-go-round

Situation: Mrs. Wallace is a 22-year-old primigravida who is 6½ months pregnant.

28. When she is seen by the physician Mrs. Wallace's BP is 150/85 and she has gained 2.27 kg (5 lb) in the last 2 weeks. The nurse should:
    ① Give Mrs. Wallace an appointment for 2 weeks hence
    ② Prepare Mrs. Wallace for a vaginal examination
    ③ Take Mrs. Wallace's temperature and pulse
    ④ Prepare the equipment for testing Mrs. Wallace's urine
29. Preeclampsia is first suspected in a pregnant woman when there is:
    ① An excessive weight gain
    ② Fluctuation of the BP

③ Progressive ankle edema
④ Presence of albuminuria

30. Mrs. Wallace has been diagnosed as having preeclampsia. When counseling Mrs. Wallace, the nurse instructs her to follow a diet that includes:
    ① Normal sodium with ample calories and protein
    ② High sodium and calories and low protein
    ③ Moderate sodium, low calories, and ample protein
    ④ Low sodium and calories and high protein
31. Later, Mrs. Wallace is admitted to the hospital and is receiving magnesium sulfate ($MgSO_4$) 10 mg IM, every 4 hours. Before giving the drug the nurse should check her:
    ① Respirations and patellar reflex
    ② Blood pressure and apical pulse
    ③ Urinary output relative to fluid intake
    ④ Temperature and pulse rate
32. When giving $MgSO_4$ IM, the nurse should:
    ① Add 1% normal saline to maximize the dispersion of the drug
    ② Add 1% procaine to minimize the pain caused by the drug
    ③ Use a large-gauge needle to expedite dispersion of the drug
    ④ Give the injection in the outer aspect of the thigh
33. In severe preeclampsia, changes in blood values include an elevation of the hematocrit. This results from:
    ① Hemodilution of pregnancy caused by increases in blood volume
    ② Vasodilation caused by an alteration in circulating fluid
    ③ Agglutination of red cells caused by membrane fragility
    ④ Hemoconcentration caused by a decrease in plasma volume

Situation: Eight-year-old Kim is admitted to the hospital for the first time with a diagnosis of diabetes.

34. Juvenile (Type I or IDDM) diabetes:
    ① Has a more rapid onset than adult diabetes
    ② Occurs more often in obese children
    ③ Does not always require insulin
    ④ Involves early vascular changes
35. The nurse plans to include the entire family in Kim's care and is especially concerned that:
    ① The parents receive immediate instruction about urine testing
    ② Kim is taught to give injections before being discharged
    ③ The parents and child be helped to understand their feelings about diabetes
    ④ Kim's activity be limited and the parents understand the need for this
36. The physician orders 20 units of NPH insulin daily for Kim. The vial reads 1 ml = 100 units of NPH which has been diluted so that the solution contains 50 units of NPH insulin per ml. The nurse does not have an insulin syringe so, using a regular syringe, gives:
    ① 0.6 ml
    ② 0.4 ml
    ③ 0.3 ml
    ④ 0.2 ml

37. A night feeding planned for a juvenile diabetic includes milk, crackers, and cheese. This will provide:
    ① High-carbohydrate nourishment for immediate utilization
    ② Nourishment with latent effect to counteract late insulin activity
    ③ Encouragement for the child to stay on a diet
    ④ Added calories to help the child gain weight

38. Before Kim goes home, the nurse reviews with the family the importance of their knowing that Kim's insulin needs will be decreased when:
    ① There is an emotional upset
    ② An infectious process is present
    ③ She reaches puberty
    ④ She participates in active exercise

Situation: Mr. Bunger, age 45, has been aware of a mass in his right cheek and upper neck for several years. Although the mass had become increasingly noticeable, he did not seek medical attention. As a result of an extensive campaign in his community, he made an appointment at a local hospital for a cancer detection examination. He was informed by the physician that he should be hospitalized for surgery immediately for a tumor involving the parotid gland.

39. Although the physician has explained the possible extent of surgery, Mr. Bunger is still quite anxious. Nursing intervention should be aimed at:
    ① Attempting to discover what is bothering him
    ② Elaborating on what the physician has already told him
    ③ Planning for postoperative communication, since a tracheostomy is likely
    ④ Teaching him to use the suction equipment preoperatively

40. At surgical intervention the tumor proves to be malignant, and a right total parotidectomy is performed. A complication, distressing to the client, is:
    ① Tracheostomy
    ② Facial nerve dysfunction
    ③ Frey's syndrome
    ④ Salivation

41. Postoperatively Mr. Bunger is kept in a high Fowler's position to:
    ① Promote drainage of the wound
    ② Prevent edema at operative site
    ③ Prevent strain on the incision
    ④ Provide stimulation for the client

42. When Mr. Bunger complains that his dressing is tight, the nurse should plan to:
    ① Check it for signs of bleeding
    ② Check it for signs of constriction
    ③ Inform him that a tight dressing is necessary
    ④ Alter it to relieve the sensation

43. Mr. Bunger's condition deteriorates, and he is in the terminal stage. The nurse must understand that in dealing with terminally ill clients perhaps the most important factor relative to therapeutic nurse-client relationships is:
    ① How the nurse feels about the situation
    ② The nurse's recognition of the family's ability to cope
    ③ The nurse's knowledge of the grieving process
    ④ Previous experiences with terminally ill clients

Situation: Mr. Kirk, pale, thin, and dehydrated, is admitted to the hospital with an exacerbation of colitis. He is placed on a residue-free, bland, high-protein diet, and vitamins B, C, and K parenterally. An IV solution containing electrolytes is also started.

44. The type of person who most frequently develops ulcerative colitis is:
    ① Hard driving and immature
    ② Sensitive and dependent
    ③ Quick tempered and hostile
    ④ Unassuming and secure

45. The nurse administers vitamins parenterally because:
    ① More rapid action results
    ② They are ineffective orally
    ③ They decrease colon irritability
    ④ Intestinal absorption may be inadequate

46. Mr. Kirk is to receive 2000 ml of IV fluid in 12 hours. The drop factor is 10 gtt/1 ml. The nurse should regulate the flow so the number of drops per minute is approximately:
    ① 27 to 29
    ② 30 to 32
    ③ 40 to 42
    ④ 48 to 50

47. The food combinations that can be included on a residue-free diet include:
    ① Lean roast beef, buttered white rice with egg slices, white bread with butter and jelly, tea with sugar
    ② Creamed soup and crackers, omlet, mashed potatoes, bran muffin, orange juice, coffee
    ③ Stewed chicken, baked potato with butter, strained peas, white bread, plain cake, milk
    ④ Baked fish, macaroni with cheese, strained carrots, fruit gelatin, milk

48. Mr. Kirk's diet is designed to reduce:
    ① Gastric acidity
    ② Colonic irritation
    ③ Electrolyte depletion
    ④ Intestinal absorption

49. In addition, the nurse encourages a high-protein diet to:
    ① Correct anemia
    ② Slow peristalsis
    ③ Improve muscle tone
    ④ Repair tissues

Situation: Sallie Gerraghty, a 36-year-old primigravida with a history of endometriosis, is admitted to labor and delivery. Her husband accompanies her as her labor coach. A fetal monitor is being used.

50. When caring for Sallie while her fetus is being monitored, the nurse must realize that:
    ① The machinery can be very frightening to the laboring couple
    ② The mother may need a mild sedative every 4 hours for comfort
    ③ Internal monitoring is usually employed when severe complications are suspected
    ④ Older primigravidas have more complications than younger women

51. Sallie, who has been successfully treated for endometriosis, completes this much-desired pregnancy with the delivery of a 4082.4 g (9 pound) baby girl. During the pregnancy the symptoms caused by endometriosis were alleviated. Sallie expresses concern that her symptoms will return now that the pregnancy is over. The most appropriate response by the nurse would be:
    ① "A hysterectomy will be necessary if the symptoms recur."
    ② "Breast-feeding your baby will delay the return of symptoms."
    ③ "Pregnancy usually cures the endometriosis."
    ④ "Endometriosis will usually cause an early menopause."

52. Four hours after delivery Sallie still has not voided. The nurse's initial action should be to:
    ① Encourage voiding by placing Sallie on a bedpan frequently.
    ② Inform the physician of Sallie's inability to void and await orders
    ③ Palpate Sallie's subrapubic area for distention
    ④ Place Sallie's hands in warm water to encourage micturition

53. The public health nurse visits Sallie at home for the first time. She is breast-feeding her infant and complains that her breasts are swollen and painful. In teaching her about breast-feeding, the nurse should include information to assist her in preventing engorgement in the future such as:
    ① "Feed the baby four times a day. This will prevent rapid filling of the breast."
    ② "Use a bottle for feeding when you are experiencing discomfort."
    ③ "Nurse the baby frequently and for at least 10 minutes on each breast."
    ④ "Limit nursing to 4 to 6 minutes on each breast, four times a day."

Situation: Mrs. Korto, 60 years old, is hospitalized for an acute episode of bronchial asthma.

54. Mrs. Korto is experiencing difficulty in breathing due to:
    ① Spasms of the bronchi, which trap the air
    ② A too rapid expulsion of air
    ③ An increase in the vital capacity of the lungs
    ④ Hyperventilation due to an anxiety reaction

55. Nursing management of Mrs. Korto is now directed toward:
    ① Raising mucus secretions from the chest
    ② Limiting pulmonary secretions by decreasing fluid intake
    ③ Curing the condition permanently
    ④ Convincing the client that her condition is emotionally based

56. The nurse administers aminophylline via suppository to Mrs. Korto as ordered. The effect of this therapy is:
    ① Rest and relaxation
    ② Evacuation of the lower bowel
    ③ Relaxation of bronchial muscles
    ④ Reduction of respiratory bacteria

57. Mrs. Korto has an IV infusion to keep the vein open for emergency medications. If the IV infusion infiltrates, the nurse should:
    ① Attempt to flush the tube
    ② Elevate the IV site
    ③ Discontinue the infusion
    ④ Apply warm, moist soaks

58. The physician orders daily sputum specimens to be collected from Mrs. Korto. It is most appropriate for the nurse to collect this specimen:
    ① On awakening
    ② Before meals
    ③ Before an IPPB treatment
    ④ After activity

59. The nurse understands that Mrs. Korto's asthmatic wheeze is thought to be:
    ① An impairment of cardiovascular function
    ② An unexpressed rejection of independence
    ③ A dilation of the bronchi
    ④ An expression of hypochondriasis

60. Mrs. Korto is found to be allergic to dust. The teaching plan for her should include the fact that:
    ① She will probably be unable to do her own housework in the future
    ② It is imperative that her entire house be redecorated, since she must live in a dust-free environment
    ③ Damp-dusting her house will help limit dust particles in the air
    ④ She may as well accept her condition, since dust cannot be avoided

Situation: Mrs. Sims is returned to her room after a radical neck dissection for a malignant tumor.

61. Mrs. Sims has an endotracheal tube still in place. The nurse should:
    ① Change the dressing to observe for covert bleeding
    ② Irrigate the tube to maintain patency
    ③ Reposition the endotracheal tube when the gag reflex returns
    ④ Have a tracheostomy set at the bedside

62. When Mrs. Sims' color improves and she is able to breathe on her own, the anesthesiologist removes the endotracheal tube. That evening the nurse decides Mrs. Sims is showing signs of respiratory embarrassment and notifies the physician immediately when Mrs. Sims demonstrates:
    ① Decreased pulse and respirations
    ② Restlessness and confusion
    ③ Cyanosis and clubbing of the fingers
    ④ Anxiety and constricted pupils

63. A tracheostomy is performed and Mrs. Sims is placed on a mechanical ventilator. For a client on a ventilator, the nurse must be sure to check the cuff of the tracheostomy tube, which:
    ① Must be inflated during suctioning
    ② Must remain deflated for 10 minutes every hour
    ③ Should allow only a slight air leak at the height of inspiration
    ④ Should create a tight seal between the trachea and the tube

64. When doing deep tracheal suction for a client after a tracheostomy, the nurse should:
    ① Be sure the cuff of the tracheostomy is inflated during suctioning
    ② Instill acetylcysteine (Mucomyst) into the tracheostomy prior to suctioning to loosen secretions
    ③ Apply negative pressure as the catheter is being inserted
    ④ Suction the client with the head turned to either side

65. When doing tracheostomy care for Mrs. Sims, the nurse must:
    ① Monitor her temperature after the procedure
    ② Use sterile gloves during the procedure
    ③ Use Betadine to clean the inner cannula when it is removed
    ④ Place Mrs. Sims in the semi-Fowler's position

66. As a result of the tracheostomy the nurse is aware that the drug that would be contraindicated for Mrs. Sims is:
    ① Pyrvinium pamoate (Povan)
    ② Atropine
    ③ Chloral hydrate
    ④ Nalorphine (Nalline)

67. Mrs. Sims' tracheostomy tube has an inner cannula. In providing tracheostomy care the nurse should plan to remove the inner cannula:
    ① And use sterile applicators to cleanse the outer cannula
    ② Only after the cuff is deflated
    ③ And cleanse it with peroxide
    ④ Only when the obturator is in place

Situation: After trying for several years, Mr. and Mrs. Gosney have succeeded in becoming parents. He is a successful lawyer, and she teaches at the local community college.

68. When Mrs. Gosney is 10 weeks pregnant, she calls the gynecologist's office and complains of morning sickness, which interferes with her job. The nurse, to promote relief, might suggest:
    ① Increasing her protein intake before bedtime
    ② Eating dry crackers before arising
    ③ Having two small meals daily and a snack at noon
    ④ Drinking more high-carbohydrate fluids with meals.

69. Mrs. Gosney complains of feeling tired. The nurse recognizes that this is probably related to the normal cardiovascular changes which:
    ① Decrease cardiac output
    ② Increase hematocrit
    ③ Increase blood volume
    ④ Increase BP

70. When Mrs. Gosney is 36 weeks pregnant, her membranes rupture spontaneously. The physician calls and informs the delivery room that her cervix is 2 cm dilated and 75% effaced and that she is being admitted. When Mr. and Mrs. Gosney arrive, the nurse should:
    ① Immediately attach an external fetal monitor to evaluate the fetal heart
    ② Have them wait in the admission room while the nurse notifies the physician that they have arrived

③ Send Mrs. Gosney to the admission room to undress while the nurse takes her history from Mr. Gosney
④ Introduce self to Mr. and Mrs. Gosney and try to make them feel welcome

71. Mrs. Gosney's labor progresses. She should be moved to the delivery room when the nurse observes:
    ① An increase in the amount of bloody discharge from the perineum
    ② That she is becoming irritable and does not follow instructions
    ③ That her perineum is beginning to bulge with each contraction
    ④ That her contractions are occurring every 2 to 3 minutes and lasting 60 seconds

72. Mrs. Gosney delivers a 2953.6 g (6½ lb) baby boy. She becomes extremely upset that her newborn son has a nevus vasculosus on the midthigh. The nurse can best respond by telling her:
    ① "This is a superficial area that will fade in a few days."
    ② "This mark will not grow or fade, but will be covered by clothes."
    ③ "The area will spread rapidly and then regress."
    ④ "Surgical removal will be necessary as soon as the infant is older."

73. Mrs. Gosney plans to breast-feed her baby. The nurse helps Mrs. Gosney understand the advantages of breast-feeding by explaining that:
    ① Allergic responses are diminished in breast-fed infants
    ② Breast milk has a larger concentration of protein than does cow's milk
    ③ Breast-fed infants adhere more easily to a 4-hour schedule
    ④ Breast-feeding inhibits ovulation in the mother

74. Mrs. Gosney is being discharged. In teaching her to care for her newborn who has just been circumcised, the nurse should instruct her to:
    ① Observe for fussy behavior
    ② Observe for yellow exudate
    ③ Apply petrolatum gauze to the penis
    ④ Leave the infant undiapered

75. After 6 months, Mrs. Gosney returns to work. Shortly thereafter, she is appointed Dean of Students. Mr. and Mrs. Gosney decide to postpone adding to their family, and Mrs. Gosney begins using an estrogen-progestin oral contraceptive. The nurse explains it is important that she observe for:
    ① Nausea, rash, and bleeding
    ② Lethargy, syncope, and tachycardia
    ③ Hypertension, calf and breast tenderness
    ④ Bradycardia, visual changes, and hypertension

Situation: Susan Langham, a 19-year-old single parent, gives birth to a 2268 g (5 lb) baby boy with severe cleft palate. The nurse brings the baby to Susan.

76. The nurse recognizes the fairly typical response to a baby with a visible birth defect when Susan states:
    ① "No, you must have brought me the wrong baby."
    ② "I'm unhappy and I guess I'm being punished."

③ "I shouldn't have had this baby. Now John will never marry me."

④ "What will my parents say? What could have happened?"

77. Susan refuses to look at her baby. The nursing approach that would be most therapeutic would be:
① Gently tell Susan that she should stop blaming herself for the child's handicap
② Explain the problem to Susan's family and encourage them to help comfort her
③ Reinforce the physician's explanation of the handicap and allow Susan time to discuss her fears
④ Wait until Susan has sufficiently recovered from the stress of delivery before bringing her the baby again

78. Susan brings her son, Steve, who is now 18 months old, to the clinic. In discussing him with the nurse, she asks why Steve is so difficult to please, has temper tantrums, and annoys her by throwing food from the table. The nurse should explain that:
① Steve is learning to assert his independence, and his behavior is considered normal for his age
② Steve needs to be disciplined at this stage to prevent development of antisocial behaviors
③ It is best to leave Steve alone in his crib after calmly telling him why his behavior is unacceptable
④ This is the usual way for a toddler to express his needs during the initiative stage of development

79. The nurse asks Susan what she does when Steve has a tantrum. The nurse should recognize that Susan understands the basis for temper tantrums when she tells the nurse she:
① Ignores and isolates Steve until he behaves properly
② Disciplines Steve by restricting a favorite food or activity
③ Partially gives in to Steve before his tantrums become excessive
④ Allows Steve to choose between two reasonable alternatives

Situation: Twenty-four-month-old Molly Brown is admitted with croup. She is clinging to her mother crying and responds negatively to all suggestions.

80. In assessing Molly, the nurse would expect to find:
① Bronchospasm, whooping cough
② Expiratory stridor, rales
③ Laryngospasm, barking cough
④ Productive cough, inspiratory stridor

81. Mr. and Mrs. Brown ask the nurse what they should do if Molly has another attack of croup at home. The nurse suggests that Molly's parents interrupt the croup attack by administering:
① Cheracol syrup
② Syrup of ipecac
③ Hydrocortisone succinate (Solu-Cortef)
④ Epinephrine

82. The nurse's teaching is based on the action of this drug, which results in:
① Dilation of the bronchi
② Reduction of the inflammation
③ Interruption of the spasm
④ Depression of the cough center

83. When Mrs. Brown returns with Molly to the physician's office for medical follow-up, she tells the nurse that Molly has been "driving her crazy," by saying no to everything she suggests. She asks the nurse for help in handling her. The nurse explains to Mrs. Brown that Molly's negativism is normal for her age and that it is helping her meet her need for:
① Discipline
② Independence
③ Attention
④ Trust

84. Mrs. Brown states, "This morning I gave Molly her juice and she said 'no' and I got angry, but she needs her fluids. What shall I do?" The nurse suggests that she:
① Be firm and hand her the glass
② Distract her with some food
③ Let her see that she is making her mother angry
④ Offer her a choice of two things to drink

85. The nurse plans to talk to Mrs. Brown about toilet training Molly, knowing that the most important factor in the process of toilet training is the:
① Child's desire to be dry
② Approach and attitude of the parent
③ Ability of the child to sit still
④ Parent's willingness to work at it

86. Before Mrs. Brown leaves the clinic, the nurse tells her that she can best help her daughter learn to control her own behavior by:
① Rewarding her for good behavior
② Allowing her to learn by her mistakes
③ Punishing her when she deserves it
④ Setting limits and being consistent

Situation: Mrs. Ivy is a 35-year-old woman who compulsively washes her hands. Her ritual includes four separate scrubs, which are carried out methodically.

87. Although the nurse becomes tense as the ritual is carried out, it should be recognized that a compulsive act is one which:
① A person performs willingly
② Is performed after long urging
③ Is purposeful but useless
④ Seems absurd but is necessary to the person

88. Mrs. Ivy's basic personality is probably characterized by:
① Marked emotional maturity
② Elaborate delusional system
③ Doubts, fears, and indecisiveness
④ Rapid, frequent mood swings

89. In caring for Mrs. Ivy it is most important that the nurse:
① Promote reality by showing that the ritual serves little purpose
② Try to ascertain the meaning of the ritual by discussing it with the client
③ Interrupt the ritual to demonstrate that the ritual does not control what happens
④ Allow the client sufficient time to carry out the ritual

90. If interrupted in the performance of the ritual, Mrs. Ivy would most likely react with:
    ① Aggression
    ② Anxiety
    ③ Withdrawal
    ④ Hostility

Situation: David Brown, 5½ years old, is admitted with a diagnosis of lead poisoning. He is listless and has had two convulsions within the last 48 hours.

91. The nurse should suspect lead-induced renal damage to the proximal tubules when a urinalysis demonstrates the presence of:
    ① Albumin, glucose, amino acids, and phosphate
    ② Protein, calcium, glucose, and amino acids
    ③ Glucose, amino acids, potassium, and calcium
    ④ Protein, calcium, phosphate, and glucose

92. David is started on a regimen of chelation therapy that consists of intramuscular injections of calcium disodium edetate (EDTA) and dimercaprol (BAL) q4h for 5 days. The nurse understands that a combination of these drugs is preferred because it:
    ① Removes lead from the blood more rapidly and decreases deposition in the bones
    ② Has fewer side effects and removes lead from the brain more effectively
    ③ Eliminates lead from the body more rapidly through the urine
    ④ Removes lead from the bone marrow more efficiently

93. Recognizing that David's mother shares characteristics in common with other mothers whose children chronically ingest lead, the nurse could help her prevent a recurrence by:
    ① Discussing with her ways to renovate her home to remove sources of lead and teaching her measures to improve her parenting
    ② Educating her about the dangers of lead ingestion and the type of treatment and medical care required
    ③ Helping her recognize factors in her maternal-child interactions and in the home environment that predispose her son to pica
    ④ Initiating referrals to appropriate social and public health service agencies for the total management of her problem

COMPREHENSIVE TEST 1: PART 2

To simulate the National Council Licensure Examination, this test should be completed within 1½ hours.

Situation: Mr. Brown, a 48-year-old man with a long history of chronic obstructive lung disease, is admitted to the hospital for a segmental resection of the right lower lobe.

94. Intermittent positive pressure breathing is given preoperatively to:
    ① Encourage respiration at a faster rate than that established by respiratory center control
    ② Provide more adequate lung expansion than could be achieved by unassisted breathing
    ③ Force air through the infected secretions that accumulated in the lung bases
    ④ Remove air and fluid from the pleural cavity

95. Because of Mr. Brown's history of COPD, the nurse should be aware of complications involving:
    ① Kidney function
    ② Peripheral neuropathy
    ③ Cardiac function
    ④ Joint inflammation

96. When scheduling intermittent positive pressure breathing treatments, the nurse should realize that the *least* appropriate time of day to receive an IPPB treatment is:
    ① On awakening
    ② Before a meal
    ③ At bedtime
    ④ After a meal

97. Immediately after Mr. Brown's arrival in the recovery room, the nurse caring for the closed chest drainage apparatus should:
    ① Secure the chest catheter to the wound dressing with a sterile safety pin
    ② Mark the time and the fluid level on the side of the drainage bottle
    ③ Raise the drainage bottle to bed level to check patency of the system
    ④ Add 3 to 5 ml of sterile saline to the water seal

98. The purpose of the water in the closed chest drainage bottle is to:
    ① Facilitate emptying bloody drainage from the chest
    ② Foster removal of chest secretions by capillarity
    ③ Prevent entrance of air into the pleural cavity
    ④ Decrease the danger of sudden change in pressure in the tube

99. Mr. Brown has a large amount of respiratory secretions. Independent nursing care should include:
    ① Turning and positioning
    ② Cupping
    ③ Clapping
    ④ Postural drainage

100. Mr. Brown requires oxygen. Although all of the following are factors to consider when determining the method of oxygen administration to be used for a specific client, the *major* concern is:
    ① Facial anatomy
    ② Pathologic condition
    ③ Age and mental capacity
    ④ Level of activity

101. A preventive measure to be taken by the nurse regarding the untoward effects of oxygen therapy is:
    ① Padding elastic bands of the face mask
    ② Humidifying the gas
    ③ Taking the apical pulse before starting therapy
    ④ Placing the client in the orthopneic position

Situation: Jason Agnew, 6 months old, is brought to the emergency room with a fever of unknown origin and projectile vomiting. Because meningitis is suspected, he is admitted to the pediatric unit.

102. The test that would be done immediately to confirm the diagnosis of meningitis is:
① Meningomyelogram
② Peripheral skin smears
③ Lumbar puncture
④ Blood cultures

103. Jason is receiving 500 ml of IV fluid per 24 hours. Using an IV set with a drop rate of 60 drops/ml, the nurse should plan to regulate the IV at:
① 8 drops per minute
② 13 drops per minute
③ 21 drops per minute
④ 24 drops per minute

104. According to Piaget's theory of cognitive development, Jason should be demonstrating:
① Beginning of object permanence
② Repetitious use of reflexes
③ Early traces of memory
④ Beginning sense of time

Situation: Mrs. Smith is admitted to the hospital with a diagnosis of possible bronchogenic carcinoma.

105. When Mrs. Smith returns to the room following a bronchoscopy and biopsy, she is fully awake. The nurse should:
① Advise her to stay flat in bed for 2 hours
② Provide ice chips to reduce swelling
③ Encourage her to cough frequently
④ Evaluate the presence of a gag reflex

106. Mrs. Smith's diagnosis of bronchogenic carcinoma is confirmed and a right pneumonectomy is performed. During the surgery the phrenic nerve is severed to:
① Produce an atonic diaphragm
② Limit the postoperative pain considerably
③ Allow the diaphragm to rise and partially fill the space
④ Permit greater excursion of the thoracic cavity

107. Mrs. Smith returns from surgery to the intensive care unit with an endotracheal tube in place. The most effective way for the nurse to loosen Mrs. Smith's secretions would be by:
① Administering oral fluids
② Pulmonary toileting
③ Administering humidified oxygen
④ Instilling a saturated solution of potassium iodide

108. In the immediate postoperative period it would be most beneficial for Mrs. Smith to be placed:
① On her right side with head slightly elevated
② In the left Sims' position with the bed elevated 45°
③ In the high-Fowler's position
④ Flat in bed with her knees flexed slightly

109. The nurse should palpate Mrs. Smith's trachea at least once a day because:
① Tracheal edema may lead to an obstructed airway
② The position may indicate mediastinal shift
③ Nodular lesions may demonstrate metastasis
④ The cuff of the endotracheal tube may be overinflated

Situation: Indira Mohamet, age 33, has difficulty becoming pregnant. She visits her gynecologist and is diagnosed as having endometriosis.

110. Endometriosis is characterized by:
① Amenorrhea and insomnia
② Ecchymoses and petechiae
③ Painful menstruation and backache
④ Early osteoporosis and pelvic inflammation

111. When obtaining a health history, the nurse would eliminate, as a possible complication of endometriosis, a history of:
① Menopause
② Metrorrhagia
③ Bowel stricture
④ Voiding difficulties

112. An antiovulatory medication of combined progestogen and estrogen is prescribed for Mrs. Mohamet. The nurse, instructing her about the medication, should include the need to:
① Have bimonthly Pap smears
② Report any vaginal bleeding
③ Temporarily restrict sexual activity
④ Increase her intake of calcium

Situation: Mrs. Evad, with a history of upper abdominal pain, nausea, and vomiting, is admitted to the hospital for a diagnostic workup of cancer of the pancreas. She has a history of hypertension and is taking antihypertensive medication.

113. As Mrs. Evad is admitted to her room, she asks the nurse, "Do you think I have anything serious—like cancer?" The nurse's best reply would be:
① "Why don't you discuss this with your doctor?"
② "Don't worry, we won't know until all the test results are back."
③ "What makes you think you have cancer?"
④ "I don't know if you do, but let's talk about it."

114. A complete blood count, urinalysis, and x-ray examination of the chest are ordered for Mrs. Evad prior to surgery. She asks why these tests are done. The nurse's best answer would be:
① "Don't worry, these tests are strictly routine."
② "They are ordered for all clients undergoing surgery."
③ "I don't know; the doctor ordered them."
④ "They determine whether it's safe to proceed with surgery."

115. An abdominal resection is to be performed on Mrs. Evad. The first priority of preoperative nursing care is directed toward:
① Teaching and answering all questions
② Maintaining proper nutritional status
③ Recording accurate vital signs
④ Alleviating the client's anxiety

116. The most significant influence on Mrs. Evad's perception of pain is her:
① Overall physical status
② Intelligence and economic status
③ Previous experience and cultural values
④ Age and sex

117. A progressive ambulation schedule is to be instituted for Mrs. Evad the morning after surgery. Morphine sulfate, 10 mg, has been ordered q4h prn for pain. When the nurse helps her out of bed, she should first sit on the edge of the bed with her feet dangling because her expected adaptation will be:
    ① Postural hypotension
    ② Respiratory distress
    ③ Initial hypertension
    ④ Abdominal pain

118. Early symptoms of morphine overdose are:
    ① Profuse sweating, pinpoint pupils, and deep sleep
    ② Slow respirations, dilated pupils, restlessness
    ③ Slow pulse, slow respirations, sedation
    ④ Slow respirations, constricted pupils, and deep sleep

119. On the second postoperative day Mrs. Evad complains of pain in her right calf. The nurse should first:
    ① Elevate the extremity
    ② Apply warm soaks
    ③ Notify the physician
    ④ Chart the symptoms

Situation: Mr. and Mrs. Monrow, a couple in their late twenties, happily receive the news that Mrs. Monrow is pregnant. A year before, Mrs. Monrow had spontaneously aborted in the sixteenth week. It is determined that she is about 8 weeks pregnant and healthy.

120. While in the office for a prenatal checkup during the twelfth week of her pregnancy, Mrs. Monrow says to the nurse, "Everyday I wonder if I'll ever have this child." The nurse's best response would be:
    ① "You have the best doctors possible. What was the problem with your previous pregnancy?"
    ② "I can understand why you're worried. You will have other chances in the future."
    ③ "Just do exactly what the doctors tell you to do. I can understand why you're worried, though."
    ④ "It's understandable for you to feel concerned that you may not carry this pregnancy to term."

121. Sixteen weeks into her pregnancy, Mrs. Monrow begins to experience heavy bleeding and severe abdominal cramping. She is admitted to the hospital with an incomplete abortion. Her doctor orders a dilation and curettage. She says to the nurse, "We wanted this baby so badly." The nurse's best response would be:
    ① "You must be disappointed, but don't feel guilty. These things sometimes happen."
    ② "It's not your fault. This is nature's way of dealing with babies that may have problems."
    ③ "It must be difficult to lose something that was important to you both."
    ④ "The D & C will give you a new start. I bet you'll become pregnant again soon."

122. Mrs. Monrow tells the nurse that her doctor explained to her that she has had an incomplete abortion, but she does not understand what was said. The nurse's best response would be:
    ① "I think it would be best if you asked your doctor for the answer to that question."
    ② "An incomplete abortion is when the fetus is expelled but part of the placenta and membranes are not."

③ "I really don't think you should focus on what happened right now."
④ "This is when the fetus dies but is retained in the uterus for 8 weeks or more."

123. The evening after the D & C, Mrs. Monrow says, "We've always wanted this pregnancy. How come this happened to us again?" The nurse is aware that Mrs. Monrow is exhibiting the usual initial reaction to a loss, which is:
    ① Apathy and sadness
    ② Shock and denial
    ③ Despair and anger
    ④ Dissociation and rationalization

124. When making rounds during the night, the nurse enters Mrs. Monrow's room and finds her crying. The most appropriate action would be to:
    ① Document on the chart that Mrs. Monrow is having difficulty accepting the loss of her baby
    ② Pull the curtain to provide privacy for Mrs. Monrow
    ③ Sit down and stay with Mrs. Monrow, allowing her to cry
    ④ Explain to Mrs. Monrow that her feelings are normal and will pass with time

Situation: Ann Julio, a newborn in distress, is admitted to the neonatal intensive care unit immediately after birth.

125. When assessing Ann, the nurse should suspect the possibility of hydrocephalus if:
    ① The infant's cry sounds high pitched
    ② The head circumference is 2 to 3 cm greater than the chest circumference
    ③ The infant's Apgar score was less than 5
    ④ The infant has a lumbosacral meningomyelocele

126. Ann is diagnosed as having communicating hydrocephalus. In explaining communicating hydrocephalus to the parents, the nurse should state:
    ① "Too much cerebrospinal fluid is produced within the ventricles of the brain."
    ② "The cerebrospinal fluid is prevented from proper absorption by a blockage in the ventricles of the brain."
    ③ "The part of the brain surface that normally absorbs cerebrospinal fluid after its production is not functioning adequately."
    ④ "There is a flow of cerebrospinal fluid between the brain cells and the ventricles, which do not empty properly into the spinal cord."

127. Several days later a ventriculoperitoneal shunt is inserted. In discharge planning, the nurse should teach the parents to observe for the most common complications after this type surgery—which include:
    ① Eyes with sclerae that are visible above the irises
    ② Fever, irritability, and decreased responsiveness
    ③ Violent involuntary muscle contractions
    ④ Excessive fluid accumulation in the abdomen

128. In teaching Ann's parents to pump the valve of the ventriculoperitoneal shunt, the nurse explains to them that the primary purpose of this procedure is to:

① Drain excessive cerebrospinal fluid rapidly
② Increase absorption of cerebrospinal fluid
③ Keep the tubing of the shunt patent
④ Divert the cerebrospinal fluid from the ventricles

129. Ann demonstrates urinary incontinence and flaccidity of the lower extremities. The teaching plan for her parents should include the fact that:
① She will probably wear diapers for a lifetime since bladder training is impossible
② An ileal bladder will be necessary once she is of school age
③ She will probably be a candidate for an intermittent straight catheterization program
④ An indwelling Foley catheter offers the best hope for bladder management

Situation: Mrs. Allen, a gravida III, para II, has an uneventful labor and delivery. After a 7-hour labor she delivers a 3692 g (8 lb 2 oz) baby girl spontaneously.

130. Two hours after delivery, the nurse finds that Mrs. Allen's fundus is firm, shifted to the right, and two fingers above the umbilicus. This would indicate:
① A normal process
② Retained secundinae
③ A full bladder
④ Impending bleeding

131. After delivery, when checking Mrs. Allen's vital signs, the nurse should normally find:
① An elevated basal temperature with a decrease in respirations
② A decided bradycardia with no change in respirations
③ A slight lowering of basal temperature with an increase in respirations
④ A decided tachycardia with a decrease in respirations

132. Eight hours after delivery the nurse notices that Mrs. Allen is voiding frequently in small amounts. Intake and output are important in the early postpartal period, since small amounts of output:
① Are commonly voided and should cause no alarm
② May be indicative of beginning glomerulonephritis
③ May indicate retention of urine with overflow
④ Are common because less fluid is excreted following delivery

133. In helping Mrs. Allen develop her parenting role, the nurse should:
① Do things for the baby in the mother's presence
② Find out what she knows about babies and proceed from there
③ Demonstrate baby bathing and care before discharge
④ Provide enough time for her and the baby to be together

134. Mrs. Allen's infant develops a cephalohematoma. The nurse should plan to explain to Mrs. Allen that:
① This condition is unusual with vaginal delivery
② It will resolve spontaneously in 3 to 6 weeks
③ The swelling may cross a suture line
④ The soft sac will bulge when the infant cries

135. Nursing care of baby Allen is directed primarily toward:
① Supporting the parents
② Applying ice packs to the hematoma

③ Recording neurologic signs
④ Protecting the infant's head

Situation: Mary Jane Lee, age 33, is admitted from the emergency room to the neurologic service with a diagnosis of myasthenia gravis.

136. Because of the involvement of the ocular muscles, a common early symptom the nurse should observe for is:
① Nystagmus
② Diplopia
③ Blurring
④ Tearing

137. A test that might be performed on Ms. Lee in diagnosing this condition involves the use of the drug:
① EDTA
② Edrophonium (Tensilon)
③ Prednisolone
④ Phenytoin (Dilantin)

138. The prognosis of myasthenia gravis is most likely to be:
① Poor, with termination in a few months
② Chronic, with exacerbations and remissions
③ Slowly progressive without remissions
④ Excellent with proper treatment

139. The sex and age most frequently affected are:
① Males ages 15 to 35
② Females ages 10 to 30
③ Both sexes ages 20 to 40
④ Children ages 5 to 15

140. Ms. Lee is receiving neostigmine bromide (Prostigmin) for control of myasthenia gravis. In the middle of the night the nurse finds her weak, unable to move, and barely breathing. Signs that would identify the problems as being related to overactivity of neostigmine bromide are:
① High-pitched, gurgling bowel sounds
② Rapid pulse with occasional ectopic beats
③ Distention of the bladder
④ Fine tremor of the fingers and eyelids

141. Ms. Lee's husband asks the nurse whether his wife will be an invalid. Recognizing the individuality of responses to disease, the best answer would be:
① "The progression is slow, so she will spend her young life with few problems."
② "Deformities will occur, but she will not be an invalid."
③ "With continuous treatment the disease progression can be controlled."
④ "There will be periods when she is confined to bed rest and times when she can have fairly normal activity."

142. The diversional activity that would meet the nursing objectives for Ms. Lee during remissions is:
① Watching selected television shows
② Swimming with the family
③ Teaching sewing classes
④ Short hikes with the family

Situation: After an uneventful labor and delivery Mrs. Handler delivers a 3181 g (7 lb) boy with a bilateral cleft lip and palate. She does not see the baby in the delivery room. Mr. Handler has been told of the defect and has seen the baby. He is very upset, but his major concern is for his wife and her reaction.

143. While looking at the baby, Mr. Handler says to the nursery nurse, "Oh, what am I going to do, how could this happen to us, what is my wife going to do? It would have been better if she had never become pregnant." The most appropriate response for the nurse to make is:
    ① "How can you say that? You have a lovely healthy baby; the cleft lip can be fixed and then the baby will be fine."
    ② "I know how hard this must be for you. But believe me, you will love the baby so much, you won't even notice that he is disfigured."
    ③ "This must be very hard on you. Would it help if I went with you when the doctor talks to your wife?"
    ④ "I know that this is very difficult for you. But you can't think of yourself now. Your wife needs you. You must be strong."

144. After the physician talks to Mrs. Handler, she seems quite composed and asks to see the baby. To assess Mrs. Handler's reaction, the nurse should:
    ① Bring the baby to her immediately
    ② Tell her exactly what the baby looks like before bringing him to her
    ③ Encourage her to express and explore her feelings; bring the baby to her and stay with her during this time
    ④ Show her some pictures and give her some literature on harelip and cleft palate and discuss the treatment with her before bringing the baby to her

145. When Mrs. Handler sees the baby, she becomes very disturbed, pushes him away, and says, "Oh, take him away, I never want to see him again." This reaction would indicate to the nurse that Mrs. Handler is:
    ① Unable to cope with the situation and that arrangements will have to be made to place the baby in a foster home, at least for the first few months
    ② Responding as most normal new mothers, who find it difficult to accept that their baby is less than perfect
    ③ Severely emotionally disturbed and is in immediate need of psychiatric help
    ④ Rejecting the baby and he will have to be placed for adoption

146. Afterward Mrs. Handler asks how she is going to feed the baby if his mouth is deformed and he cannot suck properly. The nurse teaches her carefully and gently how feedings are to be given and states:
    ① "Try using a soft nipple with an enlarged opening so that he can get the milk through a chewing motion."
    ② "Since he tires easily, it is best to have him lying in bed while he is being fed."
    ③ "He should be held in a horizontal position and fed slowly to avoid aspiration."
    ④ "Give him brief rest periods and frequent burpings during feedings to expel swallowed air."

Situation: Mrs. Acker has missed her second menstrual period and attends the prenatal clinic.

147. Mrs. Acker asks the nurse why menstruation ceases once pregnancy occurs. The nurse's best response would be that this occurs because of the:
    ① "Production of estrogen and progesterone by the ovaries."
    ② "Secretion of luteinizing hormone produced by the pituitary."
    ③ "Secretion of follicle-stimulating hormone produced by the pituitary."
    ④ "Reduction in the secretion of hormones by the ovaries."

148. When Mrs. Acker returns for her fourth-month checkup, she is very upset and indicates that her husband was recently diagnosed as having genital herpes. In teaching about sexual activity, the nurse should include the fact that:
    ① It will be necessary to refrain from all sexual contact during pregnancy
    ② Meticulous cleaning of her hands and vaginal area after intercourse is essential
    ③ Use of condoms by her husband during sexual activity will be required
    ④ Sexual abstinence should be practiced during the last 6 weeks of pregnancy

149. In the fifth month, ultrasonography is performed. The results indicate that the fetus is small for gestational age and there is evidence of a low-lying placenta. In the last trimester the nurse should use this information and assess Mrs. Acker for signs of possible:
    ① Precipitate delivery
    ② Abruptio placentae
    ③ Placenta previa
    ④ Premature labor

150. Three weeks prior to her expected date of delivery, Mrs. Acker experiences painless vaginal bleeding and is admitted to the hospital. The nurse's care plan for the client should include:
    ① Administering vitamin K to promote clotting
    ② Administering an enema to prevent contamination during delivery
    ③ Performing a rectal examination to determine cervical dilation
    ④ Placing her in a semi-Fowler's position to increase cervical pressure

151. Mrs. Acker's bleeding increases and the physician decides to perform a cesarean delivery. A premature male infant is delivered. One of the criteria the nurse should use in assessing the gestational age of Baby Acker is:
    ① The presence of reflex stability
    ② Breast bud size
    ③ The presence of simian creases
    ④ Fingernail length

152. The initial nursing action after the birth of the baby should be to:
    ① Check clamp and dress the umbilical cord
    ② Quickly dry the baby and place in a controlled, warm environment
    ③ Obtain a footprint and apply an identification band
    ④ Assist the physician with resuscitative measures

153. About 1 hour after delivery the nurse can expect Baby Acker to be:
    ① Relaxed and sleeping quietly
    ② Hyperresponsive to stimuli
    ③ Intensely alert with eyes wide open
    ④ Crying and cranky

154. Mrs. Acker is moved to the recovery room after delivery. When her dressing is examined for signs of drainage, a nursing priority should be to:
    ① Note the color and consistency of the drainage
    ② Circle the drainage on the bandage and note the date and time
    ③ Observe behind the small of the back for drainage
    ④ Reinforce the dressing if drainage is excessive

Situation: Mrs. Lobinski, a 52-year-old Polish woman, is admitted for diagnostic evaluation for arteriosclerotic heart disease. In the year since her husband's death she has lived with her son and daughter-in-law. Currently she is not physically distressed but is apprehensive and alienated.

155. Nursing care that may help Mrs. Lobinski to feel more at ease includes:
    ① Telling her that everything is all right
    ② Giving her a copy of hospital regulations
    ③ Reassuring her that staff will be available if she becomes upset
    ④ Orienting her to the environment and unit personnel

156. In understanding Mrs. Lobinski's diagnosis, the nurse knows that atherosclerosis is:
    ① A loss of elasticity in and thickening and hardening of the arteries
    ② Development of atheromas within the myocardium
    ③ A mobilization of free fatty acid from adipose tissue
    ④ Development of fatty deposits within the intima of the arteries

157. The nurse's initial approach to creating a therapeutic environment for Mrs. Lobinski should give priority to:
    ① Accepting her individuality
    ② Promoting her independence
    ③ Providing for her safety
    ④ Explaining everything that is being done for her

158. On one occasion after her family has been visiting, Mrs. Lobinski is angry and says to the nurse, "My daughter-in-law says they can't take me home until the doctor lets me go. She doesn't understand; she isn't Polish." The nurse should:
    ① Ignore the statement for the present
    ② State, "The physician makes decisions about discharge."
    ③ Reflect on her feelings about the present situation
    ④ State, "You feel she doesn't want you home."

159. Mrs. Lobinski is placed on nitroglycerine therapy for angina. In administering nitroglycerine the nurse should:
    ① Make certain the medication is stored in a dark container
    ② Discontinue the medication if the client complains of a headache
    ③ Limit the number of tablets to four daily
    ④ Replace the tablets if she complains of a sublingual tingling sensation

Situation: Mrs. White, a 73-year-old widow, lives with her daughter. While picketing for senior citizens' rights at the state legislature, she fell and fractured her right hip. Mrs. White is admitted to the hospital for reduction of the fracture and insertion of a pin. On admission her blood pressure is 180/102 with some dependent edema.

160. During the day the nurse puts Mrs. White's side rails up specifically:
    ① As a safety measure because of the client's age
    ② Because all clients over 65 years of age should use side rails
    ③ Because elderly people are often disoriented for several days after anesthesia
    ④ To be used as handholds and to facilitate the client's mobility in bed

161. Mrs. White is apprehensive about being hospitalized. The nurse realizes that one of the stresses of hospitalization is the strangeness of the environment and activity. Extension of this stress can best be limited by:
    ① Listening to what Mrs. White has to say
    ② Calling her by her first name
    ③ Visiting Mrs. White frequently
    ④ Explaining what is expected of her

162. A 1-gram sodium diet and furosemide (Lasix) IM are prescribed for Mrs. White. She does not like her diet and tells the nurse that her sister is bringing in some "good home-cooked food." The initial, most effective, nursing action should be to:
    ① Call in the dietitian for client teaching
    ② Tell Mrs. White that she cannot have salt, since it will raise her BP
    ③ Wait for Mrs. White's sister and discuss the diet with both of them
    ④ Catch Mrs. White's sister before she goes into the room and tell her about the diet

163. Since sodium is the major cation controlling fluid outside the cells, diet therapy in congestive heart failure with subsequent edema is aimed at reducing the sodium intake. In teaching Mrs. White about her diet, the nurse should encourage her to exclude:
    ① Fruits
    ② Vegetables
    ③ Grains
    ④ Processed foods

164. The nurse should explain to Mrs. White that sodium restriction is an effective therapeutic tool in the treatment of congestive heart failure because its restriction:
    ① Helps to prevent the potassium accumulation that occurs when sodium intake is higher
    ② Helps to control food intake and thus weight
    ③ Causes excess tissue fluid to be withdrawn and excreted
    ④ Aids the weakened heart muscle to contract and improves cardiac output

165. Since Mrs. White has gluteal edema in the unaffected hip, the nurse should use the deltoid muscle for administration of drugs IM, mainly because at edematous sites:
    ① Deposition of an injected drug causes pain
    ② Blood supply is insufficient for drug absorption
    ③ Fluid leaks from the site for long periods after injection
    ④ Tissue fluid dilutes the drug before it enters the circulation

166. An independent nursing action that could be used to prevent thrombus formation in the unaffected leg would be:
    ① Gentle massage
    ② Passive range-of-motion exercises
    ③ Encouraging fluids
    ④ Elastic stockings

167. While assisting Mrs. White to transfer from the bed to a wheelchair, the nurse should remember that:
    ① During a weight-bearing transfer the client's knees should be slightly bent
    ② Transfers to and from the wheelchair will be easier if the bed is higher than the wheelchair
    ③ The transfer can be accomplished by pivoting while bearing weight on both upper extremities and not on the legs
    ④ The appropriate proximity and visual relationship of wheelchair to bed must be maintained

168. To prepare Mrs. White for crutch walking, the nurse should encourage her to:
    ① Sit up straight in a chair to develop the back muscles
    ② Keep the affected limb in extension and abduction
    ③ Do exercises in bed to strengthen her upper extremities
    ④ Use the trapeze to strengthen the biceps muscles

169. When assisting Mrs. White to ambulate, the nurse should be standing:
    ① In front of her
    ② Behind her
    ③ On her left side
    ④ On her right side

170. Mrs. White is being discharged from the hospital; however, she needs assistance with activities of daily living and needs to learn how to use a cane, since her daughter works full time and cannot care for her. The most appropriate place for Mrs. White to convalesce would be:
    ① Her own home, with a public health nurse
    ② A rehabilitation center
    ③ An adult facility
    ④ A nursing home

Situation: Mrs. Sanford, 60 years old, has become increasingly forgetful and disoriented as to time and place. Her mood is labile and she doesn't take part in family discussions. Her daughter brings her to the clinic and she is hospitalized for diagnostic evaluation with a possible diagnosis of Alzheimer's disease.

171. The nurse knows that Alzheimer's disease is characterized by:
    ① Slowly progressive deficits in intellect, which may not be noted for a long time
    ② Transient ischemic attacks
    ③ Remissions and exacerbations
    ④ Rapid deterioration of mental functioning because of arteriosclerosis

172. Mrs. Sanford frequently switches from being pleasant and happy to being hostile and sad without apparent external cause. The nurse can best care for Mrs. Sanford by:
    ① Avoiding her when she is angry and sad
    ② Attempting to give nursing care when she is in a pleasant mood
    ③ Encouraging her to talk about her feelings
    ④ Trying to point out reality to her

173. The nurse should provide Mrs. Sanford with an environment that is:
    ① Challenging
    ② Nonstimulating
    ③ Variable
    ④ Familiar

174. It is important for a team working with clients who have a diagnosis of organic mental disorder to adopt a common approach of care because the clients need to:
    ① Learn that the staff cannot be manipulated
    ② Relate in a consistent manner to staff
    ③ Accept external controls that are fairly applied
    ④ Have sameness and consistency in their environment

175. Clients who have an organic mental disorder need assistance in maintaining contact with society for as long as possible. A group that might help Mrs. Sanford achieve this goal is:
    ① Psychodrama
    ② Recreation therapy
    ③ Remotivation therapy
    ④ Occupational therapy

176. The objective of remotivational therapy in psychiatry is to stimulate:
    ① Face-to-face contact with other clients
    ② Diminished psychologic faculties
    ③ Interaction with environment
    ④ Participation in educational activities

Situation: Jay Lee, age 4 years, has gained several pounds over the last month. This morning when he wakes up his eyes are swollen shut. Mrs. Lee takes Jay to his pediatrician where proteinuria is found. Jay is admitted to the hospital with a diagnosis of nephrotic syndrome.

177. Jay's doctor orders steroid therapy for him. The nurse understands that the goal of this treatment is to:
    ① Prevent infection
    ② Cause diuresis
    ③ Reduce BP
    ④ Provide hemopoiesis

178. Jay is placed on a low-sodium diet. Of the following lunches the most appropriate would be:
    ① Cheeseburger on a bun, fresh green beans, iced tea
    ② Bacon and tomato sandwich, canned chicken noodle soup, low-sodium milk
    ③ Salmon, navy beans, fresh peaches, lemonade
    ④ Macaroni and cheese, fresh pears, V-8 juice

179. Jay is placed on complete bed rest. However, as he begins to feel better he becomes interested in playing. Based on his developmental level and activity restriction the nurse should provide him with:
    ① Television viewing time
    ② Simple three- or four-piece wooden puzzles
    ③ Little cars and a shoebox garage
    ④ Squeaky stuffed animals

180. As Jay begins to improve, Mrs. Lee expresses concern that he is acting babyish. He has been toilet trained for over a year but has been wetting himself lately. The best response to Mrs. Lee would be:
    ① "This is a normal response to hospitalization. Ignore his regressive behavior and be supportive of him."
    ② "The incontinence is due to his renal disease. It will improve as he gets better."
    ③ "Jay is wetting the bed to get attention. Reprimand him when he does this."
    ④ "He is using this regressive behavior to help him cope with hospitalization; just place him in diapers and say nothing."

Situation: Mrs. Axel delivers a 3629 g (8 lb) boy.

181. At the time of delivery Baby Axel's blood is typed to determine his ABO group and the presence of the Rh factor. The nurse is aware that:
    ① The Rh factor is not genetically determined
    ② The Rh factor of the fetus is determined by the father
    ③ Not all infants of Rh positive fathers are Rh positive
    ④ During gestation, the Rh factor of the fetus may change

182. Baby Axel is Rh positive and his mother is Rh negative. He is to receive an exchange transfusion. The nurse knows that the baby will receive Rh negative blood because:
    ① Its RBCs will not be destroyed by maternal anti-Rh antibodies
    ② It is the same as his mother's blood
    ③ It eliminates the possibility of a transfusion reaction
    ④ It is neutral and will not react with his blood

183. When the nurse brings Baby Axel to his mother, she comments about the milia on his face. The nurse should:
    ① Explain that these are birthmarks which will disappear within a few months
    ② Instruct her to avoid squeezing them or attempting to wash them off
    ③ Tell her that all babies have them and they clear up in 2 to 3 days
    ④ Instruct her about proper hand washing since the milia can become infected

Situation: Mrs. Cohen brings her 3-year-old son John to the emergency room at 12:00 midnight with a temperature of 103° F (39.4° C). On examination, it is found that John has an inflamed pharynx, respiratory distress with mild retractions, a barking cough, and inspiratory stridor. John is diagnosed as having a lower respiratory tract infection with acute spasmodic laryngitis (croup) and is admitted to the pediatric unit.

184. To prepare for John's admission, the nurse on the unit should:
    ① Obtain a tracheostomy set for the bedside
    ② Pad the side rails of the Croupette
    ③ Set up a cot so that a parent can stay
    ④ Arrange for a quiet, cool room

185. When caring for John, the priority nursing function should be to:
    ① Ensure delivery of 40% humidified oxygen
    ② Constantly assess respiratory status
    ③ Initiate measures to reduce fever
    ④ Provide support to reduce apprehension

186. Two hours after John's admission, the nurse observes an increase in John's respiratory and cardiac rates, increased restlessness, and substernal and intercostal retractions. The nurse, acting on these observations, should immediately:
    ① Strike John on his back to dislodge mucus
    ② Increase the level of oxygen being delivered
    ③ Remove secretions with suction apparatus
    ④ Inform the physician of John's respiratory status

187. An emergency tracheotomy is performed, and John is placed in a Croupette. In caring for him, the nurse should suction the tracheotomy routinely, and if he:
    ① Becomes restless, pale, or his pulse increases
    ② Tells the nurse he is having difficulty breathing
    ③ Becomes restless, diaphoretic, and cyanotic
    ④ Has severe substernal retractions and stridor

COMPREHENSIVE TEST 1: PART 3

To simulate the National Council Licensure Examination, this test should be completed within 1½ hours.

Situation: Mrs. Wyer, 21 years old, is 6 months pregnant with her second child and is being visited at home by a community health nurse as part of her prenatal care. While in the kitchen with Mrs. Wyer, the nurse notes that her lunch includes salami, cheese, and a cola drink. During assessment the nurse notes increased edema in Mrs. Wyer's ankles.

188. Besides advising rest with legs elevated, the nurse discusses the foods Mrs. Wyer has been eating and gives instructions concerning her diet. In this instance:
    ① Dietary preferences must influence the food that is eaten
    ② The food selected should have low salt content
    ③ The nutritionist should be brought in to plan a diet
    ④ The client should be advised to attend the prenatal clinic to see the physician

189. Mrs. Wyer complains of constipation. The nurse should explain that constipation frequently occurs during pregnancy because of:
    ① Pressure of the growing uterus on the anus
    ② Increased intake of milk as recommended during pregnancy
    ③ The slowing of peristalsis in the gastrointestinal tract
    ④ Changes in the metabolic rate

190. Mrs. Wyer begins labor close to her expected date of delivery and is admitted to the hospital. The nurse notices a gush of fluid from the client's vagina. After checking the FHR the nurse should:
    ① Notify the physician immediately about the gush of fluid from the vagina
    ② Place the client in a modified lithotomy position and inspect the perineum
    ③ Keep the client flat in bed and elevate her legs
    ④ Place the client on her side and obtain her BP

191. After several hours of labor the physician orders oxytocin (Pitocin). When a client in labor is being infused with oxytocin, it is the nurse's responsibility to:
    ① Obtain a physician's order to slow the IV in the presence of hypertonic contractions
    ② Flush the IV tubing if the flow slows
    ③ Shut off the IV in the presence of hypertonic contractions
    ④ Monitor fetal heart tones every 2 hours

192. The nurse knows that Mrs. Wyer has begun the transitional phase of labor when she:
    ① Complains of pains in the back
    ② States that the pain has lessened
    ③ Perspires and her face flushes
    ④ Assumes the lithotomy position

193. Shortly following delivery Mrs. Wyer says she feels as if she is bleeding. On checking the fundus the nurse finds a steady trickling of blood from the vagina. The first action should be to:
    ① Call the physician immediately
    ② Hold the fundus firmly and gently massage it
    ③ Check Mrs. Wyer's BP and pulse
    ④ Take no action, since this is a common occurrence

194. While checking Mrs. Wyer's fundus 2 days postpartum the nurse observes that it is at the umbilicus and displaced to the right. This means that the client probably has:
    ① A full, overdistended bladder
    ② Overstretched uterine ligaments
    ③ A slow rate of involution
    ④ Retained placental fragments

Situation: Mrs. Lane has delivered a 3685 g (8 lb 2 oz) boy. Her first child is 15 months old. She is discharged 5 days after delivery and is referred for home care follow-up.

195. The initial visit to Mrs. Lane will be more productive if scheduled when:
    ① The nurse has more time to expend
    ② She is feeding the children
    ③ Her husband is at work
    ④ It is convenient for the family

196. The role most likely to foster sound interpersonal relationships during the first visit to the Lane home is that of:
    ① Stranger
    ② Teacher
    ③ Counselor
    ④ Surrogate

197. When the nurse first talks with Mrs. Lane, the type of interview that is likely to be most productive is:
    ① Information-giving
    ② Problem-solving
    ③ Exploratory
    ④ Directive

198. On arrival for the first visit at 10 AM, the nurse finds Mr. Lane at home. He is temporarily collecting unemployment benefits, and the family is on welfare. Mrs. Lane is worried and ill at ease in the situation. The infant is due for bottle-feeding and the toddler is playing on the floor. At this time the nurse's best action would be to ask Mr. Lane if he would mind:
    ① Giving the baby a bottle
    ② Taking the toddler for a walk
    ③ Leaving you and Mrs. Lane alone
    ④ Participating in the discussion

199. The 15-month-old child has had no inoculations. Mr. Lane says he does not believe in them. The nurse's best response to this statement would be:
    ① "Scientific evidence proves you wrong."
    ② "Have you discussed this with a doctor?"
    ③ "How can you risk the life of your child?"
    ④ "You feel they may be harmful?"

200. After discussion with the nurse, Mr. and Mrs. Lane agree to have their 15-month-old immunized. The initial immunizations on the first visit to the health clinic are:
    ① Diphtheria and tetanus toxiods and pertussis vaccine (DTP) and trivalent oral poliovirus vaccine (OPV)
    ② Measles, rubella, and mumps combined vaccines
    ③ Diphtheria and tetanus toxoids and pertussis vaccine, trivalent oral poliovirus vaccine, and tuberculin test
    ④ Combined tetanus and diphtheria toxoid (Td), trivalent oral poliovirus vaccine, and tuberculin test

Situation: Julie Syms, a 12-month-old girl, is admitted to the hospital with a diagnosis of failure to thrive. Her weight is below the third percentile, her development is retarded, and she shows signs of neglect.

201. Based on this assessment, the behaviors that might also support the possibility of parental deprivation include:
    ① Julie is cuddly, responsive to touch, and wants to be held
    ② Julie is stiff, unpliable, and uncomforted by touch
    ③ Julie is a poor eater, sleeps soundly, and is easily satisfied
    ④ Julie is responsive to adults, rarely cries but shows no interest in her environment

202. A plan of care that would best meet the needs of this child should include:
    ① A vigorous schedule of stimulation geared to the infant's present level of development
    ② A plan to have all staff members pick her up and play with her whenever they can
    ③ A schedule of care that allows the infant stimulation and physical contact by several staff members
    ④ As consistent a caregiver as possible, with stimulation that is moderate and purposeful

203. During assessment of Julie, the nurse observes that the child has good head control, can roll over, but cannot sit up without support or transfer an object from one hand to the other. Based on these facts, the nurse concludes that Julie is developmentally at age:
    ① 2 to 3 months
    ② 3 to 4 months

③ 4 to 6 months
④ 6 to 8 months

204. Based on Julie's present developmental age the nurse should avoid giving her:
① Brightly colored mobiles
② Soft stuffed animals that she can hold
③ Small rattle that she can hold
④ Snap toys, large snap beads

Situation: John Gray, a 21-year-old physical education major in college, sustained a crushing fracture of the third and fourth lumbar vertebrae with severance of the cord while practicing on the trampoline. Three days after the injury the physician explained to him that he was a paraplegic and what this diagnosis entailed.

205. The nurse understands that paraplegia involves:
① Paresis of both lower extremities
② Paralysis of one side of the body
③ Paralysis of upper and lower extremities
④ Paralysis of both lower extremities

206. When caring for John, the initial responsibility of the nurse is to:
① Prevent contractures and atrophy
② Avoid flexion or hyperextension of the spine
③ Prevent urinary tract infections
④ Prepare the client for vocational rehabilitation

207. Considering the diagnosis, the nurse knows that John must be encouraged to drink a lot of fluids to prevent:
① Urinary tract infections
② Fluid and electrolyte imbalance
③ Dehydration
④ Constipation

208. John was placed on a CircOlectric bed primarily to:
① Promote mobility
② Prevent calcium loss from long bones
③ Prevent pressure sores
④ Promote orthostatic hypotension

209. Two weeks after the accident John begins vomiting thick coffee-ground material and appears restless and apprehensive. The nurse should:
① Change the client's diet to bland
② Prepare for insertion of a nasogastric tube
③ Check laboratory reports for hemoglobin level
④ Collect a stool specimen and check for occult blood

210. While caring for John the nurse should immediately report:
① Tachycardia, diaphoresis, and cold extremities
② Complaints of thirst and warm flushed skin
③ Nausea, weakness, and headache
④ Dyspepsia, distension, and diarrhea

211. Three weeks after his injury, John explains to the nurse that he must get out of the hospital soon to practice for the upcoming intercollegiate gymnastic tournament. In light of what he is saying, the nurse should realize that John is:
① No longer able to adapt
② Extremely motivated to get well
③ Verbalizing a fantasy
④ Exhibiting denial

Situation: Baby Ginger Little is admitted to the newborn nursery. The nurse weighs her and performs a newborn evaluation.

212. The most important weak or absent reflex for the nurse to report in her initial evaluation of the newborn is:
① Moro
② Tonic neck
③ Gag
④ Babinski

213. Baby Ginger has small, whitish, pinpoint spots over her nose, which the nurse knows are caused by retained sebaceous secretions. When charting this observation, the nurse identifies it as:
① Lanugo
② Milia
③ Whiteheads
④ Mongolian spots

214. When changing Baby Ginger, the nurse notices a brick red stain on the diaper. This is:
① A normal but uncommon occurrence
② A symptom of low iron stores
③ Due to medication given to the mother
④ To be expected in female babies

215. Three days after birth, Ginger is slightly jaundiced. The nurse knows that this is due primarily to her:
① Immature liver function
② Mother's high hemoglobin level
③ High hemoglobin and low hematocrit levels
④ Inability to synthesize bile

216. The physician orders phototherapy. During the therapy the nurse should apply eye patches to Ginger's eyes to:
① Be sure the eyes are closed
② Prevent injury to conjunctiva and retina
③ Reduce overstimulation from bright lights
④ Limit excessive rapid eye movements and anxiety

Situation: Karen Sutter, 6 months old, is admitted to the hospital because of increasing head size and a possible diagnosis of hydrocephalus.

217. In preforming a developmental appraisal, the observation that would be most important to the nurse in light of the diagnosis of hydrocephalus would be:
① Absence of Moro, tonic neck, and grasp reflexes
② Presence of the Babinski reflex
③ Head lag
④ Inability to sit unsupported

218. Because of the diagnosis, the nurse is especially alert to signs of increasing intracranial pressure, such as:
① Bulging fontanel, "sunset" eyes, projectile vomiting not associated with feeding
② Depressed fontanel, bulging eyes, irritability
③ Dilated scalp veins, depressed and sunken eyeballs, decreased BP
④ High shrill cry, decreased skin turgor, elevated fontanels

219. Proper positioning of Karen is essential to prevent breakdown of the scalp. A suitable position would be:
① Prone, with her legs elevated about 30°
② Prone or supine, with her head elevated about 45°
③ Positioned on either side and flat
④ Supine and Trendelenburg

220. Hydrocephalus, if untreated, can cause mental retardation because:
    1. Hypertonic CSF disturbs normal plasma concentration, depriving nerve cells of vital nutrients
    2. CSF dilutes blood supply, causing cells to atrophy
    3. Increasing head size necessitates more oxygen and nutrients than normal blood flow can supply
    4. Gradually increasing size of ventricles presses the brain against the bony cranium; anoxia and decreased blood supply result

221. After several tests have been performed, the diagnosis of noncommunicating hydrocephalus is confirmed and a ventriculoperitoneal shunt is performed. Postoperatively the nurse should:
    1. Position her flat for about 48 hours
    2. Administer sedatives and analgesics to keep her quiet
    3. Encourage the parents to pick up Karen to prevent crying
    4. Avoid touching the valve for 24 hrs

222. Mr. and Mrs. Sutter have been very anxious during their child's admission and especially concerned about the prognosis. The nurse should explain that:
    1. The prognosis is excellent and the valve is permanent
    2. The shunt may need to be revised as the child grows older
    3. If any brain damage has occurred, it is reversible during the first year of life
    4. Hydrocephalus usually is self-limiting by 2 years of age and then the shunt is removed

Situation: John Hanes has a long history of peptic ulcer and is admitted to the hospital with gastric bleeding. On the second day in the hospital, perforation occurs and an emergency gastrectomy is performed.

223. The emotional response that most frequently contributes to peptic ulcer is:
    1. Anxiety
    2. Depression
    3. Fear
    4. Rage

224. In the immediate postoperative period John's nasogastric tube is draining a bright red liquid. The nurse should expect this drainage for:
    1. 1 to 2 hours
    2. 3 to 4 hours
    3. 10 to 12 hours
    4. 24 to 48 hours

225. John is returned to his room on the second postoperative day. An IV of 1000 ml of 5% glucose in water containing 40 mEq potassium chloride is running. Parenteral preparations of potassium are administered slowly and cautiously to prevent:
    1. Acidosis
    2. Cardiac arrest
    3. Edema of the extremities
    4. Psychoticlike reactions

226. John's IV stopped and was restarted in his other arm by the IV team. The nurse coming on duty checked the IV bottle, noting that it was practically full and seemed to be dripping adequately. She did not count the drip rate or check the site of infusion. Later in the morning it was noted that a large infiltrated area had developed, and the needle had to be removed. The area of infiltration became reddened, and ultimately sloughing of tissue occurred. In situations such as this:
    1. The staff nurse is not responsible for IVs when the hospital has an IV team
    2. The rate of flow should have been regulated and maintained at a slow rate
    3. Sloughing of tissue is a frequent complication of IV therapy
    4. The rate of flow is unrelated to the problem of infiltration

227. After the nasogastric tube is removed, John is placed on a gradually increasing diet, which he tolerates fairly well. As the diet is increased, John develops the dumping syndrome. Dumping syndrome refers to:
    1. Buildup of feces and gas within the large intestine
    2. Rapid passage of osmotic fluid into the jejunum
    3. Reflux of intestinal contents into the esophagus
    4. Nausea due to a full stomach

228. Management of the dumping syndrome is best accomplished by planning to maintain John on a:
    1. Low-protein, high-carbohydrate diet
    2. Low-residue, bland diet
    3. Fluid intake below 500 ml
    4. Small frequent feeding schedule

Situation: Mrs. Hanson is an obese 59-year-old secretary with a long history of asthma dating back to her childhood. She has varicosed veins and has been admitted to the hospital for surgery.

229. Varicosed veins are usually the result of:
    1. Atherosclerotic plaques along the veins
    2. External compression of the muscles of the legs
    3. Defective valves within the veins
    4. The formation of thrombophlebitis

230. The nurse should expect Mrs. Hanson to complain of:
    1. Continued edema of the affected extremity
    2. A positive Homans' sign
    3. Coolness and pallor of the affected extremity
    4. Cramping sensations in the calf muscle

231. A simple test for varicose veins is the:
    1. Trendelenburg test
    2. Babinski reflex
    3. Romberg's sign
    4. Arteriography

232. Mrs. Hanson is going to have a vein ligation and stripping. The nurse explains that prior to surgery the physician must be certain:
    1. She understands the need to lose weight
    2. The deep veins of the leg are not occluded
    3. The saphenous vein has no sign of aneurysms
    4. She is aware of the need for several weeks of bed rest

233. The nurse should base preoperative teaching on the fact that Mrs. Hanson:
    1. Can control and limit her asthmatic attacks if she wants
    2. Should try to limit coughing, since this causes distention of the chest

③ Can control her anxiety and decrease the severity of postoperative asthma attacks

④ Will be quite prone to respiratory tract infections

234. When Mrs. Hanson returns from the recovery room, the nurse should position her:
① Supine with legs elevated 30°
② Flat with the knee gatch engaged
③ In a semi-Fowler's position with knees slightly flexed
④ Head elevated, feet tight against the foot-board

235. The evening of surgery, after Mrs. Hanson is fully re-acted, the nurse should:
① Apply a binder for support
② Assist her out of bed to a chair
③ Perform passive range of motion exercises to legs
④ Ambulate her in the room

Situation: Maria Lory, a 12-year-old girl, is admitted to the hospital with the diagnosis of acute lymphocytic leukemia (ALL).

236. With the diagnosis of ALL the nurse should consider it unusual to observe:
① Multiple bruises, petechia
② Marked fatigue, pallor
③ Enlarged lymph nodes, spleen, and liver
④ Marked jaundice and generalized edema

237. A pathophysiologic change underlying the production of symptoms in leukemia is:
① Progressive replacement of bone marrow with fibrous tissue
② Destruction of red blood cells and platelets by over-production of white blood cells
③ Proliferation and release of immature white blood cells into the circulating blood
④ Excessive destruction of blood cells in the liver and spleen

238. To induce a remission, Maria is started on a drug regimen that includes prednisone, vincristine, and L-asparaginase. The side effect of these drugs that requires the greatest preparation of Maria is:
① Constipation
② Generalized, short-term paralysis
③ Retarded growth in height
④ Alopecia

239. A major objective of nursing care related to Maria's disease and drug regimen is to:
① Avoid contact with infected persons
② Reduce unnecessary stimuli
③ Check her vital signs every 2 hours
④ Prevent all physical activity

240. Understanding the side effects of vincristine, the nurse plans a diet for Maria that is:
① Low in residue with increased fluids
② High in iron with decreased fluids
③ High in both roughage and fluids
④ Low in fat with regular fluids

241. Because Maria's platelet count is very low, the nurse plans to observe her urine for the presence of:
① Erythrocytes
② Leukocytes
③ Casts
④ Lymphocytes

242. Maria's physician also plans a program of irradiation of the spine and skull. The nurse explains that this treatment is used mainly because:
① Leukemia cells invade the nervous system more slowly, but the usual drugs are ineffective in the brain
② Radiation will retard growth of cells in bone marrow of the cranium
③ Neoplastic drug therapy without radiation is effective in most cases, but this is a precautionary treatment
④ Radiation will decrease cerebral edema and prevent increased intracranial pressure

243. One day Mr. Lory asks the nurse whether he should tell his son, who is 7 years old, the truth about Maria. The nurse should reply:
① "A child of his age cannot comprehend the real meaning of death, so don't tell him until the last moment."
② "Your son probably fears separation most and wants to know that you will care for him, rather than what will happen to his sister."
③ "Your son probably doesn't understand death as we do but fears it just the same. He should be told the truth to let him prepare for his sister's possible death."
④ "Why don't you talk this over with your doctor, who probably knows best what is happening in terms of Maria's prognosis?"

Situation: David King is a 34-year-old sales manager. He frequently experiences weakness and difficulty in moving his right hand. A thorough medical examination reveals no physical pathologic condition. The physician now believes the symptoms are the result of a somatoform disorder.

244. A somatoform disorder is:
① A psychosomatic reaction to stress
② An unconscious means to control conflict
③ A psychologic defense against stress
④ A conscious defense against anxiety

245. A person who habitually expresses anxiety through physical symptoms is displaying the defense mechanisms known as:
① Psychoneurotic
② Psychosomatic
③ Regressive
④ Projective

246. Conversion disorder is the term used to describe the phenomenon whereby anxiety associated with stress or conflict has been repressed and converted into specific physical manifestations. One of the characteristics of the client's reaction to the physical symptom is:
① Agitation
② Indifference
③ Anger
④ Anxiety

247. The basic difference between psychophysiological disorders and hypochondria is that in psychophysiological disorders there is:
① An emotional cause
② A feeling of illness
③ An actual tissue change
④ A restriction of activities

248. David is scheduled for an occupational therapy group. While listening to instructions for the group project, he experiences the feeling of weakness and is unable to move his right arm. After a check of pulse and respirations, the nurse's best response would be:
    1. "Exactly when did the weakness begin?"
    2. "Is this similar to what you usually experience?"
    3. "What emotion were you feeling before you felt the weakness?"
    4. "Would you like to leave the group for a while?"

249. The occurrence of this pattern of behavior can be reduced if the nurse:
    1. Decreases anxiety by limiting discussion of problems with the client
    2. Provides client teaching regarding medical care
    3. Teaches the family how to decrease stress at home
    4. Assists the client in developing altered life patterns

250. During group therapy other members accuse David of intellectualizing and avoiding his feelings. He asks if the nurse agrees with the others. The nurse's best answer would be:
    1. "It seems that way to me, too."
    2. "I'd rather not give my personal opinion."
    3. "What is your perception of my behavior?"
    4. "You seem to need my opinion."

Situation: Mr. Norman, a husky 6-foot man, 30 years of age, hospitalized with a diagnosis of bipolar disorder, is active and sometimes combative. Since his admission he has been alone in a room. A 45-year-old man is admitted and placed in the room with Mr. Norman. Mr. Norman seems to accept the newcomer and the nurse pays little attention to them for the rest of the afternoon.

251. Suddenly a commotion is heard, and Mr. Norman is found beating the other client. Legally:
    1. The admitting office should not have put the client in with Mr. Norman
    2. Knowing that Mr. Norman was frequently combative, close observation was indicated
    3. Clients who are combative should never be left unsupervised
    4. A combative client like Mr. Norman should have been sedated with tranquilizers

252. Mr. Norman is receiving lithium carbonate. While the medication is being administered, it is important that the nurse:
    1. Restrict his sodium intake
    2. Test his urine weekly
    3. Withhold other medications for the first week
    4. Monitor his blood level regularly

253. While the nurse is talking with Mr. Norman in his room, his conversation becomes embarrassingly vulgar. The nurse should respond to his behavior by:
    1. Restricting Mr. Norman's contact with staff until this symptom passes
    2. Tactfully teasing him about the use of such vulgarity
    3. Asking him to limit his vulgarity and continuing the conversation with him
    4. Discreetly refusing to talk to him when he is speaking in this manner

254. Activities that would be most therapeutic for Mr. Norman and that the nurse should encourage include:
    1. Carving figures out of wood
    2. Sanding and varnishing wooden bookends
    3. Stenciling designs on copper sheeting
    4. Lacing tooled leather wallets

255. Mr. Norman is noisy, loud, and disruptive. The nurse informs him that, unless he is more quiet, he will be isolated and put in restraints, if necessary. Legally:
    1. Restraint of Mr. Norman is justified for his own protection
    2. The information given Mr. Norman is actually a threat
    3. Clients like Mr. Norman cannot be expected to understand instructions
    4. Mr. Norman's behavior is to be expected and should be ignored

256. During a period of hyperactivity, Mr. Norman demands to be allowed to go downtown to do his shopping. He has no privileges at the present time. The nurse's best response would be:
    1. "I'm sorry, Mr. Norman, you can't go. Let's look through this new catalog."
    2. "You cannot leave the ward, Mr. Norman."
    3. "You'll have to ask your doctor, Mr. Norman."
    4. "Not right now, Mr. Norman. I don't have a staff member to go with you."

257. One day while the nurse is staying with Mr. Norman, who is shaving, he states, "I have hidden a razor blade and tonight I am going to kill myself." The nurse's best reply would be:
    1. "You're going to kill yourself?"
    2. "You'd better finish shaving; it's time for lunch."
    3. "I'm sure you don't really mean that."
    4. "Things can't really be that bad."

Situation: Mrs. Loft, 42 years of age, is admitted to the hospital with a tentative diagnosis of chronic adrenal insufficiency.

258. Because of her condition, it would be unwise to place Mrs. Loft in a room:
    1. With an elderly CVA client
    2. With a middle-aged woman who has pneumonia
    3. That is private and away from the nurses' station
    4. Next to a 17-year-old girl with a fractured leg

259. Mrs. Loft complains of weakness and dizziness on arising from bed in the morning. The nurse realizes that this is most probably caused by:
    1. Postural hypertension
    2. A hypoglycemic reaction
    3. A lack of potassium
    4. Increased extracellular fluid volume

260. After a Thorn test shows an increased eosinophil count, Mrs. Loft is advised that she has Addison's disease. It is most important that the nurse discuss with her the need for:
    1. Frequent visits to the physician
    2. Restriction of physical activity
    3. A special low-salt diet
    4. Hormone replacement therapy

261. In teaching Mrs. Loft about her diet, the nurse should tell her to:
    ① Add a little extra salt to her food
    ② Limit intake to 1200 calories
    ③ Omit protein foods at each meal
    ④ Restrict her daily intake of fluids
262. In the event Mrs. Loft neglects to continue the cortisone therapy, an adrenal crisis may occur. The predominant symptom she should be advised to report is:
    ① Hypertension
    ② A high body temperature
    ③ Muscle spasms
    ④ Diarrhea
263. Clients on prolonged cortisone therapy may exhibit adaptations caused by its glucocorticoid and mineralocorticoid actions. The nurse should teach Mrs. Loft and her family to observe for:
    ① Hypoglycemia and anuria
    ② Weight gain and moon face
    ③ Anorexia and hyperkalemia
    ④ Hypotension and fluid loss
264. When Mrs. Loft shows concern about the fact that she is developing signs of masculinity, the nurse should tell her:
    ① It is a further sign of the illness
    ② That this is due to therapy
    ③ Not to worry, since it will disappear with therapy
    ④ That this is not important, so long as she gets better
265. In observing Mrs. Loft for cortisone overdose, the nurse should be particularly alert for:
    ① Behavioral changes
    ② Severe anorexia
    ③ Hypoglycemia
    ④ Anaphylactic shock

Situation: Mrs. Garvin, age 38, has cancer of the cervix. She is hospitalized for internal radiation therapy with radium.

266. When Mrs. Garvin returns to her room, after the insertion of radium, the nurse should:
    ① Immediately place her in a high Fowler's position to prevent dislodging the radium
    ② Check her voiding and catheterize her if necessary, since a distended bladder can interrupt the path of radiation
    ③ Check that a low-residue diet has been ordered to prevent bowel movements and the possibility of dislodging the radium
    ④ Stay with her for half an hour to watch for symptoms of radiation sickness
267. Six months later Mrs. Garvin is readmitted for an abdominal hysterectomy. During her preoperative care she asks how the surgery will affect her periods. The nurse should respond:
    ① "Initially your periods will increase."
    ② "You will no longer menstruate."
    ③ "Your monthly periods will be more regular."
    ④ "Your monthly periods will be lighter."
268. Mrs. Garvin is admitted to the recovery room after surgery. The observation that should be reported to the physician immediately is:
    ① Increased drainage from the Levin tube
    ② Serosanguinous drainage on the perineal pad

③ Decreased urinary output
④ Apical pulse of 90

269. Abdominal distention develops in Mrs. Garvin. The measures that would most likely provide immediate relief are:
    ① Restriction of oral intake and frequent change of position
    ② Ambulation and carbonated drinks
    ③ Insertion of a rectal tube and application of heat to the abdomen
    ④ Nasogastric intubation and administration of cholinergic agents
270. Mrs. Garvin's physician has ordered that she wear a girdle while out of bed. The nurse should explain that this is to:
    ① Prevent pooling of blood in the pelvic area
    ② Increase wound healing
    ③ Prevent feelings of nausea
    ④ Support abdominal muscles

Situation: Mrs. Grite, who is 35 weeks pregnant and a diabetic, is admitted to the hospital to await delivery.

271. Mrs. Grite's questions about why she is being hospitalized can be answered best if the nurse understands that in diabetic pregnant woman:
    ① Complete rest prior to the work of delivery is essential
    ② Fetal death usually occurs after the thirty-sixth week of gestation
    ③ Fetal development is completed and should be monitored
    ④ Insulin needs to be administered intravenously before labor begins
272. The nurse should be aware that diabetic pregnant women such as Mrs. Grite require:
    ① Increased dosage of insulin
    ② Administration of estrogenic hormones
    ③ Decreased caloric intake
    ④ Administration of pancreatic enzymes
273. Mrs. Grite asks why she cannot take the oral hypoglycemic pills she used for her diabetes. The nurse's response should be based on the fact that oral hypoglycemics are not used during pregnancy because:
    ① The fetal pancreas compensates for the mother's inability to secrete adequate insulin
    ② The effect of exogenous insulin on the fetus is uncertain
    ③ They may produce deformities in the fetus
    ④ During the latter part of pregnancy, diabetes can usually be controlled by diet alone
274. Mrs. Grite's delivery is induced and she delivers a baby girl. A sign of hypoglycemia in Baby Grite for which the nurse should be alert is:
    ① Excessive birth weight
    ② Excessive body movement
    ③ Pallor of the skin and mucosa
    ④ Poor sucking reflex
275. In caring for Baby Grite the nurse should provide:
    ① A decreased glucose intake
    ② Routine newborn care
    ③ For administration of insulin
    ④ Special high-risk care

Situation: Mr. Rudolph is admitted to the burn unit with second- and third-degree burns.

276. Fluid shifts are a great danger to the client with burns. The nurse should expect to observe:
    ① Increased fluid shifts and irreversible shock after 2 hours
    ② Loss of sodium and increase in blood potassium
    ③ Decreased capillary permeability
    ④ Rise in blood volume

277. IV fluid replacement therapy is important. An expected intake and output in the first 24 hours would be:
    ① Intake, 8000 ml; output, 480 ml
    ② Intake, 12,000 ml; output, 4500 ml
    ③ Intake, 3000 ml; output, 2400 ml
    ④ Intake, 6000 ml; output, 1200 ml

278. The rate of fluid replacement for a client with severe burns during the first 48 hours is considered satisfactory if the urinary output is approximately:
    ① Half the intake
    ② One-tenth the intake
    ③ One-third the intake
    ④ Equal to the intake

279. To maintain Mr. Rudolph's nutrition during convalescence, it is most important to:
    ① Reduce protein intake to avoid overtaxing the kidneys
    ② Limit caloric intake to decrease the work of the body
    ③ Encourage the drinking of orange juice or other fluids containing vitamin C
    ④ Encourage increased intake of sodium

280. In the recovery and convalescent periods, the nurse should be aware that:
    ① Death may still occur from septicemia
    ② The danger of physical complications is past
    ③ Because of the client's need for rest, diversional therapy must be delayed
    ④ Mirrors should be removed to decrease the client's anxiety about appearance

281. Mr. Rudolph asks why he is being given an antacid. The nurse explains that it is prophylactic during the first 2 weeks after the burn to prevent:
    ① Curling's ulcer
    ② Gastric ulcer
    ③ Colitis
    ④ Gastritis

COMPREHENSIVE TEST 1: PART 4

To simulate the National Council Licensure Examination, this test should be completed within 1½ hours.

Situation: Mrs. Coan, 9 months pregnant, is admitted to the hospital with bleeding caused by possible placenta previa. The laboratory technician takes blood samples and IV fluids are begun.

282. The nurse, following the physician's orders, begins administering oxygen by mask. The client's apprehension is increasing and she asks the nurse what is happening. The nurse tells her not to worry, that she is going to be all right and everything is under control. The nurse's statements are:
    ① Correct, since only the physician should explain why treatments are being done
    ② Proper, since the client's anxieties would be increased if she knew the dangers
    ③ Adequate, since all preparations are routine and need no explanation
    ④ Questionable, since the client has the right to know what treatment is being given and why

283. Nursing care of Mrs. Coan includes:
    ① Withholding food and fluids
    ② Encouraging ambulation with supervision
    ③ Inspecting for hemorrhage
    ④ Avoiding all extraneous stimuli

284. If a vaginal examination is to be performed on Mrs. Coan, the nurse must be prepared for an immediate:
    ① Induction of labor
    ② Cesarean delivery
    ③ Forceps delivery
    ④ X-ray examination

285. Baby Coan, weighing 2840 g (6 lb 4 oz) should have a daily intake of:
    ① 740 ml (25 oz) of fluid and 450 calories
    ② 592 ml (20 oz) of fluid and 400 calories
    ③ 532.8 ml (18 oz) of fluid and 375 calories
    ④ 888 ml (30 oz) of fluid and 500 calories

286. While working in the newborn nursery, the nurse observes a yellowish color in the skin of Baby Coan. The immediate nursing action should be to:
    ① Cover the baby's eyes with a blindfold and put the baby under the ultraviolet light
    ② Notify the physician of the development
    ③ Take a heel blood sample and send it to the laboratory
    ④ Ascertain the age of the infant

Situation: Mrs. Gold is a 50-year-old woman with a history of a mood disorder. She is diagnosed as having a bipolar disorder/depressed. She is agitated, paces in her room almost continuously, and has difficulty sleeping at night.

287. Mrs. Gold frequently states that she will die. The nurse tells her this is not true and she should not dwell on the subject. The nurse urges Mrs. Gold to go to the day room and talk with the other clients. Mrs. Gold becomes more agitated and ultimately has to be sedated. In instances such as this:
    ① The nurse must be accepting and should not try to talk a client out of a delusion
    ② The sleeplessness and agitation should have been treated as a symptom
    ③ Mrs. Gold has to be encouraged to relate to the other clients
    ④ Mrs. Gold should have been given a tranquilizer before this incident developed

288. The treatment plan for Mrs. Gold would probably include:
    ① High doses of mood elevators
    ② Psychoanalysis
    ③ Electroconvulsive therapy
    ④ Nondirective psychotherapy

289. In caring for Mrs. Gold the nurse should keep in mind that:
① Clients with simple depressions rarely attempt suicide
② Once the severe depression begins to lift, the danger of suicide is no longer a problem
③ Depressed clients are potentially suicidal during the entire course of their illness
④ Opportunities to attempt suicide are practically absent on a closed psychiatric unit

290. Mrs. Gold appears preoccupied. She remains seated when it is time for the clients to go to eat. The nurse's best approach would be to:
① Overlook her not eating and leave snacks in the room
② Tell her she must eat now, since no food will be served later
③ Ask her whether she would like to eat in her room instead of the dining room
④ Take her by the hand and accompany her to the dining room

291. Mrs. Gold is eating very little at this time. A part of the nursing care plan should be to assist her with her meals. Besides encouraging nourishment, this action also:
① Shows her she is a worthwhile individual
② Gets her out of the dining room with the rest of the clients
③ Proves to her that she can tolerate food
④ Provides her with some special attention

292. Mrs. Gold is taking lithium carbonate. It is vital that the nurse carefully monitor her
① Daily weight
② Toxicology reports
③ Psychomotor activity
④ Leukocyte count

293. Mrs. Gold is much improved and is permitted passes to leave the hospital. She is going home for a 3-day weekend. The nurse should advise her to:
① Adjust her lithium dosage if her mood changes
② Have a snack with milk before going to bed
③ Avoid participation in controversial discussions
④ Maintain her sodium intake

Situation: An incision and drainage of a rectal abscess was performed 2 days ago on Mr. Silson, 48 years of age. He is receiving meperidine hydrochloride (Demerol) for pain and sitz baths tid to promote comfort and drainage.

294. The nurse turns from preparing Mr. Silson's sitz bath and discovers he is lying on the floor. After ascertaining that he is unconscious, the nurse should:
① Help him back to bed
② Check the BP
③ Check the carotid pulse
④ Call for assistance

295. The nurse sends the nurse's aide for help and begins CPR. When there is only one person to perform cardiopulmonary resuscitation, the ratio of ventilation(s) to cardiac compressions is:
① 1:5
② 1:10

③ 2:15
④ 4:15

296. In performing external cardiac compression on Mr. Silson the nurse should exert downward vertical pressure on the lower sternum by placing:
① The heels of each hand side by side, extending the fingers over the chest
② The heel of one hand on the sternum and the heel of the other on top of it, interlocking the fingers
③ The fingers of one hand on the sternum and the fingers of the other hand on top of them
④ The fleshy part of the clenched fist on the lower sternum

297. The cardiac arrest team arrives and places Mr. Silson on a monitor. To prepare the skin area for placement of the electrodes for cardiac monitoring, the nurse:
① Uses a scrubbing motion while cleansing the skin
② Scrubs the area with povidone iodine solution
③ Makes certain the area is moistened with normal saline before applying the electrodes
④ Applies electrode paste only if the skin becomes excoriated

298. The cardiac monitor shows ventricular fibrillation. The nurse from the coronary care unit should prepare for:
① An IM injection of digoxin (Lanoxin)
② An IV line for emergency medications
③ Immediate defibrillation
④ Elective cardioversion

299. Because the cells are deprived of oxygen during a cardiac arrest, metabolic acidosis develops. The nurse should be prepared to administer:
① Potassium chloride
② Calcium gluconate
③ Sodium bicarbonate
④ Regular insulin

Situation: Mrs. Palecek, a 33-year-old housewife, is admitted to the hospital with a diagnosis of acute cholecystitis, biliary colic, and possible obstructive jaundice.

300. In addition to pain in the right upper quadrant, the nurse should expect Mrs. Palecek to have:
① An intolerance of foods high in lipids
② Vomiting of coffee-ground emesis
③ Gnawing pain when the stomach is empty
④ Melena and diarrhea

301. A cholecystectomy is scheduled. Vitamin K is administered to Mrs. Palecek prior to surgery, since it is used in the formation of:
① Bilirubin
② Prothrombin
③ Thromboplastin
④ Cholecystokinin

302. After surgery Mrs. Palecek is transferred to the recovery room with a nasogastric tube in place. She vomits 30 ml of bile-colored fluid. The nurse should:
① Administer an antiemetic
② Check the patency of the tube
③ Elevate the head of the bed
④ Encourage the client to breathe deeply

303. Once Mrs. Palecek is returned to her unit, the nurse continues to make frequent checks of the wound area to note any tendencies toward excess bleeding or hemorrhage. These observations are made because:
    ① Diaphragmatic excursion places pressure on the suture line
    ② Mrs. Palecek's temperature is slightly elevated
    ③ Blood clotting may be hindered by lack of vitamin K absorption
    ④ Mrs. Palecek is complaining of severe pain

304. Mrs. Palecek is prone to upper respiratory tract complications because of the:
    ① Proximity of the incision to the diaphragm
    ② Length of time required for surgery
    ③ Lowered resistance caused by bile in the blood
    ④ Transfer of bacteria from the biliary tract to the blood

305. Three days after the cholecystectomy Mrs. Palecek begins a full fluid diet. When the breakfast tray arrives, it has whole milk and cream for cereal. The luncheon tray includes whole milk and ice cream. When the surgeon visits at lunchtime, he notes the tray's contents and, disturbed that the diet is not low in fat, takes the tray away. In situations such as this the:
    ① Dietitian should check the diet that the client receives
    ② Physician orders the diet, and the order should be carried out as written
    ③ Nurse shares responsibility, since the physician's order was not questioned
    ④ Client should have followed the physician's directions

306. When Mrs. Palecek is ready to be discharged, the dietitian instructs her to remain on her prescribed diet for several more weeks. Afterward she asks her nurse, "Will I have to stay away from fat for the rest of my life?" The most appropriate response by the nurse would be:
    ① "You'll have to remain on a fat-free diet from now on to avoid problems."
    ② "It's too early to say. Later, when we see whether your operation is successful, we'll know the answer."
    ③ "Only the doctor can answer that. Why don't you ask him about it before your discharge from the hospital?"
    ④ "After you have fully recovered from surgery, you'll probably be able to eat a normal diet, avoiding excessive fat."

Situation: Miss Abigail Jones, age 17 years, is admitted to the obstetric unit in labor. She is 41 weeks pregnant and experiencing mild contractions every 15 minutes, lasting 10 seconds each. Vaginal examination reveals the cervix to be 1 cm dilated, membranes intact, and vertex at station 1. A fetal monitor is used.

307. One problem that confronts the client when an external indirect fetal monitor is being used is the:
    ① Restriction of movement
    ② Interference with Lamaze techniques
    ③ Increased frequency of vaginal examinations
    ④ Inability to take sedatives

308. The nurse asks about Abigail's marital status. Abigail refuses to answer and becomes very agitated, telling the nurse to leave. The nurse should:
    ① Have restricted questions to those relevant to the situation
    ② Have this information to complete the client's history
    ③ Questions the family about the marital status of the client
    ④ Refer the client to a social service organization for help

309. After an 8-hour uneventful labor Miss Jones delivers a baby boy spontaneously under epidural block anesthesia. As the nurse places the baby in her arms immediately following delivery, she asks, "Is he normal?" The most appropriate response by the nurse would be:
    ① "Of course he is; your pregnancy and labor were so normal."
    ② "Shall we unwrap him so you can look him over for yourself?"
    ③ "He must be all right, he has such a good strong cry."
    ④ "Most babies are normal; of course he is."

310. The major concern for a pregnant unmarried teenager is that she is:
    ① Socially ostracized
    ② Diabetogenic
    ③ Financially dependent
    ④ Prone to toxemia

Situation: Robert Dorn, 5 weeks old, is admitted to the hospital with a tentative diagnosis of congenital heart defect. His mother states that he tires easily and has difficulty breathing and feeding.

311. Part of the nursing care for Robert would include proper positioning. The best position in which to place Robert would be:
    ① Supine with the knees flexed
    ② Orthopneic with pillows for support
    ③ Side-lying with the head and chest elevated
    ④ Prone with the head supported by pillows

312. A cardiac catheterization is performed. Postoperatively Robert is brought back to the pediatric unit for observation. The leg used for the procedure is mottled. The nurse should immediately:
    ① Check the pulse in the extremity
    ② Notify the physician of the situation
    ③ Cover the baby with a blanket
    ④ Elevate the leg

313. Baby Robert is in the pediatric recovery room after open heart surgery for the repair of a ventricular septal defect. A nursing priority should be to:
    ① Determine the status of the operative site
    ② Ascertain Robert's pulmonary status
    ③ Check the patency of the intravenous catheter
    ④ Monitor Robert's urinary output

314. The Dorns are informed that Robert is in the recovery room and is stable. Mrs. Dorn is crying and extremely worried. The nurse can best help allay her anxiety by:

① Bringing her and her husband to the recovery room for several minutes
② Reassuring them that Robert is doing well
③ Allowing her to continue to express her feelings
④ Encouraging them to go have a cup of coffee and return in 2 hours

315. When Robert is ready to go home, Mrs. Dorn asks the nurse, "Shall I continue to scrub my baby's bottles?" Prior to replying, the nurse should remember that during early infancy:
① The gastric acidity is low and unable to provide bacteriostatic protection
② The absence of hydrochloric acid renders the stomach vulnerable to infection
③ *Escherichia coli,* the bacterium normally found in the stomach, does not act on milk
④ Infants are almost completely lacking in immunity and need sterile fluids

Situation: Mrs. Owens, a 72-year-old woman with congestive heart failure, is often troubled by edematous feet and ankles. She comes to the clinic for evaluation.

316. Mrs. Owens admits to the nurse that she has not been following her salt-restricted diet and now is experiencing markedly increased ankle edema, orthopnea, and dyspnea on exertion. The nurse should be alert for other complaints of fluid retention such as:
① Dizziness on rising
② Weak and thready pulse
③ Rhinitis and headache
④ Decreased hemoglobin count and hematocrit

317. Mrs. Owens also has osteoporosis. This is best described as:
① A decrease in bone substance
② Hyperplasia of osteoblasts
③ Pathologic fractures
④ Avascular necrosis

318. Mrs. Owens' care plan for osteoporosis includes active and passive exercises, calcium supplements, and daily vitamins. The desired effect of therapy would be noted by the nurse if Mrs. Owens:
① Had fewer bruises than on admission
② Increased her mobility
③ Developed fewer cardiac irregularities
④ Developed fewer muscular spasms

319. Two weeks after discharge Mrs. Owens experiences mild epigastric pain and is returned to the hospital by her daughter, who is very concerned. Mrs. Owens is admitted to the coronary care unit for observation. She states, "I know I'm sick but I could really take care of myself at home." The nurse recognizes that Mrs. Owens is attempting to:
① Deny her illness
② Suppress her fears
③ Reassure her daughter
④ Maintain her independence

Situation: Mrs. Jane Donnley, a 32-year-old, obese woman with a history of mild rheumatic heart disease, is in the first trimester of her first pregnancy.

320. During the seventh week of her pregnancy, Mrs. Donnley complains of dependent edema in her ankles. The nurse advises her to:
① Limit her fluid intake during the day
② Stop using salt for the next 3 months
③ Elevate her legs more frequently during the day
④ Call her physician immediately for a mild diuretic

321. Nutritional management is most important for the pregnant woman with cardiac problems. The nurse should advise Mrs. Donnley to eat a diet with:
① Increased fats
② Increased sodium
③ Decreased protein
④ Decreased calories

322. In the eighth month Mrs. Donnley is scheduled for an oxytocin challenge test (OCT). The nurse caring for her understands that the OCT is used in evaluating the:
① High-risk mother's ability to tolerate a vaginal delivery
② Fetal heart rate (FHR)
③ Contractibility of the pregnant uterus prior to delivery
④ Uteroplacental function

323. One important instruction for Mrs. Donnley prior to the oxytocin challenge test is that she should:
① Take diazepam (Valium) 5 mg po ½ hour before the test
② Empty her bladder before the test
③ Eat nothing for 2 hours before the test and 6 hours after the test
④ Be prepared to be in the hospital for 12 hours after the test

324. Prior to the start of the OCT the nurse explains to Mrs. Donnley that:
① The FHR will be monitored for 30 minutes prior to actual testing
② She will be placed in a right lateral position, which must be maintained throughout testing
③ At least 6 contractions must be observed before the test is discontinued
④ A double-voided urine specimen will be collected prior to the test

325. Mrs. Donnley gives birth to a 3124 g (6 lb 14 oz) baby boy, and the nurse is performing a newborn assessment. Baby Donnley's vital signs should be measured in the following sequence:
① Respirations, temperature, pulse
② Temperature, pulse, respirations
③ Respirations, pulse, temperature
④ Pulse, respirations, temperature

326. Mrs. Donnley is breast-feeding her son. One day when the nurse brings him to be fed, Mrs. Donnley mentions that she cannot believe her newborn wants to breast-feed again since she just fed him 2½ hours ago. The nurse should plan to teach Mrs. Donnley that a newborn usually should be nursed:
① Every hour
② Every 2 hours
③ Every 4 hours
④ Every 5 hours

327. Mrs. Donnley is afraid that her heart condition will prevent her from being able to care for her baby and her home properly when she is discharged. The most appropriate nursing intervention is to:
① Speak to her husband alone and explain how he can assist
② Ask Mrs. Donnley to explain more fully why she feels this way
③ Tell Mrs. Donnley to speak to her physician about her concerns
④ Suggest that Mrs. Donnley's husband arrange for help at home

328. Mr. Donnley tells the nurse that he is anxious about feeling like a father. The priority in planning to meet the father's needs would be to:
① Provide a demonstration on diapering, feeding, and bathing the baby
② Provide the opportunity to ask questions after viewing the film *Our New Baby*
③ Provide time for the father to be alone with and get to know the baby
④ Encourage the father's participation in a fathering class

329. On her 6-week postpartum visit, Mrs. Donnley tells the nurse she wants to feed her baby a whole milk (cow's milk) formula after 2 months since she will be returning to work. The nurse should plan to teach her that whole milk does not meet the infant's nutritional requirements because it is low in
① Thiamin and sodium
② Protein and carbohydrates
③ Fat and calcium
④ Vitamin C and iron

Situation: Mr. Dime, age 39, an unmarried executive producer for one of the major television networks, was in a serious auto accident. He is admitted with multiple fractures and deep lacerations with hemorrhage. He is in severe shock and is rushed to the operating room. A blood transfusion proves incompatible with his blood type.

330. The initial sign of such a transfusion reaction, which the nurse should observe for, is:
① Dyspnea
② Backache
③ Cyanosis
④ Bradycardia

331. As a result of this transfusion reaction, Mr. Dime suffers kidney damage. In determining kidney damage, the most significant clinical response that the nurse should assess is:
① Acute pain over kidney area
② Decreased urinary output
③ Hematuria
④ Polyuria

332. Although Mr. Dime does not request an analgesic, the nurse should be alert for a sign of an involuntary reaction to pain, which is:
① Perspiration
② Crying
③ Splinting
④ Grimacing

333. Mr. Dime's kidney function has not returned and is currently about 10% of normal. Peritoneal dialysis is ordered when his BUN begins to rise. Once instituted, peritoneal dialysis:
① Is largely a nursing responsibility
② May be maintained from 12 to 48 hours
③ Requires checking of vital signs every 15 minutes
④ Should be discontinued if the client complains of abdominal discomfort

334. The purpose of peritoneal dialysis is to:
① Reestablish kidney function
② Clean the peritoneal membrane
③ Remove toxins and metabolic wastes
④ Provide fluid for intracellular spaces

335. Mr. Dime complains of nausea, pain in the abdomen, diarrhea, and muscular weakness. The nurse notes an irregularity in pulse and signs of pulmonary edema. These are probably manifestations of:
① Calcium deficiency
② Calcium excess
③ Sodium deficiency
④ Potassium excess

336. Between dialysis treatments, Mr. Dime is maintained on a modified Giordano-Giovannetti diet. This diet is:
① High in protein
② Low in potassium
③ High in sodium
④ Low in calories

337. In caring for Mr. Dime when he is being dialyzed, the nurse should:
① Maintain him in a flat, supine position during the entire procedure
② Notify the physician if there is a deficit of 200 ml in the drainage fluid
③ Apply firm manual pressure on his lower abdomen if fluid is not draining properly
④ Remove the cannula at the end of the procedure and apply a dry, sterile dressing

338. If Mr. Dime is observed to have severe respiratory difficulty, the most immediate nursing action would be to:
① Change his position
② Drain fluid from the peritoneal cavity
③ Notify the physician
④ Discontinue the treatment

339. Mr. Dime has been immobilized in traction for 3 weeks. The nurse realizes that he may develop renal calculi as a complication because:
① He has more difficulty urinating in a supine position
② His dietary patterns have changed since admission
③ Lack of muscle action and normal tension cause calcium withdrawal from the bone
④ Fracture healing requires more calcium and thus increases total calcium metabolism

340. Mr. Dime's leg is set in a long leg cast. The nurse should observe for signs that indicate compromised circulation because of the long leg cast such as:
① Foul odor
② Swelling of the toes
③ Increased temperature
④ Drainage on the cast

341. Mr. Dime is waiting for a renal transplant. In teaching Mr. Dime, the nurse informs him that:
    ① He will require immunosuppressive drugs daily for the rest of his life
    ② He will be unable to follow a full program of work and recreation, including sports
    ③ Symptoms of rejection include fever, hypotension, and edema
    ④ Urine production will be delayed after surgery

Situation: Four-year-old Ted Corleone is admitted to the hospital with a hemoglobin count of 7 g/100 ml and a red blood cell count of 2,500,000/100 ml.

342. In addition to weakness and fatigue, the nurse should expect Ted to exhibit:
    ① Cold, clammy skin
    ② Cyanosis of the nail beds
    ③ Increased pulse rate
    ④ Elevated BP

343. Ted has never been separated from his parents. His parents should be encouraged to:
    ① Stay with him throughout the hospitalization
    ② Bring a favorite toy to the hospital for him
    ③ Visit as often as possible
    ④ Allow the nurse to be the major care giver

344. While Ted is playing in the hall, he complains of feeling "woozy." The nurse's best initial response would be to:
    ① Check his pulse and BP
    ② Assist him back to his room and place him supine in bed
    ③ Use spirits of ammonia to prevent fainting
    ④ Have him sit until the dizziness subsides

345. The nurse should recognize that the most probable cause of Ted's dizziness was:
    ① Decreased levels of serum glucose
    ② A sudden drop in BP
    ③ Insufficient cerebral oxygenation
    ④ An inflammation of the inner ear

346. The physician orders a liquid iron preparation for Ted. The nurse should:
    ① Administer this at least an hour before meals
    ② Caution Ted's mother to avoid orange juice or other citrus juice
    ③ Have Ted use a straw to take the medication
    ④ Explain that loose stools are common with iron

347. When Ted develops gastrointestinal discomfort, the physician prescribes a daily parenteral iron preparation. In administering this medication, the nurse should:
    ① Rotate injections among the four extremities
    ② Firmly massage the site after withdrawal of the needle
    ③ Change needles after drawing the drug into the syringe
    ④ Apply ice packs to the site after the injection

348. The nurse attempts to meet Ted's emotional needs. The most appropriate method would be to:
    ① Encourage Ted to draw pictures of what he is feeling
    ② Explain the procedures to Ted in simple terms at least an hour before they are scheduled

③ Allow Ted to play with a needle and syringe
④ Provide Ted with a doll and other equipment and observe his behavior

349. Because of his anemia, Ted requires multiple transfusions. He has an increased risk of developing:
    ① Pulmonary edema
    ② Allergic response
    ③ Hemolytic reaction
    ④ Serum hepatitis

Situation: Mr. Burn, 55, is admitted to the hospital with benign prostatic hypertrophy. Surgery is scheduled.

350. The night nurse reports that Mr. Burn is complaining of inability to void. On making the morning rounds it is noted that his bladder is distended. The nurse should:
    ① Force fluids to induce voiding
    ② Encourage use of a urinal
    ③ Apply pressure over the pubic area
    ④ Assist him into a warm tub bath

351. Mr. Burn has undergone a suprapubic prostatectomy. In addition to a Foley catheter, the nurse should expect Mr. Burn to have:
    ① A rectal incision and a ureteral catheter
    ② A ureterostomy with gravity drainage
    ③ A nephrostomy tube with tidal drainage
    ④ An abdominal incision and a cystostomy tube

352. The most significant complication immediately after this surgery is:
    ① Hemorrhage
    ② Impotence
    ③ Urinary incontinence
    ④ Spasms

353. Mr. Burn has just returned from the recovery room after the suprapubic prostatectomy. He accidently pulls out the urethral catheter. The nurse should:
    ① Check for bleeding by irrigating the suprapubic tube
    ② Reinsert a new catheter
    ③ Notify the physician immediately
    ④ Take no immediate action if the suprapubic tube is draining

354. In the postoperative care of Mr. Burn an important action to prevent secondary bladder infection is to:
    ① Observe for signs of uremia
    ② Attach the catheter to suction
    ③ Clamp off the connecting tubing
    ④ Change the dressings frequently

355. Mr. Burn complains of pain in the area operated upon. The initial response of the nurse should be to:
    ① Administer the prescribed analgesic
    ② Measure and record the vital signs before administering an analgesic
    ③ Inspect the drainage tubing for occlusion
    ④ Encourage intake of fluids to dilute urine

356. After a prostatectomy the nurse should:
    ① Have the client stand to void
    ② Aspirate the catheter with a bulb syringe
    ③ Discourage straining for a bowel movement
    ④ Notify the physician if the client does not void in 12 hours

Situation: Baby boy Charles Brown, 7 days old, is admitted to the pediatric unit from the nursery with a diagnosis of Down syndrome.

357. In caring for Charles, the nurse recognizes that he will have:
① A developmental lag after 1 or 2 years of age
② High incidence of circulatory problems
③ Proneness to respiratory tract infections
④ Difficulty in hearing

358. The symptom of Down syndrome most evident to the nursery nurse during the initial newborn assessment would be:
① Asymmetric gluteal folds
② Hypertonicity of the skeletal muscles
③ A rounded occiput
④ A transverse palmar (simian) crease

359. Special nursing care for Baby Brown should include:
① Frequent handling and rocking to keep him from crying
② Helping the parents learn about their child
③ Teaching infant to nipple-feed
④ Preventing aspiration of formula by frequent bubbling

360. When observing a newborn with Down syndrome, the nurse should be aware that a common defect associated with the condition is:
① Deafness
② Congenital heart defect
③ Hydrocephaly
④ Muscular hypertonicity

361. The factor that would probably be most significant for the nurse working with the Brown family is their:
① Response to family's and friends' reactions to their infant
② Ability to give physical care to their infant
③ Ability to talk about changing plans they had made for their infant
④ Understanding of the factors causing Down syndrome

362. As Charles grows, his development lags and it is found that he is moderately retarded. The suggestion that would be most helpful to his parents is that they should:
① Offer challenging, competitive situations
② Offer simple, repetitive tasks
③ Concentrate on teaching detailed tasks
④ Offer complete directions at the beginning of the task to be accomplished

363. The handicapped child has the same needs as the normal child, although his or her means of satisfying these needs are limited. This limitation frequently causes:
① Emotional disability
② Overcompensation
③ Frustration
④ Rejection

Situation: Mr. and Mrs. Halloway are expecting their first child after 10 years of marriage. In the thirty-eighth week of pregnancy Mrs. Halloway is scheduled for a nonstress test.

364. Mrs. Halloway asks if the nurse thinks the nonstress test is necessary. The nurse's best reply would be:
① "Certainly; you have had problems and we want to reduce the risks."
② "Your physician feels it is necessary so I think you should have it done."
③ "You still have doubts about this test, don't you?"
④ "It is a fast procedure and totally harmless."

365. Two weeks later Mrs. Halloway is admitted to the labor and delivery unit in active labor. When assessing her, the nurse recognizes true labor by the occurrence of:
① Regular contractions
② Cervical dilation
③ Leakage of fluid from the vagina
④ Rectal pressure

366. Mrs. Halloway's labor progresses, and she complains of low back pain. To increase comfort the nurse should recommend that Mr. Halloway:
① Place her in the supine position
② Instruct her to flex her knees
③ Apply back pressure during contractions
④ Help her perform neuromuscular control exercises

367. The nurse withholds food and limits fluids as the second stage approaches because:
① The mechanical and chemical digestive process requires energy that is needed for labor
② Undigested food and fluid may cause nausea and vomiting and limit the choice of anesthesia
③ Food will further aggravate gastric peristalsis, which is already increased due to the tension of labor
④ The gastric phase of digestion stimulates the release of hydrochloric acid and may cause dyspepsia

368. Mrs. Halloway delivers a 2721.6 g (6 lb) baby girl. As part of the physical assessment of this baby the nurse observes for the presence of an umbilical hernia. This assessment can best be accomplished when the baby is:
① Crying
② Sucking
③ Inhaling
④ Sleeping

Situation: Mrs. Johnson, a 47-year-old obese housewife, is admitted to the hospital with a diagnosis of Ménière's disease.

369. When assessing Mrs. Johnson during an attack, the nurse should expect her to experience:
① Nystagmus
② An increase in temperature
③ Diarrhea
④ A decrease in pulse rate

370. To control the disease, Mrs. Johnson is given a salt-restricted diet to reduce endolymphatic fluid. When discussing her diet with the nurse, she states that she has four favorite foods. After reviewing her list the nurse tells her she may still eat:
① Baked clams
② Grilled cheese
③ Carrot cake
④ Macaroni

371. When discussing weight loss with Mrs. Johnson, it would be most therapeutic if the nurse suggested that she:
    ① Get involved in diversionary activities when there is an urge to eat
    ② Enroll in an exercise class at the local high school
    ③ Limit intake to 900 calories a day
    ④ Keep a diary of all foods eaten each day, making certain to list everything

Situation: Mrs. Bartin, 46 years old, has a history of alcohol abuse. She is admitted to an alcohol rehabilitation center, where she is being detoxified.

372. A nursing assessment of Mrs. Bartin would probably reveal:
    ① Nausea, hypertension, and loss of appetite
    ② Hypotension and agitation
    ③ Hypertension, bradycardia, and hyperactivity
    ④ Lethargy and hypotension

373. In the initial interview with Mrs. Bartin the nurse should plan to include:
    ① An explanation of the unit's routines
    ② An explanation of the client's role on the unit
    ③ A complete list of the unit's rules and regulations
    ④ A description of acceptable behavior on the unit

374. Mrs. Bartin should be assigned to a:
    ① Room that is well lit and away from the areas of activity
    ② Room without windows and close to the nurse's station
    ③ Room with adequate lighting from the corridor
    ④ Room with dim lights shared by a quiet, withdrawn client

375. The plan that would best gain Mrs. Bartin's involvement in her own hygienic care would include:
    ① Giving her a schedule and requiring her to bathe and dress herself each morning
    ② Drawing up a schedule with her and making certain that she adheres to it
    ③ Bathing and dressing her each morning until she is willing to do it for herself
    ④ Assisting her in bathing and dressing by giving her clear, simple directions

COMPREHENSIVE TEST 2: PART 1

To simulate the National Council Licensure Examination, this test should be completed within 1½ hours.

Situation: Mrs. Dane, a gravida II para I, is admitted to the labor unit by ambulance, and delivery is imminent. She keeps bearing down, and after two contractions the baby's head is crowning.

1. The nurse should:
   1. Tell her to breathe through her mouth and pant during contractions
   2. Tell her to breathe through her mouth and not to bear down
   3. Transfer her immediately by stretcher to the delivery room
   4. Tell her to pant while supporting the perineum with her hand to prevent tearing

2. With the next contraction Mrs. Dane delivers a large baby boy spontaneously. The nurse's initial action should be to:
   1. Ascertain the condition of the fundus
   2. Establish an airway for the baby
   3. Quickly tie and cut the umbilical cord
   4. Move mother and baby to delivery room

3. The physician arrives and cares for the baby and delivers the placenta. Pitocin, an oxytocic, is administered intramuscularly. Since Mrs. Dane has had a precipitous delivery, it is important to observe for:
   1. Bleeding and infection
   2. Sudden chilling
   3. Elevation in blood pressure
   4. Respiratory insufficiency in the baby

4. If involution is progressing normally, immediately after birth the nurse should expect the fundus to be located:
   1. Three centimeters above the umbilicus
   2. At the level of the umbilicus
   3. Two centimeters below the umbilicus
   4. Two centimeters above the symphysis pubis

Situation: Mrs. Penny has delivered a 3005 g (6 lb 10 oz) baby boy. The newborn infant is taken from the delivery room to the nursery, where it is the policy for the nurse to appraise the infant.

5. During the examination the nurse notes that the temperature, pulse, and respiration are in normal range. Other physical characteristics are also normal. The nurse records all observations on the baby's chart. Which of the following statements is correct?
   1. The nurse was making a medical diagnosis
   2. Only the physician should determine the infant's physical status
   3. According to the Nurse Practice Act the nurse performed correctly
   4. Assessment by the nurse is not equivalent to the physician's assessment

6. Mr. and Mrs. Penny name their baby Andrew. At 10 hours of life he has a large amount of mucus and becomes slightly cyanotic. The nurse should:
   1. Give the infant oxygen
   2. Insert a Levin tube
   3. Note the incident on the chart
   4. Suction the mucus as needed

7. Baby Andrew must be observed carefully for the first 24 hours, particularly for:
   1. Respiratory distress
   2. Change in body temperature
   3. Frequency in voiding
   4. Duration of cry

8. When Andrew's mother removes his blanket and starts to examine her infant, she becomes concerned because he assumes a fencing position as she turns his head; the mother suspects neurologic damage. The nurse discusses with the mother that:
   1. This is a normal response
   2. The physician had been notified of this suspicious response
   3. This reflex disappears around 2 months of age
   4. Tonic neck reflex may indicate neurologic damage in the newborn

9. Supportive nursing care in the beginning mother-infant relationship should include:
   1. Encouraging Mrs. Penny to decide between breast-feeding and bottle-feeding
   2. Allowing Mrs. Penny ample time to inspect the baby
   3. Requiring Mrs. Penny to assist with simple aspects of infant's care
   4. Unobtrusive observation to pick up disturbed mother-infant relationship

Situation: Thomas James, 1 month old, has been vomiting for 1 week. His mother explains that the vomiting has been progressively more forceful and contains undigested formula. Presently he is dehydrated and has abdominal distention. A tentative diagnosis of pyloric stenosis has been made.

10. Vomiting caused by pyloric stenosis is usually not bile stained because:
    1. The obstruction is above the opening of the common bile duct
    2. The bile duct is also obstructed
    3. The obstruction of the cardiac sphincter prevents bile from entering the esophagus
    4. The sphincter of the bile duct is connected to the hypertrophied pyloric muscle

11. While doing the physical assessment of Thomas, the nurse should particularly observe for visible peristaltic waves and:
    1. An olive-shaped mass in the right upper quadrant
    2. Decreased bowel sounds
    3. Severe cramping movements in the lower intestine
    4. A boardlike abdomen

12. The physician orders a gavage tube for Thomas. To determine the distance needed to advance the gavage tube the nurse should:
    1. Advance the tube until resistance is met
    2. Measure the distance from the nose to the earlobe to the epigastric area of the abdomen
    3. Measure from the mouth to the umbilicus and add half the distance
    4. Advance the tube as far as necessary to aspirate gastric contents

13. During insertion of the tube, the nurse would evaluate that Thomas was experiencing difficulty if he demonstrated:
    ① Choking
    ② Cyanosis
    ③ Flushing
    ④ Gagging

14. A Fredet-Ramstedt procedure is performed and, postoperatively, the nurse instructs Mrs. James regarding proper feeding techniques, such as:
    ① Feed the child in the semi-Fowler's position and then afterward place prone
    ② Rock the child after feedings to reduce crying and ingestion of air
    ③ Feed the child in the supine position to reduce pressure on the sutures
    ④ Feed the child in an upright position and then place on the right side with the head slightly elevated

15. Five months after his discharge, Mrs. James brings Thomas into the pediatric clinic and asks about the introduction of new foods. The nurse suggests:
    ① "Mix the puréed food with the formula and give through the bottle to help him learn new tastes."
    ② "Offer a new food every day until he likes one."
    ③ "Offer a new food after he has had some milk when he is still hungry."
    ④ "Offer a new food after he has had his regular feeding."

16. Mrs. James also asks about what foods she should begin to introduce. A likely choice would be to start with:
    ① Rice cereal and fruit, then add egg yolk
    ② Cereal, and add a soft-boiled egg for breakfast
    ③ Fruit first, then add meat and vegetables
    ④ Sweets, such as fruits and puddings

Situation: Mrs. Mager has become increasingly anxious and tense over the last few months. She visits her physician and after examination is admitted to the hospital with a tentative diagnosis of hyperthyroidism.

17. Because of her diagnosis, the nurse should expect Mrs. Mager to exhibit:
    ① Nervousness, weight loss, increased appetite
    ② Protruding eyeballs, slow pulse, sluggishness
    ③ Increased appetite, slow pulse, dry skin
    ④ Loss of weight, constipation, listlessness

18. When teaching Mrs. Mager about the diagnostic tests to be done, the nurse should include:
    ① Radioactive iodine uptake and T_3
    ② Protein-bound iodine and SMA 12
    ③ T_4 and x-ray films
    ④ Basal metabolic rate and Po_2

19. The major nursing problem in caring for Mrs. Mager would be:
    ① Providing an adequate diet
    ② Keeping the bed linen neat
    ③ Providing sufficient rest
    ④ Modifying hospital routines

20. The purpose of propylthiouracil, which was ordered for Mrs. Mager, is to:
    ① Interfere with the synthesis of thyroid hormone
    ② Produce atrophy of the thyroid gland
    ③ Increase the uptake of iodine
    ④ Decrease the secretion of thyroid-stimulating hormone

21. The physician decides that Mrs. Mager should have a subtotal thyroidectomy. In preparation for surgery, Lugol's Iodine Solution is ordered. This medication is given to:
    ① Maintain the function of the parathyroid glands
    ② Decrease the total basal metabolic rate
    ③ Block the formation of thyroxine by the thyroid gland
    ④ Decrease the size and vascularity of the thyroid gland

22. Mrs. Mager is concerned that the thyroidectomy will interfere with her ability to become pregnant. In replying the nurse bases the response on the following information:
    ① As long as medication is taken as ordered, ovulation will occur
    ② Pregnancy is not advisable for the client with a thyroidectomy
    ③ Hyperthyroidism can cause abortions or fetal anomalies
    ④ Pregnancy will affect metabolism and will require greatly increased thyroid hormone

23. When Mrs. Mager returns to her room after surgery, the nurse should immediately:
    ① Instruct her not to speak
    ② Inspect the incision
    ③ Keep her flat in bed for 24 hours
    ④ Place a tracheostomy set at the bedside

24. Postoperatively the nurse should carefully observe Mrs. Mager for signs of thyroid storm. These include:
    ① Hypothermia
    ② Elevated serum calcium
    ③ Rapid heart action and tremors
    ④ Sudden drop in pulse rate

25. Thyroid storm is caused by:
    ① Removal of the parathyroid gland
    ② Increased amount of thyroid hormone in the blood
    ③ Increased iodine in the blood
    ④ A rebound increase in metabolism following anesthesia

Situation: May Ann Lewis, age 18, is admitted to the mental health unit of the general hospital. She has always been a shy, introverted person, but within the past few days she has retreated into a world of fantasy. She makes up her own vocabulary and talks to an imaginary person. She has taken to wearing several sets of clothing at the same time and has made up her face like a clown. The day of admission she retreats to her room, telling the family that she is wired to the television, which informed her that the family was out to kill her.

26. The initial action by the admitting nurse that would be most therapeutic for May Ann is:
    ① Taking her to the day room and introducing her to the other clients
    ② Telling her that the door is locked and no one can harm her here
    ③ Reassuring her that she will not be frightened here, away from her family
    ④ Introducing her to the primary nurse who will be working with her

27. When May Ann says, "My lacket hss kelong mon," the nurse should respond by:
    1. Trying to learn the language of the client
    2. Telling the client she is not understood
    3. Communicating in simple terms directed toward the client
    4. Recognizing that she needs a nurse who can understand her fantasies

28. May Ann, unprovoked, attacks another client. A short-term plan for her would be to:
    1. Protect others from her impulsive acts by secluding her
    2. Keep her actively participating and in contact with reality
    3. Have a staff member whom she trusts stay with her
    4. Get May Ann to apologize for her behavior

29. May Ann tells the nurse the voices have told her she is no good. She asks if the nurse heard the voices. The most appropriate response would be:
    1. "No, I do not hear your voices, but I believe you can hear them."
    2. "The voices are coming from within you and only you can hear them."
    3. "It is the voice of your conscience, which only you can control."
    4. "Oh, the voices are a symptom of your illness; don't pay attention to them."

30. May Ann holds herself aloof; she ridicules and is sarcastic to other clients. She identifies with the staff. The nursing care plan at this time should be to:
    1. Assign activities with the staff only
    2. Accept the negative emotions; praise the positive ones
    3. Explain that she should be more accepting of others
    4. Encourage group participation with withdrawn clients

31. The physician has ordered chlorpromazine (Thorazine), 300 mg po tid. To alleviate the side effects May Ann might experience the first week she takes the drug the nurse should:
    1. Have her increase her fluid intake
    2. Take her BP before giving the drug
    3. Give her coffee with the medication and meals
    4. Give her benztropine (Cogentin) with the medication

32. The major reason for treating severe emotional disorders with tranquilizers is to:
    1. Make the client more amenable to psychotherapy
    2. Prevent destructiveness by the client
    3. Reduce the neurotic symptoms
    4. Prevent secondary complications

33. May Ann is much improved and, with a group of other clients, is preparing for a social evening in town. They are to go with a staff member. The purpose of visits into the community under the supervision of a professional is to:
    1. Assist clients in adjusting to anxieties in the community
    2. Observe a client's ability to cope with a more complex society

    3. Help the clients return to reality under controlled conditions
    4. Broaden the client's experiences by providing exposure to cultural activities

Situation: Mrs. Hinch, age 20, is 37 weeks pregnant. She is admitted to the hospital with preeclampsia and sudden abdominal pain.

34. On Mrs. Hinch's admission to the unit the nurse should observe for:
    1. Decrease in size of uterus, cessation of contractions, visible or concealed hemorrhage
    2. Firm and tender uterus, concealed or external hemorrhage, shock
    3. Increase in size of uterus, visible bleeding, no associated pain
    4. Shock, decrease in size of uterus, absence of external bleeding

35. The nurse realizes that the abdominal pain associated with abruptio placentae is caused by:
    1. Hemorrhagic shock
    2. Inflammatory reactions
    3. Blood in the uterine muscle
    4. Concealed hemorrhage

36. Mrs. Hinch is given a unit of blood. The nurse realizes that this is necessary, since the bleeding following severe abruptio placentae is usually caused by:
    1. Hypofibrinogenemia
    2. Hyperglobulinemia
    3. Thrombocytopenia
    4. Polycythemia

37. Mrs. Hinch delivers a stillborn baby girl. To foster a healthy grieving response to the birth of a stillborn child, the nurse's best response to an expression of anger from Mrs. Hinch would be:
    1. "It's God's will; we have to have faith that it was for the best."
    2. "You are young; you'll have other children."
    3. "This often happens when something is wrong with the baby."
    4. "You may be wondering if something you did caused this."

Situation: Two-year-old Tommy is brought to the pediatric clinic. His mother states he has been irritable and that she noticed swollen glands on the left side of his neck. After examination a diagnosis of otitis media is made and analgesic eardrops ordered.

38. To teach the correct way to administer eardrops to a small child, the nurse should instruct the parent to position the child on the right side and instill the drops while pulling the auricle:
    1. Straight back
    2. Up and back
    3. Forward
    4. Down and back

39. Physiologically the middle ear (containing the three ossicles) serves primarily to:
    1. Communicate with the throat via the eustachian tube
    2. Amplify the energy of sound waves entering the ear
    3. Translate sound waves into nerve impulses
    4. Maintain balance

40. Tommy's condition does not improve, and he is admitted for a myringotomy. Postoperatively the nurse would expect Tommy to have:
    ① Symptoms of CNS irritation
    ② Difficulty voiding and slight hematuria
    ③ Irrigations to the lacrimal glands
    ④ Purulent drainage into the external auditory canal

41. When Tommy is ill and has temporary dietary restrictions, the best way for the nurse to avoid any future feeding problems is to have the restrictions:
    ① Limited to foods that are not essential
    ② Administered by someone other than parents
    ③ Explained to the child by the dietitian
    ④ Handled in a matter-of-fact way

42. Before discharge, while his mother is talking to the nurse about his care at home, Tommy joins the other children in the playroom. The nurse would expect him to engage in:
    ① Parallel play
    ② Competitive play
    ③ Solitary play
    ④ Tumbling-type play

43. While successfully learning autonomy and independence, Tommy would be learning:
    ① Trust and security
    ② Roles within society
    ③ Superego control
    ④ To accept external limits

Situation: As a result of an industrial accident, Mr. Jones has suffered second-degree and third-degree burns on his left leg, left arm, and face.

44. Burns classified as third degree involve destruction of the:
    ① Epidermis layer
    ② Subcutaneous tissue
    ③ Corium
    ④ Fatty layer

45. The percent of Mr. Jones' total skin surface that has been burned is:
    ① 18%
    ② 27%
    ③ 36%
    ④ 45%

46. The major objective during the early postburn phase is to:
    ① Prevent infection
    ② Replace blood loss
    ③ Restore fluid volume
    ④ Relieve pain

47. One difficult problem for the nurse to deal with concerning a recently admitted burned client is:
    ① Severe pain
    ② Alteration in body image
    ③ Frequent dressing changes
    ④ Maintenance of sterility

48. In assessing Mr. Jones for respiratory involvement during the first 2 days after the accident, the nurse should observe for sputum that is:
    ① Frothy
    ② Sooty
    ③ Yellow
    ④ Tenacious

49. The nurse should assess for symptoms of hypovolemic shock, which is often associated with burns because of:
    ① Sodium retention as a result of the aldosterone mechanism
    ② Decreased rate of glomerular filtration
    ③ A shift of proteins and water out of intravascular compartment
    ④ Excessive blood loss through the burned tissues

50. An individual with serious burns requires frequent checks of potassium levels because:
    ① Damaged cells absorb potassium, causing hyperkalemia
    ② Burned individuals excrete excessive potassium, resulting in hypokalemia
    ③ Damaged cells release potassium, causing hyperkalemia
    ④ Potassium loss from damaged skin may cause hypokalemia

Situation: Mr. Smith, 55, has had difficulty sleeping and eating. He has lost a great deal of time from work because he "wasn't feeling well." Lately he has just sat in his room staring at the floor with a sad look on his face. His one wish is that he would die.

51. Mr. Smith is brought to the general hospital after taking an overdose of phenobarbital. After a lavage, Mr. Smith states, "Let me die, I'm no good." The nurse's most appropriate response would be:
    ① "Of course you're good, we'll take care of you."
    ② "You must have been upset to try to take your life."
    ③ "Do you feel like telling me why you did this?"
    ④ "You have been through a rough time; let me take care of you."

52. Mr. Smith has been placed on suicide precautions. A therapeutic community would provide these precautions by:
    ① Removing all "cutting" objects
    ② Not allowing him to leave his room
    ③ Giving him an opportunity to ventilate his feelings
    ④ Assigning a staff member to be with him at all times

53. Mr. Smith is to receive electroconvulsive therapy (ECT). The nurse, in explaining this procedure, should emphasize that:
    ① He will have amnesia afterward
    ② The treatments will make him better
    ③ Someone will be with him all the time
    ④ He should not be afraid; it will not hurt

54. One of the side effects of ECT that Mr. Smith may experience is:
    ① Loss of appetite
    ② Postural hypotension
    ③ Confusion for a time after treatment
    ④ Complete loss of memory for a time

55. Mr. Smith is given a muscle relaxant just before the ECT. The major disadvantage of this drug is that it inhibits the:
    ① Intercostal and diaphragmatic muscles
    ② Biceps and triceps muscles
    ③ Facial and thoracic muscles
    ④ Sternocleidomastoid and abdominal muscles

56. The aspect of ECT that can result in the most serious complication is the use of:
    ① Thiopental sodium (Pentothal) to induce sleep
    ② Succinylcholine chloride to relax muscles
    ③ Positive pressure to inflate the alveoli
    ④ Electric voltage to induce convulsions

57. The staff set specific goals directed toward helping the client:
    ① Develop trust in others
    ② Express his hostile feelings
    ③ Set realistic life goals
    ④ Get involved in activities

58. The least helpful activity for a severely depressed client such as Mr. Smith would be:
    ① Allowing the client to plan his own projects
    ② Specific simple instructions to be followed
    ③ Simple, easily completed short-term projects
    ④ Monotonous, repetitive projects and activities

Situation: Mr. Sill, age 45, who has smoked three to four packs of cigarettes per day for the last 25 years, was treated with irradiation of his larynx 3 months ago for squamous cell carcinoma. For the past 2 weeks he has noted recurrent hoarseness that has progressively worsened. He now enters the hospital for evaluation and further therapy. Except for findings of hoarseness and a small mass in the left vocal cord, the remainder of his physical examination is unremarkable. Total laryngectomy with block dissection of the cervical lymph nodes is performed after appropriate diagnostic studies and preparation for surgery have been carried out.

59. An important aspect of preoperative nursing care includes:
    ① Adequate explanation of the nature of the surgery to be performed
    ② Instruction in breathing exercises and/or equipment used postoperatively to prevent complications
    ③ Basing instruction on those areas which Mr. Sill questions
    ④ Having a speech therapist visit Mr. Sill

60. The factor that would have little influence in predisposing an individual to cancer of the larynx would be:
    ① Heavy alcohol ingestion
    ② Poor dental hygiene
    ③ Air pollution
    ④ Chronic respiratory infections

61. Immediate postoperative management for Mr. Sill would include:
    ① Placing him in the orthopneic position
    ② Removing the outer tracheostomy tube prn
    ③ Suctioning the tracheostomy tube at least every 10 or 15 minutes
    ④ Instructing him to whisper

62. Mr. Sill's initial feedings are by nasogastric tube. Soon afterward he begins to develop diarrhea. A possible solution to this problem would be to:
    ① Increase the carbohydrate content of the formula to give it more energy value
    ② Decrease the protein content to make it easier to digest
    ③ Dilute the formula with water to give it more volume
    ④ Decrease the carbohydrate content of the formula and give it more slowly

63. Mr. Sill asks how long he will have to be fed through a tube. The nurse should explain that nasogastric feedings will be required:
    ① For the rest of his life
    ② Until healing has occurred
    ③ Until Mr. Sill develops the ability to belch
    ④ Until Mr. Sill can digest oral feedings

64. On the day Mr. Sill is being discharged he exhibits concern about the possibility that his laryngectomy tube might become dislodged. The nurse should teach him to:
    ① Notify the physician at once
    ② Keep calm, since there is no immediate emergency
    ③ Recognize that prompt closure of the tracheal opening may occur
    ④ Reinsert another tube immediately

65. Since Mr. Sill's tracheostomy is permanent, the nurse should include in the teaching plan:
    ① The sterile technique necessary for care of his tracheostomy tube
    ② The establishment of a regular pattern for suctioning the tube
    ③ The importance of cleanliness around the site
    ④ The importance of covering the tube opening while bathing and swimming

Situation: Mr. Leonard is an alcoholic and has cirrhosis of the liver.

66. Mr. Leonard is brought to the emergency room in the midst of protracted clonic convulsions. He is given diazepam (Valium), which decreases central neuronal activity and:
    ① Dilates the tracheobronchial structures
    ② Relaxes peripheral muscles
    ③ Slows cardiac contractions
    ④ Provides amnesia for the convulsive episode

67. Mr. Leonard's serum albumin level is low, and the physician prescribes 50 ml of salt-poor albumin IV. Albumin replacement is expected to:
    ① Decrease tissue fluid accumulation and the hematocrit level
    ② Decrease ascites and the blood ammonia level
    ③ Decrease capillary perfusion and BP
    ④ Decrease venous stasis and the blood urea nitrogen level

68. While Mr. Leonard is receiving the albumin, the planned therapeutic effect will be greater if the infusion is regulated to run:
    ① Slowly, and fluid intake is restricted
    ② Rapidly, and fluids are encouraged
    ③ Slowly, and fluids are encouraged liberally
    ④ Rapidly, and fluid intake is withheld

69. Mr. Leonard is having delirium tremens and is given paraldehyde (Paral) IM. Elimination of the drug can be assessed by monitoring:
    ① Urination
    ② Salivation
    ③ Diaphoresis
    ④ Breathing

70. Mr. Leonard is receiving neomycin sulfate (Mycifradin) orally. The purpose for administration of the drug is to:
    ① Protect against infection while immune mechanisms are deficient
    ② Suppress ammonia-forming bacteria in the intestinal tract
    ③ Increase urea digestive activity of enteric bacteria
    ④ Protect regenerative nodules in the liver from invading bacteria

71. Immediately before an abdominal paracentesis, the nurse should ask the client to void because:
    ① A urine specimen must be obtained at this time to check level of nonprotein nitrogen
    ② A full bladder increases the danger of puncture of the bladder
    ③ An empty bladder will decrease the intraabdominal pressure
    ④ A full bladder decreases the amount of fluid in the abdominal cavity

72. Mr. Leonard, participating in an alcohol abstinence program, has a cold when he comes to the clinic. He tells the nurse he plans to use elixir of terpin hydrate for his cough. The nurse would advise him not to take it while he is taking disulfiram (Antabuse) because it will cause:
    ① Abdominal cramps and muscle twitching
    ② Epigastric pain and headache
    ③ Jitteriness and nausea
    ④ Dizziness and violent vomiting

Situation: Jane Bond, a 15-year-old girl, is brought into the emergency room after being found unconscious in the locker room at school. There is a strong odor of acetone to her breath and her face is flushed.

73. After developing a relationship with the nurse, Jane admits that she has not been adhering to her diabetic regimen. As a first step in attempting to help Jane develop some understanding of the importance of a diabetic regimen, the nurse should:
    ① Give her printed material about diabetes in teenagers
    ② Impress on the parents that it is their responsibility to help and understand Jane
    ③ Allow Jane to express her feelings about diabetes
    ④ Assume that Jane has not been properly taught previously

74. When teaching Jane about diabetes and self-administration of insulin, the first step for the nurse should be to:
    ① Begin the teaching program at Jane's present level
    ② Find out what Jane knows about her health problem
    ③ Set specific and realistic short- and long-term goals
    ④ Collect all the equipment needed to demonstrate giving an injection

75. Jane exhibits a need for cognitive learning when she asks:
    ① "What is diabetes?"
    ② "How do I give myself an injection?"
    ③ "When do I test my urine for S and A?"
    ④ "Can I still be a cheerleader?"

76. After initial treatment to correct the acidosis, Jane is moved to the medical ward. Her height and weight are average—5 feet 3 inches, 114 pounds (160 cm tall, 51.8 kg)—and the diet ordered for her is 2200 calories, 75 g protein, 250 g carbohydrate, and 100 g fat. She is receiving NPH insulin mixed with regular insulin, according to need. In planning a menu for a juvenile diabetic such as Jane, the nurse considers a meal pattern that:
    ① Limits calories to encourage weight loss
    ② Allows for normal growth and developmental needs
    ③ Avoids using potatoes, bread, and cereal
    ④ Discourages substitutions on the menu pattern

77. The nurse instructs Jane and her parents to:
    ① Weigh all her food on a gram scale
    ② Eat all her meals at home
    ③ Prepare her food separately from that of the rest of the family
    ④ Always carry some form of sugar with her

78. The nurse plans an evening snack for Jane including milk, crackers, and cheese to provide:
    ① High-carbohydrate nourishment for immediate use
    ② Nourishment with latent effects to counteract late insulin activity
    ③ Encouragement for her to stay on her diet
    ④ Added calories to help her gain weight

79. A week after the nurse speaks with Jane, Mrs. Bond, whose sister died of diabetes, asks the nurse for information about her daughter's disease. The nurse should recognize that Mrs. Bond is:
    ① Too upset to learn new information
    ② Transferring attitudes about her sister to her daughter
    ③ Exhibiting readiness for learning
    ④ Expressing her attitudes through her behavior

Situation: Mrs. Rule, gravida II, para I, is admitted to the delivery room in active labor. She delivers a healthy baby girl and would like to breast-feed her infant.

80. Mrs. Rule has some doubts as to whether she will be successful breast-feeding, since her breasts are small. Concerning Mrs. Rule's statement about the size of her breasts, the nurse's best response would be:
    ① "The size of your breasts has nothing to do with the production of milk."
    ② "The amount of fat and glandular tissue in the breasts determines the amount of milk produced."
    ③ "You seem to have some concern about breast-feeding."
    ④ "Everybody can be successful at breast-feeding."

81. It is now 2 days postpartum and Mrs. Rule asks the nurse about cleansing her nipples. The nurse's best response would be:
    ① "Thoroughly scrub the nipples with soap and water before each feeding."
    ② "Cleanse the nipples with sterile water before each feeding."
    ③ "Cleanse the nipples with an alcohol sponge before and after each feeding."
    ④ "Wash the breasts and nipples daily with water."

82. On the third day following delivery Mrs. Rule states that she has a great deal of pain in her breasts and that she is afraid that the baby will hurt her when she tries to grasp the nipple. The most appropriate action for the nurse to take is to explain the reasons for the client's discomfort and to:
    ① Call the physician to obtain advice
    ② Administer a medication for pain
    ③ Express some of the milk manually before putting the baby to breast
    ④ Suggest that she limit fluids and not try to nurse the baby for the next 2 days

83. Mrs. Rule is concerned because she heard that her neighbor's breasts suddenly dried up when she got home and she had to discontinue nursing. An appropriate comment for the nurse to make is:
    ① "This commonly happens with the excitement of going home. Putting the baby to breast more frequently will reestablish lactation."
    ② "This commonly happens; however, we will give you a formula to take home so the baby won't go hungry until your milk supply returns."
    ③ "This is not true; once lactation is established, this rarely happens."
    ④ "You have little to worry about, since you already have a good milk supply."

84. Mrs. Rule has heard of demand feeding and wonders how anyone ever finds time to do anyting but feed the baby. The nurse's best response would be:
    ① "Most mothers find babies on breast do better on demand feeding, since the amount of milk ingested varies at each feeding."
    ② "Perhaps a schedule might be better, since the baby is already accustomed to hospital routine."
    ③ "Although the baby is on demand feedings, she will eventually set her own schedule, so there will be time for your household chores."
    ④ "Most mothers find that feeding the baby whenever she cries works out fine."

85. Mrs. Rule wants to know whether it is true that she will not have to use contraceptives while nursing. The nurse's most appropriate response should be:
    ① "Since lactation suppresses ovulation, you probably don't have to worry about becoming pregnant."
    ② "As long as you have no mentrual period, you won't have to worry about using contraceptives."
    ③ "It is best to use contraceptive measures, since ovulation may occur without a menstrual period."
    ④ "It is best to delay any sexual relations until you have your first menstrual period."

Situation: Mr. Gold, a 42-year-old insurance broker, is admitted to the hospital with a diagnosis of coronary occlusion and is experiencing pain and distress.

86. The nurse realizes that the pain associated with coronary occlusion is caused primarily by:
    ① Arterial spasm
    ② Irritation of nerve endings in the cardiac plexus
    ③ Ischemia of the heart muscle
    ④ Blocking of the coronary veins

87. On Mr. Gold's admission the nurse immediately gives him oxygen to:

① Prevent dyspnea
② Prevent cyanosis
③ Increase oxygen concentration to heart cells
④ Increase oxygen tension in the circulating blood

88. During the acute period of Mr. Gold's illness the nurse should make the bed by:
    ① Changing the top linen and only the necessary bottom linen
    ② Changing the linen from top to bottom without lowering the head of the bed
    ③ Sliding him onto a stretcher, remaking the bed, then sliding him back to the bed
    ④ Lifting rather than rolling him from side to side while changing the linen

89. Mr. Gold's orders include strict bed rest and a clear liquid diet. The nurse should explain that the primary reason for this diet is to reduce:
    ① Gastric acidity
    ② The metabolic work load of digestion
    ③ His weight
    ④ The amount of fecal elimination

90. Two days after admission Mr. Gold's temperature rises to 38.3° C (101° F). The nurse should realize that this elevation indicates:
    ① Possible infection
    ② Tissue necrosis
    ③ Pulmonary infarction
    ④ Pneumonia

91. In creating a therapeutic environment for Mr. Gold the nurse should provide for:
    ① Daily papers in the morning
    ② Telephone communication
    ③ Short family visits
    ④ Television for short periods

92. The monitor shows a PQRST wave for each beat and indicates a rate of 120. The rhythm is regular. The nurse should note that the client is experiencing:
    ① Atrial fibrillation
    ② Ventricular fibrillation
    ③ Sinus tachycardia
    ④ First-degree heart block

93. Mr. Gold complains of severe nausea, and his heart beat is irregular and slow. The nurse should recognize these symptoms as toxic effects of:
    ① Lanoxin
    ② Lidocaine
    ③ Morphine sulfate
    ④ Meperidine hydrochloride

COMPREHENSIVE TEST 2: PART 2

To simulate the National Council Licensure Examination, this test should be completed within 1½ hours.

Situation: Mr. Wilson, a 57-year-old man with a history of myocardial infarction, is admitted to the hospital for a hemorrhoidectomy.

94. The nurse should expect Mr. Wilson's preoperative diet to be:

① High protein
② Low residue
③ Bland
④ Clear liquid

95. Mr. Wilson is in pain on the second postoperative day. A method usually ordered to relieve pain, which the nurse uses, is:
① A medicated suppository
② Water-soluble jelly
③ Sitz baths
④ Ice packs

96. Mr. Wilson is having his first postoperative bowel movement. When cleaning the anus, Mr. Wilson should be instructed to use:
① Moist cotton balls
② Betadine pads
③ Sterile 4- × 4-inch gauze pads
④ Soft facial tissue

Situation: Roy Brown, an 18-month-old boy, is admitted to the hospital with an immunodeficiency syndrome. It is his first hospitalization and prolonged separation from his mother.

97. Based on this information, the nurse, during the initial admission, would expect him to:
① Cry when people enter the room, but respond with a smile after a few minutes
② Cry relentlessly and be consoled by no one except his mother or father
③ Withdraw, sit quietly, and not be interested in playing
④ Initially be unhappy and cry, but become contented after meeting his roommates

98. After a prolonged period of hospitalization, Roy becomes depressed, withdrawn, and apathetic toward his mother. Eventually, he begins playing with toys and relating to others, even strangers. The nurse should realize that he has:
① Accepted his hospitalization well and has matured because of his experience
② Grown out of the stage of separation and realizes that he has to depend on others
③ Probably become somewhat detached because of this traumatic separation
④ Finally recognized that the staff is not out to hurt him

99. Studies of young children institutionalized for some time indicate that they show signs of retarded development. Least affected by this type retardation is the child's:
① Neuromuscular development
② Sense of hearing
③ Ability to understand
④ Ability for self-expression

100. The major depriving factor in long-term hospitalization of which the nurse should be aware is usually the:
① Absence of interaction with a mother figure
② Lack of multisensory inputs
③ Care provided only by a mother substitute
④ Lack of play objects

101. The nurse should be aware that histories of children who have suffered prolonged maternal deprivation early in life indicate that these children:
① Are unable to love
② Establish warm relationships with a mother substitute
③ Recall past experiences vividly
④ Are particularly conscious of time

102. When Roy's mother is getting ready to take him home, she asks the nurse what kind of behavior she should expect Roy to display. The nurse informs her that Roy will probably be:
① Hostile toward her
② Making excessive demands on both parents
③ Cheerful but have a shallow attachment to all adults
④ Apathetic and withdrawn from all emotional ties to her

Situation: John and Mary June are a young married couple. John is the first of his family to attend college. Mary is supporting the family by working as a keypunch operator at a large insurance company. They have decided to postpone starting a family until John finishes his education in 2 years. Mary has therefore been taking oral contraceptives since shortly before the marriage. She has always had a regular menstrual cycle. Understandably then she is concerned when she misses her regular menstrual period. After 3 weeks pass she decides to go to a physician for a check-up. She tells the nurse interviewing her that she suspected she might be pregnant because she missed taking her contraceptive pills for more than a week when she had the flu.

103. Concerning the client's statement about her possible pregnancy, the best response by the nurse would be:
① "Contraceptive pills are very unpredictable anyhow. You probably would have become pregnant even if you had taken them regularly as prescribed."
② "You may well be correct; one of the reasons for prescribing an exact schedule is that the effect of contraceptive drugs depends on the regularity with which they are taken."
③ "Don't think about that now. It's too late to worry anyhow. First find out whether you really are pregnant. If you are, you may want to consider having an abortion."
④ "That's the trouble with using contraceptive pills. People become too careless and don't use proper restraint. If you had used the rhythm method, this probably would not have happened."

104. While Mrs. June is being prepared for the examination, she complains of feeling very tired and being sick to her stomach, particularly in the morning. The best response by the nurse would be:
① "This is a common occurrence during the early part of pregnancy and you need not worry."
② "This is a common occurrence due to all the changes going on in your body."
③ "These are common occurrences. You say your sick feelings bother you most often in the morning?"
④ "Perhaps you might discuss this with the doctor when he arrives."

105. Mrs. June asks, "Is it true the doctor will do an internal examination today?" The nurse should respond:
    ① "Yes, an internal is done on all mothers on the first visit."
    ② "Yes, an internal is done on all mothers, but it is only slightly uncomfortable."
    ③ "Are you fearful of having an internal examination done?"
    ④ "Yes, he will; have you ever had an internal examination done before?"

106. Mrs. June asks when she may expect her baby. She states that her last menstrual period was April 14. Her expected date of delivery would be:
    ① December 21
    ② January 7
    ③ January 21
    ④ February 1

107. Mrs. June is concerned because she had read that nutrition during pregnancy is important for proper growth and development of the baby. She wants to know something about the foods she should be eating. The nurse should proceed by:
    ① Giving her a list of foods to refer to in planning meals
    ② Asking her what she usually eats at each meal
    ③ Emphasizing the importance of limiting salt and highly seasoned foods
    ④ Instructing her to continue eating a normal diet

108. Mrs. June's work as a keypunch operator would necessarily have implications for her plan of care during pregnancy. The nurse should recommend that Mrs. June:
    ① Ask for time in the morning and afternoon to elevate her legs
    ② Tell her employer she cannot work beyond the second trimester
    ③ Ask for time in the morning and afternoon to obtain nourishment
    ④ Try to walk about every few hours during the workday

109. Since Mrs. June is a primigravida, she should be told to come to the hospital when:
    ① Contractions are 2 to 3 minutes apart and she cannot walk about
    ② Contractions are 10 to 15 minutes apart
    ③ She has a bloody show and back pressure
    ④ Membranes rupture or contractions are 5 to 8 minutes apart

110. During a later visit the nurse asks Mrs. June if she would like to listen to her baby's heartbeat. She is delighted and after listening comments on how rapid it is. She appears frightened and asks if this is normal. The nurse should respond:
    ① "The baby's heart rate is usually twice the mother's pulse rate."
    ② "The baby's heartbeat is rapid to accommodate the nutritional needs."
    ③ "The baby's heart rate is normally rapid, so you needn't worry."
    ④ "It is far better that the heart rate is rapid; when it is slow, there is need to worry."

111. Mrs. June spontaneously delivers a 2953.6 g (6 lb 8 oz) baby daughter. Although Mr. June expresses delight, he appears anxious and tends to avoid physical contact with the baby. One evening he says to the nurse, "My wife seems so wrapped up with the baby, I hope she has time for me when she gets home." The nurse's best response would be:
    ① "Do you think your parents will be able to help out, Mr. June?"
    ② "I can understand your concern about the changes you'll have to make."
    ③ "You seem to feel you'll have to fend for yourself."
    ④ "You'll both be so busy you won't even miss her attention."

Situation: Mrs. O'Hanlon, a childless widow born in Ireland, is employed as a cook in the sandwich shop of the local department store. She has been an outpatient in the medical clinic for 6 months, under treatment for diabetes and hypertension. Her regimen includes tolbutamide (Orinase), a low-sodium, diabetic diet, and reserpine (Serpasil) bid. On the occasion of a regular visit her urine sample shows sugar 3+ and a trace of acetone.

112. The nurse interviewing Mrs. O'Hanlon would be most concerned to find out about any changes in her:
    ① Eating habits
    ② Blood pressure
    ③ Weight range
    ④ Serum glucose

113. In discussing the client's present metabolic state, the nurse should inform her that people taking oral antidiabetic agents:
    ① Should not work where food is readily accessible
    ② Consciously or unconsciously may tend to relax dietary rules
    ③ Are not as threatened by their disease as those taking insulin
    ④ Need not be concerned about serious complications

114. Mrs. O'Hanlon tells the nurse that she cannot eat big meals and prefers to snack throughout the day. The nurse should carefully explain that:
    ① Small, frequent meals are better for digestion
    ② Large meals can contribute to a weight problem
    ③ Salt and sugar restriction is her main concern
    ④ Regulated food intake is basic to her control

115. When promoting affective learning (developing attitudes), the nurse must first consider the influence of the:
    ① Client's personal resources
    ② Type of onset of the disease
    ③ Total stress of the situation
    ④ Client's past experiences

116. Mrs. O'Hanlon complains that she finds the low-salt food very tasteless. The nurse's best response would be:
    ① "Salt can be very harmful to your health."
    ② "I know how difficult it is for you."
    ③ "You miss your ham and cabbage?"
    ④ "Ask the doctor if you can splurge occasionally."

117. Mrs. O'Hanlon is scheduled to have a serum glucose test the following morning. To ensure accuracy in the result, the nurse should instruct her to:

① Take her regular dose of tolbutamide
② Abstain from food and fluid
③ Have clear fluids for breakfast
④ Eat her usual diet

118. Mrs. O'Hanlon has a cough. She tells the nurse that she takes Robitussin (glyceryl guaiacolate) cough syrup about every 2 hours when she has a cold. The nurse should tell her that she:
① May take the cough syrup if her urine test remains negative
② Must calculate the sugar in her daily carbohydrate allowance
③ Can substitute an elixir for the syrup
④ Can increase her fluid intake and humidify her bedroom to control the cough

119. Mrs. O'Hanlon complains of difficulty seeing at night. The nurse knows this frequently occurs in client's with diabetes because of:
① Poor glucose supply to rods and cones
② Lack of glucose in the retina
③ The effect of ketones on retinal metabolism
④ Atherosclerotic changes in blood vessels within the eyes

Situation: Mrs. Carroll is admitted to the hospital with a cerebral vascular accident. Three weeks later she still has left-sided paresis but is able to ambulate fairly well with a cane. She is very frustrated and angry because of her expressive aphasia.

120. The nurse anticipates Mrs. Carroll will have difficulty with:
① Following specific instructions
② Recognizing words for familiar objects
③ Speaking and/or writing
④ Understanding speech and/or writing

121. Mrs. Carroll gets frustrated and upset when she tries to communicate with the nurse. To help alleviate this frustration the nurse should:
① Face the client and raise her voice so Mrs. Carroll can see and hear her better
② Limit Mrs. Carroll's contact with other clients to limit the frustration
③ Anticipate Mrs. Carroll's needs so she does not have to ask for help
④ Give Mrs. Carroll plenty of time so she does not have to respond under pressure

122. Although Mrs. Carroll has regained control of her bowel movements, she is still incontinent of urine. To help her reestablish bladder function, the nurse should encourage her to:
① Assume her normal position for voiding
② Void every 4 hours and attempt to hold urine between set times
③ Drink a minimum of 4000 ml of fluid equally divided among the hours she is awake
④ Attempt to void more frequently in the afternoon than in the morning

123. Mrs. Carroll is using a cane specifically to:
① Prevent further injury to weakened muscles
② Maintain balance and improve stability
③ Relieve pressure on weight-bearing joints
④ Aid in controlling involuntary muscle movements

124. When teaching Mrs. Carroll to ambulate with a cane, the nurse should instruct her to:
① Hold it in the hand on the same side as the affected lower extremity
② Lean the body toward the cane when ambulating
③ Advance the cane and the affected extremity simultaneously
④ Shorten the stride of the unaffected extremity

Situation: Melanie, a 21-year-old heroin addict, delivers a 2268 g (5 lb) baby boy. On the third day after delivery she leaves the hospital because the person caring for her 3-year-old Mary can no longer do this. She assures the staff she can care for both Mary and Baby Jesse.

125. The nurse administered vitamin K intramuscularly to Jesse immediately after birth to:
① Prevent increased levels of serum bilirubin
② Promote the synthesis of prothrombin
③ Substitute for normal bacterial flora
④ Decrease calciferol until renal clearance can take over

126. Typical signs of drug dependence in babies are due to withdrawal and usually begin within 24 hours after birth. The nurse should have observed for:
① Prolonged periods of sleep
② Hyperactivity
③ Dehydration and constipation
④ Hypotonicity of muscles

127. Nursing care of Jesse should have included:
① Increasing environmental stimuli
② Reducing elevated body temperature
③ Offering small frequent feedings
④ Administering methadone

128. In caring for Melanie prior to her discharge the nurse should:
① Keep Melanie and the baby separated until Melanie is drug free
② Refer Melanie to a drug rehabilitation program
③ Support Melanie's positive maternal responses
④ Help Melanie understand that Jesse's problems are due to her drug intake

129. Two weeks after Melanie and Baby Jesse are discharged, 3-year-old Mary is admitted with second- and third-degree burns over 30% of her body. She is placed in a warm isolation room with a humidifier, and strict sterile technique is instituted. The physician orders a Foley catheter to be inserted and IV therapy to begin immediately. One nurse is assigned to care for Mary each shift for the first 48 hours. Nursing observations in the first 48 hours of hospitalization are directed primarily toward preventing:
① Pneumonia
② Contractures
③ Dehydration
④ Shock

130. Despite Mary's physical distress and discomfort, her weight must be accurately taken because it provides a:
① Baseline for future growth
② Measure of the burned surface area
③ Basis for fluid replacement and medications
④ Guideline for dietary and fluid management

131. On the second day of hospitalization Mary has decreased urinary output with edema. The nurse, recognizing this as one sign of possible complications that commonly occur in the first 2 days, should watch for other signs including:
    ① Vomiting and bradycardia
    ② Subnormal temperature and slow pulse
    ③ High fever and disorientation
    ④ Rapid pulse and low BP

132. The nurse must accurately measure Mary's urinary output each hour to evaluate kidney function. The minimum safe output per hour for Mary is:
    ① 10 to 20 ml
    ② 20 to 40 ml
    ③ 40 to 60 ml
    ④ 60 to 80 ml

133. As Mary's burns begin to heal, the nurse attempts to involve her in therapeutic play to give her the opportunity to:
    ① Learn to accept the hospital situation
    ② Know the other children on the unit
    ③ Forget the reality of the situation for a while
    ④ Work out ways of coping with her fears

Situation: Mrs. Felton is admitted after an argument with her daughter, during which she incurred a sucking stab wound of the left thorax.

134. In the emergency room the nurse should position Mrs. Felton:
    ① On her back with her feet elevated
    ② On her left side with head elevated
    ③ In a high Fowler's position with her left side supported
    ④ On her right side flat in bed with a pillow supporting her left arm

135. When assessing Mrs. Felton the nurse should be concerned primarily with the:
    ① Quality and depth of respirations
    ② Blood pressure and pupillary response
    ③ Amount of serosanguineous drainage
    ④ Degree and level of pain

136. Mrs. Felton has a large pressure dressing over the stab wound. The nurse recognizes that the purpose of this dressing is to:
    ① Seal off major vessels
    ② Prevent additional contamination
    ③ Protect the pleura
    ④ Maintain negative intrathoracic pressure

137. Twenty-four hour IV fluids are ordered for Mrs. Felton. The fluid orders read: Bottle 1: 1000 ml 5% D/W; bottle 2: 1000 ml 5% D/0.9% NaCl; bottle 3: 1000 ml 5% D/0.33% NaCl. The drop factor of the IV set is 20 gtts/ml. The nurse should set the drop rate at:
    ① 22 gtts/min
    ② 27 gtts/min
    ③ 36 gtts/min
    ④ 42 gtts/min

138. The nurse should encourage Mrs. Felton to perform deep breathing exercises. The reason for this is that deep breathing exercises help to:
    ① Counteract respiratory acidosis
    ② Expand the residual volume
    ③ Increase blood volume
    ④ Decrease partial pressure of oxygen

139. Mrs. Felton has chest tubes attached to a Pleurevac suction. When caring for Mrs. Felton, the nurse should:
    ① Change the dressing daily using aseptic technique
    ② Palpate the surrounding area for crepitus
    ③ Empty the drainage chamber at the end of the shift
    ④ Clamp the chest tubes when suctioning the client

140. Mrs. Felton complains of severe pain 2 days following surgical repair of the wound. Initially the nurse should:
    ① Have the client rest
    ② Take her vital signs
    ③ Administer prn analgesic
    ④ Check time of her last medication

Situation: Arlene Cinton, 23 years old, is arrested after stabbing a friend and is admitted to the psychiatric unit for observation.

141. On admission Ms. Cinton has delusions of persecution and auditory hallucinations. The nurse greets her by saying, "Good evening, Arlene. How are you?" Ms. Cinton answers, "Arlene is bad." This is an example of:
    ① Dissociation
    ② Reaction formation
    ③ Displacement
    ④ Transference

142. In planning care for a confused or delusional client such as Arlene, it is most important for the nurse to:
    ① Maintain quiet, dim surroundings to minimize stimuli
    ② Encourage realistic activity considering the client's ability
    ③ Recognize the client is completely unable to differentiate fantasy from reality
    ④ Provide physical hygiene and comfort to demonstrate the client is worthy of receiving care

143. That evening Arlene appears quite upset. As the nurse approaches, Arlene states, "I am hearing voices that are saying bad things about me." The nurse should:
    ① Tell her she does not hear the voices
    ② Encourage her not to listen to what the voices are saying
    ③ Suggest she join other clients playing cards
    ④ Let her know the staff understands she is frightened and stay with her

144. One day the nurse and Arlene sit together and draw. Arlene draws a face with horns on top of the head and says, "This is Arlene. She is a devil." The nurse should respond:
    ① "Arlene, you are not a devil. Don't talk about yourself like that."
    ② "Let's go to the mirror, Arlene, and see what you look like."
    ③ "Arlene, when I look at you, I see a young woman not a devil."
    ④ "I don't see a devil. Why do you see a devil?"

145. Arlene is receiving a major tranquilizer bid. Two-thirds of the daily dose is given in the evening, one-third in the morning. This is done to:
    ① Help her sleep at night
    ② Reduce sedation during the daytime
    ③ Maintain diurnal rhythms
    ④ Reduce increased assaultiveness in the evening

146. After 2 weeks of drug therapy the nurse notices that Arlene has become jaundiced, but she continues to give the tranquilizers until the psychiatrist can be consulted. In situations such as this:
    ① Jaundice is sufficient reason to discontinue the tranquilizers
    ② The psychiatrist's order for tranquilizers should be reduced by the nurse
    ③ Jaundice is a benign side effect and has little significance
    ④ The blood level of tranquilizers must be maintained once established

147. Arlene describes her delusions to the nurse. The nurse should:
    ① Change the topic as soon as she begins to discuss her delusions
    ② Encourage Arlene to discuss her delusions
    ③ Get Arlene involved in a repetitive project
    ④ Accept this as Arlene's reality without argument

148. After a couple of weeks in the hospital the nurse notices Arlene's hair is dirty and asks if she would like to wash it. Arlene answers, "Yes, and I'd like to curl it too." The nurse uses this information to assess that Arlene:
    ① Has some feelings of self-worth
    ② Has a need for social reassurance and approval
    ③ Is quite open to suggestions
    ④ May be entering a hyperactive phase

Situation: Mrs. Donira is a 29-year-old obstetric client with a history of three spontaneous abortions.

149. Mrs. Donira is being observed in the high-risk clinic and has expressed anxiety about remaining at home during this pregnancy. The nurse should question Mrs. Donira to determine her knowledge of the:
    ① Signs and symptoms of impending labor
    ② Causes of spontaneous abortion
    ③ Mechanisms of early labor
    ④ Interrelationship among rest, normal delivery, and diet

150. Mrs. Donira complains of heartburn. When counseling her, the nurse explains that during pregnancy:
    ① The pyloric sphincter relaxes and acid is regurgitated
    ② The cardiac sphincter relaxes and acid is regurgitated
    ③ Gastric acidity and motility are increased
    ④ There is increased gastric motility, which causes acid to be regurgitated

151. When involved in prenatal teaching, the nurse should also inform the client that an increase in vaginal secretions during pregnancy is called leukorrhea and is caused by increased:
    ① Metabolic rate
    ② Functioning of the Bartholin glands
    ③ Production of estrogen
    ④ Supply of sodium chloride to the cells of the vagina

152. Mrs. Donira is trying to decide whether she should breast-feed or bottle-feed her expected baby. She asks the nurse what advantage breast-feeding has over bottle-feeding. The nurse replies that one major group of substances in human milk that are of special

importance to the newborn and cannot be reproduced in any bottle formula is:
    ① Gamma globulins
    ② Complex carbohydrates
    ③ Amino acids
    ④ Essential ions (electrolytes)

153. During labor Mrs. Donira states that she does not want "eyedrops or ointment" placed in her baby's eyes immediately after delivery. The most appropriate response by the nurse would be:
    ① "They are required and should be administered right after delivery."
    ② "The medication protects the infant, and that's why it's used."
    ③ "Is there a reason why you don't want the medication instilled?"
    ④ "You'll have to check with your doctor regarding this."

154. During labor Mrs. Donira receives continuous caudal anesthesia. When she has a sudden episode of severe nausea and her skin becomes pale and clammy, the nurse's immediate reaction is to:
    ① Notify the physician
    ② Elevate the client's legs
    ③ Monitor the FHR every 3 minutes
    ④ Check for vaginal bleeding

155. During delivery the physician performs an episiotomy. The nurse explains to Mrs. Donira that this is most commonly done to:
    ① Prevent lacerations during birth
    ② Limit postpartal discomfort
    ③ Stretch the perineum
    ④ Reduce trauma to the fetus

156. Mrs. Donira delivers a normal baby boy. When assessing the newborn's respiratory status, the nurse should expect respirations to be:
    ① Shallow and thoracic
    ② Deep and retracting
    ③ Abdominal and irregular
    ④ Stertorous and regular

Situation: Mrs. Ryan, 82 years of age, is hard of hearing and has severe painful rheumatoid arthritis. She was admitted to a nursing home when she became incontinent and her family could no longer care for her.

157. Mrs. Ryan's condition indicates that a primary consideration in her care would be her need for:
    ① Immobilization of joints
    ② Bladder control reeducation
    ③ Control of pain
    ④ Motivation and teaching

158. The nurse should be aware that the drug of choice in rheumatoid arthritis is:
    ① Methocarbamol (Robaxin)
    ② Aspirin
    ③ Cortisone
    ④ Gold salts

159. Concerning positioning, the nurse should encourage Mrs. Ryan to:
    ① Assume a position that is most comfortable
    ② Place pillows beneath her knees
    ③ Assume the Fowler's position
    ④ Maintain her limbs in extension

160. Since Mrs. Ryan's admission to the nursing home she has not been incontinent. While discussing her past and present elimination patterns she tells the nurse of her anger at being bedridden and unable to go anywhere or see anyone. The nurse deduces that her incontinence at home may have been related to:
    ① An unconscious expression of hostility
    ② A method to determine her family's love for her
    ③ A physiologic response expected with the elderly
    ④ A way of maintaining control

161. When caring for Mrs. Ryan, the nurse should:
    ① Frequently ask if she needs the bedpan to void
    ② Create an environment that prevents sensory monotony
    ③ Limit her fluid intake in the evening
    ④ Provide television or radio when Mrs. Ryan is alone

162. Mrs. Ryan uses an air-conduction hearing aid. This increases hearing sensitivity in instances of:
    ① Diminished sensitivity of the cochlea
    ② Perforation of the tympanic membrane
    ③ Immobilization of the auditory ossicles
    ④ Destruction of the auditory nerve

Situation: Mrs. Cole brings her son Johnny to the emergency room with severe gastrointestinal distress symptoms. Johnny is a normal infant who weighed 7.2 kg (16 lb) on his 6-month checkup last week.

163. The nurse immediately prepares for:
    ① Type and cross match
    ② Intestinal intubation with continuous suction
    ③ Placement in an Isolette
    ④ Insertion of an IV line

164. Johnny is admitted to the hospital. The most important clinical indication of the degree of dehydration would be:
    ① Sunken fontanel
    ② Weight loss
    ③ Decreased urine output
    ④ Dry skin

165. When observing Johnny's laboratory reports, the nurse should be especially concerned about a decrease in sodium and:
    ① Potassium
    ② Chlorides
    ③ Calcium
    ④ Phosphates

166. Johnny is receiving parenteral therapy. His IV orders are 400 ml of D 5/0.5 NS to run in 8 hours. A mini-dropper with a drop factor of 50 gtts per milliliter is used. The nurse should set the rate to deliver:
    ① 35 to 36 drops per minute
    ② 37 to 38 drops per minute
    ③ 41 to 42 drops per minute
    ④ 44 to 45 drops per minute

167. Johnny may be given liquids in small amounts. The liquid that would be most beneficial for the nurse to give Johnny is:
    ① Cranberry juice
    ② Liquefied gelatin
    ③ Ginger ale
    ④ Skim milk

168. An essential nursing action when caring for the small child with severe diarrhea is to:
    ① Force fluids orally
    ② Take daily weights
    ③ Replace lost calories
    ④ Keep body temperature below 100° F (37.7° C)

169. Johnny improves, and prior to discharge the nurse discusses Johnny's diet with Mrs. Cole. Mrs. Cole asks when Johnny should be able to drink from a cup. The nurse responds:
    ① Five months
    ② Seven months
    ③ Twelve months
    ④ Eighteen months

Situation: Mrs. Lund is admitted to a psychiatric unit. Her history shows that she has been eating and sleeping very little and has charged hundreds of dollars worth of purchases to her husband.

170. The symptoms that the nurse should expect Mrs. Lund to exhibit in the hospital would include:
    ① Decreased psychomotor activity
    ② Increased interest in the environment
    ③ Depressed mood and crying
    ④ Increased insight into her behavior

171. In view of Mrs. Lund's elated state, the nurse should arrange for her to be in a room:
    ① That will provide a great deal of stimuli
    ② With as little furniture as possible
    ③ With another client who is overactive
    ④ With another client who is very quiet

172. Mrs. Lund becomes loud and insulting and says to a staff member, "Get lost you old buzzard!" The nurse should respond:
    ① "Now, Mrs. Lund, he isn't an old buzzard."
    ② "Don't be so rude, Mrs. Lund, it isn't necessary."
    ③ "Here is something I feel you might be interested in, Mrs. Lund."
    ④ "Could you tell me why you are angry, Mrs. Lund?"

173. Mrs. Lund leaves group therapy in the middle of the session. She is obviously upset and crying when she meets the nurse. She tells the nurse that the group's discussion is too much for her. The most therapeutic nursing action would be to:
    ① Suggest kindly but firmly that she return to the group to work out the conflict
    ② Suggest that she accompany the nurse to her room so that they can talk about it
    ③ Respect her right to decline therapy at this time and simply report the incident to the rest of the health team
    ④ Ask the group leader what happened in the group and base intervention on this additional information

174. Mrs. Lund is to receive lithium carbonate. The nurse should ensure that prior to the drug's administration Mrs. Lund has:
    ① Neurologic studies
    ② Fluid and electrolye studies
    ③ Enzyme studies
    ④ Renal studies

Situation: Mrs. Lamb is 39 years of age and has three children, aged 12, 9, and 5 years. She was admitted to the hospital with the diagnosis of severe metrorrhagia and menorrhagia of 1-year duration. She was found to have a submucous myoma that had grown over the past 6 months. Mrs. Lamb was told that a hysterectomy was necessary.

175. The term *metrorrhagia* refers to:
① Episodes of bleeding between menstrual periods
② Severe bleeding during each menstrual period
③ Presence of blood in the vaginal discharge
④ Painful intercourse

176. To provide preoperative teaching the nurse should know that after a hysterectomy:
① Ovarian hormone secretion ceases, but the hypophysis continues secretion of gonadotrophic hormones
② The cyclical oscillation of hormones between the hypophysis and ovaries continues
③ Menstruation ceases and ovarian hormone secretion decreases
④ Menopause begins immediately with the cessation of ovarian hormone production

177. Mrs. Lamb is recovering from the hysterectomy. The sign that would be indicative of a developing thrombophlebitis would be:
① A reddened area at the ankle
② Pruritus on the calf and thigh
③ Pitting edema of the ankle
④ A tender, painful area on the leg

178. As the nurse walks into Mrs. Lamb's room on the fifth postoperative day, the client asks for sanitary pads because she feels as if she is going to menstruate. The nurse's response is based on knowledge that:
① Mrs. Lamb will not menstruate because her uterus was removed
② It will take several weeks before Mrs. Lamb has a normal menstrual flow
③ Mrs. Lamb is showing signs of psychosomatic responses
④ The postoperative appearance of frank vaginal bleeding is expected

179. Mrs. Lamb's roommate has undergone a hysterectomy and oophorectomy. Her therapy differs from Mrs. Lamb's in that she is receiving estrogen therapy to suppress:
① Heat intolerance
② Flushing of the face
③ Premature aging
④ Dysmenorrhea

Situation: Mr. Osgood is admitted to the hospital for surgery for an incarcerated hernia.

180. The nurse is aware that the diagnosis of incarcerated hernia means that:
① The blood supply to the intestine has been cut off
② The protruding hernia cannot be reduced
③ An erosion of the involved intestine has occurred
④ The bowel has twisted on itself

181. Prior to Mr. Osgood's hernia repair the nurse should:
① Place him in the supine position
② Periodically check his vital signs
③ Observe his bowel movements
④ Monitor his serum enzyme levels

182. The physician returns the incarcerated tissue to the abdominal cavity and uses a stainless steel mesh to reinforce the muscle wall, thereby preventing a future recurrence. This procedure is referred to as a:
① Herniorrhaphy
② Herniotomy
③ Herniectomy
④ Hernioplasty

183. Postoperatively, to help limit a common complication of this surgery, the nurse should:
① Place a rolled towel under the scrotum
② Encourage a high-carbohydrate diet
③ Have Mr. Osgood cough and deep breath frequently
④ Apply an abdominal binder

184. An important part of discharge planning is educating Mr. Osgood about body mechanics. An important concept in body mechanics is:
① Bending at the waist reduces tension on the inguinal muscles
② Keeping the body straight when lifting reduces pressure on the abdomen
③ Placing the feet apart increases the stability of the body
④ Relaxing the abdominal muscles and using the extremities to prevent strain

Situation: John McNabb has been feeling very tired and has developed anorexia and jaundice. After a diagnostic workup at the clinic, he is diagnosed as having infectious hepatitis type A.

185. His wife asks about gamma globulin for herself and other family members. The most appropriate response by the nurse would be:
① "Don't be concerned. Your husband's type of hepatitis is no longer communicable."
② "A vaccine has not yet been developed for this type of hepatitis."
③ "You should contact your physician immediately about getting gamma globulin."
④ "Gamma globulin provides passive immunity for serum hepatitis."

186. John's wife explains that he likes seafood. She asks about preparing seafood to avoid infection with hepatitis virus type A. The cooked food most likely to remain contaminated by the virus that causes infectious hepatitis is:
① Broiled shrimp
② Baked haddock
③ Canned tuna
④ Steamed lobster

187. John asks when he will be able to go back to work. The best response by the nurse is:
① "As soon as you're feeling less tired, you may go back to work."
② "Unfortunately, few people fully recover from hepatitis in less than 6 months."
③ "You cannot return to work for 6 months, since the virus will still be present in your stools for this period."
④ "Gradually increase your activities. Relapses are very common in people who return to full activity too soon."

COMPREHENSIVE TEST 2: PART 3

To simulate the National Council Licensure Examination, this test should be completed within 1½ hours.

Situation: Mrs. Jane Dooney, a 30-year-old pregnant woman, has had rheumatic heart disease since childhood. Because of her history, she can expect to experience some symptoms during her pregnancy that noncardiac clients probably would not experience.

188. A normal symptom of pregnancy that Jane will also experience is:
   ① Dyspnea at rest
   ② Tachycardia
   ③ Shortness of breath on exertion
   ④ Progressive dependent edema

189. Mrs. Dooney is concerned about the delivery of her baby and asks what she should expect. The nurse should respond that at term her care will probably include:
   ① Induction of labor to reduce stress
   ② An elective cesarean delivery
   ③ Regional anesthesia and forceps delivery
   ④ General anesthesia and forceps delivery

190. Mr. and Mrs. Dooney arrive in the delivery suite. The nurse explains to the couple that Mrs. Dooney should avoid lying on her back during labor. The nurse has based this statement on the knowledge that the supine position can:
   ① Unduly prolong labor
   ② Cause decreased placental perfusion
   ③ Interfere with free movement of the coccyx
   ④ Lead to transient episodes of hypertension

191. Mrs. Dooney delivers a healthy baby girl. The nurse should plan Mrs. Dooney's postpartum care based on the knowledge that:
   ① The first 48 hours postpartum are the most stressful on the cardiopulmonary system
   ② Mrs. Dooney is out of immediate danger because the stress of pregnancy is over
   ③ Clients with cardiac problems should be kept on bed rest for a minimum of 7 days
   ④ Mrs. Dooney should increase her fluid intake, particularly if she is breast-feeding

192. Mrs. Dooney and her baby, who is 10 weeks old, are being seen by the visiting nurse. When the nurse arrives, Mrs. Dooney appears tired and the baby is crying. The most appropriate question by the nurse would be:
   ① "Is everything all right? You look tired."
   ② "When did the baby have her last bottle?"
   ③ "Tell me a little about your daily routine."
   ④ "Oh, it looks like you two are having a bad day."

193. The nurse should strive to help Mrs. Dooney facilitate optimum growth and development for her daughter by encouraging her to provide appropriate activities such as:
   ① Playing pat-a-cake
   ② Giving the infant push-pull toys
   ③ Keeping her in the carriage in the living room
   ④ Placing her daughter in an infant seat

194. The nurse initiates nutritional anticipatory guidance with Mrs. Dooney. The sequence for introducing other foods into the baby's diet after the introduction of cereals is:
   ① Table foods, fruits, vegetables, meats
   ② Fruits, vegetables, meats, table foods
   ③ Meats, fruits, vegetables, table foods
   ④ Vegetables, table foods, meats, fruits

Situation: Mr. Manning, a 48-year-old photographer, has developed fatigue and dyspnea on exertion. His ECG shows atrial fibrillation. The physician suspects mitral stenosis.

195. The nurse is doing a physical assessment of Mr. Manning. It would be most significant if Mr. Manning presented a history of:
   ① Rubella, age 6
   ② Strep throat, age 12
   ③ Pleurisy, age 20
   ④ Cystitis, age 28

196. After the initial workup, the physician orders a cardiac catheterization for Mr. Manning. In caring for him after the procedure, the nurse should:
   ① Provide for rest
   ② Check pulse in the area distal to the cutdown
   ③ Check the ECG every 30 minutes
   ④ Administer oxygen

197. Mr. Manning undergoes a mitral replacement. Postoperatively his peripheral pulses must be checked frequently. The chief purpose of this is to detect:
   ① The existence of emboli
   ② Arteriovenous shunting
   ③ Postsurgical bleeding
   ④ Atrial fibrillation

198. Mr. Manning develops a temperature of 102.8° F (39° C). The nurse notifies the physician, because elevated temperatures:
   ① May indicate cerebral edema
   ② May be a forerunner of hemorrhage
   ③ Increase the cardiac output
   ④ Cause diaphoresis and possible chilling

199. During the first 24 hours after surgery, 1000 ml of serosanguineous fluid drains from the chest tube. The expected drainage during this period is:
   ① 800 to 1000 ml
   ② 100 to 300 ml
   ③ 750 to 900 ml
   ④ 400 to 500 ml

200. During a blood transfusion Mr. Manning develops chills and headache. The nurse's best action is to:
   ① Stop the transfusion immediately
   ② Lightly cover the client
   ③ Notify the physician STAT
   ④ Slow the blood flow to keep vein open

201. Mr. Manning's fever does not respond to ASA. He is placed on a hypothermia blanket. One reaction to hypothermia that should be prevented is:
   ① Venous stasis
   ② Hypotension
   ③ Shivering
   ④ Dehydration

202. Mr. Manning requires intravenous fluids postoperatively. To set the drip rate to deliver 125 ml/hour of D5W, the nurse must know:
① The total volume in the bottle or bag
② The size of the needle or catheter in the vein
③ The drops per milliliter delivered by the infusion set
④ The diameter of the tubing being used

Situation: Mrs. Madison is a 40-year-old, with an obsessive-compulsive disorder at the psychiatric day treatment center. She has shown a marked decrease in symptoms and has uncovered her underlying fear of incurring parental disapproval.

203. Mrs. Madison wants to get a part-time job, but on the day of her job interview, she comes in fretful, displaying symptoms. The nurse's best response is:
① "If going to an interview makes you this anxious, it seems like you're not ready to work."
② "It must be that you really don't want that job after all. I think you should think more about it."
③ "Going for your interview triggered some feelings in you. What would your mother say about you getting a job?"
④ "I know you're anxious, but make yourself go to the interview and conquer your fear."

204. The hospital or day treatment center is often indicated in the treatment of the client with an obsessive-compulsive disorder because:
① It provides the neutral environment the client needs to work through conflicts
② It prevents the client from carrying out symptomatic rituals
③ It resolves the client's anxiety, since decision making is minimal
④ It allows the staff to exert control over the client's activities

205. In developing a care plan for Mrs. Madison, the objective that would most likely increase her anxiety would be:
① Having her understand the nature of her anxiety
② Involving her in establishing the therapeutic plan
③ Providing a nonjudgmental and accepting environment
④ Permitting her ritualistic acts three times a day

206. Mrs. Madison continually walks up and down the hall, touching every other chair. If she is unable to do this, she gets quite upset. The nurse should:
① Remove all chairs from the hall, thereby relieving her of the necessity to touch every other one
② Allow her to continue to touch the chairs as long as she wants and wait for her to get tired
③ Keep talking to her to distract her so she will forget about touching the chairs
④ Allow the behavior for a specified time, letting her set the time she would prefer

Situation: Bobby, age 4 years, is admitted with a diagnosis of acute lymphocytic leukemia (ALL). He has a history of an upper respiratory infection 1 week before admission, and his complete blood count reveals a hemoglobin level of 7 g/100 ml, a hematocrit of 20, a white blood count of 39,000 and a platelet count of 130,000.

207. Platelets are ordered for Bobby, and an IV is started. The nurse should:
① Flush the line with 5% dextrose and normal saline
② Administer the platelets over 2½ hours
③ Administer the platelets rapidly
④ Check vital signs 3 hours after the transfusion

208. Bobby is scheduled to receive methotrexate. His mother asks, "Can we start Bobby on vitamin supplements? He looks so weak." The nurse's response should be:
① "That's a fine suggestion, I'll ask the doctor to order some for Bobby."
② "Vitamin supplements won't help Bobby feel any better right now."
③ "Some vitamin preparations contain folic acid, which interferes with the drug."
④ "Yes, Bobby may benefit from a vitamin supplement and will be receiving it soon."

209. Allopurinol (Zyloprim) is prescribed for Bobby. He asks, "Why do I have to take that pill?" The nurse's response should be:
① "Because your doctor ordered it. He would not order anything for you unless it was very important."
② "Because this pill helps the other medicines get rid of the things that are making you sick."
③ "To protect your body from developing other problems after your treatment has been stopped."
④ "To stop your sick white cells from going to other parts of your body."

210. Bobby looks very pale and feels warm to the touch. The nurse suspects a fever and checks Bobby's axillary and oral temperatures because:
① Rectal temperatures are too upsetting for a 4-year-old child
② Axillary temperatures alone are not accurate when fever is suspected
③ Oral temperatures alone are inaccurate in children with leukemia
④ Rectal temperatures are avoided to reduce the risk of rectal trauma

211. Bobby requires oral hygiene because of the potential for mouth lesions from the chemotherapy. The teaching should include:
① Brushing three times a day with a toothbrush
② Frequent mouth rinsing with hydrogen peroxide
③ Brushing with foam-tipped applicators
④ Frequent rinsing with undiluted mouth wash

212. Bobby is scheduled to receive cranial radiation. The teaching plan reflects the fact that this is done to:
① Reduce the risk of systemic infection
② Improve the quality of life
③ Avoid metastasis to the lymphatic system
④ Prevent central nervous system involvement

Situation: Mary Connor is in the thirty-third week of pregnancy when she begins to experience contractions. She calls her physician and is advised to come into the office to be examined. Her cervix is found to be dilated 2 cm. A decision is made to treat her at home with bed rest.

213. The teaching plan for Mary should include the information that:
    ① Mary should be on her side with her head raised on a small pillow
    ② The lower end of Mary's bed will need to be raised on blocks
    ③ Mary should assume the knee-chest position every 2 hours for 10 minutes while she is awake
    ④ Mary should sit in bed with several large pillows supporting her back

214. When the therapeutic regimen is explained to Mary, she starts to cry and says, "I have two small children at home." The nurse should reply:
    ① "You are worried about how you will be able to manage?"
    ② "You will need someone to care for the children."
    ③ "You'll be able to fix meals, and the children can go to nursery school."
    ④ "Perhaps a neighbor can help out, and your husband can do the housework in the evening."

215. The nurse should also explain to Mary that coitus:
    ① Should be restricted to the side-lying position
    ② Is prohibited, as it may stimulate labor
    ③ Is permitted as long as penile penetration is shallow
    ④ Need not be restricted in any way

216. Mary follows the prescribed regimen at home for 1 week and has only occasional mild contractions. Then the contractions begin to increase in intensity and frequency. Mary is advised by her physician to come to the hospital, where ritodrine therapy is instituted. During the initial intravenous administration of ritodrine the nurse should:
    ① Check Mary's reflexes q2h
    ② Monitor Mary's blood pressure q10 min
    ③ Insert a Foley catheter to monitor urinary output
    ④ Institute safety measures because of altered consciousness

Situation: Mrs. Carpenter enters the hospital with esophageal strictures. She has been unable to eat solid food for many weeks. Nutritional edema does not mask the emaciation and malnourishment present.

217. The nurse is aware that Mrs. Carpenter's nutritional edema is a result of the following primary homeostatic mechanism:
    ① The capillary fluid shift mechanism
    ② The aldosterone mechanism
    ③ The ADH mechanism
    ④ Nitrogen balance

218. The nurse can prevent a major reaction to total parenteral nutrition infusions by:
    ① The slow administration of the fluid
    ② Checking vital signs every 4 hours
    ③ Changing site every 24 hours
    ④ Recording intake and output

219. Later, a gastrostomy tube is inserted and Mrs. Carpenter is to be discharged with the tube in place. An advantage of gastrostomy tube feeding over naso-gastric tube feeding is that:
    ① More tube feeding mixture can be given each time
    ② The procedure does not require gravity
    ③ There is less chance of aspiration
    ④ The client can self-administer the feeding

220. The nurse administers the initial tube feeding. The observation that indicates that Mrs. Carpenter is unable to tolerate further tube feeding would be:
    ① Passage of flatus
    ② Rapid flow of feeding
    ③ Epigastric tenderness
    ④ Rise of formula in the tube

221. In teaching the tube feeding procedure to Mrs. Carpenter, the nurse advises her that she should:
    ① Heat the feeding 10° above body temperature
    ② Finish the feeding with water
    ③ Maintain a supine position the entire time
    ④ Instill fluid prior to feeding to ensure that the tube is in the stomach

222. Mrs. Carpenter must utilize a gastrostomy tube as her only route of ingestion. To maintain the pleasure of eating, the nurse may advise her to:
    ① Chew the food prior to using it for feeding
    ② Use the blender to puree favorite foods
    ③ Feed via the tube at normal mealtimes
    ④ Chew gum during gastrostomy tube feeding

Situation: Mr. Ryan is admitted to the hospital with GI bleeding and a burning epigastric pain. The initial diagnosis is peptic ulcer or gastric carcinoma.

223. To differentiate between a gastric ulcer and gastric carcinoma, the diagnostic test that would provide conclusive evidence is a:
    ① Gastric analysis
    ② GI series
    ③ Gastroscopy
    ④ Stool examination

224. Mr. Ryan is placed on a stretcher and restrained with Velcro straps for his transport to the x-ray department for an upper GI examination. While coming out of the elevator, he shifts his position, the Velcro strap breaks, and he falls to the floor, sustaining a fractured arm. He later comments that "the Velcro strap was worn, just at the very spot where the strap snapped." The nurse is:
    ① Completely exonerated, since only the hospital, as principal employer, is primarily responsible for the quality and maintenance of equipment
    ② Exempt from any law suit because of the doctrine of *respondeat superior*
    ③ Normally liable, along with the employer, for misapplication of equipment or use of defective equipment that harms the client
    ④ Totally and singly responsible for the obvious negligence because of her failure to report defective equipment

225. Barium salts in the GI series and barium enemas serve to:
    ① Give off visible light and illuminate the alimentary tract
    ② Fluoresce and thus illuminate the alimentary tract
    ③ Dye the alimentary tract and thus give it color contrast
    ④ Absorb x-rays and thus give contrast to the soft tissues of the alimentary tract

226. Peptic ulcer is diagnosed. This is considered to be a psychophysiologic disorder about which it is believed that:
    ① Structural changes have occurred as a result of psychologic conflicts
    ② Illness is a defense against psychologic conflicts
    ③ Structural changes have occurred as a result of physiologic changes caused by psychologic conflict
    ④ Physiologic changes stimulated psychologic changes

227. The nurse should be aware that the most common complication of peptic ulcer is:
    ① Perforation
    ② Hemorrhage
    ③ Pyloric obstruction
    ④ Esophageal varices

228. The foods Mr. Ryan would be permitted include:
    ① Sliced oranges, pancakes with syrup, coffee
    ② Applesauce, Cream of Wheat, milk
    ③ Orange juice, fried eggs, sausage
    ④ Tomato juice, raisin bran cereal, tea

Situation: Mrs. Reed was admitted to the obstetrical unit in active labor.

229. During a contraction the nurse observes a 15 beat per minute acceleration of the FHR above the baseline rate. The nurse's most appropriate action would be to:
    ① Prepare for immediate delivery because of fetal distress
    ② Call the physician immediately and await orders
    ③ Turn Mrs. Reed on her left side to increase venous return
    ④ Record this normal fetal response to contractions on the chart

230. Mrs. Reed begins to experience contractions 2 to 3 minutes apart that last about 45 seconds. Between contractions the nurse records a fetal heart rate of 100 beats per minute. The nurse should:
    ① Closely monitor maternal vital signs
    ② Chart the rate as a normal response to contractions
    ③ Notify the physician immediately
    ④ Continue to monitor the fetal heart

231. During delivery an episiotomy is performed. When caring for Mrs. Reed during the postpartum period, the nurse encourages sitz baths three times a day for 15 minutes. Sitz baths primarily aid the healing process by:
    ① Softening the incision site
    ② Promoting vasodilation
    ③ Cleansing the perineal area
    ④ Tightening the rectal sphincter

232. When preparing Mrs. Reed to care for her episiotomy after discharge, the nurse should include, as a priority, instructions to:
    ① Continue the sitz bath three times a day if it provides comfort
    ② Discontinue the sitz baths once she is at home
    ③ Continue perineal care after toileting until healing occurs
    ④ Avoid stair climbing for at least a few days after discharge

Situation: After a car accident Ed, an 18-year-old high school senior, is taken to the local hospital with a back injury. He did not lose consciousness and remembers that he was unable to move his legs following the accident.

233. After an accident in which there is a questionable back injury, the individual involved:
    ① May be transported in sitting position, if necessary, to secure immediate medical care
    ② May be transported in any position because position is not important, since damage to the cord has already occurred
    ③ Should be protected from flexion and hyperextension of the spine
    ④ May be transported best when placed in the side-lying position

234. After the examination the physician indicates that Ed is paraplegic. His family asks the nurse what this means. The nurse explains that:
    ① Both lower and upper extremities are paralyzed
    ② Upper extremities are paralyzed
    ③ One side of the body is paralyzed
    ④ Lower extremities are paralyzed

235. When caring for Ed, the nurse should plan to provide a high intake of fluid to help:
    ① Prevent elevation of temperature
    ② Maintain electrolyte balance
    ③ Prevent dehydration
    ④ Prevent urinary tract infection

236. Teaching Ed to care for himself while in the hospital is:
    ① Unnecessary; he will be back to normal when he leaves the hospital
    ② Avoided; it is too complicated to be undertaken by a layperson
    ③ Unnecessary; his family will be able to care for him at home
    ④ An essential part of his nursing care plan

237. The paraplegic client frequently loses calcium from the skeletal system. A factor which contributes to this condition is:
    ① Decreased activity
    ② Decreased calcium intake
    ③ Inadequate kidney function
    ④ Inadequate fluid intake

238. Sympathetic hyperreflexia is a syndrome seen in clients with spinal cord injuries. The signs and symptoms include diaphoresis, pulsating headaches, and goose bumps. This syndrome may occur when:
    ① The bowel and/or bladder is distended
    ② The myelin sheath is deteriorating
    ③ The client is upright on a tilt table
    ④ The spinal cord is crushed rather than severed

Situation: Cherri, age 6, is admitted with myoclonic seizures of the right arm and leg lasting 1 to 2 minutes and occurring with increased frequency. Seizure precautions are instituted.

239. If a child develops cyanosis early during a seizure, it is most appropriate for the nurse to:
    ① Use a padded tongue blade
    ② Insert an oral airway
    ③ Observe without intervening
    ④ Administer oxygen by mask

240. Cherri has a myoclonic seizure that progresses to a generalized seizure with clenched jaws. The nurse's best initial action would be to:
    ① Phone for assistance
    ② Attempt to open the jaws
    ③ Hyperextend the neck
    ④ Place a large pillow under the head

241. Cherri is given phenytoin (Dilantin) 75 mg orally twice a day. The activities pertinent to long-term Dilantin therapy, which the nurse should teach Cherri's parents include:
    ① Observing for reddish brown discoloration of urine
    ② Administering the drug 2 hours after breakfast and dinner
    ③ Supplementing the diet with high-calorie foods and forcing fluids
    ④ Providing oral hygiene, especially gum massage and flossing of teeth

242. Cherri's primary nurse is aware that the most common reason for the development of status epilepticus is that the prescribed dosage of Dilantin:
    ① Was ineffective for Cherri's seizures
    ② Was probably not taken consistently
    ③ Was insufficient to cover her activities
    ④ Had reached a therapeutic level

Situation: Laura Arndt is in her twenty-eighth week of pregnancy and develops thrombophlebitis of the left leg. She is admitted to the hospital, bed rest is prescribed, and she is given anticoagulant therapy.

243. The anticoagulant the nurse would expect to administer is:
    ① Heparin
    ② Warfarin (Coumadin sodium)
    ③ Dicumarol
    ④ Diphenadione (Dipaxin)

244. As part of the nursing care for Laura, the nurse checks the PPT reports daily. One morning Laura's clotting time is about 95 seconds. The nurse notifies the physician to request that the anticoagulant be:
    ① Increased for better clotting results
    ② Omitted for one dose and monitored further
    ③ Changed to a more effective anticoagulant
    ④ Discontinued, since the PPT is normal

245. Laura's thrombophlebitis improves. In her thirty-second week of pregnancy, Laura is scheduled for ultrasonography. The nurse explains the procedure and informs her that for this test she will have to:
    ① Be kept NPO for 12 hours to minimize the possibility of vomiting
    ② Be monitored closely afterward for signs of precipitate labor
    ③ Refrain from voiding for at least 3 hours before the test
    ④ Be given an enema the night before the examination

246. The sonogram demonstrates a low-lying placenta. The adaptation to this condition that would be most likely to occur first in Laura is:
    ① Sharp abdominal pain
    ② Early rupture of membranes
    ③ Increased lower back pain
    ④ Painless vaginal bleeding

247. Two weeks before delivery, Laura is scheduled for a nonstress test. The nurse explains the nonstress procedure to Laura. The nurse is satisfied with the explanation when Laura says:
    ① "If my baby's heart reacts normally during the test, he should do okay during delivery."
    ② "I hate having needles in my arm, but now I understand why it's necessary."
    ③ "I hope this test does not cause my labor to begin early."
    ④ "I hope the baby doesn't get too restless after this procedure."

Situation: Gail, 17 years old, has a history of being a loner. She made excellent grades in school, but often her thinking was highly symbolic. During her senior year in high school she refused to get out of bed, experienced loss of appetite, and displayed disorganized speech. She was hospitalized at a community hospital.

248. One of the primary goals in providing a therapeutic environment for Gail is to:
    ① Involve her in a group with her peers
    ② Remove her from the home
    ③ Foster a trusting relationship
    ④ Give her medication on time

249. While in the hospital Gail still refuses to get out of bed and becomes very hostile with the staff when approached. The most immediate therapeutic nursing approach would be:
    ① Require that she get out of bed at once
    ② Stay with her until she calms down
    ③ Give her the prn tranquilizer that is ordered
    ④ Allow her to stay in bed for now but leave her alone

250. Gail sits huddled in a chair and seldom leaves it. She occasionally lets out a scream and runs to the end of the hallway and crouches in a corner. The nurse realizes that this type of behavior is classified as:
    ① Reactive
    ② Regressive
    ③ Dissociative
    ④ Hallucinatory

251. To begin to establish a therapeutic relationship with Gail, the nurse must:
    ① Obtain a complete history from her family
    ② Ascertain what topics are of interest to her
    ③ Protect her from herself
    ④ Plan to keep her anxiety at a minimum

252. The priority goal is for Gail to develop:
    ① A sense of identity
    ② Ego strengths
    ③ Trust
    ④ An ability to socialize

253. Gail is taking chlorpromazine (Thorazine), 2000 mg, every day. She comes to the nurse complaining that her fingers are twitching. The best reply would be:
    ① "This is a temporary situation until your body adjusts to the medication."
    ② "I will get the doctor to order a medication that will help overcome this. It is a side effect of the drug you are taking."
    ③ "You need the medication that we are giving you. You will soon get used to the side effects."
    ④ "Let's wait a few days and see whether the side effects of the drug you are taking go away."

254. The symptom that would cause the nurse to stop giving chlorpromazine to Gail until further laboratory work was done is:
① Photosensitivity
② Shuffling gait
③ Yellow sclerae
④ Grimacing

255. On being discharged Gail should be encouraged to:
① Go back to her regular activities
② Continue in the aftercare clinic
③ Call the unit whenever upset
④ Find a group that has similar problems

Situation: Mr. Curan, 54 years old, has angina pectoris. He is admitted for a cardiac catheterization, which is to be done via the femoral approach.

256. The facts about this procedure that should be included as part of the nurse's teaching plan for Mr. Curan include:
① A general anesthetic will be given, and he will not be awake during the procedure
② He will be kept on bed rest, in the supine position, with the affected leg extended for 12 to 24 hours
③ He will be permitted to get up and walk around as soon as he returns to his room
④ His physician will immediately tell him about the results of the procedure

257. Following his cardiac catheterization, Mr. Curan is discharged and is scheduled to return for coronary bypass surgery. His wife asks, "When my husband gets chest pain at home, how will we know if we should call the doctor?" The nurse should teach the family to call the physician if the pain:
① Is not relieved by rest or by nitroglycerin
② Radiates to the arms, neck, or jaw
③ Is accompanied by mild diaphoresis
④ Occurs after moderate exercise

258. When obtaining the consent for surgery from Mr. Curan, the nurse should:
① Explain to Mr. Curan the risks involved in the surgery
② Evaluate whether Mr. Curan's knowledge level is sufficient to give consent
③ Witness the signature, since this is what the nurse's signature documents
④ Explain to Mr. Curan that obtaining the signature is routine for any surgery

259. Mr. Curan asks how his coronary bypass surgery will benefit him. The nurse bases her response on the knowledge that:
① Studies have consistently shown that this surgery increases an individual's life span
② Evidence substantiates that surgery can prevent progression of coronary artery disease
③ Surgery will improve his chances of returning to gainful employment
④ This surgery significantly decreases symptoms in a large percentage of individuals

260. Primary preoperative teaching for Mr. Curan before the open-heart surgery should include:
① A detailed description of the surgical procedure
② A thorough discussion of discharge plans
③ Visits by recovery room and/or ICU nursing staff
④ An explanation that just his chest and groin will be shaved

261. In the immediate postoperative period following coronary bypass surgery, the nurse should be particularly alert for the common complication of:
① Postpericardotomy syndrome with fever and audible friction rub
② Supraventricular arrhythmias, especially atrial fibrillation
③ Graft closure with recurrence of angina-like chest pain
④ Elevation of hemoglobin and hematocrit levels with risk of embolization

262. When preparing Mr. Curan for discharge, the nurse should teach him that there will be:
① No further drainage from the incisions after hospitalization
② Some increase in edema in the leg used for the donor graft with increased activity
③ Little incisional pain and tenderness after 3 to 4 weeks following surgery
④ A mild fever and extreme fatigue for several weeks following surgery

263. Mr. Curan is discharged and given propranolol (Inderal) 20 mg po, qid. The teaching plan for him should include:
① Telling him that he may drink alcoholic beverages in moderation
② Instructing him not to abruptly discontinue his medication
③ Telling him to report a pulse rate below 70 beats per minute
④ Advising him to increase the medication if chest pain occurs

Situation: Danny Lyons, 30 months old, is being admitted to the hospital for the first time for chelation therapy because of chronic lead poisoning.

264. The exact etiology of lead poisoning in children like Danny is:
① Clearly understood to be caused by the child's ingestion of nonfood substances
② Unknown, but groups at high risk include children with pica and those exposed to environmental hazards
③ Attributed to an indigent and passive mother who fails to supervise them
④ Considered to be an environment with lead available for oral exploration by unsupervised children

265. The nurse admitting Danny should be able to identify the early signs of chronic lead poisoning (plumbism) such as:
① Mental retardation
② Convulsions
③ Oliguria
④ Anemia

266. Although lead poisoning affects various organ systems, its irreversible side effects are exerted mainly on the:
① Hematological system
② Urinary system
③ Central nervous system (CNS)
④ Skeletal system

267. The nurse can determine the success of Danny's chelation therapy by monitoring for:
   ① Increased urinary excretion of lead
   ② Elevated blood lead levels
   ③ Increased fecal excretion of lead
   ④ Decreased deposition of lead in the bones
268. Danny's chelation therapy will involve receiving a total of 60 injections. To effectively prepare him to cope with this painful treatment, the nurse should give priority to:
   ① Carefully explaining the rationale for the injections so that Danny does not feel he is being punished for eating paint chips
   ② Allowing Danny to play with a syringe and a doll before the therapy is initiated and after receiving each injection
   ③ Rotating the injection sites and adding procaine to the chelating agents to lessen the discomfort
   ④ Role playing with puppets dressed as physicians and nurses to minimize Danny's fear of unfamiliar adults
269. An important nursing goal for Danny would be to relieve local discomfort from the painful injections necessitated by the chelation therapy. This can best be accomplished by:
   ① Having Danny ambulate with assistance immediately following each injection
   ② Applying warm soaks to the affected area
   ③ Massaging the affected area vigorously after each injection
   ④ Giving Danny a cool tub bath following each injection
270. The side effect which is attributed to both the lead toxicity and the primary chelating agent, Ca EDTA, is:
   ① Hypocalcemia
   ② Bone marrow depression
   ③ Increased intracranial pressure
   ④ Nephrotoxicity

Situation: Mrs. Clara Reed, 72 years of age, is admitted to the psychiatric unit with a tentative diagnosis of primary degenerative dementia.

271. The nurse understands that primary degenerative dementia results from:
   ① Cerebral atrophy specifically involving the frontal lobes
   ② A delayed response to severe emotional trauma in early adulthood
   ③ Anatomic changes in the brain that produce acute but transient symptoms
   ④ A long history of poor nutrition and associated avitaminosis
272. Mrs. Reed tells the nurse, "I am useless to everyone, even myself." The nurse recognizes that Mrs. Reed has probably failed to accomplish Erikson's developmental task of:
   ① Ego integrity versus despair
   ② Autonomy versus shame and doubt
   ③ Identity versus role diffusion
   ④ Generativity versus stagnation

273. A nurse's aide complains to the nurse that Mrs. Reed will do things, but only when she feels like doing them, and wonders how one can deal with this. The nurse's response to the aide should be based on the understanding that the elderly:
   ① Lose their ability to cooperate
   ② Are ambivalent toward authority
   ③ Lose ego flexibility
   ④ Utilize strong superego control
274. Mrs. Reed has difficulty following simple directions and selecting her clothes for the day. The nurse recognizes that these problems are the results of:
   ① Clouding of consciousness
   ② Impaired judgment
   ③ Loss of abstract thinking ability
   ④ Decreased attention span

Situation: Mr. Jones is admitted with acute gastritis secondary to alcoholism and cirrhosis.

275. When planning care, it is most important for the nurse to include assessment of Mr. Jones for:
   ① Obstipation
   ② Complaints of nausea
   ③ Blood in the stool
   ④ Specific food intolerances
276. The gastritis improves, but Mr. Jones becomes dyspneic as a result of ascites. The nurse understands that the ascites is most likely the result of:
   ① Decreased interstitial osmotic pressure
   ② Excess production of serum albumin
   ③ Inadequate secretion of bile salts
   ④ Impaired portal venous return
277. A paracentesis is ordered. Immediately before the paracentesis, the nurse should:
   ① Instruct Mr. Jones to void
   ② Have Mr. Jones sign a consent form
   ③ Position Mr. Jones on his side
   ④ Measure Mr. Jones' abdominal girth
278. The physician removes 1500 ml of fluid. It is most essential that the nurse observe Mr. Jones for:
   ① An increased pulse rate
   ② Abdominal distention
   ③ A hypertensive crisis
   ④ Dry mucous membranes

Situation: Mary Sherman, a young gravida I, comes to the health center for prenatal care.

279. In order to elicit information about Ms. Sherman's risk for exposure to DES the nurse should ask:
   ① "Were you born before 1963?"
   ② "Did your mother take hormones during her pregnancy?"
   ③ "Have you noticed any lesions in your perineal area?"
   ④ "Have you ever taken oral contraceptives?"
280. The nurse explains to Ms. Sherman that the Rh factor determination is routinely performed on expectant mothers. This test predicts whether the fetus is at risk for the development of:
   ① Physiologic hyperbilirubinemia
   ② Protein metabolism deficiency
   ③ Respiratory distress syndrome
   ④ Acute hemolytic anemia

281. Anticipatory guidance during the first trimester of pregnancy is primarily directed toward increasing Ms. Sherman's knowledge of:
① Physical changes resulting from pregnancy
② Role transition into parenthood
③ Labor and delivery
④ Signs of complications

COMPREHENSIVE TEST 2: PART 4

To simulate the National Council Licensure Examination, this test should be completed within 1½ hours.

Situation: Mrs. Winet, a 32-year-old gravida III, para II, spontaneously delivers a 4082.3 g (9 lb) baby boy en route to the hospital after a brief labor.

282. The nurse should be aware that the chief hazard to a child in precipitate delivery is:
① Brachial palsy
② Intracranial hemorrhage
③ Dislocated hip
④ Fractured clavicle

283. Perineal laceration is a common complication of precipitate delivery. In addition to regular perineal care, Mrs. Winet's nursing care should include:
① Encouraging early and frequent ambulation
② Encouraging perineal exercises to strengthen muscles
③ Telling the client to expect slower healing
④ Providing a high-protein, high-roughage diet

284. Baby Winet has sustained an intracranial hemorrhage because of a tear in the tentorial membrane. The nurse should expect the baby to display:
① Extreme lethargy
② Weak, timorous cry
③ Abnormal respirations
④ Generalized purpura

285. The nurse checks Baby Winet's Babinski reflex and finds it to be positive. A positive Babinski sign in a newborn infant is due to:
① Immaturity of the CNS
② Hypoxia during labor and delivery
③ Hyperreflexia of the muscular system
④ Neurologic impairment

286. Nursing care of Baby Winet should include:
① Stimulating frequently to monitor level of consciousness
② Elevating his head higher than his hips
③ Checking reflexes every 15 minutes
④ Weighing him daily before feeding

287. The nurse who has been caring for Baby Winet decides on a plan of care for the mother as well. The plan calls for:
① Setting up a schedule for teaching the mother how to care for her baby
② Discussing the matter with her in a nonthreatening manner
③ Showing by example how to care for the infant and satisfy her own needs
④ Supplying emotional support to the mother and encouraging her dependence

Situation: Baby Jimmy Lyle is suspected of having cerebral palsy (CP) in the newborn nursery. At 6 weeks the diagnosis is confirmed when Mrs. Lyle takes him to the health clinic.

288. When Mrs. Lyle hears that Jimmy has CP she cries, "What did we do to deserve this?" The nurse responds:
① "Why do you feel you are being punished?"
② "You didn't do anything; let me tell you about this disorder."
③ "Let's sit down and have a cup of coffee."
④ "I know you must be upset, but it's too early to tell."

289. As Jimmy Lyle develops, his vision, hearing, and speech are fine but he does have a slight general sensory loss in position, pain, and temperature in both legs. He uses braces and special appliances to provide self-care. He is admitted to the hospital at the age of 7 years for a tendon-lengthening procedure. While in bed after surgery, he must wear his braces and shoes for at least 8 hours a day. This is to:
① Continue his acceptance of physical restraints
② Maintain hip and knee alignment and prevent footdrop
③ Stretch his ligaments and strengthen muscle tone
④ Encourage ambulation as soon as possible

290. The orthopedic surgeon is anxious to get Jimmy onto crutches. In preparing Jimmy for crutch walking the nurse must determine:
① The weight-bearing ability of Jimmy's upper and lower extremities
② Whether Jimmy has the power in his trunk to drag his legs forward when erect
③ When Jimmy's circulation can tolerate an erect position
④ The ability of Jimmy's shoulder girdle to support his body weight when it leaves the floor

291. It is decided that Jimmy be taught the four-point alternate crutch gait. This gait was probably chosen because:
① There are always two points of support on the floor
② Jimmy has more power in the upper extremities than in the lower extremities
③ It provides for equal but partial weight-bearing on each limb
④ Jimmy has no power or step ability in the lower extremities

292. In view of his slight sensory loss in the legs, Jimmy and his parents should be taught to:
① Keep the braces in good repair and pad them well
② Check alignment of the braces (brace joints should coincide with body joints)
③ Select shoes which have heels that are wide and low
④ Examine the skin for evidence of pressure points

293. When teaching Jimmy to ambulate with crutches, the nurse should remember that:
① Learning progresses on a line forward and upward
② Because of his age, Jimmy's experiential background is limited
③ Learning is a result of adequate teaching
④ Jimmy must first understand normal walking patterns

294. Because of the diminished sensation in Jimmy's legs, he should be taught the following safety precautions:
    ① Test the temperature of water in any water-related activity
    ② Set the clock two times during the night to awaken and change position
    ③ Tighten straps and buckles more than usual on braces when ambulating
    ④ Look down at the lower extremities when crutch walking to determine proper positioning of the legs

295. When planning long-term care for Jimmy, it is important for the nurse to recognize that:
    ① CP is unstable and unpredictable
    ② Jimmy should have genetic counseling before planning a family
    ③ His illness is not progressively degenerative
    ④ Jimmy probably has some degree of mental retardation

Situation: Mrs. Simon, a 72-year-old with congestive heart failure, is having difficulty breathing as a result of pulmonary edema. She is being treated with digitalis and diuretic therapy and also with a 1 g sodium diet.

296. At 9 PM Mrs. Simon asks for a glass of juice. Since the only kinds of juice on the ward are pear nectar, apple, and tomato, the nurse should:
    ① Explain to Mrs. Simon that she should not have juice between meals but she may have a glass of water
    ② Ask her which she prefers, the apple juice or the pear nectar
    ③ Explain to her that the only kind she can have is tomato juice
    ④ Tell her that she cannot have any kind of juice because she is on a low-sodium diet

297. Mrs. Simon is to receive 0.2 mg of digoxin IM. The ampule is labeled 0.5 mg = 2 ml. The nurse should administer:
    ① 8 ml
    ② 0.8 ml
    ③ 1 ml
    ④ 1.2 ml

298. Mrs. Simon's ankles are swollen on admission. The nurse should prepare to:
    ① Restrict fluids
    ② Elevate the legs
    ③ Apply elastic bandages
    ④ Do range-of-motion exercises

299. Mrs. Simon is on a 1 g sodium diet. Assuming all the food involved is cooked without salt, the nurse should recognize Mrs. Simon needs further teaching if she ordered:
    ① Baked chicken, boiled potatoes, broccoli, coffee
    ② Mixed fruit salad bowl with cottage cheese; crackers, relish dish (celery, carrot, olives, sweet pickles), tea
    ③ Soft cooked egg, salt-free toast, jelly, skim milk
    ④ Fillet of sole, baked potato, lettuce and tomato salad, fresh fruit cup, milk

300. To help monitor Mrs. Simon's physical status, a central venous catheter is inserted. The nurse can take a correct central venous pressure reading when the water level in the manometer:
    ① Drops and then rises
    ② Synchronizes with the BP
    ③ Rises and stops at a specific plateau
    ④ Fluctuates with respirations

301. Mrs. Simon is receiving hydrochlorothiazide (Diuril) and furosemide (Lasix) to relieve edema. The nurse should observe for evidence of:
    ① Excessive loss of potassium ions
    ② Elevation of the urine specific gravity
    ③ Negative nitrogen balance
    ④ Excessive retention of sodium ions

302. Mrs. Simon will be taking digitalis at home. She asks the nurse why this is necessary. The nurse bases the answer on the fact that digitalis:
    ① Slows and strengthens cardiac contractions
    ② Lengthens the refractory phase of the cardiac cycle
    ③ Reduces edema in extracellular spaces
    ④ Increases ventricular contractions

Situation: Mrs. Malone, 48 years old, has discovered a lump in her breast on self-examination. It is fixed, and the physician can aspirate no fluid. She is admitted for a possible right radical mastectomy.

303. A priority of nursing intervention for Mrs. Malone in the preoperative period would be to:
    ① Teach isometric arm exercises
    ② Ascertain how client will adjust to radical mastectomy
    ③ Cleanse operative site with Betadine several times
    ④ Have a representative from Reach to Recovery visit her

304. During her morning care Mrs. Malone tells the nurse that she is worried about what she will look like after the surgery. The nurse's most appropriate *initial* response is:
    ① "Try not to think about the surgery now."
    ② "Why don't you discuss this with your husband?"
    ③ "I can understand that you'd be concerned."
    ④ "Everyone having this surgery feels the same way."

305. After a mastectomy the nurse should position Mrs. Malone's right arm:
    ① In abduction surrounded by sand bags
    ② Lower than the level of the right atrium on pillows
    ③ In adduction supported by sand bags
    ④ With the hand higher than the arm on pillows

306. When teaching Mrs. Malone postmastectomy arm exercises, it is important for the nurse to:
    ① Exercise both arms simultaneously
    ② Exercise the right arm only
    ③ Have Mrs. Malone wear a sling in between exercises
    ④ Wait until the incision has healed

307. Mrs. Malone's physician plans chemotherapy 2 weeks after the surgery. The delay in instituting the plan for drug therapy is because the drugs:
    ① Interfere with cell growth and delay wound healing
    ② Cause vomiting, which endangers the integrity of the large incisional area
    ③ Decrease red blood cell production, and the resultant anemia would add to postoperative fatigue
    ④ Increase edema in areas distal to the incision by blocking lymph channels with destroyed lymphocytes

Situation: Mrs. Clarke, 37 years old, has been complaining of headaches and difficulty with her embroidery. Her BP is elevated and her pupils react sluggishly. She is admitted to the hospital for further evaluation.

308. The finding the nurse would consider unusual when doing an assessment of Mrs. Clarke for increased intracranial pressure is:
① Jacksonian seizures
② Rapid pulse
③ Psychotic behavior
④ Nausea and vomiting

309. Mrs. Clarke's physician writes orders for her. The nurse should question an order which states:
① Administer osmotic diuretic as ordered
② Place the client in a reverse Trendelenburg position
③ Administer steroids as ordered
④ Apply rotating tourniquets

310. The nurse assists the physician in performing a lumbar puncture. When pressure is placed on the jugular vein during a lumbar puncture, there is normally a rise in the spinal fluid pressure. This is referred to as:
① Chvostek's sign
② Romberg's sign
③ Queckenstedt's sign
④ Homan's sign

311. Mrs. Clarke has a tumor of the cerebellum. In view of the functions of this organ, the nurse should expect to observe an:
① Absence of the knee-jerk and other reflexes
② Inability to execute smooth, precise movements
③ Inability to execute voluntary movements
④ Unconsciousness

312. Before preparing Mrs. Clarke for cranial surgery, the nurse should:
① Wash the client's hair with pHisoHex
② Help the client choose a wig
③ Obtain consent for shaving the head
④ Wait to shave the head until the client is anesthetized

313. In caring for Mrs. Clarke postoperatively, the nurse should:
① Take only axillary temperatures
② Encourage coughing but discourage deep breathing
③ Report yellow drainage on dressing to the physician immediately
④ Administer narcotics and sedatives at the first sign of irritability

Situation: Mrs. Janeway is 36 weeks pregnant and is attending a class in preparation for childbirth with her husband.

314. Mrs. Janeway verbalizes, "I am sick and tired of wearing these same old clothes; how I wish all this would be done and over with." The nurse's best response would be:
① "Is there something bothering you? You sound discouraged."
② "Most women feel the same way you do at this time."
③ "I understand how you feel; what do you know about labor?"
④ "Yes, this is the most uncomfortable time during pregnancy."

315. In the preparation for childbirth class the nurse would teach that labor:
① Should be painless and uneventful
② May be uncomfortable, but medication is available when needed

③ Will be painful, but clients will be taught how to tolerate it
④ Will be uncomfortable; however, medication will not be needed

316. Mrs. Janeway is admitted to the labor and delivery unit in extreme discomfort with contractions occurring 3 minutes apart. The nurse realizes that the greatest influence on the perception of pain for a woman in labor is the:
① Difficulty of the labor
② Length of the labor
③ Tension of the client
④ Parity of the client

317. The nurse takes the FHR during a contraction and finds it is 115 per minute. The next nursing action should be to:
① Notify the physician immediately
② Take second reading during decrement
③ Take a second reading during the acme of the next contraction
④ Administer oxygen immediately

318. The nurse knows that Mrs. Janeway has begun the advanced stage of labor when:
① She feels the need to move her bowels
② She complains of sudden intense back pain
③ The cervix is dilated to 6 cm
④ Restlessness and thrashing increase

319. One hour following delivery the nurse finds that Mrs. Janeway's uterus has become boggy. The initial response should be to:
① Notify the physician
② Check the BP
③ Massage it until firm
④ Observe the amount of bleeding

320. Mrs. Janeway has walked to the nursery numerous times to see her baby each day. Two days postpartum she complains of pain in her right leg. The nurse's initial response should be to:
① Encourage ambulation and exercise
② Massage the affected area
③ Apply hot soaks
④ Maintain bed rest and notify the physician

Situation: Mrs. Hosper gives birth to a baby girl with a unilateral cleft lip and palate. The physician recommends that the lip be repaired as soon as possible after birth because the baby is in otherwise good physical condition.

321. Cleft lip is usually repaired early because of:
① Emotional impact on the parents
② Feeding difficulty
③ Infection
④ Obstruction of breathing

322. Mr. and Mrs. Hosper are very concerned about the defect and ask the nurse, "What caused our baby to be born deformed?" The nurse should reply:
① "I don't know, but you don't need to worry because surgery can correct it."
② "I'm glad that you are able to ask these kinds of questions."
③ "Are you feeling guilty?"
④ "It sounds as if you are wondering what you might have done to cause this situation."

323. While informing the parents about the significance and etiology of cleft lip and palate, the nurse should:
    ① Assess the family history for presence of the defect in other siblings or relatives
    ② Emphasize that the two defects follow laws of mendelian genetics
    ③ Prepare the parents for the likelihood of mental and psychologic problems in the child
    ④ Stress that the defect is rare and will probably never happen twice in the same family

324. Before Baby Sarah was born, Mrs. Hosper had wanted to breast-feed. Now feeding will probably be:
    ① With a rubber-tipped syringe or medicine dropper
    ② Too difficult because of breathing problems
    ③ With a soft, large-holed nipple
    ④ IV fluids

325. Sarah's cleft lip predisposes her to infections primarily because of:
    ① Poor nutrition from disturbed feeding
    ② Poor circulation to the defective area
    ③ Mouth breathing, which dries the oropharyngeal mucous membranes
    ④ Waste products that accumulate along the defect

326. Baby Sarah's lip is repaired 4 days after birth. During the postoperative period the nurse should avoid:
    ① Examining the tongue, lips, and mucous membranes for swelling
    ② Placing her on her abdomen to prevent aspiration
    ③ Keeping the suture line clean and free of crusting
    ④ Encouraging the parents to visit as much as possible to prevent the infant from crying

Situation: Carrie Walsh, a 39-year-old primigravida, is admitted to labor and delivery for sonography to determine fetal age, since she appears to be large for her expected date of delivery. She is 36 weeks pregnant, but her uterus is the size expected at 40 weeks.

327. Before the test begins, Mrs. Walsh complains of severe abdominal pain. Her BP drops from 128/80 to 102/60, and her pulse rate increases from 80 to 104. Heavy vaginal bleeding begins with the onset of the pain. The nurse should suspect that Mrs. Walsh has a:
    ① Marginal placenta previa
    ② Complete abruptio placentae
    ③ Vena caval syndrome
    ④ Hydatidiform mole

328. The nurse notifies the physician of Mrs. Walsh's condition and prepares for:
    ① A high forceps delivery
    ② An immediate cesarean section
    ③ The insertion of a fetal monitor
    ④ The administration of oxytocin (Pitocin)

329. Mrs. Walsh is prepared for delivery. Nursing care should include:
    ① An abdominal prep and administration of a Fleet enema
    ② Inserting a Foley catheter and administration of a tap water enema
    ③ Obtaining an informed consent and assessment for drug allergies
    ④ Teaching coughing and deep-breathing techniques

Situation: Miss Louise Monroe, age 62, has a hiatal hernia. She tells the nurse that she wakes up frequently at night with heartburn.

330. The suggestion by the nurse that would be most likely to reduce the symptoms of heartburn is:
    ① Have a light snack of orange juice and crackers at bedtime
    ② Elevate the head of the bed on 6-inch blocks
    ③ Eat the largest meal at noontime
    ④ Take an intestinal sedative, such as hyoscyamine sulfate (Donnatal), at night

331. The physician prescribes a bland diet for Miss Monroe. She asks the nurse about foods that must be avoided on a bland diet. The nurse should instruct her to exclude:
    ① Poached eggs
    ② Roast beef
    ③ Whole wheat bread
    ④ Green beans or peas

332. Miss Monroe tells the nurse that she takes one-half teaspoon of baking soda in a glass of water for heartburn. The nurse suggests that she use an antacid preparation such as aluminum hydroxide (Maalox). This response is based on the fact that antacids:
    ① Cause few side effects such as diarrhea or constipation
    ② Are readily absorbed by the stomach mucosa
    ③ Have no direct effect on systemic acid-base balance
    ④ Contain little if any sodium

333. When teaching Miss Monroe about antacid therapy the nurse should include the fact that:
    ① Antacids should be taken only at 4-hour intervals
    ② Tablets are equally as effective as the liquid forms
    ③ Antacids interfere with the absorption of other drugs
    ④ Antacids should be taken 1 hour before meals

Situation: Mrs. Jones, a 35-year-old mother of four children, is diagnosed as having Cushing's syndrome.

334. In planning her care the nurse should take into consideration the fact that Mrs. Jones would have:
    ① Hypotension and sodium loss
    ② Hyperkalemia and edema
    ③ Muscle weakness and frequent urination
    ④ Muscle wasting and hypoglycemia

335. Mrs. Jones would probably demonstrate:
    ① Lability of mood
    ② Decrease in the growth of hair
    ③ Ectomorphism with a moon face
    ④ Increased resistance to bruising

336. Prior to Mrs. Jones' undergoing an adrenalectomy the nurse should:
    ① Withhold all medications for 48 hours
    ② Administer steroids IM or IV
    ③ Provide a high-protein diet
    ④ Collect a 24-hour urine specimen

337. Postoperatively, prior to maintenance steroid therapy, the nurse should expect to see signs of:
    ① Hyperglycemia
    ② Sodium retention
    ③ Potassium excretion
    ④ Hypotension

338. In teaching Mrs. Jones about her medications, the nurse should plan to emphasize the fact that:

① Once she is regulated, her dosage will remain the same for life

② Taking her medications late in the evening may cause sleeplessness

③ While she is taking medications, her salt intake may have to be restricted

④ Steroid therapy will be given in conjunction with insulin

339. Mrs. Jones is very upset after visiting hours. She tearfully tells the nurse that her 4-year-old son is being admitted to the hospital in the morning for a tonsilectomy. After quieting Mrs. Jones, the nurse notifies the physician, since Mrs. Jones:

① Will probably require mild sedation to ensure her rest

② Should have her steroid medication dosage reduced

③ Has a decreased ability to handle stress despite steroid therapy

④ Will have feelings of exhaustion and lethargy as a result of stress

340. Mrs. Jones is being discharged. In response to her question the nurse explains to Mrs. Jones that her therapy includes a low-sodium, high-potassium diet because:

① Excessive secretions of aldosterone and cortisone cause renal retention of sodium and loss of potassium

② Her use of salt had probably contributed to her disease

③ She is losing excess salt in her urine and requires less renal stimulation

④ She will gain excessive weight if sodium is not limited

341. After discharge Mrs. Jones begins to manifest signs of diabetes mellitus. The nurse recognizes that diabetes mellitus may develop because:

① The cortical hormones created a too rapid weight loss

② The excessive glucocorticoids secreted by the adrenal gland caused excessive tissue catabolism and gluconeogenesis

③ A negative nitrogen balance resulted from the tissue catabolism

④ The excessive ACTH damaged pancreatic tissue

Situation: Two-year-old Alex Kerr is being admitted to the hospital early in the morning for a circumcision because of phimosis.

342. Alex is being prepared for surgery. As the nurse enters his room with a preoperative injection, he begins to scream and flail about the bed. His father is sitting at his bedside and gets up to leave. The nurse's best response to this situation is to:

① Leave the room and ask another nurse to come in to hold Alex during the injection

② Allow Alex to say goodbye to his father before giving the injection

③ Tell Mr. Kerr he can return to comfort Alex after the injection is given

④ Ask Mr. Kerr to stay to comfort and hold Alex while the injection is given

343. Attendance of parents during painful procedures on their children should be:

① Based on the type of procedure to be performed

② Encouraged and permitted if the child desires their presence

③ Based on individual assessment of the parents

④ Discouraged for the benefit of the parents and the child

344. The gluteal muscle is generally not used when giving IM injections to infants and young children because they:

① Fear intrusive procedures

② Are able to wiggle and change position when placed on their abdomen

③ Have an undeveloped muscle mass in this area

④ Associate this area with punishment

345. A major nursing responsibility in caring for Alex postoperatively is to:

① Limit oral fluids

② Monitor IV fluids carefully

③ Apply ice packs to the penis

④ Observe for bleeding at the operative site

Situation: Mr. Jay is admitted to the psychiatric service by his parents, who can no longer deal with him. He is a handsome, smooth-talking, bright young man who has been married three times and has a child by each wife. He states he has never loved any of his wives, does not intend to support his children, and has no reason to be sorry for anything he has ever done.

346. The nurse would expect Mr. Jay's behavior to demonstrate a defect in:

① Id development

② Ego development

③ Superego development

④ Sexual development

347. In working with Mr. Jay the nurse should be:

① Sincere, cautious, and consistent

② Strict, punishing, and restrictive

③ Accepting, supportive, and friendly

④ Sympathetic, motherly, and encouraging

348. Mrs. Jones, one of the nurses, is taking a new client on an orientation tour of the unit when Mr. Jay rushes down the hallway and asks her to sit and talk to him. The nurse should:

① Excuse herself from the new client and speak with Mr. Jay

② Suggest to Mr. Jay that he talk with another staff member

③ Introduce Mr. Jay and suggest that he join them on the tour

④ Tell Mr. Jay that she will speak to him later

349. Mr. Jay responds by smiling broadly and saying, "Mrs. Jones you sure do look messy today." The most appropriate response by the nurse would be:

① "That's not a nice thing to say, Mr. Jay."

② "Don't you feel well today, Mr. Jay?"

③ "I didn't get a chance to set my hair last night."

④ "You're angry with me, Mr. Jay."

350. Mr. Jay takes Mrs. Jones by the shoulder, suddenly kisses her, and shouts "I like you." The most appropriate response would be:

① "I like you too but please don't do that again."

② "I wish you wouldn't do that."

③ "Don't ever touch me like that again."

④ "Thank you, I like you too."

351. Mr. Jay has just been given his first day pass from the hospital. He is due to return at 6 PM. At 5 PM Mr. Jay telephones the nurse in charge of the ward and says, "Six o'clock is too early. I feel like coming back at 7:30." The nurse would be most therapeutic by telling him to:
    ① Return immediately, to demonstrate control
    ② Return on time or he will be restricted
    ③ Come back by 6:45, as a compromise to set limits
    ④ Come back as soon as he can or the police will be sent

352. Mrs. Jones is leaving in 2 weeks and tells Mr. Jay. Mrs. Jones would recognize that he is progressing in his ability to maintain more mature relationships if he:
    ① Tells her that he must get well enough by then so that he may also leave
    ② Wishes her good luck and thanks her for helping him
    ③ Tells her that her leaving is just another loss he must adjust to
    ④ Informs her that, since she is leaving, this should be their last meeting

Situation: Mr. Walter is admitted to the psychiatric unit with a diagnosis of paranoid schizophrenia.

353. During the admission procedure Mr. Walter appears to be responding to voices. He cries out at intervals, "No, no, I didn't kill him," and states, "You know the truth, tell that policeman. Please help me!" The nurse should:
    ① Respond by saying, "Mr. Walter, I want to help you and I realize you must be very frightened."
    ② Sit there quietly and not respond at all to his statements
    ③ Respond by saying, "Whom are they saying you killed, Mr. Walter?"
    ④ Respond by saying, "Mr. Walter, do not become so upset. No one is talking to you; we are alone. This is part of your illness."

354. Mr. Walter has delusions that his food is poisoned and he refuses to eat. The nurse tells him that it is foolish for him to believe that, since his food comes from the same kitchen as for all other clients. The nurse states, "Unless you eat, you will have to be fed by other means." This response indicates that:
    ① Mr. Walter needs nourishment and therefore has to eat
    ② Mr. Walter's misinterpretations have to be corrected
    ③ Mr. Walter has to be reminded about needing to eat
    ④ The nurse really does not know how to handle the situation

355. One evening the nurse finds Mr. Walter trying to leave the unit. He says, "Please let me go. I trust you. The Mafia are going to kill me tonight." The nurse should respond:
    ① "Nobody here wants to harm you, you know that. I'll come with you to your room."
    ② "Mr. Walter, you are frightened. Come with me to your room and we can talk about it."
    ③ "Thank you for trusting me, Mr. Walter. Maybe you can trust me when I tell you no one can kill you while you're here."
    ④ "Come with me to your room. I'll lock the door and no one will get to you to hurt you."

356. In caring for Mr. Walter, whose behavior is characterized by pathologic suspicion, one of the goals of nursing care should be to:
    ① Help him realize suspicions are unrealistic
    ② Remove as much environmental stress as possible
    ③ Help him to feel accepted
    ④ Ask him to explain the reasons for his feelings

357. The nurse has been observing Mr. Walter for some time. He is quite delusional, talking about people who are out to get him. Staff notices he is pacing more than usual. One afternoon the nurse decides that Mr. Walter is beginning to lose control of himself. The best nursing intervention would be to:
    ① Allow him to use a punching bag
    ② Move him to a quiet place on the unit
    ③ Allow him to continue pacing
    ④ Suggest that he sit down for a while

358. Mr. Walter is receiving large doses of chlorpromazine (Thorazine) and the nurse is concerned, since the phenothiazine derivatives produce a wide variety of untoward side effects. The nurse should hold the drug if he exhibits:
    ① Masklike facies
    ② Blurred vision
    ③ Edema
    ④ Jaundice

359. Mr. Walter tells the nurse that he used to believe that he was God, but now he knows that this is not true. The nurse's best response would be:
    ① "You really believed that?"
    ② "You must be getting well."
    ③ "What caused you to think you were God?"
    ④ "Many people have this delusion."

360. Mr. Walter is to be discharged with orders for chlorpromazine therapy. In developing a teaching plan for discharge the nurse should include cautioning Mr. Walter against:
    ① Taking medications containing aspirin
    ② Staying in the sun
    ③ Driving at night
    ④ Ingesting wines and cheeses

Situation: Virginia Wills, age 36, visits her gynecologist to confirm a suspected pregnancy.

361. During the nursing history Mrs. Wills states that her last menstrual period began on April 11. She experienced some spotting on May 8. The nurse calculates Mrs. Wills' due date as:
    ① January 10
    ② January 18
    ③ February 12
    ④ February 15

362. The change in the hematologic system which is expected during the first trimester of pregnancy is:
    ① A decrease in sedimentation rate
    ② An increase in blood volume
    ③ A decrease in WBCs
    ④ An increase in hematocrit

363. Mrs. Wills is concerned about Down's syndrome. An amniocentesis is performed during the sixteenth week of gestation. Examination of the amniotic fluid will also provide information regarding which of the following:

① Fetal lung maturity
② Cardiac anomalies
③ Development of neural tube defects
④ Fetal diabetes

364. During the fifth month Mrs. Wills arrives for her appointment and begins to cry as she tells the nurse that her husband wants to have intercourse at least three times per week. The nurse's most appropriate response would be:
① "Intercourse is permitted during your pregnancy."
② "Have you talked with your husband about this?"
③ "I can see you're concerned; what's bothering you the most?"
④ "Have you and your husband spoken about this to the physician?"

Situation: George Brown, 4 years old, is admitted to the hospital with multiple bruises and a dislocated shoulder. Child abuse is suspected.

365. In many states, failure by the nurse to report a suspected case of child abuse is punishable by law. Child abuse is one of the major causes of death in young children. When a child is admitted to the hospital with traumatic injuries, a common clue that the child was battered is that he:
① Cries for longer periods and has large hematomas
② Ignores offers of toys and favors and cries when picked up
③ Shows no expectation of being comforted
④ Does not cry during painful procedures

366. There are many common reactions of parents who batter their children. One reaction the nurse should be aware of is that the parents:
① Seldom touch or look at the child
② Show signs of guilt about the child's injury
③ Are quick to inquire about the discharge date
④ Are very concerned about their own physical health

367. Another behavior that is most typical of the parents of the battered child is that they:
① Present many details related to how the trauma occurred
② Show concern about the child's medical condition
③ Become irritable about having the history taken
④ Give contradictory explanations about what happened

Situation: Miss Jean Bradley is admitted to the hospital for a thyroidectomy. She is 27 years old, and the physical assessment reveals no other health problems.

368. Immediately after Miss Bradley's surgery the nurse should be especially observant for:
① Signs of restlessness
② Increased BP
③ Urinary retention
④ Signs of respiratory obstruction

369. Nerve injury can occur as a result of the trauma of surgery. When assessing for this complication, the nurse should evaluate Miss Bradley's ability to:
① Swallow
② Purse her lips
③ Turn her head
④ Speak

370. On the first postoperative day Miss Bradley tolerates a full fluid diet. This is changed to soft on the second postoperative day. She then complains of a sore throat when swallowing. The nurse should:
① Reorder the full fluid diet
② Notify the physician immediately
③ Administer analgesics as prescribed prior to meals
④ Provide a humidifier to moisten the mucous membranes

Situation: Twenty-year-old Jimmy Barbino is involved in a motorcycle accident and sustains a cervical fracture. To maintain cervical immobilization, he is placed in Crutchfield tongs and on a CircOlectric bed.

371. In providing care the nurse should:
① Keep a roll behind the client's neck to provide support
② Provide for urinary elimination when in the prone position
③ Keep sand bags on each side of the head to keep it immobile
④ Monitor the vital signs before and after turning the client

372. The plan for Jimmy's care is based on the nurse's awareness that:
① Two people must be present when turning the bed
② The client is rotated from side to side to prevent decubiti
③ A receptacle for elimination is easily accessible
④ Postural hypotension after prolonged bed rest can be prevented

373. In caring for Jimmy, the nurse should:
① Avoid the cervical spine area when administering back care
② Clean the area around the tongs daily and apply antibiotic ointment
③ Relieve tension on the tongs for 5 minutes every hour
④ Remove the weights from tongs prior to rotating the CircOlectric bed

374. Jimmy asks the nurse how long it will take before he can walk out of the hospital. The nurse's reply is based on the knowledge that destroyed nerve fibers in the brain or spinal cord do not regenerate because they lack:
① A myelin sheath
② A neurilemma
③ Nissl bodies
④ Nuclei

375. Crushing of the spinal cord above the level of phrenic nerve origin will have significance for the nurse because it will result in:
① Ventricular fibrillation
② Dysfunction of the vagus nerve
③ Retention of sensation but paralysis of the lower extremities
④ Respiratory paralysis and cessation of diaphragmatic contractions

Bibliography

MEDICAL-SURGICAL NURSING

Andreoli KG: Comprehensive cardiac care: a text for nurses, physicians, and other health practitioners, ed 6, St. Louis, 1987, The CV Mosby Co.

Anthony CP and Thibodeau GA: Textbook of anatomy and physiology, ed 13, St. Louis, 1990, The CV Mosby Co.

Berne RM and Levy MN, editors: Physiology, St. Louis, 1983, The CV Mosby Co.

Berne RM and Levy MN: Cardiovascular physiology, ed 5, St. Louis, 1986, The CV Mosby Co.

Billings DM and Stokes LG: Medical-surgical approaches throughout the life cycle, ed 2, St. Louis, 1987, The CV Mosby Co.

Bowers AC and Thompson JM: Clinical manual of health assessment, ed 3, St. Louis, 1988, The CV Mosby Co.

Broadwell DC and Jackson BS: Principles of ostomy care, St. Louis, 1982, The CV Mosby Co.

Brooks Tighe SM: Instrumentation for the operating room, ed 3, St. Louis, 1989, The CV Mosby Co.

Budassi SA and Barber J: Mosby's manual of emergency care: practices and procedures, ed 2, St. Louis, 1984, The CV Mosby Co.

Byrne CJ, Saxton DF, Pelikan PK and Nugent PM: Laboratory tests: implications for nursing care, ed 2, Menlo Park, Calif, 1986, Addison-Wesley, Inc.

Canobbio M: Nursing care of patients with cardiovascular disorders, St. Louis, 1990, The CV Mosby Co.

Christensen PJ and Kenney JW: Nursing process, ed 3, St. Louis, 1990, The CV Mosby Co.

Clark JB et al.: Pharmacological basis of nursing practice, ed 3, St. Louis, 1990, The CV Mosby Co.

Conover MB: Understanding electrocardiography, ed 5, St. Louis, 1988, The CV Mosby Co.

Daily EK and Schroeder JS: Techniques in bedside hemodynamic monitoring, ed 4, St. Louis, 1989, The CV Mosby Co.

Ebersole P and Hess P: Toward healthy aging: human needs and nursing response, ed 3, St. Louis, 1990, The CV Mosby Co.

Estes NJ and Heinemann ME: Alcoholism: development, consequences, and interventions, ed 3, St. Louis, 1986, The CV Mosby Co.

Gahart BL: Intravenous medications, ed 5, St. Louis, 1989, The CV Mosby Co.

Given BA and Simmons SJ: Gastroenterology in clinical nursing, ed 4, St. Louis, 1983, The CV Mosby Co.

Groer ME and Shekleton ME: Basic pathophysiology; a conceptual approach, ed 3, St. Louis, 1989, The CV Mosby Co.

Gruendemann BJ and Meeker MH: Alexander's care of the patient in surgery, ed 8, St. Louis, 1987, The CV Mosby Co.

Holloway NM: Nursing the critically ill adult, ed 2, Menlo Park, Calif, 1984, Addison-Wesley, Inc.

Johanson BC et al.: Standards for critical care, ed 3, St. Louis, 1988, The CV Mosby Co.

Kozier BB and Erb GL: Fundamentals of nursing: concepts and procedures, ed 3, Menlo Park, Calif, 1987, Addison-Wesley, Inc.

Long BC and Phipps WJ: Medical-surgical nursing, ed 2, St. Louis, 1989, The CV Mosby Co.

Malasanos L et al.: Health assessment, ed 4, St. Louis, 1989, The CV Mosby Co.

Marriott HJL and Conover MHB: Advanced concepts in arrhythmias, ed 2, St. Louis, 1989, The CV Mosby Co.

McHenry LM and Salerno E: Mosby's pharmacology in nursing, ed 17, St. Louis, 1989, The CV Mosby Co.

Pagana KD and Pagana TJ: Diagnostic testing and nursing implications: a case study approach, ed 2, St. Louis, 1986, The CV Mosby Co.

Perry AG and Potter PA: Clinical nursing skills and techniques, ed 2, St. Louis, 1990, The CV Mosby Co.

Phipps WJ et al.: Medical-surgical nursing: concepts and clinical practice, ed 3, St. Louis, 1987, The CV Mosby Co.

Potter PA and Perry AG: Fundamentals of nursing, ed 2, St. Louis, 1989, The CV Mosby Co.

Redman BK: The process of patient education, ed 6, St. Louis, 1988, The CV Mosby Co.

Saxton DF and Ercolano-O'Neill N: Basic mathmatics and calculation of drugs and solutions, St. Louis, 1986, The CV Mosby Co.

Sundeen SJ et al.: Nurse-client interaction: implementing the nursing process, ed 4, St. Louis, 1989, The CV Mosby Co.

Thompson JM et al.: Mosby's manual of clinical nursing, ed 2, St. Louis, 1989, The CV Mosby Co.

Tilkian SM et al.: Clinical implications of laboratory tests, ed 4, St. Louis, 1987, The CV Mosby Co.

Tucker SM et al.: Patient care standards, ed 4, St. Louis, 1988, The CV Mosby Co.

Vinsant-Crawford MO and Spence MI: Commonsense approach to coronary care, ed 5, St. Louis, 1988, The CV Mosby Co.

Weldy NJ: Body fluids and electrolytes, ed 5, St. Louis, 1988, The CV Mosby Co.

Wilkins RO, Sheldon RL, and Krider SJ: Clinical assessment in respiratory care, ed 2, St. Louis, 1990, The CV Mosby Co.

Williams SR: Nutrition and diet therapy, ed 6, St. Louis, 1989, The CV Mosby Co.

Woods NF: Human sexuality in health and illness, ed 3, St. Louis, 1984, The CV Mosby Co.

PSYCHIATRIC NURSING

Aguilera DC and Messick JM: Crisis intervention: theory and methodology, ed 5, St. Louis, 1986, The CV Mosby Co.

American Psychiatric Association: Diagnostic and statistical manual of mental disorders, ed 3 (revised), Washington, D.C., 1987, The Association.

Beck CM et al.: Mental health-psychiatric nursing: a holistic life-cycle approach, ed 2, St. Louis, 1988, The CV Mosby Co.

Estes NJ and Heinemann E: Alcoholism: development, consequences, and interventions, ed 3, St. Louis, 1986, The CV Mosby Co.

Gorton J and Partridge R: Practice and management of psychiatric emergency care, St. Louis, 1982, The CV Mosby Co.

Haber J et al.: Comprehensive psychiatric nursing, ed 3, New York, 1989, McGraw-Hill, Inc.

Pasquali EA et al.: Mental health nursing: a holistic approach, ed 3, St. Louis, 1989, The CV Mosby Co.

Saxton DF and Haring PW: Care of patients with emotional problems, ed 4, St. Louis, 1984, The CV Mosby Co.

Stuart GW and Sundeen SJ: Principles and practice of psychiatric nursing, ed 3, St. Louis, 1987, The CV Mosby Co.

Sundeen SJ et al.: Nurse-client interaction, ed 4, St. Louis, 1989, The CV Mosby Co.

Taylor CM: Mereness' essentials of psychiatric nursing, ed 12, St. Louis, 1986, The CV Mosby Co.

Wilson HS and Kneisl CR: Psychiatric nursing, ed 3, Menlo Park, Calif, 1987, Addison-Wesley, Inc.

PEDIATRIC NURSING

Betz CL and Poster E: Mosby's pediatric nursing reference, St. Louis, 1989, The CV Mosby Co.

Engel JK: Pocket guide to pediatric assessment, St. Louis, 1989, The CV Mosby Co.

Hazinski MF: Pediatric critical care: a nursing perspective, St. Louis, 1984, The CV Mosby Co.

Korones SB: High-risk newborn infants: the basis for intensive nursing care, ed 4, 1986, The CV Mosby Co.

Merenstein GB and Gardner SL: Handbook of neonatal intensive care, ed 2, St. Louis, 1989, The CV Mosby Co.

Nelson NP and Beckel J: Nursing care plans for the pediatric patient, St. Louis, 1987, The CV Mosby Co.

Pipes PL: Nutrition in infancy and childhood, ed 4, St. Louis, 1988, The CV Mosby Co.

Sammons WAH and Lewis JM: Premature babies: a different beginning, St. Louis, 1985, The CV Mosby Co.

Scipien GM et al.: Comprehensive pediatric nursing, ed 3, New York, 1984, McGraw-Hill, Inc.

Whaley LF and Wong DL: Nursing care of infants and children, ed 3, St. Louis, 1987, The CV Mosby Co.

Whaley LF and Wong DL: Essentials of pediatric nursing, ed 3, St. Louis, 1989, The CV Mosby Co.

Wong DL and Whaley LF: Clinical handbook of pediatric nursing, ed 2, St. Louis, 1986, The CV Mosby Co.

MATERNITY NURSING

Bobak IM and Jensen MD: Essentials of maternity nursing, ed 2, St. Louis, 1987, The CV Mosby Co.

Bobak IM, Jensen MD, and Zalar MK: Maternity and gynecologic care, ed 4, St. Louis, 1989, The CV Mosby Co.

Gilbert ES and Harmon JS: High-risk pregnancy and delivery, St. Louis, 1986, The CV Mosby Co.

Klaus MH and Kennell JH: Parent infant bonding, ed 2, St. Louis, 1982, The CV Mosby Co.

Lawrence RA: Breastfeeding: a guide for the medical profession, ed 3, St. Louis, 1990, The CV Mosby Co.

Olds SB et al.: Obstetric nursing, ed 3, Menlo Park, Calif, 1987, Addison-Wesley, Inc.

Phillips CR: Family-centered maternity-newborn care: a basic text, ed 2, St. Louis, 1987, The CV Mosby Co.

Reeder SR, Mastroianni ML and Fitzpatrick E: Maternity nursing, ed 16, Philadelphia, 1987, JB Lippincott Co.

Riordan J: A practical guide to breastfeeding, St. Louis, 1983, The CV Mosby Co.

Tucker SM: Pocket nurse guide to fetal monitoring, St. Louis, 1988, The CV Mosby Co.

Weiner S: Clinical manual of maternity and gynecologic nursing, St. Louis, 1989, The CV Mosby Co.

Williams SR and Worthington-Roberts B: Nutrition in pregnancy and lactation, ed 4, St. Louis, 1990, The CV Mosby Co.

Woods NF: Human sexuality in health and illness, ed 3, St. Louis, 1984, The CV Mosby Co.

ANSWERS AND RATIONALES FOR CHAPTER REVIEW QUESTIONS

Letters indicating the difficulty of the questions appear next to the answers. The letter *a* signifies that more than 75% of the students answering the question answered it correctly; *b* signifies that between 50% and 75% of the students answering the question answered it correctly; and *c* signifies that between 25% and 50% of the students answering the question were correct.

Chapter 3: Medical-Surgical Nursing

1. **3** Painless enlargement of the cervical lymph nodes is often the first sign of Hodgkin's disease, a malignant lymphoma of unknown etiology. (c)
   1 Inguinal enlargement occurs later.
   2 Axillary enlargement occurs after cervical.
   4 Mediastinal involvement follows after the disease progresses.
2. **2** For reasons unknown, Hodgkin's disease occurs most frequently between 15 and 30 years of age. (b)
   1 Less common in children.
   3 Uncommon during middle years.
   4 Uncommon in later years.
3. **2** Radiation exposure may lead to depression of the bone marrow, with subsequent insufficient WBCs to combat infection. (b)
   1 Red cell production is decreased by radiation.
   3 Bone structure is not affected by treatment; pathologic fractures may occur in response to disease.
   4 There is no increase in the number of cells; therefore viscosity is not increased.
4. **1** Depression of the bone marrow interferes with hemopoiesis and results in anemia. (a)
   2 Radiation causes increased susceptibility to infection as a result of the decreased number of white blood cells.
   3 Pathologic fractures result from the disease, not the treatment.
   4 There is a decrease in the number of cells and therefore a decrease in viscosity.
5. **3** Radiation in controlled doses is therapeutic. When uncontrolled or in excessive amounts, it is carcinogenic. (a)
   1 Therapeutic doses are helpful in whatever areas are being treated.
   2 Nutritional status of the cells does not influence radiation's effect.
   4 Physical status does not affect the outcome of radiation therapy.
6. **4** A paradoxical response to a drug is directly opposite the desired therapeutic response. (c)
   1 This response involves drug combinations that enhance each other.
   2 A response to a drug that is more pronounced than the response observed in most of the population.
   3 An allergic response induces an allergen-antibody reaction.
7. **2** Many antihypertensive agents lower peripheral vascular resistance and may cause orthostatic hypotension. Therefore blood pressure should be monitored in both a supine and an upright position. (c)

1 This is too short a time for determination of the drug's effect.
   3 Change in position causes hypotension; when a position has been maintained for 5 minutes, the blood pressure has probably stabilized.
   4 Assessment prior to administration will not yield information related to effectiveness.
8. **4** Hypokalemia causes a flattening of the T wave of the ECG because of its effect on muscle function. (c)
   1 Hypokalemia widens the QRS complex.
   2 Hypokalemia depresses the ST segment.
   3 Hypokalemia does not deflect the Q wave.
9. **2** Potassium follows insulin into the cells of the body, thereby raising the cellular potassium and preventing fatal arrhythmias. (c)
   1 Potassium is not excreted as a result of this therapy; it shifts into the intracellular compartment.
   3 The potassium level has no effect on pancreatic insulin production.
   4 Insulin does not cause excretion of these substances.
10. **4** Methyldopa decreases tissue concentrations of norepinephrine and interferes with its release in response to sympathetic stimulation. Therefore the vasoconstriction caused by norepinephrine is inhibited. (c)
   1 Does not cause vasodilation.
   2 Does not affect adrenal release of epinephrine.
   3 Does not stimulate histamine release.
11. **4** Sitting on the edge of the bed before getting up is recommended because it gives the body a chance to adjust to the effects of gravity on circulation in the upright position. (b)
   1 This would not prevent episodes of orthostatic hypotension.
   2 Energetic tasks do not increase hypotension.
   3 Support hose would not be worn continuously and would not prevent hypotension.
12. **4** Unexpressed rage or anger affects the sympathetic nervous system, precipitating the release of epinephrine and norepinephrine, constricting the blood vessels, and thus raising arterial blood pressure. (b)
   1 May contribute; not the primary cause.
   2 May contribute; not the primary cause.
   3 Although the renin-angiotensin mechanism may contribute, kidney failure is not the primary cause of essential hypertension.
13. **2** If there is a decrease in urinary output with increased conservation of body fluid, the blood pressure will be increased and vice versa. (c)
   1 This may cause a short-term increase but does not have a long-term effect.
   3 These cause a rapid response; short-term effect.
   4 These cause a rapid response; short-term effect.
14. **1** Because propranolol (Inderal) competes with catecholamines at the beta-adrenergic receptor sites, the normal increase in heart rate and contractility in response to exercise does not occur. This, combined with the drug's hypotensive effect, may lead to dizziness. (c)
   2 Rapid systemic side effects do not occur with this drug.
   3 The drug does not increase heart rate.
   4 Rapid, systemic side effects do not occur.
15. **1** Adams-Stokes syndrome is a result of complete atrioventricular block. The ventricles take over the pacemaker function in the heart, but at a much slower rate than that of the SA node. As a result there is decreased cerebral circulation, causing syncope. (a)
   2 These are symptoms of a cerebrovascular accident.

3 These symptoms are unrelated to Adams-Stokes.

4 These do not occur with the Adams-Stokes syndrome.

16. **4** Both ventricular fibrillation and ventricular standstill are death-producing arrhythmias because the heart is not functioning as a pump. Immediate action is required or death will occur as a result of anoxia to the brain and other vital organs. (a)

   1 Not a lethal arrhythmia.

   2 Similar to atrial fibrillation and not lethal.

   3 May require intervention and insertion of a pacemaker but not lethal.

17. **1** Functioning pacemakers initiate impulses when the client's pulse rate falls below the preset rate. (b)

   2 The client's heart may still be irregular.

   3 The pacemaker affects the rate, not the volume of the pulse.

   4 The client's heart rate may exceed the pacemaker.

18. **4** Pulse pressure is obtained by subtracting the diastolic from the systolic readings after the blood pressure has been recorded. (a)

   1 This is not pulse pressure; it is pulse deficit.

   2 This is only a partial factor in determining pulse pressure; it is not the pulse pressure itself.

   3 This is not pulse pressure.

19. **1** Shock may have different etiologies (e.g., hypovolemic, cardiogenic, septic, anaphylactic) but always involves a drop in blood pressure and failure of the peripheral circulation because of sympathetic nervous system involvement. (b)

   2 Shock can be reversed by the administration of fluids, plasma expanders, and vasoconstrictors.

   3 Hypovolemia is only one cause; shock may also be septic, cardiogenic, or anaphylactic; always involves a drop in blood pressure.

   4 It may be a reaction to tissue injury but has many different etiologies (e.g., hypovolemia, sepsis, anaphylaxis).

20. **1** Adrenalin is used to treat shock because the induced arterial constriction reduces blood pooling (vessels cannot hold as much blood) and increases venous return and cardiac output. (c)

   2 Tourniquets constrict veins of the extremities, reduce venous return.

   3 A sympathectomy interferes with autonomic vasoconstriction; reduces venous return.

   4 Digoxin slows and strengthens the heartbeat; does not cause vasoconstriction.

21. **3** The vessels branching from the circle of Willis provide excellent collateral circulation for the brain; partial blockage of one vessel is compensated by flow through other vessels. (b)

   1 This is not collateral circulation.

   2 This is not collateral circulation.

   4 These take blood away from the brain.

22. **4** Polycythemia vera results in pathologically high concentrations of erythrocytes in the blood; increased viscosity increases the tendency toward thrombosis. (b)

   1 Hypertension is usually related to narrowing or sclerosing of arteries, not to increased number of blood cells.

   2 There is an increased number of RBCs in polycythemia; their immaturity is not related to the increased viscosity.

   3 The fragility of blood cells does not affect the viscosity of the blood.

23. **1** Viscosity, a measure of a fluid's internal resistance to flow, is increased as the number of red cells suspended in plasma increases. (a)

2 Number of cells does not affect the blood pH.

3 RBCs do not affect immunity.

4 The hematocrit would be higher.

24. **1** Desired anticoagulant effect is achieved when the accelerated partial thromboplastin time is 1.5 to 2 times normal. (b)

   2 Does not affect viscosity.

   3 While absence of bleeding is an indication that the drug has not reached toxic levels, it is not an indication of its effectiveness.

   4 Weakness and confusion are not related to anticoagulant therapy.

25. **2** After removal of an arterial obstruction by endarterectomy, adequate circulation may be monitored by observation of skin color, pulses, and skin temperature. (b)

   1 Bowel habits would not be altered after surgery.

   3 Turgor would be affected by changes in hydration.

   4 Appetite does not change as a result of vascular surgery.

26. **4** Blood albumin, a protein, establishes the plasma colloid osmotic pressure because of its high molecular weight and size, which helps prevent cerebral edema postoperatively. (b)

   1 Red cell formation (erythropoiesis) occurs in red marrow and can be related to albumin only indirectly; albumin is the blood transport protein for thyroxin, which stimulates metabolism in all cells, including those in red bone marrow.

   2 Albumin does not activate WBCs; white blood cells are activated by antigens and substances released from damaged or diseased cells.

   3 Blood clotting involves blood protein fractions other than albumin; for example, prothrombin and fibrinogen are within the alpha and beta globulin fractions.

27. **2** Plasma proteins do not easily pass through the capillary endothelium; however, the slight leakage through the capillary endothelium is important and results in edema if not corrected (one of the lymphatic system's functions is to return "leaked" plasma proteins to the blood). (a)

   1 Oxygen and carbon dioxide pass through capillary endothelium easily.

   3 Glucose, oxygen, and carbon dioxide pass through the capillary endothelium easily.

   4 Ions, amino acids, and water pass through the capillary endothelium easily.

28. **3** Because furosemide (Lasix) and aspirin compete for the same renal excretory sites, salicylate toxicity may occur even with lower dosages. (c)

   1 This response does not take into account the other drug that the client is receiving.

   2 Although furosemide has a uricosemic effect similar to that of the thiazide diuretics, it is not potentiated by aspirin.

   4 Aspirin does not affect the metabolism of Lasix.

29. **1** Congestive heart failure is the failure of the heart to pump adequately to meet the needs of the body, resulting in a backward buildup of pressure in the venous system. Adaptations by the body include edema, ascites, hepatomegaly, tachycardia, dyspnea, and fatigue. (a)

   2 These symptoms might be indicative of coronary insufficiency or infarction.

   3 These symptoms are generally not related to a specific disorder.

   4 This vague complaint is not specific to CHF; it might be indicative of a variety of pulmonary conditions.

30. **2** Right-sided heart failure causes increased pressure in the systemic venous system, which leads to a fluid shift into the interstitial spaces. Because of gravity, the lower extremities are first affected in an ambulatory client. (b)
    1 Pulmonary edema results in severe respiratory distress and peripheral edema.
    3 Myocardial infarction itself does not cause peripheral edema.
    4 Pulmonary disease would not result in varying degrees of edema.

31. **4** In right-sided heart failure blood backs up in the systemic capillary beds; the increase in plasma hydrostatic pressure shifts fluid from the intravascular compartment to the interstitial spaces, causing edema. (b)
    1 This would occur with crushing injuries or if proteins were pathologically shifting from the intravascular compartment to the interstitial spaces.
    2 Increased fluid pressures within the tissue would result in fluid shifts into the intravascular compartment.
    3 Although a decrease in colloid osmotic pressure can cause edema, it is due to lack of protein intake, not increased hydrostatic pressure associated with right-sided heart failure.

32. **3** Measuring an area is an objective assessment and is not subject to individual interpretations. (b)
    1 Assessing for pitting is a subjective technique.
    2 Although assessing fluid balance by weighing a client is important, it does not determine the degree of edema in a specific extremity.
    4 Although monitoring the intake and output helps in assessing fluid balance, it does not determine the degree of edema in a specific extremity.

33. **1** Failure of the right ventricle causes an increase in pressure in the systemic circulation. To equalize this pressure, fluid moves into the tissues, causing edema, and into the abdominal cavity, causing ascites. (c)
    2 The opposite results when there is an increase in hydrostatic pressure.
    3 Ascites is the accumulation of fluid in an extracellular space, not intracellular.
    4 There is no loss of cellular constituents of blood in right-sided heart failure.

34. **3** The CVP is a measure of the pressure within the right atrium. For an accurate reading the zero point must be level with the right atrium. This is at approximately the midaxillary line. (a)
    1 A high reading is indicative of circulatory overload.
    2 A normal CVP reading ranges from approximately 2 to 8 mm Hg.
    4 The client must be supine when the reading is taken.

35. **4** Buerger's disease (thromboangiitis obliterans) is characterized by vascular inflammation, usually in the lower extremities, leading to thrombus formation. As a result of impaired circulation, there is burning pain and intermittent claudication. (a)
    1 These symptoms are not related to thromboangiitis obliterans.
    2 These symptoms are not related to thromboangiitis obliterans.
    3 These symptoms are not related to thromboangiitis obliterans.

36. **2** Constriction of the peripheral blood vessels and the resulting increase in blood pressure impair circulation and limit the amount of oxygen being delivered to body cells, particularly in the extremities. (a)
    1 Nicotine constricts rather than dilates peripheral vessels.

3 Nicotine constricts rather than dilates peripheral vessels.
4 Nicotine constricts all peripheral vessels, not just superficial ones; its primary action is to cause spasm; will not dilate deep vessels.

37. **4** Injured tissue cannot heal properly because of cellular deprivation of oxygen and nutrients; ulceration and gangrene may result; diminished sensation decreases awareness of injury. (b)
    1 Poor hygiene is only one stress that may cause tissue trauma; not an inclusive answer.
    2 Caffeine stimulates the cerebral cortex; does not contribute to ulceration or deprivation of oxygen.
    3 Emotional stress does not cause tissue injury; however, because of vasoconstriction, it may prolong healing.

38. **3** Relaxation of muscles and facial expression are examples of nonverbal behavior; nonverbal behavior is a better index of feelings because it is less likely to be consciously controlled. (b)
    1 Increased activity may be an expression of anger or hostility.
    2 Clients may suppress verbal outbursts despite feelings and become withdrawn.
    4 Refusing to talk may be a sign that the client is just not ready to discuss feelings.

39. **2** The sympathectomy causes dilatation of the blood vessels in the lower extremities; the resulting shift in the fixed blood volume lowers systemic blood pressure. (c)
    1 While anesthesia depresses vital signs, generally there is not a sudden drop in BP postoperatively.
    3 Fluid losses associated with surgery may gradually lower BP and are compensated by endocrine and renal compensatory mechanisms.
    4 Epinephrine would increase BP by stimulating cardiac contractility.

40. **1** Myocardial infarction (MI) may cause increased irritability of tissue or interruption of normal transmission of impulses. Arrhythmias occur in about 90% of clients after MI. (b)
    2 Anaphylactic shock is due to an allergic reaction, not to MI.
    3 Cardiac enlargement is a slow process and is not a complication that can be observed.
    4 Hypokalemia may result when clients are taking cardiac glycosides and diuretics; a complication associated with therapy, not pathologic entity related to MI itself.

41. **2** LDH, CPK, and SGOT are enzymes released into the blood from cardiac muscle cells when the myocardium is damaged. (a)
    1 The Paul-Bunnell test identifies heterophilic antibodies in infectious mononucleosis; would not be specific for myocardial infarction.
    3 The sedimentation rate identifies the presence of inflammation or infection; not specific; SGPT identifies tissue destruction; more specific for liver injury.
    4 APPT refers to the ability of blood to clot, not to the presence of myocardial infarction.

42. **2** Lidocaine hydrochloride (Xylocaine) decreases the irritability of the ventricles and is used in the treatment of ectopic beats originated by a ventricular focus. (b)
    1 Digoxin slows and strengthens ventricular contractions; it will not rapidly correct ectopic beats.
    3 Furosemide (Lasix), a diuretic, does not affect ectopic foci.
    4 Levarterenol bitartrate (Levophed) is a sympathomimetic and is indicated in cases of cardiogenic shock.

43. **2** Asystole refers to the absence of atrial and ventricular contractions, which can cause death within minutes. (b)
    1 This would be tachycardia if the heart rate was 100 to 150 beats per minute.
    3 The heartbeat has ceased in asystole.
    4 This might be bradycardia (less than 60 beats per minute) or heart block (a partial or complete interruption in transmission of impulses from the sinoatrial node to the ventricles).

44. **1** Irreversible brain damage will occur if a client is anoxic for more than 4 minutes. (a)
    2 Prior heart rate is of minimal importance. Rhythm is more significant.
    3 The age of the client does not affect the code.
    4 Although a variety of emergency medications must be available, their administration is ordered by the physician.

45. **1** Resuscitative efforts are futile unless an airway is patent so that oxygen expired by the resuscitator can reach the alveoli. (a)
    2 Prior to pulmonary resuscitation, the airway must be clear; two rather than four breaths would be given.
    3 This would not be done until the airway was clear and two breaths had been given.
    4 The nurse has already checked the carotid pulse; this action would waste valuable time.

46. **4** The sternum must be depressed at least 3.7 to 5 cm (1½ to 2 inches) to compress the heart adequately between the sternum and vertebrae and simulate cardiac pumping action. (c)
    1 This distance is ineffectual.
    2 This distance is ineffectual.
    3 This distance is ineffectual.

47. **3** Blood has a narrow pH range of 7.35 to 7.45. Venous blood (pH 7.35) is more acidic and closer to 7.35 than is arterial blood, which is normally closer to a pH of 7.45. (a)
    1 This is very acidic and needs immediate treatment.
    2 This is slightly acidic for both arterial and venous blood.
    4 This is alkaline and needs treatment.

48. **2** Bundle branch block interferes with the conduction of impulses from the AV node to the ventricle supplied by the affected bundle. Conduction through the ventricles is delayed, as evidenced by a widened QRS complex. (c)
    1 P waves, produced when the SA node fires to begin a cycle, are present in bundle branch block.
    3 Changes in the T waves and/or ST segments usually occur as a result of cardiac damage.
    4 Changes in the T waves and/or ST segments usually occur as a result of cardiac damage.

49. **3** The pacemaker (PM) electrode is inserted via the venous system into the right ventricle, where PM-generated impulses can directly stimulate the ventricles. (c)
    1 The pacing catheter must directly stimulate the ventricles; this site is too far from the ventricles.
    2 The pacing catheter must directly stimulate the ventricles; the left atrium cannot transmit the impulse.
    4 Stimulation of the SA node would be inadequate because of inability of the left bundle branch to transmit the impulse to the Purkinje fibers of the left ventricle.

50. **4** The SA node is the heart's natural pacemaker. An electronic pacemaker is used in some persons to supply an impulse that stimulates the heart to more efficient action. (a)

1 Sympathetic fibers to the heart do not act as a pacemaker to initiate and regulate the heartbeat.
2 Modified cardiac muscle, which receives impulses from the SA node and conducts them to the ventricular walls via the bundle of His and Purkinje fibers.
3 Special cardiac muscle, which receives impulses from the AV node and conducts them to the ventricular walls.

51. **3** Atropine blocks vagal stimulation of the SA node, resulting in an increased heart rate. (c)
    1 Lanoxin (digoxin) slows the heart rate; hence would not be indicated in this situation.
    2 Lidocaine hydrochloride (Xylocaine) decreases myocardial sensitivity and would not increase heart rate.
    4 Procainamide hydrochloride (Pronestyl) is an antiarrhythmic drug; would not stimulate the heart rate.

52. **3** A demand pacemaker functions only when the heart rate falls below the set rate of the pacemaker. The client can detect pacemaker malfunctions by monitoring the pulse rate and noting a drop below the set rate. (b)
    1 The client need not alter previous sleeping habits.
    2 Demand pacemakers function only when the heart rate drops below a predetermined level.
    4 Normal activity may be resumed when healing has occurred.

53. **2** Five to seven liters provide enough oxygen without altering the client's blood gases, which would cause increased respiratory distress. (b)
    1 Higher concentrations of oxygen may depress CO_2 and raise O_2 concentrations, interfering with the impetus to breathe.
    3 Is insufficient for an individual with congestive heart failure and pulmonary edema.
    4 Higher concentrations of oxygen may depress CO_2 and raise O_2 concentrations, interfering with the impetus to breathe.

54. **4** An open flame or spark from static electricity (e.g., leather-soled shoes, wool, silk, nylon and Dacron blankets, ungrounded electric appliances) can initiate an explosion and fire in the presence of higher than normal oxygen levels. (a)
    1 Oxygen is not flammable; however, it increases the rate of combustion.
    2 Oxygen is not unstable.
    3 Oxygen does not increase apprehension; by reducing dyspnea and shortness of breath, it usually reduces apprehension.

55. **3** Irritability and restlessness increase the metabolic rate (and the heart rate) and blood pressure. This complicates congestive heart failure. (a)
    1 Restlessness does not affect oxygen supply.
    2 Restlessness does not interfere with respiration; if anything, it increases respirations.
    4 Restlessness alone usually does not elevate the body temperature.

56. **2** Oxygen via nasal cannula is the most comfortable and least intrusive, since the cannula extends minimally into the nose. (a)
    1 This method is oppressive, and clients complain of feeling "suffocated" when it is used.
    3 This method is oppressive, and clients complain of feeling "suffocated" when it is used.
    4 This method is oppressive, and clients complain of feeling "suffocated" when it is used.

57. **3** The client is made to feel that the nurse cares about him personally and will have time for his special emotional needs. Such an approach allays anxiety and reduces emotional stress, which is beneficial in cases of cardiovascular disease. (a)

1 Indicates a lack of interest in the client, interferes with developing an effective nurse-client relationship.

2 Does not respond to client's need, cuts off communication.

4 Does not respond to client's need, cuts off communication.

58. **2** Since digoxin slows the heart, the apical pulse should be counted for 1 minute prior to administration. If the apical rate is below 60 (bradycardia), digoxin should be withheld since its administration could further depress the heart rate. If the heart rate is above 120, digoxin should be withheld because the client may be in digitalis toxicity. (a)

1 Not as accurate as apical pulse; the client may also have an atrial arrhythmia, which would not be detected with the radial rate alone.

3 Not as accurate as apical pulse; the client may also have an atrial arrhythmia, which would not be detected with the radial rate alone.

4 This is the pulse deficit, not an indicator of heart rate.

59. **4** Bradycardia refers to a heart rate of less than 60 per minute. It may be a physiologic adaptation to long-term exercise, cardiac disease, or digitalis toxicity. (a)

1 This condition is described as an arrhythmia; whereas bradycardia is also considered an arrhythmia, the rhythm is usually regular.

2 Tachycardia is the term used for rapid heart rates.

3 This is called a bigeminal rhythm.

60. **3** Potassium is lost with the urine during diuresis. Hypokalemia, in turn, predisposes the client to digitalis toxicity. (a)

1 This electrolyte is not lost as a result of digitalis-induced diuresis.

2 This electrolyte is not lost as a result of digitalis-induced diuresis.

4 This electrolyte is not lost as a result of digitalis-induced diuresis.

61. **4** Clients adapting to illness frequently feel afraid and helpless and strike out at health team members as a way of maintaining control or denying their fear. (b)

1 There is no evidence that the client denies the existence of her health problem.

2 Although disorders such as cerebral vascular accidents and atherosclerosis, which are associated with hypertension, may lead to cerebral anoxia, there is insufficient evidence to support this conclusion in this situation.

3 Although reserpine may cause agitation or depression, the behaviors described are more likely attributable to the client's psychologic adjustment to the situation.

62. **1** Chlordiazepoxide (Librium) is an anxiolytic. It promotes muscle relaxation, reducing anxiety and facilitating rest. (b)

2 This is a side effect of Librium due to its effect on the brainstem reticular formation, which controls the overall degree of central nervous system activity.

3 This is a side effect of Librium due to its effect on the brainstem reticular formation, which controls the overall degree of central nervous system activity.

4 The antianxiety effect of Librium may indirectly reduce hostility, but this is not the goal.

63. **4** Drowsiness is a side effect of Librium and indicates excessive depression of the central nervous system. (b)

1 Although tremors are listed as a possible adverse reaction, hyporeactivity is more common.

2 Not commonly attributed to chlordiazepoxide.

3 This drug may cause hypotension.

64. **3** Reserpine is an antihypertensive because it reduces norepinephrine levels in the peripheral nerve endings. (a)

1 Reserpine is an antihypertensive not a diuretic; diuretics produce fluid excretion.

2 Reserpine is an antihypertensive not a hypnotic; hypnotics promote sleep.

4 Reserpine is an antihypertensive not a tranquilizer; tranquilizers reduce muscle tension and anxiety.

65. **4** An improper reading of the level of mercury will be obtained if the reader is not perpendicular to the column. An error of parallax results when an object is displaced by an observer's altered position. (a)

1 Too narrow a cuff can result in erroneously high readings; not an error of parallax.

2 Standing close to the manometer is not explicit; there may or may not be a resultant error of parallax depending upon whether the examiner is perpendicular to the column of mercury.

3 Elevating the arm above the level of the heart will result in an erroneously low reading; not an error of parallax.

66. **2** An honest nurse-client relationship should be maintained so that trust can develop. (a)

1 Although other health team members may need to be informed eventually, the initial action should concern only the nurse-client relationship.

3 Does nothing to establish communication about feelings or motivation behind behavior.

4 Although other health team members may need to be informed eventually, the initial action should concern only the nurse-client relationship.

67. **3** At this time the client is using this behavior as a defense. Quiet acceptance can be an effective interpersonal technique, since it is nonjudgmental. (c)

1 During periods of overt hostility, perceptions are altered, making it difficult to evaluate the situation rationally.

2 Withdrawal signifies nonacceptance and rejection.

4 The nurse may be the target of a broad array of emotions; by focusing on only behaviors that affect the nurse, the full scope of the client's feelings are not considered.

68. **2** The orthopneic position allows maximum lung expansion because gravity reduces the pressure of the abdominal viscera on the diaphragm and lungs. (b)

1 Elevation of the extremities should be avoided because it increases venous return, placing an increased workload on the heart.

3 Excessive coughing and mucus production is characteristic of pulmonary edema and does not need to be encouraged.

4 Positioning for postural drainage does not relieve acute dyspnea; furthermore, it increases venous return to the heart.

69. **3** Application of rotating tourniquets keeps blood in the extremities, decreasing venous return, which reduces pulmonary artery pressure and relieves congestion. (b)

1 Extreme dyspnea and congestion necessitate a high-Fowler's position.

2 At times oxygen must be delivered under pressure to overcome the pressure of the edema fluid, but this is less common and is generally the responsibility of the inhalation or respiratory therapist.

4 A wet phlebotomy is used only occasionally to reduce venous return to the heart; a dry phlebotomy (rotating tourniquets) is usually effective.

70. **4** Diuretic therapy generally involves use of drugs that directly or indirectly increase urinary sodium excretion. Increased urinary excretion of sodium also promotes potassium loss. (a)
 1 Sodium restriction does not necessarily accompany administration of furosemide (Lasix).
 2 Unless otherwise ordered, oral intake is unaffected.
 3 Dyspnea does not directly result in a depletion of electrolytes.
71. **1** CVP is to be recorded when the client is horizontal and the zero point of the manometer is at the midaxillary line (level of the right atrium). (a)
 2 Alters the relationship of the midaxillary line and right atrium; inaccurate readings will be obtained.
 3 Alters the relationship of the midaxillary line and right atrium; inaccurate readings will be obtained.
 4 Alters the relationship of the midaxillary line and right atrium; inaccurate readings will be obtained.
72. **2** With air conditioning, blood vessels in the skin remain partially constricted, preventing extensive skin blood flow through the skin. Such extensive skin blood flow would ordinarily occur in hot weather to promote radiation of heat from the body; however, the heart must then work to pump the blood through many extra miles of blood vessels in the skin. (a)
 1 Body temperature is maintained.
 3 There is decreased circulation to the skin, which makes it beneficial to the person with cardiopulmonary problems.
 4 There is decreased circulation to the skin, which makes it beneficial to the person with cardiopulmonary problems.
73. **3** Cardioversion involves administration of precordial shock, which is synchronized with the R wave to interrupt the heart rate. It is used for atrial fibrillation, paroxysmal atrial tachycardia (PAT), and ventricular tachycardia when pharmaceutical preparations fail. The heart is stopped by the electric stimulation, and it is hoped that the SA node will take over as pacemaker. (c)
 1 Since there are no R waves, the shock would not be delivered.
 2 Premature ventricular contractions suggest irritable myocardium and generally respond well to antiarrhythmic agents.
 4 Since there are no R waves, the shock would not be delivered.
74. **2** Ventricular fibrillation is a death-producing arrhythmia and, once identified, must be terminated immediately by precordial shock (defibrillation). This is usually a standing physician's order in a cardiac care unit. (c)
 1 CPR is instituted only when defibrillation fails to terminate the arrhythmia.
 3 Bicarbonate is administered to correct acidosis; does not take priority over defibrillation.
 4 Oxygen is administered to correct hypoxia; does not take priority over defibrillation.
75. **2** The precordial shock during cardioversion must not be delivered on the T wave, or ventricular fibrillation may ensue. By placing the synchronizer in the "on" position, the physician presets the machine so it will not deliver the shock on the T wave. (b)
 1 The energy level may be set from 50 to 400 watt-seconds.
 3 This will not ensure that the shock is not delivered on the T wave.
 4 This will not ensure that the shock is not delivered on the T wave.
76. **2** The height of the ventricular complexes must be sufficient to be picked up by the voltmeter, which will sound an alarm if the heart rate is outside the high and low parameters. (c)
 1 The oscilloscope is the screen on which the electrical signals from the heart are displayed.
 3 The pulse generator (pacemaker) may be either an internal or an external device but is generally not part of the monitor.
 4 The synchronizer is used only during cardioversion to ensure that the electric shock is delivered during the QRS complex.
77. **1** Atrial fibrillation is the rapid discharge of impulses from a focus other than the SA node. Since not all these impulses are transmitted through the AV node, the ventricular response varies. Quinidine inhibits discharge of electric impulses from such ectopic foci, whereas digoxin delays the conduction of impulses from the AV node, slowing down the rate of ventricular response to impulses from the atria. (b)
 2 Digoxin increases vagal activity to slow the heart rate, and quinidine inhibits ion exchange across the cellular membrane; thus excitability of the atrial and ventricular myocardium is decreased, intraventricular and AV nodal conduction is slowed, and the refractory period is prolonged.
 3 This is true of quinidine but does not explain the action of digoxin.
 4 This is only partially true. Digoxin increases vagal activity to slow the heart rate, and quinidine inhibits ion exchange across the cellular membrane; thus excitability of the atrial and ventricular myocardium is decreased, intraventricular and AV nodal conduction is slowed, and the refractory period is prolonged.
78. **3** The apex of the heart is between the fifth and sixth ribs at the midclavicular line. It is closest to the chest wall here, so auscultation is easier. (b)
 1 Although it may be possible to auscultate the heart in this area, it is usually easier to do so over the apex.
 2 Although it may be possible to auscultate the heart in this area, it is usually easier to do so over the apex.
 4 Although it may be possible to auscultate the heart in this area, it is usually easier to do so over the apex.
79. **1** Adverse effects of digoxin include many types of arrhythmias. An apical pulse rate less than 60 or above 120 contraindicates administration of the drug. Since the client will be taking the medication at home, he must be taught to take his own pulse and to contact the physician if the rate falls outside the parameters mentioned. (b)
 2 Since the client will be assuming responsibility for drug administration at home, teaching is more of a priority than the nurse's observations.
 3 Since the client will be assuming responsibility for drug administration at home, teaching is more of a priority than the nurse's observations.
 4 Since the client will be assuming responsibility for drug administration at home, teaching is more of a priority than the nurse's observations.
80. **4** Coumarin anticoagulants are administered orally and take 2 or 3 days to achieve the desired decrease in prothrombin level. Heparin, which must be administered parenterally, has immediate effects. (c)
 1 This does not account for the reason for the administration of both drugs because coumarin derivatives will not exert an immediate therapeutic effect.
 2 These drugs do not dissolve clots already present.
 3 Since each drug affects a different part of the coagulating mechanism, dosages must be adjusted separately.

81. **3** Warfarin sodium (Coumadin) has been shown to inhibit the metabolism of phenytoin (Dilantin), which results in an accumulation of this drug in the body. (b)
    1 This is true only if the client is receiving phenytoin to control the epilepsy.
    2 They do not have a significant effect on the metabolism of Coumadin.
    4 By potentiating the anticoagulant, phenytoin decreases clotting potential.

82. **2** Coumarin derivatives cause an increase in the prothrombin time, leading to an increased risk of bleeding. Any abnormal or excessive bleeding must be reported, since it may indicate toxic levels of the drug. (b)
    1 TIAs are not caused by bleeding, which is the primary concern in clients receiving anticoagulants.
    3 Edema is not caused by bleeding.
    4 Would not be caused by Coumadin.

83. **4** Compliance with the prescribed regimen, which includes taking the drug and having prothrombin times performed by the laboratory, is necessary for safe and effective warfarin sodium (Coumadin) therapy. The dosage of Coumadin is adjusted according to the prothrombin time (PT); and if the client fails to take the drug as prescribed, the tests are not reliable in monitoring the response to therapy. (a)
    1 Although some medications can affect the absorption or metabolism of Coumadin and also should be investigated, this is less likely to be a cause of fluctuations in laboratory values.
    2 Although some medications can affect the absorption or metabolism of Coumadin and also should be investigated, this is less likely to be a cause of fluctuations in laboratory values.
    3 Although some medications can affect the absorption or metabolism of Coumadin and also should be investigated, this is less likely to be a cause of fluctuations in laboratory values.

84. **2** Secobarbital sodium (as well as other barbiturates) decreases the body's response to warfarin sodium (Coumadin). As a result there is less suppression of prothrombin. (c)
    1 Insomnia may increase seizure incidence, but methods to promote sleep other than barbiturates should be considered.
    3 Serious withdrawal symptoms are unlikely in this situation; however, indiscriminate use of the drug should be avoided.
    4 Secobarbital is not used to control seizures although other barbiturates such as phenobarbital may be prescribed for this purpose.

85. **4** The Nurse Practice Act states that nurses diagnose human responses to actual or potential health problems. The nurse used knowledge. (b)
    1 Since the client's symptoms reflected an immediate need for oxygen, postponement of treatment could result in further deterioration of her condition.
    2 Since the client's symptoms reflected an immediate need for oxygen, postponement of treatment could result in further deterioration of her condition.
    3 Since the client's symptoms reflected an immediate need for oxygen, postponement of treatment could result in further deterioration of her condition.

86. **2** The two coronary arteries are the first branches of the aorta and carry blood with a high oxygen content to the myocardium. (c)
    1 They carry blood with high oxygen content to the myocardium.

3 Carry blood with high oxygen content to the myocardium, not the endocardium.
4 This is function of the pulmonary veins.

87. **1** Angina pectoris is the pain referred to the chest wall and caused by hypoxia of the cardiac muscle. (b)
    2 There is no cell death in angina.
    3 A coronary thrombosis is an aggregation of platelets, clotting factors, and blood cellular elements that reduces the lumen of the artery; may progress to a complete obstruction, resulting in a myocardial infarction.
    4 Mitral insufficiency refers to an incompetent mitral valve; could be only indirectly related to angina.

88. **2** Anginal pain, which can be anticipated during certain activities, may be prevented by dilating the coronary arteries immediately before engaging in the activity. (b)
    1 One tablet is generally administered at a time; doubling the dosage may produce severe hypotension and headache.
    3 The sublingual form of nitroglycerin is absorbed directly through the mucous membranes and should not be swallowed.
    4 When the pain is relieved, rest will generally prevent its recurrence by reducing oxygen consumption of myocardium.

89. **1** Nitroglycerin tablets are affected by light, heat, and moisture. A loss of potency can be detected by absence of a tingling sensation when the tablet is placed under the tongue or by its ineffectiveness in relieving pain. A new supply should be obtained immediately. (c)
    2 Does not necessarily indicate a loss of potency.
    3 Does not necessarily indicate a loss of potency.
    4 Does not necessarily indicate a loss of potency.

90. **1** Cardiac nitrates relax the smooth muscles of the coronary arteries so that they dilate and deliver more blood to relieve ischemic pain. (b)
    2 While dilatation of blood vessels and subsequent drop in BP may occur, this is not the basis for evaluating drug's effectiveness.
    3 While cardiac output may improve because of improved oxygenation of the myocardium, this is not a basis for evaluating the drug's effectiveness.
    4 While superficial vessels dilate, lowering BP and creating a flushed appearance, this is not a basis for evaluating the drug's effectiveness.

91. **4** In addition to GI disturbances, visual disturbances such as blurred vision may be evidence of digitalis toxicity. Heart rates over 120 may also indicate toxicity. (b)
    1 This is not a symptom of digitalis toxicity.
    2 This is not a symptom of digitalis toxicity.
    3 This is not a symptom of digitalis toxicity.

92. **3** Toxic levels of digitalis overstimulate the vagus nerve, leading to depressed conduction through the AV node (AV block of any degree) as well as SA node depression (sinus bradycardia). In addition, ectopic pacemakers are accelerated, leading to multiple premature beats. Such pathologic effects are enhanced by low serum potassium levels from diuretics, vomiting, and nasogastric drainage as well as by chronic arterial hypoxemia and impaired renal function. (b)
    1 Untrue statement.
    2 True but not specific to the situation described.
    4 Vitamins act as coenzymes.

93. **1** Blood samples from the right atrium, right ventricle, and pulmonary artery would all be about the same with regard to oxygen concentration. Such blood con-

tains slightly less oxygen than does systemic arterial blood. (b)

2 Contain slightly more carbon dioxide than does blood in the pulmonary vein, which has had some of its CO_2 expelled into the alveoli.

3 Contains the same amount as do samples from the right atrium and right ventricle.

4 Contain less oxygen than does the pulmonary vein, which will carry oxygenated blood to the circulation.

94. **2** The Swan-Ganz catheter is placed in the pulmonary artery. Information regarding left ventricular function is obtained when the catheter balloon is inflated. (c)

1 Information on stroke volume, the amount of blood ejected by the left ventricle with each contraction, will not be provided by a Swan-Ganz catheter.

3 Central venous pressure is measured via a catheter that is inserted through the superior vena cava into the right atrium. It is attached to a water manometer.

4 Circulation time is measured by injecting a tasteable substance into a vein and noting the time it takes to travel to the tongue.

95. **3** Sodium polystyrene sulfonate, a cation exchange resin used in the treatment of hyperkalemia, will release sodium ions in the intestines in exchange for potassium ions. Sorbital has a hyperosmotic effect in the intestinal tract concomitantly maintaining the liquid content of the feces and counteracting the constipating effect of the resin. (b)

1 Does not provide carbohydrates.

2 Does not reflect a combined effect.

4 Sorbitol counteracts the constipating effect of resin.

96. **2** Hypersensitivity to a foreign substance can cause an anaphylactic reaction. Histamine is released, causing bronchial constriction, increased capillary permeability, and dilation of arterioles. This decreased peripheral resistance is associated with hypotension and inadequate circulation to major organs. (c)

1 Dilation of arterioles occurs.

3 These are the problems that result from bronchial constriction and vascular collapse.

4 Arterioles dilate, capillary permeability increases, and eventually vascular collapse occurs.

97. **3** Hypersensitivity results from the production of antibodies in response to exposure to certain foreign substances (allergens). Prior exposure is necessary for the development of these antibodies. (c)

1 Not a sensitivity reaction to penicillin; hay fever and asthma are atopic conditions caused by atopens.

2 It would be an active immunity.

4 Antibodies have been developed in a prior exposure to the allergen, in this case penicillin.

98. **1** Since an elevated plasma bilirubin level could indicate an increased rate of red cell destruction (bilirubin is a product of free hemoglobin metabolism), the individual may have a hemolytic anemia (e.g., sickle cell anemia, glucose 6-phosphate dehydrogenase deficiency). (b)

2 Oxygen-carrying ability reflected by hemoglobin.

3 Does not involve the destruction of red blood cells with subsequent liberation of bilirubin.

4 The decreased destruction of red cells does not liberate bile pigment.

99. **3** Methyldopa is associated with acquired hemolytic anemia and should be discontinued to prevent disease progression and complications. (c)

1 Not associated with red blood cell destruction.

2 Not associated with red blood cell destruction.

4 Not associated with red blood cell destruction.

100. **1** Brief pressure is generally enough to prevent bleeding. (b)

2 Complications are rare; no special positioning required.

3 The site is cleansed prior to aspiration.

4 Complications are rare; frequent monitoring is unnecessary.

101. **3** The heart may be strained by prolonged anemia because the blood's decreased viscosity eases its return to the heart from the peripheral vessels. In accordance with Starling's law, the greater volume of blood returning to the heart will stretch it and result in greater cardiac output. The increased blood viscosity occurring in polycythemia forces the heart to strain to maintain adequate peripheral blood flow; the heart must exert greater force to propel the more viscous blood through the circulatory system. (a)

1 Pressure is not involved; the terms anemia and polycythemia both refer to the number of cells present in a given volume (viscosity).

2 Surface tension is not involved; the terms anemia and polycythemia both refer to the number of cells in a given volume (viscosity).

4 Temperature is not involved; the terms anemia and polycythemia both refer to the number of cells present in a given volume (viscosity).

102. **2** Ventricular fibrillation will cause irreversible brain damage and then death within minutes because the heart is not pumping blood. Defibrillation or CPR (until defibrillation is possible) must be initiated immediately. (a)

1 Although this condition requires prompt treatment, a client will live if treatment is withheld for several minutes.

3 Although this condition requires prompt treatment, a client will live if treatment is withheld for several minutes.

4 Although this condition requires prompt treatment, a client will live if treatment is withheld for several minutes.

103. **3** The gamma globulin fraction in the plasma is the fraction that includes the antibodies. (a)

1 Hemoglobin carries oxygen.

2 Albumin helps regulate fluid shifts by maintaining the plasma oncotic pressure.

4 Thrombin is involved in clotting.

104. **2** Platelets (thrombocytes) adhere to the intima of damaged vessels within seconds after injury, releasing substances that promote hemostasis. (b)

1 Red blood cells play no role in clotting; they carry oxygen to all body cells.

3 Play no role in clotting; they protect the body against microorganisms.

4 Erythrocytes are red blood cells; they carry oxygen and play no role in coagulation.

105. **1** Isotonic solutions are those which cause no change in the cellular volume or pressure, since their concentration is equivalent to that of body fluid. (a)

2 Contains more than 0.85 g of sodium chloride in each 100 ml.

3 Contains less than 0.85 g of sodium chloride in each 100 ml.

4 Relates to two compounds that possess the same molecular formula but that differ in their properties or in the position of atoms in the molecules; isomers.

106. **3** The pulmonary capillary beds are the first small vessels (capillary beds) that the embolus encounters once it is released from the calf veins. (b)

1 Unlikely to occur because the embolus would enter the pulmonary system first.

2 Gangrene occurs when the arterial rather than the venous circulation is compromised.

4 Unlikely to occur; the embolus would enter the pulmonary system first.

107. **4** An appendectomy is a relatively simple operation; the client is generally out of bed the same day. With an ambulatory client there is less risk of venous stasis, a condition that predisposes the individual to thrombus formation and emboli. (a)

1 May or may not be out of bed the same day depending on the surgical approach; mobility may be hampered by a Foley catheter.

2 Although generally ambulated the first day postoperatively, the client often is hampered by pain; pelvic surgery increases risk.

3 Vein ligation is performed for varicose veins; the diseased vein is removed, placing an additional burden on the deep venous system and possibly increasing the risk of thrombi.

108. **3** Thromboplastin is a substance released by platelets that initiates the clotting process by converting prothrombin to thrombin. (b)

1 Plasma does not produce thromboplastin.

2 RBCs do not produce thromboplastin.

4 Bile does not contain thromboplastin.

109. **2** Fibrinogen is a soluble plasma protein that becomes the insoluble gel, fibrin, during the clotting process. (c)

1 Fibrin is the insoluble gel formed from fibrinogen by the action of thrombin.

3 Prothrombin is the precursor of thrombin; becomes fibrinogin.

4 Thrombin is needed to convert fibrinogen to fibrin; also needed in platelet aggregation.

110. **2** Calcium acts as a catalyst to convert prothrombin to thrombin. Thrombin accelerates the formation of insoluble fibrin from the soluble fibrinogen. (c)

1 Iron is essential for the synthesis of hemoglobin, which is not involved in clotting.

3 Fluorine (F^-) is a gas of the halogen group and is not involved in clotting; sodium fluoride helps harden tooth enamel.

4 Chloride is an extracellular anion that helps regulate osmotic pressure and combines with hydrogen to form hydrochloric acid; not involved with clotting.

111. **1** Mitral stenosis impairs blood flow from the left atrium to the left ventricle. This backs up blood into the pulmonary veins and lungs. The result may be pulmonary edema. (c)

2 Tricuspid disease may cause jugular vein distension and hepatic congestion.

3 Severe arterial sclerosis of the coronary arteries narrows the arterial lumen, which can result in a decreased blood supply to the myocardium causing hypoxia and angina.

4 Pulmonic stenosis tends to cause a bulging of the intraventricular septum.

112. **4** A culture and testing of the antibiotic sensitivity of secretions or drainage identify the causative organism (culture) and the antibiotics to which the organism is particularly sensitive or resistant (sensitivity). (a)

1 A test to determine whether a pathogen is virulent.

2 A test for viral activity.

3 A test for antibody content.

113. **4** This is the causative organism of tuberculosis and is acid fast. (a)

1 Not an acid-fast organism.

2 Not an acid-fast organism.

3 Not an acid-fast organism.

114. **2** The respiratory membrane, consisting of the alveolar and capillary walls, is extremely thin. This thinness facilitates exchange of respiratory gases without the need for additional energy. (a)

1 This mechanism is utilized when energy is required to move matter against the concentration gradient.

3 A process to prevent passage of certain-sized particles.

4 Diffusion of water through a selective membrane.

115. **1** Tidal air is defined as the amount of air exhaled normally after a normal inspiration. (b)

2 This is the expiratory reserve volume (ERV).

3 The volume of air that can be forcibly inspired over and above a normal inspiration is the inspiratory reserve volume (IRV).

4 This is the residual air volume.

116. **3** The absence of bacteria in the sputum indicates that the disease can no longer be spread by droplet infection. (b)

1 Treatment is over an extended period; eventually the client may not have an active disease, but still remains infected.

2 Once an individual has been infected, the test will always be positive.

4 This is not evidence that disease will not be transmitted.

117. **2** Because of potential damage to the eighth cranial (vestibulocochlear) nerve, the dosage is regulated according to the combination of drugs prescribed and the severity of the illness. (b)

1 Dosage spacing does not increase compliance with the regimen.

3 Although rest is important, this is not the rationale behind spacing doses.

4 Injection sites may be rotated to decrease tissue trauma.

118. **3** INH (isoniazid) often leads to pyridoxine (vitamin B_6) deficiency because it competes with the vitamin for the same enzyme. This is most often manifested by peripheral neuritis, which can be controlled by regular administration of vitamin B_6. (b)

1 A vitamin does not, in and of itself, improve nutritional status.

2 Pyridoxine does not enhance the effect of INH.

4 Pyridoxine does not destroy organisms.

119. **3** Streptomycin is ototoxic and may cause damage to the auditory and vestibular portions of the eighth cranial nerve. (c)

1 The drug does not adversely affect the cerebellum.

2 The motor end plates of the peripheral nervous system are not affected.

4 These cells and tracts of the nervous system are not affected.

120. **1** The etiology of a spontaneous pneumothorax is commonly the rupture of blebs on the lung surface. Blebs are similar to blisters. (b)

2 Pleural friction rub would result in pain on inspiration, not a pneumothorax.

3 A tracheoesophageal fistula would cause aspiration of food and saliva, resulting in respiratory distress.

4 The client had no history of trauma.

121. **2** Sudden chest pain occurs on the affected side; may also involve the arm and shoulder. (b)

1 Decreased chest motion would occur because of failure to inflate the involved lung.

3 Bloody vomitus is unrelated to pneumothorax.

4 The shift is toward the unaffected side caused by pressure from the pneumothorax.

122. **3** Thoracic pressure is reduced because thoracic volume is increased as the diaphragm descends. (c)
    1 Rising pressure in the alveoli and the intrapleural space or relaxation of the diaphragm expels air from the alveoli.
    2 Rising pressure in the alveoli and the intrapleural space or relaxation of the diaphragm expels air from the alveoli.
    4 Contraction of the diaphragm causes inspiration.
123. **3** As a person with a tear in the lung (e.g., a ruptured bleb) inhales, air moves through that opening into the pleural space. This creates a positive pressure and causes partial or complete collapse of the lung. (c)
    1 Mediastinal shift occurs toward the unaffected side.
    2 There is loss of intrathoracic negative pressure.
    4 This is not an impending problem.
124. **4** Pressure within the pleural cavity causes a shift of the heart and great vessels to the unaffected side. This not only decreases the capacity of the unaffected lung but also impedes the filling of the right side of the heart and leads to a decreased cardiac output. (c)
    1 The volume of the unaffected lung may decrease because of pressure from the shift.
    2 Infection is not caused by a mediastinal shift.
    3 This complication might occur in severe chest trauma, not in mediastinal shift.
125. **3** A pneumothorax results in decreased surface area for gaseous exchange. If the unaffected pleural regions cannot compensate, carbon dioxide builds up in the blood (hypercapnia). The client becomes drowsy and may lose consciousness. The body attempts to compensate by increasing the respiratory and pulse rates and by the renal retention of bicarbonate. (c)
    1 Carbon dioxide builds up in the blood, and the PO_2 is lowered because of the decreased surface area for gaseous exchange.
    2 Acidosis occurs with elevated PCO_2.
    4 Hypokalemia causes extreme muscle weakness, abdominal distension, and changes in the ECG pattern.
126. **4** Oxygen is supplied to prevent anoxia but cannot be given in higher concentrations because, in an individual with emphysema, a low PO_2 (not high PCO_2) is the only respiratory stimulus. (b)
    1 This might increase the risk of mediastinal shift and interfere with expansion of the unaffected lung.
    2 This concentration is too high for a client with emphysema because it precipitates carbon dioxide narcosis.
    3 This dependent action would require orders as to specific electrolytes.
127. **4** Fluctuations occur with normal inspiration and expiration until the lung is fully expanded. If these fluctuations do not occur, the chest tube may be clogged. The nurse should milk the chest tube q 1 to 2 h and avoid kinking the tube. (a)
    1 The client may not be agitated; morphine depresses respirations and is usually avoided; dependent function of the nurse.
    2 The binder does not prevent tension on the tube; would be contraindicated, for it limits thoracic expansion.
    3 The tube should be clamped only if ordered or if an air leak is suspected.
128. **4** Chest x-ray films or radiographs reveal the degree to which the lung fills the pleural cavity and also the presence of any mediastinal shift. (c)
    1 The chest tubes may have minimal drainage; this is not an indicator.

2 These are not normal chest sounds and do not indicate the degree of lung expansion.
    3 This would be an indicator of expansion of both lungs, and would not be specific to expansion of the affected side.
129. **2** The tidal volume is the amount of air inhaled and exhaled while breathing normally. (b)
    1 Air that can be forcibly expired after deep inspiration.
    3 The maximum amount of air that can be inspired following the inspiration of the tidal volume.
    4 The maximum amount of air that can be expired after expiration of the tidal volume.
130. **3** The orthopneic position is a sitting position that permits maximum lung expansion for gaseous exchange, since the abdominal organs do not provide pressure against the diaphragm and gravity facilitates the descent of the diaphragm. (b)
    1 This position does not maximize lung expansion to the same degree as the orthopneic position.
    2 This position does not maximize lung expansion to the same degree as the orthopneic position.
    4 This position does not permit the diaphragm to descend by gravity, and pressure of the abdominal organs against the diaphragm limits its movement.
131. **4** Isoproterenol stimulates the beta receptors of the sympathetic nervous system, causing bronchodilation and increased rate and strength of cardiac contractions. (b)
    1 Expectorants mobilize respiratory secretions.
    2 Antihypertensives and diuretics help decrease blood pressure.
    3 Barbiturates and hypnotics produce sedation.
132. **2** Isoproterenol is a sympathomimetic catecholamine that causes increased heart contraction (positive inotropic effect) and increased heart rate (positive chronotropic effect). If toxic levels are reached, side effects occur and the drug should be withheld until the physician is notified. (c)
    1 False reassurance; this is not a true statement, and the drug will have to be withheld until the physician is notified.
    3 False reassurance; this is not a true statement, and the drug will have to be withheld until the physician is notified.
    4 Controlled breathing may be helpful in allaying a client's anxiety; however, the drug may be producing side effects and should be withheld.
133. **2** As a result of the narrowed airways, exhalation is difficult, leaving air trapped in the lung. Distention of alveolar walls to accommodate this volume leads to emphysema. (b)
    1 Atelectasis is the collapse of lung tissue.
    3 Pneumothorax is the term that describes the collapse of a lung.
    4 Pulmonary fibrosis is a condition in which fibrous connective tissue spreads over normal lung tissue.
134. **4** Destruction of the alveolar walls leads to diminished surface area for gaseous exchange and an increased CO_2 level in the blood. (b)
    1 Infectious obstructions occur in conditions in which microorganisms invade lung tissue; emphysema is not an infectious disease.
    2 Muscle paralysis may occur in diseases affecting the neurologic system; emphysema does not affect the neurologic system; therefore it is not a neurologic disease.
    3 Pleural effusion occurs when there is seepage of fluid into the thoracic cavity; this does not occur with emphysema.

135. **2** Loss of elasticity causes difficult exhalation, with subsequent air trapping. Clients who have emphysema are taught to use accessory abdominal muscles and to breathe out through pursed lips to help keep the air passages open until exhalation is complete. (b)
    1 There will be decreased vital capacity.
    3 Expiration is difficult because of air trapping and poor elasticity.
    4 Diaphragmatic breathing is a learned mechanism that is beneficial.

136. **1** Retention of carbon dioxide after exhausting the available bicarbonate ions as buffers will cause a lower pH (respiratory acidosis). (b)
    2 Tissue necrosis is due to localized tissue anoxia and will not cause the systemic response of respiratory acidosis; this is due to excessive carbonic acid resulting from a respiratory insufficiency.
    3 Hyperventilation will cause respiratory alkalosis.
    4 The loss of carbon dioxide reduces the body's level of carbonic acid, causing respiratory alkalosis.

137. **2** Since the client's condition is described as terminal, nursing priority should be directed toward providing comfort. (b)
    1 Although these are important aspects of nursing care, provision of comfort retains priority in the care of a dying client.
    3 Although these are important aspects of nursing care, provision of comfort retains priority in the care of a dying client.
    4 Although these are important aspects of nursing care, provision of comfort retains priority in the care of a dying client.

138. **4** Small meals are not as psychologically overwhelming and do not upset the stomach as easily. They are therefore better tolerated. (a)
    1 Does not ensure adequate nutrition; if the portion size is decreased, frequency must be increased.
    2 Administration of vitamins is a dependent nursing function.
    3 If no attempts are made to decrease portions at regular mealtimes, aversion will usually persist.

139. **1** Anorexia refers to loss of appetite. (a)
    2 Anoxia refers to lack of oxygen.
    3 Apathy refers to lack of concern or emotion.
    4 Dysphagia refers to difficulty swallowing.

140. **2** IPPB treatments loosen bronchial secretions and dilate the air passages, but coughing is needed to raise the secretions for expectoration. (a)
    1 A sitting position will allow secretions to remain in the lungs unless coughing is encouraged.
    3 IPPB is sometimes administered before postural drainage to loosen secretions so they can be more easily mobilized.
    4 Rest should be encouraged only after coughing to bring up secretions mobilized by postural drainage.

141. **3** Meperidine hydrochloride is the generic name for Demerol. (a)
    1 Propoxyphene hydrochloride is the generic name for Darvon.
    2 Glutethimide is the generic name for Doriden.
    4 Naloxone is the generic name for Narcan.

142. **4** Clients with COPD (chronic obstructive pulmonary disease) respond only to the chemical stimulus of low oxygen levels. Administration of high concentrations of oxygen will eliminate the stimulus to breathe, leading to decreased respirations and lethargy. (c)
    1 High concentrations of oxygen will eliminate the stimulus to breathe, so the respiratory rate would decrease.

2 Cyanosis is caused by excessive amounts of reduced oxyhemoglobin; since oxygen is being administered, cyanosis may be reduced.
    3 Rising carbon dioxide levels cause lethargy rather than anxiety.

143. **3** Since family members are old enough to understand his needs, they should be encouraged to participate in his care. (c)
    1 Deprives the client of support system.
    2 Self-care increases oxygen utilization, causing fatigue and dyspnea.
    4 Overworking the client causes undue fatigue and dyspnea; frequent rest periods should be incorporated into the plan.

144. **4** Aspirin can cause a lowered prothrombin blood level, increasing the risk of undesired bleeding that may occur with administration of anticoagulants. (a)
    1 Isoxsuprine hydrochloride is a vasodilator; it does not affect bleeding times.
    2 Chloral hydrate is a hypnotic; it does not affect bleeding times.
    3 Chlorpromazine is an antipsychotic; it does not affect bleeding times.

145. **4** The client who is immobilized must do exercises such as dorsiflexion of the feet to prevent venous stasis and thrombus formation. (a)
    1 Improves pulmonary function rather than prevents venous stasis.
    2 Actually promotes venous stasis by compressing the popliteal space.
    3 Limiting fluid intake may lead to hemoconcentration and subsequent thrombus formation.

146. **2** The high vascularity of the nose, combined with its susceptibility to trauma (e.g., sneezing, nose blowing), makes it a frequent region for hemorrhage. (a)
    1 This symptom is usually not associated with anticoagulant therapy.
    3 This symptom is usually not associated with anticoagulant therapy.
    4 This symptom is usually not associated with anticoagulant therapy.

147. **4** Hemoptysis is expectoration of blood-stained sputum derived from the lungs, bronchi, or trachea. (a)
    1 Refers to blood in the urine.
    2 Refers to vomiting of blood.
    3 Refers to a local accumulation of blood in the tissues.

148. **3** Orthopneic position refers to sitting up and leaning slightly forward. This drops the diaphragm, allowing the lungs more room for expansion. (a)
    1 The Trendelenburg position forces the diaphragm up, interfering with lung expansion.
    2 Horizontal positions do not allow the gravitational effect on the diaphragm and thus do not maximize air exchange.
    4 Horizontal positions do not allow the gravitational effect on the diaphragm and thus do not maximize air exchange.

149. **3** The tourniquets must be rotated in a clockwise direction at 15-minute intervals so venous outflow in any one extremity is not occluded more than 45 minutes at a time. (b)
    1 Arterial blood flow cannot be totally occluded, or cell death will occur.
    2 One extremity is left without a tourniquet every 15 minutes.
    4 Since tourniquets are applied to three of the four extremities, only one tourniquet is rotated at a time.

150. **3** Application of rotating tourniquets keeps blood in the extremities, decreasing venous return to reduce pulmonary artery pressure and relieve pulmonary congestion. (b)
  1 The aim is to maintain adequate arterial flow to prevent tissue hypoxia.
  2 Visceral blood flow is not primarily affected.
  4 Capillary blood flow is not primarily affected.

151. **4** The exact mode of action of morphine sulfate is unknown. However, it has a rapid onset, lowers blood pressure, decreases pulmonary reflexes, and produces sedation. (c)
  1 Hydroxyzine hydrochloride is generally used to control anxiety associated with less acute situations and is available in oral form only.
  2 Phenobarbital has a slower onset than morphine and does not affect respirations and blood pressure to the same extent as morphine.
  3 Chloral hydrate is a hypnotic but is not appropriate for the acute situation described.

152. **2** Ethacrynic acid interferes with the concentrating and diluting mechanism of the descending and ascending limbs of the renal tubule and the concentrating process in the collecting duct. It inhibits the active transport of chloride ions back into the blood. A copious and dilute urine high in chloride and sodium ions is excreted. (c)
  1 Potassium-sparing diuretic; less potent than thiazide diuretics.
  3 Although used in the treatment of edema and hypertension, this drug is not as potent as ethacrynic acid.
  4 Although used in the treatment of edema and hypertension, this drug is not as potent as ethacrynic acid.

153. **3** Aminophylline, a theophylline derivative, promotes diuresis and relaxes smooth muscles, resulting in hypotension. (b)
  1 Side effects include sinus tachycardia.
  2 Urine output is increased.
  4 Not a side effect of the drug.

154. **2** The fluid level in the manometer fluctuates with respiration because the changes in thoracic pressure affect the pressure in the right atrium. (b)
  1 The positive pressure of a ventilator alters the central venous pressure readings, so the ventilator must be removed when CVP is taken.
  3 Although the CVP line is not used routinely for blood samples, blood can be easily aspirated.
  4 To approximate the level of the right atrium, the "O" level should be even with the midaxillary line.

155. **3** Deslanoside (Cedilanid-D) can be administered slowly by IV infusion; although available IM it is usually not administered because it is too irritating. (c)
  1 This can be administered intravenously, intramuscularly, and orally.
  2 This is available only in tablet form.
  4 This is administered orally.

156. **2** Cool mist suppresses the local inflammatory response, thus helping to prevent edema and subsequent airway obstruction. (b)
  1 A local anesthetic may be used for associated sore throat discomfort; does not prevent edema.
  3 May cause aspiration if gag reflex has not returned.
  4 May cause aspiration if gag reflex has not returned.

157. **2** Cancerous lesions in the pleural space increase the osmotic pressure causing a shift in fluid to that space. (b)
  1 A bronchoscopy does not involve the pleural space.
  3 Inadequate chest expansion results from pleural effusion, is not the cause of it.

4 Excessive intake is normally balanced by increased urine output.

158. **2** Expectoration of blood is an indication that the lung itself was damaged during the procedure; a pneumothorax may occur. (b)
  1 Increased breath sounds are anticipated as the lung is closer to the chest wall after the fluid in the pleural space is removed.
  3 Increased lung expansion should improve cerebral oxygenation and decrease confusion if present.
  4 A decreased rate may be indicative of improved gaseous exchange and is not evidence that the client is in danger.

159. **3** These agents are classified as antiinflammatory or immunosuppressive. Glucocorticoids interfere with the body's response to microorganisms but do not directly promote the spread of enteroviruses. (a)
  1 Interferes with the release of enzymes responsible for the inflammatory response.
  2 Immunosuppressant action causes bone marrow depression, which decreases the number of WBCs.
  4 Interferes with antibody production.

160. **4** Many chemotherapeutic agents function by interfering with DNA replication associated with normal cellular reproduction (mitosis). The normal rapid mitoses of the stratified squamous epithelium of the mouth and anus result in their being powerfully affected by the drugs. (b)
  1 Chemotherapeutic agents affect the cells that are most rapidly proliferating, which include not only the cells of the GI epithelium but also those of the bone marrow and hair follicles.
  2 Effect not due to direct irritation; most agents are administered parenterally.
  3 State of nourishment would be applicable to all cells; although anorexia is common, this client may not be anorexic.

161. **3** Unwashed hands are considered contaminated and are used to turn on sink faucets. The use of foot pedals or a paper towel barrier prevents recontamination of washed hands. (c)
  1 They are not considered contaminated for this reason; areas cannot be sterile.
  2 Although bacterial growth is facilitated in moist environments, this is not the reason why sinks are considered contaminated.
  4 It has nothing to do with the number of people; it is related to being touched by contaminated hands.

162. **3** Bargaining is one of the stages of dying in which the client promises some type of desirable behavior to postpone the inevitability of death. (a)
  1 Rationalization is a defense mechanism in which attempts are made to justify or explain an unacceptable action or feeling.
  2 Frustration is a subjective experience, a feeling of being thwarted, but not one of the stages of dying.
  4 Classified as the fourth stage, depression represents the grief experienced as the individual recognizes his fate.

163. **2** When an individual reaches the point of being able intellectually and psychologically to accept death, anxiety is reduced and he becomes detached from his environment. (c)
  1 Although resigned to death, the individual is not euphoric.
  3 Although detached, the client is still concerned and may use this time constructively.
  4 At the stage of acceptance, the client is no longer angry or depressed.

164. **2** Since 1 oz equals approximately 30 ml and the client drank a total of 21.5 oz, 21.5 × 30 yields the answer in milliliters. (a)
    1 An incorrect calculation; too low.
    3 An incorrect calculation; too low.
    4 An incorrect calculation; too low.

165. **4** Denial, bargaining, and detachment are coping mechanisms often needed by the client, especially when facing a devastating illness, and should be accepted by the nurse. (a)
    1 Ignoring the behavior does not convey a willingness to listen and denies the client's feelings.
    2 Coping mechanisms are needed by the client as psychologic protection and must not be taken from him until he is able to replace one for another.
    3 Reinforcement of denial will inhibit the individual's transition toward acceptance.

166. **4** In the process of rocking, the Trendelenburg position facilitates venous return from the lower extremities; reverse Trendelenburg decreases the pressure of the abdominal organs on the diaphragm, allowing maximum lung expansion. (c)
    1 Refers to a force directed outward from a central point, such as the force responsible for the planets' orbiting the sun.
    2 Refers to the tendency of a body at rest to remain at rest or if in motion to remain so.
    3 Refers to the force of a moving object; equal to mass times velocity.

167. **2** The residual volume is the amount of air remaining in the lungs after maximum exhalation. (b)
    1 The force exerted by the abdominal thrust surpasses that which the individual is voluntarily capable of exerting; normally under the individual's control.
    3 The force exerted by the abdominal thrust surpasses that which the individual is voluntarily capable of exerting; normally under the individual's control.
    4 The force exerted by the abdominal thrust surpasses that which the individual is voluntarily capable of exerting; normally under the individual's control.

168. **3** After a submucosal resection (SMR), hemorrhage from the area is frequently detected by vomiting of blood that has been swallowed. (b)
    1 Headaches in the back of the head would not be a complication of a submucosal resection.
    2 The occurrence of crepitus would be caused by leakage of air into tissue spaces and is not usually a complication of SMR.
    4 The tongue is not involved in this surgery.

169. **2** The respiratory center in the medulla responds primarily to increased carbon dioxide concentration in the blood. (a)
    1 Not a stimulant for respiration; involved in transmission of neural impulses.
    3 Not a stimulant; a by-product of muscular activity.
    4 Normally not the primary stimulus to breathing; functions as a primary stimulus in individuals who have chronic hypercapnia.

170. **2** The lower the Po_2 and the higher the Pco_2, the more rapidly oxygen dissociates from the oxyhemoglobin molecule. (c)
    1 Must be associated with an increase in carbon dioxide pressure.
    3 Oxygen dissociations would be decreased in this situation.
    4 Must be associated with a decrease in oxygen pressure.

171. **1** Carbon monoxide (CO) binds with hemoglobin more avidly than does oxygen. The progressive results are dyspnea, asphyxia, and death. (b)
    2 Carbon monoxide does not block carbon dioxide transport; it binds with hemoglobin.
    3 Carbon monoxide inhibits oxygen transport, not vasodilation.
    4 Carbon monoxide does not form bubbles in the blood plasma; bubbles in tissues are due to increased nitrogen, as in decompression sickness (bends).

172. **4** With an oxygen debt, a muscle would show primarily low levels of oxygen and low levels of ATP caused by the low levels of aerobic respiration and high levels of lactic acid formation. (c)
    1 Low levels of calcium are present.
    2 High levels of lactic acid are present.
    3 Low levels of glycogen are present.

173. **1** The respiratory and urinary systems interact with the bicarbonate buffer system to preserve the normal body pH of 7.4 (7.35 to 7.45). Consider the following equation:

$$CO_2 + H_2O \rightleftharpoons H_2CO_3 \rightleftharpoons H^+ + HCO_3^-$$

    Increased respiration blows off carbon dioxide and pulls the equation to the left; this decreases H^+ and the pH rises (less acidity). Decreased respiration results in carbon dioxide buildup, which pushes the equation to the right; this increases H^+ and the pH falls (more acidity). Similarly, the kidneys either conserve or excrete bicarbonate, which respectively shifts the equation to the left or to the right, thereby helping to adjust the pH. (a)
    2 Interaction does not maintain pH.
    3 Interaction does not maintain pH.
    4 Although the circulatory system carries fluids and electrolytes to the kidneys, it does not interact with the urinary system to regulate plasma pH.

174. **3** Accumulated carbon dioxide (CO_2) will powerfully stimulate the breathing center of the brainstem, forcing resumption of respiration even if the person has fainted first. (b)
    1 Increased carbon dioxide will stimulate breathing.
    2 Rising carbon dioxide not oxygen will stimulate breathing.
    4 Unrelated; will occur with changes in pressure, as in decompression sickness.

175. **4** An Ambu Bag is a piece of equipment that can be compressed at regular intervals by hand for temporary ventilation of the client in respiratory arrest. (a)
    1 Ventricular fibrillation requires immediate defibrillation.
    2 Wound drainage bags, not an Ambu Bag, may be used for gross incisional drainage.
    3 The Ambu Bag is used to ventilate a client, not to measure respiratory output.

176. **1** During suctioning of a client, negative pressure (suction) should not be applied until the catheter is ready to be drawn out because, in addition to the removal of secretions, oxygen is being depleted. (b)
    2 A cough reflex may be absent or diminished in some clients; the catheter should be inserted approximately 12 cm (4 to 5 inches) or just past the end of the tracheostomy tube.
    3 Skin care is not involved in suctioning; may be part of tracheostomy care; tapes are untied only when being changed.
    4 The inner cannula is not removed during suctioning; it may be removed during tracheostomy care.

177. **2** The phrenic nerves conduct motor impulses to the diaphragm; cutting one phrenic nerve will paralyze the portion of the diaphragm innervated by that nerve. (c)
    1 Phrenic nerves are motor not sensory nerves.

3 Phrenic nerves take motor impulses to the diaphragm not the lungs.

4 Paralysis of the diaphragm will result on the same side.

178. **2** Intussusception is the telescoping or prolapse of a segment of the bowel within the lumen of an immediately connecting part. (a)

  1 Volvulus is a twisting of the bowel onto itself.

  3 Adhesions are bands of scar tissue that can compress the bowel.

  4 Herniation is the term that describes protrusion of an organ through the wall that contains it.

179. **3** A flat plate film of the abdomen visualizes abdominal organs as they are. (b)

  1 The client may eat and drink as tolerated.

  2 No bowel preparation is indicated.

  4 No bowel preparation is indicated.

180. **1** The semi-Fowler's position aids in drainage and prevents spread of infection throughout the abdominal cavity. (b)

  2 The Trendelenburg position would contribute to the spread of infection throughout the abdominal cavity.

  3 The Sims position is generally used for administration of enemas, or rectal examination; would not be helpful in draining the area.

  4 The dorsal recumbent position would not allow for lower body drainage.

181. **2** Paralytic ileus occurs when neurologic impulses are diminished, as from anesthesia, infection, or surgery. (a)

  1 Interference in blood supply would result in necrosis of the bowel.

  3 Perforation of the bowel would result in pain and peritonitis.

  4 Obstruction of the bowel lumen would initially cause increased peristalsis and bowel sounds.

182. **4** Thrombophlebitis is inflammation of a vein that occurs with the formation of a clot. Signs include pain (especially on dorsiflexion of the foot), redness, warmth, tenderness, and edema. (a)

  1 Pain occurs on flexion of the foot (Homan's sign).

  2 Pitting edema does not occur in thrombophlebitis.

  3 Intermittent claudication (pain and limping when walking) may occur with peripheral vascular disease.

183. **1** Coumarin derivatives are ordered day by day, based on the prothrombin time of the client. This test gives a good index of the individual's clotting ability. (b)

  2 Clotting time is the time required for blood to form a clot; not used for dosage calculation.

  3 Bleeding time is the time required for blood to cease flowing from a small wound; not used for coumarin dosage calculation.

  4 Sedimentation rate is a test used to determine the presence of inflammation or infection; not indicative of clotting ability.

184. **3** Dicumarol depresses prothrombin activity and inhibits the formation of several of the clotting factors by the liver. Its antagonist is vitamin K, which is involved in prothrombin formation. (c)

  1 Imferon is an iron supplement, not an antidote for coumarin.

  2 Heparin is an anticoagulant.

  4 Protamine sulfate is the antidote for heparin overdose.

185. **1** Carcinoma can be ruled out only by tissue biopsy, which is obtained during surgery. (c)

  2 Symptoms could have been treated medically.

  3 The complication was the reason for the second surgical intervention.

  4 Diverticulitis can in most cases be treated by diet, rest, and antibiotic therapy.

186. **2** To promote drainage of different lung regions, clients should turn every 2 hours. Deep breathing inflates the alveoli and promotes fluid drainage. (b)

  1 Coughing is a major cause of incisional pain, and its desirability in the absence of accumulated secretions is questioned.

  3 During physical efforts, individuals with abdominal incisions often revert to shallow breathing.

  4 Administration of IPPB is a dependent function of the nurse.

187. **2** Pernicious anemia is due to a lack of vitamin B_{12}. Intrinsic factor, produced by the parietal cells of the gastric mucosa, is necessary for B_{12} absorption. (b)

  1 B_{12} is absorbed in the ileum.

  3 Intrinsic factor is secreted by the stomach; the hemopoietic factor is the combination of B_{12} and intrinsic factor.

  4 Chief cells secrete the enzymes of the gastric juice.

188. **1** To ensure continued suction, the patency of the tube should be maintained. Physiologic saline is used to prevent fluid and electrolyte disturbances during irrigation. (a)

  2 Ice chips and water represent fluid intake, which must be approved by the physician; being hypotonic in nature, such intake may lower the serum electrolytes.

  3 The stomach is not considered a sterile body cavity, so medical asepsis is indicated.

  4 Care must be taken to avoid traumatizing the mucosa.

189. **3** Overbathing and use of soap can cause increased dryness and skin breakdown. Emollients help relieve dryness. (b)

  1 The need for bathing must be evaluated on an individual basis.

  2 The need for bathing must be evaluated on an individual basis.

  4 Use of emollients without simultaneous consideration of the effects of soap and excessive bathing is generally ineffective.

190. **2** After a subtotal gastrectomy, small frequent feedings are best tolerated. (a)

  1 As soon as edema subsides, the individual is generally given an ounce of fluid per hour and then diet is gradually progressed.

  3 Recuperation from gastric surgery may take up to 3 months.

  4 IV therapy is not sufficient to provide the nutrients needed for healing unless hyperalimentation is employed.

191. **1** The symptoms indicate hepatic coma. Protein is reduced according to tolerance, and calories are increased to prevent tissue catabolism. (a)

  2 This represents a high-protein diet, which is contraindicated in hepatic coma.

  3 This represents a high-protein diet, which is contraindicated in hepatic coma.

  4 This represents a high-protein diet, which is contraindicated in hepatic coma.

192. **4** The liver manufactures albumin, the major plasma protein. A deficit of this protein will lower the osmotic pressure in the intravascular space, leading to a fluid shift. (c)

  1 The enlarged liver compresses the portal system, causing increased rather than decreased pressure.

  2 The kidneys are not the primary source of the pathologic condition. It is the liver's inability to manufacture albumin that maintains the colloid oncotic pressure.

  3 Potassium is not produced by the body, nor is its major function the maintenance of fluid balance.

193. **3** With obstruction of the portal vein there is an increase in pressure in the abdominal veins, which empty into the portal system. These veins develop collaterals to circumvent the obstruction. The collaterals are usually in the paraumbilical, hemorrhoidal, and esophageal areas. (a)
    1 Although viral hepatitis may predispose to the development of cirrhosis, which in turn causes portal hypertension, most often it does not.
    2 Kupffer cells are part of the reticuloendothelial system, which helps prevent infection and does not primarily affect venous pressure.
    4 Obstruction of these ducts blocks the flow of bile, causing obstructive jaundice.

194. **2** The elevated pressure within the portal circulatory system causes elevated pressure in areas of portal systemic collateral circulation (most important, in the distal esophagus and proximal stomach). Hemorrhage is a possible complication. (a)
    1 Perforation of the duodenum is usually caused by peptic ulcers; not a direct result of portal hypertension or cirrhosis.
    3 Liver abcesses may occur as a complication of intestinal infections; not related to portal hypertension.
    4 Not related to portal hypertension; may be caused by manipulation of the bowel during surgery, peritonitis, neurologic disorders, or organic obstruction.

195. **1** Since lipoproteins, a combination of a fat and a simple protein, have not been formed because of poor protein intake, fat accumulation occurs in the liver. (c)
    2 Individuals with cirrhosis of the liver tend to have bleeding tendencies (rather than clotting) because of the decreased synthesis of prothrombin.
    3 Deficiency of protein results in the breakdown of tissue (catabolism) and a negative nitrogen balance.
    4 Elevations of bile in the blood occur as a result of obstruction of hepatic ducts by the enlarged liver.

196. **2** IV fluids do not provide proteins required for tissue growth, repair, and maintenance. Therefore tissue breakdown occurs to provide the essential amino acids. (b)
    1 Although each liter provides approximately 200 calories, additional liters can be infused to meet minimal energy requirements and prevent weight loss.
    3 Weight loss is caused by insufficient intake of nutrients, which provide calories; vitamins do not provide calories.
    4 An infusion of 5% dextrose in water may decrease the electrolyte concentration because of a fluid shift.

197. **3** When bile does not mix with foods in the intestine, emulsification of fats cannot occur and fat digestion is retarded. Stomach motility is also reduced, since increased stomach peristalsis is dependent on fat digestion in the small intestine. (b)
    1 The production of the bile is unaffected.
    2 Once emulsified by bile, fatty foods are readily broken down by digestive enzymes.
    4 Although people with cholecystitis may refrain from eating fatty foods, the basic pathologic disorder remains unaltered.

198. **2** Vitamin K, a fat-soluble vitamin, is not absorbed from the GI tract in the absence of bile. Bile enters the duodenum via the common bile duct. (a)
    1 Extrinsic factor (cyanocobalamin) is a water-soluble vitamin; bile is not necessary for its absorption.
    3 Calcium is related to rhythmic muscle contraction not coagulation.
    4 Bilirubin is formed by the breakdown of hemoglobin and RBCs and is not related to coagulation.

199. **3** Cholecystography is an x-ray examination of the gallbladder after ingestion or IV injection of a radiopaque drug that is concentrated in the normally functioning gallbladder. (b)
    1 The ampulla of Vater is not visualized.
    2 The common bile duct is examined during choledochography.
    4 In the presence of biliary obstruction, the dye is poorly absorbed by the gallbladder so visualization is generally poor.

200. **1** Cholecystokinin is a widely distributed hormone whose functions include stimulation of gallbladder contraction and the release of pancreatic enzymes. It also functions as a neurotransmitter in the CNS. (b)
    2 Promotes the production of bile by the liver and the secretion of pancreatic juice.
    3 Stimulates the secretion of gastric juice.
    4 Stimulates the secretion of intestinal juice (succus entericus).

201. **2** A drain is inserted to remove fluid, which could cause pressure on the operative site and delay healing. The nurse should anticipate drainage and reinforce the surgical dressings as needed. (a)
    1 Changing a dressing unnecessarily increases the risk of infection as well as possible dislodgement of the drain.
    3 An abdominal binder may be ordered prior to ambulation but would interfere with assessment of the dressing at this time.
    4 Montgomery straps are utilized when frequent dressing changes are anticipated; not appropriate at this time.

202. **4** Localized sensory changes may indicate nerve damage, impaired circulation, or thrombophlebitis. Activity should be limited, and the physician notified. (a)
    1 Symptoms may be indicative of a serious problem, and the physician must be notified.
    2 Rubbing or massaging the legs is contraindicated because of possible dislodging of a thrombus if present.
    3 Bed rest is indicated to prevent the possibility of further damage or creation of an embolus.

203. **1** Protein and calories are necessary for tissue building. (a)
    2 The obstruction has been corrected; dietary fat intake is dependent on the individual's tolerance.
    3 Protein and calories are necessary for tissue repair.
    4 A high-fat diet is contraindicated since fat requires bile to be absorbed; spasms in the biliary system may result in pain.

204. **4** The act of eating allows the hydrochloric acid in the stomach to work on and be neutralized by food rather than irritate the gastric mucosa. (b)
    1 These symptoms are not specific to gastric ulcers.
    2 This may indicate renal colic.
    3 Generalized symptoms not specific to gastric ulcers.

205. **1** Peptic ulcers may occur in an individual in whom there is a conflict between a strong drive for independence and an unconscious need to be dependent. (c)
    2 This psychologic state is not involved in the etiology of peptic ulcer.
    3 This psychologic state is not involved in the etiology of peptic ulcer.
    4 Does not include many feelings; involves the unconscious need to be dependent.

206. **4** The client should be encouraged to rest mind and body; sedatives may be indicated to achieve this goal. (b)
    1 False reassurance is psychologically damaging.

    2 Antibiotics will have no direct effect on the client's anxiety.

    3 Knowledge itself does not always reduce anxiety.

207. **2** Irritation of the mucosa may cause increased bleeding or perforation and therefore should be avoided. (b)

    1 Bulk and roughage may irritate the mucosa and should be decreased.

    3 All clients' diets should be nutritionally balanced; this is not specific to this client's problem.

    4 Psychologic support is not the primary goal; efforts should be made to include foods that are psychologically beneficial, but not at the expense of foods that are nonirritating to the mucosa.

208. **3** Iron is needed in the formation of hemoglobin. (b)

    1 Dextran is a plasma volume expander; does not affect erythrocytes.

    2 Cari-Tab Softabs are vitamin supplements intended to promote the development of caries-free dentition.

    4 Vitamin B_{12} is a water-soluble vitamin that must be supplemented when an individual has pernicious anemia.

209. **4** Gastroscopy permits visualization of the stomach and biopsy of the tissue. (a)

    1 Soft tissue is not visualized by x-rays unless radiopaque substance is utilized.

    2 CBC may provide a general index of the extent of occult bleeding but is not diagnostic of cancer of the stomach.

    3 Screening test of adrenocortical function based on eosinophil response to ACTH administration.

210. **4** An American relative can serve as interpreter and provide emotional support and security. (b)

    1 Translation of medical terminology does not suffice in establishing communication for reducing the strangeness of the environment, nor does it provide emotional support.

    2 Such sporadic communication is less than therapeutic because interpersonal relationships do not develop.

    3 Ongoing communication is an essential element of the nursing process.

211. **3** $\dfrac{\text{Amount to be infused} \times \text{Drop factor}}{\text{Time of infusion in minutes}}$ (a)

    1 Incorrect calculation; too rapid; would infuse in approximately 1 hour.

    2 Incorrect calculation; too rapid; would take between 2 and 3 hours to infuse.

    4 Incorrect calculation; too rapid; would infuse in approximately 4 hours.

212. **4** Approximately 42 ml of fluid per hour would be infused. This is adequate to keep the vein open without causing circulatory overload; after 24 hours there is increased risk of contamination of the solution and the container should be changed. (b)

    1 Provides fluid not needed by the client; increased risk of circulatory overload or heart failure.

    2 Provides fluid not needed by the client; increased risk of circulatory overload or heart failure.

    3 Provides fluid not needed by the client; increased risk of circulatory overload or heart failure.

213. **1** Gluten, a cereal protein, appears to be responsible for morphologic changes of the intestinal mucosa in individuals with nontropical sprue (celiac disease). (b)

    2 Folic acid, along with antimicrobial agents, is used to treat tropical sprue; causes dramatic improvement.

    3 The use of corticosteroids may be advantageous with either form of sprue; however, does not produce the same effect as specific treatments already described.

    4 Vitamin B_{12} may be administered if macrocytic anemia or achlorhydria develops; however, does not correct the major pathosis.

214. **1** Gluten is found in rye, wheat, and oat products. (a)

    2 Gluten is not found in these foods; they do not have to be avoided.

    3 Gluten is not found in these foods; they do not have to be avoided.

    4 Gluten is not found in these foods; they do not have to be avoided.

215. **2** These foods are low in gluten. (c)

    1 Flours used in the production of bread are high in gluten.

    3 Flours used in the production of noodles are high in gluten.

    4 Postum is a cereal drink high in gluten.

216. **1** The diet should be high in protein and calories, low in fat, and gluten free for individuals with nontropical sprue. Protein is needed for tissue rebuilding. (b)

    2 Diarrhea is caused by malabsorption, which accounts for the poor nutritional status; once the diarrhea is corrected, it is essential to compensate for poor nutrition.

    3 May prefer foods high in gluten, which would potentiate malabsorption.

    4 IV therapy does not provide all the necessary nutrients.

217. **4** The location of the tumor will usually indicate whether a colostomy, creation of an opening proximal to the tumor between the colon and the skin surface, is needed. (a)

    1 A cecostomy is the creation of an opening between the cecum and the skin surface; usually a temporary procedure.

    2 An ileostomy is the creation of an opening between the ileum and the skin surface; would not be done.

    3 A colectomy is the surgical removal of a portion of the colon, with creation of an anastomosis; generally used in less extensive carcinoma.

218. **3** Neomycin sulfate is poorly absorbed from the GI tract and is therefore used for sterilization of the intestines prior to bowel surgery. (a)

    1 Being poorly absorbed from the GI tract, neomycin sulfate does not affect urinary tract infections.

    2 Because intestinal bacteria are destroyed, there is a decreased production of vitamin K.

    4 Oral administration of neomycin primarily affects intestinal bacteria.

219. **3** Preparations such as aluminum paste can be used on the skin around the stoma to prevent excoriation from the ostomy drainage. (a)

    1 Petroleum jelly would interfere with adherence of any ostomy appliance.

    2 Alcohol tends to dry out the skin and mucous membranes, leading to irritation and breakdown.

    4 Mineral oil is not an effective skin protectant and could interfere with adherence of any appliance.

220. **3** Surgery on the bowel has no direct anatomic or physiologic effect on sexual performance. However, psychologic factors could hamper this function, and the nurse should encourage verbalization. (b)

    1 There is no reason why sexual relationships must be curtailed.

    2 Although his partner should understand the nature of the surgery, the focus at this time should be on the client.

    4 Although it may take several months to resume satisfying sexual relationships, the surgery has no direct physiologic effect.

221. **1** Ample time in the bathroom must be ensured for the actual irrigation process and fecal returns, which may not be immediate. (c)
    2 The availability of adequate time takes precedence over any specific timing that may be convenient.
    3 The availability of adequate time takes precedence over any specific timing that may be convenient.
    4 The availability of adequate time takes precedence over any specific timing that may be convenient.

222. **3** The rapid rate of enema administration or ostomy irrigation often causes cramping. Additional fluid leads to more discomfort. Cramping will generally subside if the enema tubing is clamped for a few minutes; the procedure can then be continued. (b)
    1 Lowering the container will decrease the rate of flow, but fluid will continue to enter the colon if the container remains above the stoma.
    2 Discontinuing the irrigation could lead to ineffective evacuation of the colon.
    4 Indiscriminate advancing of the catheter can injure the mucosa and does not affect cramping.

223. **2** This is far enough to direct the flow of solution into the bowel. (c)
    1 Inadequate; fluid may leak back around the catheter.
    3 Insertion of 6 inches may cause trauma to the mucosa.
    4 Insertion of 8 inches may cause trauma to the mucosa.

224. **1** A colostomy irrigation is much like a tap water enema. The solution must be held high enough to allow it to flow into the bowel but not so high that it flows rapidly, or it can cause cramping or mucosal injury. (b)
    2 Does not represent maximum height of the solution; may not ensure flow of solution into the bowel.
    3 Does not represent maximum height of the solution; may not ensure flow of solution into the bowel.
    4 Does not represent maximum height of the solution; may not ensure flow of solution into the bowel.

225. **3** Personality and psychologic stresses cause pathologic changes that influence the development of ulcerative colitis. (b)
    1 Although this may be another causative factor, psychologic stress is more commonly associated with this disease.
    2 Although this may be another causative factor, psychologic stress is more commonly associated with this disease.
    4 Although this may be another causative factor, psychologic stress is more commonly associated with this disease.

226. **1** Potassium, the major intracellular cation, functions with sodium and calcium to regulate neuromuscular activity and contraction of muscle fibers, particularly heart muscle. In hypokalemia these symptoms develop. (b)
    2 These symptoms would indicate hypocalcemia, which does not generally occur in colitis.
    3 Nausea and vomiting might occur with prolonged potassium deficit; however, not an early sign; leg and abdominal cramps occur with potassium excess, not deficit.
    4 These symptoms are not indicative of an electrolyte imbalance.

227. **4** To promote understanding and allay anxiety, all diagnostic tests should be explained to the client. (b)
    1 Preparations for the test may vary depending on the client's condition.
    2 Preparations for the test may vary depending on the client's condition.
    3 Preparations for the test may vary depending on the client's condition.

228. **1** To take advantage of the anatomic position of the sigmoid colon and the effect of gravity, the client should be placed in a left Sims' position for the enema. (b)
    2 This position does not facilitate the flow of fluid into the sigmoid colon by gravity.
    3 This position does not facilitate the flow of fluid into the sigmoid colon by gravity.
    4 This position does not facilitate the flow of fluid into the sigmoid colon by gravity.

229. **3** If the height of the enema fluid container above the anus is increased, the force and rate of flow also increase. If the container is raised excessively, damage to the mucosa may result and the procedure will be much more difficult for the client to tolerate. (b)
    1 The enema container can be held up to 30.5 cm above the anus and still be considered within safe limits.
    2 The enema container can be held up to 37 cm above the anus and still be considered within safe limits.
    4 This would be too high and could cause mucosal injury.

230. **3** Administration of additional fluid when a client complains of abdominal cramps adds to discomfort because of additional pressure. By clamping the tubing a few minutes the nurse allows the cramps generally to subside and the enema can be continued. (b)
    1 Slowing the rate decreases pressure but does not reduce it entirely.
    2 This will reduce the solution flow, which will decrease pressure but not reduce it entirely.
    4 Cramps are not a reason to discontinue the enema entirely; temporary clamping of the tubing usually relieves the cramps and the procedure can be continued.

231. **1** Since the soft tissues of the GI tract lack sufficient quantities of x-ray-absorbing atoms (as are naturally present in the dense calcium salts of bone), an x-ray-absorbing coating of barium is used for radiologic studies. (c)
    2 Barium does not color the intestinal wall.
    3 Barium absorbs x-rays.
    4 No interaction with electrolytes.

232. **2** Milk and the caffeine in cola are chemically irritating to the intestinal mucosa. They also promote secretion of gastric juice. (b)
    1 These are absorbed slowly and are not irritating.
    3 Salt helps retain water and rice produces bulk, both of which aid elimination.
    4 Too general; except for those that contain lactose sugars, products containing sugar generally are not irritating to the mucosa; protein also is not irritating.

233. **3** The parasympathetic nervous system (a branch of the autonomic nervous system) causes increased GI motility and secretions. The adrenal cortex releases glucocorticoids, which also stimulate the GI tract, increasing the acidity of the secretions. (b)
    1 They do not affect involuntary muscles of the colon.
    2 The stress function of the pancreas is not directly related to the intestines but is related to glycogen release from the liver. The sympathetic nervous system decreases GI motility.
    4 These do not affect involuntary muscles of the colon.

234. **2** The nurse must actively try to understand his or her own feelings and prejudices, since these will affect the ability to assess a client's behavior objectively. (b)
    1 Understanding a client's emotional conflict can be accomplished only after dealing with one's own feelings.
    3 Information from significant others is beneficial, but only after a nurse is able to deal with his or her own feelings.
    4 The health team members should work together for the benefit of all clients.

235. **3** Ulcerative colitis is linked to psychoemotional stress and generally is exacerbated when conflicts exist. (c)
  1 There is no physiologic change that can be made surgically to alter the disease; an ileostomy may be done to rest the small intestine.
  2 This may be only one factor that is causing psychologic conflict.
  4 Endocrine activity is not the only causative factor.
236. **1** Glucocorticoids and acetylcholine tend to increase peristalsis, causing cramping and diarrhea with subsequent weight loss. As ulceration occurs, loss of blood leads to anemia. (b)
  2 Hemoptysis (coughing up blood from the respiratory tract) is not a related symptom.
  3 Fever may not be a symptom and leukopenia (deficiency in number of leukocytes) does not occur.
  4 Leukocytosis or increased leukocytes in the blood is not common in this disease.
237. **2** Occult blood in the stool could indicate active bleeding; the stool should also be examined for microorganisms to detect early infections that could easily become systemic by spread through the damaged intestinal mucosa. (b)
  1 This situation does not warrant culturing.
  3 No indication that parasites are present; situation does not warrant this examination.
  4 Situation does not warrant these examinations.
238. **2** As a result of chronic irritation, the colon becomes thin and may perforate. (b)
  1 Bleeding may vary from a small amount to hemorrhage; this is not the most serious complication.
  3 Obstruction would not occur as the result of this disease.
  4 Paralytic ileus may be a complication of surgical interventions involving the intestines or of perforation.
239. **4** This is a low-residue diet and is necessary in the acute phase of ulcerative colitis to prevent irritation of the colon. (c)
  1 The juice in this diet contains cellulose, which is not absorbed and irritates the colon; cream soup contains lactose, which is irritating to the colon.
  2 Milk contains lactose, which is irritating to the colon and contraindicated in colitis.
  3 Milk contains lactose, which is irritating to the colon and contraindicated in colitis.
240. **3** Gamma globulin, an immune globulin, contains most of the antibodies circulating in the blood. When injected into an individual, it prevents a specific antigen from entering a host cell. (b)
  1 Does not stimulate antibody production.
  2 Does not stimulate antibody production.
  4 Does not affect antigen-antibody function.
241. **4** Phenobarbital depresses the CNS, particularly the motor cortex, producing side effects such as lethargy, loss of appetite, depression, and vertigo. (b)
  1 These are not side effects of phenobarbital.
  2 These are not side effects of phenobarbital.
  3 These are not side effects of phenobarbital.
242. **3** The virus is present in the stool of clients with infectious hepatitis, so special handling is required. The virus may also be present in the urine and in the nasotracheal secretions of such clients. (b)
  1 Bringing food to a client requires no precautions; however, disposable utensils should be used because the client's nasotracheal secretions contain the virus.
  2 Infectious hepatitis is not usually transmitted via the air.
  4 Infectious hepatitis is not usually transmitted via the air.

243. **3** Proximity to the nurses' station is vital. The client must be observed frequently, since behavior is unpredictable. (a)
  1 The client may be unable to ambulate safely to the bathroom; this choice does not indicate proximity of the room to the nurses' station.
  2 Sharing a room with another client would be disturbing to the other client; a room far from the nurses' station would prevent close observation.
  4 Sharing a room with another client would be disturbing to the other client.
244. **4** Paraldehyde is a sedative that is ordered to reduce psychomotor stimuli. (b)
  1 Fluid and electrolyte balance is unaffected by this drug.
  2 Detoxification is a slow process and is not affected by sedation.
  3 Emotional problems are masked, not resolved, through sedation.
245. **2** Protein helps correct severe malnutrition; moderate fat limits the need for bile; a high-calorie, high-vitamin diet prevents tissue breakdown. (b)
  1 A diet high in protein, carbohydrates, and calories is needed to improve nutritional status.
  3 This diet does not offer enough fat or calories.
  4 A high-protein diet is essential in repairing tissues and restoring nutritional status.
246. **2** The liver detoxifies alcohol and is the organ most often damaged in chronic alcoholism. The high-calorie diet prevents tissue breakdown, which produces additional amino acids and nitrogen. (a)
  1 These organs are not involved in detoxification of alcohol.
  3 This organ is not involved in detoxification of alcohol.
  4 These glands are not involved in detoxification of alcohol.
247. **2** Thiamine and nicotinic acid help convert glucose for energy and therefore nerve activity. (a)
  1 These vitamins are not related to circulatory activity.
  3 Vitamin K, not thiamine and niacin, is essential for the manufacture of prothrombin in the liver.
  4 These vitamins do not affect elimination.
248. **4** Intact skin is the first line of defense against entry of microorganisms. A surgical incision is a portal of entry, so a technique that requires the absence of all microorganisms (surgical asepsis) is essential. (c)
  1 Concurrent disinfection refers to measures initiated to control the spread of infection while an infection is present; concurrent asepsis is incorrect terminology.
  2 Medical asepsis utilizes clean technique to minimize the spread of microorganisms; when there is a break in the skin, such technique is insufficient.
  3 Wound asepsis is incorrect terminology.
249. **1** These symptoms result from failure of bile to enter the intestines, with subsequent backup into the biliary system and diffusion into the blood. The bilirubin is carried to all body regions, including the skin (itching) and kidneys (excretion of bile-colored urine). The absence of bilirubin in the intestine results in clay-colored stools. (c)
  2 If bile levels in the bloodstream are high, there would be bile in the urine, causing it to have a dark color.
  3 Signs refer to objective findings of an examiner; the signs of inadequate absorption of vitamin K include ecchymosis, hematuria, and other bleeding.
  4 The urine would be dark, reflecting increased serum bilirubin levels, and the stools would not be brown because the bile pigments would not be present in the GI tract.

250. **1** Vitamin C (ascorbic acid) plays a major role in wound healing. It is necessary for the maintenance and formation of strong collagen, the major protein of most connective tissues. (b)
  2 Phytonadione (e.g., Mephyton) is vitamin K, which plays a major role in blood coagulation.
  3 Vitamin B$_{12}$ is needed for red blood cell synthesis and a healthy nervous system.
  4 Vitamin A is important for the healing process; however, vitamin C cements the ground substance of supportive tissue.

251. **3** The location of the incision results in pain on inspiration or coughing. The subsequent reluctance to cough and deep breathe facilitates respiratory complications from retained secretions. (b)
  1 Bile does not impair inflammatory or immune responses.
  2 A cholecystectomy is usually performed to treat cholelithiasis or cholecystitis; there is generally an inflammatory, not an infectious, process.
  4 The duration of surgery is not longer than for other abdominal surgery.

252. **4** Bile, a natural antioxidant, helps stabilize the vitamin and prevents destruction by oxygen. In addition, it serves as a transport vehicle for fat through the intestinal wall. (c)
  1 Digestive enzyme for lipids.
  2 Digestive enzyme for starch.
  3 Stomach acid.

253. **4** This position maximally exposes the rectal area and facilitates entry of the sigmoidoscope. It is preferred. (b)
  1 Although prone refers to a face-down position, the rectal area is not exposed.
  2 The lithotomy position is appropriate for gynecologic examinations.
  3 The Sims' position does not expose the rectal area to the same extent as the knee-chest position does but can still be used for a sigmoidoscopy if the client is unable to maintain the knee-chest position.

254. **3** To permit adequate visualization of the mucosa during the sigmoidoscopy, the bowel must be cleansed with a nonirritating enema before examination. (a)
  1 Since only the lower bowel is being visualized, keeping the client npo is unnecessary and debilitating; clear liquids and a laxative may be given the day before to limit fecal residue.
  2 The client does not drink such a substance in preparation for a sigmoidoscopy.
  4 Stool should be eliminated from the colon by an enema before the examination.

255. **4** The nurse should pick up all clues to client anxiety and allow for verbalization. This response recognizes the client's feelings. (a)
  1 This response negates the client's feelings and presents a negative connotation about the procedure.
  2 This response negates the client's feelings and presents a negative connotation about the procedure.
  3 This response focuses on the task rather than on the client's feelings.

256. **4** Because neomycin is poorly absorbed from the GI tract, most remains in the intestines and exerts its antibiotic effect on the intestinal mucosa. In preparation for GI surgery the level of microbial organisms will be reduced. (a)
  1 Neomycin is mainly effective in suppression of intestinal flora.
  2 Since it is poorly absorbed from the GI tract, the systemic effect is minimal.
  3 Neomycin is nephrotoxic.

257. **2** If the area is not kept both clean and dry, drainage from the colostomy can quickly cause a breakdown of the skin around the stoma. This, in combination with a warm moist surface, also predisposes the individual to infection. (a)
  1 The client is often unable to accept the altered body image and must be given time to adjust before participating actively in dressing changes.
  3 Although oral fluids are withheld until peristalsis returns, it is essential that parenteral fluids be administered to replace the losses incurred by surgery.
  4 Although oral fluids are withheld until peristalsis returns, it is essential that parenteral fluids be administered to replace the losses incurred by surgery.

258. **3** The stoma of a colostomy must be dilated with a lubricated, gloved finger to prevent strictures and subsequent obstruction. (b)
  1 Clothing need not be special but should be nonconstricting.
  2 Once healing has occurred, activity is not limited.
  4 Diet should be as close to normal for the individual as possible; gas-forming foods should be avoided.

259. **1** Although foods that produce gas are generally avoided, the diet of an individual with a colostomy should be as close to normal as possible for optimal physiologic and psychologic adaptation. (b)
  2 A high-protein diet is important until healing occurs; but a balanced diet generally meets nutritional needs for protein.
  3 There is no need to limit fiber; it provides bulk necessary for unconstipated stools.
  4 Since absorption of nutrients is unaffected, there is no need to increase carbohydrate intake.

260. **2** Cirrhosis of the liver results in the development of extensive scar tissue within the liver structure; such scar tissue contracts around hepatic blood vessels, impeding blood flow and raising the pressure in the hepatic portal system. The physiologic response to slowly developing portal circulatory obstruction is the growth of collateral vessels linking portal veins with esophageal veins; as destruction progresses, the collaterals become so large that they bulge into the esophageal lumen and are called esophageal varices. (b)
  1 The varicosities are the result of increased portal pressure.
  3 Ascites and edema are the result of the liver pathophysiologic process, not the cause; the fluid is present in the interstitial spaces and abdominal cavity as a result of portal hypertension and decreased plasma protein.
  4 The liver regenerates; but in the case of cirrhosis, scar tissue is formed.

261. **3** Gastric suctioning provides an estimate of the extent of bleeding but does not control it. (a)
  1 Aminocaproic acid inhibits the fibrinolysis that may accompany hepatic cirrhosis.
  2 Balloon tamponade (Sengstaken-Blakemore tube) may be used to apply pressure against the bleeding varices.
  4 Iced saline is instilled via a nasogastric tube to control hemorrhage; cold promotes blood vessel constriction.

262. **2** Neomycin destroys intestinal flora, which breaks down protein and in the process gives off ammonia. Ammonia at this time is poorly detoxified by the liver and can build up to toxic levels. (b)
  1 Urea is a by-product of protein metabolism; formed in the liver as it detoxifies ammonia. The production of urea is hampered by severe liver damage and is unaffected by neomycin.

3 Bile levels may be elevated because of biliary obstruction by the enlarged liver but are unaffected by neomycin.

4 Hemoglobin levels may be lowered as a result of cirrhosis and bleeding but are not increased by administration of neomycin.

263. **1** This tube has an esophageal balloon that on inflation exerts pressure, which retards hemorrhage. (b)

    2 This is used for intestinal decompression.

    3 This is used for intestinal decompression.

    4 This is used for gastric decompression, gavage, or lavage.

264. **2** The client's breath has a sweet odor because the liver is not metabolizing the amino acid methionine. (b)

    1 Anuria is characteristic of renal failure.

    3 Sensation of a lump in the throat associated with acute anxiety; unrelated to liver disease.

    4 Refers to spasm of the eyelid associated with anxiety or cranial nerve pathosis; unrelated to liver disease.

265. **1** Since protein breakdown gives off ammonia, which cannot be detoxified by the liver, protein should be eliminated from the diet. (b)

    2 Carbohydrates are unrelated to protein breakdown and rising ammonia levels; eliminating carbohydrates would have no effect.

    3 A Fleet enema would not affect ammonia levels, which are associated with hepatic coma; a neomycin enema would limit intestinal flora, which breaks down protein, giving off ammonia.

    4 No surgical intervention would affect ammonia levels associated with hepatic coma.

266. **2** Low sodium controls fluid retention, blood pressure, and consequently edema; low protein controls ammonia formation in proportion to the liver's ability to detoxify ammonia in forming urea; moderate fat and high calories and vitamins help repair a long-standing nutritional deficit. (b)

    1 High-protein diets are contraindicated because of the liver's inability to detoxify ammonia.

    3 Regeneration of tissue requires a high-calorie diet; 1200 calories is too low.

    4 Since protein is required for tissue regeneration, restriction is based on the liver's ability to detoxify ammonia; a high-fat diet is avoided because of the related cardiovascular risks and increased need for bile.

267. **1** Because of the liver's inability to detoxify ammonia to urea, protein intake should be further restricted when coma is inevitable. (b)

    2 Normal intake of protein is 55 to 60 g; this high-protein diet will further increase blood ammonia levels.

    3 Normal intake of protein is 55 to 60 g; this high-protein diet will further increase blood ammonia levels.

    4 Normal intake of protein is 55 to 60 g; this high-protein diet will further increase blood ammonia levels.

268. **1** Almost all peptic ulcers in the stomach develop along the lesser curvature of the antral (pyloric) region. About 85% of all peptic ulcers occur within the first 2 cm of the duodenum. These regions are most exposed to acid conditions. (b)

    2 Less exposed to gastric secretions.

    3 Less exposed to gastric secretions.

    4 Less exposed to gastric secretions; however, erosion may occur after repeated episodes of gastric reflux.

269. **4** Propantheline bromide (Pro-Banthine) reduces the motility of the GI tract and thereby facilitates healing. (c)

    1 It does not affect the pH of gastric secretions.

    2 It decreases motility.

    3 It does not affect the pH of gastric secretions.

270. **1** Physiologic normal saline is used in gastric irrigation to prevent electrolyte imbalance. Because of the fresh gastric sutures, slow and gentle irrigation should be performed. Most surgeons, however, prefer gastric instillations. (a)

    2 The purpose of irrigation is to maintain the patency of the tube for gastric decompression; with disconnection from suction a buildup of secretions and air can occur or the tube can become blocked by viscous drainage.

    3 The purpose of irrigation is to maintain the patency of the tube for gastric decompression; with disconnection from suction a buildup of secretions and air can occur or the tube can become blocked by viscous drainage.

    4 Increasing the pressure may cause damage to the suture line.

271. **4** The vagus nerve stimulates the stomach to secrete hydrochloric acid. When it is severed, this neural pathway is interrupted and there will be a decrease in stomach secretions. (b)

    1 The portion of the vagus nerve that was severed innervated the stomach, not the heart; therefore the heart rate would not be affected.

    2 The vagus nerve controls hydrochloric acid secretion, not gastric emptying; this is determined by the nature of foods being digested.

    3 The vagus nerve is not a sensory nerve.

272. **4** To calculate the rate of fluid infusion:

$$\frac{\text{Amount of fluid to be infused} \times \text{Drop factor}}{\text{Number of hours} \times 60 \text{ minutes}}$$

$$\frac{1000 \times 15}{8 \times 60} = \frac{15000}{480} = 31.25 \text{ drops/min} = 31 \text{ drops} \qquad (b)$$

    1 Incorrect calculation, resulting in excessive administration of fluid.

    2 Incorrect calculation, resulting in inadequate administration of fluid.

    3 Incorrect calculation, resulting in inadequate administration of fluid.

273. **2** Since IV solutions enter the body's internal environment, all solutions and medications utilizing this route must be sterile to prevent the introduction of microbes. (b)

    1 The medication can be mixed with the IV solution in many ways; sterility takes priority.

    3 The amount and type of solution depend on the medication; sterility takes priority.

    4 The needle does not have to be changed if sterility is maintained.

274. **1** Symptoms of dumping syndrome occur to some degree in about 50% of all individuals who have undergone gastrectomy or vagotomy. They include weakness, faintness, heart palpitations, and diaphoresis. It is therefore important to explain to the client that such symptoms can be minimized by resting after meals in the semi-Fowler's position and eating small meals, omitting concentrated and highly refined carbohydrates. (b)

    2 Gas-forming foods affect the intestines, not the stomach.

    3 Eating habits must be modified to prevent rapid emptying of the stomach.

    4 Modification of roughage is part of the management of intestinal rather than gastric disorders.

275. **3** In hepatic coma there is an accumulation of nitrogenous wastes, which affect the nervous system. In the second stage of this disease there are flapping tremors and generalized twitching. (b)

    1 Elevated cholesterol levels not necessarily present.

2 Hepatic coma includes CNS disturbances; the stool is often clay colored as a result of biliary obstruction by a cirrhotic liver.

4 As encephalopathy progresses to coma, all reflexes are absent.

276. **4** Bile deposits will impart a yellowish tinge (jaundice or icterus) to the skin, often first observed in the sclerae. (c)

1 Uremic frost is characteristic of renal failure.

2 Urticaria (or hives) is generally characteristic of an allergic response.

3 Hemangioma is a benign lesion composed of blood vessels.

277. **3** In cirrhosis of the liver, fibrous scarring within the liver parenchyma, most often from alcohol toxicity, compresses the portal veins and causes a backup of blood and increased pressure within the portal system. Fluid forms in excess and seeps into the abdominal cavity (ascites), mainly from the surface of the liver. (b)

1 Plasma osmotic pressure is decreased because of decreased albumin production.

2 Lymph does not escape from the liver sinusoids.

4 Secretion of ADH and aldosterone increases as renal blood flow decreases.

278. **2** The increased plasma hydrostatic pressure in the extremities resulting from heart failure or liver cirrhosis, possibly combined with a genetic weakness in the vein walls, may lead to varicose veins. (c)

1 Toxins are not responsible for varicose veins.

3 Decreased plasma protein causes fluid to move out of the vascular compartment into the interstitial spaces.

4 Distention of venous walls occurs as a result of increased rather than decreased pressure.

279. **4** Increased ammonia levels indicate the inability of the liver to detoxify protein by-products. Neomycin reduces the amount of ammonia-forming bacteria in the intestines. (c)

1 Culture and sensitivity testing would identify the presence of a microorganism and the medication that would be effective in its eradication; would not be indicated in cirrhosis.

2 Serum glutamic-pyruvic transaminase (SGPT) is a test to assess for liver disease but has no relationship to the need for neomycin enemas.

3 White blood cells may indicate the presence of infection; however, this would have no relationship to the need for neomycin enemas.

280. **3** Fluid and electrolytes are lost through intestinal decompression; on a daily basis about one-fifth the total body water is secreted into and almost completely reabsorbed by the GI tract. (a)

1 Since the client is kept npo, there would be no stimulus to cause enzymes to be secreted into the GI tract.

2 Dextrose in IV supplies some carbohydrates as a source of energy; would not be drawn from storage by intestinal decompression.

4 Since the client is being kept npo, vitamins and minerals are not entering the GI tract and therefore are not lost.

281. **1** Dehydration is a danger because of fluid loss in GI suction. (b)

2 Based on data provided, these symptoms are not likely to occur.

3 Based on data provided, these symptoms are not likely to occur.

4 Based on data provided, these symptoms are not likely to occur.

282. **2** Isotonic saline most closely resembles normal body fluids; will not cause an imbalance by pulling extra fluids and electrolytes out of the circulation. (a)

1 Hypertonic solutions would draw fluids out of the circulation into the GI tract; glucose provides a medium for bacterial growth.

3 Hypotonic solutions would allow absorption of fluid into the circulation, resulting in dilution of electrolytes and possible circulatory overload.

4 Hypotonic solutions would allow absorption of fluid into the circulation, resulting in dilution of electrolytes and possible circulatory overload.

283. **1** Open communication lines are always important in relieving anxiety and reducing stress, which might interfere with postoperative recovery. (b)

2 Reassurances do not allow for open communication, invalidating the emotions experienced by the client.

3 Learning does not occur when anxiety levels are too high.

4 Does not acknowledge the client's feelings and therefore does not deal with the source of her anxiety.

284. **2** The client must be ready to accept changes in body image and function; this acceptance will facilitate mastery of the techniques of colostomy care, special diets, and optimistic utilization of community resources. (b)

1 Specific knowledge can be imparted only when an individual is ready to learn; requires acceptance of a new body image.

3 Specific knowledge can be imparted only when an individual is ready to learn; requires acceptance of a new body image.

4 Specific knowledge can be imparted only when an individual is ready to learn; requires acceptance of a new body image.

285. **2** A transverse colostomy is an opening created in the transverse colon. The rectal tube should be pointed to the proximal intestine to evacuate the bowels. (b)

1 A water-soluble lubricant is generally used to facilitate insertion.

3 Continual force may traumatize the mucosa; lack of nerve endings diminishes sensation.

4 There are no sphincters so bearing down is unnecessary.

286. **3** Weight is valuable objective data that can be helpful in determining the extent of ascites. (a)

1 Pain is subjective data.

2 Diet history will not help in monitoring a client's condition.

4 Bowel sounds are objective data but do not help monitor the liver.

287. **1** The high-Fowler's position promotes optimal entry into the esophagus aided by gravity. (c)

2 Position does not take full advantage of the effect of gravity.

3 Position does not take full advantage of the effect of gravity.

4 Position does not take full advantage of the effect of gravity.

288. **3** In the liver a simple protein combines with a lipid to form a lipoprotein. Lipoproteins circulate freely in the blood and can be utilized easily and quickly in various metabolic processes. (c)

1 The liver does not phosphorolyze fat.

2 The liver does not oxidize fat.

4 Fat is stored in adipose tissue.

289. **1** The liver stores carbohydrates as glycogen, which is a polymer of glucose. (a)

2 Glycerol is a by-product of lipids and combines with three fatty acids to form triglyceride molecules.

3 Fat is not stored in the liver.

4 Not a ready form of energy; combination of amino acids from protein.

290. **3** Fatty acids are insoluble and must combine with bile to form water-soluble substances. (a)

1 Lipase is a pancreatic enzyme.

2 Amylase, which digests starch, is found in saliva and pancreatic juice.

4 A component of bile. It is produced in the liver and stored in the gallbladder, but it is not the component of bile that emulsifies fats.

291. **4** Leukoplakia is present from the precancerous stage of cancer of the tongue. (b)

1 Halitosis would not be expected in mouth cancer.

2 Bleeding gums occur in gingival diseases.

3 Pain is not a common symptom of cancer of the tongue.

292. **2** Heavy alcohol ingestion predisposes an individual to the development of oral cancer. (b)

1 Gum chewing is not a contributing factor to development of oral cancer.

3 Nail biting has no effect on the development of oral cancer.

4 Dental hygiene does not affect the development of oral cancer.

293. **4**

Intake (ml)		Output (ml)	
IV fluid	350	Voiding	
NG tube feeding	600	8:30 AM	150
		1:00 PM	220
Water	150	3:15 PM	235
Vitamin	30	Aspirated stomach contents	25
	1130		630

(c)

1 Represents a miscalculation; too little intake and too much output.

2 A miscalculation; too little intake and too much output.

3 A miscalculation; too little intake and output.

294. **2** Rebound tenderness is a classic subjective sign of appendicitis. (a)

1 There generally are decreased bowel sounds below an inflamed appendix.

3 Hyperacidity causes epigastric, not lower right quadrant, pain.

4 Urinary retention does not cause acute lower right quadrant pain.

295. **3** When circulation to the appendix is interfered with by a fecalith or foreign body, inflammation occurs. (b)

1 Diet patterns do not predispose the individual to the development of appendicitis.

2 Bowel infections are rare and do not predispose the individual to the development of appendicitis.

4 Hypertension may cause generalized edema; local edema would not occur.

296. **2** Muscular rigidity over affected area is a classic sign of peritonitis. (a)

1 Nausea is a common occurrence when peritonitis occurs.

3 Urinary retention may occur following surgery, as a complication of anesthesia.

4 Malaise, rather than hyperactivity, is often associated with peritonitis.

297. **2** A rectal catheter should be inserted approximately 10 cm (4 inches) since this will be far enough to pass the rectal sphincter. (b)

1 Five-centimeter (2-inch) insertion will not allow the tube to pass the sphincter.

3 Deep insertion may cause damage to the intestinal mucosa.

4 Deep insertion may cause damage to the intestinal mucosa.

298. **2** A rectal tube promotes maximum benefits in 30 minutes. This allows adequate time for gas to escape. (b)

1 Fifteen minutes is not adequate time to permit removal of flatus.

3 After 30 minutes there would be minimal release of flatus.

4 After 30 minutes there would be minimal release of flatus.

299. **1** Since stomach distention after eating results in contractions of the colon (gastrocolic reflex) promoting defecation, establishing some regularity of meals that include adequate bulk or fiber will help establish routine patterns of defecation. (b)

2 Although increased fluid intake and activity facilitate elimination, in general, they do not help establish a pattern.

3 Although increased fluid intake and activity facilitate elimination, in general, they do not help establish a pattern.

4 Increased potassium is not needed for normal elimination.

300. **2** Fiber absorbs water, swells, and consequently stretches the bowel wall, promoting peristalsis, mass movements, and defecation. Smooth muscle tends to contract when stretched because of the reflex activity of stretch receptors. (c)

1 Does not irritate the bowel wall.

3 There is no chemical stimulation.

4 Bacterial action is not involved in the process by which bulk stimulates defecation.

301. **2** Rectal bleeding is a common problem when hemorrhoids are present. (a)

1 Pruritus is not a symptom that can be observed.

3 Anal stenosis is not a complication of hemorrhoids.

4 Flatulence is unrelated to hemorrhoids.

302. **3** The client must be advised to avoid straining and constipation. (b)

1 Enemas may be ordered several days after surgery if the client has not had a bowel movement.

2 Light dressings of witch hazel may be used to promote drainage and healing.

4 Baths are advised to promote healing and cleaning of the area.

303. **4** Constipation and prolonged standing may cause this problem. (a)

1 Spicy foods may irritate hemorrhoids but do not cause them.

2 Bowel control is unrelated to the development of hemorrhoids.

3 Hypertension does not contribute to the development of hemorrhoids.

304. **2** The hepatic portal vein carries blood from the capillary beds of the viscera (small and large intestinal walls, stomach, spleen, pancreas, gallbladder) to the sinusoids of the liver. The hepatic veins drain the liver sinusoids into the inferior vena cava. (b)

1 Takes blood to the liver; the hepatic veins drain the liver sinusoids into the inferior vena cava.

3 Enters from the capillary beds of the viscera.

4 Enters from the capillary beds of the viscera.

305. **4** Alcohol stimulates pancreatic enzyme secretion and an increase in pressure in the pancreatic duct. The backflow of enzymes into the pancreatic interstitial spaces results in partial digestion and inflammation of the pancreatic tissue. (b)

1 Although blockage of the bile duct with calculi may precipitate pancreatitis, this is not associated with alcohol.

2 Alcohol does not deplete insulin stores; the demand for insulin is unrelated to pancreatitis.

3 Although the volume of secretions increases, the composition remains unchanged.

306. **1** Prothrombin, which is normally present in the plasma, is synthesized in the liver in the presence of vitamin K from the amino acid glutamine. Vitamin K initiates the vital process of coagulation. (b)

2 Needed for hemoglobin synthesis.

3 Involved in calcium absorption and metabolism.

4 Plays a role in collagen formation.

307. **4** Vitamin K is a fat-soluble vitamin and needs bile salts for its absorption from the upper segment of the small intestine. It is a catalyst in the carboxylation of glutamine to prothrombin. (c)

1 Bile salts do not affect prothrombinase (thromboplastin).

2 Bile salts do not inhibit the synthesis of prothrombin.

3 The liver does not synthesize vitamin K; intestines do.

308. **2** This is negligence. The client should have been informed. Also the nurse was responsible for collecting the specimen. (b)

1 The physician prescribes the diagnostic test, but the proper collection and handling of specimens are the nurse's responsibility.

3 Staff are liable for negligent actions.

4 The hospital should assume the added expense incurred as a result of the negligent actions of its employees.

309. **1** Vomiting may result in aspiration of vomitus, since it cannot be expelled; this could cause pneumonia or asphyxia. (b)

2 This is not a life-threatening problem.

3 This is not a life-threatening problem.

4 This is not a life-threatening problem.

310. **1** The aerobic oxidation of glucose occurring in the mitochondrion produces 38 moles of ATP for every mole of glucose oxidized. (b)

2 Digestion not hydrolysis of fats.

3 This activity involves gaseous exchange.

4 This is the formation of peptide bonds.

311. **2** Milk and milk products are not tolerated well because they contain lactose, a sugar that is converted to galactose by lactase. (c)

1 Sucrose is not a milk sugar.

3 Maltose is not a milk sugar.

4 This enzyme assists digestion of starch, which is not a milk sugar.

312. **3** The salts in bile act as detergents to break large fat droplets into smaller ones (emulsification), providing a larger surface area for the enzymatic action of fat-splitting enzymes (lipases). (a)

1 Does not have an acid pH.

2 No vitamins are present in bile; it emulsifies fat and thus assists in absorption of fat soluble vitamins.

4 Does not act on proteins.

313. **2** This is the organism that causes botulism. (a)

1 *Salmonella,* a gram-negative rod, is not anaerobic.

3 An anaerobic organism that causes tetanus.

4 A normal inhabitant of intestines; not anaerobic.

314. **2** Orange juice has a higher proportion of simple sugars, which are readily available for conversion to energy. (c)

1 Bread contains carbohydrates, which require longer time to digest since they must be converted to simple sugars.

3 Milk contains fat and protein, which require longer digesting time, and lactose, which is a disaccharide.

4 Candy bars do not contain the high proportion of simple sugars found in orange juice; also contain fat, which takes longer to digest.

315. **2** Phospho-Soda is a saline cathartic, increasing the osmotic pressure within the intestines so that body fluids are drawn into the bowel, stimulating bowel stretching, peristalsis, and defecation. (c)

1 Bulk-forming laxatives are cellulose derivatives that remain in the intestinal tract and absorb water; cause bulk, which stimulates peristalsis.

3 Emollients have a detergent action, softening the stool by facilitating its absorption of water.

4 Stimulants irritate the mucosa so that peristalsis is increased.

316. **2** Amino acids are absorbed into the blood in the intestinal capillaries with the aid of vitamin B_6 via the energy-dependent system, active transport. (b)

1 Proteins are fairly large molecules; do not passively diffuse.

3 Osmosis refers to the movement of water across a semipermeable membrane; does not apply to proteins.

4 Osmosis refers to the movement of water across a semipermeable membrane; does not apply to proteins.

317. **2** Complete proteins contain sufficient amounts of all essential amino acids and are of animal origin. (b)

1 Not all 22 but rather the 8 essential and 2 semiessential (arginine and histidine) are needed during growth.

3 Sufficient amounts of all 8 essential must be present plus 2 semiessential (arginine and histidine), which are essential only during periods of growth.

4 The body cannot make the essential amino acids; they must be present in foods ingested.

318. **1** These amino acids are needed to maintain life and are not produced by the body. (a)

2 All amino acids are needed for metabolism; however, arginine and histidine are necessary for growth, but not during adulthood.

3 The essential amino acids cannot be made by the body.

4 The body does not synthesize these amino acids; they must be ingested in the diet.

319. **3** *Entamoeba histolytica,* the organism that causes amebic dysentery, is transmitted through excreta. (a)

1 Organism not passed via milk.

2 Organism not transmitted by gnats.

4 Not a tick-borne disease.

320. **2** Excessive loss of gastric juice results in excessive loss of hydrochloric acid (HCl) and can lead to alkalosis; the HCl is not available to neutralize the sodium bicarbonate ($NaHCO_3$) secreted into the duodenum by the pancreas. The intestinal tract absorbs the excess HCO_3^-, and alkalosis results. (a)

1 Loss of HCl will move the pH to a basic level.

3 Gastric juice does not regulate osmotic pressure in the blood; the volume of blood would be altered not by loss of gastric juice but by severe dehydration.

4 Oxygen is not drawn from the blood by gastric lavage.

321. **3** Sleeping on pillows raises the upper torso and prevents reflux of the gastric contents through the hernia. (a)

1 Milk would be digested early in the night and symptoms might return.

2 This would have no effect on the mechanical problem of the stomach's entering the thoracic cavity.

4 The effect of antacids is not long lasting enough to promote a full night's sleep.

322. **4** Vitamin K is synthesized by intestinal bacteria but is also found in liver, egg yolks, cheese, tomatoes, and green leafy vegetables. (b)
    1 Vitamin K is found in a small variety of foods.
    2 Vitamin K is not easily absorbed; it is fat soluble and requires bile salts for its absorption.
    3 It is found in enough foods that a natural deficiency usually does not occur.

323. **2** Prevention of serum hepatitis from blood transfusions can be accomplished through screening donors. (b)
    1 Enteric precautions are indicated for individuals with infectious hepatitis.
    3 This is not a preventive measure.
    4 Isolation is not indicated for individuals with serum hepatitis.

324. **1** This is an enzyme that is released early in the course of liver damage. (c)
    2 This is not an early sign of liver damage.
    3 This is not an early sign of liver damage.
    4 This is not an early sign of liver damage.

325. **3** Vincent's angina (trenchmouth) is an infection of the mouth resulting in bleeding gums, pain on swallowing and talking, and fever. (c)
    1 This symptom is related to angina pectoris, resulting from insufficient oxygenation of myocardial tissue, not Vincent's angina.
    2 This symptom is related to angina pectoris, resulting from insufficient oxygenation of myocardial tissue, not Vincent's angina.
    4 This symptom is related to angina pectoris, resulting from insufficient oxygenation of myocardial tissue, not Vincent's angina.

326. **1** Pain and swelling should subside prior to 1 week postoperative. Continued pain may indicate infection. (b)
    2 Tenderness is expected during the postoperative period.
    3 Painful swallowing may occur because of generalized trauma resulting from surgery and is to be expected.
    4 The breath may have an odor because of dried blood in the oral cavity; this is to be expected during the postoperative period.

327. **4** Vitamin C is an intercellular cement substance. (c)
    1 Function of vitamin A.
    2 Function of vitamin K.
    3 Function of vitamin D.

328. **2** A triglyceride comprises three fatty acids and a glycerol molecule. When energy is required, the fatty acids are mobilized from adipose tissue for fuel. (b)
    1 This is not the function of adipose tissue in fat metabolism.
    3 This is not a function of adipose tissue; cholesterol produced in liver.
    4 This is not the function of adipose tissue; its main function is storage.

329. **2** A coenzyme is a nonprotein substance that, in the presence of a suitable enzyme, serves as a catalyst in chemical changes. (a)
    1 A coenzyme is a nonprotein that combines with an apoenzyme to form a complete enzyme.
    3 A series of complex changes is not involved in formation of the enzyme controlling a particular reaction.
    4 The coenzyme does not neutralize the enzyme.

330. **4** Lipoproteins are simple proteins combined with lipid to facilitate circulation of fat in the blood. (b)
    1 A triglyceride is insoluble in water.
    2 Plasma proteins do not contain fat.
    3 A phospholipid is insoluble in water.

331. **4** Fruits contain less natural sodium than do other foods. (b)
    1 Meat is higher in natural sodium than is fruit.
    2 Milk is higher in natural sodium than is fruit.
    3 Vegetables are higher in natural sodium than is fruit.

332. **3** Saturated fats found in animal tissue are more dense than unsaturated fats, which are found in vegetable oils. (c)
    1 This characteristic of food has no bearing on fat content.
    2 This characteristic of food has no bearing on fat content.
    4 The denseness of fat has nothing to do with digestibility.

333. **4** Animal fats are high in dense saturated fats. (a)
    1 Vegetable oils contain unsaturated fats.
    2 Fruits do not contain saturated fats.
    3 Grains do not contain saturated fats.

334. **4** Since triglycerides are made up of fatty acids bonded (esterified) to glycerol, their breakdown releases fatty acids as well as glycerol. (a)
    1 Triglycerides do not contain urea nitrogen.
    2 Triglycerides do not contain amino acids.
    3 Triglycerides do not contain simple sugars.

335. **3** Cholesterol is an absolutely essential structural and functional component of most cellular membranes. That it is associated with atherosclerotic plaques does not detract from its essential functions in membrane structure and steroid hormone metabolism. (b)
    1 Not essential for bone formation; calcium, phosphorus, and calciferol are.
    2 Not necessary for blood clotting; calcium and vitamin K are.
    4 Not involved in muscle contraction; potassium, sodium, and calcium are.

336. **2** Cholesterol is a sterol found in tissue; is attributed in part to diets high in saturated fats. (a)
    1 Cholesterol is needed for the synthesis of bile salts, adrenocortical and steroid sex hormones, and provitamin D.
    3 Only animal foods furnish dietary cholesterol.
    4 Cholesterol is also produced by the body.

337. **3** Emotional stress of any kind can stimulate peristalsis and thereby increase the volume of drainage. (b)
    1 The stoma will start to drain within the first 24 hours after surgery.
    2 Ileostomy drainage is liquefied and continuous, so irrigations are not indicated.
    4 The client should be encouraged to eat a diet as normal as possible.

338. **1** Vitamin B_{12} (extrinsic factor) combines with intrinsic factor, a substance secreted by the parietal cells of the gastric mucosa, forming hemopoietic factor. Hemopoietic factor is only absorbed in the ileum, from which it travels to bone marrow and stimulates erythropoiesis. (c)
    2 Folic acid is not absorbed in the terminal ileum.
    3 Iron absorption does not occur in the ileum.
    4 Trace elements are not absorbed in the ileum.

339. **4** Trauma to the abdominal wall and to the stoma should be avoided, so contact sports are contraindicated. (a)
    1 Trauma to the abdominal wall is a minimal risk in this sport.
    2 Trauma to the abdominal wall is a minimal risk in this sport.
    3 Trauma to the abdominal wall is a minimal risk in this sport.

340. **3** Vitamin A is a fat-soluble vitamin that accumulates in the body and is not significantly excreted even if extremely large amounts are ingested. After prolonged ingestion of extremely large doses, toxic effects can occur. (b)
   1 Vitamin A can be stored in the liver.
   2 Vitamin A is toxic only after prolonged large dosages.
   4 Vitamin A cannot by synthesized by the body.

341. **4** Pitressin is a vasoconstrictor that is used with great success in controlling GI bleeding. (c)
   1 Aquamephyton is vitamin K; it promotes formation of prothrombin in the liver; although this action would be helpful, it would take too long to be of value in an emergency situation.
   2 Neostigmine inhibits cholinesterase, permitting acetylcholine to function; used primarily for myasthenia gravis.
   3 Pro-Banthine is a gastrointestinal anticholinergic; it decreases motility but has no effect on bleeding.

342. **2** Removal of the fundus of the stomach destroys the parietal cells that secrete intrinsic factor (needed to complex with vitamin B_{12} as a preliminary to its absorption in the ileum). (c)
   1 Diabetes has no effect on intrinsic factor.
   3 Hemorrhaging may cause anemia; however, pernicious anemia occurs when intrinsic factor is not produced.
   4 Dietary intake has no effect on the production of intrinsic factor.

343. **3** The antrum is responsible for gastrin production, which stimulates hydrochloric acid (HCl) secretion; its removal reduces HCl secretion and thus reduces irritation of the gastric mucosa. (c)
   1 A resection of the fifth cranial nerve would be done in trigeminal neuralgia.
   2 A stapedectomy, mobilization of the stapes, or a prosthetic implant would be used with otosclerosis.
   4 Removal by means of a laser beam, cryotechnique, or surgery is used when cataracts occur.

344. **2** A pseudocyst of the pancreas is an abnormally dilated space that contains blood, necrotic tissue, and enzymes and is surrounded by connective tissue. (c)
   1 Incorrect definition of a pseudocyst.
   3 Incorrect definition of a pseudocyst.
   4 Incorrect definition of a pseudocyst.

345. **4** That is the unique function of pancreozymin, which is secreted by the duodenal mucosa. It particularly affects the production of amylase. (a)
   1 Cholecystokinin stimulates the flow of bile from the gallbladder.
   2 Enterocrinin increases intestinal juice secretion.
   3 Enterogastrone causes a lessening of gastric secretion and motility.

346. **2** Lipase is a pancreatic enzyme that aids in the digestion of fat. (c)
   1 Does not break down all dietary fat.
   3 Does not synthesize triglycerides.
   4 This is the function of bile.

347. **1** The duodenum secretes several digestion-related hormones, including secretin, which elicits sodium bicarbonate secretion from the pancreas, and pancreozymin, which elicits enzyme secretion from the pancreas. It also brings about gallbladder contraction and secretion of bile; in this function it is known as cholecystokinin. (b)
   2 The pancreas produces the hormone insulin.
   3 The adrenals produce glucocorticoids, mineralocorticoids, epinephrine, etc.
   4 The liver produces bile, which aids in the digestion of fat, but does not produce any hormones.

348. **1** Whole milk is high in saturated fat. (a)
   2 High in unsaturated fat.
   3 High in unsaturated fat.
   4 Low fat content.

349. **4** Vegetable oils, like most lipids from plants, are high in unsaturated fats. (b)
   1 Meats are high in saturated fats.
   2 Animal-derived products such as milk are high in saturated fats.
   3 Meats are high in saturated fats.

350. **4** Vitamin K, synthesized by the bacterial flora of the intestine, promotes the liver's synthesis of prothrombin, an important blood clotting factor. (c)
   1 Vitamin K does not affect calcium ionization.
   2 Vitamin K does not promote platelet aggregation.
   3 Vitamin K does not promote fibrinogen formation.

351. **3** Pancreatic amylase (which enters the small intestine at the sphincter of Oddi) and sucrase, lactase, and maltase (which are released by epithelial cells covering the villi in the small intestine) are responsible for carbohydrate digestion. (c)
   1 Because of the presence of ptyalin in saliva, some starch digestion occurs in the mouth.
   2 Limited carbohydrate digestion occurs in the stomach; pepsin begins the digestion of proteins.
   4 Digestion of carbohydrates is completed prior to their arrival in the large intestine, which is concerned primarily with fluid reabsorption.

352. **2** Bicarbonate buffering is limited, hydrogen ions accumulate, and acidosis results. (c)
   1 The rate of respirations increases in metabolic acidosis to compensate for a low pH.
   3 The fluid balance does not significantly alter the pH.
   4 The retention of sodium ions is related to fluid retention and edema rather than to acidosis.

353. **1** The kidneys are ultimately responsible for maintaining fluid and electrolyte balance by excretion or retention based on the body's needs. (b)
   2 The lungs eliminate water and carbon dioxide only if excess carbonic acid (H_2CO_3) is present; their role in fluid and electrolyte balance is less extensive than the kidneys'.
   3 Antidiuretic hormone has a direct effect on the nephrons, resulting in water retention.
   4 Aldosterone will cause the retention of sodium ions by the nephrons and subsequent fluid retention.

354. **4** The Giordano-Giovannetti diet includes very low protein (20 g) and controlled potassium (1500 mg) daily. (b)
   1 The diet used in the management of renal failure is low in protein because the kidneys are unable to eliminate the waste products from the body.
   2 The body is able to synthesize the nonessential amino acids.
   3 Urea is a waste product of protein metabolism; the body is able to synthesize the nonessential amino acids.

355. **3** In renal failure, as the glomerular filtration rate decreases, phosphorus is retained. As hyperphosphatemia occurs, calcium is excreted. Calcium depletion (hypocalcemia) causes tetany. (b)
   1 The symptoms described are not characteristic of this condition.
   2 The symptoms described are not characteristic of this condition.
   4 The symptoms described are not characteristic of this condition.

356. **1** An elevated blood urea nitrogen, indicating uremia, is toxic to the central nervous system and causes mental cloudiness, confusion, and loss of consciousness. (a)
   2 Hypernatremia is associated with firm tissue turgor, oliguria, and agitation.
   3 If decreased fluid intake results in dehydration, it can cause fatigue, dry skin and mucous membranes, and rapid pulse and respiratory rates.
   4 Hyperkalemia is associated with muscle weakness, irritability, nausea, and diarrhea.

357. **4** Since an external shunt provides circulatory access to a major artery and vein, special safety precautions must be taken to prevent disconnection of the cannulas. Disconnection can cause unimpeded excessive blood loss and death. Clamps should be carried at all times by the client in case this emergency should arise. (c)
   1 Although a potential complication, this does not pose the same immediate threat to life as does exsanguination.
   2 Although a potential complication, this does not pose the same immediate threat to life as does exsanguination.
   3 Although a potential complication, this does not pose the same immediate threat to life as does exsanguination.

358. **2** Urine is strained to determine whether any calculi or calcium gravel has been passed. (a)
   1 Blood pressure assessment is of no particular importance to the client with kidney stones.
   3 Fluids should be encouraged to promote dilute urine and facilitate passage of the calculi.
   4 Administration of analgesics is a dependent function.

359. **4** Dietary intake of calcium, as well as parathormone excretion, will increase calcium blood levels. (c)
   1 Calcium intake through the diet may affect the blood calcium levels.
   2 Parathyroid hormone controls the serum calcium levels.
   3 This is not conclusive evidence that parathyroidism is the cause.

360. **4** Roast beef and a baked potato have only moderate amounts of calcium compared with the other choices. (b)
   1 Ice cream is made with milk and is high in calcium.
   2 Cheese is high in calcium.
   3 Pudding is made with milk and is high in calcium.

361. **2** Cystolithectomy refers to the removal of bladder stones. (c)
   1 Cystolithiasis denotes the presence of stones in the bladder.
   3 Cystometry is the process of measuring the bladder's pressure and capacity.
   4 Cryoextraction refers to the use of subfreezing temperatures in the removal of tissue; generally used in cataract extraction.

362. **4** Calcium and phosphorus are components of these stones and should therefore be avoided. Also an acid environment is not favorable to their development. (a)
   1 Diets high in calcium must be avoided.
   2 Diets high in calcium must be avoided.
   3 This diet is indicated for clients with gout.

363. **1** To prevent crystal formation, the client should have sufficient intake to produce a liter of fluid per day while taking this drug. (b)
   2 Straining urine is not indicated when a client is taking a urinary antibiotic.
   3 The drug need not be taken at a strict time daily.

4 Urinary decrease is of concern, since it may indicate urinary failure. If fluids are forced, the client's output should increase.

364. **1** Calcium oxalate renal stones can be prevented by adhering to a diet low in calcium and oxalate and high in acid ash. (b)
   2 Diet should be high in acid, not alkaline, ash to control production of these stones.
   3 Methionine is an essential amino acid and must be included in the diet.
   4 Purines are catabolized to uric acid and must be avoided in gout.

365. **4** When two compatible drugs are being mixed, if one is a narcotic it should be drawn up first. This prevents contaminating the bottle of narcotic with atropine. (c)
   1 Separate injections will cause undue discomfort to the client and break the skin unnecessarily.
   2 These drugs are not available in powdered form; no need to dilute.
   3 The atropine may contaminate the Demerol vial, which is undesirable.

366. **4** Because of the anatomic position of the incision, drainage would flow by gravity and accumulate under the client lying in the supine position. (b)
   1 Nail beds would indicate peripheral perfusion, not early hemorrhage.
   2 Blood pressure decreases in hemorrhage, and pulse increases.
   3 Respiratory hemorrhage is not common after kidney surgery.

367. **3** A drop in blood pressure, rapid pulse, cold clammy skin, and oliguria are all signs of shock, which, if not treated promptly, can lead to death. (a)
   1 An expected response; the client will push out the airway as the effects of anesthesia subside.
   2 Shallow respirations are common because of the depressant effects of anesthesia.
   4 Snoring respirations are common because of the depressant effects of anesthesia.

368. **2** Maintenance of a patent airway is always the priority, since airway obstruction impedes breathing and may result in death. (c)
   1 This is important in the client's postoperative care; however, oxygenation is the priority.
   3 This is important in the client's postoperative care; however, oxygenation is the priority.
   4 This is important in the client's postoperative care; however, oxygenation is the priority.

369. **3** Dressings retain an undetermined amount of drainage, which would lead to an inaccurate reading. (c)
   1 Counting of saturated pads allows for some degree of objectivity in the assessment, but it is not the most accurate.
   2 Measuring drainage that has seeped through is not as accurate as weighing; however, it does allow for more objective measurement.
   4 Weighing dressings is the most accurate method of estimating postoperative drainage. The nurse must subtract the dry weight of the dressings to determine fluid loss.

370. **1** Cystitis is an inflammation of the bladder that causes frequency, urgency, pain on micturition, and hematuria. (a)
   2 Pyelitis is an inflammation of the pelvis of the kidney, causing flank pain, chills, fever, and weakness.
   3 Nephrosis is a kidney condition in which there is proteinuria, hypoalbuminemia, and edema.

4 Pyelonephritis is a diffuse pyogenic infection of the pelvis and parenchyma of the kidney that causes flank pain, chills, fever, and weakness.

371. **1** Ammonium chloride causes metabolic acidosis. As a result the kidneys secrete the excess hydrogen ions, increasing the acidity of the urine. An acid urine is essential for the antibacterial action of methenamine mandelate (Mandelamine). (c)
  2 Ammonium chloride is an acidifier and thus does not promote healing.
  3 There is no effect on uric crystal stone formation by combining these drugs.
  4 By acidifying the urine this drug enhances the antibacterial action of methenamine mandelate; it does not decrease bladder irritation.

372. **2** Since the female urethra is shorter than the male urethra, the bacteria can more easily invade the bladder. (a)
  1 Hormonal secretions have no effect on the development of bladder infections.
  3 The position of the bladder is the same in males and females.
  4 Urinary pH is within the same range in both males and females.

373. **2** Protein breakdown liberates cellular potassium ions (K^+), leading to hyperkalemia, which can cause cardiac arrhythmia and standstill. The failure of the kidneys to maintain a balance of K^+ is the main indication for dialysis. (b)
  1 Dialysis is not a treatment for hypertension; this is usually controlled by antihypertensive medication and diet.
  3 Ascites occurs in liver disease and is not an indication for dialysis.
  4 Dialysis is not the usual treatment for acidosis. This usually responds to administration of alkaline drugs.

374. **4** Hemodialysis exposes the blood to a solution that contains normal concentrations of nutrients and low concentrations of waste products; the blood and dialyzing solution are separated by a selectively permeable membrane. The diffusion of small molecules (wastes) from the blood to the dialyzing solution is an example of dialysis. (c)
  1 Use of hydrostatic pressure to pass water and solute through a permeable membrane.
  2 Osmosis is the diffusion of water through a selectively permeable membrane.
  3 Movement of solute particles in the direction of a pressure gradient from an area of greater concentration to an area of lesser concentration.

375. **4** Serum hepatitis is transmitted by blood or blood products. The hemodialysis and routine transfusions needed for a client in renal failure constitute a great risk of exposure. (b)
  1 Peritonitis is a danger in peritoneal dialysis.
  2 Renal calculi are not a complication of hemodialysis; they often occur in clients confined to prolonged bed rest because of demineralized bones.
  3 Dialysis does not involve the bladder and would not contribute to the development of a bladder infection.

376. **2** Insertion of an arteriovenous shunt represents a break in the first line of defense against infection, the skin. An infection of an arteriovenous shunt can be avoided by strict aseptic technique. (a)
  1 A bruit is normally auscultated by virtue of the increased arterial pressure in the area.

3 An elastic bandage would interfere with examination of the site.
  4 To prevent damage to the shunt, blood pressure should not be measured in the affected arm.

377. **3** Homologous serum hepatitis is caused by the B virus and is transmitted by contact with the blood of carriers of the disease. (c)
  1 Infectious or type A viral hepatitis is spread by contaminated food or water.
  2 Infectious or type A viral hepatitis is spread by contaminated food or water.
  4 This is a fictitious disease.

378. **1** Frequency and sense of urgency occur because of the irritation of the stone. (a)
  2 Pyuria may occur when infection is present; skin problems do not occur.
  3 Pain radiates from the flank to the groin area.
  4 Irritability may occur because of discomfort; twitching does not occur.

379. **3** Refrigeration retards the growth of bacteria and may preserve the specimen for several hours. (b)
  1 Represents an unnecessary waste of time, effort, and money.
  2 Growth of bacteria will alter the pH and the glucose and protein levels in the urine; must be refrigerated to retard growth.
  4 Growth of bacteria will alter the pH and the glucose and protein levels in the urine; must be refrigerated to retard growth.

380. **2** The method of preservation can affect the test results. Depending on the purpose of the 24-hour study, the urine may be iced, kept with preservatives, or stored in a routine collection bag. (b)
  1 Not necessary unless specifically ordered.
  3 Although some specimens are preserved with this method, others require chemical preservative.
  4 Not necessary unless specifically ordered.

381. **1** Paralysis of the sympathetic vasomotor nerves after administration of spinal anesthesia results in dilation of blood vessels, which causes a subsequent drop in blood pressure. (c)
  2 These receptors are sensitive to oxygen and carbon dioxide tension; not related to postural hypotension; not affected by spinal anesthesia.
  3 The cardiac accelerator center neurons in the medulla regulate heart rate; not related to postural hypotension; not affected by spinal anesthesia.
  4 Strength of cardiac contractions not affected by spinal anesthesia and postural hypotension.

382. **3** Uric acid stones are controlled by a low-purine diet. Foods high in purine, such as organ meats and extracts, should be avoided. (c)
  1 Calcium stones are controlled by a low-calcium, low-phosphate diet; milk, fruits, and vegetables need not be avoided with uric acid stones.
  2 Cystine, not uric acid, stones are controlled by a low-methionine diet, which excludes meat, milk, eggs, and cheese from the diet.
  4 Only organ meats must be avoided; vegetables do not need to be controlled.

383. **4** The causative organism should be isolated prior to institution of antibiotic therapy. (a)
  1 Catheterization is not a routine procedure for urethritis.
  2 This test will not determine the infective organisms causing the problem.
  3 The bowel is not affected by the diagnosis; enemas are not required.

384. **2** Clarity of urine must be assessed to determine the effectiveness of treatment. Cloudy urine usually indicates infection that could be due to purulent drainage from the urethral infection. (b)
  1 Specific gravity yields information related to fluid balance.
  3 Sugar and acetone are not affected by urethral problems.
  4 Viscosity is a subjective characteristic that would not be measurable.

385. **3** The prostate gland is a tubuloalveolar gland shaped like a ring, with the urethra passing through its center. (a)
  1 Lies below the prostate.
  2 Lies along the top and sides of the testes.
  4 On the posterior surface of the bladder.

386. **2** Chlorothiazide (Diuril) affects electrolyte absorption in the nephron, causing an increased excretion of sodium and chloride. (b)
  1 Loop diuretics (e.g., furosemide, ethacrynic acid) inhibit the reabsorption of sodium and chloride at the ascending loop of Henle.
  3 Most diuretics cause loss of potassium; however, potassium-sparing diuretics, such as spironolactone, decrease this loss.
  4 Osmotic diuretics affect the glomerular filtration rate.

387. **3** Occurrence of bladder tumors is related to smoking, radiation, and schistosomiasis. (b)
  1 Jogging is unrelated to the development of tumors.
  2 Vibrations may result in musculoskeletal or kidney problems; unrelated to bladder tumors.
  4 Ingestion of cola has not been linked to bladder tumors.

388. **1** Preoperative cleansing of the bowel is mandated prior to surgical resection and formation of a urinary conduit. (a)
  2 Fluids should not be restricted until after midnight of the operative day.
  3 Muscle tightening exercises have no effect on this procedure.
  4 The stoma of an ileal conduit is not irrigated.

389. **4** The ureters are implanted in a segment of the ileum, and urine drains continually because there is no sphincter. (b)
  1 No feces are present in an ileal conduit.
  2 Nutrients are not normally absorbed from urine as it passes from the kidneys.
  3 Ileal conduits are not neurologically innervated; therefore no peristalsis exists.

390. **1** Methotrexate is a folic acid antagonist that can cause depression of bone marrow. This serious toxic effect is sometimes prevented by administration of folic acid. Some physicians advocate its administration after a course of methotrexate therapy so as not to interfere with methotrexate activity. (c)
  2 Folic acid is a metabolite and does not destroy cancer cells.
  3 Folic acid is a metabolite and does not destroy cancer cells.
  4 Methotrexate does not increase the production of phagocytes.

391. **4** Prolonged chemotherapy may slow the production of leukocytes in bone marrow and lymph nodes, thus suppressing the activity of the immune system. Antibiotics may be required to help counter infections that the body can no longer handle easily. (b)
  1 Although leukocytes are circulating in both blood and lymph, these cells are more mature and thus more resistant to the effects of chemotherapy.

  2 Although leukocytes are circulating in both blood and lymph, these cells are more mature and thus more resistant to the effects of chemotherapy.
  3 The liver does not produce leukocytes.

392. **1** Approximately 25 of the 40 L of body fluid are in the cells. (c)
  2 Makes up 20%.
  3 Makes up 4%.
  4 Makes up 16%.

393. **1** Blood plasma and interstitial fluid are both part of the extracellular fluid and are of the same ionic composition. (b)
  2 Composition is the same.
  3 Osmotic pressure is the same.
  4 Ionic composition the same; the main cation of both would be sodium.

394. **4** Since the plasma colloid osmotic pressure (COP) opposes glomerular filtration, a decrease in blood proteins will increase the glomerular filtration rate (GFR). (b)
  1 Glomeruli are clusters of capillaries, not arteries.
  2 Volume is determined by the amount of water reabsorbed in the tubules.
  3 Does not affect the glomerular filtration rate.

395. **2** A balloon tube is inserted into the renal pelvis to drain urine, necessitating an incision into the kidney (nephrostomy). (c)
  1 Ileostomy is the surgical implantation of the ileum into the abdominal wall; it is not related to urinary disease.
  3 Cecostomy is the surgical creation of a temporary opening into the cecum to relieve obstruction; not done for urinary problems.
  4 Ureterostomy is the surgical implantation of the ureter in the abdominal wall; would be performed if the bladder was involved.

396. **3** A 1 molar (1 M) solution contains 1 gram-molecular weight of solute per liter of solution. Molarity is not as informative as normality because the latter is based on the actual chemical-combining properties of the substance involved. (c)
  1 Deals with the osmotic pressure of two liquids; isotonic solutions have equal osmotic pressure.
  2 A 1 normal (1 N) solution is defined as containing 1 gram-equivalent weight of solute per liter of solution. In human body fluids the milliequivalent ($\frac{1}{1000}$ of the gram-equivalent) is a more convenient term for expressing concentration, since the gram-equivalent is rather large.
  4 A solution holding all the solute it can at a given temperature and pressure.

397. **3** Osmosis is the diffusion of water through a selectively permeable membrane. Such membranes include cellular membranes and capillary walls. Osmosis occurs in the kidney tubules and in all capillary beds. (a)
  1 Dialysis is the diffusion of small molecules, other than water, down their concentration gradients through a selectively permeable membrane.
  2 Active transport is the movement of molecules against a concentration gradient and requires energy input; osmosis and diffusion are passive processes.
  4 Diffusion is the process by which particulate matter in a fluid moves from an area of greater concentration to an area of lesser concentration.

398. **3** The excreted ammonia combines with hydrogen ions (H^+) in the glomerular filtrate to form ammonium ions (NH_4^+), which are excreted from the body. This mechanism helps rid the body of excess H^+, maintaining acid-base balance. (b)

1 Ammonia is formed by the decomposition of bacteria in the urine; ammonia excretion is not related to the process and does not control bacterial levels.

2 Osmotic pressure is not affected by excretion of ammonia.

4 Ammonia excretion does not affect hemopoiesis.

399. **2** Oxygen perfusion is impaired during prolonged edema, leading to tissue ischemia. (b)

1 This is not a complication resulting from long-term edema.

3 This is not a complication resulting from long-term edema.

4 This is not a complication resulting from long-term edema.

400. **1** The presence of excess solute (Na^+) in the nephric tubules effectively decreases the water concentration of the glomerular filtrate and urine; water passively diffuses (osmosis) from the kidney tubule cells into the urine to equalize the water concentration. (b)

2 Diffusion is not specific to fluid; osmosis is.

3 Filtration refers to solutes; none are being passed.

4 Active transport requires energy; water is passively diffused from the tubule cells to the urine.

401. **2** The length of the urethra is shorter in females than in males; therefore microorganisms have a shorter distance to travel to reach the bladder. The proximity of the meatus to the anus in females also increases this incidence. (b)

1 Hygienic practices can be poor in males or females; however, the anatomic length of the urethra in females predisposes them to infection.

3 Mucous membranes are continuous in both males and females and would not make a difference.

4 Fluid intake may be adequate in both males and females and would not account for the difference.

402. **2** Since the plasma colloidal osmotic pressure (COP) is the major force drawing fluid from the interstitial spaces back into the capillaries, a drop in COP due to albuminuria results in edema. (c)

1 Hydrostatic pressure is influenced by the volume of fluid and the diameter of the blood vessel, not by the presence of protein such as albumin.

3 Hydrostatic tissue pressure is unaffected by alteration of protein levels; colloidal pressure is.

4 The osmotic pressure of tissues is not affected.

403. **2** The average adult human body is about 60% water. A newborn infant's body is about 80% water and reaches the 60% figure approximately 1 year after birth. (a)

1 The percent for a newborn infant.

3 The percent for the elderly may be as low as 40%.

4 This represents complete dehydration of tissues.

404. **1** The osmoreceptors are located in the hypothalamus. Under conditions of dehydration they stimulate the neurohypophysis to release ADH into the blood. (b)

2 This is the posterior lobe of the pituitary gland and is the source of antidiuretic hormone (ADH).

3 The kidney tubules are the target organ for ADH; they reabsorb more water from the glomerular filtrate.

4 Not a receptor for alterations in osmotic pressure.

405. **2** The kidneys regulate fluid balance by adjusting the amount of fluid reabsorbed from the glomerular filtrate. (b)

1 Primarily a pump for the movement of blood.

3 Does not play a major role in fluid balance.

4 The role of the lungs is minimal.

406. **1** Interstitial fluid constitutes about 16% of body weight, which is 10 to 12 L in an adult male of 68 kg (150 lb). (b)

2 4% of body weight (2.8 L).

3 This is derived from extracellular fluid and is calculated as part of the 20% of the total body weight.

4 Part of the intracellular component.

407. **3** The concentration of potassium is greater inside the cell and is extremely important in establishing a membrane potential, a critical factor in the cell's ability to function. (b)

1 Calcium is the most abundant electrolyte in the body; 99% is concentrated in the teeth and bones.

2 Sodium is the most abundant cation of the extracellular compartment.

4 Chloride is an extracellular anion.

408. **2** The client still had the right to make decisions regarding hours of sleep and time of medication. The concept of invasion of rights or intrusion applies. (b)

1 *Respondeat superior* (let the master respond) indicates that employers may be liable for torts committed by employees within their employment. In this case the client has the right to make decisions about his care.

3 Although this statement may be true, it has no bearing on the legality of the situation.

4 Sleeping medications are to be given at the client's bedtimes, not at the convenience of the nursing staff.

409. **1** A definitive diagnosis of the cellular changes associated with benign prostatic hypertrophy is made by biopsy with subsequent microscopic evaluation. (c)

2 This test would not yield a definitive diagnosis because malignant cells might not be present in the fluid.

3 Palpation of the prostate gland is not a definitive diagnosis; it only reveals size and configuration.

4 This would give information as to the activity of phosphorus in the body; however, no definitive diagnosis could be made.

410. **1** The phenolsulfonphthalein test (PSP) and urea clearance test evaluate the kidneys' ability to excrete a particular substance from the blood. The urine concentration or specific gravity is an indicator of the kidney's ability to concentrate urine. (b)

2 These tests are not generally ordered (as grouped) to determine kidney disease.

3 These tests are not generally ordered (as grouped) to determine kidney disease.

4 These tests are not generally ordered (as grouped) to determine kidney disease.

411. **2** Inability to empty the bladder, as a result of pressure exerted by the enlarging prostate on the urethra, causes a backup of urine into the ureters and finally the kidneys (hydronephrosis). (b)

1 It is uncommon for BPH to become malignant.

3 BPH develops over the client's life span; it is not congenital.

4 This level is elevated in prostatic carcinoma.

412. **3** The total amount of irrigation solution instilled into the bladder is eliminated with urine and therefore must be subtracted from the total output to determine the volume of urine excreted. (b)

1 An accurate specific gravity cannot be obtained when irrigating solutions are being instilled into the bladder.

2 Hourly outputs are indicated only if there is concern about renal failure or oliguria.

4 Twenty-four hour urine tests would not be accurate if the client was receiving continuous irrigations.

413. **1** Any abnormal sign of vaginal bleeding may be indicative of cervical cancer and must be checked by a physician. (c)

2 Discharge becomes foul smelling only after there is necrosis and infection.

3 There are few nerve endings, so pain is a late symptom.

4 If pressure occurs, it is not an early symptom because the cancer must be extensive to cause pressure.

414. **4** During radiation therapy with radium implants the client is placed in isolation so exposure to radiation by family and staff will be decreased. (a)

1 Excess exposure to radiation is hazardous to personnel.

2 An indwelling catheter is left in place to prevent bladder distention.

3 Rubber gloves will not protect the nurse from radiation.

415. **2** Radium atoms are unstable and spontaneously disintegrate into other atomic species. This disintegration produces potentially harmful radiation, which is absorbed by lead. (a)

1 Heat is not produced during spontaneous disintegration; radiation is.

3 Radium is not a heavy substance but an unstable one.

4 Disintegration of radium occurs in the lead containers.

416. **3** Time, distance, and shielding are the important factors in determining the amount of radiation the individual receives. Restriction of each visitor to a 10-minute stay minimizes the risk of exposure. Many institutions will not allow visitors while an implant is in place. (c)

1 Urine is not radioactive, so no precautions are indicated.

2 Lead aprons are effective shields against x-rays but not against rays emitted by internal sources of radiation.

4 Radium implants will not affect the location of IM injections.

417. **3** Prior to discharge it is important for the nurse to instruct the client to follow through with medical care at specified intervals. (b)

1 Although increased calories may be required, high-fat diets are not encouraged because of associated cardiovascular risks.

2 If diet is adequate, multivitamins are unnecessary.

4 Fluids are not reduced unless other cardiac or renal pathosis is present.

418. **4** *Trichomonas vaginalis* is a protozoan that favors an alkaline environment. (c)

1 A fungus is a simple parasitic plant; does not cause trichomonal infections.

2 A yeast is a unicellular, usually oval, nucleated fungus; does not cause trichomonal infections.

3 A spirochete is a motile spiral-shaped bacterium; does not cause trichomonal infections.

419. **2** Since *Trichomonas vaginalis* favors an alkaline environment, vinegar, an acid, is utilized to decrease the pH of the vagina. (c)

1 Normal saline will not alter the pH.

3 An increase in pH would create an environment conducive to the growth of microorganisms.

4 An increase in pH would create an environment conducive to the growth of microorganisms.

420. **3** Metronidazole (Flagyl) is a potent amebicide. It is extremely effective in eradicating the protozoan *Trichomonas vaginalis*. (c)

1 Gentian violet is a local antiinfective that is applied topically and may cause discoloration of the skin; particularly effective against *Candida albicans*.

2 Penicillin is administered for its effect on bacterial, not protozoal, infections.

4 Nystatin is an antifungal used for infections caused by *Candida albicans*.

421. **2** Most chemotherapeutic agents interfere with mitosis. The bone marrow consists of rapidly dividing cells, and therefore its activity is depressed. (a)

1 If bleeding occurs, the hemoglobin and hematocrit may be decreased because of the decreased number of thrombocytes.

3 The ESR generally increases in the presence of tissue inflammation or necrosis.

4 Because of bone marrow depression, leukopenia rather than leukocytosis can occur.

422. **3** Doxorubicin hydrochloride (Adriamycin) is a chemotherapeutic agent classified as an antibiotic. It achieves its therapeutic effect by inhibiting the synthesis of RNA. This effect blocks protein synthesis and cell division. (c)

1 Not a physiologic action of Adriamycin.

2 Not a physiologic action of Adriamycin.

4 Not a physiologic action of Adriamycin.

423. **1** Doxorubicin hydrochloride (Adriamycin), an antitumor antibiotic, causes nausea, diarrhea, and cardiac toxicity because it interferes with cell division. (c)

2 Hair loss occurs but is temporary and does not represent a life-threatening complication.

3 Anorexia may occur but is not a life-threatening complication; local necrosis not common.

4 Blood pressure and vital capacity are not directly affected but may be compromised secondarily to cardiomyopathy or arrhythmias.

424. **2** Gonorrhea is caused by a gram-negative diplococcus, *Neisseria gonorrhoeae*. (a)

1 Spirochete of syphilis.

3 Staphylococci are constantly present on the skin and in the upper respiratory tract; commonly cause suppurating infection.

4 A lactobacillus found in the vagina; does not cause gonorrhea.

425. **2** In males the inflammatory process associated with the infection may lead to destruction of the epididymis. In females the gonorrheal infection causes destruction of the tubal mucosa and eventually tuboovarian abscesses. (a)

1 Gonorrhea is difficult to treat.

3 Gonorrhea is a common sexually transmitted disease.

4 *Neisseria gonorrhoeae* will invade internal structures, particularly the epididymis in males and the fallopian tubes in females.

426. **3** Gonorrhea is a highly contagious disease transmitted through sexual intercourse. The incubation period varies, but symptoms usually occur 2 to 10 days after contact. Early effective treatment prevents complications. (a)

1 Contracting venereal disease is not necessarily indicative of promiscuity.

2 The parents may be unaware that their daughter has gonorrhea; the nurse knows the etiology of the disease.

4 Most birth control measures do not protect against the transmission of venereal disease.

427. **1** Penicillin inhibits the synthesis of bacterial cell walls. It is effective against *Neisseria gonorrhoeae*, a gram-negative diplococcus. (b)

2 Actinomycin is an antineoplastic agent.

3 Chloramphenicol is a broad-spectrum antimicrobial agent; however, it can cause bone marrow depression, so its use is limited to severe infections that do not respond to less toxic drugs.

4 Colistin sulfate is effective against most gram-negative enteric pathogens such as *Escherichia coli*.

428. **1** Penicillin is specific for *Neisseria gonorrhoeae* and eradicates the microorganism. (a)
  2 If the disease progresses before diagnosis is made, complications such as sterility, valve damage, or joint degeneration may occur.
  3 The individual may still contract gonorrhea.
  4 If tubal structures, valves, or joints degenerate, the pathologic changes will not be reversed by antibiotic therapy.

429. **1** The serum acid phosphatase is elevated when the cancer extends beyond the prostate, whereas the serum alkaline phosphatase is elevated in bony metastasis. (b)
  2 Elevated creatinine levels may be caused by impaired renal function as a result of blockage by an enlarged prostate but do not indicate that metastasis has occurred.
  3 Elevated BUN levels may be caused by impaired renal function as a result of blockage by an enlarged prostate but do not indicate that metastasis has occurred.
  4 Nonprotein nitrogen refers to waste products from metabolism of protein and includes urea, creatinine, uric acid, and ammonia.

430. **4** Dysuria, nocturia, and urgency are all signs of an irritable bladder after radiation therapy. (b)
  1 Not an indication of bladder irritability.
  2 Not an indication of bladder irritability.
  3 Not an indication of bladder irritability.

431. **3** An enlarged prostate constricts the urethra, interfering with urine flow and causing retention. When the bladder fills and approaches capacity, small amounts can be voided. (b)
  1 The urge to void is caused by stimulation of the stretch receptors as the bladder fills with urine; in renal failure little or no urine is produced.
  2 Edema does not cause the client to void frequently in small amounts because of decreased production of urine.
  4 The urge to void is caused by stimulation of the stretch receptors as the bladder fills with urine; in suppression little or no urine is produced.

432. **1** Catheter patency ensures drainage and prevents bladder distention and other complications. Therefore patency of a catheter should be established prior to notifying the physician. (a)
  2 Assessment is necessary prior to consultation with the physician.
  3 Milking a catheter is appropriate when viscous rather than clear drainage is present (e.g., with chest tubes).
  4 Irrigation is a dependent function and is avoided if possible because of associated risk of infection.

433. **2** Cleansing the urinary meatus and adjacent skin removes accumulated bacteria, limiting the possible introduction of microbes into the urinary tract. (c)
  1 Although forcing fluids helps prevent urinary stasis and subsequent infection, the most common source of infection is microorganisms from the perineal area.
  3 Cranberry juice helps acidify the urine to discourage the growth of bacteria but does not eliminate the potential source of infection as cleansing would.
  4 Irrigations require opening the closed drainage system and allowing the entry of microorganisms; increases the risk of infection.

434. **4** The Foley catheter is always positioned so the level of the bladder with catheter inserted is higher than the level of the drainage container; gravity causes urine flow. (a)
  1 Refers to a property of matter.

2 Passage of molecules from high concentration to low concentration.
  3 Diffusion of water across a semipermeable membrane; not responsible for the flow of urine through a catheter.

435. **1** An indwelling catheter dilates the urinary sphincters, keeps the bladder empty, and short-circuits the normal reflex mechanism based on bladder distention. When the catheter is removed, the body must adapt to functioning once again. (b)
  2 Although retention may result from any interruption in normal voiding habits, there is no data presented in this situation to draw the conclusion that this is involved.
  3 Although retention may result from any interruption in normal voiding habits, there is no data presented in this situation to draw the conclusion that this is involved.
  4 Although retention may result from any interruption in normal voiding habits, there is no data presented in this situation to draw the conclusion that this is involved.

436. **2** This recognizes that the client is upset and by indirect questioning helps facilitate communication. (b)
  1 An assumption is being made about the basis for the behavior; does not focus on the client's feelings.
  3 False reassurances block communication.
  4 The client has not verbally indicated that she is upset and may be unaware of or unable to verbalize the actual cause of her emotions.

437. **4** This recognizes the client's feeling of anxiety as valid; informing her honestly of a fact may help decrease the anxiety. (b)
  1 The polyps may be cancerous; this is false reassurance and may inhibit the expression of feelings.
  2 The polyps may be cancerous; this is false reassurance and may inhibit the expression of feelings.
  3 Does not focus on the client; feelings exist and will not disappear on command.

438. **1** Polyps are usually benign but should undergo biopsy, since epidermoid cancer occasionally arises from cervical polyps. (a)
  2 Untrue; polyps are usually benign.
  3 Bleeding may occur whether they are malignant or not.
  4 Untrue; polyps are rarely the precursors of uterine cancer.

439. **1** When the cancerous cells are completely confined within the epithelium of the cervix without stromal invasion, it is stage 0 and called carcinoma in situ or preinvasive carcinoma. (c)
  2 Stage I; lymph node metastasis about 10%.
  3 Stage Ia; minimal stromal invasion.
  4 Stage IIb; involves area around the broad ligaments but not the pelvic wall; extension to the corpus of the uterus.

440. **3** The endocervical surface is frequently altered by metaplasia or covered by a variant of squamous epithelium. It is thus called the transitional zone. This area is often distorted by eversion and laceration, especially in pregnancy. Therefore it is a frequent site for carcinoma. Erosion in this area most frequently leads to squamous cell carcinoma, accounting for 95% of cervical cancer. (c)
  1 Adenocarcinoma, accounting for only 5% of cervical cancers, may be found in the endocervical glands.
  2 Extension to lymph nodes is a later stage.

4 The cervix is the lower portion of the uterus; the juncture of the uterine body with the cervical canal is called the internal os; erosion most frequently occurs distal to this point, between the external and internal, closer to the external.

441. **3** Conization (conical excision of the lesion), cryosurgery, and hysterectomy can be used in the treatment of squamous cell carcinoma in situ. If treatment is initiated during the preinvasive stage, it is 100% curable. (b)

 1 Although the postponement of surgery gives the client time to cope, the decision should not be delayed; conization would be done if later pregnancy is desired. Hysterectomy would preclude that possibility.

 2 Although it may take 5 to 10 years for preinvasive carcinoma to progress to invasive carcinoma, the prognosis is excellent if therapy is initiated during the preinvasive stage. The decision should not be delayed.

 4 Conization does not predispose to abortion and can be done during pregnancy.

442. **4** Changes in the pH of the vaginal tract cause cellular alteration and destruction. (c)

 1 The direct effects of labor and delivery will not cause cervical erosion; erosion involves continuous inflammation or ulceration.

 2 The direct effects of labor and delivery will not cause cervical erosion; erosion involves continuous inflammation or ulceration.

 3 The direct effects of labor and delivery will not cause cervical erosion; erosion involves continuous inflammation or ulceration.

443. **3** Douches with acidic solutions such as vinegar and water bring back the normal pH of the vaginal tract. (a)

 1 The use of vinegar will only indirectly affect bacterial growth because it acidifies the environment.

 2 Although this may be a secondary benefit, a vinegar and water solution would not be required.

 4 Comfort may be enhanced by correcting the pathologic disorder, but it is not the main goal of the treatment.

444. **3** Dorsal recumbency takes advantage of the anatomic position of the vaginal tract and prevents undue retention or too rapid return of the douche. (a)

 1 Promote retention of the douche.

 2 Promote retention of the douche.

 4 Promotes rapid return of the douche before the therapeutic effect is achieved.

445. **3** This is the anatomic direction of the vaginal tract in the back-lying position. (b)

 1 The vaginal tract may be injured when the douche nozzle is not directed with consideration of normal anatomy.

 2 The vaginal tract may be injured when the douche nozzle is not directed with consideration of normal anatomy.

 4 The vaginal tract may be injured when the douche nozzle is not directed with consideration of normal anatomy.

446. **2** Erosion of the cervix frequently occurs at the squamocolumnar junction, the most common site for carcinoma of the cervix. (a)

 1 Infection may occur in the cancerous area accompanied by profuse, malodorous discharge; treatment of the erosion is done to prevent cancer, not the secondary infection.

 3 This may be present as erosion develops into carcinoma; however, spotting may be the earliest sign; will be eliminated when the cancer is treated; treatment of the erosion done to prevent cancer from developing.

 4 Even though a cervical erosion is treated, another may occur and repeat treatment may be necessary.

447. **4** Negative pressure such as suction should never be exerted on the bladder, since this might injure the sensitive tissue. The solution should be allowed to drain by force of gravity alone. (b)

 1 Since the bladder is a sterile body cavity, surgical asepsis is required.

 2 The solution is introduced by compressing the bulb of the irrigating syringe or by gravity; to prevent trauma, excessive pressure is avoided.

 3 The solution is normally used at room temperature.

448. **1** Although other solutions may be ordered, irrigations of the bladder usually employ normal saline (0.9% NaCl), which is a solution of approximately the tonicity of normal body fluids. (b)

 2 This is a hypotonic solution, which may be absorbed by body tissues.

 3 This is a hypotonic solution, which may be absorbed by body tissues.

 4 Genitourinary irrigants usually contain an antimicrobial agent such as neosporin; indiscriminate use of such agents leads to the emergence of resistant strains of microorganisms.

449. **2** The bladder is a sterile body cavity. Any time a solution or catheter is introduced into the urinary meatus, strict surgical asepsis is required. (b)

 1 Excessive pressure can traumatize the lining of the urinary tract.

 3 The negative pressure exerted during aspiration may cause trauma.

 4 The solution is generally administered at room temperature.

450. **2** As the uterus drops, the vaginal wall relaxes. When the bladder herniates into the vagina (cystocele) and the rectal wall herniates into the vagina (rectocele), the individual feels pressure or pain in the lower back and/or pelvis. When there is an increase in intraabdominal pressure in the presence of a cystocele, incontinence results. (b)

 1 Not indicative of cystocele and rectocele.

 3 Not indicative of cystocele and rectocele; common with infection.

 4 Not indicative of cystocele and rectocele.

451. **1** Relaxation of the pelvic musculature causes the uterus to drop, with a subsequent relaxation of the vaginal walls, most often as a result of childbirth. A rectocele is protrusion of the rectal wall into the vagina, whereas a cystocele is protrusion of the bladder into the vaginal wall. (b)

 2 Does not cause either a rectocele or a cystocele.

 3 Does not cause either a rectocele or a cystocele.

 4 Does not cause either a rectocele or a cystocele.

452. **4** Since the client is past the childbearing age, plastic surgical repair designed to tighten both the anterior and the posterior vaginal wall will probably be performed. (b)

 1 A pessary is a device employed for a prolapsed uterus.

 2 A hysterectomy is performed only if there is uterine disease.

 3 A hysterectomy is performed only if there is uterine disease.

453. **1** The effects of anesthesia and the inflammatory process may impede voiding, leading to urinary retention; a Foley catheter empties the bladder continuously, preventing retention. (c)

 2 Distention causes discomfort; this is avoided by preventing retention.

3 Distention places pressure on the suture line; this is avoided by preventing retention.

4 Because the bladder is continually empty when an indwelling catheter is in place, it loses tone. This is an expected but undesirable effect.

454. **2** Radium, a radioactive isotope, is used to destroy or delay the growth of malignant cells. Special care is taken to maintain normal tissue and not allow it to come closer to the radioactive substance than is necessary. Distance, along with time and shielding, is a way of limiting exposure. (b)

1 This is not true.

3 This is the physician's decision; it may be reinserted.

4 Not the purpose of vaginal packing; there should be no active bleeding with radium implants although there may be cellular sloughing.

455. **2** Normal activity must be limited so the implant will not become dislodged. (b)

1 Not necessary; all bed linens must be examined carefully for dislodged radium prior to sending to the laundry.

3 Not necessary; adherence to principles of time and distance will protect the nurse from excessive exposure.

4 While the client is receiving therapy, alpha, beta, and gamma rays will be emitted. Therefore the nurse should employ the principles of time and distance when providing care. Extent of exposure to the client must be monitored and kept within safe limits depending on the type and amount of rays emitted.

456. **2** Pain and elevated temperature may indicate toxic effects. Excessive sloughing of tissue can cause hemorrhage or infection. (b)

1 Expected side effects of internal radiotherapy.

3 Associated with need to maintain position, not with radium itself.

4 Expected side effects of internal radiotherapy.

457. **1** Radium should be handled with long-handled forceps since distance helps limit exposure. (b)

2 A nurse is not responsible for cleaning radium implants.

3 The amount and duration of exposure are important in assessing the effect on the client; however, will not affect safety during removal.

4 Foil-lined rubber gloves do not provide adequate shielding from the gamma rays emitted by radium.

458. **2** The Fowler's position facilitates localization of the infection by pooling pelvic drainage. (b)

1 This position does not make use of gravity to promote drainage of exudate.

3 This position does not make use of gravity to promote pelvic drainage.

4 This position does not make use of gravity to promote pelvic drainage.

459. **3** The time between ovulation and the next menstruation is relatively constant, about 14 days; variations in the total cycle time are due to variations in the preovulatory phase. Within a 30-day cycle the first 15 days are preovulatory, ovulation occurs on day 16, and the next 14 days are postovulatory. Ovulation therefore occurs on January 17. (b)

1 This is within the first 15 days and is the preovulatory phase.

2 This is within the first 15 days and is the preovulatory phase.

4 This is within the last 14 days of the cycle and is postovulatory.

460. **4** Although the usual incubation period of syphilis is about 3 weeks, clinical symptoms may appear as early as 9 days or as long as 3 months after exposure. (b)

1 The normal incubation period is 21 days.

2 The normal incubation period is 21 days.

3 The normal incubation period is 21 days.

461. **4** The FTA-ABS test utilizes fluorescent treponemal antibody to confirm a diagnosis of syphilis. (c)

1 Although convenient for screening, a complement fixation test using nonspecific antigen may give false-positives (e.g., glandular fever, SLE) and false-negatives with late syphilis.

2 A nonspecific (nontreponemal) antibody test convenient for screening; may give false-positives (e.g., glandular fever, SLE) and false-negatives with late syphilis.

3 A nonspecific (nontreponemal) antibody test convenient for screening; may give false-positives (e.g., glandular fever, SLE) and false-negatives with late syphilis.

462. **2** The tertiary stage is noncontagious; tertiary lesions contain only small numbers of treponemes; fatal cases involve the aorta, CNS, or eye. (c)

1 The primary stage lasts 8 to 12 weeks; the chancre is teeming with spirochetes, and the individual is contagious.

3 Duration of secondary stage variable (about 5 years); skin and mucosal lesions contain spirochetes, and the individual is highly contagious.

4 The incubation stage lasts 2 to 6 weeks; spirochetes proliferate at entry site, and the individual is contagious.

463. **1** Bleeding between periods is abnormal. The occurrence of bleeding other than during the menstrual period is known as metrorrhagia. (b)

2 Menorrhagia is the term used to describe excessive bleeding during menstruation.

3 The amount varies from spotting to frank bleeding; it is not occult.

4 Bleeding may not be limited to ovulation.

464. **4** A hysterectomy involves only removal of the uterus. The ovaries, which secrete estrogen and progesterone, are not removed. Therefore menopause will not be precipitated but will occur naturally. (b)

1 If the ovaries were being removed, older women might have less severe symptoms than younger women; however, in this instance there would be no symptoms.

2 The nurse should serve as a resource person; the comment does not answer the question.

3 Incorrect; fails to point out the difference between myth and reality.

465. **3** The prescribing of medications is the legal responsibility of the physician. In addition, the use of hormones is controversial and depends on the physician's beliefs and the client's needs. (b)

1 This is an evasive response; the client is left without direction.

2 Hormones may be used to prevent the development of severe symptoms.

4 This is an evasive response; does not answer the client's question.

466. **1** This response reflects and verbalizes the client's feelings in a nonjudgmental way. (a)

2 Demonstrates a lack of acceptance of the client's feelings.

3 The husband did not indicate this; the client's perception is altered by her own feelings.

4 Such feelings are common and need to be verbalized; surgery should not be postponed.

467. **2** Ulcerations may occur when the vagina and uterus are inverted. (b)
  1 Exudate would not be present with procidentia.
  3 The vagina would be inverted, and therefore discharge would not be present.
  4 Development of ulcerations, not edema, is usually the problem.

468. **3** Warm compresses may be indicated to prevent ulcerations. (b)
  1 Ambulation would encourage the development of ulcerations.
  2 The tissue should be protected, and manipulation, which causes irritation, should be avoided.
  4 Would be ineffective; gravity alone does not correct the procidentia.

469. **1** Turning the client to the side promotes drainage of secretions and prevents aspiration, especially when the gag reflex is not intact. This position also brings the tongue forward, preventing it from occluding the airway in the relaxed state. (a)
  2 This position is sometimes used in shock to increase venous return, not generally for a postoperative client.
  3 Increases the risk of aspiration; this position may flex the neck in an individual who is not alert, interfering with respirations.
  4 The risk of aspiration is increased when this position is assumed by a semialert client.

470. **2** A sharp rise in luteinizing hormone production triggers the rupture of the follicle and ovulation. (c)
  1 FSH stimulates the development of the graafian follicle.
  3 Estrogen stimulates the thickening of the endometrium.
  4 Progesterone prepares the endometrium for the implantation of the fertilized ovum.

471. **1** The function of progesterone is to relax the uterus and maintain a succulent endometrium to foster implantation of the fertilized ovum. (c)
  2 Menstruation is controlled by regulating factors from the hypothalamus and pituitary (FSH-RH, FSH, LH-RH, LH); these hormones stimulate the production of ovarian follicles, ovulation, estrogen, and progesterone by the ovarian cells.
  3 Ovulation is stimulated by increases in the levels of luteinizing hormone (LH) and estrogen.
  4 Capillary fragility is often associated with deficiency of vitamin C (ascorbic acid); progesterone is not responsible.

472. **2** Estrogen is found in the follicular fluid of the ovaries and aids in the growth of the endometrium. (b)
  1 Luteinizing hormone promotes the development of ovarian follicles as well as stimulates ovulation and the production of estrogen and progesterone; progesterone prepares the endometrium for implantation and the breasts for lactation.
  3 These hormones prepare the breasts for milk secretion (lactation).
  4 Luteinizing hormone promotes the development of ovarian follicles as well as stimulates ovulation and the production of estrogen and progesterone by the ovarian cells.

473. **2** Persistent pain of any kind is usually a symptom, and the client should seek medical attention. (b)
  1 Voluntary relaxation of the abdominal muscles does not cause cessation of uterine contractions.
  3 Although diversion is a method to alter pain perception, the presence of pain requires investigation of possible causes.
  4 Although a nutritious diet is beneficial, iron does not prevent the pain of dysmenorrhea.

474. **1** A generous supply of blood is carried by the uterine arteries (branches of the internal iliac arteries). The vaginal and ovarian arteries also supply the uterus with blood by anastomosing with the uterine vessels. (b)
  2 The hypogastric or internal iliac arteries supply the pelvic wall and viscera.
  3 The aorta does not supply the uterus directly.
  4 The hypogastric arteries (internal iliac) supply the pelvic wall and gluteal area, and the external branches (called uterine arteries) supply the uterus and genitalia; the aorta doesn't supply the uterus directly.

475. **4** The gonadotropins, follicle-stimulating hormone (FSH) and luteinizing hormone (LH), are concerned with ovarian changes that produce ovulation. Estrogen levels are high between the end of menses and ovulation because of secretion from the developing follicle. Progesterone levels are high between ovulation and the onset of menses because of secretion from the corpus luteum. The hormones work in concert to stimulate the menstrual cycle. (a)
  1 Without FSH and LH there is no cycle.
  2 The gonadatropins must work in concert with estrogen and progesterone for the cycle to be completed.
  3 Progesterone is required for the menstrual cycle to be completed.

476. **1** The *Candida* genus consists of several species of fungi commonly found in the mouth, sputum, vagina, and stools of otherwise normal people. Candidiasis (*Candida* infection) arises in certain individuals when local resistance is decreased through prolonged antibiotic therapy or with certain diseases (e.g., diabetes) and debilitating conditions (e.g., drug addiction). (a)
  2 *Streptococcus* organisms would be responsive to antibiotic therapy and are not considered part of the normal flora.
  3 *Coxiella burnetii,* a rickettsia, is not part of the normal flora; spread by contact with infected animals, drinking contaminated milk, or the bite of a vector tick.
  4 Herpes is not part of the normal flora.

477. **1** *Neisseria gonorrhoeae* is a gram-negative diplococcus commonly infecting the urogenital tract of both males and females. (b)
  2 Associated with infections of the brain and spinal cord.
  3 Associated with infections of the respiratory tract.
  4 A spirochete that causes syphilis.

478. **2** Laparoscopy involves direct visualization of the uterus via fiberoptics. The procedure is carried out through a stab wound below the umbilicus. (a)
  1 This test would give information on tissue abnormalities.
  3 This procedure involves blowing air through the fallopian tubes to test for patency.
  4 This test yields data on hormone levels; usually done prior to delivery.

479. **1** Some spermatozoa will remain viable in the vas deferens for a variable time after vasectomy. (c)
  2 Although it is considered a permanent form of sterilization, there has been some success reversing the procedure.
  3 Precautions must be taken to prevent fertilization until absence of sperm in the semen has been verified.
  4 The procedure does not affect sexual functioning.

480. **1** When the testes are twisted, a decrease in their blood supply occurs. This can result in gangrene. (c)
  2 Pain can be alleviated through the use of medication.
  3 Although edema occurs, the testes do not rupture.
  4 Sperm are continually produced, so their destruction is not the concern.

481. **3** Primitive sex cells, called spermatogonia, are present in newborn males. At puberty these cells mature and form spermatozoa (spermatogenesis). (b)
    1 Only immature cells are found during this period.
    2 Spermatogonia or primitive sex cells are found at this time.
    4 Does not occur until puberty.
482. **3** Sperm cells are very fragile and can be destroyed by heat, resulting in sterility. (b)
    1 Sperm are motile, achieving this by motion of their flagella; they move from the epididymis to the vas deferens to the ejaculatory ducts to the urethra.
    2 Sperm do not move through the urine; are found in semen.
    4 During this period the testes are not suspended.
483. **1** Mild hypocalcemia sometimes occurs during menstruation. An increase in dietary calcium just before and during menstruation may eliminate or relieve the occasional abdominal cramps resulting from this temporary disorder. (c)
    2 Hyperglycemia (elevated blood glucose levels) is evidenced by polyuria, polydipsia, polyphagia, weight loss, and urine that is positive for sugar and acetone.
    3 Hypernatremia (elevated sodium levels) is evidenced by agitation, tissue turgor, and oliguria.
    4 Hypokalemia (lowered potassium levels) is evidenced by malaise and muscle weakness.
484. **1** Condylomata acuminata are variably sized cauliflower-like warts occurring principally on the genitals or the anogenital skin or mucosa of both females and males; they are generally associated with poor hygiene. (c)
    2 Condylomata acuminata are warts occurring on the genitals or the anogenital skin or mucosa of both males and females; the epididymis is part of the male reproductive system and is an internal structure.
    3 Herpes zoster is an acute vesicular skin infection caused by the varicella-zoster virus (VZV).
    4 Scabies is an infestation of the skin by *Sarcoptes scabiei* (itch mite).
485. **3** The gonococcus *Neisseria gonorrhoeae* possesses fastidious growth requirements that are met by the columnar epithelium of the urethra, prostate, seminal vesicles, and epididymis in males and the urethra, endocervix, fallopian tubes, and Skene and Bartholin glands in females. (b)
    1 The causative organism is *Vibrio cholerae*.
    2 The causative organism is *Treponema pallidum*.
    4 The causative organism is *Haemophilus ducreyi*.
486. **2** Gonorrhea frequently is an ascending infection and affects the fallopian tubes. (b)
    1 Would not cause inflammation of the fallopian tubes.
    3 Not an infection, an aberrant growth; would not cause inflammation of the fallopian tubes.
    4 If untreated, may spread to the nervous system via the bloodstream; does not usually cause ascending infection of the fallopian tubes.
487. **3** Massive doses of penicillin may limit CNS damage if treatment is started before neural deterioration from syphilis occurs. (c)
    1 Paresis is not a behavior and is therefore not suitably treated with behavior modification.
    2 Tranquilizers used to modify behavior, not treat general paresis.
    4 Electroconvulsive therapy is used in the treatment of certain psychiatric disorders.
488. **2** Oral hypoglycemics may be helpful when some functioning of the beta cells exists, as in adult-onset (NIDDM) diabetes. (a)

1 Rapid-acting regular insulin is needed to reverse ketoacidosis.
    3 Juvenile-onset (IDDM) diabetics have no function of the beta cells.
    4 Obesity as a symptom does not offer enough information to determine the status of beta-cell function.
489. **2** Many people are ashamed or have a distorted body image when they know they have a long-term disorder. (b)
    1 Diabetes does not constitute a valid reasoning for not hiring an individual.
    3 The stress is his feelings about diabetes, not the diabetes itself.
    4 Lapses in memory are not common in diabetes until advanced vascular changes occur in the brain.
490. **2** Ketones are given off when fat is broken down for energy. (a)
    1 Diabetes does not interfere with removal of nitrogenous wastes.
    3 Carbohydrate metabolism is hampered in the diabetic.
    4 Sodium bicarbonate may be administered to correct the acid-base imbalance resulting from ketoacidosis; acidosis is due to excess acid not excess base bicarbonate.
491. **1** Infection increases the body's metabolic rate, and insulin is not available for increased demands. (b)
    2 Increased insulin dose will lead to insulin shock if diet is not increased as well.
    3 This would result in insulin shock.
    4 Although emotional stress will affect glucose levels, diabetic ketoacidosis will rarely result.
492. **2** IV fluids are given to combat dehydration in acidosis and to keep an IV line open for administration of medications. When the electrolyte levels have been evaluated, potassium may be added if needed. (b)
    1 In acidosis potassium ions (K^+) initially shift from intracellular to extracellular fluids, which results in hyperkalemia; as acidosis is corrected, hypokalemia may occur and then potassium may be administered.
    3 This is an intermediate-acting insulin; rapid-acting insulin such as regular insulin is indicated in an emergency.
    4 Not indicated; abnormally high serum potassium levels will revert once dehydration is corrected.
493. **2** To increase compliance with treatment, all clients should have an adequate understanding of their disease. (b)
    1 The precipitating cause must be investigated immediately rather than be postponed until recovery.
    3 Teaching does not ensure acceptance.
    4 Individual knowledge varies; must be assessed before a teaching plan is established.
494. **1** Glucagon, produced by the alpha cells in the islets of Langerhans, is an insulin antagonist. It mobilizes glycogen storage in the liver, leading to an increased blood glucose level. (c)
    2 Glucagon does not compete with insulin; it promotes the conversion of glycogen to glucose.
    3 Glucagon is not a glucose substitute.
    4 Stimulates an increase in blood glucose, not glycogen.
495. **3** During treatment for acidosis the client may develop hypoglycemia; careful observation for this complication should be made by the nurse, even without an order. (b)
    1 The regulation of insulin is dependent on the physician's orders for coverage.
    2 Withholding all glucose may cause insulin shock; monitoring glucose is indicated to prevent this.

4 Whole milk and fruit juices contain large amounts of carbohydrates, which are contraindicated in this period immediately following ketoacidosis.

496. **2** Hypokalemia promotes mental confusion and apathy with poor muscle contractions and weakness; these effects are related to the diminished magnitude of the neuronal and muscle cell resting potentials. Abdominal distention results from flaccidity of the intestine and abdominal musculature. (b)
   1 These are signs of sodium excess.
   3 These are signs of diabetic ketoacidosis.
   4 These are signs of hyperkalemia.

497. **2** Each client should be given an individually devised diet selecting commonly used foods from the American Diabetic Association exchange diet; family members should be included in the diet teaching. (b)
   1 Nutritional requirements are different for each individual depending on activity.
   3 Rigid diets are difficult to comply with; substitutions should be offered.
   4 Seasonings do not affect diabetics.

498. **3** Mineralocorticoids, such as aldosterone, cause the kidneys to retain sodium ions (Na^+). With Na^+, water is also retained, serving to elevate blood pressure. Absence of this hormone thus causes hypotension. (b)
   1 The major effect of glucocorticoids, such as hydrocortisone, is on glucose, not on sodium and water metabolism; absence of this hormone would not cause significant hypotension.
   2 Androgens are produced by the adrenal cortex; they have an effect similar to that of the male sex hormones; they do not affect blood pressure.
   4 Estrogen is a female sex hormone produced by the ovaries; does not affect blood pressure.

499. **2** Because of a deficit of glucocorticoids, clients with Addison's disease have decreased ability to resist infection. (b)
   1 Because of diminished glucocorticoid production, there is a decreased inflammatory effect.
   3 Glucocorticoids are involved with metabolism; however, they do not affect susceptibility to infection.
   4 In this disorder there is hyponatremia and hyperkalemia; however, these do not alter the defense against infection.

500. **1** Glucocorticoids help maintain blood sugar and liver and muscle glycogen content. A deficiency of glucocorticoids causes hypoglycemia, resulting in breakdown of protein and fats as energy sources. (c)
   2 Emaciation results from diminished protein and fat stores and hypoglycemia, not from an alteration in electrolytes.
   3 The diurnal rhythm of blood concentrations of cortisone, which start to rise around midnight and peak at 6 AM, has no effect on emaciation.
   4 Masculinization does not occur in this disease.

501. **4** Exertion, either physical or emotional, places additional stress on the adrenal glands, which may precipitate an addisonian crisis. (b)
   1 Low levels of adrenocortical hormones will cause fatigue, and exercise may result in crisis due to increased metabolic demands.
   2 Diversional activities are important to all clients, not just those with Addison's disease.
   3 Because of the limits imposed by the adrenal disease, the amount of exercise that the client may desire may not be consistent with the amount she can tolerate.

502. **1** Lack of mineralocorticoids causes hyponatremia, hypovolemia, and hyperkalemia. Dietary modification, as well as administration of cortical hormones, is aimed at correcting these electrolyte imbalances. (a)
   2 Although glucocorticoids are involved in metabolic activities, including carbohydrate metabolism, the primary aim of therapy is to restore electrolyte imbalance. Lack of electrolyte balance is life threatening.
   3 Lymphoid tissue does not change in this disease.
   4 There is no disturbance in the eosinophil count.

503. **1** Lack of mineralocorticoids (aldosterone) leads to loss of sodium ions in the urine and subsequent hyponatremia. (a)
   2 Vitamins are not energy producing.
   3 This disease is caused by idiopathic atrophy of the adrenal cortex; tissue repair of the gland is not possible.
   4 Potassium intake is not encouraged since hyperkalemia is a problem because of insufficient mineralocorticoids.

504. **1** Hydrocortisone is a glucocorticoid that has antiinflammatory action and aids in metabolism of carbohydrate, fat, and protein, causing elevation of blood sugar. Thus it enables the body to adapt to stress. (b)
   2 Lack of angiotensin II is not the cause of hypotension in this disorder.
   3 Potassium salts are retained in Addison's disease.
   4 Cardiac arrhythmias are due to electrolyte imbalances, and dyspnea is due to hypovolemia and decreased O_2 supply; neither is affected by hydrocortisone.

505. **3** Fludrocortisone acetate (Florinef) has a strong effect on sodium retention by the kidneys, which leads to fluid retention (weight gain and edema). (a)
   1 Fatigue may occur in Addison's disease and is not related to cortisone therapy.
   2 Fluid retention, and hence decreased urination, may occur.
   4 Mood swings frequently occur with fludrocortisone therapy; not an indication of a problem.

506. **3** Because water is not being reabsorbed, urine is dilute, resulting in a low specific gravity. (a)
   1 As fluid is lost from the vascular compartment, serum osmolarity increases.
   2 Diabetes insipidus is not a disorder of glucose metabolism; blood levels are not affected.
   4 Loss of fluid may actually lower blood pressure.

507. **1** Vasopressin replaces the ADH, facilitating reabsorption of water and consequent return of normal urine output and thirst. (b)
   2 While a correction of tachycardia is consistent with correction of dehydration, the client is not dehydrated if he has had adequate fluid intake.
   3 Glycosuria is a sign of diabetes mellitus, not diabetes insipidus; fractional urines are not indicated.
   4 The mechanisms that regulate pH are not affected.

508. **4** Antidiuretic hormone (ADH), from the posterior pituitary, promotes water uptake by the kidney tubules; the result is decreased urinary output—an antidiuretic effect. (c)
   1 Does not produce ADH.
   2 Does not produce ADH; the antidiuretic effect from the aldosterone that is secreted by the adrenal cortex is a secondary, osmotic effect of sodium reabsorption and not a direct antidiuretic effect (as is caused by ADH).
   3 Does not produce ADH.

509. **3** Reabsorption of sodium and water in the tubules decreases urinary output and retains body fluids. (c)
   1 No effect on filtration; increases reabsorption.
   2 Potassium reabsorption is not increased.
   4 Urine concentration increases as water is reabsorbed.

510. **3** Antidiuretic hormone aids the body in retaining fluid by causing the nephrons to reabsorb water. (b)
    1 The glomeruli are not affected.
    2 The glomeruli are not affected.
    4 Reabsorption of glucose is not affected, only the reabsorption of water.

511. **4** The ketones produced excessively in diabetes are acetoacetic acid, beta-hydroxybutyric acid, and acetone. The major ketone, acetoacetic acid, is an alpha-ketoacid; lowers the blood pH (acidosis). (c)
    1 Not an acid; does not change the pH.
    2 Produced as a result of muscle contraction; not unique to diabetes.
    3 This is a product of protein metabolism.

512. **2** Insulin stimulates cellular uptake of glucose and also stimulates the membrane-bound pump for sodium and potassium ions (Na^+ and K^+), leading to influx of K^+ into insulin's target cells. The resulting hypokalemia is offset by parenteral administration of K^+. (c)
    1 Hypokalemia may occur because the K^+ moves back into the cells as dehydration is reversed.
    3 Hypokalemia may be caused by the movement of K^+ back into the cells as dehydration is reversed.
    4 Anabolic reactions are stimulated by insulin and glucose administration; K^+ is drawn into the intracellular compartment, necessitating a replenishment of extracellular potassium.

513. **4** The urinary catheter and drainage bag should always remain a closed sterile system; fractional urine should be drawn only from the catheter, not the collection bag. (a)
    1 This would not yield a fresh specimen indicating present sugar and acetone levels.
    2 The system should remain closed so there will be fewer microorganisms entering the urinary system.
    3 The system should remain closed so there will be a decreased possibility of urinary system infection.

514. **1** Since the brain requires a constant supply of glucose, hypoglycemia triggers the response of the sympathetic nervous system which causes these symptoms. (b)
    2 Symptoms are consistent with dehydration, often associated with hyperglycemic states.
    3 Hypoglycemia causes the compensatory mechanism of hunger. Since blood glucose is low, the renal threshold is not exceeded, and there is no glycosuria.
    4 Associated with hyperglycemia; symptoms caused by the breakdown of fats as a result of inadequate insulin supply.

515. **3** The adrenal glands, stimulated by the sympathetic nervous system, secrete epinephrine during stressful situations. The ensuing alarm reaction involves rapid adjustment of the body to meet the emergency situation. (a)
    1 There may be modification in secretion of pituitary hormones, but it is not directly related to meeting emergency situations.
    2 There may be modification in secretion of thyroid hormones, but it is not directly related to meeting emergency situations.
    4 There may be modification in secretion of pancreatic hormones, but it is not directly related to meeting emergency situations.

516. **4** Liquids containing simple carbohydrates are most readily absorbed and thus increase blood sugar quickly. (a)
    1 Will not alter current situation.
    2 Complex carbohydrates and cheese take longer to elevate blood glucose, so they should be administered after simple carbohydrates.
    3 While a solution of 50% dextrose may be given if the client is comatose, 5% dextrose does not supply sufficient carbohydrates.

517. **2** A combination of diet, exercise, and medication is necessary to control the disease; the interaction of these therapies is reflected by the serum glucose. (b)
    1 Insulin alone is not enough to control the disease.
    3 Weight loss may occur with inadequate insulin.
    4 Acquisition of knowledge does not guarantee its application.

518. **3** Hyperplasia of the adrenal cortex leads to increased secretion of cortical hormones, which causes signs of Cushing's syndrome. (c)
    1 Cushing's syndrome results from excessive cortical hormones.
    2 ACTH stimulates production of adrenal hormones. Inadequate ACTH would result in addisonian symptoms.
    4 This malfunction of the pituitary would result in Simmond's disease (panhypopituitarism), which has symptoms similar to Addison's disease.

519. **3** Glucocorticoids (e.g., cortisone) and mineralocorticoids (e.g., aldosterone) are secreted by the adrenals. (a)
    1 The pancreas secretes insulin and glucagon.
    2 The anterior hypophysis secretes STH, FSH, LH, LTH, TSH, and ACTH.
    4 The gonads secrete testosterone (primarily in males) and estrogen and progesterone (primarily in females).

520. **1** Cushing's syndrome results from excess adrenocortical activity. Signs include slow wound healing, buffalo hump, hirsutism, weight gain, hypertension, acne, moon face, thin arms and legs, and behavioral changes. (c)
    2 Menorrhagia (excessive menstrual bleeding) and dehydration do not occur; menses may cease or be scanty because of virilization; water balance is maintained by mineralocorticoid production.
    3 Pitting edema does not occur except when congestive heart failure is present and severe. There is no increase in frequency of colds since the ability to adapt to pathogens is not affected.
    4 Menses may become irregular or scanty, and headaches are not caused by this syndrome.

521. **1** Adrenal steroids help an individual adjust to stress. Unless received from external sources, there would be no hormone available to cope with surgical stresses after adrenalectomy. (c)
    2 The inflammatory effect of the adrenals would be obliterated after removal.
    3 Glucose stores (glycogen) will be utilized after surgery to adapt to surgery. Insulin is the hormone that facilitates conversion of glucose to glycogen.
    4 Steroids would result in fluid retention, not loss.

522. **3** Hydrocortisone succinate (Solu-Cortef) is a glucocorticoid. A client undergoing bilateral adrenalectomy must be given adrenocortical hormones so that adjustment to the sudden lack of these hormones which occurs with this surgery can take place. (c)
    1 Insulin is produced by the pancreas, and its function is not altered by this surgery.
    2 Since adrenal glands are removed, ACTH will have no target gland on which to act.
    4 Since the surgery is on the adrenals, not the pituitary gland, secretion of pituitary hormones will not be affected.

523. **4** Adrenal insufficiency results after an adrenalectomy, causing hypotension due to fluid and electrolyte alterations. (b)

1 Hypoglycemia may be a problem stemming from the loss of glucocorticoids.

2 Hyponatremia may occur because of the lack of mineralocorticoid production.

3 Potassium ions (K^+) may be retained because of the lack of mineralocorticoids.

524. **4** In the absence of insulin, which facilitates the transport of glucose into the cell, the body breaks down proteins and fats to supply energy ketones, a byproduct of fat metabolism. These accumulate, causing metabolic acidosis (pH < 7.35). (b)

1 Cholesterol level has no effect on the development of acidosis.

2 The pH of food ingested has no effect on the development of acidosis.

3 This would indicate a state of alkalosis.

525. **3** In the absence of insulin, glucose cannot enter the cell or be converted to glycogen; so it remains in the blood. Breakdown of fats as an energy source causes an accumulation of ketones, which results in acidosis. The lungs, in an attempt to compensate for lowered pH, will blow off CO_2 (Kussmaul respirations). (c)

1 Hyperglycemia and increased acidity would be present.

2 High acidity and a low CO_2 combining power would be present.

4 Hyperglycemia and a low CO_2 combining power would be present.

526. **2** Regular insulin is rapid acting and is used to meet a client's current insulin needs, as in diabetic coma or in coverage for fractional urine or fingerstick results. (b)

1 This is an intermediate-acting insulin, which has an onset of 4 to 8 hours; in diabetic acidosis the individual needs rapid-acting insulin.

3 This is an intermediate-acting insulin, which has an onset of 4 to 8 hours; in diabetic acidosis the individual needs rapid-acting insulin.

4 PZI is a long-acting insulin, with an onset of 4 to 8 hours and a peak of 14 to 20 hours.

527. **1** Once treatment with insulin for diabetic ketoacidosis is begun, potassium ions reenter the cell, causing hypokalemia; therefore potassium, along with the replacement fluids, is generally supplied. (b)

2 Treatment with potassium would not correct this.

3 Flaccid paralysis would not occur in diabetic ketoacidosis; potassium replaces that which has reentered the cell after insulin therapy.

4 Knowing the relationship of insulin and potassium, the nurse should recognize that treatment with KCl is prophylactic, aborting any development of arrhythmias.

528. **1** Ice milk is a dairy product, whereas bread is not. (b)

2 This exchange is from the same food group and supplies approximately equal amounts of nutrients.

3 This exchange is from the same food group and supplies approximately equal amounts of nutrients.

4 This exchange is from the same food group and supplies approximately equal amounts of nutrients.

529. **2** Glucagon is an insulin antagonist produced by the alpha cells in the islets of Langerhans. It causes the breakdown of glycogen and protein to glucose. (b)

1 Acidosis occurs when there is a high sugar level; therefore glucagon is not indicated.

3 Glucagon is not indicated in idiosyncratic reactions to insulin.

4 Glucagon would be ineffective in the pathologic condition indicated.

530. **2** The Nurse Practice Act states that the nurse will do health teaching and administer nursing care supportive to life and well-being. (a)

1 Health teaching is an independent function of the nurse.

3 The teaching was essential prior to discharge.

4 The client is responsible for her own care.

531. **1** Somatotropin promotes growth by accelerating amino acid transport into cells. Oversecretion after full growth and epiphyseal closure results in acromegaly, with enlargement of bones and overlying soft tissue in the feet, hands, lower jaw, and cheeks. This growth hormone also increases blood glucose levels. (b)

2 This causes hyperthyroidism; not produced by hypophysis.

3 Would increase stimulation of the thyroid gland.

4 Oversecretion would affect secondary sexual characteristics.

532. **4** The hypophysis cerebri (pituitary) does not directly regulate insulin release. This is controlled by blood glucose levels. Since somatotropin release will stop after the hypophysectomy, any elevation of blood glucose caused by somatotropin will also stop. (a)

1 This effect may be expected after a hypophysectomy since follicle-stimulating hormone and follicle-stimulating hormone releasing factor will no longer be present to stimulate spermatogenesis.

2 ACTH, which stimulates glucocorticoid secretion by the adrenal glands, is absent and cortisone will have to be administered.

3 Thyroid-stimulating hormone will not be present; extrinsic thyroxin will have to be taken.

533. **1** ACTH is released in response to decreased blood levels of cortisol. The ACTH then stimulates release of more adrenocortical hormone. (c)

2 Cortisol assists the body in adapting to stress.

3 Cortisol has antiinflammatory properties, which delay wound healing.

4 As a glucocorticoid it increases gluconeogenesis in the liver.

534. **3** Because of the location of the pituitary gland, there is swelling in the brain after the gland's removal. This edema may result in increased intracranial pressure. (c)

1 This may follow any surgery and is not a specific occurrence following cranial surgery.

2 This may follow any surgery and is not a specific occurrence following cranial surgery.

4 Although this may be the result of pressure on the medulla caused by increased intracranial pressure, it is not an initial sign of ICP.

535. **2** Endocrine gland secretions (hormones) are inactivated by the liver and other tissues fairly rapidly; continuous hormonal secretion by the endocrine glands is regulated by immediate feedback controls, and the body's metabolism is always close to being suitable to the body's immediate needs. (b)

1 This time interval does not represent secretory patterns of the endocrine glands.

3 This time interval does not represent secretory patterns of the endocrine glands.

4 This time interval does not represent secretory patterns of the endocrine glands.

536. **2** The pH of blood is maintained within the narrow range of 7.35 to 7.45. When there is an increase in hydrogen ions (H^+), acidosis results and is reflected in the lower pH. (a)

1 This is too acidic.

3 This is within the normal range for pH.

4 This is slightly alkaline.

537. **3** Sodium bicarbonate is a base and one of the major buffers in the body. (b)
  1 Carbon dioxide is carried in aqueous solution as carbonic acid (H_2CO_3); an acid does not buffer another acid.
  2 Potassium is not a buffer; only a base can buffer an acid.
  4 Sodium chloride is not a buffer; it is a salt.
538. **4** The sodium bicarbonate-carbonic acid buffer system helps maintain the pH of the body fluids. In metabolic acidosis there is a decrease in bicarbonate due to retention of metabolic acids. Since there is a decrease in bicarbonate, the carbonic acid will increase to maintain the balance between these two buffers. (c)
  1 The pH will become more acidic.
  2 The pH will decrease, indicating an increased acid content.
  3 The carbonic acid content increases as sodium bicarbonate decreases.
539. **4** Regular insulin is rapid acting and should be used when immediate action is desired. (b)
  1 Long-acting insulin; not indicated in an emergency.
  2 Not a form of insulin; a simple protein.
  3 Intermediate-acting insulin; not indicated in an emergency.
540. **1** There are 100 units of insulin in 1 ml (or in 15 minims); 6 minims must be administered to provide the client with 40 units of insulin. (b)

$$\frac{40\ U}{100\ U} = \frac{x\ \text{minims}}{15\ \text{minims}}$$
$$100x = 600$$
$$x = 6\ \text{minims}$$

  2 This reflects a miscalculation and would be an overdose.
  3 This reflects a miscalculation and would be an overdose.
  4 This reflects a miscalculation and would be an overdose.
541. **2** Glucagon, an insulin antagonist produced by the alpha cells in the islets of Langerhans, leads to the conversion of glycogen to glucose in the liver. (b)
  1 Does not stimulate the storage of glucose but rather its release by conversion of glycogen to glucose.
  3 It is an insulin antagonist.
  4 Stimulates glycogenolysis, the conversion of glycogen to glucose.
542. **1** Different types of insulin are compatible and are administered in the same syringe. However, the regular insulin is generally drawn up first because it is fast acting; and the possibility that a slower-acting insulin will enter the multidose vial is eliminated. (c)
  2 Ratio does not affect compatibility.
  3 Ratio does not affect compatibility.
  4 Unnecessary injections increase the risk of infection as well as cause additional discomfort.
543. **3** An individual treated for a thyroid problem by intake of radioactive iodine (^{131}I) becomes mildly radioactive, particularly in the region of the thyroid gland, which preferentially absorbs the iodine. Such clients should be treated with standard precautions. (b)
  1 Since radioactive iodine is internalized, the client becomes the source of radioactivity.
  2 The amount of radioactive iodine utilized is not enough to cause high radioactivity.
  4 Since radioactive iodine is internalized, the client becomes the source of radioactivity.

544. **1** Because of the individual's increased metabolic rate, a high-calorie diet is needed to meet the energy demands of the body and prevent weight loss. (b)
  2 GI motility is increased and does not require the additional stimulus of increased roughage.
  3 Nutritional needs are increased by increased metabolism; additional calories are needed.
  4 Modification of the consistency is unnecessary.
545. **3** Lugol's solution adds iodine to the body fluids, exerting negative feedback on the thyroid tissue and decreasing its metabolism and vascularity. (a)
  1 This drug interferes with production of thyroid hormone but causes increased vascularity and size of the thyroid.
  2 This is a synthetic thyroid hormone; its use is contraindicated because there is already an excessive production of thyroid hormone.
  4 This is a topical antiseptic.
546. **3** During surgery, if the laryngeal nerves are injured bilaterally, the vocal cords will tighten, interfering with speech. If one cord is affected, hoarseness develops. This can be evaluated simply by having the client speak every hour. (b)
  1 This ability is not influenced by laryngeal nerve damage.
  2 This ability is not influenced by laryngeal nerve damage.
  4 This ability is not influenced by laryngeal nerve damage.
547. **3** These signs may indicate tetany from calcium depletion. If this occurs after a thyroidectomy, one might suspect inadvertent removal of the parathyroids. (c)
  1 Symptoms associated with hypokalemia include muscle weakness and malaise.
  2 Symptoms associated with hypomagnesemia include tremor, neuromuscular irritability, and confusion.
  4 Symptoms associated with metabolic acidosis include deep rapid breathing, weakness, and disorientation.
548. **1** Parathyroid removal eliminates the body's source of parathyroid hormone, which functions to increase blood calcium. Consequently, normal decreases in blood calcium cannot be balanced by additions to the blood from calcium reservoirs in bone, increased calcium reabsorption from the kidney tubules, or increased intestinal calcium absorption. Low body fluid calcium tetanizes muscles, including the diaphragm, resulting in dyspnea, asphyxia, and death. (a)
  2 The parathyroids do not regulate the adrenal glands.
  3 Loss of the thyroid gland would upset thyroid hormone balance and might cause myxedema.
  4 The parathyroids are not involved in regulating plasma volume; the pituitary and adrenal glands are.
549. **1** Parathyroid hormone increases osteoclastic activity, resulting in breakdown of bone substance and release of calcium into the blood. (b)
  2 It increases blood calcium and thereby will prevent tetany.
  3 Although blood calcium does increase, blood phosphate also increases.
  4 The hormone calcitonin, released by the thyroid gland, increases calcium incorporation into the bones.
550. **4** Parathormone increases blood calcium by accelerating calcium absorption from the intestine and kidneys and releasing calcium from bone. Vitamin D promotes calcium absorption from the intestine. (b)
  1 Vitamin A and thyroid hormone do not interact to regulate calcium levels. Vitamin A is essential for the normal function of epithelial cells and visual purple; calcitonin, from the thyroid gland, lowers serum calcium.

2 Ascorbic acid (vitamin C) and growth hormone do not interact to regulate calcium levels. Vitamin C promotes collagen production and the formation of bone matrix; growth hormone, produced by the anterior pituitary, controls the rate of skeletal growth.

3 Phosphorus and ACTH do not interact to regulate calcium levels. Phosphorus is a component of bone; ACTH, produced by the anterior pituitary, stimulates the adrenal cortex to secrete the corticosteroid hormones.

551. **2** Calcitonin, a thyroid gland hormone, prevents the reabsorption of calcium by bone. It also inhibits the release of calcium from bone. The net result is lowered serum calcium levels. (a)

1 Aldosterone regulates fluid and electrolyte balance by promoting the retention of sodium and water and the excretion of potassium.

3 Parathyroid hormone promotes the intestinal absorption of calcium and mobilizes calcium from the bones to increase blood calcium levels.

4 Although calcitonin lowers serum calcium levels, the other thyroid hormones (thyroxine and triiodothyronine) control the body's metabolic rate.

552. **3** Hyperparathyroidism causes calcium release from the bones, leaving them porous and weak. (b)

1 Tetany is the result of low calcium; in this condition serum calcium is high.

2 Seizures are caused by increased neural activity, a condition not related to this disease.

4 Grave's disease is the result of increased thyroid, not parathyroid, activity.

553. **2** Fluids help prevent the formation of renal calculi associated with high serum calcium. (c)

1 Rest is contraindicated because bone destruction is accelerated.

3 Seizures are associated with low, not high, serum calcium.

4 Additional calcium intake could raise already high levels of serum calcium.

554. **1** Myxedema is the severest form of hypothyroidism. Decreased thyroid gland activity causes a reduced production of its hormones. (b)

2 Results from excess growth hormone in adults once the epiphyses are closed.

3 Results from excess glucocorticoids.

4 Results from excess, not a deficiency, of thyroid hormones.

555. **1** Decreased production of thyroid hormones lowers metabolism, which leads to decreased heat production and cold intolerance. (b)

2 Lethargy, rather than irritability, is expected.

3 Skin is dry and coarse, not moist.

4 Decreased metabolism results in decreased oxygen utilization, so pulse rate is generally slower.

556. **2** The thyroid gland produces thyroxine (T_4) and triiodothyronine (T_3), which help regulate oxidation in all body cells. (a)

1 Involved in secondary regulation by its secretion of TSH, which stimulates thyroid production of thyroxine and triiodothyronine.

3 The primary regulator is the thyroid; the adrenals exert an influence on metabolism of carbohydrates in times of stress.

4 Regulates glucose metabolism by secretion of insulin.

557. **3** Glucose catabolism is the main pathway for cellular energy production. (b)

1 Glucose is not used directly for this process; ATP is the energy source.

2 Glucose is not used directly for this process; ATP is the energy source.

4 Glucose is not used directly for this process; ATP is the energy source.

558. **3** Ingested glucose not used immediately for energy needs is stored in the liver as glycogen and broken down when the blood glucose level falls (glycogenolysis). (a)

1 Not all foods provide glucose; ingested glucose may meet immediate needs but must be converted to glycogen for storage; glycogen is converted to glucose as needed.

2 This is digestion.

4 Formation of glucose from protein or fat.

559. **4** Insulin functions by facilitating the transport of glucose through the cell membrane and by increasing the deposits of glycogen in muscle. Both cellular glucose and muscle glycogen can be utilized for energy. (a)

1 Stimulates rate of oxygen consumption and thus the rate at which carbohydrates are burned; not the main controlling hormone.

2 Accelerates protein anabolism and stimulates growth.

3 Stimulates glyconeogenesis.

560. **3** Since oral hyperglycemics stimulate the islets of Langerhans to produce insulin, a regular interval between doses should be maintained. (a)

1 Manifestations of toxicity should be taught but not emphasized because occurrence of toxicity is low and the nurse may needlessly cause anxiety.

2 Untoward reactions should be taught but not emphasized because occurrence of untoward reactions is low and the nurse may needlessly cause anxiety.

4 The dosage should be regulated by the physician.

561. **1** In starvation there are inadequate carbohydrates available for immediate energy, and stored fats are used in excessive amounts. (a)

2 There is no fat in alcohol; no fat oxidation occurs.

3 Does not require use of great amounts of fat.

4 Does not require use of great amounts of fat; calcium is deposited to form callus.

562. **1** Increased intracranial pressure places tension on the brain stem, causing signs such as increased systolic blood pressure, slow bounding pulse, elevated temperature, and changes in the respiratory pattern. (b)

2 These combinations of symptoms are not found when vital brain centers are subjected to increased pressure.

3 These combinations of symptoms are not found when vital brain centers are subjected to increased pressure.

4 These combinations of symptoms are not found when vital brain centers are subjected to increased pressure.

563. **2** An unconscious individual loses voluntary control of the sphincters surrounding the urethra and anus. (b)

1 Unconscious clients may react to various degrees of pain.

3 Motion (although often purposeless) is possible in coma.

4 This cannot be assumed; hearing is often the last sense to be lost.

564. **3** It is important to help the client who has expressive aphasia regain maximum communicative abilities early during the hospital stay; this action provides reinforcement. (b)

1 Some abilities do return, and therefore he should be encouraged to participate.

2 This approach may increase client frustration and anxiety.

4 Although expectations should be realistic, improvements are possible and should be encouraged.

565. **2** Atony permits the bladder to fill without being able to empty. As pressure builds within the bladder, the urge to void occurs and just enough urine is eliminated to relieve the pressure and the urge to void. The cycle is repeated as pressure again builds. Thus small amounts are voided without emptying the bladder. (c)
   1 Total amount of urine produced and voided would be unchanged.
   3 Continual incontinence would not occur if urine were retained.
   4 These might be signs of renal failure.
566. **4** A strange environment, as well as the anxiety associated with private body functions like elimination, interferes with the client's ability to relax the urinary sphincter to void. (a)
   1 This method might be helpful in some situations; however, it does not take into account the common anxiety of voiding in a strange environment.
   2 This might be helpful in some situations; however, it does not take into account the common anxiety of voiding in a strange environment.
   3 This might be helpful in some situations; however, it does not take into account the common anxiety of voiding in a strange environment.
567. **3** All nursing intervention aims to assist an individual in maximizing capabilities and coping with modifications in life-style. (b)
   1 Rehabilitation is a commonality in all areas of nursing practice.
   2 Rehabilitation is necessary to help clients return to a previous level of functioning after both illness and surgery.
   4 Too limiting; all resources, including the private physician, acute care facilities, etc., that can be beneficial to client rehabilitation should be utilized.
568. **3** Rehabilitating exercises carried out underwater minimize strain on the partially atrophied and painful joints. The buoyant force of the water makes the limbs easier to move. (b)
   1 Exercises are carried out near the surface of the water, where the water pressure would have little effect.
   2 Vapors are produced above water as a result of evaporation; do not facilitate exercise.
   4 Water temperature would not assist movement.
569. **4** This is considered a routine procedure to meet basic physiologic needs and is covered by a consent signed at the time of admission. (c)
   1 This treatment does not require special consent.
   2 The catheter is inserted to aid the health team in assessing the client.
   3 This treatment does not require special consent.
570. **4** After a CVA the client should be repositioned frequently, and passive ROM exercises should be instituted to prevent deformity. (b)
   1 The nurse is not directly assisting the client.
   2 This would increase deformities and atrophy.
   3 Active exercises require a physician's order.
571. **1** Footboards provide a broad flat surface that helps to keep the foot in a position of dorsiflexion. (a)
   2 Blocks elevate the frame of the bed and have no effect on position of the feet.
   3 Cradles keep linen off of the client's abdomen and legs but do nothing to position the feet.
   4 Sandbags help prevent lateral movement of an extremity or the head.
572. **1** Although the client who has suffered a CVA is expected to be emotionally labile, the major factors determining the reaction to illness are past experiences and coping mechanisms. (a)

   2 The site of the CVA may influence behavior but would not affect the client's emotional response to the disease.
   3 Although care is important, basic coping mechanisms and personality are already established.
   4 Emotional response is not dependent on one's ability to understand the underlying physiologic causes of disease.
573. **2** Change of position every 2 hours helps prevent the respiratory, urinary, and cutaneous complications of immobility. (a)
   1 Turning may raise intracranial pressure; doing it this frequently may be contraindicated in the early stages.
   3 Too protracted a period in one position increases the potential for respiratory, urinary, and neuromuscular impairment; prolonged physical pressure increases the possibility of skin breakdown.
   4 Too protracted a period in one position increases the potential for respiratory, urinary, and neuromuscular impairment; prolonged physical pressure increases the possibility of skin breakdown.
574. **2** To aid in motivation, the nurse should focus on the positive aspects of the client's progress. (c)
   1 Having individuals actually perform is more beneficial than telling or showing them what to do.
   3 Short-term attainable goals provide positive reinforcement for the client, goal setting should be done by the client or shared with the nurse.
   4 This negative reinforcement may result in discouragement.
575. **1** As part of the rehabilitative process after a CVA, clients must be encouraged to participate in their own care to the extent to which they are able and to extend their abilities by establishing short-term goals. (b)
   2 Making the client feel helpless discourages independence.
   3 A client with a CVA may have dysphagia, and rapid feeding may cause aspiration as well as indigestion.
   4 Unrealistic; daughter may not be available because of other responsibilities.
576. **2** Some weight-bearing on the uninvolved leg helps maintain its muscle tone. (c)
   1 This is an unacceptable rationale for care.
   3 Speed is not important when ambulating.
   4 There is less danger of injury when the "good leg" is maintaining strength.
577. **1** Supports the fracture site; the involved leg must be maintained in alignment, avoiding adduction. (a)
   2 Comfort is not the most important reason for positioning.
   3 Adduction, not flexion contractures, are of most concern after surgery.
   4 Although friction is decreased when skin does not interface with skin, this is not the reason for separating the thighs and lower limbs.
578. **3** To prevent nerve damage in the axillary area, the palms should take all the weight. (a)
   1 Pressure in the axillary area causes nerve damage to the brachial plexus.
   2 Pressure in the axillary area causes nerve damage to the brachial plexus.
   4 Not explicit as to what extremities are being referred to; weight-bearing on the affected lower extremity is initially contraindicated.
579. **3** After a fracture, if blood supply is cut off or impaired, necrosis of the bone may occur from lack of oxygen and nutrient perfusion. (c)
   1 *Aseptic* indicates that infection is not present.

2 Immobilization does not cut off circulation to the bone; it may cause contractures.

4 Early weight-bearing at the fracture site might result in trauma to bone; circulation would not be impaired.

580. **3** This type of contracture frequently occurs when the client lies in bed with knees bent and thighs not abducted. (b)

   1 Although foot-drop is a problem for all clients confined to bed rest, hyperextension of the knee is not possible.

   2 These two anatomic positions cannot occur at the same time.

   4 This does not describe a contracture.

581. **1** Intramedullary nails are used to maintain bone alignment and provide support along the femur's length. (c)

   2 Since these orthopedic problems do not affect the shaft of a long bone, an intramedullary nailing device is not appropriate.

   3 Since these orthopedic problems do not affect the shaft of a long bone, an intramedullary nailing device is not appropriate.

   4 Since these orthopedic problems do not affect the shaft of a long bone, an intramedullary nailing device is not appropriate.

582. **3** Since pain is an all-encompassing and often demoralizing experience, the client should be kept as pain free as possible. (b)

   1 Motivation is difficult when a client is in severe pain.

   2 Concentration on learning something is difficult when a client is in severe pain.

   4 Pain can usually be managed medically; surgery is used to correct deformity and facilitate movement.

583. **1** A latex test can determine autoimmune rheumatoid factor in the blood. (a)

   2 Lipase is an enzyme that catalyzes the breakdown of lipids; test used to diagnose pancreatic problems.

   3 Bence Jones protein is a urine test helpful in diagnosing multiple myeloma.

   4 Alkaline phosphatase is a blood test to determine phosphorus activity; generally used in diagnosing liver and biliary tract disorders and identifying periods of active bone growth or metastasis of cancer to bone.

584. **3** Heat causes muscles to relax, and therefore injury during exercise can be minimized. (c)

   1 Active or passive exercises may be indicated depending on the client's tolerance.

   2 Avoiding exercise will increase the destructive effects of immobility.

   4 Active or passive exercises may be indicated depending on the client's tolerance.

585. **1** The nurse's positive attitude encourages and motivates the client. (a)

   2 This attitude on the part of the nurse may discourage the client's ability to attain highest goals.

   3 This attitude on the part of the nurse may discourage the client's ability to attain highest goals.

   4 Care plans should contain as many objectives as necessary.

586. **1** A long-range goal should be to involve the client in many activities of daily living; such a program can help reestablish the client in former life-style. (b)

   2 There is no indication that the client is unemployed or unable to work.

   3 There is no indication that the client needs an assistive device; if necessary, a walker would be safer.

   4 There is no indication that the client is unable to care for herself or live with her family.

587. **2** Braces would restrict movement of the joint, causing increased deformity. (a)

   1 This activity increases functional use of the affected part.

   3 This activity increases functional use of the affected part.

   4 This activity increases functional use of the affected part.

588. **2** The pain may prevent the client from ingesting anything by mouth. (b)

   1 This would initiate an acute attack of trigeminal neuralgia.

   3 Exercises may precipitate an attack.

   4 Hot or cold foods or compresses should be avoided because they may trigger a painful attack.

589. **2** Tic douloureux, also referred to as trigeminal neuralgia, is an inflammation of the fifth cranial (trigeminal) nerve, which innervates the midline of the face and head. (c)

   1 The oculomotor (or third, not the fifth) cranial nerve innervates the eyelid.

   3 Pain, not weakness, occurs in this disease.

   4 Petechiae are minute subcutaneous hemorrhages; not present in this disorder.

590. **1** Severe constant pain, emotional stress, muscle tensing, and diminished nutritional intake can lead to exhaustion and fatigue. (c)

   2 The client may be very quiet for fear of precipitating an attack.

   3 Pain medications do not normally cause hyperactivity.

   4 Because clients are apprehensive and feeling pain, prolonged periods of sleep usually do not occur.

591. **1** The nurse should avoid swiftly walking past the client since drafts or even slight air currents can initiate pain. (c)

   2 Oral hygiene is important in preventing infection.

   3 Massaging may trigger an attack and should be avoided.

   4 The client may assume any position of comfort, but pressure on the face while in the prone position may trigger an attack.

592. **1** Carbamazepine (Tegretol) is a nonnarcotic analgesic, anticonvulsive drug used to control pain in trigeminal neuralgia and to abort future attacks. It sometimes eliminates the need for surgery. (c)

   2 Allopurinal is used in the treatment of gout.

   3 Morphine is a narcotic analgesic that will relieve severe pain but will not prevent its recurrence; prolonged frequent use is contraindicated because of possible addiction.

   4 Ascorbic acid is vitamin C. This vitamin is found in high concentrations in the adrenal gland and is utilized when the body is subject to stress as occurs with pain.

593. **2** Recurrence of pain would be unusual since the nerve is severed, resulting in permanent anesthesia. (a)

   1 Herpes simplex may develop because of injury to the gasserian ganglion, hyperthermia, or dehydration.

   3 These symptoms can result when the sensory root of the trigeminal nerve is sectioned.

   4 Severance of the nerve interferes with muscle innervation.

594. **2** Since neurectomy eliminates sensations, the client must be counseled to get regular dental checkups to prevent local infection from becoming systemic. (c)

   1 Facial exercises are not indicated for clients with this disease.

   3 Stressful situations should have no effect on the condition after surgery.

4 Food should be chewed on the unaffected side, since after surgery chewing would be difficult on the affected side.

595. **3** Rectal temperature is the most accurate. (a)
  1 Oral temperature is contraindicated since dysphagia may cause excessive salivation.
  2 Groin temperature is less accurate since it is affected by room temperature.
  4 Axillary temperature is less accurate since it is affected by room temperature.

596. **1** Dysphagia is difficulty in swallowing. (a)
  2 Focusing with the eyes is unrelated to dysphagia and dysarthria (difficulty speaking).
  3 Writing is unrelated to dysphagia and dysarthria.
  4 Understanding information is unrelated to dysphagia and dysarthria.

597. **3** Clients with dysarthria have difficulty communicating verbally, and alternate means may be indicated. (b)
  1 An important aspect of care but not related to dysarthria.
  2 An important aspect of care but not related to dysarthria.
  4 An important aspect of care but not related to dysarthria.

598. **3** The paralyzed side has decreased muscle tone, which affects blood pressure readings. (b)
  1 Taking blood pressure does not precipitate the formation of thrombi.
  2 Return of function to the affected extremity is not affected by taking blood pressure; if it occurs, it is due to resolution of inflammation or resorption of blood in the area of the infarct.
  4 There is no difference when pressure is exerted on the brachial artery in either arm.

599. **2** To prevent distention and/or aspiration, the maximum amount of fluid administered at the first tube feeding is 250 ml. (c)
  1 More fluid than this can be administered safely.
  3 This amount of fluid would be excessive for initial tube feedings.
  4 This amount of fluid would be excessive for any tube feeding.

600. **2** Although tube feedings are often administered at room temperature, formula at body temperature is tolerated best. (b)
  1 Chilled feedings may cause gastric distress.
  3 Room temperature feedings are tolerable, but those at body temperature are better received.
  4 Hot feedings may cause gastric distress.

601. **2** Since the cardiac sphincter of the stomach is slightly opened because of the nasogastric tube, rapid feeding could result in regurgitation. (b)
  1 Indigestion is not hazardous to the client.
  3 Speed of feeding does not cause flatulence; administration of air may.
  4 Distension can be diminished by avoiding the instillation of air with the feeding.

602. **1** Decadron is a corticosteroid that acts on the cell membrane to prevent the normal inflammatory responses as well as stabilize the blood-brain barrier. (c)
  2 This is not an effect of corticosteroid therapy.
  3 This is not an effect of corticosteroid therapy.
  4 This is not an effect of corticosteroid therapy.

603. **2** Dexamethasone (Decadron) increases gluconeogenesis, which may cause hyperglycemia. (c)
  1 The renal threshold for glucose is not affected by Decadron.

3 Protein breakdown is not accelerated by Decadron.
  4 Decadron does not contain a glucose component.

604. **2** Decadron increases the production of hydrochloric acid, which may cause GI ulcers. Clients should also be instructed to take Decadron with meals. (c)
  1 Decadron is not irritating to the mucosa.
  3 Stomach emptying time may be increased by Decadron.
  4 Decadron does not affect the pepsin-induced erosion of the mucosa.

605. **4** To help prevent ulcer formation in the gastric mucosa, peristalsis and gastric motility should not be increased. (c)
  1 This statement regarding Maalox and dexamethasone is not true.
  2 This statement regarding Amphojel is not true.
  3 This statement regarding Amphojel is not true.

606. **3** Prolonged use of sodium bicarbonate may cause systemic alkalosis as well as retention of sodium and water. (a)
  1 This statement is inaccurate in describing the effects of sodium bicarbonate.
  2 This statement is inaccurate in describing the effects of sodium bicarbonate.
  4 This statement is inaccurate in describing the effects of sodium bicarbonate.

607. **2** Any hormone normally produced by the body must be withdrawn slowly to allow the appropriate organ to adjust and resume production. (b)
  1 Production of ACTH is not affected.
  3 Although important, this is not the reason for gradual withdrawal of the drug.
  4 Although important, this is not the reason for gradual withdrawal of the drug.

608. **2** Prolonged use of steroids may cause leukopenia as a result of bone marrow depression. (c)
  1 Sedimentation rate is elevated when infection is present; not associated with the medications.
  3 CRP (C-reactive protein) is present in acute inflammatory diseases and necrosis; not associated with the medications.
  4 This is the term given anemias that are characterized by decreased concentration of hemoglobin in erythrocytes; not a sequela of the use of aspirin or steroids.

609. **4** Open-ended questions provide a milieu in which people can verbalize their problems rather than be placed in a situation of forced response. (a)
  1 Direct questions do not open or promote communication.
  2 False reassurance is detrimental to the nurse-client relationship and does not promote communication.
  3 This can be threatening to the client, who may not have the answer to these questions.

610. **4** Rheumatoid arthritis is a chronic systemic disease with inflammatory and degenerative changes in the body's connective tissue. (c)
  1 Bones are not the focus of this disease.
  2 It is connective tissue in the area of the joints that is affected.
  3 Purine metabolism is affected in gout.

611. **2** Gold salts, bound to plasma proteins, are distributed irregularly throughout the body; but the highest concentration occurs in the kidneys. The slow excretion of gold salts cannot keep up with their intake; they accumulate in the kidneys, causing damage. (b)
  1 This is not a side effect associated with gold salts, such as Myochrysine.

3 This is not a side effect associated with gold salts, such as Myochrysine.

4 This is not a side effect associated with gold salts, such as Myochrysine.

612. **2** Open-angle glaucoma has an insidious onset, with increased intraocular pressure causing pressure on the retina and blood vessels in the eye. Peripheral vision is decreased as the visual field progressively diminishes. (b)

 1 Occlusions of the central retinal artery would cause a sudden loss of vision.

 3 Pain occurs in acute angle closure, not open-angle glaucoma.

 4 This may be accompanied by untreated acute angle closure glaucoma.

613. **1** In glaucoma the intraocular pressure is elevated and must be returned to normal. (b)

 2 Dilation of the pupils may cause a further increase in pressure by obstructing the canal of Schlemm; increased pressure reduces the visual field and leads to blindness.

 3 Resting has no effect on this condition, for it will not decrease the pressure.

 4 Increased intraocular pressure can lead to blindness; reducing pressure is the priority.

614. **4** The contraction permits the lens to return to its normal bulge, decreasing focal length and allowing focus on near objects. (c)

 1 The rectus and oblique muscles of the eye are involved in convergence.

 2 The ciliary muscles are intrinsic (within the eyeball); the third cranial nerve (oculomotor), an extrinsic nerve, controls movements of the eyelid.

 3 In this case the ciliary muscles would relax.

615. **1** Sedatives have no effect on the intraocular pressure. (b)

 2 Would raise the intraocular pressure.

 3 Would raise the intraocular pressure.

 4 Would raise the intraocular pressure.

616. **3** Since continued use of eyedrops is indicated, an extra supply should always be available. (b)

 1 Eyewashes (collyria) have no effect on the disease.

 2 Laxatives should not be taken on a routine basis.

 4 Since treatment must be maintained for life, extra medication should be available so the supply does not run out.

617. **1** Eye medications are applied directly to the eye. (a)

 2 Intraocular drugs are given for severe infections by an ophthalmologist.

 3 This route is not used for ocular medications.

 4 This route is not used for ocular medications.

618. **1** Acetazolamide (Diamox) is a carbonic anhydrase inhibitor that decreases the inflow of aqueous humor and controls intraocular pressure. (c)

 2 This diuretic has no effect on the eye.

 3 This diuretic has no effect on the eye.

 4 This strong miotic does not affect the production of aqueous humor.

619. **4** Cortisone, a steroid, stabilizes lysosomal membranes, inhibiting the release of proteolytic enzymes during inflammation. This antiinflammatory drug also maximizes vasoconstrictor effects. (b)

 1 An antibiotic, which would not decrease an inflammatory reaction.

 2 An antibiotic, which would not decrease an inflammatory reaction.

 3 An antibiotic, which would not decrease an inflammatory reaction.

620. **4** Cerebral damage on one side of the cortex causes alterations on the opposite side, since three-fourths of the fibers originating in the cortex decussate (cross over) in the medulla before extending down the spinal cord. When there is cranial nerve damage, the same side of the body is affected, since the cranial nerves do not decussate but leave the cranial cavity by way of the small foramina in the skull. (c)

 1 Hemiplegia refers to paralysis of one side of the body; affects both extremities.

 2 Facial muscles on the same side as the cerebral lesion are paralyzed because they are innervated by the cranial nerves, which originate above the points where the spinal nerves decussate.

 3 Hemiplegia refers to paralysis of one side of the body; affects both extremities.

621. **2** Because of the profound effect of paralysis on body image, the nurse should provide the client with an environment that permits exploration of feelings without judgment, punishment, or rejection. (a)

 1 An important part of nursing care; but not specific to the situation described.

 3 Attempts to distract the client may be interpreted as denial of the client's feelings and will not resolve the underlying conflict.

 4 An important part of nursing care; but not specific to the situation described.

622. **4** Bowel training is a program for the development of a conditioned reflex that controls regular emptying of the bowel. The key to success in a conditioning program is adherence to a strict time for evacuation based on the client's individual schedule. (c)

 1 Although this should be considered, the cerebrovascular accident affects the responses of the client by altering mobility, peristalsis, and sphincter control despite adherence to previous habits.

 2 The passage of food into the stomach does stimulate peristalsis but is only one factor that should be considered when planning a specific time for evacuation.

 3 The indiscriminate use of laxatives can result in dependency.

623. **3** Success is a basic motivation for learning. People receive satisfaction when a goal is reached. The more frequent the success, the greater is their satisfaction, which in turn motivates them to continue striving toward realistic goals. (b)

 1 An important part of teaching; but will not necessarily motivate the client to attempt them.

 2 Progress toward long-range goals is often not readily apparent and may tend to discourage a client.

 4 Constructive criticism is an important aspect in client teaching; but if not tempered with praise, is discouraging.

624. **3** Reasonably prudent behavior in dealing with an immobile client is to change the client's position at least every 2 hours to relieve pressure on tissues and promote circulation. The nurse is negligent in not doing this. (b)

 1 When a capable client refuses necessary health care despite explanation, her rights must be respected but she must also sign a document absolving health professionals of liability.

 2 Although decubitis ulcers may occur, nursing care must include preventive measures.

 4 The family is included in the health team.

625. **4** The absorbent action of Debrisan (dextranomer) helps clean decubitus ulcers and promotes healing. (c)
    1 Although the action has not been established, this drug is used to resolve inflammation resulting from accidental or surgical trauma.
    2 Used to promote diffusion of fluids in tissue during hypodermoclysis.
    3 Enzyme capable of inactivating penicillin.

626. **3** Because of the presence of feces in the colon, a client with a fecal impaction has the urge to defecate but is unable to. (a)
    1 Anorexia may occur with an impaction but may also be due to other conditions.
    2 Flatulence may occur as a result of immobility or obstruction; clients with impactions may be able to pass flatus along with liquid stool around the fecal mass.
    4 The frequency of bowel movements varies for individuals; it may be normal for this individual not to have a BM for several days.

627. **3** When the bowel is impacted with hardened feces, there is often seepage of liquid feces around the obstruction and thus uncontrolled diarrhea. (a)
    1 The bowel may become distended if completely obstructed, but this is a late symptom if it occurs at all.
    2 There are often frequent liquid bowel movements in the presence of an impaction.
    4 This is indicative of lower GI bleeding.

628. **2** As a result of the muscles' contracting and pulling on the two portions of bone, there is a characteristic shortening of the femur with external rotation of the extremity. (c)
    1 The extremity externally rotates as the muscles contract.
    3 Lateral motion of the leg does not occur.
    4 Lateral motion of the leg does not occur; the leg externally rotates.

629. **3** A fracture in the neck of the femur will cause shortening of the femur and external rotation. To correct this malalignment, the client's leg should be extended and maintained in slight internal rotation. (c)
    1 To reduce the fracture, it is necessary to maintain the leg in extension, counteracting the contraction of the quadriceps, which may cause overriding of bone fragments. External rotation of the thigh as a result of muscle contraction tends to misalign the bone fragments; therefore slight internal rotation or normal alignment is preferred.
    2 External rotation of the thigh as a result of muscle contraction tends to misalign the bone fragments; therefore slight internal rotation or normal alignment is preferred.
    4 To reduce the fracture, it is necessary to maintain the leg in extension, counteracting the contraction of the quadriceps, which may cause overriding of bone fragments.

630. **1** Buck's traction is frequently used in the treatment of a fractured hip to align the bones (reduction of fracture). If such traction were not employed, the muscles would go into spasm, shifting the bone fragments and causing pain. (b)
    2 Although the affected extremity must be properly aligned, turning and moving the client is still necessary.
    3 Buck's traction is usually a temporary measure prior to surgery; contractures result from a shortening of the muscles by prolonged immobility.
    4 External rotation is contraindicated and prevented by the use of sandbags or trochanter rolls.

631. **3** Assessment of any peripheral pulse should include the characteristics of the pulse (e.g., amplitude, rhythm, rate). Symmetry, the correspondence of homologous parts on opposite sides of the body, provides a way of assessing data that should be identical. (b)
    1 Contractility is not a characteristic of pulse but of the vessel.
    2 Color of skin and type of spasm are not pulse characteristics.
    4 Local temperature is not a characteristic of pulse.

632. **4** The three-point gait, which requires considerable arm strength, is used when a limb cannot bear weight. The affected leg and crutches are advanced together, and the strong leg swings through. (c)
    1 Requires weight bearing on both feet.
    2 Requires weight bearing on both feet.
    3 Used for individuals who cannot move their lower extremities; does not simulate normal ambulation.

633. **3** In the four-point gait the client brings the left crutch forward first, followed by the right foot; then the right crutch is brought forward, followed by the left foot. Thus both legs must be able to bear some weight. (c)
    1 Pressure on the axillae may damage nerves in the area.
    2 Although the arms are extended to allow the hands to bear weight, the elbows are not maintained in this position.
    4 Both extremities must be able to bear weight.

634. **1** Because of its great blood supply and general fragility, the spleen, when ruptured, must be removed to prevent possible hemorrhage. (b)
    2 Although rupturing of the spleen may be a sequela of certain diseases (e.g., mononucleosis) the situation described involves trauma, which is a more common cause.
    3 Does not explain the reason for removal.
    4 Splenomegaly may not be associated with discomfort; functions of purification, antibody production, and erythrocyte storage are important but not essential.

635. **1** Because the spleen has such vascularity, hemorrhage may occur and result in abdominal distention. (c)
    2 The incidence is not higher after splenectomy than after other abdominal surgery.
    3 Although an elevated temperature is common, it is usually not the result of infection; the incidence of infection is not higher after splenectomy, except in children.
    4 The incidence of obstruction is not higher than for other abdominal surgery.

636. **1** Head injuries can cause trauma to the brain; and the client should be observed for signs of increased intracranial pressure (e.g., headache, dizziness, visual disturbances). (b)
    2 The Trendelenburg position should be avoided because it will increase intracranial pressure.
    3 Not indicated in this situation.
    4 The intracranial pressure may increase after trauma because of bleeding and edema.

637. **4** Release of the adrenocortical steroids (cortisol) by the stress of surgery causes renal retention of Na^+ and excretion of K^+. Potassium can also be depleted by nasogastric suction. (b)
    1 Although sodium may be depleted by nasogastric suction, retention by the kidneys generally balances this loss.
    2 Not depleted by surgery or urinary excretion.
    3 Not depleted by surgery or urinary excretion.

638. **2** Because of the location of the spleen, expansion of the thoracic cavity during inspiration causes pain at the operative site. (b)

1 This is not to be expected; accumulation of secretions can be avoided by coughing and deep breathing.

3 Since limited activity decreases oxygen consumption, shortness of breath is not a common complaint.

4 Pain does not occur on expiration, for the lungs deflate and decrease pressure on the operative site.

639. **3** Changes in the amount of blood in the urine may indicate progressive increases in kidney damage. (b)

1 This is unrelated to hematuria.

2 This is unrelated to hematuria.

4 This is unrelated to hematuria; associated with breakdown of adipose tissue.

640. **1** Hematuria occurs when there is kidney damage with leakage of erythrocytes through the glomerular filtration membrane. (b)

2 Although lesions of the ureters may be responsible for hematuria, blunt trauma to the kidneys is more common because of their proximity to the rib cage.

3 Although injury to the bladder is possible, blunt trauma to the kidneys is more common because of their proximity to the rib cage.

4 Although injury to the urethra is possible, blunt trauma to the kidneys is more common because of their proximity to the rib cage.

641. **3** Phenytoin (Dilantin) is an anticonvulsant, most effective in controlling grand mal seizures. Data collection before planning nursing care for a client with epilepsy should always include a history of seizure incidence (type and frequency). (c)

1 Although protection is important, restraints during a seizure often cause injury as a result of violent muscle contractions.

2 Although these may be removed during a seizure, the client's normal routines should be respected.

4 Increased restlessness may be evidence of the prodromal phase in some individuals, but symptoms vary so widely that the history of the client should be obtained.

642. **4** To achieve the anticonvulsant effect, therapeutic blood levels of phenytoin must be maintained. If the client is not able to take the prescribed oral preparation, the physician should be questioned about alternate routes of administration. (b)

1 The client is kept npo.

2 The route of administration cannot be altered without physician approval.

3 Omission would result in lowered blood levels, possibly below the necessary therapeutic level to prevent a seizure.

643. **2** When an oral medication is available in a suspension form, the nurse should use it for clients with dysphagia. (c)

1 Since a palatable suspension is available, it is a better alternative than opening the capsule.

3 Intramuscular injections should be avoided because of related risks of tissue injury and infection.

4 The route of administration cannot be altered without physician approval.

644. **1** Gingival hyperplasia is a frequently occurring adverse effect of long-term phenytoin (Dilantin) therapy. The incidence can be decreased by meticulous oral hygiene. (c)

2 This is not a direct effect of Dilantin.

3 Alkalinity is not related to Dilantin or to the gingival hyperplasia caused by Dilantin. The incidence can be decreased by meticulous oral hygiene.

4 Plaque and bacterial growth at the gum line is unrelated to Dilantin or to the hyperplasia caused by it. The incidence can be decreased by meticulous oral hygiene.

645. **4** Phenytoin inhibits folic acid absorption and potentiates the effects of folic acid antagonists. Folic acid therapy is often helpful in correcting certain anemias that can result from administration of phenytoin. (*Note:* dosage must be carefully adjusted because folic acid diminishes the effects of phenytoin.) (c)

1 Neurologic side effects include an elevation of the excitability threshold of neurons; not prevented by folic acid.

2 Although folic acid plays a role in the formation of heme in hemoglobin, its prescription in this case is related to Dilantin.

3 The description of this situation does not provide data to arrive at this conclusion.

646. **4** Lesions affecting the seventh cranial (facial) nerve cause paralysis of the eyelids. (c)

1 The optic nerve is concerned with vision; lesions result in visual field defects and loss of visual acuity.

2 The oculomotor nerve is concerned with pupillary constriction and eye movements; lesions result in ptosis, strabismus, and diplopia.

3 The trochlear nerve is concerned with eye movements; lesions result in diplopia, strabismus, and head tilt to the affected side.

647. **2** The third cranial (oculomotor) nerve contains autonomic fibers that innervate the smooth muscle responsible for constriction of the pupils. (c)

1 The optic nerve is concerned with vision; lesions result in visual field defects and loss of visual acuity.

3 The trochlear nerve is concerned with eye movements; lesions result in diplopia, strabismus, and head tilt to the affected side.

4 The facial nerve is concerned with facial expressions; lesions result in loss of taste and paralysis of the facial muscles and the eyelids (lids remain open).

648. **1** The facial nerve (seventh cranial) has motor and sensory functions. The motor function is concerned with facial movement, including smiling and pursing the lips. Nonconduction of either right or left will cause drooping on that side. (c)

2 Nonconduction of the facial nerve on the right side would cause that side of the face to droop.

3 Nonconduction of the left abducent nerve would prevent abduction of the left eye.

4 Nonconduction of the trigeminal nerve would cause problems in mastication.

649. **1** Anterior horn neurons are also known as lower motoneurons. Their cell bodies are located in the anterior gray columns and are part of the reflex arc. (c)

2 Basal ganglia are islands of gray matter in each cerebral hemisphere; not part of the reflex arc.

3 Pyramidal tracts are motor nerve pathways from the brain that pass down the spinal cord to motor cells in the anterior horn; not part of the reflex arc.

4 Upper motoneurons are neurons in the cerebral cortex that conduct impulses to the spinal cord or the motor nuclei of the cerebral nerves.

650. **1** Extrapyramidal or motor pathways assist in maintaining muscle tonus; injury usually involves some spasticity. (c)

2 These are also known as anterior horn neurons; disruption causes flaccid paralysis.

3 These make up sensory tracts.

4 Pyramidal tract disorders result in either spastic or flaccid paralysis; spasticity if upper motor neurons involved, flaccidity if lower.

651. **3** This is the space between the arachnoid and the pia mater. It is filled with cerebrospinal fluid. (b)

1 The cerebral aqueduct, between the third and fourth ventricles, in the midbrain.

2 An opening in the atrial septum in the fetal heart.

4 The innermost of the three meninges covering the brain and spinal cord.

652. **1** Pain and temperature sensations enter the posterior horns of the spinal cord, cross to the contralateral side, and travel upward via the spino-thalamic tracts to the thalamus. There they synapse with other sensory neurons for transmission to the cortex. (c)

   2 The location of the fasciculus gracilis, which is involved with pressure sensation.

   3 Descending motor tracts. The lateral tracts facilitate impulse transmission to the skeletal muscles; the medial tracts inhibit transmission to the skeletal muscles.

   4 Ascending tracts. They conduct impulses of crude touch, pain, and temperature.

653. **2** Parkinson's disease involves destruction of the neurons of the substantia nigra, caudate nucleus, and globus pallidus of the basal ganglia. The cause of this destruction is unknown. (b)

   1 This pathologic condition is associated with multiple sclerosis.

   3 This condition is believed to be associated with myasthenia gravis.

   4 This condition would result in auditory and visual problems; not associated with Parkinson's disease.

654. **3** Destruction of the neurons of the basal ganglia results in decreased muscle tone. The masklike appearance and monotonous speech patterns can be interpreted as flat. (b)

   1 Not associated with Parkinson's disease.

   2 Not associated with Parkinson's disease.

   4 Not associated with Parkinson's disease.

655. **2** Levodopa is the metabolic precursor of dopamine. It reduces sympathetic outflow by limiting vasoconstriction, which may result in orthostatic hypotension. (b)

   1 Should be administered with food to minimize gastric irritation.

   3 Although periodic tests to evaluate hepatic, renal, and cardiovascular therapy are required for prolonged therapy, whether these tests should be done on a weekly basis has not been established.

   4 May produce either symptom, but no established pattern of such responses exists.

656. **1** Levodopa is the precursor of dopamine. It is converted to dopamine in the brain cells, where it is stored until needed by axon terminals; functions as a neurotransmitter. (b)

   2 Not an action of L-dopa; neurons do not regenerate.

   3 Not an action of L-dopa.

   4 Not an action of L-dopa; once myelin is destroyed, it does not usually regenerate.

657. **3** The cerebellum coordinates muscular activity and promotes balance. The other brain regions govern motor, sensory, and higher integrative functions. (a)

   1 Controls the heartbeat, blood pressure, and reflexes such as vomiting and coughing.

   2 Involved in temperature regulation; controls and integrates the autonomic nervous system; intermediary between the nervous and endocrine systems; associated with feelings of rage and aggression.

   4 Controls conscious recognition of pain, temperature, and crude touch and pressure.

658. **2** Rheumatoid spondylitis (Marie-Strümpell disease) is a chronic, progressive polyarthritis. Ossification of cartilage, particularly of the spine, causes fixation of the involved joints. (a)

   1 Redness and swelling are symptoms of local inflammation; do not indicate irreversible damage.

3 Inflammation and thickening of the synovial membrane are characteristic of arthritis.

4 Although rest is essential, complete immobility would result in a loss of joint motion.

659. **1** ROM exercises must be instituted to maintain mobility of joints. However, overuse may prevent resolution of the inflammation. (a)

   2 Pain may persist but cannot be allowed to legitimize inactivity.

   3 Severely damaged joints may require prosthetic replacement.

   4 Activity will not prevent the inflammatory process; may aggravate it.

660. **3** As a result of the normal stresses on the body, the incidence of chronic illness increases in the elderly population. (a)

   1 Younger individuals have greater physiologic reserves.

   2 Younger individuals have greater physiologic reserves.

   4 Younger individuals have greater physiologic reserves.

661. **3** A balanced diet, consisting of the basic four food groups, is essential in maintaining good nutrition. (b)

   1 Limiting the diet to particular foods does not provide all essential nutrients.

   2 Limiting the diet to particular foods does not provide all essential nutrients.

   4 If nutritional intake is adequate, multivitamins are unnecessary.

662. **2** Osteoarthritis affects the hips and knees first because they are the weight-bearing joints and undergo the most stress. (b)

   1 Although the distal interphalangeal joints are frequently affected, the remaining interphalangeal joints and metacarpals are not.

   3 Although these are weight-bearing joints, normal motion is not as great as in the hips and knees; thus there is less degeneration.

   4 These are not weight-bearing joints.

663. **1** The Stryker frame provides for horizontal changes of position to prone or supine while maintaining proper body alignment. (a)

   2 Although the frame itself does not directly promote body functions or prevent deformities, it does enable the nurse to turn the client, which helps prevent complications of immobility.

   3 Vertical turning is not possible with a Stryker frame.

   4 Does not prevent deformities; only provides for horizontal turning.

664. **3** The main nursing principles in turning a client on the Stryker frame are the maintenance of alignment and safety. Securing all bolts and straps ensures that the client is snug yet comfortably wedged between the frames. (b)

   1 Many clients who require special beds such as the Stryker frame or an electric circular bed are not able to use their arms.

   2 Since the client is being turned horizontally, hypotension is not a major problem.

   4 The procedure does not require two nurses unless such a protocol is established by the institution.

665. **2** Progressive client care is based on the precept that different levels of client needs require different services and facilities. The care provided is specialized and individualized to meet the client's needs in an appropriate, continuous, and dynamic pattern. (b)

   1 This explanation does not focus on the changing needs of the client, which is inherent in progressive client care.

3 It is only part of answer; does not recognize specialized needs; change does not always mean less intensive care.

4 Progressive care makes use of these; but they are only part of what is involved in progressive care, which adapts itself to specialized and changing needs of the individual.

666. **4** During prolonged inactivity bone reabsorption proceeds faster than bone formation, and lack of therapeutic weight bearing on bone results in disuse atrophy. A tilt table provides gradual progressive weight-bearing, which counters these effects. (c)

1 Lateral turning is possible and necessary if a client is immobile, but a tilt table does not make this possible.

2 The tilt table is used for scheduled periods in physical therapy; the nursing care required to prevent decubiti must be consistently performed frequently throughout all shifts.

3 The tilt table does not cause hyperextension of the spine; the spine remains in normal body alignment.

667. **1** Clients with quadriplegia do not have and never will have the muscle innervation, strength, or balance needed for ambulation. (b)

2 Orthostatic hypotension can be prevented by any upright positioning and does not necessarily require a wheelchair.

3 Quadriplegia refers to paralysis of all four extremities.

4 Bracing and crutch walking require muscle strength and coordination that a quadriplegic individual does not have.

668. **3** Clients with aphasia must be encouraged to speak so that communication ability is regained. (b)

1 Despite difficulty speaking, individuals with expressive aphasia can understand what is said to them.

2 To avoid frustration, needs should be anticipated.

4 Speech can usually be improved through therapy.

669. **2** A client who is comatose loses voluntary control of elimination. (a)

1 Since there are different levels of coma, the individual may respond to intense stimuli such as pain.

3 Since cerebral functioning is depressed, purposeful or voluntary movement is absent.

4 Twitching motions may be evidence of abnormal cerebral electrical activity; such seizure-like activity is present often in comatose individuals.

670. **1** Absence of a gag reflex is common after a CVA. To prevent aspiration, the client is positioned on the side to allow gravity to drain mucus in the nasopharyngeal area away from the trachea. (b)

2 Chest expansion is hindered in the prone position.

3 This position allows the tongue to occlude the airway and encourages the aspiration of secretions if the gag reflex is not intact.

4 This position allows the tongue to occlude the airway and encourages the aspiration of secretions if the gag reflex is not intact.

671. **2** Passive ROM exercises prevent the development of deformities and yet do not require any energy expenditure by the client who is confined to bed. Instituting ROM exercises is an independent nursing function. (b)

1 Bed rest is prescribed to decrease oxygen demands; active exercises markedly increase oxygen consumption.

3 Bed rest is prescribed to decrease oxygen demands; active exercises markedly increase oxygen consumption.

4 Bed rest is prescribed to decrease oxygen demands; active exercises markedly increase oxygen consumption.

672. **3** Changes in self-image and family role can initiate a grieving process with a variety of emotional responses. (a)

1 This cannot be assumed from the situation described unless the client's feelings are elicited.

2 The ability to cope successfully with an illness varies widely between individuals.

4 This cannot be assumed from the situation described unless the client's feelings are elicited.

673. **4** To foster communication and cooperation, family members should be involved in planning and implementing care. (a)

1 This intervention does not focus on the client's feelings or needs.

2 This intervention does not focus on the client's feelings or needs.

3 The nurse remains responsible; the client may promote dependency of her husband to satisfy her own needs.

674. **2** The brachial plexus is a maze of nerves extending from the axilla to the neck in the shoulder area; trauma to the arm may also injure this plexus. (a)

1 The basilar plexus is a venous plexus over the basilar part of the occipital bone; unrelated to the arms.

3 The celiac plexus (solar plexus) is where the splanchnic nerves terminate; unrelated to the arms.

4 The solar plexus, also known as the celiac plexus, is where the splanchnic nerves terminate; unrelated to the arms.

675. **1** The medulla contains the vital respiratory, cardiac, and vasomotor centers. (a)

2 The midbrain deals with sensory input from the eyes and ears.

3 Conducts impulses; reflex centers for cranial nerves V, VI, VII, VIII (trigeminal, abducent, facial, vestibulocochlear).

4 Relays sensory impulses to cerebral cortex.

676. **1** The hypothalamus connects with the autonomic area for vasoconstriction, vasodilation, and perspiration and with the somatic centers for shivering; therefore it is an important area for regulating body temperature. (a)

2 The pallidum is part of the basal ganglia; also called the globus pallidus. Together with the putamen, it compresses the lenticular nucleus; concerned with muscle tone, which is required for specific body movements.

3 The temporal lobe is concerned with auditory stimuli; may also be involved with the sense of smell.

4 Receives all sensory stimuli, except taste, for transmission to the cerebral cortex; also involved with emotions and instinctive activities.

677. **2** The eighth cranial nerve has two parts—the vestibular nerve and the cochlear nerve. Sensations of hearing are conducted by the cochlear nerve. (a)

1 Cranial nerve VI (abducent) is concerned with abduction of the eye.

3 The frontal lobe is concerned with thinking, skeletal muscle tone, and biorhythms.

4 The occipital lobe is concerned with sight, particularly shape and color.

678. **2** The primary site of action is the motor cortex, where seizure activity is limited by maintaining the sodium ion gradient of the neurons. (b)

1 This incorrectly describes the pharmacologic action of Dilantin.

3 This incorrectly describes the pharmacologic action of Dilantin.

4 This incorrectly describes the pharmacologic action of Dilantin.

679. **4** The respiratory tract can be obstructed during a seizure, and therefore a plastic airway should be available at all times for clients with convulsive disorders. (b)
 1 Taking a blood pressure reading will not protect the client; maintaining a patent airway is a priority.
 2 Oxygen does not prevent seizures, nor would it be used during a seizure because the individual does not breathe; if an airway is maintained, room air is usually sufficient after a seizure.
 3 A tongue blade is no longer considered appropriate because of the danger of airway occlusion when the blade is forced into place.
680. **3** Seizure disorders are usually associated with marked changes in the electrical activity of the cerebral cortex, requiring prolonged or life-long therapy. (b)
 1 Absence of seizures would probably be due to medication effectiveness rather than to correction of the pathophysiologic condition.
 2 A therapeutic blood level must be maintained through consistent administration of drug.
 4 Seizures may occur despite drug therapy; the dosage may need to be adjusted.
681. **3** The precentral gyrus is the most posterior convolution of the frontal lobe and the primary motor area. Other gyri also contain motor neurons. (c)
 1 The basal ganglia are islands of gray matter within the cerebral hemispheres; one activity with which they are concerned is muscle tone, required for specific body movement.
 2 The parietal lobes translate nerve impulses into sensations such as taste, touch, and temperature.
 4 The postcentral gyrus is the primary sensory area of the cerebral cortex; unrelated to motor activity.
682. **3** There are no dietary restrictions, but iron and vitamins should be encouraged to normalize any underlying nutritional deficiencies. (b)
 1 A normal protein intake should fulfill nutritional needs.
 2 Sodium retention is not a major complication, so a salt-free diet is not indicated.
 4 Bland diets are usually prescribed for clients with gastric disturbances.
683. **2** Because of its antiinflammatory effect, aspirin is useful in treating arthritis symptoms. (a)
 1 Narcotics should be avoided because they promote dependency and do not affect the inflammatory process.
 3 Narcotics should be avoided because they promote dependency and do not affect the inflammatory process.
 4 Pentobarbital sodium (Nembutal) is a hypnotic not an analgesic; normal adult dosage is 100 to 200 mg po hs.
684. **3** Exercise of involved joints is important to maintain optimal mobility and prevent buildup of calcium deposits. (c)
 1 Immobilization causes loss of joint mobility and contractures.
 2 Immobilization causes loss of joint mobility and contractures.
 4 Immobilization causes loss of joint mobility and contractures.
685. **2** Steroids have an antiinflammatory effect, which can reduce arthritic pannus formation. (c)
 1 Ankylosis refers to fusion of joints. It is only indirectly influenced by steroids, which exert their major effect on the inflammatory process.
 3 Not a use for the drug; steroids can cause mood swings.
 4 The relief of pain is incorporated into the antiinflammatory actions of steroids.

686. **3** Sneezing, as well as lifting and straining, causes an increase in the intraspinal pressure, resulting in pain. (c)
 1 Does not affect the intraspinal pressure.
 2 Maximizes the intervertebral spaces, relieving pressure and pain.
 4 Although pain may increase as a result of compression of the vertebrae, the increase is gradual, not sudden.
687. **4** Compresses are not required after a spinal puncture. (c)
 1 Careful assessment is required to detect possible injury to the spinal cord.
 2 To prevent severe headache, which may accompany the procedure, the head of the bed is not elevated and fluids are encouraged.
 3 To prevent severe headache, which may accompany the procedure, the head of the bed is not elevated and fluids are encouraged.
688. **3** Ambulation may be postponed for several days. The use of back braces or body casts varies. (b)
 1 The bed is generally kept flat; prevents strain on the operative site.
 2 The client is log rolled from side to side; will prevent complications of immobility while vertebral alignment is maintained.
 4 To detect damage or compression of the spinal cord, assessment of motor and sensory status is necessary.
689. **3** A laminectomy that involves the removal of portions of one or more vertebrae is generally done in conjunction with removal of a herniated disc. Inflammation from the trauma of surgery could lead to compression of the spinal cord, with consequent motor or sensory dysfunction. (b)
 1 Urinary retention rather than spasticity may occur if pressure on the cord occurs as a result of edema or bleeding.
 2 Pain is usually experienced at the operative site and in the legs as a result of edema around the cord.
 4 Cerebral edema does not occur.
690. **2** Sore throat and oral secretions are additional problems of the client after cervical laminectomy. (c)
 1 Limited range of motion occurs after both operations.
 3 To prevent strain on the operative site, flexion of the head is avoided.
 4 The head of the bed may be only slightly elevated after a cervical laminectomy.
691. **2** Decubiti easily develop when a particular position is maintained; the body weight, directed continuously in one region, restricts circulation and results in tissue necrosis. (a)
 1 Clients often state that they are comfortable and wish to remain in one position.
 3 Since turning is usually done laterally, the circulation to the lower extremities is not dramatically affected.
 4 Proper positioning with supportive devices and ROM are more effective measures to prevent contractures.
692. **4** The paraplegic client is unable to exercise actively. (c)
 1 Changing a position involves moving the extremities. Contractures develop as a result of prolonged immobility.
 2 The use of pillows, splints, and other supportive devices helps maintain alignment and prevent the shortening of muscle fibers associated with contractures.
 3 Passive ROM helps maintain joint mobility and muscle tone.
693. **3** Calcium leaves the long bones during periods of prolonged bed rest. The tilt table places the client in an upright position, which provides for weight bearing. (b)

1 The tilt table is used to prevent orthostatic hypotension by gradually allowing an individual who has been immobilized to adjust to an upright position.

2 Although the pressure on bony prominences is altered, the use of the tilt table is not frequent enough to prevent the development of decubiti.

4 The client is carefully strapped to the table so that mobility is actually impaired to ensure safety.

694. **4** Calcium that has left the bones as a response to prolonged inactivity enters the blood and may precipitate in the kidneys, forming calculi. (b)

1 Increased fluid intake is helpful in avoiding this condition by preventing urinary stasis.

2 Calcium intake is usually limited to prevent the increasing risk of calculi.

3 Calculi may develop despite adequate kidney function; kidney function may be impaired by the presence of calculi and the high incidence of urinary tract infections associated with urinary stasis or repeated catheterizations.

695. **1** To promote optimism and facilitate smooth functioning, all rehabilitation should begin on admission to the hospital. (a)

2 Since paralysis is permanent, alterations in normal lifestyle are required.

3 The client and family are often unaware of options available in the health care system; the nurse should be available to provide necessary information and support.

4 Since the paralysis is permanent, rehabilitation plans should be made.

696. **4** Because of the location of the micturition reflex center (in the sacral region of the spinal cord), bladder function may be impaired with lower spinal cord injuries. (b)

1 Since there is no voluntary control over the lower extremities mobility is usually accomplished through the use of a wheelchair rather than ambulation.

2 Plans for education are usually postponed until the client has had a chance to deal with his feelings; high anxiety interferes with learning.

3 These exercises require motor control, which the client does not have.

697. **1** Correct positioning prevents the client from assuming incorrect positions, which could result in contracture formation. (a)

2 The tilt board is used primarily to prevent orthostatic hypotension or bone demineralization.

3 Since he is paralyzed, active exercises are not possible.

4 Deep massage may dislodge thrombi that have formed as a result of venous stasis.

698. **1** The acetabulum is the socket in the pelvis with which the head of the femur articulates. (b)

2 Does not articulate with the acetabulum; long bone of the femur (longest and strongest bone in the body).

3 No articulation with the acetabulum; part of bone between the head and shaft; commonly fractured in the elderly.

4 The greater and lesser trochanters bulge at the proximal end of the femur shaft; serve as attachment points for some buttock and thigh muscles.

699. **2** Nails, pins, plates, and screws maintain bone alignment while bone replacement (healing) occurs. (a)

1 A prosthesis can be used if an intracapsular fracture cannot be reduced satisfactorily with the use of pins or nails; internal fixation is used instead of traction, which would require prolonged immobilization.

3 A hip spica cast requires prolonged immobilization and increases the risk of complications associated with immobility.

4 Skeletal traction requires prolonged immobilization and increases the risk of complications associated with immobility.

700. **3** Turning and periodic deep breathing promote drainage of and circulation in the lung alveoli, which helps prevent circulatory and pulmonary complications. To prevent strain and possible misalignment or pressure at the fracture site, clients should not be turned onto the affected side. (b)

1 The client must be turned at least every 2 hours to help prevent the complication of immobility; 5 hours is too long to keep a client in one position.

2 The client is generally not allowed out of bed until at least 1 day postoperative, and then weight bearing is not permitted on the affected extremity.

4 The client is generally not allowed out of bed until 1 to 3 days postoperative.

701. **1** Pressure on the operative site may cause unnecessary pain and impair circulation necessary for healing. (c)

2 Supine or on the unaffected side is the position of choice; however, a wedge, thigh spreader, or pillows must be used to maintain abduction of the affected thigh; adduction can result in displacement of the prosthesis.

3 This is acceptable since there is no stress placed on the operative site.

4 This is acceptable since there is no stress placed on the operative site.

702. **3** Prune juice and warm water can be administered prophylactically by the nurse to promote defecation. Prune juice irritates the bowel mucosa, stimulating peristalsis. Increased fiber in the diet may also improve intestinal motility. (b)

1 Routine use of enemas should be avoided because they promote dependency and can result in electrolyte imbalance.

2 Routine use of enemas should be avoided because they promote dependency and can result in electrolyte imbalance.

4 Routine use of laxatives promotes dependency.

703. **2** Bones become more fragile with advancing age because of osteoporosis, often associated with lower circulating levels of estrogens or testosterone. (a)

1 Carelessness is a characteristic applicable to certain individuals rather than to a developmental level.

3 Rheumatoid diseases certainly can affect the skeletal system but do not increase the incidence of hip fractures.

4 Although prolonged immobility is associated with bone demineralization, hip fractures occur in elderly individuals who are active.

704. **3** Flexion contracture of the hip can be prevented by routinely placing the client in a prone position to extend the hip. (b)

1 This can cause flexion of the hip, which will result in a hip contracture and affect balance.

2 Lying in the supine position does not allow for full extension of the hip.

4 This can cause flexion of the hip, which will result in a hip contracture and affect balance.

705. **1** This position offsets the development of hip deformities due to contractures. It also maintains the correct center of gravity when the client is upright. (b)

2 Promotes flexion contracture of the hip.

3 May alter the center of gravity and cause a loss of balance.

4 A prosthesis may be applied early in the postoperative period but requires a rigid dressing (cast) to prevent edema; ambulation can be facilitated by the use of a walker, crutches, parallel bars, or cane.

706. **2** Preparing muscles that will do the work in crutch walking is imperative. (b)
  1 The biceps are not the major muscles required for crutch walking.
  3 Strengthening the hamstring muscles will not assist in the use of crutches.
  4 The condition of the limb will not have a great influence on the ability to use crutches.

707. **2** A four-point gait provides for weight bearing on all four extremities and maximum support during ambulation. (b)
  1 A three-point gait is used when one extremity cannot bear weight.
  3 A three-point gait is used when one extremity cannot bear weight.
  4 A swing-through gait does not simulate ambulation; it is used when the individual can bear weight but lacks the muscular control needed for ambulation without an assistive device.

708. **2** Practicing ambulation without proper preparation of ambulation techniques and strengthening the involved muscle groups would not be helpful in the rehabilitation process and could exhaust the client. (a)
  1 Prior to ambulation the individual must be able to maintain balance.
  3 The muscles used for crutch walking are different from those used in normal ambulation; therefore they must be strengthened by active exercises prior to ambulation.
  4 Since different muscle groups are utilized, the client must be instructed even about what seems to be simple maneuvers; transfer from a sitting to a standing position must be accomplished before ambulation.

709. **1** Rehabilitation should begin on admission; this includes preoperative discussion of the nature of the operation and rehabilitation techniques. (b)
  2 Too late; valuable time to rehabilitate is not utilized.
  3 Too late; valuable time to rehabilitate is not utilized.
  4 Too late; valuable time to rehabilitate is not utilized.

710. **3** A cataract is a clouding of the crystalline lens or its capsule. (b)
  1 Not included in the pathophysiology related to cataracts.
  2 Not included in the pathophysiology related to cataracts.
  4 Not included in the pathophysiology related to cataracts.

711. **2** Activities such as rigorous brushing of hair and teeth cause increased intraocular pressure and may lead to hemorrhage in the anterior chamber. (b)
  1 Coughing and deep breathing can increase intraocular pressure.
  3 The client is generally permitted out of bed as soon as the effects of anesthesia have worn off.
  4 Weakening of the eye musculature is not related to cataracts.

712. **2** Retinal detachment is a separation between the sensory retina and the retinal pigment epithelium. These layers are not attached by any special structures and can separate as a result of various pathologic processes. (c)
  1 The statement does not explain the disease process involved.

3 The statement does not explain the disease process involved.
  4 The statement does not explain the disease process involved.

713. **1** Scar formation seals the hole and promotes attachment of the two retinal surfaces. (c)
  2 This is not the treatment used; treatment is formation of a scar by the use of lasers or surgical "buckling."
  3 The retina is part of the nervous system; does not regenerate or grow new cells.
  4 The sclera is not involved; the retina adjoins and is nourished by the choroid.

714. **2** Although sympathetic impulses usually control most visceral effectors in times of stress, parasympathetic fibers likewise stimulate increased gastric contractions and increased peristalsis. Sympathetic fibers also inhibit organs such as the bladder and cause relaxation of this organ. (c)
  1 This statement is accurate.
  3 This statement is accurate.
  4 This statement is accurate.

715. **2** The sympathetic nervous system constricts the smooth muscle of blood vessels in the skin when a person is under stress. (a)
  1 Not under sympathetic control; the parasympathetic system constricts the pupils.
  3 The sympathetic system stimulates rather than inhibits secretion by the sweat glands.
  4 The parasympathetic system (vagus nerve) slows the pulse, and the sympathetic increases it.

716. **2** Parasympathetic nerves increase peristalsis and secretion of gastric hydrochloric acid. (b)
  1 Epinephrine is sympathomimetic.
  3 The parasympathetic nervous system increases intestinal motility, which would result in diarrhea.
  4 Goosebumps, caused by contraction of the musculi arrectores pilorum, are under sympathetic control; vasoconstriction is also under sympathetic control.

717. **4** The woman is unconscious. Although her husband can consent, he has no legal power to refuse a treatment for her unless he was previously given power of attorney; the court can make a decision for her. (b)
  1 This alternative does not have a legal basis, and the nurse could be held liable.
  2 This alternative does not have a legal basis, and the nurse could be held liable.
  3 This alternative does not have a legal basis, and the nurse could be held liable.

718. **3** Sensory impulses from temperature, touch, and pain travel via the spinothalamic pathway to the thalamus and then to the postcentral gyrus of the parietal lobe, the somatosensory area. (a)
  1 Area of abstract thinking and muscular movements.
  2 Area where nerve impulses are translated into sight.
  4 Area where nerve impulses are translated into sound.

719. **4** The thalamus receives sensory impulses from the spinothalamic tract and relays them to the cerebral cortex. (c)
  1 Conducts impulses between the cord and brain.
  2 Relays between the cortex and autonomic centers.
  3 Involved in motor activity and coordination.

720. **3** The autonomic nervous system functions to regulate visceral effectors and maintain internal equilibrium. (b)
  1 Conveys information from peripheral receptors to the central nervous system and information from the CNS to muscles and glands.
  2 Concerned with overall control; consists of the brain and spinal cord.

4 Transmits impulses from the periphery to the brain and from the brain to the periphery; also integrates reflexes.

721. **2** Since their mental status prevents total awareness of reality, confused or delirious clients may protect themselves by assimilating small amounts of information at a time. (b)

   1 Confusion or delirium is not synonymous with brain destruction.

   3 A client may be aware of surroundings; but perception may be inaccurate.

   4 Although this statement is true, teaching principles must be altered when dealing with a confused client who can not handle the complex.

722. **4** Prolonged immobility results in bone demineralization becuase there is decreased bone production by osteoblasts and increased resorption by osteoclasts. (c)

   1 Estrogen helps prevent bone demineralization.

   2 Decreased calcium intake or absorption may precipitate osteoporosis.

   3 Hypoparathyroidism causes a low serum calcium, decreasing calcium resorption from bones.

723. **2** Pathologic fractures occur as a result of minimal injury to an already weakened bone; osteoporosis causes this weakening. (b)

   1 Fatigue fractures occur when muscles are so fatigued that they no longer act as shock absorbers to protect the bone, a condition not related to osteoporosis.

   3 Compound fractures refer to the protrusion of the bone fragments through the skin, not related to osteoporosis.

   4 Greenstick fractures occur in soft bones, usually just in children.

724. **3** Turnip greens are high in calcium, but not in phosphorus. (c)

   1 High in phosphorus, may interfere with calcium absorption from GI tract.

   2 High levels of nitrogen from protein breakdown may increase calcium resorption from bone to serve as a buffer of the nitrogen.

   4 High in phosphorus; may interfere with calcium absorption from GI tract.

725. **2** Weakened muscles result in ineffective coughing; secretions are retained and provide a medium for bacterial growth. (b)

   1 Airways are not narrowed.

   3 Immune mechanisms are not directly impaired.

   4 Viscosity of secretions depends on fluid intake and humidity.

726. **3** A tracheostomy set may be necessary to establish an emergency airway in case of respiratory crisis. (b)

   1 An IV may or may not be started; does not represent the critical nature of airway obstruction.

   2 Tensilon effects are brief; used primarily for diagnostic purposes.

   4 Not indicated; client is not febrile.

727. **4** Tensilon, an anticholinesterase drug, causes temporary relief of symptoms of myasthenia gravis in clients who have the disease and is therefore an effective diagnostic aid. (b)

   1 There is a decrease in symptoms.

   2 Excessive salivation may occur.

   3 Hypotension may occur.

728. **2** Only axon terminals secrete acetylcholine, so nerve impulse propagation occurs in one direction only: from axon terminal to dendrite or cell body of the next neuron, or from axon terminal to effector organ (muscle or gland). The action of cholinesterase (to inactivate acetylcholine) has physiologic meaning only at the synapse, where acetylcholine is active; its presence all along the axon would not affect the direction of the nerve impulse. (b)

   1 Does not affect direction; polarization refers to the resting potential of the neuron when one side of the membrane is negatively and the other side positively charged.

   3 Does not affect the duration of the impulse; refers to the active movement of sodium ions into the cell and back across the membrane to the opposite side.

   4 Cholinesterase acts only at the synapse, inactivating acetylcholine at the myoneural junction.

729. **1** Axon terminals release acetylcholine at the myoneural junctions. As acetylcholine contacts the sarcolemma, it stimulates the muscle fiber to contract. (a)

   2 ATP is not produced by axons; it is a nucleotide that gives off energy when it loses a phosphate radical.

   3 Cholinesterase is released by muscle cells.

   4 Epinephrine is produced by the adrenal medulla and released by axons of the autonomic nervous system.

730. **2** Neostigmine, an anticholinesterase, inhibits the breakdown of acetylcholine, thus prolonging neurotransmission. (c)

   1 Action is at myoneural junction, not cortex.

   3 Prevents neurotransmitter breakdown but is not a neurotransmitter.

   4 Action is at myoneural junction, not sheath.

731. **4** Tensilon improves muscle strength in myasthenic crisis; weakness persists if symptoms are due to cholinergic crisis, which can result from toxic levels of neostigmine. (c)

   1 The diagnosis has already been established and treatment initiated.

   2 Same type of drug as neostigmine; no resistance indicated.

   3 Is not used for synergistic effect; duration of effect is brief.

732. **2** Allopurinol interferes with the final steps in uric acid formation by inhibiting the production of xanthinoxidase. (a)

   1 This drug acts to prevent the formation of uric acid.

   3 This drug acts to prevent the formation of uric acid.

   4 Allopurinol has no effect on swelling of the synovial membranes.

733. **2** Colchicine decreases the formation of lactic acid, which may promote the deposition of uric acid in the joints. It also decreases the inflammatory response. (b)

   1 Hydrocortisone is an antiinflammatory; not used to treat gout.

   3 Butazolidin (phenylbutazone) is a nonsteroid antiinflammatory agent.

   4 Benemid (probenecid) acts to inhibit the reabsorption of urate in the kidneys and, therefore, decreases uric acid in the blood; not useful in the treatment of acute gout but rather of chronic gout.

734. **1** Laminar air flow decreases the risk of bone infection, since potentially contaminated air continuously flows away from the sterile field, decreasing the concentration of airborne pathogens. (c)

   2 The procedure is performed at one time.

   3 The lithotomy position is used for gynecologic procedures; the side-lying position is generally used for hip surgery.

   4 Surgery is generally considered when destruction of the femoral head and acetabulum is extensive.

735. **4** Warm compresses (at or slightly above body temperature) dilate blood vessels, increasing blood flow to the area and decreasing edema. (c)

1 This temperature is too cool to increase blood flow to the area.

2 This temperature is too cool to increase blood flow to the area.

3 This temperature is too cool to increase blood flow to the area.

736. **4** Marie-Strümpell disease is synonymous with rheumatoid spondylitis, which involves fixation of joints (usually vertebral). (c)

1 As the cartilage of the joints degenerates, there are hypertrophic changes of the bone edges, which eventually replace the articular cartilage.

2 Ankylosis occurs in rheumatoid arthritis, not in hypertrophic or degenerative arthritis.

3 Heberden nodules are the bony or cartilaginous enlargements of the distal interphalangeal joints that are associated with degenerative arthritis.

737. **2** Synovial fluid minimizes friction at joints by providing lubrication for the moving parts. (b)

1 Synovial fluid increases the speed of movements.

3 Synovial fluid increases the efficiency of joint movements.

4 Synovial fluid increases work output.

738. **3** The client has a right to know what medication she is receiving (informed consent). This also constitutes an invasion of the client's rights. (b)

1 The client has a right to refuse treatment and a right for an explanation of treatment prior to its administration; that client's right takes precedence over the physician's order.

2 This cannot be determined from the situation described; the client should have been questioned about her reasons for refusing the drug to determine her level of understanding.

4 The physician should have been notified only after the nurse had interviewed the client to determine the reasons for her decision; this would have been the time to impart the appropriate information.

739. **2** Synovial joints, like the knee, shoulder, or articulations between the middle ear bones, are lined with synovial membrane. (a)

1 Serous membrane does not line joints but rather areas such as the thoracic and abdominal cavities.

3 Mucous membrane lines passages that open to the exterior of the body such as the mouth and the genitourinary tract.

4 Epithelium covers the internal and external organs of the body, including the skin.

740. **4** The greater density of compact bone makes it stronger than cancellous bone. Compact bone forms from cancellous bone by the addition of concentric rings of bone substance to the marrow spaces of cancellous bone; the large marrow spaces are reduced to haversian canals. (a)

1 Not related to strength.

2 Overall size does not determine strength.

3 Weight alone is not a factor.

741. **2** The ache in muscles that have been vigorously worked without adequate oxygen supply is caused in part by the buildup of lactic acid. During rest the lactic acid is oxidized completely to carbon dioxide and water, providing ATP for further muscular contraction. (a)

1 Butyric acid is not a product of muscle contraction; it is a fatty acid occurring in feces, urine, and perspiration.

3 Acetoacetic acid is not a product of muscle contraction; it is a ketone body resulting from incomplete oxidation of fatty acids. It is also produced by the metabolism of lipids and pyruvates.

4 Acetone is not a product of muscle contraction; it is a ketone body and a by-product of acetoacetic acid metabolism.

742. **4** Electrodes are attached to sensory nerves or over the dorsal column; a transmitter is worn externally and, by electric stimulation, may be used to interfere with the transmission of painful stimuli as needed. (c)

1 Clients may bathe when the transmitter is disconnected.

2 The device should not interfere with a remote control apparatus.

3 The client may need analgesics in conjunction with the transmitter.

743. **3** A rhizotomy is the resection of posterior nerve roots to eliminate nerve impulses associated with severe pain from the thoracic area (as in lung cancer). (c)

1 A chondrectomy is the surgical excision of a cartilage.

2 A cordotomy is the surgical interruption of pain-conducting pathways in the spinal cord.

4 This is a fictitious procedure.

744. **1** Vitamin A is used in the formation of retinene, a component of the light-sensitive rhodopsin molecule. (a)

2 Vitamin A does not influence color vision, which is centered in the cones.

3 The cornea is a transparent part of the anterior portion of the sclera; a cataract is an opacity of the normally transparent crystalline lens. Vitamin A does not prevent cataracts.

4 Melanin is a pigment of the skin.

745. **2** Deep green and yellow vegetables contain large quantities of the pigments α-, β-, and γ-carotene; β-carotene is the major chemical precursor of vitamin A in human nutrition. (a)

1 Levels of vitamin A are higher in whole milk than in skim milk.

3 Oranges are considered a good source of both vitamin C and potassium.

4 Tomatoes are a good source of vitamin C.

746. **4** Malignant melanoma of the eye is an intraocular tumor that metastasizes rapidly; therefore enucleation—removal of the eye—is the treatment of choice. (c)

1 Only palliative at best.

2 Only palliative at best.

3 Only palliative at best.

747. **3** The optic chiasm is the point of crossover of some optic nerve fibers in the cranial cavity at the base of the brain. The optic tracts conduct nerve impulses from the optic chiasm to other brain regions. (b)

1 Optic tracts conduct nerve impulses from the optic chiasm.

2 This is the vitreous body.

4 The orbit is the cavity in which the eyeball is fixed.

748. **3** Vagal stimulation slows the heart. The vagus is the principal nerve of the parasympathetic portion of the autonomic nervous system, and its axon terminals release acetylcholine. The response of the viscera to acetylcholine varies, but in general the organ is in a relaxed state. (c)

1 Function of the sympathetic nervous system (accelerator nerve); release of norepinephrine.

2 Stimulation of the sympathetic nervous system dilates bronchioles in the lungs; the vagus constricts them.

4 No parasympathomimetic fibers to the coronary blood vessels; sympathetic impulses dilate these vessels.

749. **4** The thalamus associates sensory impulses with feelings of pleasantness and unpleasantness; therefore it is partly responsible for emotions. The cortical limbic system is also involved in expression of emotions. (c)

1 Located in the cerebrum; controls all conscious functions.

2 Outer layer of the cerebrum; controls mental functions.

3 Controls body temperature and serves as a neural pathway.

750. **3** The arteries communicating (anastomosing) at the base of the brain are referred to as the circle of Willis. (b)

   1 Anastomosis of blood vessels located in the palm of the hand.

   2 A single large branch of the aorta.

   4 Nerve communication network in the region of the neck and axilla.

751. **3** Gliomas account for about 45% of all brain tumors. (c)

   1 An adenoma is a tumor involving glandular tissue; may occur in the pituitary.

   2 Neurofibroma is a tumor of nerve tissue but is more common in the peripheral nervous system.

   4 Meningioma, which occurs in the meninges of the brain, accounts for about 20% of all brain tumors.

752. **1** Dendrites of the cochlear nerve terminate on the hair cells of the organ of Corti in the cochlea. (a)

   2 Contains bones (malleus, incus, stapes).

   3 Part of the middle ear that contains the auditory ossicles; area between the tympanic membrane and the bony labyrinth.

   4 A membranous sac that communicates with the semicircular canals of the ear.

753. **3** The ear bones that transmit and amplify air pressure waves from the tympanic membrane to the oval window of the cochlea, which is in the inner ear. The tympanic membrane separates the outer from the middle ear. (b)

   1 Consists of the pinna and outer ear canal.

   2 The organ of Corti, chochlea, and semicircular canals are found in the inner ear.

   4 Connects the middle ear and nasopharynx; helps maintain the balance of air pressure.

754. **1** Since the organ of hearing is the organ of Corti, located in the cochlea, nerve deafness would most likely accompany damage to the cochlear nerve. (b)

   2 The vestibular nerve would affect balance.

   3 The trigeminal nerve would affect chewing movements.

   4 The vagus nerve would affect voice production.

755. **4** The medulla, part of the brainstem just above the foramen magnum, is concerned with vital functions. (b)

   1 Sexual development controlled by the hypothalamus (through releasing hormones) and the pituitary at puberty.

   2 Temperature and water balance are controlled by the hypothalamus.

   3 Voluntary movements are mediated through the somatomotor area of the frontal cerebral lobe. The opercular-insular area of the parietal cerebral lobe is concerned with taste sensations. (a)

756. **1** One of the centers for reflex control of respiration is in the medulla. Another important reflex respiratory center is in the pons. The other brain regions—cerebral cortex, hypothalamus, and cerebellum—may influence respiration but not so directly as the centers in the medulla and pons. (a)

   2 Center of control for all conscious functions.

   3 Control and integration of higher autonomic functions; influences respiration but not so directly as the centers in the medulla and pons.

   4 Center for coordination and equilibrium.

757. **2** The labyrinth is the inner ear and consists of the vestibule, cochlea, semicircular canals, utricle, saccule, cochlear duct, and membranous semicircular canals. A labyrinthectomy is performed to alleviate the symptom of vertigo but results in deafness, since the organ of Corti and cochlear nerve are located in the inner ear. (b)

   1 There is no pain associated with Ménière's syndrome.

   3 Anosmia is loss of the sense of smell and would not be affected by surgery to the ear.

   4 Ménière's syndrome does not produce tinnitus.

758. **4** In otosclerosis there is an overgrowth of bone in the middle ear, fusing the three ossicles. Removal of the stapes eliminates this obstruction. (b)

   1 All tones are diminished or lost in otosclerosis, not just the base tones.

   2 Bone conduction is better than air conduction in otosclerosis.

   3 Since the ossicles can no longer vibrate and conduction is impaired, hearing aids are of little value.

759. **4** A subjective symptom such as ringing in the ears can be felt only by the client. (b)

   1 The term is not generally used to describe a symptom; a functional disease is one in which there is alteration in function without physiologic changes.

   2 Prodromal refers to symptoms that are early indications of a developing disease; there is insufficient information to decide this from the situation described.

   3 An objective symptom refers to signs that can be assessed through direct physical examination.

760. **2** An autograft is one taken from an uninjured area of the same person's body. (b)

   1 A homograft is skin taken from the same species.

   3 A heterograft or xenograft is skin taken from a different species.

   4 An allograft is skin taken from the same species.

761. **3** A heterograft or xenograft involves the grafting of tissues from a different species. (b)

   1 A homograft is skin taken from the same species.

   2 An allograft is skin taken from the same species.

   4 This type of graft does not exist.

762. **3** An increased hematocrit level indicates hemoconcentration secondary to fluid loss. (b)

   1 The pH levels reflect acid-base balance.

   2 The sedimentation rate is not used as an indicator of fluid loss; indicates the presence of an inflammatory process.

   4 May be used to indicate dehydration from burns, but interpretation can be complicated by other conditions accompanying burns that also cause elevation of the BUN.

763. **1** As the amount of tissue involved increases, there is greater extravasation of fluid into the tissues. Thus the relationship of fluid loss to body surface is directly proportional. Several formulas (e.g., the Evans, the Baxter, the Brooke Army Hospital) are used to estimate fluid loss based on percent of body surface burned. (b)

   2 Incorrect; relationship is proportional.

   3 Incorrect; relationship is proportional.

   4 Incorrect; relationship is proportional.

764. **3** *Clostridium tetani* can develop in wounds in which there is dead tissue. (b)

   1 Indicated for hypoprothrombinemia caused by deficiency of vitamin K; not related to burns.

   2 Although provides passive immunity against certain infectious agents, not specifically indicated in the treatment of burns.

4 Adrenergic drug used in the treatment of broncho-spasm and heart block.

765. **3** Mafenide (Sulfamylon) interferes with the kidneys' role in hydrogen ion excretion, resulting in metabolic acidosis. (c)
   1 Not indicated as an adverse effect of this drug.
   2 Not indicated as an adverse effect of this drug.
   4 Not indicated as an adverse effect of this drug.

766. **4** A second-degree burn over 30% of the body is considered critical. Shock, infection, electrolyte imbalance, and respiratory distress are life-threatening complications that can occur. (a)
   1 Burns involving less than 30% of the body surface of older children and adults under 50 years of age are generally less severe; the condition would be rated accordingly.
   2 Burns involving less than 30% of the body surface of older children and adults under 50 years of age are generally less severe; the condition would be rated accordingly.
   3 Burns involving less than 30% of the body surface of older children and adults under 50 years of age are generally less severe; the condition would be rated accordingly.

767. **3** The leukocyte count would not be affected in the first few hours. (b)
   1 Inhalation of hot air can cause tracheal edema.
   2 Replacement of fluids and electrolytes is essential in all burned clients.
   4 Pain is present in first-degree and second-degree burns, since the sensory nerves are not damaged.

768. **3** Potassium replacement is generally not indicated in the management of burns because hyperkalemia results from the liberation of potassium ions (K^+) from the injured cells. (c)
   1 This will be given with Ringer's and dextrose solutions in various combinations depending on the client's needs.
   2 This will be given with colloidal and glucose solutions in various combinations depending on the client's needs.
   4 This will be given with colloidal Ringer's solution in various combinations depending on the client's needs.

769. **3** Tetanus immune globulin provides antibodies against tetanus. This is used if the client has never received tetanus toxoid or antitoxin, which confer active immunity (the body makes its own antibodies in response to the antigen). (c)
   1 Administration would produce active immunity.
   2 Administration would produce active immunity.
   4 DPT vaccine—diphtheria and tetanus toxoid combined with pertussis vaccine—produces active immunity.

770. **4** Sulfisoxazole (Gantrisin) is a short-acting sulfonamide. It has an antibacterial effect by acting as an antimetabolite and interfering with the microorganism's ability to manufacture folic acid. (a)
   1 Gantrisin is an antimicrobial not an antiseptic.
   2 Gantrisin is an antimicrobial; does not relieve pain.
   3 Gantrisin is an antimicrobial; does not inhibit the reabsorption of uric acid.

771. **1** Bethanechol chloride (Urecholine) improves the muscle tone of an atonic bladder, facilitating micturition. (c)
   2 Pilocarpine hydrochloride is a miotic, used in the treatment of glaucoma.
   3 Carbachol is a miotic, used in the treatment of glaucoma.

4 Neosporin is a urinary tract antibiotic; does not aid in increasing bladder muscle tone.

772. **2** Lymphadenopathy occurs in clients with malignancies that have metastasized. (b)
   1 Skin is generally dry and itchy.
   3 Nikolsky's sign occurs in clients with pemphigus.
   4 Erythema of the palms is not a symptom of melanoma.

773. **3** A sarcoma is defined as a malignant tumor whose cells resemble those of the supportive (connective) tissues of the body. (c)
   1 Osteoblastomas are benign tumors of the bone.
   2 Although collagen is the substance used to form the connective tissue, the term collagenoma is incorrect.
   4 Carcinoma refers to a malignant neoplasm of epithelial tissue.

774. **1** Seeking other opinions to disprove the inevitable to a form of denial employed by individuals having illnesses with a poor prognosis. (b)
   2 Indiscriminate use of the call bell is often indicative of a fear of being alone, not denial, which is the first coping mechanism generally used.
   3 Criticism that is unjust is often characteristic of the stage of anger.
   4 Sleeping long periods is common during the depression experience as one moves toward acceptance.

775. **4** In the stage of acceptance the client frequently detaches the self from the environment and may become indifferent to family members. In addition, the family may take longer to accept the inevitable death than does the client. (c)
   1 Denial is often exhibited by both client and family at the same time.
   2 Although the family may not understand the anger, dealing with the resultant behavior may serve as a diversion.
   3 During this stage the family is often able to offer emotional support, and sometimes false reassurances, thus fulfilling one of their needs.

776. **2** The nurse's presence communicates concern and provides an opportunity for the client to initiate communication if needed. Silence is an effective interpersonal technique that permits the client to direct the content and extent of her verbalizations without the nurse's imposing on her privacy. (b)
   1 During acceptance the client may not wish to have visitors, preferring time for personal reflection.
   3 Detached from her environment, the client may find the details of various hospital procedures lose significance.
   4 Crying, which is so much a part of depression, usually ceases when the individual reaches acceptance.

777. **1** Psoriasis is characterized by dry, scaly lesions that occur most frequently on the elbows, knees, scalp, and torso. (a)
   2 Pruritis, if present at all, is generally mild.
   3 Petechiae are not characteristic.
   4 Erythematous flat spots on the skin as in measles; no scales are present.

778. **3** Steroids are applied locally and usually covered with plastic (or Sara Wrap) at night to reverse the inflammatory process. (b)
   1 Solar rays are used in the treatment of psoriasis.
   2 Potassium permanganate is an antiseptic astringent used on infected, draining, or vesicular lesions.
   4 The plaques are not necrotic and therefore do not require debriding.

779. **1** Scabies is caused by the itch mite *(Acarus scabiei),* the female of which burrows under the skin to deposit eggs. It is intensely pruritic and is transmitted by direct contact or, in a limited way, by soiled sheets or undergarments. (b)
   2 It is caused by the itch mite, a parasite.
   3 It is an infectious disease and is unrelated to allergies.
   4 Scabies is an acute infection.

780. **4** Pemphigus is primarily a serious disease characterized by large vesicles called bullae. Although potentially fatal, it has been relatively controlled by steroid therapy. (b)
   1 Pemphigus is a disease of the skin.
   2 Pemphigus is a disease of the skin.
   3 Pemphigus is a disease of the skin.

781. **3** Application of a solution of sodium bicarbonate (a mild alkali) after a thorough flushing with water is the best way to treat acid-splashed skin, since the alkali will neutralize residual acid on the skin. (b)
   1 Although sodium hydroxide is also an alkali and would neutralize acid, it is too strong and can also cause burns.
   2 Sodium chloride is a neutral salt, which would serve no immediate first-aid benefit.
   4 Sodium sulfate is a neutral salt, which would serve no immediate first-aid benefit.

782. **1** This first-aid treatment will chemically neutralize residual alkali still on the skin. It will not reverse the chemical damage already done by the alkali (burns) but will minimize additional chemical change. (a)
   2 A weak base will not neutralize alkaline substance.
   3 This is a neutral substance; will not neutralize base.
   4 This is a neutral substance; will not neutralize base.

783. **1** The connective tissue degeneration of SLE leads to involvement of the basal cell layer, producing a butterfly rash over the bridge of the nose and in the malar region. (b)
   2 This occurs in polyarteritis nodosa, a collagen disease affecting the arteries and nervous system.
   3 This occurs in muscular dystrophy, which is characterized by muscle wasting and weakness.
   4 This occurs in scleroderma and may advance until the client has the appearance of a living mummy.

784. **3** Scleroderma is an immunologic disorder characterized by inflammatory, fibrotic, and degenerative changes. (c)
   1 This is not involved in a development of scleroderma.
   2 This is not involved in the development of scleroderma.
   4 This is not involved in the development of scleroderma.

785. **3** Not only the skin but also the major organs are affected, including the heart, lungs, liver, kidneys, and intestine. Death usually occurs from cardiac arrest, renal failure, or cachexia. (c)
   1 The disease is fatal, with no known cure. Treatment with corticosteroids may prove helpful.
   2 Depending on the client's condition, death does not come rapidly since the disease spreads slowly to major organs.
   4 The disease is fatal, with no known cure. Treatment with corticosteroids may prove helpful.

786. **3** According to the Nurse Practice Act, a nurse may independently treat human responses to actual or potential health problems. (c)
   1 Providing supportive care is an independent, not dependent, function of the nurse.
   2 Active exercises must be ordered by the physician.
   4 Wound debridement is performed by the physician.

787. **1** Malaria is caused by the protozoan parasite *Plasmodium.* Plasmodium appear in the bloodstream during chills and fever. (b)
   2 White blood cells are not affected; this is not an infectious process but an infestation.
   3 Malaria is not an inflammation or infection but an infestation of parasites.
   4 Parasites in various stages are most easily identified in a smear of erythrocytes. The spleen enlarges because of destruction of the parasitized erythrocytes and accumulation of pigment.

788. **1** Parasites invade the erythrocytes, subsequently dividing and causing the cell to burst. The spleen enlarges from the sloughing of red blood cells. (c)
   2 WBCs (leukocytes) are not increased in number.
   3 Malaria is an infestation, not an infection or inflammation.
   4 RBCs (erythrocytes) are not increased in number.

789. **3** Although it is not possible to prevent infection once an individual is bitten by an infected mosquito, early treatment with quinine sulfate, a selective parasiticide, can arrest disease and prevent recurrence. (b)
   1 No vaccine is available.
   2 Isolation is not required; contracted by bite of infected *Anopheles* mosquito.
   4 Antibiotic therapy is ineffective against this parasite.

790. **4** *Plasmodium falciparum* in persons who have been treated with quinine causes hemoglobinuria, intravascular hemolysis, and renal failure as a result of destruction of red blood cells. (c)
   1 This symptom is unrelated to the development of blackwater fever.
   2 This symptom is unrelated to the development of blackwater fever.
   3 This symptom is unrelated to the development of blackwater fever.

791. **3** Fluid and electrolyte disturbances occur because of fever, profuse diaphoresis, vomiting, and diarrhea. (c)
   1 These symptoms are not associated with complications of malaria.
   2 This symptom is not associated with complications of malaria.
   4 This symptom is not associated with complications of malaria.

792. **3** Maintaining adequate nutritional and fluid balance is essential to life and must be accompanied during periods when intestinal motility is not too excessive so absorption can occur. (b)
   1 Peritoneal dialysis is not generally used in the treatment of malaria.
   2 The client should receive maximum rest and be given nourishment upon awakening.
   4 Infection may occur only through direct serum contact or a bite from an infected *Anopheles* mosquito.

793. **4** $\dfrac{1000 \text{ ml} \times 20 \text{ drops per ml}}{8 \text{ hr} \times 60 \text{ min}} = \dfrac{20,000}{480} = 42 \text{ drops/min}$ (a)
   1 This rate would be too slow.
   2 This rate would be too slow.
   3 This rate would be too slow.

794. **2** Signs of cinchonism, such as tinnitus, headache, dizziness, and nausea, indicate that the maximum therapeutic level of quinine has been attained. (c)
   1 Tinnitus and auditory status are affected by maximum levels of quinine; however, nausea not a symptom.
   3 These are not signs of cinchonism.
   4 These are not signs of cinchonism.

795. **2** Quinine administered orally can cause gastric irritation, resulting in nausea and vomiting. By administering such a medication after meals the nurse minimizes its irritating effect. (c)
  1 Absorption of the drug is not significantly affected by administration after meals.
  3 Appetite is not affected by this drug as long as gastric irritation is avoided.
  4 Quinidine sulfate or gluconate, also derived from cinchona bark, is given as an antiarrhythmic.

796. **1** Quinine sulfate is used in malaria when the plasmodia are resistant to the less toxic chloroquine. However, a new strain of *Plasmodium,* resistant to quinine, must be treated with a combination of quinine (quick acting), pyrimethamine, and sulfonamide (slow acting). (b)
  2 This would not occur if drug therapy is successful.
  3 The aim of therapy is to eliminate the asexual erythrocytic parasite, which is responsible for the symptoms, not to control them.
  4 Reinfestation can occur with a different species or strain of *Plasmodium.*

797. **4** Toxins from the bacillus invade nervous tissue; respiratory spasms may result in respiratory failure. (c)
  1 Muscle rigidity can occur; however, this generalized condition is not life threatening.
  2 Voluntary muscles may contract because of toxins from the bacillus; however, this is not life threatening.
  3 These subjective symptoms are not life threatening.

798. **3** Any product containing aluminum, magnesium, or calcium ions should not be taken in the hours before or after an oral dose, since it decreases absorption by as much as 25% to 50%. (c)
  1 Citrus juice has no influence on this drug.
  2 Antacids will interfere with absorption of this drug.
  4 Food interferes with absorption; should be given 1 hour before or 2 hours after meals or snacks.

799. **4** Diphenhydramine hydrochloride (Benadryl), like other antihistamines, competes with histamine at receptor sites. This alleviates the effects of histamine, which include increased dilation and permeability of capillaries (the cause of urticaria). (c)
  1 Benadryl does not destroy histamine; it competes with histamine at receptor sites.
  2 Benadryl does not have these actions; histamine dilates capillaries.
  3 Benadryl does not metabolize histamines.

800. **3** Penicillinase alters the structure of the penicillin molecule so it loses its antibiotic and allergenic capabilities. (c)
  1 Not the action of penicillinase; penicillins' molecular structure is altered by this drug.
  2 Penicillinase does not counteract tissue effects; it inactivates circulating penicillin.
  4 Drug is used only to inactivate circulating penicillin.

801. **2** Tetanus antitoxin provides antibodies, which confer immediate passive immunity. (c)
  1 Antitoxin does not stimulate production of antibodies.
  3 This is an example of passive immunity.
  4 Passive immunity, by definition, is not long lasting.

802. **2** Cardiac arrhythmias leading to heart failure can result in death of the client. (c)
  1 Although thirst may be a complaint, excessive salivation is the common problem.
  3 Hematuria does not occur in this disease.
  4 Double vision does not occur in rabies.

803. **1** Hydrophobia (fear of water) is a symptom associated with rabies. (c)
  2 The central nervous system is affected; diarrhea is not a concern.
  3 Urinary stasis is not a potential problem; catheterization can be employed.
  4 Memory is not affected by this disease.

804. **4** Accidents are common during young adulthood. (a)
  1 Glaucoma is a common health problem in the older adult.
  2 Cardovascular disease is a common health problem in middle adulthood.
  3 Kidney dysfunction is not a problem particular to any one stage of growth.

805. **4** Antibodies produced against group A beta-hemolytic streptococci sometimes interact with antigens in the heart's valves, causing damage and symptoms of rheumatic heart disease; early recognition and treatment of streptococcal infections has almost eliminated the occurrence of rheumatic heart disease. (b)
  1 Rheumatoid arthritis is thought to be an autoimmune disease; it is not caused by microorganisms such as beta-hemolytic streptococci.
  2 Hepatitis, an inflammation of the liver, is caused by the hepatitis A virus (HAV) or the hepatitis B virus (HBV), not by bacteria; there is also a non A-non B hepatitis.
  3 The most common causes of meningitis, an infection of the membranes surrounding the brain and spinal cord, include *Streptococcus pneumoniae, Neisseria meningitides,* and *Haemophilus influenzae.*

806. **2** Streptococcal organisms are present on the skin, mucous membranes, and in the environment at all times. The most frequent portals of entry are the respiratory tract and breaks in the skin. (b)
  1 Vaccinations are not available for most of these conditions; there is an antitoxin for scarlet fever, but antibiotics are now used.
  3 All are caused by streptococci.
  4 Bacteria are not classified as parasites.

807. **1** In gangrene the release of iron from hemoglobin as erythrocytes disintegrate in necrotic tissue results in ferrous sulfide formation, causing darkening of the tissues. (c)
  2 Ferric chloride is used as a reagent; it is also used topically as an antiseptic and as an astringent; not related to gangrene.
  3 Heme constitutes the pigment portion of the hemoglobin molecule, which gives blood its red color; does not cause the darkening of tissue associated with gangrene.
  4 Proteins are not insoluble.

808. **1** In active immunity, plasma cells provide antibodies in response to a specific antigen. (c)
  2 Eosinophils are involved in phagocytosis of antigen-antibody complexes.
  3 Lymphocytes are white blood cells that become plasma cells.
  4 Erythrocytes (red blood cells) carry oxygen in the bloodstream.

809. **2** *Clostridium welchii,* which causes muscle-decay-releasing gas, is the specific causative agent for gas gangrene. (a)
  1 *Clostridium tetani* enters the body via puncture of the skin and affects the nervous system; no development of gas occurs in tissue.
  3 *Clostridium botulinum* contaminates food which is ingested causing botulism.
  4 Caused by *Bacillis anthracis,* not *Clostridium.*

810. **1** The first action should be to remove the victim from a source of further injury. (b)
   2 This wound would be treated after patency of the airway is verified and the victim is moved from danger.
   3 Breathing is the priority once further injury is avoided.
   4 Preventing further injury and reestablishing breathing are the priorities.

811. **2** To avoid additional spinal cord damage, the victim must be moved only with great care. Moving a person whose spinal cord has been injured could cause irreversible paralysis. (b)
   1 A back injury is suspected; therefore the person should not be moved.
   3 A back injury precludes changing the person's position.
   4 A flat board would be indicated; however, one rescuer could not move the person alone.

812. **4** This position is useful in treating shock since it promotes gravity-induced venous return. Warmth and fluids are also supportive to the person. (a)
   1 These are not methods used in the treatment of shock.
   2 This is not a method used in the treatment of shock; may also cause burns.
   3 Promotes venous pooling, which compounds shock.

813. **3** People in panic could initiate the panic reaction in those who appear to be in control. (c)
   1 Depressed people will be calm and not affect others.
   2 Euphoric individuals would not adversely affect others.
   4 Comatose individuals will not cause panic in others.

814. **2** This group would succumb quickly to severe blood loss if dressings as indicated were not applied. (c)
   1 These individuals could wait for treatment per the triage routine.
   3 These individuals could wait for treatment per the triage routine.
   4 These individuals could wait for treatment per the triage routine.

815. **4** This may occur because of the high osmotic pressure of the aspirated water. (c)
   1 Hypovolemia occurs because fluid is drawn to the lungs by the hypertonic salt water.
   2 Not a sequela of near drowning.
   3 Hypoxia and acidosis may occur after a near drowning.

816. **2** May occur after hypothermia due to slowed metabolic processes. (c)
   1 Temperature would be low; however, pulse would be irregular.
   3 Blood pressure and respirations would be lowered.
   4 Temperature would be below 94° F; pallor, not erythema, would be present.

817. **1** Core rewarming with heated oxygen and administration of warmed fluids is the preferred method of treatment. (b)
   2 The victim would be too weak to ambulate; ambulation would expend energy.
   3 Warmed oral feedings are advised; gastric gavage would be unnecessary.
   4 Rectal or esophageal temperature is monitored.

818. **4** Nursing diagnosis defines an actual or potential health problem faced by the client. (a)
   1 Intervention follows the nursing diagnosis; it is part of the nursing process but not part of the nursing diagnosis.
   2 Plan of care made prior to implementation; it follows the nursing diagnosis but is not part of it; a step in the nursing process.
   3 Part of data collection prior to making nursing diagnosis; first step of nursing process.

819. **4** The primary nurse provides or oversees all aspects of care, including assessment, implementation, and evaluation of that care. (b)
   1 Title given to a specially prepared nurse for one very specific clinical role.
   2 The head nurse oversees all the staff and clients on a unit and coordinates care.
   3 A clinician is an expert teacher or practitioner in the clinical area.

820. **2** Immunization programs prevent the occurrence of disease and are considered a primary intervention. (b)
   1 This is a secondary intervention.
   3 This is a tertiary intervention.
   4 This is a tertiary invertention.

821. **4** Specimens can be analyzed for specific information which is objective. (c)
   1 Direct observations without precise measurements are subjective.
   2 The history from a client's family is subjective data.
   3 The client's verbal history of the illness is subjective data.

822. **4** When a plan does not adequately produce the desired outcome, the plan should be changed. (b)
   1 Client response is the determinant, not the nursing hypothesis.
   2 Various methods may have the same outcome; effectiveness is most important.
   3 Time is not relevant in the revision of a care plan.

823. **3** The nursing process is more than identifying a nursing problem. It is a step-by-step process that scientifically provides for client's nursing needs. (b)
   1 Incomplete; the nursing process goes beyond identification of a problem.
   2 Incomplete; goal establishment is one aspect of the nursing process.
   4 Incomplete; implementation of care is one aspect of the nursing process.

824. **3** The initial step in any process using problem solving is the collection of data. (a)
   1 Nursing needs can be determined only after assessment.
   2 Goals are set after nursing needs are established.
   4 Evaluation is the last phase of the process.

825. **3** Feedback permits the client to ask questions and express feelings and allows the nurse to verify client understanding. (b)
   1 Team conferences are subject to all members' evaluations of a client's status.
   2 Medical assessment does not necessarily include nurse-client relationships.
   4 Nurse-client communication should be evaluated by the client's verbal and behavioral responses.

826. **3** Soap helps by reducing surface tension of water, but friction is necessary for the removal of microorganisms. (b)
   1 Although water flushes some microorganisms from the skin, without friction it has minimal value.
   2 Although soap reduces surface tension, without friction it has minimal value.
   4 Although this aspect of hand washing is important, without friction it has minimal value.

827. **2** The fluid in a bottle hung over a person lying down possesses potential energy. When that fluid is allowed to drip into the person intravenously, its potential energy is then converted to kinetic energy (energy of motion). (c)
   1 No chemical reaction occurs when fluid drips into a vein.

3 No chemical reaction or formation of new substances occurs when fluid drips into a vein.

4 Energy is not being stored in this action; rather stored energy is converted to energy of motion.

828. **2** Since pressure is force developed per unit of area over which the force is applied, as the area decreases the pressure increases. The tip of a needle or the point of a knife has an extremely small area, and consequently a very high pressure can be developed for a given force. (c)

1 Although some energy is required to insert the needle, the amount is very little because the area at the tip of the needle is so small.

3 Although a factor, texture relationship is not the primary reason for ease of insertion; the small point in relation to energy developed at the point of insertion is the prime factor.

4 The length and shape of the needle have no relevance to ease the penetration; the small point in relation to energy developed at the point of insertion is the prime factor.

829. **1** $C° = \frac{5}{9} (F° - 32)$
$= \frac{5}{9} (99.8 - 32)$
$= \frac{5}{9} (67.8)$
$= 37.7$ (b)

2 $38.2° C = 100.8° F$

3 $37.0° C = 98.6° F$

4 $36.5° C = 97.7° F$

830. **3** The pulse increases to meet increased tissue demands for oxygen in the febrile state. (a)

1 Fever may not cause difficulty breathing.

2 Blood pressure is not necessarily elevated in fever.

4 Pain is not related to fever.

831. **2** REM (rapid eye movement) sleep is necessary for psychologic coping. The nurse should be aware that some medications affect this sleep stage and thereby alter emotional health. (b)

1 The individual is just drifting off to sleep; alpha brain waves are present.

3 The individual is in a light sleep and can be readily wakened; delta waves are interspersed with alpha waves.

4 The individual is in a deep sleep and is difficult to arouse; delta brain waves predominate; stages 1 and 4 are associated with physiologic rest.

832. **3** The absorption of fluids by gauze is due to the adhesion of water to the gauze threads. The surface tension of water causes contraction of the fiber, pulling fluid up the threads. (c)

1 This is movement of molecules from high to low concentration.

2 This refers to diffusion of water through a semipermeable membrane.

4 Separation of substances in solution utilizing their differing rates of diffusion through a membrane.

833. **1** The temperature range for tepid applications is somewhat below body temperature. (c)

2 This temperature is too cool to be considered tepid.

3 This temperature is too cool to be considered tepid.

4 This temperature is too cool to be considered tepid.

834. **4** Conduction is the conveyance of energy such as heat, cold, or sound by direct contact. (a)

1 Direct contact is not necessary to convey heat by radiation.

2 This is the transfer of heat by air circulation (e.g., by fans or open windows).

3 This refers to retention of heat, not its transfer.

835. **4** Cold reduces the sensitivity of receptors for pain in the skin. In addition, local blood vessels constrict, limiting the amount of interstitial fluid and its related pressure and discomfort. (b)

1 Local cold applications do not depress vital signs.

2 Local blood vessels constrict.

3 Local cold applications increase blood viscosity.

836. **3** An individual is held legally responsible for actions committed against another indiviudal or his property. (c)

1 This is the definition of negligence.

2 This is related to battery, which involves physical harm.

4 This is the definition of a crime.

837. **2** False imprisonment and battery are wrongs committed by one person against another in a willful intentional way without just cause and/or excuse. (c)

1 Malpractice, which is professional negligence, is classified as an unintentional tort; assault, which is knowingly threatening another, is an intentional tort.

3 Negligence, which is classified as an unintentional tort, involves exposure of another's person or property to unreasonable risk of injury by acts of commission or omission; invasion of privacy is an intentional tort.

4 Malpractice and negligence are both unintentional torts.

838. **1** The reporting of possible child abuse is required by law, and the nurse's identity can remain confidential. (b)

2 Although the Good Samaritan Act protects health professionals, the nurse would still be responsible for acting as any reasonably prudent nurse would in a similar situation.

3 Although the Good Samaritan Act protects health professionals, the nurse would still be responsible for acting as any reasonably prudent nurse would in a similar situation.

4 The nurse is functioning in a professional capacity and therefore can be held accountable.

839. **1** Each state or province is charged with the responsibility of protecting the health and welfare of its populace, which it does by regulating nursing practice. (b)

2 Although the members of the profession can also benefit from a clear description of their role, this is not the primary purpose of the law.

3 Professional standards are established by the profession to assure quality care for the public.

4 The employing agency does assume rsponsibility for its employees and therefore benefits from maintenance of standards, but this is not the purpose of the law.

840. **1** The description of the situation provides no evidence of incompetence. Since the client has not been certified as incompetent, he retains the right of informed consent. (c)

2 Since the description of the situation provides no evidence of incompetence, the client should sign his own consent.

3 Since the description of the situation provides no evidence of incompetence, the client should sign his own consent.

4 The client can sign his own consent, and his signature requires only one witness.

Chapter 4: Psychiatric Nursing

1. **4** The unconscious stores past experiences and the emotional feelings associated with them. These emotional feelings influence one's perceptions, attitudes, and behavior. (c)
   1 There is no such thing as the foreconscious level.
   2 Material in the conscious is in a state of immediate awareness.
   3 Material in the conscious is in a state of immediate awareness.

2. **1** Mild anxiety motivates one to action, such as learning or emotional changes. Higher levels of anxiety tend to blur the individual's perceptions and interfere with functioning. (b)
   2 The perceptual field is narrowed.
   3 The perceptual field is greatly reduced.
   4 Attention is severely reduced.

3. **2** The individual using sublimation attempts to fulfill desires by selecting a socially acceptable activity rather than one which is socially unacceptable (e.g., pursuing a career in nursing as a means of giving and receiving love). (b)
   1 This would be an example of reaction formation.
   3 This would be regression not sublimation.
   4 This would be an example of repression.

4. **3** When acting out against the primary source of anxiety creates even further anxiety or danger, the individual may use displacement to express feelings on a safer object. (a)
   1 An example of denial.
   2 This would be fantasy.
   4 An inability to mature and accept responsibility.

5. **2** The parameters set by birth, psychologic experiences, and the environment make each individual unique. Although other factors may impinge to a slight degree, these factors form the personality. (b)
   1 Autoimmunity plays no part in personality development.
   3 Not inclusive; limited to only some aspects of personality development.
   4 Not inclusive; limited to only some aspects of personality development; race plays no part.

6. **3** When the individual experiences a threat to self-esteem, anxiety increases and the normal defense mechanisms are used to protect the ego. (a)
   1 Ritualistic behavior is not a normal aspect of the developmental process.
   2 Withdrawal patterns are an abnormal way of coping with stress; if carried to an extreme, can become pathologic.
   4 Affective reactions are mood disorders.

7. **4** Incorporation of parental and societal values into the superego leads to the development of a sense of right and wrong. Guilt and shame are experienced when these values are broken. Thus the superego is the conscience. (b)
   1 The self is the total of the id, ego, and superego.
   2 The ideal self is how a person perceives the self to be or strives to be.
   3 Narcissism involves an excessive love of self with strong dependency needs that are impossible for others to meet.

8. **1** The child views his or her own worth by the response received from the parents. This sense of worth sets the basic ego strengths and is vital to the formation of the personality. (a)
   2 Although important, it is not as important as the parent-child relationship.

   3 Peer groups come later in a child's development, but the parent-child relationship is still the most important.
   4 This comes later in life, after the basic personality has been formed.

9. **4** The sympathetic nervous system reacts to stress by releasing epinephrine, which prepares the body to fight or fleet by increasing the heart rate, constricting peripheral vessels, and increasing oxygen supply to the muscles. (b)
   1 Although the brain responds to stress, it is the sympathetic nervous system that is primarily affected.
   2 The sympathetic and parasympathetic nervous systems are both part of the peripheral nervous system; the sympathetic nervous system is primarily affected; the parasympathetic nervous system does not play a role in the fight or flight reaction.
   3 This has an effect opposite to that of the sympathetic nervous system.

10. **3** Conscience and a sense of right and wrong are expressed in the superego, which acts to counterbalance the id's desire for immediate gratification. (b)
    1 This is the id seeking satisfaction.
    2 A healthy ego can delay gratification and is in balance with reality.
    4 This does not reflect any part of the self.

11. **4** Learning from others occurs in a group setting and is reinforced by group acceptance of the norms. Group pressure is peer pressure, which is more easily accepted if the individual wants to stay in the group. (a)
    1 Groups do not go through the same developmental phases as individuals.
    2 One member of a group can be the target of hostility.
    3 Not necessarily so; the group may not be easily identified by its members, and identification does not play a role in emotional development.

12. **2** Socialization, values, and role definition are learned within the family and help develop a sense of self. Once established in the family, the child can more easily move into society. (a)
    1 Only a very small aspect of the family's influence.
    3 This is true, but not as important as identity and roles in relation to emotional development.
    4 This is true, but not as important as identity and roles in relation to emotional development.

13. **3** Socialization occurs through communication with others. Without some form of communication there can be no socialization. (a)
    1 People interact with other social beings, not with inanimate objects.
    2 People interact with other social beings, not with inanimate objects.
    4 People interact with other social beings, not with inanimate objects.

14. **3** Before this age the infant has not developed enough ego strength to have an identity or personality. (c)
    1 Too early; has not developed enough ego strength to have a personality.
    2 Self-concept is nonexistent.
    4 The primary emergence of the personality has already occurred.

15. **2** The toddler learns to say "no" and to express independence, yet because of human nature he or she is both physically and emotionally dependent on the parents. (c)
    1 The major task during infancy is development of trust.
    3 This stage deals with developing a sense of initiative.
    4 This stage deals with the task of industry and developing skills for working in and relating to the world.

16. **1** The toddler is struggling to identify his or her own needs. Too early and too strict toilet training results in ambivalence because the child's needs and physical abilities are in conflict with the parental demands. The child is faced with giving up these needs or risking parental disapproval. (b)

    2 A child is involved from birth in satisfying the parent's needs, but toilet training is really the first time a conflict develops.

    3 A toddler has no interest in society's expectations.

    4 A child is involved from birth in satisfying his or her own needs.

17. **2** Testing the self both physically and psychologically occurs during the toddler stage after trust has been achieved. (c)

    1 Trust is the task of infancy.

    3 Between the ages of 3 and 6, a child starts to identify with the parent of the same sex.

    4 This task is accomplished between the ages of 6 and 12.

18. **1** The infant and toddler are dependent on significant others and react strongly to separation and loss, which they view as rejection and abandonment. These needs are strongest during the "taking in" or oral phase of development. (c)

    2 The child begins to exert control over the environment rather than be concerned with separation.

    3 Sexual drives for the opposite sex are dealt with and repressed; the child has already developed a sense of autonomy and is no longer as concerned with separation.

    4 The child between the ages of 6 and 12 learns a sense of self-worth through dealings with others in the environment; this age is concerned with task of industry, developing skills, and relating to the world; separation is not the major concern.

19. **3** A sense of one's self and a feeling of belonging form the basis for mental health, since it provides comfort with self and group. (c)

    1 A person could have emotional balance without all three.

    2 A person needs to have biologic needs met; does not need social acceptance; the group providing acceptance may not be acceptable to society or to the individual.

    4 A person needs security but can do without social recognition.

20. **1** Rivalry between siblings is normal and arises because one child resents the care and attention given another child. One child unconsciously wishes the other would disappear and frequently acts out negatively against him or her. (a)

    2 These conflicts are directed not toward siblings but toward parents.

    3 This would deal more with thoughts and desires.

    4 The superego would be involved more with making amends.

21. **2** The individual who cannot communicate cannot test reality. Without this connection to others or reality, severe emotional problems will develop. (b)

    1 Without the stimulation of communication, mental dullness or slowness will occur, not mental deficiency.

    3 There is a frustration and inability to foster communication.

    4 Lack of communication can lead to isolation and withdrawal but this response is too narrow since a variety of problems usually develop.

22. **1** Feelings of resentment toward children by parents is a normal response. To relieve feelings of guilt and shame, it is vital to help parents realize this. (a)

    2 This is an untrue generalization.

    3 These are normal feelings.

    4 The first child causes the greatest amount of adjustment in one's life.

23. **3** During the oedipal stage (between 2½ and 6 years of age) the child has many fears about his or her body. Any invasive techniques done at this time can create severe emotional problems. (c)

    1 If a sense of trust has been established and a caring person is allowed to spend time with the child, no damage should occur.

    2 There will probably be some regression in motor skills, but the outcome is favorable upon return home.

    4 The child is older and better able to deal with the surgery.

24. **1** The mature personality does not respond to the immediate gratification demands of the id or the oppressive control of the superego because the ego is strong enough to maintain a balance between them. (a)

    2 There would be no healthy resolution of conflicts if the superego were always in control.

    3 With society in control there would be chaos, rather than maturity.

    4 This would create a rigid personality who made impossible demands on the self.

25. **3** Values and beliefs from parents and society are expressed through the child's play world. These values become part of the child's system through the process of internalization (introjection). (c)

    1 If this happened, the child would be learning to blame others for his or her own faults.

    2 This would occur at a later age.

    4 The environment and others in it, rather than play, influence independence.

26. **4** Freud's theory is that a child develops a sexualized love for the parent of the opposite sex and become jealous of the parent of the same sex. These thoughts result in feelings of guilt, anxiety, fear, and hate toward the parent of the same sex, which are repressed. (a)

    1 The child loves the parent of the opposite sex and hates the parent of the same sex.

    2 The child loves the parent of the opposite sex but fears and hates the parent of the same sex.

    3 In the normal stage of development, ambivalence does not occur.

27. **2** The child resolves oedipal conflicts by leaning to identify with the parent of the same sex and accomplishes this by mimicking the role of this parent. (b)

    1 This is the earliest stage of development and operates solely on the pleasure principle, largely id oriented; concerned with development of trust.

    3 There is increasing sex role development; concerned with peer group identification.

    4 Interest shift from the anal region to the genital region, and questions about sexuality arise.

28. **1** When props are needed to blur reality, the individual is not able to rely on the self to test out situations and therefore dependence on others or props increases. (c)

    2 The person who mistrusts has not learned to trust the environment; however, does not necessarily need props.

    3 Role blurring is not a problem requiring a prop.

    4 The person with an ego ideal would not need props to blur reality.

29. **4** During a crisis one may regress to a stage provoking less anxiety in an attempt to cope with an unacceptable situation. (b)
    1 A client may use denial during an illness, but this would not make him or her dependent and demanding.
    2 This is a normal defense mechanism; not used specifically during times of illness.
    3 This compensatory mechanism would cause a person to try to make amends, not become more dependent and demanding.

30. **4** The defense mechanism is called conversion because the individual actually reduces emotional anxiety by converting it to a physical disability. (b)
    1 In dissociation there is separation of certain mental processes from the consciousness as though they belonged to another; a dissociative-type reaction is expressed as amnesia, fugue, multiple personality, aimless running, depersonalization, sleep walking, etc.
    2 This just identifies the term used to describe mind and body; not a defense mechanism.
    3 This is a mechanism used to make up for a lack in one area by emphasizing capabilities in another.

31. **2** By developing skills in one area the individual compensates or makes up for a real or imagined deficiency, thereby maintaining a positive self-image. (a)
    1 This person is not trying to make amends for unacceptable feelings (reaction formation) but rather for a felt deficiency and a poor self-image.
    3 This would deal more with unacceptable impulses that would pose a threat.
    4 If the boy incorporated the qualities of the college athlete, that would be introjection.

32. **3** An illusion is a misperception or misinterpretation of actual external stimuli. (b)
    1 This is a false believe that cannot be changed even by evidence; a fixed false belief.
    2 This would deal with imaginary, not real, stimuli.
    4 A belief that others are talking about the person is not a visual distortion.

33. **3** Mediating frustration within the real world is an ego function and requires ego strengths. (b)
    1 The id is unable to tolerate frustration since it is totally involved with gratification.
    2 The superego is involved with putting pressure on the ego because of the id's not tolerating frustration.
    4 The unconscious does not deal with frustration.

34. **1** The ego develops during childhood as a result of positive experiences. When the situation in childhood is such that severe anxiety is unresolved, the ego seems to be permanently traumatized and is unable to recover totally. (b)
    2 This would have no effect.
    3 This is a normal occurrence; children are often unable to verbalize their feelings and play therapy is utilized for that reason.
    4 This in itself would not necessarily be traumatic unless abuse was also present.

35. **3** The child realizes that the parent of the same sex cannot be bested in a struggle for the affection of the parent of the opposite sex. The role and behavior of the same-sex parent are therefore assumed by the child to attract the parent of the opposite sex. (b)
    1 This would be a conflict not a resolution.
    2 This would be in conflict with heterosexual drives.
    4 Doing this would give rise to greater conflict and leave a fragmented self.

36. **1** Any behavioral therapy or learning of new methods of dealing with situations requires modifications of approach and attitudes; hence personality is always capable of change. (b)
    2 Acccepting this theory would close the door on all future growth and development.
    3 The capacity for change exists throughout the life cycle.
    4 Certain personality traits are established by age 2, but not the total personality.

37. **2** The superego incorporates all experiences and learning from external environments (society, family, etc.) into the internal environment. (b)
    1 The id with its drives is a source of creative energy.
    3 This is the function of the id.
    4 This is the function of the id.

38. **2** Slips of the tongue, also called "Freudian slips," are material from the unconscious that slips out in unguarded moments. (a)
    1 There is no evidence linking these experiences to the unconscious.
    3 Material in the unconscious cannot deliberately be brought back to awareness.
    4 Free-floating anxiety is linked to the unconscious, but the best evidence of the unconscious is slips of the tongue.

39. **4** Poor interpersonal relationships, inappropriate behavior, and learning disabilities prevent these children from emotionally adapting or responding to the environment despite possible high level of intelligence. (b)
    1 It is the lack of response to stimulus that is the clue to a child's being emotionally disturbed.
    2 The exact opposite is true.
    3 This is true but not *most* characteristic.

40. **1** From infancy the child is nonresponsive. Not wanting to eat demonstrates a further withdrawal. (c)
    2 This is not indicative of an autistic child.
    3 This would not be characteristic of autism.
    4 An autistic child would not be labeled autistic if he or she enjoyed being with people.

41. **3** The drug of choice in this diagnosis. It appears to act by stimulating release of norepinephrine from nerve endings in the brainstem. (b)
    1 Thorazine is an antipsychotic medication.
    2 Haldol is an antipsychotic medication.
    4 This is a muscle relaxant.

42. **3** When the individual consciously pretends an illness with no physical basis, it is called malingering. (c)
    1 A person out of contact with reality is unable to pretend an illness.
    2 A neurotic person really believes he or she is sick.
    4 The use of conversion defenses is not a conscious act.

43. **4** Everyone has the right to personal sexual preference, but limits must be set on acting out behavior within the hospital. (c)
    1 This would be a punishing attitude, especially for the client who would be transferred.
    2 Not a realistic approach to the situation.
    3 Limits would need to be set, not punishment.

44. **3** Clients with these sexual disorders usually have many other emotional problems which may be overt or covert in nature. (b)
    1 There is normal development of sexual organs in individuals with paraphilic sexual disorders.
    2 There is no proof of a deficiency of these hormones.
    4 This has no basis in fact.

45. **3** This medication can be given IM every 2 weeks for clients who cannot be relied upon to take oral medications; allows them to live in the community while keeping the symptoms under control. (b)
    1 This medication must be taken on a daily basis.
    2 This medication must be taken on a daily basis.
    4 This medication is not used for the treatment of schizophrenia.

46. **4** When individuals use these defense mechanisms to blur the pains of reality, they are unable to test out their feelings or differentiate the real world from their personal intrapsychic perceptions. (b)
    1 The thought process is only one aspect of reality testing.
    2 Association is only one part of reality testing.
    3 Logic is only one part of reality testing.

47. **3** A delusion of persecution is a fixed and firm belief or feeling of being harassed, in danger, or at the mercy of others. (a)
    1 Hallucinations are perceived experiences that occur in the absence of actual sensory stimulation.
    2 In this instance the person blamed himself for an act that was never committed.
    4 An error in judgment can be corrected by pointing out reality, but a delusion cannot.

48. **2** Nursing care involves a steady attempt to draw the client into some response. This can best be accomplished by focusing on nonthreatening subjects that do not demand a specific response. (b)
    1 Questions like these do not allow a person to explore his own feelings.
    3 Client is not ready yet to discuss his feelings, so the first step is to focus on nonthreatening subjects.
    4 By doing this, the nurse is showing acceptance of him but is doing nothing to encourage communication.

49. **3** Keeping the withdrawn client oriented to reality prevents him from withdrawing even further into his private world. (a)
    1 This would be futile at present.
    2 A gradual involvement in selected activities would be best.
    4 The client would be unable to tell anyone why this is so.

50. **1** By observing behavior, the nurse is able to understand the client's feelings better. Behavior usually serves a purpose and is directed toward satisfaction of needs. (b)
    2 It is only one of the many aspects that are part of making a diagnosis; true in the care of all clients not just the withdrawn individual.
    3 It is more important to have insight into what the person may be feeling rather than the degree of depression.
    4 Observation alone is insufficient to make this judgment; however it would allow the staff to individualize the nursing care plan to suite the client's needs.

51. **3** A one-to-one trusting relationship is essential to help the client become more involved and interested in interpersonal relationships. (a)
    1 Selected activities, rather than a large variety of activities, are best.
    2 Specific routines are normally a part of any unit, for all clients.
    4 A very withdrawn individual needs to start with a one-to-one relationship before progressing to group involvement.

52. **1** Depression is a disturbance in the mood or affect (classified as a mood disorder) that usually develops when the ego suffers a real or imagined loss. (c)

2 There is not a total loss of control, and the loss of control may be only part of the clinical picture.
    3 The degree of depression will determine the extent to which a person can function.
    4 This may also be true, but it is not the most accurate description.

53. **3** No organic pathology has yet been identified in schizophrenia. Behavioral responses learned in childhood cause the individual to distort events and relationships and lose the ability to relate to the world. (a)
    1 This would be an organic rather than a functional illness.
    2 This would be an organic rather than a functional illness, and there is no evidence that the brain undergoes any change.
    4 This might be a factor, but there is no proof that it is true since we do not know what causes schizophrenia.

54. **2** Disinterest in or fear of personal involvement creates distancing behavior and lack of response to the environment. (b)
    1 This would be symptomatic more of the manic phase of a bipolar disorder.
    3 May or may not be present.
    4 May or may not be present.

55. **1** Mental illness is characterized by the use of abnormal defense mechanisms or the abnormal use of normal defense mechanisms. These defenses build a wall and interrupt interpersonal relationships. (a)
    2 It is the ability or inability to handle periods of high anxiety that gives evidence of mental illness.
    3 Possible, but may be just one factor.
    4 Possible, but not a common factor.

56. **4** Shows acceptance for the client yet sets firm limits on the behavior. This response also points out reality to the client. (b)
    1 This statement not only rejects the behavior but also attacks the client.
    2 The nurse accepts the client but should not accept physical abuse from the client.
    3 Puts the focus on the nurse rather than on what is behind the outburst.

57. **2** Family interaction patterns and role identification and definition lay the foundations for the child's future emotional response. (b)
    1 This, as yet, has not been proved.
    3 This would be organic not functional.
    4 This is a part of organic mental disorders.

58. **3** Inner psychic stress and environmental difficulties can interfere with the function of organically sound organs, resulting in a loss of ability to communicate. (a)
    1 This would have an organic basis.
    2 Mental deficiency has an organic basis.
    4 This has an organic basis.

59. **2** The nurse's response really was a threat by attempting to put pressure on the client to speak or be left alone. (b)
    1 Reward and punishment are used in behavior modification therapy, not for severe depression.
    3 The statement reflects an insensitivity to rather than a recognition of the client's rights.
    4 She is not ready yet at this stage for group involvement; she must start with a one-to-one relationship.

60. **3** Clients who are out of control are seeking control and frequently respond to simple directions stated in a firm voice. (b)
    1 This would be done only after an attempt at calming him down had failed.

2 This would not be helping the client gain control of his actions and might be frightening to other clients in the day room.

4 "Be quiet" is an order that is nontherapeutic and is, furthermore, demeaning behavior on the part of the nurse.

61. **4** The nurse's response provides an example to the client that feelings can be expressed by words rather than by action. This response also demonstrates that the nurse cares enough to set limits on behavior. (b)

1 The nurse is punishing the client rather than trying to focus on what is happening at this time to cause the behavior.

2 The nurse would be accepting physical abuse, which is never done.

3 The client won't need the nurse to talk to her when she is better; she needs limits set on her behavior now.

62. **2** Acting out anxiety with antisocial behavior is most commonly found in individuals with personality rather than anxiety disorders. (c)

1 An example of a conversion disorder.

3 An example of a phobic disorder.

4 Regression is an attempt during periods of stress to return to behavior that has been satisfying and is appropriate at an earlier stage of development.

63. **4** In phobias the individual transfers anxiety to a rather safe inanimate object. Therefore the anxiety and resulting feelings will only be precipitated when in direct contact with the object. (b)

1 It is not thinking about the feared object that caused anxiety; it is the thought of having to come into contact with it.

2 It is the guilt or fear within the person, not the object, that must be dealt with.

3 Not possible to introject the feared object within the body.

64. **2** The longer the child stays out, the more difficult it is to get him or her to return to school, since more fantasies and fears develop. (c)

1 This approach rarely accomplishes anything.

3 This will feed into the fear that the phobia is realistic.

4 This would increase, not decrease, the fear.

65. **3** Having poor superego control, these individuals cannot set limits for themselves and require an environment in which appropriate limits for behavior are set for them. (a)

1 This person has too much freedom of expression and is unable to control impulses.

2 This would be too stimulating for a person with socially aggressive behavior.

4 An environment that can be manipulated teaches the client nothing; encourages a continuation of maladjustive behavior.

66. **3** Accepting the client and the symptomatic behavior sets the foundation for the nurse-client relationship. Setting limits provides external controls and helps lower anxiety. (c)

1 This will only increase the anxiety and increase the behavior.

2 Restricting a person's movements would have no effect other than to increase anxiety.

4 Unrealistic.

67. **1** Clients prevented from using ritualistic behavior to control anxiety will be deprived of their defense and have no way of relieving tension. (a)

2 Preventing ritualistic behavior will only increase anxiety.

3 This would not decrease the ritualistic behavior.

4 Such clients' behavior should never be ignored; it is important to accept and support these clients during this time.

68. **4** The problem is psychologic. Therefore the initial approach by the nurse should be directed toward establishing trust. (a)

1 She is convinced that she is overweight; telling her she has a lovely figure would not change per perception of herself.

2 The client is not ready for this information.

3 This would be an initial nursing intervention after trust had been established.

69. **3** If seizures were physiologically based, the client would not be able to continue to chew gum. This "attack" should be reported as a behavioral response, with the precipitating factors noted. (c)

1 The chewing gum is not a danger when the client is not having a true attack.

2 This would probably not be necessary now.

4 Not necessary since there is no danger of the tongue's blocking the airway as it would in a true attack.

70. **3** Accept the client as a person of worth rather than being cold or implying rejection. However, the nurse maintains a professional rather than a social role. (a)

1 The client is aware that he is a client and the nurse is a nurse.

2 This is shifting responsibility from the issue at hand to the institution.

4 This is avoiding the real issue and elevates the nurse to a higher social order.

71. **1** Individuals with this personality disorder tend to be self-centered and impulsive. They lack judgment and superego controls and do not profit from their mistakes. (c)

2 Generally, just the opposite is true.

3 These people are too self-centered to have a sense of responsibility to anyone.

4 These people never learn from their mistakes, experiences, and punishment.

72. **4** The lack of superego control allows the ego and the id to control the behavior. Self-motivation and self-satisfaction are of paramount concern. (c)

1 They count on others to extricate them from the problems they find themselves faced with.

2 These people are extremely dependent on others.

3 These people are usually charming on the surface and can easily "con" people into doing what they want.

73. **4** The liquid concentrate is a highly irritating substance on contact with skin and eyes and can cause uncomfortable dermatologic conditions. (c)

1 No indication for this precaution.

2 Not necessary; and leaving it unmixed provides greater assurance that the client will ingest the full dose of Thorazine.

3 Not necessary.

74. **3** Acute dystonic reactions, parkinsonian syndrome, dyskinesia, and akathisia are observable side effects of chlorpromazine hydrochloride therapy. (b)

1 After the first few days of treatment, Thorazine has no effect on concentration or other mental abilities.

2 Not a side effect of Thorazine.

4 Not a side effect of Thorazine.

75. **1** This checks functioning of the liver, since liver damage may occur from use of the drug. Cholestatic hepatitis with obstructive jaundice is the most frequent form of liver disturbance and can be identified by yellow sclerae and clay-colored stools. (c)

2 Anorexia is not a side effect of Thorazine; the client frequently gains weight.

3 Not a side effect of Thorazine.
4 Not a side effect of Thorazine.
76. **1** The physician is responsible for medication orders but depends on the nurse's observations in making decisions. (b)
2 This would not be a severe enough symptom to warrant withholding the drug.
3 It is reaction to the Thorazine and must be treated.
4 This would have no effect on the tremors.
77. **3** Occurs as a late and persistent extrapyramidal complication of long-term chlorpromazine therapy. Can take many forms (e.g., torsion spasm, opisthotonos, oculogyric crisis, drooping of the head, protrusion of the tongue). (c)
1 Reversible with administration of Cogentin and Benadryl.
2 Reversible with administration of Cogentin and Benadryl.
4 Reversible with administration of Cogentin and Benadryl.
78. **4** Lithium carbonate does not impair intellectual activity, consciousness, or range or quality of emotional life. However, it can control the manic phase of a bipolar disorder. (b)
1 Liithium is not used for schizophrenia.
2 Lithium is not used for an agitated paranoid state.
3 Lithium is not used for major depressions.
79. **2** Unintentional tremors are one of the extrapyramidal side effects of the major tranquilizers and are considered common and manageable. (a)
1 Not a common occurrence, but periodic liver function tests should be done.
3 Not a common side effect.
4 Not applicable; an excessive number of melanocytes is not a side effect.
80. **3** The monoamine oxidase inhibitors can cause a hypertensive crisis if food or beverages that are high in tyramine are ingested. (b)
1 An elixir base only makes the medications more palatable.
2 This would be important for clients taking one of the phenothiazines.
4 No contraindication.
81. **1** Clients taking chlorpromazine should be told to stay out of the sun. Photosensitivity makes the skin more susceptible to burning. (b)
2 Reported as being extremely rare.
3 Not reported with the use of Ritalin.
4 Not a side effect of lithium.
82. **4** The major tranquilizers modify the behavior of psychotic clients so they can more effectively cope with the environment and benefit from therapy. (a)
1 Contraindicated.
2 Antidepressants are used for depression.
3 The action is to decrease the severity of psychotic symptoms more than to sedate; Ritalin is used to treat hyperkinetic children.
83. **1** These drugs are used to control the extrapyramidal (parkinsonism-like) symptoms that often develop as a side effect of major tranquilizer therapy. (b)
2 No documented use with minor tranquilizers because they do not have extrapyramidal side effects.
3 Barbiturates do not have extrapyramidal side effects, which would respond to these drugs.
4 Antiparkinson drugs (e.g., Cogentin) are not usually prescribed in conjunction with antidepressants; gastrointestinal tract depression can result in paralytic ileus.

84. **3** These drugs control the extrapyramidal (parkinsonism-like) symptoms associated with the major tranquilizers and are classified as antiparkinsonian drugs. (b)
1 Does not potentiate phenothiazine derivatives.
2 Has no effect on postural hypotension.
4 Has no effect on depression.
85. **3** The nurse's failure to observe what was brought in for the client constituted negligence. The nurse's knowledge of the alcoholic would warrant checking to see what the client was consuming. (b)
1 Not on a substance abuse unit.
2 This is true, except the nurse might have felt that the friend herself had a good effect on the client.
4 Also true, but the client has no manifestations of a psychosis.
86. **4** Thiamine is a coenzyme in producing energy from glucose. If thiamine is not present in adequate amounts, nerve activity is diminished and damage or degeneration of myelin sheaths occurs. (b)
1 Used only in the acute phase to control delirium tremens.
2 Use of these has a higher risk of toxic side effects in older persons.
3 A diet high in the B vitamins would be included in the care plan.
87. **1** Polydrug users abuse a variety of drugs in their search for the ultimate "high." They usually will include alcohol in their search and frequently combine their abuses. (b)
2 Not necessarily true.
3 Has been mentioned as a possible causative factor but with no evidence to support it.
4 Not necessarily so, some become very happy and outgoing.
88. **1** The nurse's major tool in psychiatric nursing is the therapeutic use of self. Psychiatric nurses must learn to be aware of their own feelings and how they affect the situation. (c)
2 This may be true but is not part of the nurse-client relationship.
3 This implies that the nurse is working alone in planning care for the client.
4 This may be true, but an awareness of self still seems to be the most difficult.
89. **2** The therapeutic milieu is directed toward helping the client develop effective ways of dealing with interpersonal situations. (b)
1 This would accomplish nothing in regard to a long-term goal of functioning in society.
3 This would be a means of achieving the goal.
4 The hospital atmosphere should be more structured and accepting than the client's home.
90. **2** Permits the client to see that his feelings are not unique but are shared by others. (a)
1 A nonsupportive remark to a realistic fear of leaving the safe hospital and going back to where he has to deal with his problem.
3 Makes the client worry why he does not feel happy.
4 How the others feel about whether he is ready to be discharged is totally irrelevant.
91. **1** By sensing, supporting, and verbalizing the emotional feelings of others the individual emerges as the leader. (a)
2 This is a role filled by many group leaders, but it does not permit focus on feelings.
3 The group members do this themselves.
4 Designation of group members may be done by many people in various ways.

92. **3** Sharing problems with others who have similar problems, thoughts, and feelings help the individual learn new ways of coping. (b)
    1 Emotional illness is not enough; the person must recognize that a problem exists and help is necessary.
    2 All people are dependent on others to some degree; this would not be a criterion for group therapy.
    4 This might be partly true, but the person should still feel he needs help in coping with a problem.

93. **1** The group setting provides the individual with the opportunity to learn that others share the same problems and needs. The group also provides an arena where new methods of relating to others can be tried. (c)
    2 It has the opposite effect.
    3 The focus is still on the individual, but on the individual's learning how to relate to others.
    4 This may happen from time to time with support given to the individual by the group, but it is not a main function of the group.

94. **2** Group therapy should focus on the present and how current problems and feelings are affecting current behavior. In the group setting the individual members have the opportunity to receive feedback on their behavior. (b)
    1 The focus is the feelings behind the behavior with which others can identify.
    3 Not the stress itself, but how to deal with the stress.
    4 The nurse must protect individual group members from confrontation until certain that they are strong enough to deal with it.

95. **3** A person able to cope with life situations usually has developed fairly strong ego defenses. In a crisis situation the individual frequently just needs support to regroup strengths and reestablish the ability to cope. (b)
    1 Not possible or realistic.
    2 Socialization would be part of recovery, not the crisis stage.
    4 This might have the effect of increasing anxiety, thereby making the crisis situation worse.

96. **2** The current trend in psychiatry is to treat the client and maintain him or her in the community. This trend includes the family and community in the plan and has reduced the number of clients in psychiatric hospitals. (a)
    1 This possibly would have the effect of masking the symptoms and should be used only in conjunction with psychotherapy.
    3 This would follow when the client was ready.
    4 Might be part of the overall treatment plan but not the only aspect.

97. **1** The day hospital provides the client with a therapeutic setting for a few hours daily during the transitional stage between hospital and total discharge. (b)
    2 This would have little or no effect on social skills.
    3 This does help during the transition stage, but it is not the primary goal of day care.
    4 Day-care treatment would meet this goal, but that is not its primary purpose.

98. **1** Her stated feelings of distrust of others and her inability to mix socially can best be defined in these terms. (a)
    2 Nothing in the situation indicates this.
    3 Before she became sick she held a responsible job.
    4 It was her later personality that took on schizoid qualities.

99. **4** Demonstrating that the staff can be trusted is a vital initial step in the therapy program. (b)

1 Even proof would not convince the client that her delusion is false.
2 The client is not ready to enter group activities yet and will not be until trust is established.
3 This would not be realistic even if it were possible; limiting contact does not develop trust.

100. **1** Clients cannot be argued out of delusions, so the best approach is a simple statement of reality. (c)
    2 This may reinforce her delusion that the hospital food is poisoned.
    3 This would be a form of entering into her delusions; client would only feel that particular part was free of poison.
    4 Threats are always poor nursing intervention no matter how exasperated the nurse feels.

101. **2** It is important to help the client focus on her feelings, and this is the only response that does so. (c)
    1 "Why" calls for a conclusion rather than exploring the issue; the client may not have the answer.
    3 Although this is true, it is not something the client is ready to understand; it is a closed statement.
    4 This is false reassurance and not realistic; the client is still concerned as to what she will do when the nurse is not there.

102. **4** If clients feel a need to be punished, it is best to permit them to engage in controlled activities that expiate guilt feelings. (b)
    1 A procedure such as this would reinforce her belief of the need to be punished.
    2 This would do nothing to interrupt the delusional system; it would support the hallucination.
    3 The client cannot be talked out of her delusion; she must believe within herself that she has nothing to atone for.

103. **1** Bringing another client into a set situation would be the most therapeutic, least threatening approach. (b)
    2 Transfers nursing responsibility to the physician.
    3 At this point in time, it would not be therapeutic to allow her to remain with solitary pursuits.
    4 Someone has already pointed this out to her, with no results.

104. **1** Since the client has feelings that people are trying to harm her, assignment to a four-bed room would be very threatening. (b)
    2 This seems unlikely since it appears to have started with the transfer to a four-bed room.
    3 This is possible but not likely; schizophrenics have difficulty working out problems.
    4 This is also possible but unlikely; planning an escape is not usually part of a schizophrenic pattern.

105. **2** The client is too anxious to sleep in a four-bed room and should simply be told she is being moved to a private room. (c)
    1 This is false reassurance; does not get to the reason for the problem.
    3 This would not help since she has delusions of being poisoned.
    4 Quietly moving her to a private room would be better intervention at this time.

106. **3** Sitting quietly gives the client the message that the nurse accepts her feelings and cares. (a)
    1 This in effect closes the door on any further communication of feeling.
    2 This is negating her feelings and her right to cry if she is upset.
    4 Helping her explore the reason is more therapeutic than giving advice.

107. **4** Needing to be dependent while wanting to be independent creates a struggle that makes all movement psychologically difficult. Symptoms develop and remove psychologic choice, making movement physically impossible. (b)
    1 It is unlikely the feelings would involve his home; rather the people in the home.
    2 This is part but not all of it.
    3 This is also a part of the picture but not the total picture.

108. **3** This type of defense (conversion) tends to be a learned behavioral response that the individual will use when put under stress. (b)
    1 This is not a likely occurrence if he learns to deal with his problems.
    2 Psychiatric treatment may be needed at different times throughout life but usually not on a continuous basis.
    4 Based on what we know of this disorder, it usually returns when the client is under severe stress.

109. **1** The client is caught between two equally compelling needs, and movement is impossible. Paralysis justifies to the client the inability to move. (b)
    2 It is an unconscious method of solving a conflict.
    3 It is necessary for the client to focus on the problem causing the disorder, not on other things.
    4 It is more important that he learn how to deal with his own feelings before dealing with his wife and mother.

110. **2** From the history the nurse can determine that the client's contacts were limited, her schedule fixed, and her demands on self quite rigid. (b)
    1 The situation gives no evidence of this.
    3 The situation gives no evidence of this.
    4 The situation gives no evidence of this.

111. **2** Her suicidal impulses take priority, and she must be stopped from acting on them while her treatment is in progress. (b)
    1 Safety is the primary responsibility.
    3 This is an internal process; reassurance will not necessarily make it happen; safety is the priority.
    4 This has a very low order of priority.

112. **1** These clients can usually be fairly easily distracted by planned involvement in repetitious simple tasks. (b)
    2 This would be abusive treatment for a client with a need to pace and would reinforce her belief that she should be punished.
    3 This should be employed only if her restlessness could not be controlled with other measures.
    4 She may perceive this isolation as a punishment, and it would not allow for observation by the staff.

113. **4** Points out reality while accepting the fact that the client believes they are real. (b)
    1 Does the nurse know this to be a fact? They may not.
    2 The opposite is true; she does believe she is a bad woman.
    3 This is reality but not supportive.

114. **2** The nurse's response again urges the client to reflect on feelings and encourages communication of feeling tones. (c)
    1 "Why" asks her to draw a conclusion, which she may not be able to do.
    3 This is not what she is asking the nurse; closes the door to further communication.
    4 This is shifting responsibility from the nurse to the doctor; is an evasion technique.

115. **3** Clients frequently report suicidal feelings so the staff will have the chance to stop them. They really ask, "Do you care enough to stop me?" (c)

    1 This may be true; but, more important, she is seeking help and protection.
    2 This could be true but is an unlikely motivation for the behavior.
    4 This could be true but is an unlikely motivation for the behavior.

116. **4** The client is using this compulsive behavior to control anxiety. She needs to continue with it until the anxiety is reduced and more acceptable methods are developed to handle it. (b)
    1 This would greatly increase anxiety; compulsive behavior is a defense that cannot be interrupted until new defenses are learned.
    2 This would not reduce the client's anxiety since she is aware that doorknobs are not contaminated but cannot stop the compulsive act.
    3 This would not reduce the client's anxiety since she is aware that doorknobs are not contaminated but cannot stop the compulsive act.

117. **2** By carrying out the compulsive ritual, the client unconsciously tries to control the situation so that unacceptable impulses and feelings will not be acted on. (b)
    1 This mechanism does not operate on a conscious level.
    3 Hallucinations are not part of a phobic disorder.
    4 They feel no need to punish others.

118. **2** Helping clients understand that a behavior is being used to control impulses usually make them more amenable to psychotherapy. (b)
    1 This would only mask symptoms and would not get at the root of what is bothering her.
    3 Part of her treatment may be with activities to help herself, not others.
    4 The client usually understands this already.

119. **3** The client with an organic mental disorder rarely expresses any concern about personal appearance. The staff must meet most of the needs in this area. (a)
    1 Resistance to change is a symptom of this disorder.
    2 The past is where they feel more comfortable as opposed to the threatening present.
    4 Typical of this disorder is a short attention span and little or no interest in new activities.

120. **1** When an elderly person's brain atrophies, some unusual deposits of iron are scattered on nerve cells. Throughout the brain, areas of deeply staining amyloid, called senile plaques, can be found; these plaques are end stages in the destruction of brain tissue. (c)
    2 It is a chronic deterioration, not one with remissions and exacerbations.
    3 This may or may not be part of the disorder.
    4 Senile psychosis may also be caused by multiple infarcts of the brain.

121. **1** Clients with this disorder need a simple environment. Because of brain cell destruction, they are unable to make choices. (b)
    2 A well-balanced diet is important throughout life not just during senescence; a diet high in carbohydrates and protein may be lacking other nutrients such as fats.
    3 Physical and emotional needs must be met on a continuous basis, not just at a fixed time.
    4 The client is incapable of making choices; this will only increase her anxiety.

122. **3** The senile client attempts to utilize defense mechanisms that have worked in the past but uses them in an exaggerated manner. Because of brain cell destruction such clients are unable to focus on one defense mechanism or develop new ones. (b)
    1 The client is incapable of developing new defense mechanisms at this time.

2 The senile client will depend on old familiar defense mechanisms.

4 The client is not capable of focusing on one defense mechanism.

123. **2** Damaged brain cells do not regenerate. Care is therefore directed toward preventing further damage and providing protective and supportive care. (b)

1 The deterioration of the brain cells makes an extensive reeducation program unrealistic.

3 A client with this disorder may not be able to grasp, understand, or enjoy new leisure activities.

4 It is beyond the scope of her ability to function in a group therapy session.

124. **1** The client who has an organic mental disorder will be most comfortable with the familiar and repetitive daily routine since it creates less anxiety. (b)

2 Cognitive changes would make this unrealistic.

3 It would be beyond her capabilities to develop new social skills.

4 The memory impairment might make this impossible.

125. **3** Simply states facts without getting involved in role conflict. (b)

1 Being a doctor is a big part of his self-esteem, and by her remark the nurse is threatening that self-esteem.

2 Firm consistent limits need to be set and the nurse-client role established.

4 Threats will only make the situation worse and set the tone for future nurse-client interactions.

126. **2** The client has the right to decide how he will be introduced, and the staff should accept his wishes. (b)

1 For whom is it better—the staff, the other clients, or the client?

3 It gives dignity to clients to allow them to be addressed as they wish.

4 The client is a doctor, and the nurse is attacking his concept of himself.

127. **2** A client out of control needs controls set for him. Staff must understand that the client is not deliberately setting out to disrupt the unit. (c)

1 Ignoring him will not stop his disruptive behavior; the nurse has a responsibility to the other clients.

3 This is demeaning him in the eyes of the other clients, not dealing with the problem directly.

4 This may be a last resort taken to solve the problem but should not be used until other alternatives are explored.

128. **4** The hyperactive client is usually rather easily distracted, so the excess energy can be redirected into constructive channels. (a)

1 The client will talk a great deal with no encouragement.

2 There is nothing to indicate at this time that he is not in touch with reality.

3 He will not be able to stay long enough with one thing to finish it.

129. **1** This will help reduce the client's anxiety, thereby reducing hyperactivity. (b)

2 It is not possible physically to control his hyperactivity.

3 He is not capable of choosing activities at this time.

4 He is not capable of controlling his overactive behavior; setting verbal limits will not be effective.

130. **4** Hyperactive clients frequently will not take the time to sit down to eat because they are over-involved in everything that is going on. (b)

1 This is indicative of a depressive episode.

2 The client probably gives no thought to food; he is involved with activity in the environment.

3 He is unable to sit long enough with the other clients to eat a meal; this is not conscious avoidance.

131. **3** The hyperactive client will frequently eat hand foods that do not require sitting down to eat. (b)

1 He will most likely ignore the tray.

2 Unworthy feelings are part of a depressive episode.

4 Unlikely that the client would understand or care about this piece of information.

132. **1** Hyperactive behavior in individuals such as this is typical of the hypermanic flight into reality associated with mood disorders. (a)

2 A flat affect and apathy are more indicative of a schizophrenic disorder.

3 The symptoms are more indicative of a mood than a personality disorder.

4 Depression, loss of interest in usual activities, and poor appetite are more indicative of a major depression than of a personality disorder.

133. **3** Recognizing it as part of the illness makes it easier to tolerate, but limits must be set for the benefit of the staff and other clients. Setting limits also demonstrates to the client that the nurse cares enough to stop her. (b)

1 This statement shows little understanding or tolerance of the illness.

2 This statement demonstrates a rejection of the client and little understanding of the illness.

4 Ignoring the behavior is a form of rejection; client is not using the behavior for attention.

134. **2** Hyperactive clients burn up large quantities of calories, which must be replenished. Since these clients will not take the time to sit down to eat, providing them with food they can carry with them sometimes helps. (b)

1 An exercise in futility for the nurse.

3 The client will probably not be aware of any hunger and could go without food for a dangerously long time.

4 She is not presently capable of preparing her own food.

135. **1** Physical activity will help utilize some of the excess energy without requiring her to make decisions or forcing other clients to deal with her. (c)

2 The client needs guidance herself; would not be able to guide others.

3 She would greatly disrupt the unit with her excess activity and bossiness.

4 Her extreme activity would limit her ability to sit and write or concentrate.

136. **4** Having her wear her own clothes helps keep her more in touch with reality. (b)

1 The client will need help with her makeup, since she will probably go to extremes with it.

2 This is not helping her learn new and better ways to deal with situations.

3 This may set her up as a target of ridicule by the other clients.

137. **3** Behavior demonstrates increased anxiety. Since it was directed toward the new staff, it was probably precipitated by their arrival. (b)

1 This is also possible, but the remark is more indicative of increased anxiety.

2 The client is aware of where she is and who she is at this time.

4 The client is not filling her "life-of-the-party" role; is resorting to previous coping behavior in the face of extreme stress.

138. **3** The nurse must base nursing intervention on a client's problems. Since major depression is due to the client's feelings of self-rejection, it is important for the nurse to have the client identify these feelings before a plan of action can be taken. (b)
    1 This is asking the client to draw a conclusion; he may be unable to do so at this time.
    2 Asking why does not let a client explore his feelings; usually elicits an "I don't know" response.
    4 This is beyond the scope of his abilities at present; he would rather have the nurse tell him how staff can help him help himself.

139. **4** This attitude conveys to others that the client feels he is not really significant enough for anyone to listen to. (b)
    1 Indicative of his feelings of sadness not self-effacement.
    2 Initiative and self-effacement are two different factors.
    3 The gestures and affect as described are appropriate to his inner feelings of depression.

140. **2** Directness is the best approach at the first interview, since this sets the focus and concern and lets the nurse know what the client is feeling now. (b)
    1 This would be one resource for input; but regarding suicide, it is best to approach the client directly.
    3 This may be helpful during the course of treatment, but initially the direct approach with the client is best.
    4 At this point he is most likely unable to think past the present much less deal with future plans; too general a question.

141. **4** This is the most therapeutic approach. The staff member also provides the client with special attention to meet his dependency needs and reduce his self-defeating attitude. (c)
    1 This would be part of intervention; but, in addition, he will need 24-hour observation.
    2 This is negating his feelings and cutting off further communication.
    3 This is unrealistic since the nurse cannot be with him constantly until his depression lifts.

142. **1** Routines should be kept simple and no demands should be made that the client cannot meet. The client is depressed, and all his reactions will be slow. Putting pressure on him will only increase his anxiety and feelings of worthlessness. (c)
    2 This would feed into his feelings of unworthiness and his frustration.
    3 The client will have to focus on his own strengths, not on family strengths.
    4 Feelings of worth must come from within the individual; the nurse must reassure the client through actions not words.

143. **2** The client is expressing his hostility symbolically by not being cooperative. He has a right to feel this way. If members of the staff criticize him, it will only increase his feelings of guilt. (c)
    1 This will not change his mind about the activities; does not show an understanding of his needs.
    3 This will only serve to increase his feelings of guilt since he is unaware of the hostility.
    4 This would be allowing him to manipulate the environment.

144. **3** The client is very dependent, and such individuals can never get enough attention to fill their dependence. This unfulfilled need causes anger, which he has problems expressing for fear of losing the person on whom he is dependent. (c)
    1 He is well able to express his feelings of low self-esteem.

    2 He is well able to express remorse and guilt.
    4 He is expressing the need for comfort.

145. **1** Clients fear this therapy because of the expected pain. If they are reassured that they will be asleep and have no pain, there will be less anxiety and more cooperation. (b)
    2 No treatment requiring anesthesia is totally safe.
    3 He may not be able to realize his fears and thus not ask questions; statement cuts off future communication.
    4 This is not true.

146. **3** The development of glaucoma is one of the side effects of imipramine (Tofranil), and the client should be alerted to these symptoms. (c)
    1 Tofranil is not an MAOI.
    2 This is true of MAOIs.
    4 This would be essential for a person being treated with lithium.

147. **2** This response demonstrates understanding that the newly discharged client needs to have the support of the therapeutic unit when he goes home. He needs to feel that in a crisis he can turn to them for his support. (b)
    1 The role of the nurse was not to become a good friend but to aid the client in becoming a functioning being again.
    3 Unprofessional and blurs the roles of nurse and client.
    4 False reassurance.

148. **4** The client is in the hospital for treatment and evaluation, not judgment of behavior. Since he feels people will judge him. it is important to point out that at this time he is the only one filling this role. (c)
    1 The nurse would be ignoring his feelings and not helping him deal with the situation.
    2 This may or may not be true and could be false reassurance.
    3 The nurse does not know this to be a fact.

149. **4** Lets the client know the nurse realizes he is having difficulty without asking direct questions or focusing on his specific behavior. (a)
    1 This is an avoidance technique.
    2 This would be negating his feelings.
    3 Stated more like an order rather than offering an opportunity to express his feelings.

150. **3** By staying physically close, the nurse conveys to the client the message that someone cares enough to be there and that she is a person worth caring for. (c)
    1 The client is incapable of telling anyone what is bothering her.
    2 Sitting still will increase the tension she is experiencing.
    4 This would not be an initial nursing intervention.

151. **2** When tension is reduced, anxiety diminishes and the person feels more comfortable, safe, and secure. (b)
    1 This action would have an effect on psychologic rather than physical discomfort.
    3 This is what the person hopes will happen but does not.
    4 There would be less anxiety if they were able to deny the situation.

152. **2** Anxiety is a normal human response, causing both physical and emotional changes that everyone experiences when faced with stressful situations. (b)
    1 The fear may be related to a specific aspect of rather than the total environment.
    3 Anxiety is experienced to a greater or lesser degree by every person.
    4 Anxiety does not operate from the conscious level.

153. **1** Providing support, understanding, and acceptance of feelings that the client is experiencing is essential for reducing stress. (b)
    2 This would most likely have the effect of increasing anxiety.
    3 What would happen on the nurse's day off? Concern about this would increase anxiety.
    4 The hospital provides the client with a safe, accepting environment in which to face problems and discuss emotionally charged areas.
154. **1** The "fight or flight" responses of the autonomic nervous system would be stimulated and result in these findings. (b)
    2 The "fight or flight" response is not aided by constricted pupils and bronchioles and hypoglycemia.
    3 The pulse rate would be increased, and blood sugar would increase not decrease.
    4 The pupils would dilate not constrict, and the blood sugar would increase not decrease.
155. **4** Learning a variety of coping mechanisms helps reduce anxiety in stressful situations. (a)
    1 Prolonged exposure would increase anxiety to possibly uncontrollable levels.
    2 Fearful situations can never be viewed as pleasurable.
    3 A person must learn to cope with unpleasant objects and events.
156. **3** The client with a conversion disorder literally converts the anxiety to the symptom. Once the symptom develops, it acts as a defense against the anxiety and the client is diagnostically almost anxiety free. (b)
    1 In a conversion disorder the reactions the nurse would expect to encounter are not in proportion to the disability; therefore the client would not be greatly depressed.
    2 The conflict is resolved by the paralysis in her legs; therefore the anxiety is under control.
    4 Just the opposite is true.
157. **2** The physical symptoms are not the client's major problem and therefore should not be the focus for care. This is a psychologic problem, and the focus should be on this level. (b)
    1 This would be focusing on the physical symptoms of her conflict; the client is not ready to give this up.
    3 The disorder operates on an unconscious level but is very real to the client; denies feelings.
    4 Psychotherapy would have to come before physical therapy.
158. **2** The client's anxiety results from being unable to choose psychologically between two conflicting actions. The conversion to a physical disability removes the choice and therefore reduces the anxiety. (c)
    1 The anxiety is put under control by the conversion to a physical disability.
    3 The anxiety is decreased, and the conversion disorder operates on an unconscious level.
    4 The anxiety is internalized into a physical symptom.
159. **3** The symptoms are problematic to the client and thus have caused emotional pain that is beyond conscious control. (a)
    1 Ignoring the client's complaints will increase anxiety.
    2 Willpower does not enter into it; conversion disorder operates on an unconscious level.
    4 There is no evidence that this is so.
160. **3** Recognizes the importance of feelings and provides an opening so the client may talk about her feelings. (b)
    1 The client is not going to believe this, and it is not helping the client express her feelings.
    2 The nursing goal is to help people function outside the hospital environment, not be afraid to leave it.

4 A statement like this avoids the real issue and solves nothing.
161. **2** Puts focus on the feelings, not on a statement of what did or did not happen. (b)
    1 This statement does not give him an opportunity to explore his feelings.
    3 Implies that the client may have had some part in causing Sally's death.
    4 This statement closes the door to any further communication of feelings or fears.
162. **2** Ambivalence about life and death plus the introspection commonly found in clients with emotional problems would lead to increased anxiety and fear in the group members. (b)
    1 This will probably be a secondary goal of the group leader.
    3 These feelings must be handled within the support system of other staff members.
    4 It is not a primary goal; but this lack of concern should also be explored later on to see what is behind such apparent indifference, which may be a mask to cover feelings.
163. **2** The first step in a nursing care plan should be the establishment of a meaningful relationship because it is through this relationship that the client can be helped. (b)
    1 The situation states that she was admitted when she refused to get out of bed; encouraging this behavior would not be therapeutic.
    3 Reduction of stimuli may help in regard to the hallucinations, but there is no evidence she is not eating her meals.
    4 This would be a long-term goal.
164. **2** Assisting clients with grooming keeps them in contact with reality and allows them to see that staff members care enough to help. It also places value on appearance. (a)
    1 A one-to-one relationship would be best initially.
    3 This would be a long-term goal.
    4 She may withdraw even more.
165. **4** Sets limits on her behavior as well as shows the client that staff care enough to protect her. It accepts the client but rejects the behavior. (c)
    1 It would be unrealistic as well as cruel to do this.
    2 The nurse has a responsibility to the other clients to limit the behavior.
    3 This is a punishment rather than a setting of limits.
166. **3** Echolalia is repetition of another person's remarks, words, or statements. It occurs when individuals are fearful of saying their own words and therefore just echo the words of others. (b)
    1 This is a thought process connected with associative looseness.
    2 Echopraxia is the reflecting of observed movements rather than of speech.
    4 This is when new words are coined or old words take on private symbolic meanings.
167. **3** The client is voiding on the floor not to express hostility but because she is confused. Taking her to the toilet frequently limits the voiding in inappropriate places. (b)
    1 A form of punishment for something the client cannot control.
    2 Not realistic; will have no effect on the problem.
    4 If the client were doing this to express hostility, such action would be useful; but not when the client is unable to control herself.

168. **1** The client needs limits set. This response by the nurse sets limits and rejects the behavior but accepts the client. (b)
  2 A degrading remark; serves no useful purpose.
  3 A punishing action; shows no support or acceptance of the client.
  4 Does not help raise the client to a functioning level.

169. **3** Lets the client know the nurse is available if needed. It also demonstrates an acceptance of her. (b)
  1 Although it is important to note the incident on the chart, it does not take precedence over letting the client know the nurse is there if needed.
  2 Another client's perception of the incident may or may not be valid.
  4 An avoidance technique; shows a lack of acceptance of the client as a person.

170. **4** A delusion is a fixed, false personal belief that is not founded in reality. (a)
  1 A distortion in thought process associated with schizophrenic disorders.
  2 This would be a misinterpretation of a sensory stimulus.
  3 A perceived experience that occurs in the absence of an actual sensory stimulus.

171. **2** The nurse's response reflects on the client's feelings rather than focuses on verbalization. (b)
  1 Puts the client on the defensive, asks for verification that the nurse is indeed a good person; fails to focus on the feeling behind the statement.
  3 Focuses on the statement rather than on the feeling behind the statement.
  4 Dismisses the client's feelings.

172. **2** Clients are confused when they awaken after electroconvulsive therapy. They have a loss of recent memory, so it is important to orient them to time, place, and situation. (b)
  1 This would not be appropriate for a client who has just awakened after a treatment.
  3 This would be a later action, if the client asked for food.
  4 This is not necessary.

173. **2** The anniversary frequently reemphasizes the feeling of loss and abandonment and serves to heighten the current feelings of depression and hopelessness. (c)
  1 Length of time has less influence than the anniversary of a loss.
  3 Suicide risk may still be a factor at this time but less than at the anniversary of a loss.
  4 This would be an important consideration, but the anniversary of the loss of a loved one would take precedence.

174. **3** Gives the client the nonverbal message that someone cares and that she is worthy of attention and concern. (b)
  1 She is incapable of making decisions at this time.
  2 Depressed clients often have too much thinking time.
  4 The concentration required for chess is too much for the client at this time.

175. **2** Telling the client the nurse will spend time with her communicates that she is worthy of the nurse's time and that the nurse cares. (c)
  1 It is unlikely that she would respond to the nurse since she feels so unworthy and depressed.
  3 Does not show the acceptance and care that sitting with her would.
  4 She may be unable, at this point, to expend energy on anything outside herself.

176. **3** Depression is usually both emotional and physical, so a simple daily routine is the least stressful and least anxiety producing. (b)
  1 A depressed client has limited interest in simple activities; too many may increase the anxiety.
  2 Too many stimuli increase the anxiety in a depressed client.
  4 Such a client may be incapable of making even simple decisions.

177. **2** Naloxone hydrochloride (Narcan) is a narcotic antagonist that counteracts and reverses the respiratory depressive action of narcotics without causing sedation or analgesia; nalorphine (Nalline) could also be used but can precipitate a severe withdrawal reaction. (b)
  1 A CNS stimulant with no therapeutic use for a narcotic overdose.
  3 A CNS stimulant with no therapeutic use for a narcotic overdose.
  4 A CNS stimulant with no therapeutic use for a narcotic overdose.

178. **3** Narcan is used when narcotic-induced apnea occurs. It competes for CNS receptor sites, thus acting as a narcotic antagonist. (c)
  1 An adverse reaction is cardiovascular irritability.
  2 Narcan does not accelerate the metabolism of heroin; competes for CNS receptor sites.
  4 Not the specific action of this drug; it is given to prevent respiratory arrest.

179. **3** When Narcan is metabolized and its effects are diminished, the respiratory distress caused by the original drug overdose returns. (b)
  1 Narcan counteracts the respiratory depression from heroin overdose.
  2 No known report of this.
  4 Not a known effect after use of Narcan.

180. **4** The strength of this drug is controlled and remains constant from dose to dose, which is uncertain in illicit drugs. (c)
  1 Methadone is a synthetic narcotic and can cause dependence; it is only used in the treatment of heroin addiction.
  2 Not known to have this action.
  3 Used in the medically supervised withdrawal period to treat physical dependence on opiates; substitutes a legal for an illegal drug.

181. **3** The drug is not taken for medical reasons but for the favorable, pleasant, unusual, or desired effects it produces. It is often taken in doses that would be fatal if the individual had not established a tolerance to it. (b)
  1 True but also with psychologic dependence on the drug.
  2 True but also with physiologic need for the drug.
  4 It is a physiologic and psychologic need to take the drug rather than a compulsion.

182. **3** The addict tries to avoid stress and reality. The drug produces a blurring of these feelings to the point that the addict becomes dependent on it. (a)
  1 Later on the psychologic effect is usually more important than the ability to ease pain.
  2 Large doses of narcotics can cause a dreamlike state.
  4 Hard drugs such as cocaine can increase motor activity.

183. **3** The symptoms of withdrawal reach a peak on the third day. (c)
  1 Symptoms begin within 8 hours.
  2 Symptoms become more severe 24 hours later.
  4 Symptoms begin to subside.

184. **1** The addictive personality is marked by low self-esteem, fear of stress, and dependence with poor self-boundaries and the need for immediate gratification. (b)

2 He would be operating on the pleasure principle; would be unable to delay gratification.

3 No evidence to support this.

4 He would have a strong id drive; usually the ego is weak.

185. **1** When methadone is reduced, a craving for narcotics may occur. Without narcotics anxiety will increase, agitation will occur, and the client may try to leave the hospital to secure drugs. (b).

2 Not related to methadone hydrochloride reduction.

3 Not related to reduced methadone hydrochloride dosage.

4 May occur with methadone hydrochloride overdose.

186. **4** Alcoholics have a low self-image and overwhelming guilt feelings. They drink to relieve these feelings, but the drinking only adds to them. (b)

1 It is not with whom but with what that they have the difficulty.

2 The problem is with low self-esteem rather than dependence/independence.

3 There is no evidence of this.

187. **3** Addresses the emotional impact of this hallucination. The nurse's presence can reduce anxiety and provide comfort. (c)

1 This would be entering into the hallucination.

2 This is presenting reality but not offering the comfort of the nurse's presence.

4 Presenting reality but not offering the comfort of the nurse's presence.

188. **2** The individual is unaware of gaps in memory, so the use of stories is an unconscious attempt to deny or cover up the gaps. (a)

1 Denying is blocking out of conscious awareness rather than a coverup for loss of memory.

3 Lying is a deliberate attempt to deceive rather than a face-saving device for loss of memory.

4 Rationalizing would be used to explain and justify his behavior rather than cover up his loss of memory.

189. **4** The client is using denial as a defense against feelings of guilt. (a)

1 May be part of the reason, but the bigger motivating factor is to decrease guilt feelings.

2 Denial would deal more with his own expectations of himself.

3 It would help make him seem more stable rather than independent.

190. **3** Focuses on the client's feelings rather than the organization itself. Organization is effective only when the client is able to discuss feelings openly. (a)

1 It may be too late by that time.

2 False reassurance; AA may give him insight but may not be able to help him cope with his problem.

4 This may or may not be true.

191. **2** Sharing problems with others who are also open and concerned because of similar problems can reduce guilt and shame and begin to increase ego strengths. (a)

1 AA is viewed by some as a crutch in itself.

3 His problems are caused by how he feels about himself.

4 AA is a support group, a self-help group.

192. **4** Members find sympathy, patience, and understanding in the group. They are able to have their dependence needs met while helping others who are even more dependent than themselves. (a)

1 Important for the detoxification stage not overall therapy.

2 Helpful, but does not have the success rate of AA.

3 Not getting at what is causing the alcohol problem.

193. **4** Self-help groups are successful because they support a basic human need for acceptance. A feeling of comfort and safety and a sense of belonging may be achieved in a nonjudgmental, supportive, sharing experience with others. (b)

1 AA would not meet the client's need to be trusted.

2 If the client had a need to grow, AA would not be able to meet this need.

3 On the contrary, AA meets dependency needs rather than focusing on independence.

194. **1** Self-help groups deal with behavior and changes in behavior rather than the underlying causes of behavior. Small steps are encouraged and when attained are reinforced by the group. (c)

2 Help to identify with the people in the group is not necessary since they all share the same problem and identify readily.

3 On the contrary, they deal with 1 day at a time.

4 This is not the purpose of this group.

195. **4** According to the philosophy of Alcoholics Anonymous, the alcoholic must identify his or her own need to seek help and is thus the primary rehabilitator. (a)

1 The nurse can give support but is not the primary rehabilitator.

2 The physician can give direction but is not the primary rehabilitator.

3 The entire health team works for the client, but in dealing with alcoholism the client is the primary rehabilitator.

196. **1** Intrinsic motivation, stimulated from within the learner, is essential if rehabilitation is to be successful. Often the client is most emotionally ready for help when he has "hit bottom." Only then is he motivationally ready to face reality and put forth the necessary energy and effort to change his behavior. (a)

2 An important factor but not the most important one.

3 An important factor and a helpful one but not the most important one.

4 An important factor but not the most important one.

197. **4** Past level of success demonstrates ego strengths that can be built on. (b)

1 This constitutes only a crisis situation, not necessarily a poor prognosis.

2 His premorbid personality must be fairly sound since he is in his second year of college and thus has achieved some success.

3 Intelligence has little to do with his recovery, but his ego strengths play a big part.

198. **3** Helps the client realize that staff members care about him and that he is worthy of care. (b)

1 An evasive tactic by the nurse.

2 A response that places the client on the defensive.

4 An inappropriate response to a rather obvious situation.

199. **3** Encourages the client to talk about feelings without really setting the focus for the discussion. (b)

1 Would make the client wonder where the nurse had been for 4 days.

2 Shifts the responsibility of care to the doctor rather than dealing with it directly.

4 Cuts off any further communication of feelings; ignores what he has expressed to the nurse.

200. **4** The nurse failed to use knowledge regarding suicidal clients and did not protect the client from this everpresent danger. This failure could be legally defined as negligence. (b)

1 If the unit was left unlocked, this would not be constant supervision.

2 Clients are in more danger of suicide when they are coming out of depression.

3 Clients need observation even after depression has lifted, especially when plans for discharge are pending.

201. **1** Improvement is usually seen within 48 hours to 3 weeks with this monamine oxidase inhibitor. (b)

2 May need a longer time to see an effect from this medication.

3 Not true; this monamine oxidase inhibitor works within 48 hours to 3 weeks.

4 Not true; this monamine oxidase inhibitor works within 48 hours to 3 weeks.

202. **2** Wine, aged cheese, and other foods with a high tyramine level must be avoided. (b)

1 Not true for this medication.

3 No photosensitivity reported in clients on this medication.

4 This is not an expected side effect but can occur as an adverse reaction.

203. **3** An art project that she could work on successfully at her own pace would be important. (b)

1 Used mostly for severely regressed clients and at this point may not be appropriate for this client.

2 This would require too much concentration and increase the client's feelings of despair.

4 This would require too much concentration and increase the client's feelings of despair.

204. **4** A major part of depression involves an inability to accept ourselves as we are, which leads to making unrealistic demands on others to meet our needs. (c)

1 She needs to develop a more effective manner of coping, not new defense mechanisms.

2 Not important or crucial to her recovery.

3 A short-term goal would be to talk about her depressed feelings; a long-term goal would be to look at what is causing those feelings.

205. **4** A reflection of her feelings that allows her to either validate or correct the nurse. (b)

1 A response that gives advice and does not allow the client to explore her feelings.

2 An uncalled for statement that does not allow the client to explore her feelings.

3 Delays confronting the problem and avoids exploring her feelings.

206. **3** An occipital headache is the beginning of a hypertensive crisis that results from excessive tyramine. (b)

1 It would be a rise in blood pressure, not a drop.

2 Unrelated to ingestion of tyramine.

4 Unrelated to ingestion of tyramine.

207. **4** The withdrawal regimen is usually gradually decreasing doses of a barbiturate in order to prevent the severe symptoms associated with barbiturate withdrawal. (c)

1 Used for narcotic addiction withdrawal.

2 Used in the treatment of affective disorders.

3 Contraindicated in the presence of central nervous system depressants.

208. **1** A serious side effect that may happen with abrupt withdrawal from barbiturates. (b)

2 Not associated with barbiturate withdrawal.

3 Not associated with barbiturate withdrawal.

4 Not associated with barbiturate withdrawal.

209. **3** An important aspect of the role of the psychiatric nurse is primary, secondary, and tertiary intervention to prevent emotional disequilibrium. (b)

1 Only a small part of the role of the psychiatric nurse; a role usually shared with others on the health team.

2 Only a small part of the role of the psychiatric nurse; a role usually shared with others on the health team.

4 Only a part of the role of the psychiatric nurse, since psychiatry is concerned with people with varying degrees of mental and emotional disorders.

210. **2** It is the inability to meet these needs that will cause a person to become mentally ill. (b)

1 Not necessary to be mentally healthy.

3 To be considered mentally healthy a person must be more than just free from illness.

4 This would rule out most of the population.

Chapter 5: Pediatric Nursing

1. **4** Play during infancy (solitary) promotes physical development. For example, mobiles strengthen eye movement, large beads promote fine finger movement, and soft toys encourage tactile sense. (a)

1 Play during infancy is usually initiated by the parent.

2 Children do not begin to share until the preschool years.

3 Play is important throughout childhood.

2. **3** Walking is the primary developmental task of this age group. The other choices are not applicable to this age group. (b)

1 A child learns to climb stairs at around 18 months of age.

2 The ability to drink from a cup is not developed until 18 months.

4 Learning to walk takes precedence over learning to talk; speaking is not a primary task at this age.

3. **1** Role playing encourages expression of feelings through behavior, since children's ability to verbalize feelings is limited. (b)

2 The preschooler is too young to think about careers.

3 This may occur, but it is not a purpose of role playing.

4 Although preschoolers may try to imitate adults, providing guidelines for adult behavior is premature.

4. **1** Although there is a time range, there is no specific time for a developmental task. (b)

2 Children differ in the ages at which they learn tasks.

3 Tasks are more often learned in spurts than at a uniform rhythm.

4 The entire life cycle requires the learning of developmental tasks.

5. **2** If food is used early as praise or punishment, the older child or adult will either undereat or overeat at times of stress to decrease anxiety. (b)

1 Eating is a social as well as a nutritional process.

3 This does not usually cause nutritional problems.

4 This is important for teaching good eating habits in later life and, therefore preventing certain nutritional problems.

6. **1** The early school-age child has become a cooperative member of the family and will mimic parents' attitudes and food habits readily. (b)

2 The peer group does not become highly influential until later school age and during adolescence.

3 This does not have a major influence on later eating habits.

4 This certainly has some influence, though not major, on later eating habits.

7. **4** When the causative organism is isolated, it is tested for antimicrobial susceptibility (sensitivity) to various antimicrobial agents. When an organism is sensitive to a medication, the medication is capable of destroying the organism. (b)

1 Inappropriate answer.

2 Although this is considered, the selection of drugs is based primarily on the ability of the drug to destroy the specific organism.

3 Although the physician's preference is considered, the selection of drugs is based primarily on the ability of the drug to destroy the specific organism.

8. **2** The tetracyclines are not recommended during periods of tooth development (children under 8 years of age or in pregnant women during the later half of pregnancy) because they may permanently discolor teeth yellow, gray, or brown. (b)

1 This is not an expected complication of tetracycline.

3 Anemia is not a common condition for 6-year-olds; thrombocytopenia is a very rare complication.

4 Tetracycline does not interfere with bone structure of school-age children or pregnant women.

9. **1** Rubeola, or measles, is generally a viral-induced childhood disease, diagnosed on or about the second day by the presence of Koplik's spots on the oral mucosa. (a)

2 Rubella is manifested by a rash but not by Koplik's spots.

3 Chickenpox is manifested by a maculopapular rash; no Koplik's spots are present.

4 Neither a rash nor Koplik's spots occur with mumps.

10. **3** Invasion of the posterior (dorsal) root ganglia by the same virus that causes chickenpox can result in herpes zoster, or shingles. This may be due to reactivation of a previous chickenpox virus that has lain dormant in the body or by fresh contact with an individual who has chickenpox. (a)

1 Athlete's foot is caused by a fungus.

2 Infectious hepatitis is caused by a virus, but not the herpesvirus.

4 German measles is caused by a virus, but not the herpesvirus.

11. **4** Corticosteroids (e.g., cortisol) cause involution of lymphatic tissue and resultant depression of the immune response. Antineoplastic drugs or high-energy radiation preferentially destroys tissues with high mitotic rates, including lymphatic tissue and bone marrow, where antibody production and other immune responses take place. (a)

1 Inappropriate answer; no more true for these than for other children.

2 This is not a reason to withhold immunizations.

3 The measles vaccine does not contain rabbit serum.

12. **1** The injected bacteria in the vaccine have been so modified that they do not cause active infection but still elicit an immune response. (b)

2 This is an antibody capable of neutralizing a specific toxin.

3 This is a modified toxin, whose poisonous properties are destroyed but that is still capable of producing antibodies.

4 This is a poisonous substance released from bacterial cells.

13. **4** In passive artificial immunity an antibody made in another organism is injected into the infected or presumed infected person to provide immediate immunity to the invading organism. (b)

1 This type of immunity takes too much time to develop; this client needs immediate protection.

2 This type of immunity takes too much time to develop; this client needs immediate protection.

3 This type of immunity is probably not applicable in this case, for passive natural immunity is acquired from the mother and is effective only during the first few months of the child's life.

14. **1** In active natural immunity the infected person's immune system responds to the invading organism by producing antibodies specific for the invader. (c)

2 Active artificial immunity is acquired by the injection of antigens, after which the individual develops antibodies.

3 Passive natural immunity is acquired by the fetus from the mother.

4 Passive artificial immunity is acquired through injection of antibodies.

15. **1** Rubeola, or measles, produces coldlike respiratory symptoms and, after 3 or 4 days, a dark red macular or maculopapular skin rash. Complications include convulsions in young children and secondary infection with hemolytic steptococci, pneumococci, or staphylococci. Such infection can result in otitis media and pneumonia, which are especially dangerous in children under 2 years of age. (c)

2 This is the most benign communicable disease of childhood; complications are rare.

3 Yellow fever does not have respiratory complications.

4 Chickenpox does not usually include respiratory inflammation, although pneumonia may occur as a complication.

16. **1** Adequate immunizations for normal preschool children include DTP and OPV at 4 to 6 years. (c)

2 Measles vaccine is normally given between 12 and 15 months of age.

3 Rubella vaccine is normally given between 12 and 15 months of age.

4 The tuberculin test is not an immunization.

17. **2** Antibodies received in utero through the placenta and in the newborn through the mother's milk provide the baby with immunity against most bacterial, viral, and fungal infections during the first several weeks after birth. Then, as the titer of maternal antibodies drops and is not replaced by the child's own antibodies, prolonged and repeated infection occurs. (a)

1 This probably does not occur in children born without an immune system.

3 Bacteria do not produce antibodies.

4 This is not enough to prevent infection in these children.

18. **1** Since part of a nurse's responsibility is to foresee potential harm and prevent risks, it is imperative that the nurse not only take a health history and perform a physical assessment on each client, but also ensure the safety of the client. (c)

2 This is not true and cannot be accepted as a rationale for inaction.

3 High temperatures are common in children but are nonetheless a valid cause for concern.

4 The nurse and physician share interdependent roles in the assessment and care of clients.

19. **2** A common side effect of long-term phenytoin (Dilantin) therapy is hyperplasia of the gingiva. (c)

1 Dilantin does not affect urinary output.

3 Dilantin does not influence pupillary response.

4 Dilantin does not cause flushing.

20. **1** Chickenpox, mumps, and rubeola are all caused by a virus and may be followed by encephalitis. (c)

2 Pertussis is caused by a bacterium and does not result in encephalitis.

3 Although polio is caused by a virus, it does not result in encephalitis.

4 Scarlet fever is caused by a bacterium and does not result in encephalitis.

21. **3** The virus for polio damages the anterior horn cells of the spinal cord with a typical irregular and asymmetric pattern. The cervical and lumbar regions contain more anterior horn cells, and therefore the extremities are more frequently affected than the trunk. (b)

 1 The virus for rubeola does not affect the motor cells of the anterior horn of the spinal cord.

 2 The virus for rubella does not affect the motor cells of the anterior horn of the spinal cord.

 4 The virus for chickenpox does not affect the motor cells of the anterior horn of the spinal cord.

22. **4** Rheumatic fever is an inflammatory disease involving the joints, heart, CNS, and subcutaneous tissue. It is believed to be an autoimmune process that causes connective tissue damage. (b)

 1 Whooping cough is not caused by a streptococcus and does not include the symptoms listed.

 2 Measles is caused by a virus and does not include the symptoms listed.

 3 Tetanus is not caused by a streptococcus and does not include the symptoms listed.

23. **4** Impetigo is a bacterial infection of the skin caused by streptococci or staphylococci. Group A hemolytic streptococci cause rheumatic fever and glomerulonephritis. (b)

 1 This is a viral condition; not associated with rheumatic fever or glomerulonephritis.

 2 This infectious condition of the skin is a result of infestation by mites; not associated with rheumatic fever or glomerulonephritis.

 3 Intertrigo is a superficial dermatitis in the folds of the skin; not associated with rheumatic fever or glomerulonephritis.

24. **3** Respiratory tract obstructions usually occur in the larynx, trachea, or major bronchi (usually right). Hoarseness may indicate vocal cord injury. Unintelligible speech may indicate an interference in the flow of air out of the respiratory tract and/or obstruction or injury to the larynx. (b)

 1 Acute respiratory infection usually has a gradual onset.

 2 In view of the sudden onset of clinical signs and the age of the child, this is unlikely.

 4 A retropharyngeal abscess would not produce the clinical signs listed.

25. **2** Thrush, also called moniliasis, usually affects the mucous membranes of the oral cavity, causing painful white patches. Individuals with immunologic deficiencies or those receiving prolonged antibiotic therapy are particularly susceptible to this organism. (b)

 1 This is not caused by yeast, nor does it occur often in infants.

 3 This is not caused by yeast and is not common in the United States or in infants.

 4 This is usually caused by an amoeba or a bacterium; is not common in infants.

26. **2** Grunting and rapid respirations are abnormal behaviors in the infant. Grunting is a compensatory mechanism whereby the infant attempts to keep air in the alveoli to increase arterial oxygenation; increased respirations increase the amount of oxygen and carbon dioxide exchange. (b)

 1 This is not necessarily a sign of illness.

 3 Sweating in infants is usually scanty because of immature functioning of the exocrine glands; profuse sweating is rarely seen in the sick infant.

 4 This is not necessarily indicative of illness.

27. **4** In heart failure there is a decrease in the blood flow to the kidneys, causing sodium and water reabsorption and resulting in peripheral edema. The peripheral edema indicates severe cardiac decompensation. (b)

 1 This may be an early attempt by the body to compensate for decreased cardiac output.

 2 This may be an early attempt by the body to compensate for decreased cardiac output.

 3 This may be an early attempt by the body to compensate for decreased cardiac output.

28. **2** Crying increases the amount of air being brought into the lungs. The flow of air coming into the lungs creates an increase in positive pressure, which helps expand the alveoli and improve gaseous exchange, thereby decreasing cyanosis. In atelectasis some of the alveoli do not expand, which is evidenced by a lack of chest expansion on the affected side. (c)

 1 Decreasing cyanosis with crying is not indicative of neurologic damage.

 3 The heart rate will not provide information about atrioventricular septal defects.

 4 The signs of respiratory distress syndrome are much more severe than transient cyanosis.

29. **3** Chalasia is an incompetent cardiac sphincter, which allows a reflux of gastric contents into the esophagus and eventual regurgitation. Placing the infant in an upright position keeps the gastric contents in the stomach by gravity as well as limits the pressure against the cardiac sphincter. (b)

 1 This will promote regurgitation.

 2 This will probably have little effect on chalasia.

 4 This will promote vomiting since it is too much formula for a week-old infant.

30. **2** Assault is a threat or an attempt to do violence to another. (c)

 1 This is not the appropriate legal definition of assault.

 3 Assault implies harm to persons rather than property.

 4 This definition is too broad to describe assault.

31. **3** Battery means touching in an offensive manner or the actual injuring of another person. (b)

 1 This definition is too broad to describe battery.

 2 Battery refers to harm against persons instead of property.

 4 Battery refers to actual bodily harm rather than threats of physical or psychologic harm.

32. **1** Because phenylalanine is an essential amino acid, it must be provided in quantities sufficient for promoting growth while maintaining safe blood levels. (c)

 2 Phenylalanine is an essential amino acid and cannot be totally removed from the diet.

 3 In PKU phenylalanine accumulates in the blood, causing irreversible CNS damage; additional phenylalanine must be avoided.

 4 All proteins do not contain phenylalanine.

33. **2** Congenital cretinism is the result of insufficient secretion by the thyroid gland due to an embryonic defect. The decreased thyroid hormone has been affecting the infant since before birth during cerebral development, so it is likely that mental development will be retarded. Treatment prior to 3 months will limit damage. (b)

 1 Myxedema is the adult form of cretinism.

 3 Treatment corrects abnormal responses.

 4 This is a term for hyperthyroidism.

34. **2** $\dfrac{0.35\ \text{mg}}{0.25\ \text{mg}} \times \dfrac{x\ \text{ml}}{1\ \text{ml}} = 1.4\ \text{ml}$ (b)

 1 This is too low.

 3 This is too low.

 4 This is too low.

35. **3** This is due to the fact that celiac clients have a gluten-induced enteropathy and are unable to absorb fats from the intestinal tract. (b)
    1 Although stools are large and frothy, they lack color because of incomplete absorption.
    2 Stools are large and fatty or frothy, not mucoid.
    4 Stools are foul smelling, in large quantities, and without color because of incomplete absorption.
36. **1** Rubeola signs and symptoms include a high fever, photophobia, Koplik's spots (white patches on mucous membranes of the oral cavity), and a rash. Rubella usually does not cause a high fever, runs a 3-to-6-day course, and never causes Koplik's spots. (c)
    2 Some symptoms may be similar to those of a severe cold, but are associated with high fever.
    3 These symptoms are not associated with rubeola.
    4 The rash spreads over most of the body.
37. **1** Tap water enemas are hypotonic and are contraindicated; they may cause increased absorption of fluid via the bowel and may upset the balance of fluid in the body. It could also interfere with potassium ion balance, the electrolyte that can be lost via the large intestine. (a)
    2 Preschoolers fear intrusive procedures.
    3 The temperature of the water should be regulated so this does not occur.
    4 The enema would remove only waste products from the bowel.
38. **2** Steroids have an antiinflammatory effect. It is believed that resistance to certain viral diseases, including chickenpox, is greatly decreased when the child is taking steroids regularly. (b)
    1 Since chickenpox is viral, antibiotics would have no effect.
    3 There is no known correlation between chickenpox and these drugs.
    4 There is no known correlation between chickenpox and insulin.
39. **3** Mumps can cause orchitis (inflammation of the testes) in males and oophoritis (inflammation of the ovaries) in females. Although rare, both can render the postpubescent child sterile. (b)
    1 This symptom is not associated with mumps.
    2 This symptom is not associated with mumps.
    4 This symptom is not associated with mumps.
40. **3** Assault is a threat or an attempt to do violence to another, and battery means touching an individual in an offensive manner or the actual injuring of another person. (a)
    1 Although the behavior (scratching) needs to be decreased, this can be done through mittens so as not to immobilize a child of this age.
    2 A 3-year-old does not have the capacity to understand cause (scratching) and effect (bleeding).
    4 The nurse's behavior demonstrates anger and has not taken into account the growth and developmental needs of this age.
41. **4** Tetracycline is potentially hepatotoxic, especially in anyone with liver dysfunction, since it is metabolized in the liver. Signs of hepatotoxicity are lethargy, anorexia, behavioral changes, jaundice, and fatty necrosis. (c)
    1 The decreasing fever and secretions indicate that the infectious process is under control.
    2 Anemia may cause fatigue but is unassociated with withdrawal and irritability.
    3 Common symptoms of bladder infection include burning upon urination, frequency or hesitancy, abdominal pain, and low-grade fever.

42. **3** Decision making fosters and supports independence, a developmental need of the adolescent. It also increases a sense of self-worth and control. (b)
    1 Although this may be true, it is not motivating.
    2 This does not ensure movement but social interaction.
    4 Limit setting meets the security needs of young children.
43. **3** A plaster cast is not flexible and can inhibit circulation. Cold toes, loss of sensation in toes, pain, and inability to move toes should be reported to the physician immediately. (b)
    1 The normal pulse for a 9-year-old ranges from 70 to 110.
    2 It takes 24 to 48 hours for a plaster cast to dry.
    4 This may be related to increased fluid intake.
44. **4** Mineral oil coats the mucosal lining of the stomach and retards absorption of the poison. (c)
    1 Soap, baking soda, and milk of magnesia are all chemical antidotes that neutralize ingested acids.
    2 Strong tea only dilutes the substance to be absorbed and wastes precious treatment time.
    3 A weak salt solution provides no effective immediate treatment.
45. **3** Lye, a basic solution, is neutralized by administration of a weak acid such as vinegar. (c)
    1 This induces vomiting and would cause further burning of tissue when the lye was vomited back through the esophagus.
    2 Milk is useful to soothe irritated mucous membrane but will not inactivate the poison.
    4 Bicarbonate is used to neutralize acids.
46. **2** Ipecac exerts its effect through direct stimulation of the vomiting control center and local irritation of the gastric mucosa, which is enhanced through dilution of the drug in large quantities of fluid. (c)
    1 Resting has no effect on drug efficiency.
    3 The child should be kept calm and quiet.
    4 Ipecac works by stimulating the vomiting control center and local gastric irritation.
47. **3** Prednisone is a synthetic glucocorticoid that has an active antiinflammatory effect by stabilizing lysosomal membranes and thus inhibiting proteolytic enzyme release. (b)
    1 Prednisone has an antiinflammatory effect, which inhibits proteolytic enzyme release.
    2 Prednisone's antiinflammatory effects include inhibiting phagocytosis and preventing or suppressing other clinical evidence of inflammation.
    4 Increased appetite and aggravation of preexisting psychiatric conditions are adverse reactions of prednisone.
48. **1** Vincristine is highly neurotoxic, causing paresthesias, muscle weakness, ptosis, diplopia, paralytic ileus, vocal cord paralysis, and loss of deep tendon reflexes. (c)
    2 Alopecia is reversible with cessation of the drug.
    3 Hematologic effects are rare with vincristine.
    4 The most severe problems associated with vincristine are neurologic and neuromuscular.
49. **4** Excessive crying and clinging are the usual responses of an infant who expects to be comforted, not one who has been separated from a parent because of illness. (a)
    1 Prolonged hospitalization and separation from parenting can cause delayed growth or even death in infants.
    2 Inattentiveness to focus may be learned from failure to gain response from humans in previous experiences.
    3 Withdrawing active attention is the infant's way to "turn off" and may be learned from multiple failure in interactions with stimuli.

50. **2** Infants who have experienced maternal deprivation usually exhibit failure to thrive (i.e., weight below third percentile, developmental retardation, clinical signs of deprivation, and malnutrition). These physical and emotional factors predispose the infant to a variety of illness. (b)
    1 Infants who have experienced maternal deprivation are usually quiet and nonresponsive.
    3 Responsiveness to stimuli is limited or nonexistent.
    4 Weight below the third percentile is characteristic.

51. **2**
$$\frac{20\ mg}{50\ mg} \times \frac{x\ ml}{1\ ml}$$
$$50\ x = 20$$
$$x = 0.4\ ml \qquad (a)$$
    1 This calculation is too high.
    3 This calculation is too high.
    4 This calculation is too high.

52. **1** This defect interferes with the normal diaphragmatic respirations of the newborn. Respirations are further affected by stomach and intestinal distension, a mediastinal shift, atelectasis, and the presence of abdominal organs in the thoracic cavity. Oxygen should be administered via positive pressure by a nonintrusive means such as mask or hood. (c)
    2 An endotracheal tube would be used when there is a concern of upper respiratory or other interference with oxygen reaching the lungs adequately.
    3 The least intrusive method which adequately delivers oxygen should be used.
    4 The defect interferes with normal respirations so oxygen is needed.

53. **4** Following a thoracotomy, negative intrathoracic pressure is reestablished and the alveoli reexpand within 12 to 48 hours. (b)
    1 This time is inadequate for reexpansion to occur.
    2 In some instances, reexpansion will occur sooner than 48 hours.
    3 This time is inadequate for expecting reexpansion.

54. **3**
$$\frac{\text{Total milliliters to be infused} \times \text{Drop factor}}{\text{Total time to be infused in minutes}}$$
$$\frac{1000 \times 60}{1440} = \frac{60,000}{1440} = 41.6\ \text{drops/minute} \qquad (a)$$
    1 Calculations show this is too low to deliver 1000 ml in 24 hours.
    2 Calculations show this is too low to deliver 1000 ml in 24 hours.
    4 Calculations show this is too low to deliver 1000 ml in 24 hours.

55. **3** When the nurse takes a health history, any areas of concern should be explored fully before a nursing diagnosis is made. (a)
    1 Data are inadequate to focus immediately on nutrition.
    2 The nurse needs to gather more data to be able to determine the basis for the problem.
    4 More data are needed before recommendations can be made.

56. **2** Normally there may be a weight gain caused by the influence of hormones prior to the growth spurt. Also, 10-to-12-year olds eat an adult-size meal without the increased metabolic needs of adolescence. (b)
    1 This weight gain is normal and adequate calorie intake is needed for the growth spurt occurring in adolescents.
    3 Before advising increased activity, the nurse would need to assess the client's present activity level.

    4 Family eating patterns have more effect on weight than do genetics.

57. **1** Hepatitis virus B is in the blood during the late incubation and acute stages of the disease. It may also persist in the carrier state for years. It is transmitted when the blood of an infected individual comes in contact with the blood or mucous membranes of another individual. Posttransfusion hepatitis has been reduced now that the surface antigen of hepatitis B (HBsAg) and the antibody to hepatitis B core antigen tests are performed on blood donors and on the blood of carriers of type B virus (a).
    2 Hepatitis A is principally transferred through oral-fecal routes.
    3 Hemophilia treatment products are now safer.
    4 Oral and venereal transmission is a less frequent mode of transmission.

58. **3** Positioning on the right side after feeding facilitates digestion because the pyloric sphincter is on this side and gravity aids in emptying the stomach. (c)
    1 The usual height for elevation of the gastrostomy tube when feeding an infant is 6 to 8 inches.
    2 It is standard procedure to flush the tube after the feeding to ensure that all the formula gets into the stomach.
    4 Feeding may proceed immediately after opening the tube.

59. **3** A pacifier should be given during the feeding to help the infant associate sucking with feeding and the sense of fullness. (b)
    1 Instilling water after the feeding clears the tube.
    2 Although aspiration may be used to ascertain residual stomach content before feeding, it is not necessary when feedings are well tolerated.
    4 Upright positioning is essential to prevent regurgitation or reflux and subsequent aspiration.

60. **3** Isotonic saline is compatible with body fluids. It is neither hypertonic nor hypotonic so it does not cause a change in osmotic pressure and upset the balance of intracellular and extracellular fluid and electrolytes. (b)
    1 Soap suds enemas are water with added soap products and therefore usually hypotonic; this can cause fluid shifts and overloads.
    2 This solution would cause excess fluid loss and therefore be dangerous.
    4 This hypotonic solution might cause fluid and electrolyte imbalances.

61. **4** Amblyopia is reduced visual acuity that may occur when an eye weakened by strabismus is not forced to function. (c)
    1 Only vision in the affected eye will be diminished.
    2 Depth and spatial perceptions are impaired when vision in one eye is severely impaired.
    3 The lack of binocularity could result in impaired depth and spatial perceptions, not dyslexia.

62. **2** Common developmental norms of the toddler, who is struggling for independence, are inability to share easily, egotism, egocentrism, and possessiveness. (b)
    1 This task is too advanced for toddlers and more accurate for preschoolers.
    3 This is true of 4-year-olds.
    4 One characteristic of toddlers is their short attention spans; 15 minutes is too much to expect.

63. **1** Four-year-olds boast, exaggerate, and are impatient, noisy, and selfish. (c)
    2 The tendency toward tantrums and negativism should have waned by the age of 4.

3 Four-year-olds engage in more advanced cooperative play.

4 This is highly unusual for 4-year-olds as they are striving toward more initiative and less dependence.

64. **4** Children 9 to 12 months of age can stand alone with support. By 15 months strength and balance improve, and they can stand and walk alone. (b)

1 This is not usually true until the child is 2 years old.

2 A 10-month-old is capable of this task.

3 Infants are very capable of this.

65. **2** Six-year-olds are aware of their hands as tools and enjoy building simple structures. (b)

1 This is more useful for an older, school-age child, with a longer attention span and a better ability to follow instructions.

3 This is more useful for an older, school-age child, with a longer attention span and a better ability to follow instructions.

4 This is more appropriate for preschoolers.

66. **2** Helps and encourages parents to put their fears and feelings into words. Once these sentiments are expressed, they can at least be examined and dealt with. (b)

1 This would not assist the parents in coping with the problem. Neither would it demonstrate the supportive and empathetic roles of the nurse.

3 This response lacks insight. Parents will worry about their infant anyway.

4 This may or may not be helpful.

67. **1** These children frequently have difficulty in handling secretions as well as breathing after surgery. Nursing measures such as using the partial side-lying position or gently aspirating secretions from the mouth or nasopharynx may be necessary to prevent aspiration and respiratory complications. (a)

2 This is not necessary.

3 Fluids are usually administered carefully by mouth.

4 Although this is important, maintaining a patent airway is essential.

68. **2** Crying should be prevented, since it places tension on the suture line. Frequently an appliance called a Logan bow is taped to the cheeks to relax the operative site, which helps prevent trauma. (b)

1 May also be positioned on the side and on the back with surveillance.

3 The feeding method of choice is by a rubber-tipped syringe or medicine dropper.

4 This is not necessary or desirable.

69. **4** The 2-year-old is still attached to and dependent on the parents. Fear of separation is a great stress. (b)

1 Most likely these will not be remembered accurately.

2 This is neither possible nor desirable.

3 This is not possible in a health care setting.

70. **1** A priority during the immediate postoperative period is protecting the operative site. (a)

2 Two-year-olds can brush their teeth.

3 Normal 2-year-olds have about 16 teeth; although tooth development may not be normal in these children, they usually have them.

4 A toothbrush should be a familiar sight to a 2-year-old and therefore not frightening.

71. **4** David is anemic. A diet of milk only is not sufficient to meet iron needs. Raisins and meat are high in iron, and finger foods are appropriate for toddlers. (b)

1 This is not appropriate for a 1-year-old, nor is it necessary or desirable.

2 Although medical care and monitoring will be required, the metabolic clinic is not the appropriate referral.

3 Weaning from the bottle is not the issue; supplementary iron intake is.

72. **1** Fetal iron reserves are depleted by the fourth to fifth month in the full-term infant and considerably earlier in the premature infant. When exogenous sources of iron are not supplied after depletion of fetal iron stores, iron-deficiency anemia results. (a)

2 Although this is true, it is not an important reason for starting solid foods earlier with this child.

3 The problem is not with bone marrow production of cells but with the production of hemoglobin.

4 Weight control by itself is not the major reason for starting solid foods; the overingestion of milk often seen in anemia frequently causes the infant to be overweight.

73. **1** Milk is a very poor source of iron. If fed in large amounts to the exclusion of solid foods after 4 to 6 months of age, iron-deficiency anemia results. (b)

2 Maternal iron stores are usually adequate for the infant's first 4 to 5 months.

3 This is not a major cause of anemia.

4 Lack of absorption and early introduction of solid foods are not commonly found as problems producing anemia in infants.

74. **4** Folic acid acts as a necessary coenzyme in the formation of heme, the iron-containing protein in hemoglobin. (c)

1 The production of red blood cells does not involve carbohydrates.

2 This is a coenzyme in carbohydrate metabolism.

3 Calcium is not involved in the production of red blood cells.

75. **3** A rich source of iron and is easily digested by infants. (a)

1 This does not contain iron.

2 This contains iron in smaller amounts and is not as easily digestible as cereal.

4 Milk is a poor source of iron.

76. **3** The child should be taken to the dentist between 2 and 3 years of age, when all 20 deciduous teeth have erupted. (a)

1 This is too soon.

2 This is too late.

4 This is too late.

77. **3** Proteins are essential for the synthesis of the blood proteins, albumin, fibrinogen, and hemoglobin. Ascorbic acid influences the removal of iron from feritin (making more iron available for production of heme) and influences the conversion of folic acid to folinic acid. (b)

1 These are not involved in building red blood cells.

2 These are not involved in building red blood cells.

4 These are not involved in building red blood cells.

78. **4** The adult pinworm lives in the rectum or colon and emerges onto the peri-rectal skin during hours of sleep, depositing her eggs during this time. (b)

1 Pinworms attach to the bowel wall and do not emerge from the rectum at this time.

2 Pinworms attach to the bowel wall and do not emerge from the rectum at this time.

3 Pinworms attach to the bowel wall and do not emerge from the rectum at this time.

79. **4** The worm attaches itself to the bowel wall in the cecum and appendix and can damage the mucosa, causing appendicitis. (c)

1 The pinworm does not migrate to the respiratory system.

2 Although pinworms (and their ova) are ingested by mouth, they do not attach there; inflammation of the mouth is not a complication of pinworm.

3 The pinworm does not migrate to the liver.

80. **1** Forty pounds = 18 kg; therefore 5 mg per kilogram × 18 kg = 90 mg. (b)

2 This is an inadequate dose.

3 This is an inadequate dose.

4 This is an overdose.

81. **3** Pyrvinium pamoate (Povan), a cyanine dye, is a deep red, relatively insoluble crystalline powder that stains the stool, vomitus, and most materials. (b)

1 Incorrect answer; does not cause a brown color.

2 Incorrect answer; does not cause a green color.

4 Incorrect answer; does not cause a blue color.

82. **2** Pyrvinium pamoate (Povan), a cyanine dye, is a deep red relatively insoluble crystalline powder that stains the stool, vomitus, and most materials. In this instance, red-stained excreta would not be significant. (b)

1 These complications do not occur with pinworms.

3 This does not occur.

4 Intestinal bleeding does not occur as a result of Povan administration.

83. **4** School-age children lose their primary teeth, which could be aspirated during surgery. The anesthesiologist must take special precautions to maintain client safety. (a)

1 This is important but not essential and not always possible.

2 This is a comforting gesture but is not essential.

3 There is no reason to obtain an ASO titer on the client.

84. **4** The seeping of blood from the operative site increases secretions, which the child adapts to by swallowing frequently. (b)

1 Snoring can be expected in a child who is postoperative from a tonsillectomy.

2 This may be a later sign of hemorrhage. Frequent swallowing would be an initial sign.

3 The child has been NPO for an extended time and is not able to ingest fluids easily because of his sore throat; as a result he will probably be thirsty.

85. **2** Acetaminophen relieves pain and does not cause bleeding tendencies, as does aspirin. The correct dose for this age is 300 mg. (c)

1 Aspirin increases the clotting time and should be avoided.

3 Phenobarbitol will not relieve the pain; it will only sedate the client.

4 Demerol may be given, although a narcotic is not usually necessary for children after tonsillectomy; however, 50 mg would be the normal dose for an adult.

86. **3** A meningomyelocele sac is thinly covered and can be partially open, allowing a portal of entry for organisms directly to the CNS. The sac should be protected. (b)

1 A meningomyelocele will influence the client's ability to control these functions, but control is not developed until the toddler and preschool years.

2 Although this is always an important nursing measure, care of the sac is even more important.

4 Although observation of paralysis is an important nursing measure, care of the meningomyelocele sac is of primary importance.

87. **3** The surgical closure of the sac eliminates the route by which the spinal fluid drains. Skull bones are soft and will expand as fluid increases, causing hydrocephalus. (b)

1 There is no reason to decrease environmental stimuli for infants with hydrocephalus unless they also have seizures.

2 Most infants with meningomyelocele are partially or completely paralyzed in the lower extremities; careful range of motion exercises are one of the important parts of nursing care for these infants.

4 This is not expected since damage to the meninges of the brain is not a factor in the surgical treatment of meningomyelocele.

88. **2** Sucking meets oral needs, which are primary during infancy. (c)

1 Two-day-old infants are not yet developmentally capable of enjoying a soft, cuddly toy.

3 This is not a developmental need.

4 An infant of a few days is probably too young to focus well on a mobile; in addition, he will be placed in a prone or side-lying position postoperatively and thus would not be able to focus on the mobile.

89. **3** Fluids prevent dehydration. Under conditions of decreased oxygen, dehydration promotes the sickling of erythrocytes. (c)

1 This is not necessary.

2 Rigorous exercise will cause sickling.

4 This is not necessary or helpful in sickle cell anemia.

90. **1** High levels of fetal hemoglobin prevent sickling of red blood cells. The newborn has from 44% to 89% fetal hemoglobin, but this rapidly decreases during the first year. (c)

2 These will not affect the diagnosis of sickle cell anemia.

3 Respiratory difficulties are not associated with sickle cell anemia except as a consequence of hypoxia during a crisis.

4 The diagnosis of sickle cell anemia is made on the basis of hematologic tests; general health and growth are not affected initially.

91. **2** Under conditions of decreased oxygen the relatively insoluble hemoglobin S changes its molecular structure to form long slender crystals and eventually the crescent, or sickled, shape. (b)

1 Hemodilution helps prevent sickling and is accomplished by encouraging fluids.

3 The platelets are not involved in sickle cell anemia.

4 This will not influence the sickling process.

92. **2** Sickling is related to the concentration of hemoglobin within the cell. Since hypertonicity of the blood plasma increases the intracellular concentration of hemoglobin, dehydration promotes sickling. (c)

1 This will not prevent thrombus formation.

3 The condition determines his activity level; although bed rest may be necessary during a crisis, complete bed rest is rarely necessary.

4 Anticoagulants do not help prevent the thrombus formation in sickle cell anemia.

93. **2** Both cause poor resistance. With sickling it is due to low oxygen levels, and with celiac disease it is due to malnourishment and immunologic defects. (b)

1 Activity does not need to be limited in celiac disease; strenuous activity should be limited in sickle cell anemia.

3 This specific diet is not particularly helpful for either sickle cell anemia or celiac disease.

4 Vital signs will not be abnormal except during a crisis in either condition.

94. **2** The recommended immunization schedule for infants is administration of the combined diphtheria, pertussis, and tetanus vaccine and the trivalent oral polio virus at ages 2, 4, and 6 months. (b)

1 Measles and rubella vaccines are not usually given until 15 months of age; tuberculosis vaccine is not given routinely to children.

3 Measles, mumps, and rubella vaccines are not given until 15 months; tuberculosis vaccine is not routinely administered to children.
4 Measles vaccine is not usually administered until the child is 15 months old.

95. **3** The body's immune system constructs proteins called antibodies that possess a specificity toward another protein called the antigen. The antibody may neutralize or damage the antigen and thus render it harmless. (c)
   1 Antigens are harmful to the body.
   2 Antibodies are produced to fight antigens.
   4 Antibodies are protein substances.

96. **2** Maternal antibodies to measles infection persist in the infant until approximately 15 months of age. (b)
   1 Side effects are no more common for infants than for toddlers.
   3 This has not been found to be true.
   4 This is true, but it is due to the presence of maternal antibodies.

97. **4** An attenuated virus is an antigen that causes a protective active response in the individual, the development of antibodies. (b)
   1 An immunization contains antigens, not antibodies.
   2 An immunization contains antigens, not antibodies.
   3 Passive antibodies are produced by another person; for example, maternal antibodies that cross the placenta to the fetus.

98. **2** Because of the infant's increasing mobility, high level of oral activity, and relative lack of fear or appreciation for danger, accidents are the primary cause of death in children above 1 year of age. (c)
   1 This is best discussed with the mother prenatally or soon after delivery.
   3 This is too early for discussions of psychosexual development.
   4 This is too early for discussions about toilet training.

99. **2** Rest reduces the need for oxygen and minimizes metabolic needs during the acute, febrile stage of the disease. (a)
   1 This is not a priority, and the child will be anorexic during the febrile phase.
   3 The child with pneumonia is usually confined to bed and needs to reduce activity to conserve oxygen.
   4 Elimination is not usually a problem except as a result of immobility.

100. **4** Nonstrenuous, diversional activities involving interpersonal relationships with another person provide better support and resting conditions than does more active play. (a)
   1 A jigsaw puzzle is too complicated for a 5-year-old and does not provide her the human contact she needs.
   2 This will probably increase her fretfulness and does not provide the human contact she needs.
   3 Although a doll is appropriate for a 5-year-old, it does not provide the human contact she needs.

101. **3** A bland high-protein, high-carbohydrate diet provides adequate nutrition in the face of infection and fever. (a)
   1 This does not provide the protein needed for the healing process.
   2 These are empty calories.
   4 This is too heavy for a between-meal snack and contains fats, which are not helpful in the healing process.

102. **4** A few minutes will be enough time for the child to begin to feed herself. The nurse should provide both physical and emotional support, since the child's request for help indicates the need for dependence during a period of stress. (a)

1 This does not provide the child the help she may need.
2 A nurse should never make a statement like this; it can cause stress, feelings of guilt, and embarrassment to a sick child.
3 It may be a while until the child feels better; in the meantime, she needs adequate nourishment to provide for healing.

103. **3** Regression is the retreat to a past level of behavior as a way of minimizing stress or controlling anxiety. Increased dependence, such as being fed by another person, is a form of regression. (a)
   1 Her statement does not reflect immaturity.
   2 Although loneliness may be a factor, it is not the key one in her response.
   4 Her statement can hardly be construed as a temper tantrum.

104. **3** Dinner is frequently a family activity. Having her parents visit during mealtime may provide her with additional emotional, social, and physical support, resulting in an improved nutritional intake. (a)
   1 This will further inhibit her nutritional intake.
   2 This may not influence her overall intake.
   4 If given full rein, 5-year-olds will not select the most nutritional foods.

105. **3** In PKU the absence of the hepatic enzyme phenylalanine hydroxylase prevents normal metabolism (hydroxylation to tyrosine) of the amino acid phenylalanine. The increased fluid levels of phenylalanine in the body and the alternate metabolic by-products (phenylketones) are associated with severe mental retardation (exact mechanism not known). (b)
   1 PKU is transmitted by an autosomal recessive gene.
   2 Testing for PKU cannot be done until after several days of milk ingestion.
   4 Children are usually treated until they are 8 years old, when most of the growth and development of the brain are complete.

106. **1** The Guthrie blood test reliably detects abnormal phenylalanine levels as early as 4 days of age, provided the infant has been fed a milk diet. (a)
   2 This is not used since it takes too long for the phenylpyruvic acid to appear in the urine. By this time (10 to 14 days), brain damage may have occurred.
   3 This is used for screening large groups of infants but cannot be used until after 6 weeks of age.
   4 This is an inappropriate test for PKU.

107. **3** It is hoped that reducing dietary phenylalanine will prevent brain damage. Diets are planned to attempt to maintain the serum phenylalanine level between 5 and 10 mg/100 ml. (c)
   1 Phenylalanine is essential for normal growth and development of the brain.
   2 There are no substitutes; phenylalanine is one of the essential amino acids.
   4 It is not possible to do this.

108. **3** Maintaining low phenylalanine levels is recommended until brain growth is almost completed, usually by 6 to 8 years of age. (b)
   1 Dietary management is necessary until the child is 8 years old.
   2 Dietary management is necessary until the child is 8 years old.
   4 This is untrue and is not helpful to the parents.

109. **4** Shivering increases the metabolic rate, which intensifies the body's need for oxygen and raises the body temperature. (c)
   1 Monitoring vital signs is not as important as taking affirmative action to prevent increases in fever.

2 Forcing fluids is contraindicated because the child is vomiting.

3 Although monitoring output will provide information about the client's level of hydration, it is more important to take affirmative action toward preventing increases in fever.

110. **3** Since the child is in his crib, remain, observe, and protect him from injury to his head or extremities during the seizure activity. (a)

   1 Once jaws have closed, attempts at inserting a tongue blade are futile; this could damge the child's teeth.

   2 Never leave the child having a seizure alone; put on the call light to obtain assistance if needed.

   4 Never restrain an individual during a seizure; fractured bones or torn muscles and ligaments can result.

111. **3** Febrile convulsions are not necessarily associated with major neurologic problems but often accompany fever. Such convulsions may be partially accounted for by the overall brain immaturity in children. (b)

   1 Febrile convulsions are more common in the infant and young toddler.

   2 The cause of febrile convulsions is still uncertain.

   4 Boys are affected about twice as often as girls.

112. **4** Perform the computation for the correct dosage:

$$\frac{150 \text{ mg}}{80 \text{ mg}} \times \frac{x \text{ tablets}}{1 \text{ tablet}}$$
$$80\, x = 150$$
$$x = 1.8 \text{ or } 2 \text{ tablets} \qquad \text{(b)}$$

   1 This is an insufficient dose.

   2 This is an insufficient dose.

   3 This is an insufficient dose.

113. **1** Meningococcal meningitis is identified by its epidemic nature and purpuric skin rash. It is treated with sulfadiazine. (c)

   2 This is not characteristic of meningococcal meningitis.

   3 The fever of meningitis is usually high.

   4 This is not characteristic of meningococcal meningitis.

114. **3** Peripheral circulatory collapse (the Waterhouse-Friderichsen syndrome) is a serious complication of meningococcal meningitis due to bilateral adrenal hemorrhage. The resultant acute adrenocortical insufficiency causes profound shock, petechiae and ecchymotic lesions, vomiting, prostration, and hypotension. (b)

   1 Although this may occur, it is rare and not as serious as peripheral circulatory collapse.

   2 Although this may occur, it is not as serious a complication as peripheral circulatory collapse.

   4 Although this may occur, it is controllable and not as serious as peripheral circulatory collapse.

115. **3** Pain is paroxysmal due to peristaltic action. Abdominal distention pushes up the diaphragm, causing respiratory distress characterized by grunting respirations. (c)

   1 The pain of intestinal obstruction is paroxysmal.

   2 These symptoms do not usually accompany intestinal obstruction.

   4 These symptoms are not characteristic of intestinal obstruction.

116. **1** Sucking is a primary need of infancy. It decreases anxiety and does not interfere with gastric decompression. (b)

   2 This will probably not help to calm him.

   3 This will probably increase his pain from abdominal distension.

   4 This would be more helpful if client were a toddler.

117. **3** If the circulation is overloaded with too much fluid or the rate is too rapid, the stress on the heart becomes too great and cardiac embarrassment may occur. (b)

   1 This is important, but an infiltrated IV is not a serious complication.

   2 This is not a primary consideration in intestinal obstruction.

   4 Although fluid replacement is important, prevention of cardiac problems from fluid overload is critical.

118. **2** By 4 months of age infants are able to turn over and can easily fall from an inadequately guarded height. (a)

   1 Although infant is capable of putting small things in his mouth, he is not yet able to crawl and would probably not be placed on the floor.

   3 At 4 months of age infants are not yet able to explore the environment to the point that electric outlets pose a problem.

   4 Infant is still too small and has not yet developed motor capabilities to get into containers of poison.

119. **3** The decreased filtration of plasma in the glomeruli results in an excess accumulation of water and sodium, producing edema that is first evident around the eyes. Hypertension is thought to be due to the hypervolemia, although its exact cause is unclear. (b)

   1 Neither of these is a sign of acute glomerulonephritis.

   2 Although hematuria is found, dehydration is not a sign of acute glomerulonephritis.

   4 Oliguria is not found with acute glomerulonephritis. The client is usually hypertensive.

120. **4** During the acute stage, anorexia and the loss of protein lower the child's resistance to infection. (b)

   1 Bed rest is necessary only during the most acute stage; 4 weeks is too long.

   2 A bland diet is not necessary, and high protein should be avoided.

   3 Antibiotics are not necessary for all children with acute glomerulonephritis, only those with persistent streptococcal infections.

121. **3** Piaget stresses that age 7 is the turning point in mental development. New forms of organization appear at this age that mark the beginning of logic, symbolism, and abstract thought. (a)

   1 A toddler is capable of making simple decisions.

   2 A 5-year-old is capable of tying his shoes.

   4 An infant is capable of hand-eye coordination.

122. **2** When urinary test findings are normal, such as no evidence of hematuria or proteinuria, the child is allowed to resume his pre-illness activities. (b)

   1 Bed rest is unnecessary at this stage.

   3 This restriction is unnecessary.

   4 This restriction is unnecessary.

123. **1** Cystic fibrosis is characterized by overproduction of viscid mucus by exocrine glands in the lungs. The mucus traps bacteria and foreign debris that adheres to the lining and cannot be expelled by the cilia, thus obstructing the airway and favoring growth of organisms and infection. (a)

   2 Although there is increased sodium and chloride in the saliva, it does not irritate or necrose mucous membranes.

   3 Neuromuscular irritability of the bronchi does not occur in cystic fibrosis.

   4 Cardiac defects are not associated with cystic fibrosis.

124. **2** The first usual indication of cystic fibrosis is meconium ileus. The small intestine is blocked with a thick, tenacious, mucilaginous meconium, usually near the ileocecal valve. This causes intestinal obstruction with abdominal distention, vomiting, and fluid and electrolyte imbalance. (b)

   1 This is not an early sign of cystic fibrosis.

3 This does not have special significance in cystic fibrosis.

4 This is not an early sign of cystic fibrosis.

125. **2** Production of tenacious mucus in the pancreatic ducts prevents the flow of digestive enzymes into the intestines. Thus fats, proteins, and (to a lesser extent) carbohydrates cannot be digested and absorbed. (b)

1 Anorexia is not a usual problem found with cystic fibrosis.

3 Cystic fibrosis does not influence the secretion of growth hormone.

4 These are not problems associated with cystic fibrosis.

126. **1** In cystic fibrosis the mucous glands secrete thick mucoid secretions that accumulate, reducing ciliary action and mucus flow. Expectoration is greatly hindered. Postural drainage promotes the removal of mucopurulent secretions by means of gravity. (b)

2 The nurse should encourage activities appropriate for the child's physical capacity; this will include helping him conserve energy during acute phases of illness.

3 Coughing should be encouraged.

4 This is not necessary with cystic fibrosis.

127. **3** Because of a lack of the pancreatic enzyme lipase, fats remain unabsorbed and are excreted in excessive amounts in the stool. (a)

1 This does not cause the foul smell of stools.

2 This does not cause the foul smell of stools.

4 These are the pancreatic enzymes, whose passage into the intestine is prevented by blocked pancreatic ducts.

128. **3** Pancreatic enzymes are given as replacement because of the lack of their production by the pancreas. Antibiotics are prescribed to prevent and control respiratory tract infection. (a)

1 These are not indicated in the treatment of cystic fibrosis.

2 These may be used but are not specific for cystic fibrosis.

4 Mists and expectorants may be used; fat-soluble vitamins must be given in water-miscible preparations.

129. **4** Rectal prolapse is the most common GI complication and is due to wasting of perirectal supporting tissues, secondary to malnutrition. (c)

1 Intussusception is not associated with cystic fibrosis.

2 Anal fissures may or may not occur with cystic fibrosis.

3 Meconium ileus is associated with cystic fibrosis in newborns and prevents the passage of stools.

130. **2** The nurse recognizes the child's protest over his mother's absence and tries to comfort him by staying near him until he feels more relaxed. The bathing can be postponed until he has had time to test out his environment and is less anxious. (b)

1 This may frighten him more.

3 This is probably true, although the nurse has not attempted to reduce anxiety.

4 This action does not attempt to relieve the child's anxiety and will probably cause it to increase.

131. **4** The second stage of separation anxiety is despair, in which the child is depressed, lonely, and disinterested in his surroundings. (b)

1 The third stage of separation, denial or detachment, is a more advanced stage than that demonstrated in the situation.

2 The nurse must recognize that the child is suffering from separation anxiety, which does not include a stage of mistrust.

3 The nurse must recognize that the child is suffering from separation anxiety, which does not include a stage of rejection.

132. **1** Detachment is the result of trying to escape the emotional pain of desiring the mother by repressing feelings for her. (c)

2 This interpretation is not appropriate to the situation cited.

3 This response lacks insight.

4 This conclusion cannot be drawn from the situation cited.

133. **4** When the child has progressed to detachment as a method of coping with the separation, reunion of child and mother necessitates a period of reconciliation before the child is again willing to experience his emotional feelings because of his memory of the pain during their separation. (a)

1 Mike will not miss the nurses or the hospital routine.

2 Because he has suffered extreme separation anxiety, Mike will have some difficulty readjusting to his home.

3 Mike will probably demonstrate difficulty in his readjustment to his family.

134. **2** The hyperextension required in swimming aids in strengthening back muscles and increases deeper respirations, both of which are necessary prior to surgery and/or wearing a brace or cast. (a)

1 This will not be especially therapeutic for Sara.

3 This will not be especially therapeutic for Sara.

4 This will not be especially therapeutic for Sara.

135. **1** Continuing growth causes changes in muscle and bone structure and position. Adolescent girls have a rapid growth spurt. The brace is worn for 6 months after physical maturity, which is proved by x-ray examination to show cessation of bone growth. (b)

2 The Milwaukee brace is used to halt the progression of the curvature, not correct it.

3 Pain is not usually a symptom with scoliosis.

4 This is not an appropriate criterion for removal of the Milwaukee brace.

136. **4** The hypothalamic-pituitary-gonadal-adrenal mechanism is responsible for the physiologic and structural changes that occur at puberty. In girls the adrenal glands secrete androgens that are responsible for the appearance of axillary and pubic hair, generally between 11 and 14 years of age. Menarche usually occurs 2 years after initial pubescent changes. (b)

1 This is not a reliable indicator of sexual maturity.

2 This is not an indicator of sexual maturity.

3 This is not an appropriate indicator of sexual maturity in females or males.

137. **1** Hypertrophy of the pyloric sphincter, at the distal end of the stomach, causes partial and then complete obstruction. Nonprojectile vomiting progresses to projectile vomiting, which rapidly leads to dehydration. (c)

2 This can be expected with a tracheoesophageal fistula but not with pyloric stenosis.

3 The infant's cry is not affected by pyloric stenosis; there does not appear to be pain associated with this condition, except for the pain of hunger.

4 The quality of the stool is not usually affected by pyloric stenosis.

138. **2** In excessive vomiting there is an increased loss of hydrogen ions (hydrochloric acid), which leads to a lowered serum pH (metabolic alkalosis) and an excess of base bicarbonate. (b)

1 Although some calcium is lost through vomiting, it is highly unusual that the infant would develop tetany.

3 This is caused by a retention of hydrogen ions and a loss of base bicarbonates. In vomiting, base bicarbonates are retained and hydrogen ions are lost.

4 Hyperactivity is not associated with pyloric stenosis.

139. **4** The newborn's proportion of total body water is 20% greater than the adult's. It rapidly diminishes in the neonatal period and continues to decline steadily until about 2 years of age, when it almost equals that of the adult. In addition, infants have very little fluid volume reserve. (c)
   1 Renal function is immature during infancy only.
   2 Cellular metabolism in children is not less stable than in adults.
   3 The proportion of total body water in children (up to 2 years) is 20% greater than in adults.

140. **1** An infant's intravascular compartment is fairly limited and cannot accommodate large volumes of fluid administered in a short time. Equipment such as mini-droppers, volume control chambers, and infusion pumps should be used, since they help control or limit the volume of fluid to be infused. (b)
   2 IV fluids can be administered at room temperature.
   3 This is the physician's role.
   4 This is important for everyone receiving IV fluids.

141. **4** Initial feedings of glucose in water or electrolyte solutions are given 4 to 6 hours after surgery. When clear fluids are retained, usually within 24 hours, diluted formula feedings are begun. (c)
   1 This is not necessary.
   2 This is not necessary.
   3 The formula should be diluted 24 hours after surgery in a gradual attempt to return the infant to a full feeding schedule.

142. **2** Tetralogy of Fallot classically consists of four defects. Three of them are anatomic: ventricular septal defect, pulmonic stenosis, and overriding aorta. The fourth defect, right ventricular hypertrophy, is secondary to increased resistance to blood flow in that ventricle. (b)
   1 Although right ventricular hypertrophy is correct, the other anomalies are not.
   3 These are the characteristics of transposition of the great vessels.
   4 Although the right ventricular hypertrophy is correct, the other anomalies are not.

143. **4** Oxygen is necessary for growth of cells. Decreased oxygen in the developing child causes a slow growth rate. (b)
   1 Mental retardation is not a common finding in children with congenital heart disease.
   2 Cyanosis and clubbing are not characteristic of most children with cardiac anomalies, only of those with the more serious forms.
   3 Cardiac anomalies are more often a result of prenatal, rather than genetic, factors.

144. **2** The purpose of digoxin (Lanoxin) is to slow and strengthen the apical rate. The normal apical rate for a child of 5 years is 90 to 110 beats per minute. If the apical rate is already slow (10 to 20 beats below normal), administration of the drug could lower the apical rate to an unsafe level. (a)
   1 This rate is well below that which necessitates withholding Lanoxin for children; it is the correct rate for withholding Lanoxin in adults.
   3 This is within the normal range of the heart rate of 5-year-olds and does not necessitate withholding Lanoxin.
   4 This is within the normal range of the heart rate of 5-year-olds and does not necessitate withholding Lanoxin.

145. **4** Decreased tissue oxygenation stimulates erythropoiesis, resulting in excessive production of red blood cells. (a)
   1 This would not be a direct cause of polycythemia.

2 This may or may not affect the production of red blood cells.
   3 This would not be a direct cause of polycythemia.

146. **1** Forceful evacuation results in the child's taking a deep breath, holding it, and straining (Valsalva maneuver). This increased intrathoracic pressure puts excessive strain on the heart sutures. (b)
   2 Activity is gradually increased postoperatively.
   3 Crying is not a problem after cardiac surgery; it may, in fact, help prevent respiratory complications.
   4 Coughing and deep breathing are essential for the prevention of postoperative respiratory complications.

147. **3** The nurse's data collection was not adequate because no questions were asked concerning the recency of the previous tetanus inoculation. The nurse failed to support the life and well-being of a client. (c)
   1 It was essential to determine the recency of the immunization; for a "tetanus prone" wound like a puncture from a rusty nail some form of tetanus immunization is usually given.
   2 The nurse's assessment was not thorough in regard to determining the recency of immunization.
   4 This is usually a clinical decision.

148. **4** The slightest stimulation sets off a wave of very severe and very painful muscle spasms involving the whole body. Nerve impulses cross the myoneural junction and stimulate muscle contraction due to the presence of exotoxins produced by *Clostridium tetani*. (c)
   1 Body alignment is not an important consideration in tetanus.
   2 Oral intake of fluids may not be possible because of excessive secretions and laryngospasm.
   3 Monitoring output is not a major nursing concern with tetanus.

149. **4** Gluteal folds should be symmetric, as should all planes and folds of the body. An abnormality of the hips will cause asymmetry and/or a shorter leg on the affected side. (a)
   1 In congenital hip dysplasia there is usually a limited abduction of the leg at the hip.
   2 The affected side is shorter.
   3 The dance reflex is not affected.

150. **1** Hypostatic pneumonia can develop from decreased activity. Also the cast prevents full chest expansion. (a)
   2 Cast damage, although problematic, is not a serious complication.
   3 Soiling of the cast with excreta, although problematic, is not a serious complication.
   4 This is not necessary or desirable.

151. **2** Pillows under the head or shoulders of a child in a spica cast will thrust the chest forward against the cast, causing discomfort and respiratory distress. Therefore, when elevation of the head is desired, the entire mattress and spring should be raised at the head of the bed. (b)
   1 There is no reason to place a time limit on this position.
   3 This will thrust the chest forward against the cast, causing discomfort and respiratory distress.
   4 This will not help in any way.

152. **2** Polycythemia, reflected in an elevated hematocrit level, is a direct attempt of the body to compensate for the decrease in oxygenation to all body cells due to the mixture of oxygenated and unoxygenated circulating blood. (c)
   1 Edema is not a common finding in cyanotic heart disease.
   3 This is characteristic of coarctation of the aorta, an acyanotic heart disease.

4 This is not characteristic of cyanotic heart disease in children.

153. **3** In the fetus, oxygenated blood is shunted directly into the systemic circulation via the ductus arteriosus, a connection between the pulmonary artery and the aorta. Normally after birth the increased oxygen tension causes a functional closure of the ductus arteriosus. Occasionally, particularly in premature infants, this vessel remains open and is known as patent ductus arteriosus. (c)
 1 This is known as pulmonic stenosis.
 2 Patent ductus arteriosus does not involve ventricular septal defects.
 4 This is not the problem in patent ductus arteriosus.

154. **4** In acyanotic heart disease there is a narrowing of the vessels and/or pinpoint holes in the septum of the heart that cause a murmuring sound as the blood is pumped through. (c)
 1 This is not a common clinical finding in acyanotic heart disease.
 2 Clubbing is a common finding in cyanotic heart disease.
 3 This is not a common finding in acyanotic heart disease, for tissue perfusion is usually adequate.

155. **2** Coarctation of the aorta is a narrowing, usually in the thoracic segment, causing decreased blood flow below the constriction and increased blood volume above it. (c)
 1 In coarctation of the aorta, radial pulses would be full and bounding.
 3 In coarctation of the aorta, femoral pulses would be weak or absent and blood pressure in the lower extremities would be decreased.
 4 This has nothing to do with coarctation of the aorta.

156. **1** Hemophilia is carried on the X chromosome but is recessive. Therefore the female is the carrier (a normal Xo and an affected XH). If the male receives the affected XH(XHYO), the disease is manifest. (a)
 2 Hemophilia is a sex-linked recessive disorder.
 3 Hemophilia is carried by the female. Regular laws of Mendelian inheritance are not sex-specific.
 4 Only females carry the trait; only males have the disease.

157. **2** The mating of a carrier female (XoXH) and an unaffected male (XoYo) results in the following possible offspring: a carrier female (XoXH), a normal female (XoXo), a normal male (XoYo), or an affected male (XHYo). (b)
 1 For each child there is a 50% chance of being normal.
 3 For each child there is a 50% chance of being affected.
 4 Males cannot carry the trait; females have a 50% chance of being carriers.

158. **4** Bleeding is greatly influenced by activity. Therefore hemorrhage into weight-bearing joints, especially the knees, is the most common site. (b)
 1 This area is fairly well protected by the skull and less likely to be injured.
 2 Bleeding from bones themselves is not common without other associated trauma.
 3 This area is usually protected from the trauma of direct force.

159. **2** Salicylates in large doses cause irritation of the gastric mucosa (gastric distress, nausea, vomiting) and also affect the CNS (tinnitus, dizziness, disturbance in hearing and vision). (a)
 1 Although nausea and dizziness and severe headache may be associated with salicylate ingestion, edema is not.

3 Constipation is not a common problem associated with salicylates.
 4 Edema is not a problem associated with salicylates.

160. **2** Salicylates act as analgesics by protecting peripheral pain receptors from bradykinin, a component in the inflammatory process. Salicylates act as antipyretics by affecting the heat-regulating center in the hypothalamus and increasing the elimination of heat through peripheral blood vessel dilation and evaporation of increased perspiration. (a)
 1 Salicylates have no capacity to destroy or control a microorganism's effect.
 3 Salicylates have no capacity to act as a sedative and calm individuals.
 4 Salicylates have no capacity to act as a hypnotic and induce sleep.

161. **2** School-age children have an interest in hobbies or collections of various kinds as a means of gathering information and knowledge about the world in which they live. (b)
 1 This is too advanced for a normal 8-year-old.
 3 These would probably not interest an 8-year-old.
 4 This would not interest an 8-year-old.

162. **1** Choanal atresia is a lack of an opening between one or both of the nasal passages and the nasopharynx. (c)
 2 Atresias associated with the GI tract include esophageal and intestinal atresia involving the ileum, jejunum, or colon.
 3 An atresia involving the pharynx and larynx is not commonly seen.
 4 Rectal atresia involves the rectum's ending in a pouch and the normal anal canal's opening into the other (nonconnected) end of the rectum.

163. **2** Since there is little or no opening between the nasal passages and the nasopharynx, the infant can breathe only through the mouth. When feeding, the infant cannot breathe without aspirating some of the fluid; this causes choking. (b)
 1 The swallowing reflex is normal.
 3 Since it is difficult if not impossible to eat, she will be very hungry.
 4 If choanal atresia is unilateral, there may be no symptoms and infant will eat normally; if bilateral, sucking will be almost impossible.

164. **4** An Apgar score of 3 indicates neonatal distress and should signal the nurse that the infant requires close supervision and support. (b)
 1 Average birth weight is about 3200 g.
 2 Infants often swallow in utero.
 3 A positive Babinski is normal through the age of 2 years.

165. **4** Infection is a constant threat because of poor general state of nutrition, tendency toward skin breakdown in edematous areas, corticosteroid therapy, and lowered immunoglobulin levels. (c)
 1 Fluid monitoring is important in determining whether restriction is indicated.
 2 Rather than regulating diet, the nurse should encourage intake of proteins and foods with high nutritional value.
 3 Bed rest may be used for severe stages, but generally ambulation is encouraged.

166. **3** Children with nephrosis have a characteristic pale, overweight appearance from the malnutrition and edema. They may become very sensitive about these changes as they grow older. (b)
 1 Engaging in usual childhood activities between attacks should promote normal development of fine muscle coordination.

2 Sterility is not associated with nephrosis.

4 Although this may be indicated, body image problems pose a much greater threat.

167. **1** Bed-wetting accidents are not uncommon in this age group, especially during hospitalization when regression may occur. Therefore the best approach is to ignore the event. (b)

2 This may tend to make child feel guilty for his action.

3 He may interpret this as punishment. Punishment for regressive behavior is inappropriate.

4 Since skin breakdown is a concern, rubber sheets are contraindicated; they would hold moisture close to the skin.

168. **2** Fear of mutilation and intrusive procedures is most common at this age because of fantasies and active imagination. These children also connect illness with being bad and view intrusion as punishment. (c)

1 Fear of isolation from peers is a problem for school-age children and adolescents.

3 Death is seen as reversible and not final.

4 A child this age usually has little previous contact with pain and therefore little experience upon which to base fear.

169. **2** The restricted ventilation accompanying an asthmatic attack limits the body's ability to blow off carbon dioxide. As carbon dioxide accumulates in the body fluids, it reacts with water to produce carbonic acid (H_2CO_3); the result is respiratory acidosis. (b)

1 Asthma is a respiratory problem causing carbon dioxide retention. Respiratory alkalosis is caused by exhaling large amounts of carbon dioxide.

3 The problem basic to asthma is respiratory, not metabolic.

4 Asthma is a respiratory problem, not a metabolic one; metabolic acidosis can be produced by a gain of nonvolatile acids or a loss of base bicarbonate.

170. **2** Prednisone causes atrophy of the thymus, decreases the number of lymphocytes, plasma cells, and eosinophils in the blood, and decreases the formation of antibodies. Therefore it reduces the individual's resistance to certain infectious processes and viral diseases. Also, prednisone is an antiinflammatory drug that masks infection. (b)

1 Eosinophil counts are often consistently elevated in children with asthma.

3 Child will need adequate hydration to assist with loosening and removing mucus from the lungs.

4 Child will limit her own activity based upon her respiratory status.

171. **2** Aminophylline relaxes the smooth muscle of the vasculature, causing peripheral vasodilation that can lead to hypotension. (b)

1 Temperature changes will not be related to aminophylline administration.

3 Oxygen therapy is not associated with drug administration.

4 Epinephrine, also used in the treatment of asthma, may cause tachycardia.

172. **1** Cold can precipitate bronchospasm, and increased exercise depletes oxygen. (b)

2 Asthma is a chronic condition. Return to usual activities after the acute stage is essential for normal growth and development.

3 Although increased calories may be needed to support the child during a coexisting bacterial infection in the acute stage, by discharge a return to usual habits is indicated.

4 Treatment of asthma does not involve a high-fat diet.

173. **2** Peak crying times are early evening and night, which exhaust the mother. She needs time away from the baby to rest and should be encouraged to hire a sitter or make some arrangements for time alone. (a)

1 Many treatments, including this one, may not be effective; children do outgrow colic, so parents need support to help them manage until that time.

3 Treatment is usually based on relieving abdominal cramping by stimulating peristalsis; quiet environments may help prevent, not treat, the problem.

4 Providing warmth through a hot water bottle or heating pad over the abdomen may be helpful for some children but not for others.

174. **3** The traditional efforts to explain and treat colic center around control of gas in the intestinal tract that is causing the paroxysmal pain. (a)

1 Colic is thought to be due to excessive fermentation and gas production.

2 The exact cause of colic is not known.

4 Excessive intake of carbohydrates may cause flatus, but diet changes rarely prevent colic attacks.

175. **3** Muscular coordination and perception are developed enough at 6 months so the infant can roll over. If unaware of this ability of the infant, the mother could leave the child unattended for a moment to reach for something and the child could roll off the crib. (b)

1 Sitting up unsupported is accomplished by most children at 7 to 8 months.

2 Standing by holding on to furniture is accomplished by most children between 8 and 10 months.

4 Crawling takes place at about 9 months of age.

176. **3** Touching the palms of the hands causes flexion of the fingers (grasp reflex); this usually lessens after 3 months of age. An unexpected loud noise causes abduction of the extremities and then flexion of the elbows (startle reflex); this usually disappears by 4 months of age. Persistence of primitive reflexes usually is indicative of a cerebral insult. (b)

1 These changes are consistent with normal growth and development.

2 The data do not support making this comment and would cause needless concern.

4 Sensory stimulation at this age is directed toward experiences to add new motor, language, and social skills.

177. **4** By law, a nurse cannot administer medications without a prescription from a physician. This is a dependent function of the nurse. (a)

1 The nurse cannot distribute medication without a physician's order.

2 The nurse must get a physician's order for the medication and cannot accept the parent's information alone.

3 The nurse should not assume that the physician is aware of the problem.

178. **1** An individual is legally unable to sign a consent until age 18 years. The only exception is the emancipated minor, a minor who is self-sufficient or married. (a)

2 Although the adolescent is capable of intelligent choices, it is the legality, not the acceptability or intelligence of the choice, that is at issue.

3 Parents or guardians are legally responsible under all circumstances unless the adolescent is an emancipated minor.

4 Adolescents have the capacity to choose between alternatives, but not the legal right in this situation.

179. **4** The nurse made the assessment that the medication was ineffective in relieving child's pain for the duration ordered. This information should be communicated to the physician for evaluation. (a)

1 The physician's order is for administration only every 3 to 4 hours. Legally it can be given only within these guidelines.

2 The nurse should not ignore the client's need for pain relief.

3 There are no data to support this. The amount of medication was probably inadequate for her pain tolerance level.

180. **1** Chlorpheniramine (Chlor-Trimeton) is an antihistaminic that prevents histamine from reaching its site of action by competing for the receptors. (b)

2 Nitrofurazone is a bactericidal agent used especially with burns.

3 This is a salicylate-like agent.

4 Hyaluronidase is a mucolytic enzyme that promotes diffusion and absorption of injected fluids, exudates, and transudates.

181. **3** The principle of Bryant's traction is bilateral 90° hip flexion. It is skin traction applied to the legs to decrease the fracture, maintain alignment, and immobilize both legs. (a)

1 Bryant's traction requires the supine position.

2 Bryant's traction is always applied bilaterally.

4 Skeletal traction is applied to a pin in the affected extremity.

182. **3** No more than 350 ml of solution should be administered to an infant or child unless specifically ordered, since fluid and electrolyte balance in an infant or child is easily disturbed. (c)

1 This quantity may be ordered for a small infant.

2 This quantity may be ordered for an older or larger infant.

4 This quantity is too large for small children.

183. **3** A client cannot legally be locked in a room (isolated) unless there is a threat of danger involved either to the client or to other clients. (b)

1 Crying, although irritating, will not harm the other children.

2 The child is probably reacting to separation from her mother, which is common at this age.

4 Legal limits rarely include time parameters.

184. **2** A pounding board is a safe toy for toddlers, since it is fairly large, easy to manipulate, and sturdy. A pounding board provides a way for anger to be sublimated. (b)

1 The child's motor and hand-eye coordination is too immature for using this.

3 This is not as safe since toddlers may eat clay or Play-Doh.

4 This would be appropriate for an older child with more mature motor coordination to compensate for a moving object.

185. **1** Using the formula, convert grains to milligrams (gr 1/300 = 0.2 mg); then use the formula:

$$\frac{0.2 \text{ mg}}{0.4 \text{ mg}} \times \frac{x \text{ ml}}{1 \text{ ml}}$$
$$0.4x = 0.2$$
$$x = 0.5 \text{ ml (This will contain the desired}$$
dose of 0.2 mg atropine.) (c)

2 This amount is too much according to calculations.

3 This amount is too little according to calculations.

4 This amount is too much according to calculations.

186. **3** Since young children have difficulty verbalizing their fears or anxiety, play is a therapeutic way for these feelings to be expressed. The school-age child also likes to role play. (b)

1 Young school-age children are still somewhat egocentric and therefore interested in their own experiences and sensations.

2 A child this age is unable to express feelings entirely through words.

4 This may be helpful for a toddler or preschooler.

187. **3** Regression is normal in times of stress. It is a transient need that should be accepted, since it helps reduce anxiety. (a)

1 This behavior is unrelated to medical progress.

2 Distraction works only as long as it is employed.

4 Cause (thumb sucking) and future effect (buckteeth) will not be meaningful to a 7-year-old.

188. **2** To maintain the desired blood level, the drug must be given in the exact amount at the times directed. If the blood level of the drug falls, the organisms have an opportunity to build up resistance to the drug. (b)

1 Weighing a client is important with drugs that affect fluid balance such as Lasix.

3 Giving medication with milk or meals is important with drugs, such as Mandelamine, that cause GI distress.

4 Monitoring temperature would be important with antipyretic drugs.

189. **3** Isoniazid (INH) is the most potent tuberculostatic drug available at this time. It is given in conjunction with paraaminosalicylic acid (PAS), since PAS potentiates the action of INH as well as limits bacterial resistance to the drug. (b)

1 Old tuberculin is one type of skin test used to detect tuberculosis.

2 Bacille Calmette Guérin (BCG) vaccine is the only successful vaccine for tuberculosis to date, but greater protection is afforded by daily prophylactic administration of INH.

4 Purified protein derivative (PPD) is a widely used skin test for detecting tuberculosis.

190. **3** Tubercle bacilli multiply in caseous lesions, which have a poor vascular supply. These areas receive lower levels of the drugs, and as a result therapy must be prolonged. (b)

1 The length of therapy is insufficient to erradicate the bacilli.

2 Because lower levels of drug reach caseous lesions, longer treatment periods are needed.

4 Treatment for infected persons is usually 2 years.

191. **2** Family members who have been exposed are at high risk and should receive prophylactic therapy with INH and PAS. (b)

1 Symptoms generally do not contribute significantly to a diagnosis of tuberculosis.

3 Tubercle bacilli are not responsive to penicillin treatment.

4 Prophylactic treatment is given to children with a high probability of exposure to tuberculosis.

192. **2** One practically universal characteristic of minimally brain damaged children is distractibility. They are highly reactive to any extraneous stimuli such as noise and movement and are unable to inhibit their responses to such stimuli. (c)

1 Learning disabilities associated with minimal brain dysfunction are manifested in a variety of ways; loss of abstract thought is not a universal characteristic.

3 Repetition in language or movement may be seen; rituals are uncommon.

4 Delayed development of language skills is seen in varying degrees and may include dyslexia (reading difficulty), dysgrammatism (speaking difficulty), dysgraphia (writing difficulty), or delayed talking.

193. **2** Because of short attention span and distractibility, the specific limit setting consistently employed is crucial toward providing an environment that promotes concentration, prevents confusion, and minimizes conflicts for the child. (a)
    1 Some children have difficulty reading.
    3 Questions are appropriate as long as alternatives are limited.
    4 Parents need to manipulate the child's environment so it is simplified, controlled, and predictable.

194. **3** The extensive growth of lymphoblasts suppresses the normal growth of red cells, white cells, and platelets. (b)
    1 Internal bleeding does not cause neutropenia.
    2 Infection is a result of, not the cause of, leukopenia.
    4 Iron-intake deficit will not result in neutropenia.

195. **2** Because of the increased capillary fragility and decreased platelet counts that accompany leukemia, even the slightest trauma can cause hemorrhage. Therefore the toothbrush can produce gingival hemorrhage, and the physician should be informed of this happening; this may also assist in defining the diagnosis. (b)
    1 It cannot be assumed that a 4-year-old would follow such direction.
    3 Wiser to eliminate the use of a toothbrush and use a sponge-type applicator; therefore this is not necessary.
    4 Appropriate if oral mucosal bleeding continues or oral ulcers develop, not for a one-time incident.

196. **3** Euphoria and mood swings may result from steroid therapy. (b)
    1 Alopecia does not result from steroid therapy.
    2 An increased appetite, not anorexia, results from steroid therapy.
    4 Weight gain, not weight loss, results from steroid therapy.

197. **2** Generally, antineoplastic drugs act by interfering with, or inhibiting, synthesis of DNA in malignant cells. (c)
    1 This is the activity of the malignant cells themselves.
    3 Malignant cells are not infected, in the normal sense of the term; therefore no drug acts in this manner.
    4 Bone marrow depression is a side effect of this drug, not a desired action.

198. **4** The child is having an allergic reaction, and flow of blood should be stopped immediately. (b)
    1 Dangerous as an initial action because degree of allergic reaction cannot be determined at this time; blood must be stopped.
    2 Physician should be called after blood has been stopped.
    3 Slowing rate of infusion will not halt the allergic reaction to the blood.

199. **4** Fear of mutilation is typical of the older preschooler. (b)
    1 Toddlers and younger preschoolers fear separation from parents.
    2 Preschoolers do not view death as final.
    3 Preschoolers do not associate death with a supernatural being as does the school-age child.

200. **2** Three vessels; one vein carries oxygenated blood to fetus, and two arties return deoxygenated blood to placenta. (a)
    1 The umbilical cord has three vessels; a cord with two vessels is frequently associated with congenital abnormalities.
    3 Right number of vessels, but there are two arteries and one vein.
    4 The umbilical cord has three vessels, not four.

201. **3** The angle the wrist forms with the arm decreases as gestation increases; the angle is zero at term. (c)
    1 Sole creases develop progressively, covering the entire foot at term.
    2 In immature infants the testes are undescended; rugae develop progressively.
    4 In immature infants the ears contain little cartilage and are very springy when folded.

202. **2** This is usually sufficient if no problems exist with sucking or palate; too frequent burping is confusing. (a)
    1 Sucking too long without burping may result in regurgitation because of swallowed air.
    3 Excessive burping may confuse a new infant.
    4 Excessive burping may confuse a new infant.

203. **4** This allows air to circulate around the drying cord and permits the drainage of secretions if the infant regurgitates. (a)
    1 This could result in aspiration if regurgitation occurs.
    2 This could result in aspiration if regurgitation occurs.
    3 This may prevent aspiration if the infant regurgitates but would interfere with drying of the cord.

204. **1** She is in the stage of industry and stives to complete assigned tasks. (b)
    2 This is true of an older age group (adolescent).
    3 Peer influences increase rather than decrease as child grows.
    4 This is true in period of adolescence.

205. **3** Peak action of regular insulin is 2 to 4 hours; peak action of NPH insulin is 6 to 8 hours. (b)
    1 Regular insulin duration is 6 to 8 hours.
    2 Regular insulin onset is ½ to 1 hour; NPH insulin onset is 1 to 2 hours.
    4 The opposite is true; peak action of regular insulin is 2 to 4 hours; peak action of NPH insulin is 6 to 8 hours.

Chapter 6: Maternity Nursing

1. **3** The chorion is the outermost membrane that helps form the placenta. It develops villi and, through its interaction with the endometrium, becomes part of the placenta. (c)
    1 The amnion is the inntermost lining, from which amniotic fluid is secreted.
    2 The yolk sac is part of the inner structure of the blastocyst and is lined by inner layer of cells, the entoderm; unrelated to placental formation.
    4 The allantois is a tubular diverticulum of the posterior part of the embryo's yolk sac; fuses with the chorion to form the placenta.

2. **1** Progesterone is secreted mainly by the corpus luteum. It helps prepare the endometrium for possible implantation of a fertilized ovum. (b)
    2 Adrenal cortex secretions contain only minute quantities of progesterone.
    3 Endometrium is influenced by progesterone secretion but does not secrete it.
    4 Pituitary gland secretions stimulate the target gland (e.g., corpus luteum of the ovary) to secrete progesterone.

3. **4** Gestation is divided into three stages—blastocyst, embryo, and fetus. (b)
    1 Known as a fetus until birth.
    2 At the time of implantation the group of developing cells is called a blastocyst.
    3 The fetal heart is heard between the eighteenth and twentieth weeks; known as a fetus at the end of the eighth week.

4. **4** A determination of the station (descent) of the fetus is based on the relationship of the presenting part and the spine. If too small, delivery cannot occur. (c)
   1 The measurement of pelvic floor is not involved with the fetus' descent into the birth canal.
   2 It is a measurement of the pelvic outlet.
   3 It is the narrowest measurement.

5. **2** Progressive dilation of the cervix is the most accurate indication of true labor. (c)
   1 Contractions may not begin until 24 to 48 hours later.
   3 Contractions of true labor persist in any position.
   4 Conversely, contractions will increase with activity.

6. **1** To allow for the larger intake of air, the normal adaptation is to increase the size of the thoracic cavity. (c)
   2 There is no change in the height of the rib cage.
   3 Upward displacement would decrease tidal air volume.
   4 Blood volume is not related to tidal air volume.

7. **4** By this time the fetus and placenta have grown, expanding the size of the uterus. The extended uterus expands into the abdominal cavity. (b)
   1 The uterus is still within the pelvic area at this time.
   2 The uterus has already risen out of the pelvis and is expanding further into the abdominal area.
   3 The uterus is still within the pelvic area.

8. **2** About 75% of all spontaneous abortions take place between 8 and 12 weeks of gestation and show embryonic defects. (b)
   1 Though possible, physical trauma rarely causes an abortion.
   3 Unresolved stress may lead to congenital defects but is rarely associated with abortion.
   4 Congenital defects are asymptomatic during pregnancy and do not usually cause abortion.

9. **4** Laminaria is a seaweed that expands in a moist environment. It is a natural and safe method of dilating the cervix. (b)
   1 Untrue: may not be as strong but certainly less traumatic.
   2 It takes 24 hours for the laminaria to expand.
   3 Anesthesia is not used in the dilation phase of abortion.

10. **1** The amnion encloses the embryo and the shock-protective amniotic fluid in which the embryo floats. (a)
    2 The yolk sac contains the stored nutrients of the ovum.
    3 The chorion is the outermost membrane; does not secrete fluid.
    4 This is another name for the umbilical cord.

11. **4** The word originates from the Middle English word *quik,* which means alive. (c)
    1 Ballottement is the bouncing of the fetus in the amniotic fluid against the examiner's hand.
    2 Engagement is when the presenting part is at the level of the ischial spine.
    3 Lightening is the descent of the fetus into the birth canal.

12. **4** This is the period in which the fetus stores deposits of fat. (b)
    1 This is the period of the blastocyst, when initial cell division takes place.
    2 The first trimester is the period of organogenesis, when cells differentiate into major organ systems.
    3 Growth is occurring, but fat deposition does not occur in this period.

13. **4** Progesterone stimulates differentiation of the endometrium into a secretory type of tissue. (b)
    1 Secondary male characteristics are influenced by testosterone.
    2 Influenced by high levels of luteinizing hormone.
    3 Influenced by estrogen.

14. **2** There is a sensitive period in the first minutes or hours after birth during which it is necessary, for later interpersonal development to be normal, that the mother and father have close contact with their new infant. (b)
    1 Rooming-in is not immediate; it occurs once the mother is in the postpartal unit.
    3 Taking-in is a psychologic behavior described by Reva Rubin that occurs during the first 2 postpartal days.
    4 Taking-hold is a psychologic behavior described by Reva Rubin that occurs after the third postpartal day.

15. **1** Because mothering is not an inborn instinct, almost all mothers, including multiparas, report some ambivalence and anxiety about their ability to be good mothers. (a)
    2 Untrue; very often the maternal instinct is nurtured at the sight of the infant.
    3 Untrue; ambivalent feelings are universal in response to the infant.
    4 Untrue; may take a much longer time.

16. **2** About two-thirds of neonatal deaths are caused by prematurity; there appears to be a correlation with teenage pregnancy, lack of prenatal care, nonwhite mothers, and chronic health problems. (c)
    1 Atelectasis may occur from respiratory distress, which in turn is associated with prematurity, the leading cause of death.
    3 Usually occurs as a result of prematurity, the leading cause of death.
    4 Most babies with congenital heart disease die after the neonatal period.

17. **1** Perinatal morbidity and mortality are greatly increased in multiple pregnancy because the high metabolic demands increase the potential for medical and obstetric complications. (b)
    2 Maternal mortality during the prenatal period is not increased in the presence of multiple gestation.
    3 Multiple gestation is usually identified prior to delivery; the mother would have this time for adjustment.
    4 Although postpartum hemorrhage does occur more frequently after multiple births, it is not a routine occurrence.

18. **2** This is the result of a reduced chromosome number, from 46 to 23, readying the sex cells for fertilization. (c)
    1 The diploid number (46 chromosomes) is reached when fertilization occurs.
    3 They each have one set of chromosomes (23).
    4 They are only 23 pairs.

19. **2** Follicle-stimulating hormone is secreted from the anterior pituitary gland. (c)
    1 Chorionic gonadotropin is secreted by the trophoblastic tissue, which makes up part of the placenta.
    3 Chorionic gonadotropin is a precursor of progesterone and is secreted by the trophoblastic tissue.
    4 Produced by syncytiotrophoblastic tissue, a preplacental tissue.

20. **2** When placental formation is complete, around the twelfth week of pregnancy, it produces progesterone and estrogen. (b)
    1 FSH is secreted by the anterior hypophysis, but it is not secreted during pregnancy.
    3 This is not the chief source of progesterone and estrogen; only small amounts are secreted.
    4 The corpus luteum supplies the estrogen and progesterone needed to sustain the pregnancy until the placenta is ready to take over.

21. **3** The umbilical vein carries blood high in oxygen from the placenta and empties it into the fetal vena cava by way of the ductus venosus. (a)

1 The blood in the umbilical artery is more deoxygenated.

2 Contains a mixture of arterial and venous blood.

4 The pulmonary artery carries only small amount of oxygenated blood since the lungs are not functioning.

22. **1** Two umbilical arteries arise from the fetus and go to the placenta, where waste products are exchanged for oxygen and nutrients and then returned via one umbilical vein to the baby. (a)

2 This is an anomalous number; there are two arteries and one vein.

3 This is an anomalous number; there are two arteries and one vein.

4 This is an anomalous number; there are two arteries and one vein.

23. **3** If the fetus is in a compromised state, it does not contribute to the synthesis of estriol; consequently estriol levels fall, indicating a need for intervention. (c)

1 Untrue; elevated estriol levels indicate healthy fetal placental functioning.

2 Chorionic gonadotropin is the hormone tested for in pregnancy tests.

4 Fetal demise is generally preceded by lowered estriol levels.

24. **1** There is a 30% to 50% increase in maternal blood volume at the end of the first trimester, leading to a decrease in the concentration of hemoglobin and erythrocytes. (b)

2 This is not physiologic but is caused by lack of iron intake.

3 Erythropoiesis is increased.

4 Detoxification demands are unchanged during pregnancy.

25. **1** The greatest danger of drug-induced malformation is during the first trimester of pregnancy, since this is the period of organogenesis. (b)

2 May cause problems, but organogenesis has already taken place by the second trimester.

3 The fetus is totally formed at this time, and drug damage would not be likely.

4 Drugs should be avoided, but the first trimester (period of organogenesis) is the most critical.

26. **1** A symptom of sudden rupture of a fallopian tube is pain on the affected side, usually sudden, excruciating, and spreading over the lower abdomen; sometimes the pain is associated with nausea, vomiting, and diarrhea. (a)

2 Pain is exquisite, sharp, and sudden.

3 There may be some vaginal bleeding with ruptured tubal pregnancy; usually severe pain is present.

4 There are no contractions since the pregnancy is not uterine.

27. **2** The proliferation of trophoblastic tissue filled with fluid causes the uterus to enlarge more quickly than it would with a normally growing fetus. (b)

1 There may be slight vaginal bleeding without pain.

3 Hypertension, not hypotension, often occurs with molar pregnancy.

4 There is generally no living fetus with a hydatidiform mole.

28. **1** Prolactin is the hormone from the anterior pituitary that stimulates mammary gland secretion. Progesterone and estrogen are ovarian hormones that influence breast development and other female sexual characteristics. (a)

2 Oxytocin, a posterior pituitary hormone, stimulates the uterine musculature to contract and causes the letdown reflex.

3 Not a pituitary hormone; secreted by the corpus luteum of the ovary.

4 Not a pituitary hormone; secreted by the ovaries and placenta.

29. **1** During pregnancy, secretion of milk is inhibited; sucking can cause uterine contractions. (c)

2 Breast feeding is not always contraindicated with this disorder.

3 Breast feeding is not contraindicated with inverted nipples, since a breast shield can provide mild suction to help pull out a nipple.

4 Not always contraindicated; the baby already has the organism in the mouth, and nursing will decrease the mother's discomfort.

30. **3** Toxemia does not interfere with uterine involution, return of uterine tone, or constriction of vessels at the placental site. (c)

1 Overdistension of the uterus may lead to delayed or poor uterine myometrial contraction at the placental site after delivery.

2 Retained placenta inhibits uterine myometrial contractions; also manual removal of placenta may cause uterine trauma.

4 May inhibit myometrial contraction of the uterus at the placental site.

31. **3** The term "stillborn" is used to describe a dead fetus of more than 24 weeks gestation, weighing 600 or more grams. (c)

1 Incomplete information given for this conclusion; only the fetus is mentioned.

2 A fetus of 24 weeks gestation or more is considered viable.

4 This length is indicative of a previable fetus, which is not classified as stillborn.

32. **2** Based on the family's decision, extraordinary care does not have to be employed; the child's basic needs are met, and nature is allowed to take its course. (b)

1 Euthanasia is a deliberate intervention to cause death.

3 If the child's physical needs are met and comfort is provided, the child's rights are not ignored; "extraordinary," not "all," care is being withheld.

4 It is neither unethical nor illegal to withhold extraordinary treatment; once such treatment is started, it becomes a legal issue.

33. **1** Immaturity of the diaphragm and the intercostal and abdominal musculature inhibits adequate ventilation, which causes lung expansion to be inadequate; consequently the infant must use tremendous effort. (c)

2 Cyanosis is a later manifestation; more common with congenital heart defects.

3 Rapid respirations are normally present in newborns.

4 Grunting more commonly occurs when the baby is chilled or cold.

34. **1** Hypertension in toxemia leads to vasospasms; this in turn causes the placenta to tear away from the uterine wall (abruptio placentae). (c)

2 Generally does not affect the circulation to the placenta.

3 May cause endocrine disturbance in the infant but does not affect the blood supply to the uterus.

4 This may affect the delivery of the fetus but does not affect the placenta.

35. **1** Overdistension of the uterus because of a large baby, multiple gestation, or hydramnios predisposes a woman to uterine atony, which may cause postpartum hemorrhage. (b)

2 Unless uterine atony is present, hemorrhage should not occur; a grand multipara is at risk for placenta previa.

3 This leads to precipitous delivery (potentially harmful to the fetus) but does not affect uterine contractions after delivery.

4 Not a factor in involution of the uterus.

36. **2** In a breech delivery the head is not the presenting part bearing the brunt of the pressure against the pelvic floor during delivery. (b)

   1 May occur if there is difficulty in delivering the head after the body is born.

   3 The cord may prolapse; and pressure of the baby can cause cord compression, resulting in fetal hypoxia.

   4 This commonly occurs in breech deliveries.

37. **2** Observation and recordkeeping of bleeding are independent nursing functions and necessary for implementing safe care, since hemorrhage and shock can be life threatening. (a)

   1 The client should be restricted to complete bed rest until bleeding stops.

   3 Vital signs should be checked more often if bleeding persists.

   4 This is absolutely forbidden, since it may cause further separation of the placenta.

38. **2** A fallopian tube is unable to contain and sustain a pregnancy to term; as the fertilized ovum grows, there is excessive stretching or rupture of the fallopian tube, causing pain. (c)

   1 Pain is sudden, intense, knifelike, and usually located on one side.

   3 Leukorrhea and dysuria may be indicative of a vaginal or bladder infection.

   4 This would be difficult for the client to identify correctly.

39. **3** A position in which the mother's head is below the level of the hips helps decrease compression of the cord and therefore increase blood supply to the infant. (a)

   1 This does not relieve the pressure of the oncoming head on the cord.

   2 This may increase the pressure of the presenting part on the cord.

   4 The pressure of the presenting part on the cord is not relieved in this position.

40. **1** Blood loss depletes the normal cellular response to infection; trauma provides an excellent medium for bacteria to grow. (c)

   2 Toxemia is generally not a predisposing cause of postpartum hemorrhage.

   3 May create problems if hemorrhage occurs since the hemoglobin and hematocrit are already low.

   4 Endogenous infection is rare; infection usually caused by outside contamination; trauma and the denuded placental site do contribute to the development of infection.

41. **3** Heart development occurs between the second and eighth weeks of gestation. (b)

   1 This is a neural tube defect not associated with rubella.

   2 Associated with intake of teratogenic drugs not rubella.

   4 Generally occurs later in life; not caused by rubella; rubella may cause nerve deafness from eighth cranial (vestibulocochlear) nerve or hearing center involvement.

42. **2** The increased pulmonary blood flow raises the pressure in the left atrium and functionally forces the septum to close the foramen ovale. (c)

   1 There is an increased aortic blood flow.

   3 Caused by increased pressure in the left atrium.

   4 There is decreased pressure in the right atrium.

43. **3** There is anatomic obliteration of the lumen by fibrous proliferation, leading to the term "ligamentum arteriosum." (b)

   1 Descriptive term meaning long and round ligament.

   2 This refers to the ductus venosus.

   4 There is no such vessel.

44. **1** Bacteria, especially *Escherichia coli,* produce and synthesize prothrombin. (c)

   2 Manufactured in the liver, not synthesized by bacteria.

   3 Secreted by the gastric glands, not synthesized by bacteria.

   4 An orange bile pigment produced by the breakdown of hemoglobin.

45. **3** The immunity is that which has developed from an antigen-antibody response in the mother and is passed to the fetus. (b)

   1 Acquired by an individual in response to a disease or an infection.

   2 Acquired by an individual in response to small amounts of antigenic material (e.g., vaccination).

   4 Conferred by the injection of antibodies already prepared in another host.

46. **4** The congenital absence of a vessel in the umbilical cord is often associated with life-threatening congenital anomalies. (b)

   1 If the Apgar score 5 minutes later showed marked improvement, there would be no need for placing the infant in the ICU.

   2 This is the average weight for a full-term newborn.

   3 The fetus may have swallowed some amniotic fluid; not unusual or dangerous.

47. **1** Medical supervision requires treatment with an appropriate antibiotic for 2 to 3 weeks until two negative cultures are obtained; re-treatment may be necessary if there is a recurrence; recurring pyelitis often leads to preterm birth. (c)

   2 Signs of toxemia occur spontaneously; not preceded by specific infections.

   3 Pelvic inflammatory disease is associated with infections of the genital not the urinary tract.

   4 A low-protein diet would inhibit good fetal development and is contraindicated in pregnancy.

48. **1** The pressure exerted anywhere in a mass of fluid in a closed container is transmitted undiminished throughout all parts of the fluid and in all directions. (c)

   2 A principle dealing with the displacement of fluid not pressure.

   3 Laws dealing with motion not pressure.

   4 Theory dealing with relativity not pressure.

49. **4** Progesterone acts to reduce contractility of the uterine musculature and to maintain the decidual bed. (b)

   1 Elevated progesterone levels would inhibit contractility of the uterine musculature.

   2 Progesterone, not estrogen, inhibits contractions.

   3 Would tend to stimulate contractions but is inhibited by progesterone, not estrogen.

50. **3** Concentration of the polypeptide, a melanocyte-stimulating hormone, rises from the end of the second month of pregnancy until term. (a)

   1 High levels of chorionic gonadotropin, secreted by the chorion, are associated with nausea and vomiting.

   2 Related to advancing growth and pressure of the uterus on the bladder.

   4 Due to increased mucoidal secretions.

51. **2** If the woman had a hemophilic father, she must have had his X chromosome, which carries the recessive gene for hemophilia (if she had had his Y chromosome, she would have been male); since her blood

clots normally, her other X chromosome carries the dominant gene for normal blood clotting. She is represented by H_1h (the H_1 being the affected gamete); her normal mate is represented by HY. The cross:

Father

	H	Y
H₁	H_1H	H_1Y
h	Hh	hY

(Mother: H₁, h)   (c)

  1 Could happen only if both parents were hemophiliacs.
  3 Fifty percent of the male children could be normal.
  4 Fifty percent of the offspring are affected—male hemophiliacs or female carriers.

52. **1** Anemia decreases the capacity of the blood to carry oxygen and thus increases the demands on the heart. (b)
  2 This is due to disturbance in the conduction of impulses not the oxygen-carrying capacity of blood.
  3 Cardiac irregularity not associated with anemia.
  4 A diseased heart is not capable of further cardiac compensation; decompensation would result.

53. **2** Subsequent to IUD insertion, menstrual periods may have an excessive flow for several cycles; this is probably because of an increase in the blood supply (inflammatory process), since the IUD is really a foreign body. (c)
  1 This may occur upon insertion but is fairly uncommon.
  3 This may occur but is not classified as a side effect.
  4 No documentation of this.

54. **1** Oral contraceptives contain varying kinds and dosages of synthetic estrogen and progestogen compounds that mimic natural cyclic hormone changes and prolong the menses. (c)
  2 Untrue; since pills contain estrogen, they will minimize menopausal symptoms that are caused by lowered estrogen content.
  3 This would be symptomatic of disease not of oral contraceptive usage.
  4 It tends to prolong menses by supplying estrogen.

55. **3** Untreated ophthalmia neonatorum becomes apparent on the third or fourth postnatal day and is evidence that the mother has gonorrhea. (b)
  1 Conjunctivitis from silver nitrate instillation develops on the first day.
  2 Ophthalmia neonatorum does not develop until the third day.
  4 The incubation period for the gonococci that cause ophthalmia neonatorum is 3 to 4 days after birth.

56. **1** *Chlamydia trachomatis* transmitted from the mother is usually manifested in the infant as an eye infection; it becomes apparent on the third or fourth postnatal day.
  2 Acquired transplacentally, not via the genital tract.
  3 *Monila*, not *Neisseria gonorrhoeae*, causes thrush.
  4 Usually acquired by aspiration, not exposure to gonococci.

57. **1** Because congenital syphilis is difficult to detect at birth, the infant should be screened immediately to determine if treatment is necessary. (c)
  2 This defect occurs in first trimester; *Treponema pallidum* does not affect a fetus before the sixteenth week of gestation.
  3 This does not become manifest in the syphilitic infant until about 3 months of age.
  4 This is found in children with Down's syndrome, not congenital syphilis.

58. **1** Uninformed consent constitutes an artificial consent; sufficient information was not given. (b)
  2 The surgeon may do what is necessary if an informed consent is obtained for all eventualities.
  3 This is not sufficient to cover invasive procedures or surgery.
  4 Informed consent covers only that which is covered by the consent.

59. **1** The ovaries are responsible for producing the female sex hormones estrogen and progesterone; a bilateral oophorectomy causes an abrupt cessation in the production of most of these hormones (the adrenal cortex produces small quantities of female sex hormones) and results in surgical menopause. (b)
  2 Hysterectomy is the removal of the uterus, and ovarian function is unaffected.
  3 Salpingectomy is the removal of the fallopian tubes, and ovarian function is unaffected.
  4 Tubal ligation is the surgical severing of the fallopian tubes to produce sterility, and ovarian function is unaffected.

60. **4** Alteration of ovarian hormones cause vasomotor instability; periodic systemic vasodilation is then triggered by the sympathetic nervous system, causing the feeling of warmth. (c)
  1 Hot flashes may be associated with understimulation of the adrenals.
  2 Acetylcholine does not cause hot flashes; it is the chemical mediator of cholinergic nerve impulses.
  3 Gonadotropins do not cause hot flashes; they stimulate the function of the testes and ovaries.

61. **3** The lack of utilization of gonadotropin by the ovaries causes an elevation of gonadotropin in the blood; ovarian function is diminished; there is little or no follicular activity. (c)
  1 There would be a decrease in secretion of progesterone.
  2 There would be an increase in prostaglandins.
  4 There would be an increase in gonadotropin in the blood, for it is not used by the ovaries.

62. **1** It is the surge of LH secretion in midcycle that is responsible for ovulation. (a)
  2 When the endometrial wall is built up.
  3 When the progesterone level is low.
  4 Not related; this stimulates ejection of milk into the mammary ducts.

63. **2** High levels of plasma estrogen inhibit pituitary secretion of FSH; this effect appears to be mediated by the hypothalamus and its releasing factors. (c)
  1 LH (luteinizing hormone) causes ovulation.
  3 Low concentrations of estrogen may precipitate demineralization of bone.
  4 Lactogenic hormone (prolactin) stimulates lactation.

64. **2** Naegle's rule is an indirect noninvasive method for estimating the date of delivery:

$$EDC = LMP + 7 \text{ days} - 3 \text{ months} + 1 \text{ year} \quad (b)$$

  1 Miscalculation.
  3 Miscalculation.
  4 Miscalculation.

65. **2** True; allows the client to discuss her feelings and participate in her care. (b)
  1 Cuts off communication; denies the client's feelings.
  3 Client has already told the nurse how she feels.
  4 Within the scope of the nurse's information; also may cause the client to worry that something is seriously wrong.

66. **4** A frequent change from the sitting position is important for good circulation; walking is an excellent form of exercise to promote circulation. (b)
  1 Elevation of the legs does not promote arterial circulation; merely fosters venous return.
  2 Not true; clients may work until the day of delivery.
  3 Added nourishment can be part of her regular mealtimes; in addition, nourishment will not promote circulation.
67. **1** Although pure types are unusual, the normal female pelvis is one most favorable for normal delivery; characteristics include well-rounded inlet, straight sidewalls, well-formed sacrosciatic notches, good sacral curvature and inclination, movable coccyx, moderately sized ischial spines, and well-rounded suprapubic arches. (b)
  2 The normal female pelvis is gynecoid; this describes an android pelvis.
  3 The normal female pelvis is gynecoid; this is descriptive of an anthropoid pelvis.
  4 The normal female pelvis is gynecoid; this describes a platypelloid pelvis.
68. **2** By taking a diet history, the nurse can assess the woman's level of nutritional knowledge and gain clues for appropriate methods of counseling. (a)
  1 These foods may be too expensive and different from her normal choices, leading to noncompliance.
  3 Salt is no longer limited in normal pregnancy.
  4 Normal is too vague a term; the client will need increased protein and caloric intake.
69. **3** A sudden sharp increase near the twentieth week of pregnancy may indicate water retention and the beginning of preeclampsia. (b)
  1 Untrue; weight gain is necessary to ensure adequate nutrition for the fetus.
  2 Closes off communication; does not allow the client to ask more questions about weight gain.
  4 There is no hard-and-fast number of pounds that the client should gain, and low-calorie diets may be harmful.
70. **2** The saline may have gotten into the vascular system rather than into the amniotic sac. (c)
  1 A serious manifestation of water intoxication occurring when oxytocin is used in the saline abortion; not a consequence of saline administration.
  3 Bradycardia may occur with the use of spinal or regional anesthesia, not salinization.
  4 Edema may occur as a result of water intoxication when oxytocin is used in the saline abortion.
71. **4** The saline causes puffing of the placenta, fetal death, placental separation, release of fibrin, and then labor and paradoxical hemorrhaging. This takes at least 24 hours in most cases. (c)
  1 Normally labor starts 24 to 72 hours after the procedure.
  2 Too quick; it takes 24 to 72 hours for labor to begin.
  3 Too quick; usually takes 24 to 72 hours, unless oxytocin is used to hasten labor.
72. **3** Because of the irritation, the uterine lining is not receptive to the implantation of the fertilized egg. (c)
  1 A diaphragm blocks the cervical os.
  2 Mobility of the uterus is not related to contraception.
  4 The sperm can reach the fallopian tube; implantation of the fertilized egg is impaired.
73. **3** The IUD may cause irritability of the myometrium, inducing contraction of the uterus and expulsion of the device. (c)
  1 Increased vaginal infections are not reported with use of IUD.
  2 Clients do not complain of discomfort during coitus when an IUD is in place.
  4 This is a rare rather than a common occurrence.
74. **1** The first trimester is the period when all major organs are being laid down; drugs, alcohol, and tobacco may cause major defects. (a)
  2 Drugs, unless absolutely necessary, should be avoided throughout pregnancy; but the first trimester is most significant.
  3 Cutting down is insufficient; these teratogens should be eliminated.
  4 Aspirin is known to cause severe hemolysis in the fetus, and even 1 oz of alcohol is considered harmful.
75. **1** The physical principle is surface tension; since the lung tissue of the infant lacks the group of detergents known as surfactant, water molecules strongly interact with each other by hydrogen bonding and the alveolar sacs and respiratory passages do not easily expand; the result is extremely labored, if not impossible, breathing. (b)
  2 This is related to the equal distribution of external pressure throughout a fluid in a closed vessel.
  3 This has to do with the relationship between heat and mechanical energy.
  4 This has to do with a body in water being buoyed by force equal to the weight of the fluid displaced.
76. **2** Humidity may liquefy the tenacious secretions, making gas exchange possible. (b)
  1 Side lying, rather than prone, since the babies may be too immature to raise their heads from the prone position.
  3 This is not a routine action; oxygen concentration will depend on the babies' blood gases.
  4 Actually the caloric intake will be increased; the amount, number, and type of feedings will be related to the metabolic rate.
77. **4** Bonding between parent and baby is most successful when interaction is possible right after birth; if the child is ill, contact is limited. (c)
  1 Though certainly a factor, more important is the physical condition of the twins.
  2 Relative; but most important is the physical condition of the twins.
  3 May be relative; but most important is the physical condition of the twins.
78. **3** The overdistended uterus from the twin pregnancy does not contract readily. (b)
  1 This can occur in any delivery (not just twins) if careful inspection of the placenta is not done.
  2 This is unusual and may occur with improper use of forceps; not indicated in this situation.
  4 Cause systemic responses other than hemorrhage.
79. **3** The posterior vaginal wall is pushed forward by the herniation of the rectum; this protrusion increases rectal pressure and causes the bearing-down sensation. (c)
  1 This is the primary symptom of a cystocele.
  2 A rectocele is not accompanied by abdominal pain.
  4 A cystocele is associated with urinary tract infections.
80. **2** Heart rate is vital and the most critical observation in Apgar scoring at birth. (c)
  1 Respiratory effort rather than rate is included in the Apgar score; the rate is very erratic.
  3 May or may not be present at this time and not part of Apgar scoring.
  4 Should be assessed later, but not part of Apgar scoring.
81. **3** The rate varies with activity; crying will increase the rate, whereas deep sleep will lower it; a rate between 120 and 160 is within normal range. (b)

1 Rates below 120 are considered bradycardia; above 180, tachycardia.

2 The normal rate is between 120 and 160.

4 Below 120 is considered bradycardia.

82. **3** Rate is associated with activity and can be as rapid as 60 breaths per minute; over 60 breaths per minute is considered tachypneic in the infant. (b)

1 Considered to be tachypneic in the newborn.

2 Any rate above 60 considered to be tachypneic.

4 May go up to 60 with activity.

83. **2** Changes in equilibrium stimulate this neurologic reflex in an infant under the age of 6 months; the movements should be bilateral and symmetric; a loud noise causes the same reaction (startle reflex), but using noise as a stimulus really tests hearing. (c)

1 Tests the baby's hearing not the Moro reflex.

3 Tests for the Babinski reflex not the Moro.

4 Tests for the grasp reflex not the Moro.

84. **4** The Moro reflex is a sudden extension and abduction of the arms at the shoulders and spreading of the fingers, with the index finger and thumb forming the letter "c"; this is followed by flexion and adduction; the legs may weakly flex, and the infant may cry vigorously. (b)

1 Only part of the normal Moro response; should be accompanied by abduction and spreading of the fingers.

2 Legs generally flex weakly.

3 The reflex is abduction.

85. **3** Injury to the brachial plexus, clavicle, or humerus prevents the abductive and adductive movements of the upper extremities. (b)

1 These injuries usually cause a symmetric loss of the Moro reflex.

2 Not usually associated; however, if the cochlea is undeveloped or the eighth cranial (vestibulocochlear) nerve were injured, it would affect equilibrium and response to the test.

4 Children with Down's syndrome exhibit a normal Moro reflex.

86. **2** The Committee on Maternal Nutrition of the National Research Council recommends a weight gain of at least 25 lb (11.3 kg) during pregnancy; inadequate nutrition results in underweight babies. (a)

1 Dieting is absolutely forbidden during pregnancy and can result in congenital anomalies.

3 The cause of stillbirth is not actually known; dieting is not recommended.

4 There is a theory that an inadequate intake of protein is related to toxemia, but it has not been totally proved.

87. **2** The nurse should become informed about the cultural eating patterns of clients so that foods containing the essential nutrients, which are part of these dietary patterns, will be included in the diet. (c)

1 Pregnancy diets are not specific; merely composed of the essential nutrients.

3 Fluid retention is only one component of weight gain; growth of the baby, placenta, breasts, etc. also contribute to weight gain.

4 Calories and nutrients are increased during pregnancy.

88. **2** Fluids and salt should not be restricted, for they are necessary to the well-being of the mother and fetus; elevation of the extremities several times daily is recommended to decrease the edema. (b)

1 Salt is not limited during pregnancy.

3 Salt is not limited during pregnancy.

4 Diuretics can be harmful and are not used during pregnancy.

89. **3** As the lower uterus contracts and dilates, the edge of the low-lying placenta separates from the walls of the uterus, opening placental sinuses and allowing blood to escape. (b)

1 Abruptio placentae is usually accompanied by intense pain.

2 Highly unlikely unless placenta previa is present.

4 Previa, a low-implanted placenta, causes painless vaginal bleeding; alcohol ingestion does not.

90. **1** Gravitational pull on an already-stressed placenta may cause further bleeding. (b)

2 Unless FHR is decelerating, this is not necessary.

3 Provides for fetal assessment; does not delay delivery date.

4 Provides for fetal assessment; does not delay delivery date.

91. **1** Frequently high levels of chorionic gonadotropin are associated with severe vomiting of pregnancy, especially in the presence of hydatidiform mole and often in twin pregnancy. (b)

2 This is associated with vomiting; undigested food remains in the stomach, which leads to a reflexive action and vomiting; common but not severe in early pregnancy.

3 Unrelated; due to HCG.

4 Polyhydramnios (excessive amniotic fluid) is associated with multiple gestation; maternal dehydration is generally associated with hyperemesis gravidarum.

92. **3** Intact membranes act as a barrier against organisms that may cause an intrauterine infection. (b)

1 Common because of increased production of mucus containing exfoliated vaginal epithelial cells; intercourse is not contraindicated.

2 Intercourse is not contraindicated if membranes are intact; modification of sexual positions may be needed because of an enlarged abdomen after the thirtieth week.

4 This may be occurring, but there is no literature indicating that it is harmful for the fetus.

93. **2** Transcervical amniotomy (artificial rupture of the membranes) requires that the cervix be soft, partially effaced, and slightly dilated with the presenting part engaged or engaging; this client would meet these criteria, as demonstrated by the bloody show and the head at +1. (c)

1 IM injection of oxytocin is extremely dangerous because of the physician's inability to control the effects of the drug; oxytocin by intravenous infusion is considered safe as long as maternal and fetal monitoring is continuous.

3 Prostaglandins are effective for inducing labor, but they are expensive and produce unpleasant side effects.

4 A tap water enema would be ineffective for inducing labor.

94. **2** The client is experiencing the expected discomforts of labor; the nurse should initiate measures that will promote relaxation. (b)

1 There is no evidence at this time that the client is losing excessive blood (hemorrhage).

3 During the pushing phase, straining is unavoidable.

4 The client is not receptive to teaching at this time; all energy is being directed inward.

95. **3** Diaphoresis is a normal adaptation of the postpartum period and does not relate to bladder distension; it is caused by the reduction of antidiuretic hormone, leading to profuse perspiration. (b)

1 This may follow anesthesia and cause retention.

2 Stasis of urine and infection can occur when urinary retention is present.

4 Postpartum bleeding may occur if the uterus is impeded from involuting because of a full bladder.

96. **1** A respiratory rate below 40 in the newborn is not within the normal range; normal is 40 to 60 breaths per minute; a drop to 35 per minute is a significant change and should have been reported. (b)

2 Any significant change should be reported immediately because it may be indicative of brain damage.

3 Untrue; more likely respirations will accelerate when activity is increased.

4 The respiratory tract is fully developed, and respiratory rate is a cardinal sign of the infant's well-being.

97. **3** The mother has completed the taking-in phase (mother's needs predominate) and has moved into the taking-hold phase (active maternal involvement with self and infant) when she calls the baby by name. (c)

1 This is part of the taking-in phase.

2 Initial early action of the taking-in phase.

4 This may occur in either phase.

98. **2** Determines the number and condition of sperm aspirated from the cervix within 2 hours after coitus. (b)

1 The Rubin test determines the patency of the fallopian tubes.

3 The Papanicolaou test is used for the early diagnosis of cervical cancer.

4 The Friedman test is done to establish the diagnosis of pregnancy.

99. **4** This test enables the examiner to visualize the uterus and fallopian tubes and the pelvic organs for reproduction. (a)

1 Cystoscopy is used to evaluate the urinary bladder.

2 Biopsy is the surgical excision of tissue for diagnostic purposes.

3 Culdoscopy is the direct examination of female pelvic viscera using an endoscope introduced through a perforation in the vagina.

100. **3** The ovum is capable of being fertilized for only 24 to 36 hours following ovulation; after this time it travels a variable distance between the fallopian tube and uterus, disintegrates, and is phagocytized by leukocytes. (b)

1 The ovum is viable for 24 to 36 hours.

2 It is viable a longer time.

4 It is not fertilizable after 48 hours.

101. **2** Sperm motility is increased at pH values near neutral or slightly alkaline; a sodium bicarbonate douche will reduce the acidity of fluids in the vagina and help optimize the pH. (c)

1 Sulfur does not change the pH in any way.

3 This would increase the acid content and kill the sperm.

4 Estrogen does not alter the pH.

102. **3** The action of Enovid is to inhibit ovulation and establish regular menstrual cycles; this is one of the first steps in treating infertility problems. (b)

1 Vallestril is used for management of estrogen deficiency; no action on the ovaries.

2 Ergotrate is used to contract the uterus.

4 Relaxin is used for dysmenorrhea; causes relaxation of the symphysis pubis.

103. **3** Oxytocin is a small polypeptide hormone normally synthesized in the hypothalamus and secreted from the neurohypophysis during parturition or suckling; it promotes powerful uterine (smooth muscle) contractions and thus is used to induce labor. (c)

1 Ergonovine can lead to sustained contractions, which would be undesirable in labor.

2 Progesterone builds up the endometrium; does not initiate uterine contractions.

4 Preludin or phenmetrazine is an appetite suppressant; not used in pregnancy.

104. **1** Since oxytocin promotes powerful uterine contractions, exogenous administration of this hormone may induce uterine tetany, which does not optimize progression of labor and may restrict fetal blood flow. (b)

2 Severe pain is associated with intense contractions.

3 Not likely to occur unless the baby is in breech position.

4 Unlreated to uterine contractions.

105. **4** Contractions are stronger and more regular when the woman is standing; also, during walking the diameter of the pelvic inlet increases and allows for easier entrance of the head into the pelvis. (b)

1 Untrue; contractions of true labor are enhanced when the mother walks about.

2 Denies the nurse's understanding of the physiology of labor.

3 Timing can continue even if the client walks around.

106. **1** When the membranes rupture, there is always the possibility of a prolapsed cord leading to fetal distress, which would manifest itself in a slowed fetal heartbeat. (b)

2 Unnecessary, unless there is a marked change in the FHR.

3 This is regularly done before and after the membranes rupture; however, fetal status takes priority.

4 Done routinely throughout the entire labor process; at this point, fetal status takes priority.

107. **3** By 36 weeks gestation, normal amniotic fluid is colorless with small particles of vernix caseosa present. (a)

1 Dark amber suggests the presence of bilirubin, an ominous sign.

2 Greenish yellow may indicate the presence of meconium and suggests fetal distress.

4 Cloudy suggests the presence of purulent material, and greenish yellow may indicate the presence of meconium.

108. **2** This slow deep breathing expands the spaces between the ribs and raises the abdominal muscles, allowing room for the uterus to expand and preventing painful pressure of the uterus against the abdominal wall. (a)

1 Panting is used to halt or delay the pushing out of the baby's head before complete dilation.

3 Pelvic rocking is used during pregnancy and the puerperal period; it is not feasible during labor.

4 Athletic chest breathing is not one of the exercises used in this stage of labor.

109. **1** The contractions become stronger, last longer, and are erratic during this stage; the intervals during the contractions are shorter than the contractions themselves; much concentration and effort are needed by the mother to pace herself with each contraction. (b)

2 Not true; administration of analgesic or anesthetic at this point could reduce the effectiveness of labor and depress the fetus.

3 There is no indication that any abnormality is developing.

4 Even clients who have been adequately prepared will experience these behaviors during the transition stage.

110. **4** Both the father and the mother need additional support during the transitional stage of labor. (b)

1 This does not encourage him to fulfill his role in supporting the mother during labor.

2 He should be present throughout labor to support his wife; he should be assisted in this role.

3 Judgmental; this approach suggests that he will be failing his wife.

111. **2** The contractions in this phase of labor are expulsive in nature; having the client push or bear down with the lips closed will hasten expulsion. (a)
  1 Contractions are now frequent and intense; the client is anxious to complete the labor process; she will be unable to relax.
  3 The client should be pushing; panting will prevent this.
  4 Blowing is encouraged to slow down pushing; she should be encouraged to push.

112. **4** The heart rate increases by about 10 beats per minute in the last half of pregnancy; this increase plus the increase in total blood volume can strain a damaged heart beyond the point at which it can efficiently compensate. (c)
  1 The number of RBCs does not decrease during pregnancy; plasma volume increases, simulating lowered hemoglobin.
  2 Cardiac output begins to decrease by the thirty-fourth week of gestation.
  3 The increased size of uterus is related to growth of the fetus not to any hemodynamic change.

113. **1** The side-lying position takes the weight off large blood vessels, and blood flow to the heart is increased; elevating the shoulders relieves pressure on the diaphragm. (c)
  2 Potassium chloride is contraindicated unless lowered potassium levels indicate the need.
  3 Sodium leads to increased fluid retention; contraindicated in the cardiac client.
  4 Contraindicated unless some uterine inertia occurs.

114. **2** Any medication that might further depress a premature infant is given with extreme caution. (b)
  1 False reassurance; there is no absolute control of premature labor.
  3 At the proper time the client is encouraged to bear down.
  4 If the client is kept NPO, it is done to lessen the risk of aspiration should anesthesia become necessary.

115. **2** An early symptom of congestive heart failure is respiratory distress. (c)
  1 Although pulse is important, the primary observation should be for respiratory distress, which suggests impending congestive heart failure.
  3 Increased vaginal bleeding is not caused by alterations in cardiac status.
  4 Signs of congestive failure, not hypovolemic shock, might develop.

116. **3** Unnecessary; baby's Apgar (8/9) does not indicate need for oxygen. (b)
  1 All newborns are evaluated immediately.
  2 Poor thermoregulation necessitates keeping the baby warm to stabilize body temperature.
  4 This is an important part of record keeping on all newborns.

117. **2** Immaturity of the respiratory tract in preterm infants can be evidenced by a lack of functional alveoli, smaller lumina with increased possibility of collapse of the respiratory passages, weakness of respiratory musculature, and insufficient calcification of the bony thorax leading to respiratory distress. (a)
  1 Not a primary concern unless severe hypoxia occurred during labor; difficult to diagnose at this time.
  3 May be a problem, but generally the air passageway is well suctioned at birth.
  4 Not a common occurrence at the time of birth unless trauma has occurred.

118. **3** Neonates are unable to shiver; they use the breakdown of brown fat to supply body heat; the premature baby has a limited supply of brown fat available for this breakdown. (c)
  1 The breakdown of glycogen into glucose does not supply body heat.
  2 Newborns are unable to use shivering to supply body heat.
  4 The pituitary gland does not supply body heat.

119. **2** The premature infant has a reduced glomerular filtration rate and reduced ability to concentrate urine or conserve water. (c)
  1 Untrue; all systems of the preterm baby are less developed than in the full-term infant.
  3 The fluid and electrolyte balance of preterm infants is easily upset.
  4 The opposite occurs; urine is very dilute.

120. **2** Characteristics of the midphase of labor for the primiparous client include regular contractions 30 to 45 seconds long and 3 to 5 minutes apart, station of the presenting part at +1 to +2, and pink to bloody show in moderate amount. (c)
  1 Contractions are less frequent in the early phase, and dilation is not so advanced.
  3 In this phase, dilation is 8 to 10 cm and contractions more frequent.
  4 This terminology is not appropriate for a phase of labor.

121. **1** In reporting progress in the descent of the presenting part, the level of the tip of the ischial spines is considered to be zero and the position of the bony prominence of the fetal head is described in centimeters—minus (above the spines) or plus (below the spines). (b)
  2 Minus one (−1) would indicate that the head is above the ischial spines.
  3 This is designated by the term "floating," meaning that the presenting part has not yet engaged.
  4 This would be referred to as crowning and would be designated as +5.

122. **2** Meperidine (Demerol) is classified as a narcotic analgesic drug and is effective for the relief of pain; promethazine (Phenergan) can be classified as an analgesic potentiating drug that permits the effective use of analgesics in lower dosages. (a)
  1 This is an undesirable effect because the mother could not participate in the delivery process.
  3 These medications do not induce amnesia.
  4 There is no indication that anesthesia will be used.

123. **3** The physiologic intensification of labor occurring during transition is caused by a greater energy expenditure and increased pressure on the stomach; this results in feelings of fatigue, discouragement, and nausea. (b)
  1 This stage is from full dilation to expulsion; a heavy bloody show and pushing are evident at this time.
  2 Unclear terminology; does not indicate the specific time of labor.
  4 This stage is from delivery of the fetus to delivery of the placenta; the mother does not experience any physiologic symptoms.

124. **4** Some maternal oxytocin crosses the placenta and induces the secretion of fluids that have accumulated in the fetal breasts (sometimes called witch's milk). (a)
  1 Usually manifested in the oral mucosa as thrush (white adherent patches).
  2 An uncommon and usually undetectable occurrence in the newborn period.

3 Evidence of infection would not appear so rapidly after birth.

125. **2** The fundus descends one finger breadth per day from the day after delivery; lochia serosa begins to flow on the fifth day. (b)
  1 The fundus would be one to three fingers below the umbilicus (one finger breadth per day).
  3 The fundus would be descending into the pelvis at this time.
  4 The fundus would be within the pelvis and indiscernible at this time.

126. **2** Magnesium sulfate has a CNS depressant effect; therefore toxic levels will be reflected in decreased respiration and the absence of the knee-jerk reflex. (c)
  1 May be caused by increased potassium, not magnesium sulfate.
  3 There is a decrease in respirations with excessive magnesium sulfate.
  4 This may happen from sedation, not from magnesium sulfate.

127. **2** Absolute bed rest, a quiet room, and minimal stimulation are essential to reducing the risk of a convulsion. (b)
  1 This would be contraindicated, since fluid retention is a problem in preeclampsia.
  3 She will need constant observation and should not be isolated.
  4 This may cause temporary supine hypotension with resultant bradycardia in the infant; could also result in aspiration should a convulsion occur.

128. **1** This is a sign of CNS involvement that the nurse can observe without obtaining subjective data from the client. (c)
  2 This is a subjective sign and is not obvious to the nurse.
  3 These are subjective symptoms; the client must indicate their presence.
  4 Pain and nausea are subjective symptoms and are not directly observable.

129. **3** Increased electric charges in the brain during a convulsion may disturb the cerebral thermoregulation center. (b)
  1 One elevated reading is not a conclusive sign of infection.
  2 There is no rapid fluid loss during a convulsion; actually this client has fluid retention.
  4 Excessive muscular activity usually causes perspiration leading to a drop in body temperature.

130. **4** The danger of convulsion in a woman with eclampsia ends when postpartum diuresis has occurred, usually 48 hours after delivery. (c)
  1 Untrue; the danger of convulsion in eclampsia ends when postpartum diuresis occurs about 48 hours after delivery.
  2 Untrue; the danger of convulsion in eclampsia ends when postpartum diuresis occurs about 48 hours after delivery.
  3 Untrue; the danger of convulsion in eclampsia ends when postpartum diuresis occurs about 48 hours after delivery.

131. **1** In Erb-Duchenne paralysis there is damage to spinal nerves C_5 and C_6, which causes paralysis of the arm. (c)
  2 There would be a negative Moro reflex on the affected side only.
  3 The grasp reflex is intact since the fingers usually are not affected; if C_8 is injured, paralysis of the hand results (Klumpke's paralysis).

4 There is no interference with turning of the head; injury usually results from excessive lateral flexion of the head during delivery of the shoulder.

132. **3** Range-of-motion exercises must be done to prevent contractures. (c)
  1 Dangerous since it would lead to permanent contractures.
  2 The muscle action usually improves spontaneously when edema subsides.
  4 The length of the arm will not change on a daily basis.

133. **4** Heavy cigarette smoking or continued exposure to a smoke-filled environment causes both maternal and fetal vasoconstriction, resulting in fetal growth retardation and increased fetal and infant mortality. (a)
  1 The fetal and maternal circulations are separate; the answer is not related to the question.
  2 Smoking causes vasoconstriction; permeability of the placenta to smoke is irrelevant.
  3 There is no concrete evidence that smoking relieves tension; this is not a factor in the situation described.

134. **4** This pigmentation is caused by the anterior pituitary hormone melanotropin, which increases during pregnancy. (c)
  1 Hyperactivity of the adrenal glands is manifested by symptoms of Cushing's syndrome.
  2 Hyperthyroidism is manifested by increased temperature, pulse, and respirations and a fine hand tremor.
  3 During pregnancy ovarian activity is very quiet because of the feedback mechanism.

135. **4** Chorionic gonadotropin, secreted in large amounts by the placenta during gestation, and the metabolic changes associated with pregnancy can precipitate nausea and vomiting in early pregnancy. (b)
  1 Estrogen is elevated throughout pregnancy; symptoms of morning sickness disappear after the first trimester.
  2 Progesterone is elevated throughout pregnancy; symptoms of morning sickness disappear after the first trimester.
  3 Luteinizing hormone is present during ovulation only.

136. **4** Nausea and vomiting of pregnancy can be relieved with small snacks of dry crackers or toast before rising, since the ingestion of carbohydrates helps settle the stomach. (a)
  1 Unsound advise, since both fetus and mother need nourishment.
  2 An antacid may affect electrolyte balance; also this will not help morning sickness.
  3 Medications in the first trimester are contraindicated; this is the period of organogenesis, and congenital anomalies could result.

137. **4** When the client signs herself and the baby out of the hospital, she is legally responsible for her infant and must be given the baby. (c)
  1 The baby belongs to the mother and can leave with the mother when she signs them out.
  2 The mother is the baby's guardian and may take the baby with her when she leaves.
  3 The baby is under the guardianship of the mother and may leave with the mother.

138. **4** Sonography, based on sound wave reflection and detection, locates the position of the fetus prior to insertion of the needle in amniocentesis; this minimizes the potential for fetal damage during the procedure. (b)
  1 X-ray examinations are contraindicated during pregnancy except at term to determine cephalopelvic disproportion.
  2 This is visualization of fetus through cervix; does not aid in placing needle into sac.

3 Formerly done; however, now sonography is the procedure of choice.

139. **2** The client must feel comfortable enough to verbalize her feelings of guilt if she is to be able to complete the grieving process. (b)
1 This is a false assumption.
3 Studies show that contraceptive counseling at this time is most important, since the client may not return after the abortion.
4 This is a sterile procedure and should not predispose the client to postoperative infection.

140. **1** RH$_0$D globulin attacks fetal red cells that have gained access to the maternal bloodstream at the time of delivery; it prevents antibody formation. (b)
2 Contraindicated, since antibody formation is undesirable; it sensitizes the mother and contributes to fetal red cell destruction in future pregnancies.
3 Irrelevant; there is no production of immune bodies.
4 RH$_0$D provides passive temporary immunity and prepares the fetal red blood cells for destruction before the mother's immune system can respond by producing antibodies against Rh-positive blood.

141. **4** Although support will help minimize guilt, it will not eliminate it; however, support will sustain family cohesion and unity. (a)
1 May help, but cannot completely relieve pressure.
2 Support may help, but in no way completely alleviates guilt feelings.
3 Support does not affect legal responsibility of the parents.

142. **3** Sneezing is the way in which the newborn clears mucus from the nose; breathing is normally rapid and irregular. (a)
1 This would discourage the mother from taking responsibility and slow the mothering process; it also implies that something could be wrong.
2 More explanation is needed, and it also shuts off communication; the mother needs to express her feelings of anxiety.
4 These are normal newborn responses and indicate no respiratory distress.

143. **2** Normally the newborn's breathing is diaphragmatic and irregular in depth and rhythm; the rate ranges from 40 to 50 breaths per minute. (b)
1 Infants' respirations are irregular and abdominal in origin.
3 Infants' respirations are irregular.
4 Infants' respirations are abdominal in origin.

144. **4** Opens up an area of communication to get at what really is troubling the mother about feeding the baby. (a)
1 Since the nurse is aware that this is not the best method, the problem of time should be explored with the mother.
2 Holding can be accomplished at times other than feeding periods; does not explore the client's feelings.
3 True, but mother should not be frightened; a more gentle explanation should be used.

145. **3** Early decelerations, with onset before the peak of the contraction and low point at the peak of the contraction, are due to fetal head compression; FHR rarely drops below 100 bpm. (c)
1 This is not a deceleration; it is within normal limits.
2 This is not a deceleration; it is within normal limits.
4 This is marked bradycardia.

146. **3** As the uterus rises into the abdominal cavity, the uterine ligaments become elongated and hypertrophied; raising both legs at the same time limits the tension placed on these ligaments. (b)

1 There is no effect on the fascia with this maneuver.
2 There is already pressure on the perineum from the baby's head; this maneuver places tension on the uterine ligaments.
4 Lifting the legs simultaneously does not negatively affect circulation in the legs.

147. **2** Because this was an uneventful labor to this point with no prior deceleration problems and the client just assumed the supine position on the delivery table, there is compression of the inferior vena cava reducing venous return and maternal cardiac output; the reduced FHR may indicate fetal hypoxia because of deficient perfusion. (c)
1 The nurse cannot assume that this is just an early deceleration (Type 1 dip); delay in intervention could lead to fetal hypoxia or death.
3 There is no indication that oxytocin has been infusing.
4 The client is in the lithotomy position and cannot be turned on her side.

148. **3** Soap irritates, cracks, and dries breasts and nipples, making it difficult for the baby to suck. (b)
1 She should empty the breast at each feeding to keep milk flowing.
2 This is a permissible and often used technique of breast feeding.
4 The breasts should be washed before feeding to remove encrustations and microorganisms.

149. **4** The most likely cause is a disturbance in the ratio of calcium to phosphorus, with the amount of serum calcium reduced and the serum phosphorus increased; milk is an excellent source of calcium. (a)
1 Leg cramps are usually related to low calcium intake not hypercalcemia.
2 A low potassium level is not an usual occurrence; not improved by ingestion of leafy vegetables.
3 Elevated potassium levels are very serious; not manifested by leg cramps.

150. **1** Cow's milk is diluted with water and has sugar added to make it resemble human milk. (c)
2 Contains more protein and more calcium.
3 Contains more protein and less calcium.
4 Contains more calcium.

151. **1** The term "premature" describes a newborn delivered at 37 weeks' gestation or less, regardless of weight. (a)
2 An infant weighing less than 1136 g (2½ lb) and considerably underdeveloped at birth.
3 Nonviable would be before the twenty-fourth week of gestation.
4 Means low birth weight for related gestational age.

152. **3** Gavage feeding is preferred for immature and weak infants, those with respiratory distress or poor sucking-swallowing coordination, and those who are easily fatigued. (b)
1 Feeding the infant quickly is not desirable; vomiting with aspiration may occur.
2 This is not a reason for instituting gavage; however, vomiting may be lessened with gavage feeding since the amount and rapidity of feeding can be controlled.
4 The amount can be regulated with bottle-feeding as well.

153. **2** Much of a full-term infant's birth weight is gained during the last month of pregnancy (almost a third), and most of this final spurt is subcutaneous fat, which serves as insulation; the premature baby has not had the time to grow in the uterus and has a paucity of this insulating layer. (a)
1 There is a relatively larger surface area per body weight.

3 There is an extremely limited shivering and sweating response in the premature infant.

4 Unrelated to the maintenance of body temperature.

154. **1** Prolonged oxygen administration at relatively high concentrations in a premature infant whose retina is incompletely differentiated and/or vascularized may result in retrolental fibroplasia; when oxygen therapy is discontinued, capillary overgrowth in the retina and vitreous body may result and include capillary hemorrhage, fibrosis, and retinal detachment. (b)

2 Though true, temperature and humidity are not factors in the development of retrolental fibroplasia.

3 Oxygen concentration of more than 40% is dangerous and a factor in the development of retrolental fibroplasia.

4 Phototherapy is used to decrease hyperbilirubinemia; unrelated to retrolental fibroplasia; however, the eyes are covered to prevent ocular damage.

155. **3** Flaccid muscle tone is the only abnormal finding; all other choices indicate a normal newborn response and would be higher on the Apgar scale. (b)

1 Apgar rating of 7 to 10 usually indicates this.

2 Present with an Apgar rating of 7 to 10.

4 Usually much slower in an infant whose Apgar score is 4.

156. **2** Intracranial bleeding may occur in the subdural, subarachnoid, or intraventricular spaces of the brain, causing pressure on vital centers; clinical signs are related to the area and degree of cerebral involvement. (a)

1 This is caused by hypocalcemia; manifested by exaggerated muscular twitching.

3 This is an obvious defect of the spinal column; easily recognized.

4 Elevated potassium causes cardiac irregularities.

157. **1** Development of jaundice in the first 24 hours indicates erythroblastosis fetalis. (c)

2 Normal; serum bilirubin normally accumulates in the neonatal period because of the short life span of fetal erythrocytes, reaching levels of 7 mg/100 ml the second to third day, when jaundice appears.

3 May or may not be present in first 24 hours; dependent on bilirubin level.

4 May or may not be present during first 24 hours of life; usually develops later.

158. **2** The tonic neck reflex (fencing position) is a spontaneous postural reflex of the newborn that may or may not be present during the first days of life; once apparent, it persists until the third month. (a)

1 Demonstration of muscle tone while held prone and suspended in midair.

3 This is the "startle" reflex.

4 This is a normal, expected reflex in the neonate.

159. **3** Informing parents of the birth of an abnormal child as early as possible, and preferably in the delivery room when staff is present to support and assist them in mobilizing resources, prevents fantasizing about the problem. (b)

1 Crisis intervention should not be delayed; immediately informing the parents improves coping abilities.

2 May be too much of a shock if the mother has no awareness of the defect.

4 Parents may not ask.

160. **4** Ovulation is anticipated approximately 14 days prior to menstruation; however, it is more reliable to avoid using a specific number of days and to calculate on the basis of an individual's cycle rather than an average 28-day cycle. (c)

1 Ovulation occurs 14 days before the onset of menstruation.

2 This may not be true in females with menstrual cycles longer than 28 days.

3 Ovulation occurs 14 days prior to the onset of menstruation.

161. **2** As ovulation approaches, there may be a drop in the basal temperature because of an increased production of estrogen; when ovulation occurs, there will be a rise in the basal temperature because of an increased production of progesterone. (b)

1 At ovulation the temperature drop is slight, not marked.

3 At ovulation the temperature drops slightly and then rises.

4 At ovulation the temperature rises after a slight drop.

162. **3** Stress or infection alters the body's metabolism, causing an elevation in temperature; a rise in temperature from these causes may be misinterpreted as ovulation. (b)

1 Frequency of intercourse may affect the volume of sperm but does not alter the female's basal temperature.

2 Age is not a factor concerning efficiency of the rhythm method.

4 This may increase sperm volume but does not affect the female's basal temperature.

163. **2** Ectopic pregnancy is one of the leading causes of first trimester bleeding; unless an embryo and placenta happen to be located in the abdominal cavity, they cannot grow outside the uterus for more than 10 to 12 weeks without showing the classic signs of pressure and bleeding. (b)

1 Abdominal cramping pain is present with an incomplete abortion.

3 Abruptio placentae is accompanied by sharp abdominal pain with or without bleeding.

4 This occurs monthly during ovulation without pain or vaginal bleeding; occasionally pain occurs when the follicle ruptures (mittelschmerz), but bleeding does not.

164. **1** Staining in the first trimester may indicate that the pregnancy is in jeopardy; bed rest, sedation, and avoidance of physical and emotional stress are recommended; abortion is usually inevitable if the bleeding is accompanied by pain with dilation and effacement of the cervix. (a)

2 This can be confirmed only if vaginal examination reveals cervical dilation.

3 Usually accompanied by severe pain radiating to the shoulder on the affected side.

4 May not exhibit any outward symptoms; only the signs of pregnancy disappearing.

165. **2** After a spontaneous abortion the fundus should be checked for firmness, which would indicate effective uterine tone; if the uterus is not firm, it is hypotonic and hemorrhage may occur; nonfirmness may also indicate retained placental tissue. (a)

1 Unnecessary; fetal and placental contents are small and expelled easily in bed.

3 The nurse would do this if necessary after checking for fundal firmness.

4 The priority action is to check for firmness of the fundus and possible bleeding.

166. **2** Hemorrhage may be due to retained placental tissue or uterine atony; infection may occur from the introduction of contamination into the warm moist environment, which is favorable to microbial growth. (a)

1 No indication at this time that the client has been deprived of fluids or has lost large amounts of blood.

3 Subinvolution usually occurs after a full term delivery and may not be obvious for several days.

4 Too early in pregnancy for toxemia.

167. **4** Allows the husband and wife to comfort each other while letting them know the nurse is available and recognize and accept their feelings of loss. (b)

1 Telling the client not to be upset cuts off communication and wrongly implies that it prolongs recovery.

2 Grieving for the unborn child will and should occur during any period of pregnancy.

3 An assumption that another pregnancy will ensue; also cuts off further communication.

168. **2** Infertility is the inability of a couple to conceive after at least 1 year of adequate exposure to the possibility of pregnancy. (b)

1 This may or may not be true; it is possible that there is a problem with both.

3 May be; however, statistics show that physiologic problems are more often the cause.

4 Untrue; infertility may be corrected, but sterility is irreversible.

169. **2** At this time, because of increased estrogen levels, the cervical mucus is abundant, and its quality changes in such a way as to optimize sperm survival time. (b)

1 The cervical mucus at this time is not receptive to spermatozoa.

3 Cervical mucus at this time is still thick and not yet receptive to spermatozoa.

4 Cervical mucus is destructive to spermatozoa at this time and sperm penetration cannot occur.

170. **1** A past infection may cause tubal occlusions, most of which are due to postinfection adhesions. (c)

2 This is a tumor of the uterus and does not affect the tube.

3 Rare; anomalies of the uterus are more common than those of a tube.

4 Possible; but infections in the tube are more common.

171. **2** Human chorionic gonadotropin (HCG), an LH-like hormone, is produced by the trophoblasts of the early embryo to promote continued metabolism of the corpus luteum (source of estrogen and progesterone); HCG can be detected as early as 6 days after fertilization (by nonroutine immunofluorescent techniques) and appears in measurable amounts in the urine within about 14 days. (b)

1 Not found in the urine of pregnant women.

3 Estrogen is present in females all the time.

4 Not indicative of pregnancy; found in the urine of all women, especially after ovulation.

172. **4** A bluish color results from the increased vascularity and blood vessel engorgement of the vagina. (a)

1 Softening of the lower uterine segment.

2 Increased vascularity and cervical softening.

3 Softening of the cervix.

173. **4** The average weight gain during pregnancy is 9 to 11.25 kg (20 to 25 lb); of this, the fetus accounts for 3.4 kg (7½ lb), the blood volume 0.9 to 1.8 kg (2 to 4 lb), fluid retention 2.3 kg (5 lb), amniotic fluid 0.9 kg (2 lb), uterus 1.13 kg (2½ lb), and breasts 1.36 kg (3 lb); the remainder of weight gain is fat. (c)

1 Do not cause a weight gain.

2 Accounts for about 20% of weight gain.

3 Accounts for about 12% of weight gain.

174. **1** Statistically CPD (cephalopelvic disproportion) is the most common indication. (a)

2 This may be improved by rest and hydration followed by an infusion of oxytocin (Pitocin), leading to vaginal delivery.

3 Not done unless complete placental separation occurs before delivery.

4 A nonexistent condition.

175. **1** The diagonal conjugate is an estimation of the true conjugate with the lower edge of the symphysis pubis used as its anterior point and the sacral promontory posteriorly; the true conjugate uses the upper ridge of the symphysis pubis anteriorly but cannot be measured on a living woman. (c)

2 Diameter between the ischial tuberosities.

3 Distance from the upper margin of the symphysis to the sacral promontory.

4 Widest diameter at the inlet.

176. **2** X-ray pelvimetry is more definitive than digital pelvimetry; but because of radiation hazards it should be limited to clients in labor, in whom it is clearly essential to the outcome of pregnancy. (b)

1 This is done by external measurement; is not an accurate assessment.

3 This is a test of amniotic fluid; does not reveal actual size of the fetus or diameters of the pelvis.

4 This is done to determine fetal acidosis.

177. **1** Asymmetry of the gluteal dorsal surface of the thighs and inguinal folds indicates congenital dislocation of the hip; folds on the affected side appear higher than those on the unaffected side. (a)

2 This would be manifested by limpness or flaccidity of extremities.

3 Evidenced by protrusion of the intestine into the inguinal sac.

4 Impaired reflex behavior and a shrill cry, etc. would indicate CNS damage.

178. **3** Human milk contains 42% carbohydrate, and cow's milk 30% carbohydrate; the carbohydrate in cow's milk is further diluted when water is added to the formula, so additional sugar is required to supplement it. (b)

1 The calorie content is about the same, 20 calories/ounce.

2 It is assimilated well.

4 It is lactose, a simple sugar.

179. **4** The oxytocin challenge test provides data concerning the circulatory-respiratory reserve of the fetoplacental unit; a positive OCT usually indicates uteroplacental insufficiency; an OCT is contraindicated unless there is a specific indication of a problem. (b)

1 This is not an indication; the OCT would be of no help in diagnosing a recurrence.

2 An OCT would be contraindicated in placenta previa.

3 Contraindicated; might accelerate the labor further.

180. **1** Administration of oxytocin too early in pregnancy can cause induced labor and premature delivery. (c)

2 May be indicated to determine the fetus' response to labor.

3 May be indicated because of hypertensive influence on the placental circulation.

4 May be indicated to determine the fetus' response to labor.

181. **1** Respiratory depression occurs with the use of meperidine (Demerol) and produces significant depression of the infant at birth if circulating levels are high at delivery. (a)

2 Scopolamine induces amnesia and forgetfulness in the mother but does not cause respiratory depression.

3 Promazine (Sparine), a tranquilizer, augments the effects of Demerol, thereby lessening the amount of drug needed.

4 Promethazine (Phenergan), a tranquilizer, does not cause respiratory depression.

182. **1** Brachial palsy results from excessive stretching of the nerve fibers that run from the neck, through the shoulder, and down toward the arm; the muscles of the upper arm are involved, and the infant holds the arm at the side with the elbow extended and the hand rotated inward. (b)
  2 Signs of CNS disturbance would be present.
  3 There would be signs of dislocation and evidence of pain with a fractured clavicle.
  4 An inborn error of metabolism relating to the body's handling of bilirubin.

183. **3** There is extensive activation of blood clotting factor after delivery; this, together with immobility, trauma, or sepsis, encourages thromboembolization, which can be limited through activity. (b)
  1 Tone would be improved by regular emptying and filling of the bladder.
  2 This can be accomplished by turning the client from side to side and encouraging her to deep breathe and cough.
  4 Abdominal muscle tone will be improved with exercise over the next 6 weeks.

184. **2** Mothering is not an inborn instinct but rather a learned bheavior based on past experiences. (c)
  1 Untrue; mothering is learned not inborn.
  3 This knowledge does not assure "motherliness."
  4 Marriage is not essential for good mothering.

185. **2** The pregnant woman's increased hormones, metabolic rate, and increased blood volume place additional demands on the pancreas, thus altering carbohydrate and lipid metabolism. (b)
  1 The hormones of pregnancy act as antagonists to insulin, thus reducing its effect.
  3 The diabetic mother's glucose tolerance does not differ from that in her prepregnant state.
  4 Pregnancy lowers renal threshold for glucose in nondiabetics as well.

186. **1** Since spillage of glucose into the urine occurs in normal women who are pregnant, dietary or insulin management in a diabetic who is pregnant must be based on blood glucose levels rather than on urine glucose values. (c)
  2 Depends on body needs; pregnancy per se does not speed it up.
  3 This would be no problem if action of insulin was not antagonized by pregnancy hormones.
  4 Difficulty in regulation is unrelated to the absorption of insulin.

187. **4** Increased metabolic demands on the body during pregnancy require an increased ingestion of glucose; appropriate levels of insulin must be administered to permit normal glucose utilization by the body. (c)
  1 This type of diet is contraindicated; would not meet the demands of pregnancy and growing fetus.
  2 The caloric content is increased, not decreased, during pregnancy.
  3 This diet would not be sufficient to prevent ketosis; insulin would be necessary to cover carbohydrate intake.

188. **2** In diabetic mothers the fetal pancreas responds to the mother's hyperglycemia by secreting more than normal amounts of insulin; this leads to infant hypoglycemia after birth. (b)
  1 In response to the increased glucose received from the mother, the islets of Langerhans in the fetus may have become hypertrophied; are not congenitally depressed.
  3 There may be a generalized edema, but not specific to the CNS.

4 Increased insulin production by the fetus diminishes the glucose content of the blood; babies are most often hypoglycemic.

189. **2** The higher-than-normal glucose level in a fetus of a diabetic mother leads to increased fat synthesis and deposition; increased glucose utilization is also promoted by the combined presence of pituitary growth hormone and placental somatotropin. (c)
  1 False; glucose utilization is increased, with resultant macrosomia.
  3 False; somatotropin concentration is increased and glucose utilization is increased.
  4 False; somatotropin concentration is increased during pregnancy.

190. **1** Normal periods of marked change and adjustment are called developmental crises and predispose the woman to a situational crisis. (a)
  2 These occur throughout the life cycle of a mature woman and should not now be classified as a crisis.
  3 These are transient; similar to previous mood changes and should not affect the mother's ability to cope.
  4 Becomes a crisis only if the husband withdraws support.

191. **2** The ability to express one's feelings is often a first step in the recognition and resolution of a crisis. (b)
  1 Until the mother shows a readiness for learning (e.g., accepts the pregnancy), she would not benefit from classes.
  3 Not a priority need; may come later in the nurse-client interactions.
  4 The father, as well as the mother, must indicate a readiness for learning before beginning classes.

192. **2** Chorionic gonadotropin is present in the urine during early pregnancy and is the basis for pregnancy tests; since this hormone appears only during early pregnancy, its presence is taken as a sure sign of pregnancy. (a)
  1 Prolactin initiates milk production and is secreted after delivery.
  3 Estrogen is secreted throughout the ovulatory cycle, not just pregnancy.
  4 Secreted into the bloodstream at the time of ovulation.

193. **2** Nurses with positive attitudes toward abortion should counsel women who are thinking of undergoing the procedure; they should know what services are available and the various methods that are used to induce abortion. (b)
  1 The nurse should give the client only the information requested; should not state personal feelings.
  3 The nurse is capable of giving information about abortion; need not defer to the physician.
  4 Good nursing practice necessitates scientific knowledge; statements must be based on fact, not personal feelings or beliefs.

194. **2** The uterus and bladder occupy the pelvic cavity and lie very closely together; as the uterus enlarges with the growing fetus, it impinges on the space normally occupied by the bladder and thereby diminishes bladder capacity. (a)
  1 Atony would not cause frequency; more likely would lead to retention.
  3 An unlikely occurrence; the uterus would not impinge on that area.
  4 Would lead to incontinence rather than frequency.

195. **2** Because of changes in the hormone levels, morning sickness seldom persists beyond the first trimester. (a)
  1 Still present at this time; related to the high level of chorionic gonadotropin.

3 Usually ends at end of the third month, when the chorionic gonadotropin level falls.

4 Usually ends at end of the third month, when the chorionic gonadotropin level falls.

196. **4** Multiple pregnancy thins the uterine wall by overstretching; thus the efficiency of contractions is reduced. (b)
  1 Toxemia may bring about premature labor; does not cause hypotonic uterine dysfunction.
  2 May cause fatigue in the mother; does not affect uterine contractility.
  3 This may lead to difficult delivery because of cephalopelvic disproportion; does not affect uterine contractions.

197. **3** A fruity odor may indicate that the client is becoming acidotic. (c)
  1 This would be indicative of cardiac difficulties rather than exhaustion.
  2 Maternal exhaustion is usually accompanied by dehydration with a resultant temperature elevation.
  4 This would occur later if there were a severe electrolyte imbalance.

198. **3** This response provides the client with a comfort measure while giving her an opportunity to verbalize her fears about having an abnormal labor. (b)
  1 This can be answered "yes" or "no" and leaves no further avenue for discussion.
  2 Of no help to the client; she is concerned with what is happening to her.
  4 Closes off communication with the client.

199. **3** The oxytocic effect of Pitocin increases the intensity and durations of contractions; prolonged contractions will jeopardize the safety of the fetus and necessitate discontinuing the drug. (c)
  1 This is important throughout labor.
  2 Since she is only 3 to 4 cm with head floating, there will be no bulging.
  4 There is no indication at this time that a cesarean delivery is necessary.

200. **3** IV oxytocin (Pitocin) is used to enhance postpartum uterine contractions after cesarean delivery, since massage of the fundus is difficult and painful after surgery; the drug produces effective clamping down on the vessels. (c)
  1 This may be difficult because of the new incision.
  2 This is done routinely for all postoperative clients.
  4 This is done for all postoperative clients.

201. **1** Normal infants require about 73 ml (2 to 3 oz) of fluid per pound and 60 calories a day per pound for growth. (b)
  2 Too little; normal infants require 2 to 3 oz of fluid per pound, 18 oz/24 hr.
  3 Too much; 18 oz/24 hr is required or about 3 oz every 4 hours.
  4 Too much; 18 oz/24 hr is required or about 3 oz every 4 hours.

202. **1** The cardiac sphincter in the newborn is poorly developed; if the stomach is too full, formula backs up through the sphincter and the infant regurgitates. (b)
  2 This would be manifested by projectile vomiting, not regurgitation.
  3 This may cause cramping or colic; usually does not cause regurgitation.
  4 Nondescriptive answer; position not described; might happen if the baby were upside down.

203. **4** Clotting mechanisms are not fully effective in the infant before the eighth day of life. (a)
  1 Too soon to observe for signs of infection.

2 If gauze is not wrapped too tightly around the penis, this should be no problem.

3 Generally the baby is not too uncomfortable after circumcision; this may, with other signs, be indicative of CNS difficulty.

204. **4** This conjunctivitis occurs about 3 to 4 days after birth; if it is not treated with tetracycline, chronic follicular conjunctivitis with conjunctival scarring will occur. (b)
  1 This chemical conjunctivitis occurs within the first 48 hours and is not purulent in nature.
  2 AIDS in the newborn does not manifest itself in any type of conjunctivitis.
  3 This is due to the scarring that occurs in infants who have contracted gonorrheal infections from the maternal vaginal tract.

205. **2** *Chlamydia trachomatis* is associated with development of pneumonia in the newborn infant. (c)
  1 Purulent conjunctivitis at this time suggests a chlamydial infection not an allergic response.
  3 Physician's order required; bathing eyes with solution will not stem the infection; the infant will be put on intensive systemic antibiotic therapy.
  4 This is done at all times; the first priority here is to monitor for pneumonia, which is often associated with chlamydial infections.

206. **3** Semi-Fowler's position facilitates easier oxygen exchange, and side lying promotes better venous return. (b)
  1 Supine gravid uterus may inhibit venous return and result in placental congestion and supine hypotension.
  2 At full term, clients are placed in left side-lying position to enhance venous return.
  4 Too straight and uncomfortable; gravid uterus will impede venous return from legs.

207. **1** Clients with cardiac problems are prone to congestive heart failure in this stage of labor. (b)
  2 Not necessary; clients are maintained on left side to facilitate venous return.
  3 Done for all laboring clients; with cardiac problems priority is monitoring for congestive heart failure.
  4 Done for all laboring clients; with cardiac problems priority is monitoring for congestive heart failure.

208. **3** Clients who have had rheumatic fever are placed on prophylactic ampicillin therapy to minimize the development of streptococcus infections. (b)
  1 This would be used only if client was in congestive heart failure.
  2 This would be used only if client was in congestive heart failure.
  4 This would be used only if thrombophlebitis develops.

209. **2** Pyelonephritis often causes premature labor, leading to increased neonatal morbidity and mortality. (b)
  1 Fluids should be increased; inflammatory process may lead to fever, dehydration, and accumulation of toxins.
  3 Albuminuria occurs with pregnancy-induced hypertension (toxemia) and is not accompanied by pain or flank tenderness; client's symptoms are indicative of a kidney infection.
  4 There is no data to indicate that client has hypertension of pregnancy; an inflammatory, not a degenerative, kidney process is present.

210. **4** No known teratogenic effect associated with penicillin. (b)
  1 Nitrofurantoin may cause megaloblastic anemia.
  2 Sulfonamides may cause hemolysis in fetus.
  3 Tetracycline causes permanent yellow staining of child's teeth.

ANSWERS AND RATIONALES FOR COMPREHENSIVE TESTS

The letters following the rationales for the correct answers represent an analysis of each question. Following is a key to the letters.

A. The letter in parentheses refers to the *level of difficulty*. The letter *a* signifies that more than 75% of the students answering the question answered it correctly; *b* signifies that between 50% and 75% of the students answering the question answered it correctly; *c* signifies that between 25% and 50% of the students answering the question were correct.

B. The first set of capital letters refers to *steps in the nursing process:* AS, assessing; AN, analyzing; PL, planning; IM, implementing; EV, evaluating.

C. The second set represents the *cognitive level* of the question: KN, knowledge; CP, comprehension; AP, application; AN, analysis.

D. The third set refers to the *clinical area:* ME, medical; SU, surgical; OB, obstetrical; PS, psychiatric; PE, pediatric.

E. The fourth set refers to *client needs:* PA, physiological and anatomical equilibrium; TC, safe and therapeutic environment; ED, education and health promotion; PE, psychosocial and emotional equilibrium.

F. The last set refers to the *category of concern.*
   1. In *medical, surgical, and pediatric nursing* the abbreviations are CB, cardiovascular and blood; EI, endocrine and integumentary; GI, gastrointestinal; MN, musculoskeletal and neurologic; RE, respiratory; RG, reproductive and genitourinary.
   2. In *obstetrical nursing* the abbreviations are FS, fertility, sterility, and family planning; HP, high-risk pregnancy; PN, prenatal period; IP, intrapartal period; PP, postpartal period; NH, normal and high-risk neonate.
   3. In *psychiatric nursing* the abbreviations are MD, mood disorders; CS, crisis situations; DD, developmental disorders; PD, personality, anxiety, somatoform, and dissociative disorders; SA, substance abuse and related disorders; SD, schizophrenic disorders.

G. Two worksheets for self evaluation follow the answers and rationales for each part of the comprehensive tests.

Comprehensive Test 1: Part 1*

1. **1** Glaucoma is a disease in which there is increased intraocular pressure resulting from narrowing of the aqueous outflow channel (canal of Schlemm). This can lead to blindness caused by compression of the nutritive blood vessels supplying the rods and cones. (a); AN; CP; ME; PA; MN
   2 Pupil dilation increases intraocular pressure because it narrows the canal of Schlemm.
   3 Intraocular pressure is not affected by activity of the eye.
   4 Increased intraocular pressure can result in blindness and, therefore, must be reduced; although secondary infections are not desirable, the priority is to maintain vision.

2. **2** Retinal damage caused by the increased intraocular pressure of glaucoma is permanent and is progressive if the disease is not controlled. (b); PL; CP; ME; PE; MN

   1 One eye may be affected, and there is no restriction in the use of the eyes.
   3 Blindness may be prevented if treatment is early.
   4 Surgery can open up drainage and permanently reduce pressure.

3. **3** In chronic glaucoma there is a loss of peripheral vision long before the central vision is affected. The client may also complain of seeing halos around light. (b); AS; CP; ME; PA; MN
   1 This occurs when there is damage to the central retina; peripheral vision is affected in glaucoma.
   2 Acute glaucoma causes pain; chronic glaucoma is usually insidious.
   4 Blurred vision may be due to a refractive error; peripheral vision is affected in glaucoma.

4. **4** Atropine causes the pupils to dilate, leading to increased intraocular pressure in the client with glaucoma. Any such order must be questioned because permanent damage might result. (b); EV; AP; SU; TC; MN
   1 Administration of medication is a dependent function; the drug may not be withheld but must be changed by the physician.
   2 The nurse cannot give a medication knowing its effect will harm the client; would be an act of negligence.
   3 Pilocarpine is often used when preoperative atropine is indicated but must be ordered by the physician; administration of medication is a dependent function.

5. **2** The prone position stretches the flexor muscles, thus preventing hip flexion contractures. (b); IM; AP; SU; PA; MN
   1 Elevating the stump would cause hip flexion, which could result in a hip flexion contracture.
   3 The stump should be elevated during the first 24 hours; elevating the head of the bed would cause hip flexion, which could result in a hip flexion contracture.
   4 Sitting flexes the hips, which could result in a hip flexion contracture.

6. **2** Muscles that originate at the vertebrae or pelvic girdle and insert on the femur act to abduct, adduct, flex, extend, and rotate the femur. Normal body alignment should be maintained because it facilitates the safe and efficient use of muscle groups for balance and stability. (b); IM; AP; SU; PA; MN
   1 This position does not approximate normal body alignment; abduction of the stump will alter the center of gravity.
   3 This position does not approximate normal body alignment; hip flexion will alter the center of gravity and promote the development of a hip flexion contracture.
   4 This will interfere with the development of a normal gait; muscles that originate at the vertebrae and pelvic girdle should be used to move the stump.

7. **3** Subcutaneous fat is reduced by the pressure of the initial constrictive bandage and the socket of the prosthesis. (c); AN; KN; SU; PA; MN
   1 Edema is limited and contributes minimally to the size of the postoperative stump.
   2 Restoration of skin turgor does not affect stump size.
   4 Tissue and bone excised remain constant; after surgery there is no additional loss.

8. **4** The client is usually instructed to push forcefully yet gently over the bone to toughen the limb for weight bearing. This process is begun by pushing the stump against increasingly harder surfaces. (a); IM; AP; SU; PA; MN
   1 Abduction of the stump does not maintain normal alignment and should be avoided; does not prepare the stump end for a prosthesis.
   2 Dangling the stump does not help prepare it for a prosthesis and may impede venous return, which would prolong healing.

---

*A key to the letters following the correct rationale can be found in discussion above.

3 This procedure would soften the stump, impeding its potential for weight bearing.

9. **2** Since Mrs. Kraft has severe diabetes, it is essential that her urine be tested before meals for sugar and ketones to evaluate the success of control of diabetes and the possible need for insulin coverage. (c); EV; AP; ME; PA; EI
   1 Raising the head of the bed flexes the hips, which could result in hip flexion contratures.
   3 To prevent flexion contractures of the hip, the client should not sit in a chair for a prolonged time.
   4 Salt restriction is not indicated for this client.

10. **4** Exercise should not include bending and the Valsalva maneuver, which might increase intraocular pressure. (b); PL; AP; ME; ED; MN
    1 Mydriatics are contraindicated in glaucoma because they dilate the pupil, which increases intraocular pressure.
    2 Fluids may be taken as desired because they have no effect on intraocular pressure.
    3 Lighting conditions have no effect on intraocular pressure.

11. **3** Inactivity over an extended time increases stiffness and pain in joints. (a); PL; CP; PE; PA; MN
    1 The latex fixation test is positive when the rheumatoid factor is found in blood serum; this factor is present in many conditions, including rheumatoid arthritis, aging, narcotic addiction, and SLE.
    2 Not a factor; cold packs may decrease joint discomfort.
    4 Assistive exercises help maintain joint mobility.

12. **3** Polyarthritis of rheumatic fever is transitory and does not cause deformity. Rheumatoid arthritis is chronic and causes changes in joints. (a); AN; CP; PE; PA; MN
    1 Cardiac damage is often associated with rheumatic fever.
    2 Juvenile rheumatoid arthritis involves chronic inflammation of the joints; exacerbations are most often related to stress.
    4 The etiology of rheumatic fever is related to a previous occurrence of strep throat; rheumatoid arthritis is unrelated.

13. **2** Aspirin interferes with platelet aggregation, thereby lengthening bleeding time. (b); EV; CP; ME; TC; MN
    1 Urate excretion is enhanced by high doses of aspirin.
    3 Aspirin is readily broken down in the GI tract and liver.
    4 Aspirin inhibits platelet aggregation.

14. **1** Ten-year-old boys prefer the company of the same sex and age group. Also, Marc needs to avoid stressful situations that would tend to increase exacerbations. (b); EV; AN; PE; PE; MN
    2 Same-sex roomates are desirable for companionship and to maintain privacy needs.
    3 Asthmatic children may have severe respiratory difficulties; this may be too stressful for Marc, who needs rest.
    4 Same-sex roomates are desirable for companionship and to maintain boy/girl separateness of this age group.

15. **3** A diagnosis of cancer and a colostomy both drastically alter a person's self-image and body image. People react differently to this stress, often finding it difficult to express their concerns verbally; however, their actions may demonstrate an awareness of the situation. (b); EV; AN; PS; PE; CS
    1 Not enough information to determine this.
    2 Not enough information to determine this.
    4 Not enough information to determine this.

16. **4** Insomnia is often caused by anxiety. By stating an observation about the client's activity, the nurse communicates both concern and a recognition that the client may have more covert problems that he wishes to verbalize. (a); IM; AP; PS; PE; CS
    1 Denies the client's request and serves to cut off communication.
    2 Denies the client's request and serves to cut off communication.
    3 Denies the client's request and servies to cut off communication.

17. **4** Client's who have radical changes in their body image as a result of surgery are usually best able to relate to someone who has faced the same stress and successfully adapted. (b); IM; AN; PS; PE; CS
    1 Would provide information but do little to aid acceptance.
    2 Would do little to aid acceptance.
    3 The client cannot learn to do colostomy care until he psychologically accepts its presence.

18. **2** A diet as close as possible to normal after a colostomy is recommended for the stated reason that individuals will discover their own food intolerances and should eat accordingly. (b); PL; CP; SU; ED; GI
    1 A low-residue diet is not necessary; once healing occurs, a diet with adequate residue promotes peristalsis and colostomy functioning.
    3 Each person is an individual and reacts differently to foods.
    4 Rigid dietary regulations usually increase anxiety; return to normally tolerated foods provides security.

19. **4** Rapid instillation of fluid into the colon may cause abdominal cramps. By clamping off the tubing, the nurse allows the cramps to subside so the irrigation can be continued. (b); EV; AP; SU; TC; GI
    1 Contraindicated; this will increase the force of flow, which will increase the abdominal cramps.
    2 Emotional support will not interrupt the physical adaptation of abdominal cramps; the irrigation must be temporarily discontinued.
    3 Although this may reduce the force of the fluid, it will not eliminate the flow of fluid completely; the irrigation should be temporarily discontinued.

20. **1** A colostomy located on the left side of the abdomen would be in the descending colon. Since most but not all of the fluid would be absorbed, the stool would be moist and formed. (c); AS; KN; SU; PA; GI
    2 This would be associated with conditions that narrow the intestinal lumen; not usually associated with a colostomy.
    3 This would be associated with a colostomy involving the ascending colon.
    4 Stools are not usually covered with mucus; they may be moist but not mucoid.

21. **1** Colostomy irrigations done daily at the same time help establish normal patterns of bowel evacuation. The diet should be as close as possible to normal. (b); IM; AP; SU; ED; GI
    2 A soft low-residue diet is not necessary; it should be as close to normal as possible.
    3 Although fluid is important to prevent hard stools, it will not help the client regain bowel control; a daily regimen is the priority.
    4 Initially after surgery, protein promotes healing; protein intake has no relationship to bowel control.

22. **3** By 2 years of age the child should demonstrate an interest in others, communicate verbally, and possess the

ability to learn from the environment. Before these skills develop, autism is difficult to diagnose. (b); AS; KN; PS; PE; DD

1 Infantile autism can occur at this age but is difficult to diagnose.

2 Infantile autism can occur at this age but is difficult to diagnose.

4 Autism can be diagnosed long before this age.

23. **2** Autistic behavior turns inward. These children do not respond to the environment but attempt to maintain emotional equilibrium by rubbing and manipulating themselves and displaying a compulsive need for behavioral repetition. (a); PL; AP; PS; PE; DD

1 These children do seem to respond to music, but not necessarily loud cheerful music.

3 Part of the autistic pattern is the inability to interact with others in the environment.

4 Large group (or small group) activity would have little effect on the autistic child's response.

24. **3** One begins by trying to enter the world where the child's attention is currently focused; this is a way of making human contact, since the child's usual contacts are inanimate objects. (b); IM; AP; PS; PE; DD

1 Autistic children generally cannot tolerate cuddling and will become rigid when anyone attempts to do so.

2 The autistic child is unable to participate in group activities.

4 This would have no effect on the nurse's ability to reach Johnny; rather it would reinforce his withdrawal.

25. **2** Isolated unrelated activities predominate. The child's behavior reflects withdrawal or feelings of destructive rage. (b); AS; KN; PS; PE; DD

1 The facial expression is blank; sadness would be a response to the external world, from which the child has withdrawn.

3 The autistic child rarely if ever smiles.

4 The autistic child seems to overrespond to stimuli in the environment.

26. **2** Self-isolation and disinterest in interpersonal relationships lead the autistic child to find security in nonthreatening, impersonal objects. (c); IM; AP; PS; PE; DD

1 This would be too threatening to an autistic child.

3 Touching him might prove to be too threatening.

4 These children do not respond to bright-colored toys and blocks as other children do unless there is movement involved.

27. **4** The rhythmic movement of the merry-go-round provides soothing and nonthreatening comfort to the autistic child who cannot reach out to his environment. (c) IM; KN; PS; PE; DD

1 The autistic child rejects cuddling and anything that feels cuddly.

2 The child would prefer a mechanical object over a colored block.

3 The child would prefer a mechanical object over a colored block.

28. **4** Albumin in the urine is a sign of toxemia, as are an elevated BP and a weight gain of more than 2 pounds per week. (c); EV; AN; OB; PA; HP

1 Signs indicate that pregnancy-induced hypertension may be present; the client may be seen more frequently than every 2 weeks.

2 These signs indicate pregnancy-induced hypertension; treatment of this does not require vaginal examination.

3 BP and weight are more relative; changes in the pulse rate and temperature are not associated with pregnancy-induced hypertension.

29. **1** Weight gain caused by fluid retention is the earliest objective sign of mild preeclampsia. (c); AS; CP; OB; PA; HP

2 Continued elevations are significant; emotional upset, anxiety, and other factors may cause fluctuations or variations in blood pressure.

3 Edema progresses as the signs of preeclampsia worsen due to abnormal retention of fluid.

4 May occur; however, it usually becomes evident after weight gain and a progressive increase in BP.

30. **1** The latest concept concerning preeclampsia or eclampsia is that this condition is a consequence of salt loss during pregnancy and poor protein intake. The recommendations therefore call for a diet containing normal sodium, high protein, and a sufficient number of calories. (c); IM; AP; OB; ED; HP

2 Low protein is contraindicated for normal fetal growth; no indication for increasing sodium.

3 There is an additional daily requirement of 500 calories during pregnancy.

4 Lowering the intake of calories and sodium is detrimental to both fetus and mother.

31. **1** The cumulative effects of magnesium sulfate include depressed respirations and an absent or weak knee-jerk reflex. (b); EV; AN; OB; PA; HP

2 BP is monitored after administration of $MgSO_4$; apical pulse is not relative.

3 Urinary output is increased after administration of $MgSO_4$.

4 Temperature and pulse are not affected by administration of $MgSO_4$.

32. **2** Magnesium sulfate given by deep IM injection is very painful. One percent procaine hydrochloride may be mixed with the drug by physician's order or as established hospital protocol. (c); IM; AN; OB; PA; HP

1 One percent procaine hydrochloride, not 1% normal saline, is added to the fluid to be injected; normal saline would not maximize dispersion of the drug.

3 May be additionally traumatic; the drug is dispersed by turning the needle.

4 Tissue in this area may not be deep enough for the injection of $MgSO_4$.

33. **4** In severe preeclampsia, fluid is drawn from the plasma into the tissues and the blood becomes more concentrated. This is reflected in the elevated hematocrit level. (b); AN; CP; OB; PA; HP

1 The hemodilution results in a reduced hematocrit since there is more blood volume than there are cells.

2 Vasodilation would not alter the ratio of cells to fluid volume.

3 $MgSO_4$ does not cause agglutination of cells.

34. **1** One of the characteristic differences between juvenile and adult diabetes is the rapid onset of the disease in children. Diabetes is often first diagnosed during acute ketoacidosis. (a); AS; KN; PE; PA; EI

2 Although adult-onset diabetes (Type II or NIDDM) often occurs in obese individuals, juvenile diabetes occurs in children of thin or normal build.

3 Juvenile diabetics are insulin dependent.

4 Vascular changes are a complication associated with longstanding diabetes.

35. **3** Helping families understand their feelings about juvenile diabetes is essential in assisting them to develop positive attitudes for optimal control of the disease and promotion of a normal life for the child. (a); PL; AP; PE; PE; EI

1 Instruction in specific psychomoter tasks should be preceded by an assessment of the family's acceptance of the diagnosis and knowledge about the disease.

2 Important; however, if feelings are not dealt with first, compliance with insulin injections is less likely.

4 Kim should participate in the activities normal for her and her age group. Adequate exercise is an important part of the treatment regimen for diabetes.

36. **2**
$$50 \text{ units}:1 \text{ ml} = 20 \text{ units}:x$$
$$50x = 20$$
$$x = 0.4 \text{ ml}$$

(b): EV; AP; PE; TC; EI

1 Too large.

3 Too small.

4 Too small.

37. **2** A bedtime snack is needed for the evening. NPH insulin lasts for 24 to 28 hours. Protein and carbohydrate ingestion prior to sleep prevents hypoglycemia during the night, when the action of NPH insulin will still be high. (a); PL; AN; PE; PA; EI

1 The snack contains mainly protein-rich foods to help cover the long-acting insulin during sleep.

3 The snack is important for diet/insulin balance during the night.

4 There are no data to indicate such a need; a bedtime snack is routinely provided to help cover long-acting insulin during sleep.

38. **4** Exercise reduces the body's need for insulin. Increased muscle activity accelerates the transport of glucose into the muscle cells, thus producing an insulin-like effect. (b); PL; AN; PE; ED; EI

1 An emotional upset is a stress that requires insulin.

2 An infectious process, if severe enough, may require increased insulin.

3 With increased growth and associated dietary intake, the need for insulin increases.

39. **1** Various aspects of hospitalization and diagnosis could cause the client anxiety. The nurse should determine what disturbs the client most. (b); PL; AP; PS; PE; CS

2 An anxious client will not be receptive to learning.

3 A tracheostomy may not be performed, depending on the extent of the surgery and edema.

4 This may cause the client unnecessary anxiety.

40. **2** The facial nerve may be damaged during surgery. Drooping of the area results from loss of muscle tone. (b); AS; AN; SU; PA; MN

1 A tracheostomy may not be performed; it is not a complication but rather a preventive measure.

3 This is also called auriculotemporal syndrome; may follow infection and suppuration of the parotid gland; not a surgical complication.

4 The parotid is a salivary gland; its removal would decrease salivation.

41. **2** This position minimizes the discomfort associated with venous engorgement. It also promotes venous drainage by gravity. (c); IM; AP; SU; PA; CB

1 Drainage from the wound would not be affected.

3 This position would neither increase nor decrease strain on the suture line.

4 Providing stimulation would not be a priority item; this position would not affect the degree of stimulation.

42. **2** If the dressing is too tight, impaired cerebral circulation may result. (b); EV; AP; SU; PA; CB

1 Bleeding would not cause the client to complain of tightness.

3 Untrue; impaired cerebral circulation may result from a tight dressing.

4 The dressing may be removed only if indicated by the physician.

43. **1** To be truly effective in the relationship with the client, the nurse must know and understand personal feelings about terminal illness and death. (b) AN; CP; PS; PE; CS

2 Although the family is an important part of the client's support system, the client's feelings are more important to the relationship.

3 In dealing with terminal illness, knowledge alone is not enough to assure a good nurse-client relationship.

4 Previous experiences could be positive or negative and would not guarantee an effective nurse-client relationship.

44. **2** The sensitive and dependent individual who has a conflict accepting the need for dependence frequently develops ulcerative colitis. The exact neural mechanism resulting in colonic inflammation is unknown. (c); AN; CP; ME; PA; GI

1 These characteristics are associated with peptic ulcer disease.

3 Since the individual directs hostility outward, visceral changes may not occur.

4 An individual who is secure is not predisposed to developing visceral disorders as the result of psychologic stress.

45. **4** Since the mucosa of the intestinal tract is damaged, its ability to absorb vitamins taken orally is greatly impaired. (a); IM; CP; ME; PA; GI

1 Although this is true, the risks associated with IV administration will outweigh the benefits unless other factors are considered.

2 Vitamins are effective orally unless there is disease involving the GI tract that hampers absorption.

3 IV vitamins do not decrease colonic irritability.

46. **1**
$$\frac{\text{Amount to be infused} \times \text{Drop factor}}{\text{Amount of time (in minutes)}}$$
$$\frac{2000 \times 10}{12 \times 60} = \frac{20,000}{720} = 27.77 \text{ drops/min}$$

(b); EV; AP; ME; TC; GI

2 Incorrect calculation; would result in excessive fluid administration.

3 Incorrect calculation; would result in excessive fluid administration.

4 Incorrect calculation; would result in excessive fluid administration.

47. **1** This grouping of foods does not contain high-residue fruits, vegetables, or whole grains, which are irritating to the intestinal mucosa, cause bulk, and increase peristalsis. (c); PL; AN; ME; PA; GI

2 Includes whole grain foods, which leave increased residue.

3 Includes vegetables and grain, which leave increased residue.

4 Includes vegetables and grain, which leave increased residue.

48. **2** The key in treatment of this disease is to prevent spastic intestinal activity. (a); AN; CP; ME; PA; GI

1 Reduction of gastric acidity is the aim of bland diets used in the treatment of peptic ulcers.

3 Electrolyte depletion may be prevented by reducing colonic irritation, but this is a secondary benefit.

4 By reducing colonic irritation, motility, and spasticity, it is hoped that absorption will increase.

49. **4** The affected areas of the intestine are in need of repair. Protein is required in the building and repairing of tissues. (a); PL; CP; ME; ED; GI

1 Anemia may result from chronic bleeding; it usually is corrected, however, with increased iron and normal intake of protein.

2 Increased protein will not significantly affect peristalsis.

3 Protein is given to promote healing; once tissues are repaired, muscle tone may improve.

50. **1** Nurses can become very blasé about the equipment used in labor and forget that it may be frightening for the layperson. (b); EV; AN; OB; PE; IP

  2 Sedation is never given on a routine basis to the client in labor.

  3 External monitoring is now being used with much greater frequency, even on high-risk clients.

  4 Not universally true; older primigravidas may have totally uncomplicated labors.

51. **2** Lactation delays ovarian function after delivery. It will also therefore delay the symptoms of endometriosis. (b); IM; AP; OB; PA; PP

  1 Conservative medical therapy will be used first; a hysterectomy is only a last resort.

  3 Pregnancy temporarily suppresses ovarian function; the aberrant endometrial tissue is still present.

  4 Endometriosis may lead to sterility; does not cause menopause.

52. **3** Physical assessment is a form of data collection. It is the first step in planning care. (a); AS; AP; OB; TC; PP

  1 Implementation is not the initial action.

  2 Too soon for medical intervention; other nursing measures should be tried first.

  4 Implementation is not an initial action.

53. **3** Frequent nursing reduces the possibility of engorgement. A 10-minute period provides for complete emptying of the breast. (a); PL; AP; OB; ED; PP

  1 Will not decrease engorgement.

  2 A relief bottle will prevent emptying of the breast; will increase pain and swelling.

  4 Does not provide for complete emptying of the breasts.

54. **1** Asthma involves spasms of the bronchi and bronchioles as well as an increased mucus production. This decreases the size of the lumina, interfering with inhalation and exhalation. (b); AN; CP; ME; PA; RE

  2 Not a mechanism involved in asthma, in which there is interference with both inhalation and exhalation.

  3 There will be a decrease in the vital capacity.

  4 The client cannot hyperventilate because of mucosal edema, bronchoconstriction, and secretions, all of which cause airway obstruction. Emotional stress is only one precipitating factor that has been identified; allergens, temperature changes, odors, chemicals, and other irritants may also be causative factors.

55. **1** In addition to dilation of bronchi, treatment is aimed at expectoration of mucus. Mucus interferes with gas exchange in the lungs. (a); PL; AP; ME; PA; RE

  2 Increased fluid intake helps liquefy secretions.

  3 This is an unrealistic goal; asthma is a chronic illness.

  4 Asthma is psychosomatic, which does not imply that emotions are the only etiologic factor; there is an interaction between the psyche and the soma.

56. **3** Aminophylline relaxes the smooth muscles, causing bronchodilation and thereby relieving respiratory distress and promoting rest. (a); EV; CP; ME; PA; RE

  1 Aminophylline is not a skeletal muscle relaxant.

  2 Aminophylline is not a cathartic.

  4 Aminophylline is not an antibiotic.

57. **3** When an IV infusion is infiltrated, it should be removed to prevent swelling of the tissues and pain. (b); EV; AP; ME; TC; EI

  1 This would add to the infiltration of fluid.

  2 Elevation does not change the position of the IV cannula; the infusion must be discontinued.

4 Soaks may be applied, if ordered, after the IV is removed.

58. **1** During sleep mucus secretions in the respiratory tract move more slowly toward the throat. On awakening, increased ciliary motion raises such secretions more vigorously; this facilitates expectoration and the collection of sputum specimens. (a); PL; AP; ME; PA; RE

  2 Sputum may leave an unpleasant taste in the mouth, which could interfere with eating.

  3 Sputum would more likely be collected after an IPPB treatment because this mobilizes secretions due to positive pressure.

  4 Although activity mobilizes secretions, there may not be any secretions present at the time of activity; sputum is most plentiful upon arising.

59. **2** Individuals who have difficulty asking for help may "cry for help" through a psychophysiologic illness. (b); AN; CP; ME; PE; RE

  1 A wheeze is related to the respiratory system, not the cardiovascular system.

  3 It is due to a constriction of the bronchi.

  4 Hypochondriasis is a chronic abnormal concern about one's health; not part of the psychopathology of asthma.

60. **3** Although dust cannot be avoided completely, use of a damp cloth helps eliminate the amount of airborne particles that might be inhaled. (a); PL; AP; ME; ED; RE

  1 This is unrealistic.

  2 Redecorating will not eliminate dust; it is a part of our environment.

  4 Untrue; there are ways to limit the amount of airborne particles.

61. **4** If a tracheostomy is not performed with radical neck surgery, tracheal edema may cause obstruction of the airway after the endotracheal tube is removed. (a); PL; AP; SU; TC; RE

  1 Fresh postoperative dressings should be removed by the surgeon.

  2 An endotracheal tube is not irrigated to maintain patency, as is a nasogastric tube; the endotracheal tube is in the trachea, leading to the lungs.

  3 It is not necessary to reposition the endotracheal tube if the gag reflex returns; when the client is able to breathe on her own, the anesthesiologist will remove the tube.

62. **2** Inadequate oxygenation of the brain may produce restlessness or behavioral changes. The pulse and respiration rates increase as a compensatory mechanism for hypoxia. (b); EV; CP; SU; PA; RE

  1 The pulse and respiration rates increase with hypoxia.

  3 Clubbing of the fingers, the result of increased vascularization, is an adaptation to prolonged hypoxia.

  4 The pupils dilate with cerebral hypoxia.

63. **3** The cuff should be inflated to the minimum occlusive volume, which allows the desired volume to be achieved but does not press against the trachea, constricting circulation. This can be judged by using a stethoscope to listen for a slight air leak at the back of the throat. (c); IM; AP; SU; TC; RE

  1 The cuff is usually deflated during suctioning to prevent tracheal necrosis; secretions just above the cuff drop by gravity and can also be removed by suctioning.

  2 Several minutes per hour is recommended; some high-volume, low-pressure cuffs need minimal deflation.

  4 The seal should be minimally occlusive; a tight seal could result in tracheal necrosis.

64. **4** To facilitate entry of the suction catheter into the bronchi, the client's head should be turned from side to side. For entry into the left bronchus the head should be turned to the right; for entry into the right bronchus, to the left. (c); IM; AP; SU; TC; RE

 1 The cuff should be deflated during suctioning.

 2 When ordered, this drug is usually given by inhalation not instillation.

 3 Negative pressure is applied as the catheter is withdrawn.

65. **2** The tracheostomy site is a portal of entry for microorganisms. Sterile technique must be used. (c); IM; AP; SU; TC; RE

 1 Body temperature is not related to the suctioning procedure.

 3 The cannula is generally cleaned with peroxide and saline.

 4 High-Fowler's position promotes maximum aeration of the lungs.

66. **2** Drugs such as atropine and opiates are contraindicated because the effects of drying secretions and depressing the cough reflex are undesirable. (c); AN; AN; SU; TC; RE

 1 Pyrvinium pamoate (Povan), a drug for pinworms, is not contraindicated in persons with a tracheostomy.

 3 Chloral hydrate, a hypnotic, is not contraindicated in persons with a tracheostomy.

 4 Nalorphine (Nalline), a synthetic narcotic analgesic antagonist, is not contraindicated in persons with a tracheostomy.

67. **3** The inner cannula must be removed, cleaned with peroxide, and rinsed with saline to prevent mucus accumulation and occlusion of the tube. (b); IM; AP; SU; TC; RE

 1 The outer cannula is left in place, its patency maintained through suctioning.

 2 The status of the cuff has no effect on tracheostomy care.

 4 This is used only for inserting the outer cannula.

68. **2** Nausea and vomiting in the morning occur in almost 50% of all pregnancies. Eating dry crackers before getting out of bed in the morning is a simple remedy that may provide relief. (a); IM; AP; OB; ED; PN

 1 Increasing protein intake does not relieve the nausea.

 3 Two small meals and a snack at noon would not meet the nutritional needs of a pregnant woman; nor would it relieve nausea. Some women find that eating five or six small meals daily instead of three large ones is helpful.

 4 This is not helpful; separating fluids from solids at mealtime is more advisable.

69. **3** The nurse should expect to see an increase in blood volume by as much as 40% above prepregnant levels. During pregnancy, fluid in all body compartments increases. (c); AN; AN; OB; PA; PN

 1 An increase in cardiac output is seen as early as the end of the first trimester; due to increased blood volume.

 2 The hematocrit decreases as a result of the hemodilution of pregnancy.

 4 BP remains essentially unchanged throughout pregnancy.

70. **4** Mrs. Gosney is in early labor, and the first priority of care is to establish a trusting relationship with her and her husband. This will help to allay their anxiety. (a); IM; AP; OB; PE; IP

 1 May be necessary later; however, not of the first priority.

 2 Also not an initial priority item; the physician knows she is on her way.

3 The history should be taken from the client as long as she is capable of providing it.

71. **3** The bulging perineum indicates that the fetal head is on the pelvic floor and birth is imminent. (a); EV; CP; OB; PA; IP

 1 This is a sign that occurs during transmition or the beginning of the second stage; the second stage lasts approximately 1 hour in a primipara, and Mrs. Gosney would be more comfortable in the labor room until then.

 2 This is a sign that occurs during transition or the beginning of the second stage; the second stage lasts approximately 1 hour in a primipara, and Mrs. Gosney would be more comfortable in the labor room until then.

 4 This is a sign that occurs during transition or the beginning of the second stage; the second stage lasts approximately 1 hour in a primipara, and Mrs. Gosney would be more comfortable in the labor room until then.

72. **3** This is the usual pattern that a nevus vasculosus follows. (b); IM; CP; OB; ED; IP

 1 False; a nevus vasculosus involves the dermal and subdermal layers.

 2 False; a nevus vasculosus grows and fades. Saying it will be covered by clothes gives little reassurance.

 4 Surgical removal is not recommended.

73. **1** The antibody system is not functioning in neonates. Antibodies are transferred from the mother in the milk. (a); IM; CP; OB; ED; PP

 2 Breast milk has 1.1 g protein/100 ml; cow's milk has 3.5 g/100 ml.

 3 Because of the higher carbohydrate content of breast milk, infants wake more easily; carbohydrate is digested more rapidly.

 4 Lactating mothers rarely ovulate for the first 9 weeks postpartum; however, they may any time after that.

74. **3** Petrolatum gauze helps control bleeding, and prevent adherence of the diaper. (b); IM; AP; OB; ED; NH

 1 Fussy behavior is normal for a few hours after the procedure.

 2 Yellow exudate is normal; not part of an infectious process.

 4 Not practical with a male infant.

75. **3** The woman must watch closely for symptoms associated with side effects of these medications. Estrogen-progestin contraceptives have been associated with thrombophlebitis (calf pain) and breast malignancy (breast tenderness from estrogen-supported tumors) as well as cardiovascular changes (hypertension). (c); EV; AP; OB; ED; FS

 1 Nausea and rash are not associated with using estrogen-progestin contraceptives; however, breakthrough bleeding is a major side-effect.

 2 Lethargy, syncope, and tachycardia are not side effects of oral contraceptives.

 4 Bradycardia and visual changes are not side effects, hypertension is a major side effect.

76. **1** Denial or disbelief and shock are considered initial responses of grieving. There is a feeling of guilt and inadequacy when a child is born with a defect or abnormality. (a); AS; CP; PS; PE; CS

 2 It would be unusual for a client initially to verbalize feelings of punishment or guilt so directly.

 3 It would be unusual for a client to use rationalization and voice it so obviously.

 4 A sense of shame and guilt is voiced later; after denial, disbelief, and shock.

77. **3** This approach allows for ventilation of feelings and clarifies explanations that probably were not heard or understood because of anxiety. (b); IM; AP; PS; PE; CS
    1 Closes off communication by not allowing free expression of grief.
    2 Excludes the client from facing the problem, thereby increasing her feelings of loss of control.
    4 Supports avoidance of the reality of the situation; does not help the problem.
78. **1** The psychosocial need during the early toddler age is the development of autonomy. The toddler objects strongly to discipline. (b); AN; CP; PE; ED; MN
    2 Untrue; excessive discipline leads to feelings of shame and self-doubt, the major crisis at this stage of development.
    3 It is frightening for a child to be left alone; leaves him with feelings of rejection, isolation, and insecurity.
    4 The sense of initiative is attained during the preschool age, not during the toddler age.
79. **4** This action of Susan's gives her child more control by allowing him to make a decision. It also shows an understanding of what the toddler can and cannot do safely. (c); EV; CP; PS; PE; CS
    1 Although tantrums as attention-getting devices largely must be ignored, ignoring the child will produce feelings of isolation and insecurity.
    2 Boredom, hunger, and insecurity can lead to additional frustration and anger.
    3 This could lead to the development of more manipulative tactics, since the action brought a degree of success initially.
80. **3** A predominant clinical sign of croup is reactive spasms of the laryngeal muscles, which produces partial respiratory obstruction. Cough is tight, with a barking metallic sound. (b); AS; CP; PE; PA; RE
    1 Children with croup experience spasm of the larynx rather than the bronchi; whooping cough (pertussis) is a separate communicable disease.
    2 Children with croup experience inspiratory rather than expiratory stridor.
    4 The cough of croup is tight and nonproductive.
81. **2** Syrup of ipecac is a nonprescription emetic causing vomiting. Vomiting interrupts the laryngospasm characteristic of croup. (c); IM; AN; PE; ED; RE
    1 This does not interrupt the laryngospasm associated with croup.
    3 This is a prescription drug; not something parents can give to interrupt the attack.
    4 This is a prescription drug; although it will cause bronchodilation, it will not help laryngospasm.
82. **3** Ipecac causes forceful vomiting. The reversal of peristalsis puts pressure on the glottis and interrupts the spasm. (b); EV; AP; PE; PA; RE
    1 Ipecac does not cause bronchodilation.
    2 Ipecac does not reduce inflammation.
    4 Ipecac does not influence the cough center.
83. **2** The toddler is in Erikson's stage of acquiring a sense of autonomy. The negativism is the result of Molly's need to express her will and test out her environment. (a); AN; AP; PE; ED; MN
    1 She does not assert herself to obtain discipline.
    3 Although this is a factor, toddlers assert themselves in an attempt to attain more autonomy.
    4 This is the developmental task achieved in infancy.
84. **4** Children who are expressing negativism need to have a feeling of control. One way of achieving this within reasonable limits is for the parent or care giver to provide a choice of two items, rather than force one on the child. (a); IM; AN; PE; ED; MN

1 Will probably not be successful with a toddler; will probably end in disaster.
2 Will not achieve the goal of giving her fluids.
3 Will only complicate the situation and further inhibit the child's willingness to take fluids.
85. **2** The parents' attitude, approach, and understanding of the child's physical and psychologic readiness are essential to letting the child proceed at her own pace with appropriate interventions by the parent. (a); PL; CP; PE; ED; RG
    1 This will not be the major motivation for toilet training.
    3 Although this will definitely be a factor, it is not a major one.
    4 This, of course, is a factor; but the major factor is the child herself, who is strongly influenced by the parents' attitudes and approach.
86. **4** Children learn socially acceptable behavior when consistent reasonable limits that provide guidelines are established. (b); IM; AP; PE; ED; MN
    1 Rewards should not always be necessary for good behavior; will become expected.
    2 Not always safe or reasonable for very young children.
    3 Authorities vary on their attitudes about punishment; it should not, however, become the major means of teaching children to control their behavior.
87. **4** The client's exact compliance in carrying out the compulsive ritual relieves anxiety, at least temporarily. Furthermore, it meets a need and is necessary to the client. (a); AN; CP; PS; PE; PD
    1 The person cannot stop the activity; it is not under voluntary control.
    2 Urging has no effect on trying to have the client start or stop the ritualistic behavior.
    3 The compulsive act is purposeless repetition and useful only in that it decreases anxiety for the client.
88. **3** The anxiety disorders are characterized by anxiety and minor distortions of reality. The anxiety results in an inability to reach a decision, since all alternatives are threatening. (a); AS; CP; PS; PE; PD
    1 Just the opposite is true; part of emotional maturity is the ability to relate to people, and these people have difficulties in this area.
    2 Would be indicative of severe emotional illness, not an anxiety disorder.
    4 Would be indicative of an affective disorder.
89. **4** Rituals are a means for the individual to control anxiety. If not permitted to carry out ritual, the client will probably experience unbearable anxiety. (c); IM; AP; PS; PE; PD
    1 The client understands this already but is unable to stop the activity.
    2 The client has no idea what the ritual means; only that she must continue with it.
    3 This would have the effect of increasing anxiety in the client, possibly to panic levels.
90. **2** Since the compulsive ritual is used to control anxiety, any attempt to prevent the action would greatly increase the anxiety. (c); EV; CP; PS; PE; PD
    1 Possible only if the anxiety reached panic levels and caused the person overtly to express anger.
    3 Not a pattern of behavior associated with this disorder.
    4 Underlying hostility is considered to be part of the disorder itself; not a reaction to an interruption of the ritual.
91. **1** Albumin is not normally excreted in the urine. When found, it indicates renal disease. (a); EV; AN; PE; PA; RG
    2 Excess calcium is normally excreted.

How to Use Worksheet 1: Errors in Processing Information

Common errors in processing information are listed in the left-hand column of this worksheet. At the top of the worksheet is a row of blank spaces for inserting the number of the question missed. Directly below each number, check any errors you made in answering that question. You may have made more than one type of error in an answer.

Worksheet 1: Errors in processing information

Question number																					
Did not read situation/question carefully																					
Missed important details																					
Confused major and minor points																					
Defined problem incorrectly																					
Could not remember terms/facts/concepts/principles																					
Defined terms incorrectly																					
Focused on incomplete/incorrect data in assessing situation																					
Interpreted data incorrectly																					
Applied wrong concepts/principles in situation																					
Drew incorrect conclusions																					
Identified wrong goals																					
Identified priorities incorrectly																					
Carried out plan incorrectly/incompletely																					
Was unclear about criteria for evaluating success in achieving goals																					

How to Use Worksheet 2: Knowledge Gaps

Types of common knowledge gaps are listed along the top of this worksheet. Write a brief description of topics you want to review in the spaces provided. For example, if you missed a question on administration of a particular drug, write the drug name and problem (e.g., dosage) in the appropriate space under the column labeled *Pharmacology*.

Worksheet 2: Knowledge gaps

Basic science	Skills/ procedures	Basic human needs	Growth & develop- ment	Normal nutrition	Psycho- social factors	Clinical area/ topic	Stressors/ coping mechanisms	Patho- physiology	Pharma- cology	Therapeutic nutrition	Legal implications	Other

3 Potassium is normally excreted by the kidneys to maintain electrolyte balance.

4 Excess calcium is normally excreted.

92. **2** Fewer side effects mean better elimination of the lead, which means that further irreversible damage can be prevented. (b); EV; CP; PE; TC; MN

1 Each drug is able to accomplish this, but singly given each can cause more side effects; may be fatal if rapidly infused.

3 No marked difference in the rate of elimination when these agents are used together.

4 The combination is preferred because it removes lead more effectively from the brain rather than from bone marrow.

93. **1** Active sharing of responsibility will prove most helpful. It will contribute to the success of the mother's efforts to overcome dependency and passivity and assure that lead sources are removed. (c); IM; AP; PE; ED; MN

2 Will not resolve etiologic factors or accomplish prevention.

3 Omits the need to remove lead from the environment; therefore will not assure prevention.

4 A good idea, but does not guarantee action; concrete action should be taken first.

Comprehensive Test 1: Part 2*

94. **2** Intermittent positive pressure breathing (IPPB) is used to provide full expansion of the lungs, to loosen secretions, and to administer medication. (a); AN; CP; SU; PA; RE

1 By improving the efficiency of respiration, IPPB should ultimately decrease the respiratory rate.

3 IPPB is used prophylactically before infection occurs.

4 Positive pressure forces air into the lungs; negative pressure or suction is not involved.

95. **3** As a result of COPD, there is increased pressure in the pulmonary circulation. The right side of the heart hypertrophies (called cor pulmonale), and congestive heart failure may ensue. (b); AN; CP; SU; PA; RE

1 This system is not as closely related to the pulmonary system as the cardiac system is; kidney problems do not usually occur.

2 Peripheral nerves are not as closely related to the pulmonary system as the cardiac system is; peripheral neuropathy does not occur.

4 The skeletal system is not truly related to the pulmonary system; joint inflammation does not occur.

96. **4** Productive coughing induced by IPPB can cause nausea and vomiting. (b); EV; CP; ME; PA; RE

1 Upon awakening, mucus secretions are plentiful and tenacious; an IPPB treatment at this time would be most beneficial.

2 Approximately 1 hour before meals is a preferred time for IPPB; the resulting cough and mucus production will be less likely to affect dietary intake.

3 Since coughing must be encouraged after treatment, sleep is postponed; but as breathing is facilitated, sleep may then be more restful.

97. **2** The fluid level and time must be marked so the amount of drainage in a closed drainage system (e.g., with chest tubes) can be evaluated. (a); EV; AP; SU; TC; RE

1 The catheter is secured by skin sutures, not to the dressing itself.

3 The drainage system must be kept below chest level to promote drainage of the pleural space so the lung can expand.

4 The amount of sterile water used to create a water seal depends on the drainage system used and is usually more than 3 to 5 ml; once the water seal is created, the nurse does not add additional water.

98. **3** Atmospheric pressure is greater than the pressure inside the pleural space. If a chest tube were not attached to underwater seal drainage, air would enter the pleural space and collapse the lung (pneumothorax). (b); AN; AP; SU; TC; RE

1 The water seal does not affect the amount of suction used.

2 Capillarity is the tendency of cohesive liquid molecules to rise in a tube; not the purpose of water in a closed chest drainage system.

4 The concern is not primarily for pressure within the tube itself but to prevent atmospheric pressure from collapsing the lung.

99. **1** Turning and positioning prevent pooling of secretions in lungs as well as maximize lung expansion. (c); IM; AP; SU; PA; RE

2 Cupping is a dependent nursing function.

3 Clapping is a dependent nursing function.

4 Postural drainage is a dependent nursing function.

100. **2** There are several modes for the administration of oxygen. Selection is based upon the disease and the client's adaptation. (b); AN; CP; ME; TC; RE

1 Although anatomy may be one factor considered, selection depends on the therapeutic effect relative to the client's disease and needs.

3 Although these will be taken into consideration, the ultimate decision is based on the pathologic condition and therapeutic needs.

4 Although consideration may be given to activity, selection is based on the pathologic condition and therapeutic needs.

101. **2** Oxygen can dry the mucous membranes of the respiratory tract and must be humidified for administration. Drying of mucous membranes can predispose to infection. (a); IM; CP; ME; PA; RE

1 Padding is required because of irritation by some equipment; not related to the untoward effects of oxygen therapy.

3 Although vital signs should be assessed so the effect of treatment can be evaluated, an apical pulse is not necessary.

4 The orthopneic position promotes lung expansion and is often used in conjunction with oxygen therapy; not an untoward effect.

102. **3** A culture of CSF obtained would reveal the presence of a causative organism (e.g., the pneumococcus, tubercle bacillus, meningococcus, or streptococcus). (b); AN; CP; PE; PA; MN

1 Used to detect the presence of abnormalities by the injection of a contrast medium into the subarachnoid space; does not identify the organism.

2 Would demonstrate the presence of bacteria on the skin, not identify organisms in the cerebrospinal fluid.

4 Not a definitive test, although advisable; occasionally will prove positive when a CSF culture is negative.

103. **3**
$$\frac{\text{Amount of fluid} \times \text{Drop rate}}{\text{Time (in minutes)}}$$
$$\frac{500 \times 60}{24 \times 60} = 21 \text{ drops}$$

(a); EV; AN; PE; PA; MN

1 Too slow to infuse the desired amount.

2 Too slow to infuse the desired amount.

4 Too rapid; the fluid would run out before 24 hours had elapsed.

104. **1** The concept of object permanence begins to develop around 6 months of age. (c); AS; CP; PE; ED; MN

    2 Occurs during the first several months of life.

    3 Occurs between 13 and 24 months.

    4 Occurs between 13 and 24 months.

105. **4** After administration of a local anesthetic during a bronchoscopy, fluids and food should be withheld until the gag reflex returns. (a); EV; AP; SU; TC; RE

    1 To allow drainage and minimize possibility of aspiration, the client should be kept in a semi-Fowler's position.

    2 Ice chips must not be given until the gag reflex returns.

    3 Coughing should not be encouraged; it might initiate bleeding from the site of the biopsy.

106. **3** The phrenic nerve stimulates the diaphragm. After destruction of the nerve on the operative side, the diaphragm will move upward, decreasing the size of the empty space and helping prevent mediastinal shift. (b); AN; KN; SU; PA; RE

    1 Would occur if both nerves were severed.

    2 Since the phrenic nerve stimulates the diaphragm, its effect on postoperative pain would be negligible.

    4 There is less excursion because the nerve has been severed.

107. **3** Because Mrs. Smith has just undergone major surgery, she has an endotracheal tube in place. Secretions can be loosened by the administration of humidified oxygen and by frequent turning. (b); PL; AN; SU; PA; RE

    1 A client with an endotracheal tube in place is not permitted fluids by mouth.

    2 Would be too vigorous for a client in the immediate postoperative period.

    4 Potassium is never instilled into the lungs.

108. **1** To maintain normal expansion of the remaining lung after a pneumonectomy, the client should be positioned on the operative side or the back. (c); IM; AP; SU; PA; RE

    2 The client should not be placed on the unaffected side; will impede lung expansion.

    3 A high-Fowler's position may cause the client to slip down in the bed, diminishing thoracic excursion.

    4 Keeping the client flat will decrease lung expansion; gatching a bed may cause peripheral circulatory complications.

109. **2** After a pneumonectomy the mediastinum may shift toward the remaining lung, or the remaining lung could shift toward the empty space, depending on the pressure within the empty space. Either of these shifts would cause the trachea to move from its normal midline position. (The trachea is palpated above the suprasternal notch.) (c); EV; AP; SU; PA; RE

    1 Tracheal edema cannot be assessed through palpation; edema is not a concern when the endotracheal tube is in place.

    3 Metastatic lesions would not appear rapidly.

    4 The cuff of the endotracheal tube cannot be assessed through palpation of the trachea.

110. **3** Endometriosis is the presence of aberrant endometrial tissue outside the uterus. The tissue responds to ovarian stimulation, bleeds during menstruation, and causes severe pain. (a); AS; KN; OB; PA; FS

    1 Not symptoms of endometriosis.

    2 Ecchymoses and petechiae are not characteristic of this disorder.

    4 Osteoporosis may be a complication of menopause due to the decreased estrogen levels; pelvic inflammation usually results from infection.

111. **1** Menopause is a normal developmental adaptation. It is not caused by endometriosis, the abnormal bleeding of aberrant tissue outside the uterus. (c); AS; AP; OB; PA; FS

    2 Bleeding between periods is due to the bleeding of endometrial tissue outside the uterus.

    3 Excessive tissue may impinge on the colon and cause ribbonlike stools.

    4 Excessive tissue may impinge on the bladder and ureter; can cause voiding difficulties.

112. **2** Antiovulatory drugs suppress menstruation. Breakthrough bleeding is abnormal and will lead to recurrence of symptoms. (b); EV; CP; OB; TC; FS

    1 There is no indication for increased Pap smears; once a year is sufficient.

    3 No restriction of sexual activity is indicated when one is taking oral contraceptives.

    4 Increased calcium to counteract osteoporosis from menopause is not indicated for this client.

113. **4** The nurse should demonstrate to the client a recognition of her concern and a willingness to listen. (c); IM; AP; PS; PE; CS

    1 Avoiding the question indicates that the nurse is unwilling to listen.

    2 Could increase anxiety and would not reduce worry; furthermore, it cuts off communication and denies feelings.

    3 The client did not state directly that she thought she had cancer; this response forces her to defend her feelings.

114. **2** Certain diagnostic tests (e.g., CBC, urinalysis, chest x-ray examination) are done preoperatively to rule out the existence of other health problems that could increase the risks involved with surgery. (c); IM; AP; SU; ED; RE

    1 Feelings would not be dispelled by this response; also blocks further communication.

    3 Lack of knowledge without a statement of plans to obtain the information suggests incompetence on the part of the nurse.

    4 False information; surgery poses a risk despite test results.

115. **4** Anxiety experienced by a preoperative client can be a disruptive force affecting the client's ability to adapt psychologically and physiologically. For other nursing measures to be effective, it must be alleviated. (b); PL; AP; SU; PE; GI

    1 Learning is hampered by high anxiety levels.

    2 Diet is limited prior to surgery so residue in the intestines will be decreased.

    3 Vital signs must be recorded, for they will serve as a baseline in postoperative assessment; however, reduction of anxiety is the first priority.

116. **3** Interpretation of pain sensations is highly individual and is based on past experiences, which include cultural values. (b); AN; CP; PS; PE; CS

    1 Overall physical condition may affect one's ability to cope with stress; but unless the nervous system were involved, it would not greatly affect perception.

    2 Intelligence is a factor in understanding pain, so it can be better tolerated, but does not affect the perception of intensity; economic status has no affect on pain perception.

    4 Age and sex affect pain perception only indirectly because they generally account for past experience to some degree.

117. **1** Following the administration of certain antihypertensives or narcotics, the client's neurocirculatory reflexes may have some difficulty adjusting to the force of gravity when assuming an upright position. Postural or orthostatic hypotension occurs, and there is a temporarily decreased blood supply to the brain. (a); PL; AP; SU; TC; GI
    2 Respiratory distress is an adverse effect of morphine but is not prevented by the intervention described.
    3 Hypertension does not occur.
    4 Abdominal pain will not be prevented by the intervention described.

118. **4** Used for its analgesic effects, morphine is a CNS depressant. Its major adverse effect is respiratory depression. It can also cause lethargy, pupillary constriction, and depressed reflexes, and it could lead to coma and death. (b); EV; KN; SU; TC; GI
    1 Although diaphoresis may accompany hypotension, it is only indirectly related to the drug and is not profuse.
    2 Overdose causes miosis rather than dilated pupils.
    3 These occur to some extent with therapeutic doses because of their effect on the CNS; however, not symptoms of an overdose.

119. **3** Pain in the calf may be a sign of thrombophlebitis, a possible postoperative complication. If the thrombus becomes dislodged, it may lead to pulmonary embolism. Any client with this complaint should immediately be confined to bed, and the physician notified. (a); AN; AN; SU; TC; GI
    1 The leg should not be elevated above heart level without a physician's order; gravity may dislodge the thrombus, creating an embolism.
    2 Application of heat is a dependent nursing function.
    4 Charting does not take precedence over notifying the physician of a potentially serious complication.

120. **4** This response recognizes fearful feelings. It also permits further communication. (a); IM; AP; PS; PE; CS
    1 Does not recognize feelings of fear; changes the focus of the conversation.
    2 Does not recognize feelings; instills fear by implying that this pregnancy may not go to term, for which there is no evidence.
    3 Closes off communication and may increase anxiety and guilt.

121. **3** This response acknowledges the loss and the grieving process. It also encourages ventilation through acceptance. (a); IM; AP; PS; PE; CS
    1 Guilt feelings were never expressed by the client; this response may reflect the nurse's feelings.
    2 Minimizes the loss; may reflect the nurse's feelings. It also plants thoughts of a less than perfect fetus.
    4 Does not recognize the loss; cuts off communication.

122. **2** A correct and simple definition answers the question and fulfills the client's need to know. (b); IM; AP; OB; ED; FS
    1 The nurse can independently reinforce and clear misconceptions.
    3 Denies the client's right to know.
    4 This is the definition of a missed abortion.

123. **2** Initial disbelief and denial help protect the ego from the pain of reality in a stressful situation. (c); EV; AN; PS; PE; CS
    1 Once the initial shock is over, these are the usual results as the self realizes the loss.
    3 May result from guilt or feelings of inadequacy because of the loss; but occurs later.
    4 There is no evidence of either dissociation or rationalization.

124. **3** This action demonstrates recognition of the client's behavior as a normal response to the situation. (a); IM, AN; PS; PE; CS
    1 May be done later; the need to respond to the client's feelings is the priority at this time.
    2 May make her feel that she is doing something wrong or is annoying others.
    4 Closes off communication; does not allow the client to talk about her feelings.

125. **4** Hydrocephalus complicates approximately 90% of lumbosacral meningomyeloceles. (b); AS; CP; PE; PA; MN
    1 A shrill high-pitched cry often accompanies progressive hydrocephalus; however, may also indicate other neurologic problems.
    2 Normal for a newborn.
    3 Hydrocephalic infants may or may not have a low Apgar score.

126. **3** This is what occurs in communicating hydrocephalus. (c); IM; AP; PE; ED; MN
    1 This is often caused by a choroid plexus tumor and does not interfere with the flow of cerebrospinal fluid through the ventricles.
    2 This reflects the pathophysiologic process of noncommunicating hydrocephalus.
    4 Inaccurate answer; brain cells and the spinal cord are not involved.

127. **2** These are associated with infection, the greatest postoperative hazard for children with shunts for hydrocephalus. (b); PL; AN; PE; ED; MN
    1 Occur with progressively increasing intracranial pressure, usually before shunt insertion; considered a sign, not a complication.
    3 May be a complication, sometimes as a result of an infected shunt; however, not the most common complication.
    4 The peritoneum absorbs cerebrospinal fluid adequately; ascites is not a problem.

128. **3** Periodic pumping of the valve ensures the patency of the tubing and allows the fluid to move through. (b); IM; AN; PE; ED; MN
    1 Bleeding results if cerebrospinal fluid is drained too rapidly; the pump may be used for this purpose, but this is not its primary function.
    2 Pumping the shunt does not affect the absorption of cerebrospinal fluid.
    4 This is the purpose of the shunt itself; pumping the valve only keeps the tubing patent.

129. **3** Most children with spinal cord damage from communicating hydrocephalus can be managed successfully with this approach. (b); PL; AP; PE; ED; MN
    1 This is a devastating and inaccurate statement to make to any young infant's parents.
    2 Most children with spinal cord damage from this defect can be managed succcessfully with intermittent straight catheterization.
    4 Inaccurate statement, and the least desirable approach because of recurrent urinary tract infections.

130. **3** A distended bladder usually displaces the fundus upward and toward the right. (a); EV; CP; OB; TC; PP
    1 The normal position of the fundus is at the level of the umbilicus, or below, in the midline rather than shifted to the right.
    2 If parts of the placenta and/or membranes were retained, bleeding would be present.
    4 The fundus is firm; therefore bleeding at this time is not a problem.

131. **2** In the immediate postpartum period a slower than normal pulse rate can be anticipated as a result of a combination of factors—horizontal position, emo-

tional relief and satisfaction, enforced rest after labor and delivery. (c); AS; AP; OB; PA; PP

1 The temperature may rise slightly, but respirations generally are unchanged.

3 The temperature may rise, but respirations generally are unchanged.

4 Bradycardia more likely; respirations generally are unchanged.

132. **3** Retention of urine with overflow will be manifested in small, frequent voidings. The bladder should be palpated for distention. (a); AN; CP; OB; PA; PP

1 There should be large amounts of urine voided because of the increased fluid volume at this time.

2 An elevated temperature with urinary symptoms would be indicative of impending infection.

4 Untrue; more circulating fluid is present, causing an increased output.

133. **4** Parenting can begin only when the baby and mother get to know each other. To promote normal development, the nurse should provide time for parent-child interaction. (b); PL; AP; OB; ED; PP

1 This may make the mother feel incompetent and retard her mothering.

2 Ineffective; knowledge does not ensure good mothering. Time with the infant is more important.

3 Time must be provided for the mother with baby to return demonstrations and ask questions.

134. **2** Cephalohematoma is a collection of blood between the skull bone and its periosteum as the result of trauma. It resolves spontaneously in 3 to 6 weeks. (c); PL; CP; PE; ED; CB

1 This is trauma caused by pressure of the head against the birth canal; can occur in vaginal delivery.

3 Caput succedaneum, rather than cephalohematoma, crosses the suture line.

4 This is a hard indurated area; remains immobile even when the infant cries.

135. **1** Parents need support and reassurance that their child is not permanently damaged. (c); AN; CP; PE; PE; CB

2 Cephalohematomas resolve spontaneously; no ice is applied.

3 Cephalohematomas do not cause impaired neurologic functioning.

4 No special protection of the head is required; routine safety measures are adequate.

136. **2** In myasthenia gravis the effectiveness of acetylcholine is reduced, interfering with muscle contraction. Inadequate contraction of the ocular muscles results in double vision (diplopia). (b); AS; AP; ME; PA; MN

1 Nystagmus is a common symptom of multiple sclerosis.

3 Not a symptom of myasthenia gravis.

4 Not a symptom of myasthenia gravis.

137. **2** Tensilon is an anticholinesterase compound that drastically increases muscle strength when administered to an individual with myasthenia gravis. (c); AS; CP; ME; PA; MN

1 EDTA is a calcium chelating agent sometimes used in the treatment of digitalis intoxication.

3 Prednisolone is a steroid; not used to diagnose this disease.

4 Dilantin is an anticonvulsant; not used to test for myasthenia.

138. **2** Myasthenia gravis is a chronic degenerative disorder with exacerbations that are precipitated by emotional stress, ingestion of alcohol, and physical stress such as infection. (a); AN; CP; ME; PA; MN

1 The disease is chronic; death does not occur within a short period but usually after the muscles of respiration are affected.

3 The disease is characterized by exacerbations and remissions.

4 The prognosis is not excellent; there is no cure.

139. **3** Myasthenia gravis is a degenerative disease that occurs equally in both sexes during adulthood. (b); AN; KN; ME; PA; MN

1 Occurs equally in both sexes.

2 Occurs equally in both sexes.

4 Not a disease common in childhood.

140. **1** Neostigmine bromide (Prostigmin) is an anticholinergic that increases the peristaltic activity of the intestines. The result is hyperactive bowel sounds. (b); EV; AP; ME; PA; MN

2 Bradycardia and hypotension may occur with neostigmine.

3 Bladder distension is not associated with neostigmine.

4 These are not side effects associated with neostigmine.

141. **4** The response should be kept as optimistic as possible while still being realistic. (b); IM; CP; ME; ED; MN

1 The individual response varies; gives false reassurance.

2 False reassurance; her status will depend on her individual response.

3 Medication does not affect progression; only treats the symptoms.

142. **2** Swimming would help keep the muscles supple, without requiring fine motor activity. (b); AN; AP; ME; ED; MN

1 Sedentary activities are not helpful in maintaining muscle tone.

3 Sewing requires find motor activity; would be difficult for the client.

4 Might prove too rigorous for the client.

143. **3** Identifying feelings and providing support during stressful times are both ways of demonstrating concern during a crisis. (a); IM; AN; PS; PE; CS

1 Not a supportive or insightful reply.

2 Lacks insight and supportiveness.

4 Inappropriate reply that may instill guilt feelings; the father as well as the mother needs support through this crisis.

144. **3** Allowing the client time to talk about her feelings and staying with her when she sees the baby for the first time provide support, acceptance, and understanding. (c); AS; AP; PS; PE; CS

1 This does not give the nurse a chance to assess the mother's feelings.

2 This does not give the nurse a chance to assess the mother's feelings; anomalies are difficult to describe accurately in words.

4 Showing pictures may not be helpful, and discussing treatment is premature.

145. **2** The usual initial response to a crisis situation such as this is denial that it could occur and that she and her husband could produce a less than normal child. Mrs. Handler's response is her way of dealing with the reality of the situation. (a); EV; AN; PS; PE; CS

1 First reactions to a child with a congenital anomaly cannot be judged as final.

3 The mother's reaction is a normal part of the grief response.

4 Although the mother initially rejected her baby, time, coping, and love will help her accept his anomaly.

146. **4** The congenital defect prevents the infant from creating a tight seal with his lips to promote sucking. As a result he swallows large amounts of air when feeding. The mother should be taught to provide frequent rest periods and to bubble the infant often to expel the excess air in the stomach. (b); IM; AP; PE; ED; GI

1 Newborn infants cannot chew.

2 Infants with cleft lip and palate should be held upright during feedings.

3 Infants with cleft lip and palate should be help upright during feedings.

147. **4** Menstruation during pregnancy is interrupted because secretion of the ovarian hormones ceases. This response answers the client's question is understandable terms. (b); IM; CP; OB; ED; PN

1 These hormones are needed to rebuild the layers of cells lining the uterus that are sloughed off during menstruation.

2 LH stimulates the maturation of a primitive follicle into a vesicular graafian follicle; also promotes secretion of estrogen by the ovary.

3 This brings about the development of the ova.

148. **4** Abstinence 4 to 6 weeks prior to delivery is the best way to avoid contracting the virus and having an outbreak prior to delivery. (c); AN; AP; OB; ED; PN

1 Abstinence is necessary only when disease symptoms are present in the partner and during the last 4 to 6 weeks.

2 Washing is not enough to prevent contraction of this virus; contact has already been made.

3 Since the herpesvirus is smaller than the pores of a condom, this kind of protection has limited effectiveness.

149. **3** Placenta previa is defined as an abnormally implanted placenta (i.e., low lying or covering the cervical os). (a); PL; AN; OB; PA; HP

1 Can occur without a low-lying placenta; factors such as poor muscular tone of the uterus and excessive oxytocin during induction may cause this to occur.

2 Premature separation of the placenta can occur with normally implanted placentas

4 Can occur at any time; not specific to low-lying placentas.

150. **4** Placing the expectant mother in a semi-Fowler's position forces the heavy uterus to put temporary pressure on the blood vessels at the site of the separating placenta. This controls bleeding to some extent. (b); PL; AN; OB; TC; HP

1 No indication that the clotting mechanism is disturbed.

2 Contraindicated in any client admitted with vaginal bleeding.

3 Contraindicated when placenta previa is suspected; may further dislodge the placenta.

151. **2** The size of the breast bud is an indication of gestational age. Small underdeveloped nipples reflect prematurity. (c); AS; KN; OB; ED; NH

1 Not a good indication of gestational age; reflexes may be impaired in full-term infants also.

3 Not present in normal newborns; a clinical manifestation of Down's syndrome.

4 Not related to gestational age.

152. **2** Cold stress produces hypoxia and acidemia. Because of physiologic factors, the premature infant is more vulnerable to cool temperatures. (b); IM; AP; OB; TC; NH

1 Not a priority; keeping the baby warm is more important.

3 Not a priority; keeping the baby warm is more important.

4 No indication that this is necessary.

153. **3** This is the first period of reactivity. The newborn is alert and awake. (c); AN; AP; OB; ED; NH

1 First sleep usually occurs more than 1 hour after delivery.

2 This occurs after the first sleep.

4 Untrue; after the initial cry, the baby will settle down and become quiet and alert.

154. **3** Excessive drainage flows down the sides of the abdomen to the small of the back by gravity. Observing for hemorrhage is the priority. (b); EV; CP; OB; TC; HP

1 Color and consistency should also be noted; however, for client safety, recording the amount takes precedence.

2 This might also be done, but assessing the total amount of drainage would be the priority.

4 If drainage is excessive, the physician should be notified first.

155. **4** Orienting the client to the hospital provides knowledge that may reduce the strangeness of the environment, whereas introducing staff members lets the client know who will be caring for her as well as providing a personal touch. (b); IM; AP; PS; PE; CS

1 This may be false reassurance since no one can guarantee that everything will be all right.

2 This would be part of orienting her to the unit.

3 This implies that staff members are available to her only if she becomes upset.

156. **4** Atherosclerosis begins with the accumulation of fatty deposits (plaques) within the inner lining (intima) of the arteries, leading to a narrowing of the lumen. Later the plaques enlarge, cause greater occlusion, and harden by deposition of calcium (atheroaterioscleriosis), eventually increasing the work of the heart. (b); AN; KN; ME; PA; CB

1 This is arteriosclerosis.

2 Atheromas develop within the intima of arteries, not in the cardiac muscle.

3 Although atheromas or plaques are deposited from circulating fat, mobilization from adipose storage is not a prerequisite.

157. **1** Each person is unique. The nurse should avoid making the client feel dehumanized. (b); PL; AP; PS; PE; CS

2 This would be a later nursing action.

3 The client is in the hospital for tests; although safety is important, it is not a priority need.

4 It is important that the client understand what is happening to her; however, her individuality must be considered first.

158. **4** Identifying and accepting feelings helps to open lines of communication. (b); IM; AP; PS; PE; CS

1 This does not allow the client to explore her feelings with an accepting person.

2 This is avoiding the real issue.

3 Focuses on only one aspect of the statement; does not allow her to explore her real feelings.

159. **1** Nitroglycerine is sensitive to light and moisture and must be stored in a dark airtight container. (b); IM; AP; ME; TC; CB

2 This may be an expected side effect.

3 This medication is usually taken prn. The daily number may be as high as 12 to 15 tablets; if more than three are necessary in a 15-minute period, the doctor should be notified.

4 Expected response; if it does not occur, tablets should be replaced.

160. **4** Devices such as side rails can help clients increase their mobility by facilitating movement in bed. Side rails are an immovable object and provide a handhold for leverage when changing positions. (c); IM; AP; SU; TC; MN

1 The need to use side rails for safety must be evaluated for each individual based on the mental and physical status.

2 The need to use side rails must be evaluated for each individual based on the mental and physical status.

3 The need to use side rails for safety must be evaluated for each individual based on the mental and physical status.

161. **4** Explaining procedures and routines decreases the client's anxiety about the unknown. (a); IM; AP; PS; PE; CS

   1 Although therapeutic, this does not change the fact that the hospital environment is strange to her.

   2 The nurse should not confuse the role of professional with that of being a friend; the client should be called Mrs. White unless she requests use of her first name.

   3 The nurse should not confuse the role of professional with that of being a friend; "visiting" has a social connotation.

162. **3** Clients and their families should be included in dietary teaching. (a); PL; AP; ME; ED; CB

   1 The dietitian is a resource person who can give specific information about diet and food preparation that is more practical once the client has a basic understanding of the reasons for the diet.

   2 Foods high in sodium will also have to be restricted; this teaching is inadequate.

   4 The client should be included in her own care; she will ultimately assume the responsibility.

163. **4** Processed foods generally have sodium (usually in the form of sodium chloride) added to enhance the taste and help preserve the food. (a); PL; AP; ME; ED; CB

   1 Most fruits have a low sodium content.

   2 Most vegetables have a low sodium content; carrots and celery should be avoided.

   3 Although grain products contain sodium, the content is much less than in processed food.

164. **3** A lowered concentration of extracellular sodium brings about a decrease in the release of ADH. This leads to increased excretion of urine. (b); AN; CP; ME; ED; CB

   1 Potassium is inefficiently retained by the body; an adequate intake of potassium is needed.

   2 The sodium restriction does not control the volume of food intake; weight is controlled by a low-calorie diet and by prevention of fluid retention.

   4 The resulting elimination of excess fluid reduces the workload of the heart but does not improve contractility.

165. **2** Fluid in the interstitial spaces impairs circulation, leading to poor absorption of drugs as well as predisposing skin breakdown. (b); AN; CP; ME; TC; EI

   1 The pain caused by injection is influenced by the type and volume of the drug, not the site.

   3 Interstitial fluid may leak from edematous tissue, but this is not the rationale for altering sites.

   4 The dilution of the drug does not significantly affect absorption.

166. **2** Range-of-motion exercises keep muscles in good tone and prevent venous stasis through physical compression of veins; such compression propels venous blood toward the heart, facilitated by venous one-way valves. (b); IM; AP; ME; PA; MN

   1 Massage may dislodge a thrombus causing a fatal embolus.

   3 Fluids do not affect venous return and thus do not prevent thrombi.

   4 Application of elastic stockings is a dependent function.

167. **4** The wheelchair should be angled close to the bed so the client will have to make only a simple pivot on the stronger leg. When the wheelchair is within the client's visual field, the client will be aware of the distance and direction that the body must navigate to transfer safely and avoid falling. (c); IM; CP; SU; TC; MN

   1 If the client's knees are flexed she may be unable to support her weight on her unaffected leg.

   2 Moving a client back to bed in this situation would encompass moving against gravity.

   3 The large muscles of the legs rather than the arms should be used to prevent muscle strain.

168. **3** In crutch walking the client uses the triceps, trapezius, and latissimus muscles. A client who has been in bed may need to implement an exercise program to strengthen these shoulder and upper arm muscles before initiating crutch walking. (a); IM; AP; SU; PA; MN

   1 Back muscles are not used in crutch walking.

   2 Keeping the leg in abduction alters the center of gravity which impedes ambulation.

   4 This activity does not strengthen muscles used in crutch walking.

169. **3** When ambulating a client, the nurse walks on the client's stronger or unaffected side. This provides a wide base of support and therefore increases stability during the phase of ambulation that calls for weight-bearing on the affected side as the unaffected limb moves forward. (c); IM; AP; SU; TC; MN

   1 This tends to change the center of gravity from directly above the feet and may cause instability.

   2 This tends to change the center of gravity from directly above the feet and may cause instability.

   4 The nurse should stand on the client's stronger or unaffected side (left side).

170. **4** A nursing home would best meet the client's convalescent needs, since a wide range of services beyond acute care are provided at a lower cost than hospital care. Its health services are more appropriate for this client because they are greater than those provided in an adult facility but less than those provided in a rehabilitation center (a); PL; AN; ME; TC; MN

   1 This would be appropriate only if the client were capable of some activities of daily living and did not require continuous supervision.

   2 A rehabilitation center provides a level of nursing care that this client does not require.

   3 Residents in an adult facility are generally responsible for their own activities of daily living.

171. **1** Alzheimer's disease is an insidious atrophy of the brain. The individual maintains the ability to make socially correct comments, but the intellect is diminished. (c); AN; KN; PS; PA; DD

   2 TIAs may precede a cerebral vascular accident; unrelated to Alzheimer's disease.

   3 Alzheimer's is a progressive, deteriorating disease.

   4 It is a slow chronic deterioration.

172. **2** Since these clients do experience a lability of mood, it is best to attempt to establish a relationship and give care when they are feeling receptive. (c); PL; AN; PS; PE; DD

   1 This rejects the client when she needs the nurse most.

   3 This may be of limited help; she may be unable to do it.

   4 Clients with this disorder have limited contact with reality.

173. **4** Sameness provides security and safety and reduces stress for the client. (b); IM; AP; PS; PE; DD

   1 A challenging environment would increase anxiety and frustration.

   2 A nonstimulating environment would add to her diminishing intellect.

   3 Clients with this disease do not do well in a constantly changing environment.

174. **4** A consistent approach and consistent communication from all members of the health team help the client who has a chronic brain syndrome remain a bit more reality oriented. (b); PL; AP; PS; PE; DD
    1 Clients who have this disorder do not attempt to manipulate the staff.
    2 It is the staff members who need to be consistent.
    3 Not needed in working with clients who have this disorder; consistency is most important.

175. **3** Clients with long-term psychiatric problems who have limited contact with reality can usually still become involved with a remotivation therapy group. The demands of this type of group are limited and self-confining. (c); AN; CP; PS; PE; DD
    1 This is suitable for working through emotional problems; these clients are unable to follow the dramatization of emotions.
    2 The object of such therapy is to develop social skills; these goals are inappropriate for clients with this disorder.
    4 The object of such therapy is to develop social skills; these goals are inappropriate for clients with this disorder.

176. **3** Remotivation therapy is designed to encourage clients to interact with their environment by focusing their attention on some common "emotionally safe" article that most clients can recognize and talk about. (b); AN; CP; PS; PE; DD
    1 They do have face-to-face contact with other clients, but that is not the objective of the group.
    2 More appropriate for clients who have a schizophrenic disorder than for those with an organic brain disorder.
    4 The focus is on interpersonal skills and becoming competent in the activities of daily living.

177. **2** Although the exact mechanism is unknown, steroids produce diuresis in almost all children with nephrotic syndrome. (b); IM; KN; PE; PA; RG
    1 Steroids will not prevent infection and will in fact mask the symptoms of infection and delay treatment.
    3 Hypertension is not a common finding in nephrotic syndrome.
    4 Steroids have no effect on the production of blood cells.

178. **3** Fresh vegetables and meat are lower in sodium compared to canned foods and cured meats. (c); PL; KN; PE; ED; RG
    1 Cheese is a high-sodium food; the bun would not be allowed unless it was low-sodium.
    2 Bacon, bread, and canned soup all have high sodium content and should be avoided.
    4 Cheese and canned juices have high sodium content and should be avoided.

179. **3** Allows active 4-year-old movement within restrictions and encourages use of imagination. (c); IM; AN; PE; ED; RG
    1 Unless carefully selected, many shows are inappropriate and uninteresting for a 4-year-old.
    2 May provide him with rest but, this activity is too simple for him and will not promote his developmental level.
    4 Although a 4-year-old may still cling to a security toy, it would not allow him to expend energy.

180. **1** Regression frequently occurs during and after hospitalization; guilt about his regression should be avoided, but this behavior should not be encouraged. (b); IM; AP; PE; ED; RG
    2 Nephrotic syndrome is not associated with neurogenic control of the bladder.

3 Although punishment is a form of attention, it will not help the child overcome the problem causing the behavior.
    4 This will shame him; accepting his regressive behavior but not encouraging it is the best response.

181. **3** A heterozygous father Rr (Rh positive) coupled with Rr (Rh positive) or rr (Rh negative) mother may produce an rr (Rh negative) infant. (c); PL; CP; OB; PA; NH
    1 Rh factor is a genetically determined trait; it cannot be altered by time.
    2 Rh factor is a genetically determined trait; it is influenced by both parents.
    4 Rh factor is a genetically determined factor; it is not altered over time.

182. **1** Giving Rh-positive cells would lead to further hemolysis; Rh-negative cells are not attacked by maternal antibodies. (c); PL; AN; OB; PA; NH
    2 Not relevant, since the blood cells usually do not come from the mother.
    3 A reaction to other antigens in the cross matched blood could still occur.
    4 Not really neutral; it is only a temporary safe-guard from further hemolysis.

183. **2** These are tiny plugged sebaceous glands, and attempts to remove them will further irritate them; they will disappear by themselves. (a); IM; CP; OB; ED; NH
    1 Not a birthmark; they result from maternal hormonal influences and are temporary.
    3 Not true, since many infants do not have them; mother may look for validation of this statement in other babies.
    4 The white material is not pus and is not infectious.

184. **1** A patent airway is the first priority, and necessary equipment must be immediately available. (b); PL; CP; PE; PA; RE
    2 Convulsions are not necessarily associated with croup; respiratory promotion is the priority.
    3 Although appropriate, this is not the priority.
    4 Although this would be helpful, it is not the priority.

185. **2** Laryngeal spasms can occur abruptly; patency of airway is determined by constant assessment for symptoms of respiratory distress. (b); EV; AP; PE; PA; RE
    1 This is important, but maintenance of respiration has priority.
    3 The fever should be treated, but it is not critical at 103° F; maintenance of respiration has priority.
    4 This is important, but maintenance of respiration has priority.

186. **4** Tracheostomy may be necessary to maintain open airway. (b); EV; AP; PE; TC; RE
    1 Ineffective for laryngeal spasms.
    2 Increased O_2 therapy can induce carbon dioxide narcosis.
    3 Symptoms not indicative of increased secretions; suctioning can precipitate sudden laryngospasm.

187. **1** These are some of the first signs of hypoxia; airway must be kept patent to promote oxygenation. (c); IM; AP; PE; PA; RE
    2 The client will not be able to communicate verbally after a tracheotomy.
    3 These are late signs of hypoxia; suctioning should have been done well before this time.
    4 These are late signs of respiratory difficulty; suctioning and other measures should have been done well before this time.

How to Use Worksheet 1: Errors in Processing Information

Common errors in processing information are listed in the left-hand column of this worksheet. At the top of the worksheet is a row of blank spaces for inserting the number of the question missed. Directly below each number, check any errors you made in answering that question. You may have made more than one type of error in an answer.

Worksheet 1: Errors in processing information

Question number																				
Did not read situation/question carefully																				
Missed important details																				
Confused major and minor points																				
Defined problem incorrectly																				
Could not remember terms/ facts/concepts/principles																				
Defined terms incorrectly																				
Focused on incomplete/incorrect data in assessing situation																				
Interpreted data incorrectly																				
Applied wrong concepts/principles in situation																				
Drew incorrect conclusions																				
Identified wrong goals																				
Identified priorities incorrectly																				
Carried out plan incorrectly/incompletely																				
Was unclear about criteria for evaluating success in achieving goals																				

How to Use Worksheet 2: Knowledge Gaps

Types of common knowledge gaps are listed along the top of this worksheet. Write a brief description of topics you want to review in the spaces provided. For example, if you missed a question on administration of a particular drug, write the drug name and problem (e.g., dosage) in the appropriate space under the column labeled *Pharmacology*.

Worksheet 2: Knowledge gaps

Basic science	Skills/ procedures	Basic human needs	Growth & develop- ment	Normal nutrition	Psycho- social factors	Clinical area/ topic	Stressors/ coping mechanisms	Patho- physiology	Pharma- cology	Therapeutic nutrition	Legal implications	Other

Comprehensive Test 1: Part 3*

188. **2** The nurse fulfilled the expectation set forth in the Nurse Practice Act, which includes teaching. In this case the nurse had knowledge of dietary needs and their relation to the client's well-being during pregnancy. (b); EV; AP; OB; ED; PN
    1 False; low-salt foods would be recommended if a diagnosis of preeclampsia was made.
    3 Immediate planning based on the nurse's knowledge of proper diet is better intervention.
    4 Unless the nurse though there was a need for medical intervention, the nurse could supervise prenatal care.

189. **3** The growing uterus exerts pressure on the mesentary slowing peristalsis; more water is reabsorbed, and constipation results. (b); AN; CP; OB; ED; PN
    1 The growing uterus tends to exert pressure on the bladder; it is way above the anus.
    2 Milk is not constipating.
    4 The metabolism increases but does not affect the bowel.

190. **2** Rupture of the membranes and the gush of fluid can carry the umbilical cord downward. Immediate placement in the lithotomy position and inspection may lead to identification of prolapse and prevention of fetal distress. (b); EV; AN; OB; TC; IP
    1 Fluid is due to rupture of membranes; unless it is meconium stained or followed by the cord, this is normal and needs no medical intervention.
    3 Supine position may decrease blood flow and cause hypoxia in the fetus as well as hypotension in the mother.
    4 This is done routinely in labor, not just after membrane rupture.

191. **3** Hypertonic contractions of the uterus, if allowed to continue, can lead to uterine rupture. Therefore the infusion should be discontinued so the hypertonic contractions cease. (b); EV; AP; OB; PA; IP
    1 The resulting delay could lead to uterine rupture; the nurse should discontinue the IV.
    2 The IV should be carefully monitored with an automatic pump to ensure a regulated and continuous flow.
    4 Fetal heart tones should be monitored more frequently (q 15 min.) if a fetal monitor is not used.

192. **3** As cervical dilation nears completion, labor is intensified with an increase in pain and energy expenditure. (b); AN; CP; OB; PA; IP
    1 Back pain usually indicates a posterior-lying position of the infant.
    2 Pain is increased since contractions are more frequent and intense and they last longer.
    4 The client is usually very restless and thrashes about, assuming no particular position.

193. **2** A relaxed uterus is the most frequent cause of bleeding in the early postpartum period. The uterus can be returned to a state of firmness by intermittent gentle fundal massage. (a); EV; AN; OB; PA; IP
    1 Immediate action is directed toward the client's safety; the physician is called if uterine massage does not control bleeding.
    3 Assessment of the uterus and massage take priority; then the vital signs are checked.
    4 Steady bleeding is neither common nor normal and must be attended to immediately.

194. **1** A distended bladder will easily displace the fundus upward and laterally. (a); AN; CP; OB; PA; PP
    2 From this assessment the nurse can make no judgment about overstretched uterine ligaments.
    3 This would be manifested by slow contractions and uterine descent into the pelvis.
    4 If this were true, in addition to being displaced the uterus would be soft and boggy and vaginal bleeding would be present.

195. **4** Forcing the family to be involved at the nurse's convenience would interfere with the development of a productive relationship and affect cooperation of the family. (a); PL; AP; OB; ED; PP
    1 May be at a time that would be inconvenient for the family and thus interfere with productivity.
    2 This would be an inconvenient time for the mother and interfere with productivity.
    3 The father should be included in the visit if at all possible.

196. **1** The role of stranger is the initial role in any relationship. (a); PL; KN; PS; PE; CS
    2 If the nurse moves in too quickly, future relationships may be severely hampered.
    3 If the nurse moves in too quickly, future relationships may be severely hampered.
    4 If the nurse moves in too quickly, future relationships may be severely hampered.

197. **3** The first step in the problem-solving process would be exploration so family needs could be identified. (b); AS; CP; PS; PE; CS
    1 Without exploring family needs first, the nurse would not know what information was needed.
    2 Without exploring family needs first, the nurse would not know the problems that needed solving.
    4 Without exploring family needs first, the nurse would not know what direction the family needed.

198. **4** Inclusion in the interview will avoid a feeling of ostracism by Mr. Lane and will foster his cooperation. (b); IM; AN; PS; PE; CS
    1 Observing Mrs. Lane feed the baby provides the nurse a valuable opportunity to assess interaction.
    2 Removing Mr. Lane from the situation decreases his participation.
    3 Mr. Lane is part of the family and his feelings will affect Mrs. Lane as well.

199. **4** This allows Mr. Lane to express his feelings and is nonjudgmental. (a); IM; AP; PE; PE; CB
    1 Direct contradiction often causes defensive reactions and decreases future cooperation.
    2 Mr. Lane, as the parent, has a right to make his own decisions; this question will place him on the defensive.
    3 This value-laden statement will place him on the defensive.

200. **3** The schedule for immunization of children not immunized in early infancy is altered and adapted from the schedule followed for infants. The tuberculin test normally given at 1 year is added to the first of the DTP and OPV series. (c); PL; KN; PE; ED; CB
    1 The TB test usually given at 1 year will be added to the first series of immunizations.
    2 MMR is never given before 15 months; this will be given 1 month after the initial series is begun.
    4 The Td toxoid is given to children 6 years and older.

201. **2** These children have difficulty reaching out to the environment and tend to be withdrawn. They get little response from parents and do not learn how to respond to others. (b); AS; CP; PE; PE; GI

---

*A key to the letters following the correct rationale can be found on p. 633.

1 The infant suffering from maternal deprivation is non-responsive or only poorly responsive to human contact.

3 These children are very difficult to comfort; show little satisfaction.

4 These children do not respond readily to human contact.

202. **4** A consistent caregiver enhances the formation of a trusting and mutually satisfying relationship between child and nurse. (b); PL; AP; PE; PE; GI

1 Stimulation should proceed gradually and be geared to the present level of development.

2 Overstimulation should be avoided.

3 A consistent caregiver enhances the development of trust.

203. **3** Head control and rolling over are acheived at 4 and 5 months, respectively. Transferring objects from one hand to another and sitting unsupported are achieved at 7 and 8 months. (b); AS; CP; PE; ED; MN

1 The ability to roll over is achieved by approximately 5 months of age.

2 The ability to roll over is achieved by approximately 5 months of age.

4 Transferring objects from hand to hand is usually achieved at 6 to 7 months.

204. **4** Fine motor coordination is inadequately developed to manipulate snap toys. (a); PL; CP; PE; ED; MN

1 These are appropriate to stimulate visual attention.

2 These provide the sense of touch; and since voluntary grasp appears at about 3 to 4 months, they would be handled satisfactorily.

3 Voluntary grasp will allow her to hold this, and the rattling sound will stimulate the auditory system.

205. **4** Paraplegia is the paralysis of both lower extremities and the lower trunk resulting from damage to the spinal cord from the thoracic to the lumbar segments. (b); AN; KN; ME; PA; MN

1 Paresis is a slight or partial paralysis; paraplegia is paralysis of both lower extremities.

2 This is hemiplegia.

3 This is quadriplegia.

206. **2** The priority of care at this time is to protect the spinal area from strain to prevent additional damage to the traumatized area while it heals. (c); IM; AP; ME; PA; MN

1 Although an important aspect of care, it is not the priority item in the immediate postinjury period.

3 This usually results from prolonged immobility; although important, it is not the immediate priority.

4 Survival and safety take priority; vocational rehabilitation will assume greater importance after the client's condition stabilizes.

207. **1** Client's with early spinal cord damage experience an atonic bladder, which is characterized by the absence of muscle tone, an enlarged capacity, no feeling of discomfort with distension, and overflow with a large residual. This leads to urinary stasis and infection. High fluid intake limits urinary stasis and infection by diluting the urine and increasing urinary output. (b); IM; CP; ME; PA; MN

2 A fluid and electrolyte imbalance is not a major problem after spinal cord injury.

3 Dehydration is not a major problem after spinal cord injury.

4 Constipation may occur because of the lack of neural stimulation, not decreased fluids.

208. **3** The CircOlectric bed facilitates frequent vertical turning of the client to prevent decubiti, which can form within 24 hours because of pressure. (b); IM; CP; ME; PA; MN

1 The client with paraplegia is immobile, and the special bed does not increase mobility.

2 Because of the lack of weight bearing on bones, calcium is generally lost in clients confined to bed; the special bed does not prevent this from occurring.

4 Orthostatic hypotension is not desired; the movement of the bed may allow for gradual changes of position that would prevent it from developing.

209. **2** The client should have a nasogastric tube inserted to prevent aspiration and keep the stomach decompressed. (b); AN; AN; ME; PA; GI

1 Diet change requires a physician's order; clients who are vomiting may have food withheld.

3 This information is important; however, prevention of aspiration takes priority.

4 This would be indicated at the next bowel movement; however, maintenance of vital functions is most important.

210. **1** These signs could be indicative of hemorrhage from perforation and require immediate surgical intervention. (a); EV; AN; ME; TC; GI

2 These complaints should be noted since they may indicate early signs of diabetes mellitus; however, the nurse's primary observation should be for symptoms of perforation and shock.

3 These complaints should be noted; however, they are not indicative of potential priority problems.

4 These complaints should be noted, but they do not indicate an emergency situation that would threaten life.

211. **4** John's denial is a pattern of defense often demonstrated in the self-protective stage of adaptation to illness. His thoughts and feelings are so painful and provoke such anxiety that he rejects the existence of his paraplegia. (b); AS; AN; PS; PE; CS

1 Denial is a method of psychologic adaptation.

2 Motivation must have realistic goals in mind; the client is in denial.

3 From information available, one cannot assume that the client is fantasizing; a fantasy is the transformation of undesirable experiences into imagined events to fulfill an unconscious wish or need.

212. **3** Absent or diminished gag reflex could be life threatening. The infant might aspirate mucus or formula. (b); AN; KN; OB; ED; NH

1 Important but may be delayed because the mother has been anesthetized; the gag reflex is of primary importance.

2 Important but may be delayed because the mother has been anesthetized; the gag reflex is of primary importance.

4 Important but may be delayed because the mother has been anesthetized; the gag reflex is of primary importance.

213. **2** Milia occur commonly, are not indicative of any illness, and eventually disappear. (a); AN; KN; OB; ED; NH

1 Lanugo is fine dark hair.

3 This is a lay term for milia; not used in charting.

4 These are bluish black spots on the buttocks that present on darkly pigmented infants.

214. **1** The brick-red color is caused by albumin and urates that are concentrated because of dehydration, which is normal in the first 10 days. (c); AN; CP; OB; ED; NH

2 Iron is eliminated via the gastrointestinal tract.

3 No medication used in delivery would cause this discoloration.

4 Unrelated to sex of infant; not hormonally based.

215. **1** Jaundice occurs because of the normal physiologic breakdown of fetal red blood cells and the immaturity of the infant's liver. (a); AN; CP; OB; ED; NH

2 Unrelated to the infant hemoglobin level; the mother and baby have separate circulations.

3 The baby has high hemoglobin and high hematocrit levels.

4 Conjugation and excretion, not synthesis of bile, are compromised because of the immature liver.

216. **2** Eye patches are applied to prevent drying of the conjunctiva, injury to the retina, and alterations in biorhythms. (c); IM; CP; OB; TC; NH

 1 The baby will automatically close her eyes in response to bright lights and application of a patch.

 3 The baby should be exposed to bright lights periodically so normal rhythms will become established.

 4 These are automatic during sleep phases and will not be affected by eye patches.

217. **3** Head lag in an infant 6 months old is abnormal and is frequently a sign of cerebral damage. (c); AS; AN; PE; ED; MN

 1 The tonic reflex and grasp reflex usually disappear at 2 and 3 months, respectively.

 2 The Babinski reflex is normally present until 2 years of age.

 4 The ability to sit unsupported is achieved at 7 to 8 months.

218. **1** Increased intracranial pressure results in pressure exerted against the cranium. This is especially evident in areas with less confinement, such as the fontanel (which bulge), the orbits (which are pushed forward so the eyelids are pulled taut and upper lids are above the irides [sunset eyes]), and the brain (vomiting center stimulated regardless of activity of eating). (b); AS, CP; PE; PA; MN

 2 The fontanel will show signs of increased fluid volume in the skull and therefore bulge.

 3 The eyeballs will show signs of increased fluid volume in the skull and be pushed forward, pulling the lids taut; systolic pressure is elevated and diastolic is the same or lower, creating a widening pulse pressure.

 4 A high shrill cry and decreased skin turgor are not signs associated with increased intracranial pressure.

219. **2** The child can be positioned on the back or abdomen to allow for a routine change of head position. The head is elevated to decrease the intracranial pressure by gravity. (b); IM; AP; PE; TC; MN

 1 The head is elevated to decrease the intracranial pressure by gravity.

 3 The head is elevated to minimize the increased pressure through gravity.

 4 Trendelenburg positioning would be contraindicated since it might aggravate the ICP.

220. **4** Cellular destruction occurs as the brain is pressed against the unyielding skull. This occludes blood vessels and deprives the cells of oxygen. (a); AN; CP; PE; PA; MN

 1 Hydrocephalus results when CSF is produced in too great quantities or is not adequately circulated or absorbed; no change in the fluid tonicity.

 2 Pressure may cause occlusion of the blood supply in hydrocephalus.

 3 Oxygen deprivation occurs when blood vessels are occluded secondary to the pressure in the skull caused by hydrocephalus.

221. **1** A flat position helps prevent problems associated with too rapid reduction of intracranial fluid. (c); IM; AN; PE; TC; MN

 2 Sedatives and analgesics are avoided. They can mask signs of impending loss of consciousness.

 3 Initially, positioning flat is important to preventing serious complications.

 4 Checking and pumping the valve provide a means of assessing and promoting function of the shunt.

222. **2** Shunts need to be revised; as child grows, the length of tubing needs to be changed. The shunts are also prone to malfunction and may need revision. (a); IM; AP; PE; ED; MN

 1 Although treatment of hydrocephalus by shunt replacement is quite successful, there is danger of malfunction and infection of the shunt.

 3 Damage to brain cells is irreversible.

 4 Hydrocephalus necessitates treatment for the life of the child.

223. **1** Anxiety causes an increase in body secretions, which stimulates tissue changes. (c); AN; KN; PS; PE; CS

 2 This emotional response does not cause an alteration in tissue.

 3 Fear is usually not a prolonged emotional response; would not cause an alteration in tissue.

 4 Rage is usually not a prolonged emotional response; would not cause an alteration in tissue.

224. **3** The trauma of surgery results in some seeping or oozing of blood into the remaining gastric area, which is being immediately suctioned out of the body via the nasogastric tube. (c); AN; AP; SU; PA; GI

 1 The trauma of surgery will result in some blood loss, which will continue until coagulation takes place; this is too short a time for this to occur.

 2 The trauma of srugery will result in some blood loss, which will continue until coagulation takes place; this is too short a time for this to occur.

 4 If bright red liquid is still draining 24 to 48 hours after surgery, it is abnormal; the physician should be notified.

225. **2** Too rapid administration can result in hyperkalemia, which can cause a long refractory period in the cardiac cycle and result in cardiac arrhythmias and arrest. (c); IM; AP; SU; PA; GI

 1 This statement is too general; no indication of whether it is respiratory acidosis or metabolic acidosis. Metabolic acidosis can cause hyperkalemia.

 3 Hyperkalemia usually causes nausea, vomiting, and diarrhea, which may result in dehydration; in this instance fluid would shift from interstitial spaces to the intravascular compartment. With edema the fluid shift is in the opposite direction.

 4 This reaction does not occur in hyperkalemia.

226. **4** The nurse should not only count the rate but also inspect the infusion site, no matter who started the IV. Failure to do so constitutes negligence. (c); EV; AN; SU; TC; EI

 1 The staff nurse is always responsible for meeting the client's nursing needs regardless of whether other members of the health team are available; the nurse was negligent.

 2 The rate of flow should have been maintained at the rate ordered by the physician; the infusion site should also be monitored routinely.

 3 This is untrue; it occurred because the nurse was negligent.

227. **2** When high-osmotic fluid passes rapidly into the small intestine, it causes hypovolemia. This results in a sympathetic response with tachycardia, diaphoresis, and dizziness. The symptoms are also attributed to a sudden rise and subsequent fall in blood sugar. (b); AN; CP; SU; PA; GI

 1 This is usually associated with paralytic ileus; dumping syndrome leads to increased intestinal motility.

3 This could occur with intestinal obstruction; dumping syndrome is associated with increased motility originating in the jejunum. Reflux would need reverse peristalsis.

4 The stomach is not full; its contents rapidly empty into the jejunum.

228. **4** Small feedings reduce the amount of bulk passing into the jejunum and therefore reduce the fluid shifting into the jejunum. (b); PL; AP; SU; PA; GI

1 Concentrated sweets pass rapidly out of the stomach and increase fluid shifts; consequently the diet should be low in carbohydrates. Protein is needed to promote tissue repair.

2 Although a diet high in roughage may be avoided, a low-residue bland diet is not necessary.

3 Total fluid intake does not have to be restricted; however, fluids should not be taken immediately before, during, or after a meal because they promote rapid stomach emptying.

229. **3** Varicosed veins are dilated veins that occur as a result of incompetent valves. Varicosities may be due to numerous factors, including heredity, prolonged standing (which puts strain on the valves), and abdominal pressure on the large veins of the lower abdomen. (b); AN; CP; ME; PA; CB

1 Atherosclerotic plaques usually occur in arteries not veins.

2 This is the rationale for elastic stockings; their action limits venous pooling.

4 Thrombophlebitis is usually a sequela of varicosed veins.

230. **4** Because of the dilation in the veins and concomitant decrease in arterial flow, the client may experience heaviness or muscle cramps in the legs. Edema, if present, can be relieved by elevating the legs. (b); AS; CP; ME; PA; CB

1 Edema may be decreased when the extremity is elevated.

2 Homan's sign is present in deep vein thrombosis.

3 These signs may indicate early arterial occlusion.

231. **1** The Trendelenburg test evaluates the backflow of blood through defective valves. If, after raising the legs to empty the veins, the client stands and the veins fill from above the site of the suspected varicosity, the diagnosis is supported. (c); AS; CP; ME; PA; CB

2 This test is used to determine injury of the pyramid tract in adults; if present, it is obtained by firmly stroking the lateral aspect of the sole of the foot.

3 This is a test for position sense; the client loses balance when standing erect with feet together and eyes closed.

4 This is not a simple test that the nurse can perform.

232. **2** Since the superficial vein (saphenous) will be ligated, it is first necessary to determine whether the deep veins will be capable of supporting the return circulation. (a); AS; CP; SU; PA; CB

1 Weight loss is desired; however, it is not a prerequisite for surgery.

3 This vein is generally ligated in surgery.

4 Bed rest would promote stasis and thrombus formation.

233. **4** Hypersecretion of the mucous glands provides an excellent, warm, moist medium for microorganisms. (b); PL; AP; SU; PA; RE

1 Asthma is not a disease that is voluntarily controlled.

2 Coughing must be encouraged; prevents retention of mucus, which is an excellent medium for microorganisms. Excessive secretions also limit gaseous exchange.

3 Anxiety is not willfully controlled.

234. **1** The legs should be elevated to promote venous return by gravity. (a); IM; AP; SU; PA; CB

2 This position increases pressure on the popliteal space, which may interfere with venous return from the legs.

3 Flexion of the knees and hips with the legs lower than the heart interferes with venous return.

4 Dorsiflexion of the feet places tension on the suture line and should be avoided, placing the legs lower than the level of the heart will not promote venous return.

235. **4** Muscle contraction of the legs promotes venous return and prevents thrombus formation. (c); PL; AP; SU; PA; CB

1 Binders are used after abdominal surgery.

2 Sitting in a chair is generally avoided; flexes the hip and keeps the legs dependent, which diminishes venous return.

3 Active exercises are more beneficial after vein ligation.

236. **4** Marked jaundice generally indicates liver damage or excessive hemolysis and is not a sign of leukemia, unless hepatic damage from late effects of the disease or drugs has occurred. Edema is not a manifestation of the disease, since the pathophysiology does not involve transport of fluids. (a); AS; CP; PE; PA; CB

1 Multiple bruises and petechiae are due to thrombocytopenia associated with leukemia.

2 Marked fatigue and pallor are the result of anemia associated with leukemia.

3 Enlarged lymph nodes, spleen, and liver are due to the infiltration of these organs with leukemic cells.

237. **3** Acute leukemia is an excessive uncontrolled production of immature white blood cells that complete for nutrients and eventually crowd the bone marrow, preventing formation of other blood cells. (b); AN; CP; PE; PA; CB

1 Proliferating cells depress bone marrow production of the formed elements of blood.

2 RBCs and platelets are crowded out by proliferation of leukemic cells

4 The liver and spleen are invaded by leukemic cells.

238. **4** A side effect of vincristine is alopecia. To adolescents, who are very concerned with identity, this represents a tremendous threat to their self-image. (a); PL; AN; PE; PE; EI

1 Constipation, though possibly uncomfortable, can be minimized with medication and diet.

2 A temporary paresis may occur; not as much of a concern as alopecia to an adolescent.

3 This will not be immediately obvious.

239. **1** Infection from lowered resistance is a constant threat from the disease and from the immunosuppressant drugs, both of which affect white blood cells. (b); IM; AN; PE; TC; CB

2 Maria needs normal stimuli for a 12-year-old except when acutely ill from drug therapy.

3 Although vital signs need to be checked to assess for changes in pulse or BP, unless there is other clinical evidence of bleeding, q 2 hour frequencies are not needed.

4 Maria needs to maintain the physical activity she can tolerate.

240. **3** Constipation from adynamic ileus can be prevented with high-fiber foods and liberal fluids. These will keep the stool bulky and soft, promoting evacuation. (c); PL; AP; PE; PA; GI

1 Vincristine causes constipation; roughage and fluids are needed.

2 Treatment of constipation, a common side effect of vincristine, calls for roughage and fluids.

4 Roughage and fluids are recommended to help minimize the constipation associated with vincristine.

241. **1** Low platelet count predisposes to bleeding, which may be evident in the urine. Red blood cells are seen microscopically in the sediment. (b); EV; CP; PE; PA; CB

   2 White blood cells occur in the urine when there is a urinary tract infection.

   3 Casts are seen in the urine in some kidney disorders.

   4 Lymphocytes are not normally found in the urine.

242. **1** The protective blood-brain barrier initially screens leukemic cells from the CNS. However, in advanced stages leukemic infiltration occurs. The chemotherapeutic agents, also screened out by the blood-brain barrier, are ineffective. (c); IM; CP; PE; ED; CB

   2 Radiations destroys leukemic cells.

   3 Irradiation of the cranium is needed because chemotherapy does not pass the blood-brain barrier.

   4 Radiation does not decrease cerebral edema.

243. **3** Children at early school age are not yet able to comprehend death's universality and inevitability but fear it, often personifying death as a bogey-man or death-angel. They need an opportunity to prepare for this. (b); IM; AP; PS; PE; CS

   1 A child this age needs to know the seriousness of the illness and that recovery may not be possible.

   2 Children of this age interpret death as separation and punishment; they fear this in addition to death itself.

   4 This response only avoids the question.

244. **2** The individual cannot resolve the conflict consciously because of emotional pressure pulling him in both directions. As anxiety increases, the unconscious seeks a solution. The conversion selected usually resolves the initial conflict by making action impossible, thus removing the need to select one or the other choice. (c); AN; KN; PS; PE; PD

   1 There are no physical changes involved with this unconscious resolution of a conflict.

   3 It is a psychologic response to stress, not a defense against it.

   4 The conversion to physical symptoms operates on an unconscious level.

245. **1** The development of physical symptoms without a physical cause is an anxiety-reducing mechanism specific to the psychoneurotic pattern of behavior. (b); AN; KN; PS; PE; PD

   2 This would be the body's response to stress.

   3 Going back to an earlier state when one felt safer and more secure is not converting anxiety into physical symptoms.

   4 Blaming others in the environment for failure and mistakes is not converting anxiety into physical symptoms.

246. **2** The development of the symptoms is the unconscious method of reducing the anxiety. Because the symptom is meeting this need, it does not create anxiety itself but is passively accepted. (b); AN; CP; PS; PE; PD

   1 There is no agitation; symptoms are passively accepted.

   3 There is no anger; symptoms are passively accepted.

   4 There is no anxiety; the conflict is resolved by the physical symptom.

247. **3** The psychophysiologic response (hyperfunction or hypofunction) creates actual tissue change. Hypochondria is an exaggerated body concern unrelated to organic changes. (b); AN; CP; PS; PE; PD

   1 There is an emotional component in both instances.

   2 There is a feeling of illness in both instances.

   4 There may be a restriction of activities in both instances.

248. **3** This response focuses the client on the relationship between emotion and physical symptoms in a nonthreatening accepting manner. (b); AS; AN; PS; PE; PD

   1 The nurse knows when the weakness began; redundant to ask.

   2 This does not help pinpoint what the person was feeling when the weakness happened.

   4 This would be a secondary gain since he elicits sympathy and gets out of doing something that he apparently does not wish to do.

249. **4** Until the client learns new ways of dealing with anxiety, he will continue to use this pattern of behavior. Learning new ways to operate will break the pattern. (b); IM; AN; PS; PE; PD

   1 This would be unrealistic since the client must learn to cope with problems.

   2 This would reinforce the sick role.

   3 There is a certain amount of stress in everyday family situations and the client, not the family, must learn new coping mechanics.

250. **4** Helps the client identify behavior and feelings in a nonthreatening manner. (c); IM; AP; PS; PE; PD

   1 This would be ganging up on the client.

   2 This evasion and refusal to answer would have the psychologic effect of removing the nurse from the group.

   3 The nurse's behavior is not the issue; the situation should be turned back to the client's behavior.

251. **2** The nurse was negligent in not providing close supervision, since she knew Mr. Norman was combative. A reasonable, prudent nurse would have closely observed Mr. Norman to protect him from himself as well as to protect others. (a); EV; AP; PS; PE; MD

   1 The admittting office may have had no knowledge of the situation; therefore it was the nurse's responsibility.

   3 This is true of all clients, not only those who are combative.

   4 It would be unrealistic to keep him sedated at all times.

252. **4** Lithium carbonate alters sodium transport in nerve and muscle cells and causes a shift toward intraneuronal metabolism of catecholamines. Since the range between therapeutic and toxic levels is very small, the client's serum lithium level should be monitored closely. (b); EV; AN; PS; PA; MD

   1 Sodium restriction may cause electrolyte imbalance and lithium toxicity.

   2 Not necessary or useful.

   3 Not necessary; would depend on what the client was receiving.

253. **3** This sets appropriate limits for the client who cannot set them for himself. It rejects the behavior but accepts the client. (b); IM; AP; PS; PE; MD

   1 This does not show acceptance of the client or help him control his behavior.

   2 May have the effect of reinforcing behavior rather than decreasing it.

   4 Does not deal with problem directly; can confuse the client, since he may be unaware of why the nurse refuses to talk to him.

254. **2** Activities that release tension and use up energy can decrease anxiety. (b); PL; AP; PS; PE; MD

   1 Requires too much concentration, and he may hurt himself in the process.

   3 Requires too much concentration.

   4 Requires sitting still and a dexterity that he would probably find impossible at this time.

255. **2** A threat is a type of assult that is an intentional tort. (c); EV; AN; PS; PE; MD

1 Restraints would be cruel, illegal, and unnecessary for this client.

3 This draws a conclusion that may not be true.

4 The behavior can be expected but should not be ignored; behavior should be dealt with directly.

256. **1** Clients who are hyperactive are easily diverted. It is best to use this characteristic behavior rather than precipitate a confrontation. (a); IM; AP; PS; PE; MD

2 Shows no consideration of how he may feel.

3 Shifts responsibility to the physician; the nurse should know that a shopping trip is unrealistic at this time.

4 Only postpones having to deal directly with the problem; does not deal with reality.

257. **1** The client is asking for help to prevent suicide. This response focuses on feelings and does not challenge or deny them. (a); IM; AN; PS; PE; MD

2 The nurse is ignoring a cry for help and not following through on what he is expressing.

3 The nurse is denying the client's feelings and what he is saying.

4 The nurse is negating his feelings and interpreting the situation for him.

258. **2** Exposure to infection, cold, or overexertion in a client with chronic adrenocortical insufficiency (Addison's disease) can cause circulatory collapse. (b); PL; AN; ME; TC; EI

1 This would be an appropriate room assignment.

3 This would be an appropriate room assignment.

4 This would be an appropriate room assignment.

259. **2** Deficiency of the glucocorticoids causes hypoglycemia in the client with Addison's disease. Signs of hypoglycemia include weakness, dizziness, cool moist skin, hunger, tremors, and nervousness. (c); AN; CP; ME; PA; EI

1 Weakness with dizziness on arising is called postural hypotension, not hypertension.

3 Hypokalemia is evidenced by nausea, vomiting, muscle weakness, and arrhythmias.

4 This would be evidenced by edema, increased BP, and moist rales in the lungs.

260. **4** Clients with Addison's disease must take glucocorticoids regularly to enable them to adapt physiologically to stress and prevent an Addisonian crisis, a medical emergency similar to shock. (b); PL; AN; ME; ED; EI

1 Frequent visits are not indicated after control is established.

2 Activity is permitted as tolerated.

3 Sodium should be taken as desired since hyponatremia frequently occurs from diminished mineral corticoid secretion.

261. **1** Because of diminished mineralocorticoid secretion, clients with Addison's disease are prone to development of hyponatremia. Therefore the addition of salt to the diet is advised. (c); IM; AP; ME; ED; EI

2 Caloric intake is determined on an individual basis; diet is not necessarily restricted to 1200 calories.

3 Protein is not omitted from the diet; ingestion of essential amino acids is necessary for normal metabolism.

4 Fluids are not restricted in Addison's disease.

262. **2** When there are not enough circulating glucocorticoids and mineralocorticoids to sustain normal functioning of the body, the following symptoms occur: hypotension, fever, pallor, tachycardia, cyanosis; an Addisonian crisis. (b); EV; AP; ME; ED; EI

1 This is not a sign of an Addisonian crisis; hypotension is.

3 Muscle spasms do not occur in an Addisonian crisis; the client usually progresses into a coma.

4 This does not occur in an Addisonian crisis.

263. **2** Prolonged steroid therapy may produce Cushing's syndrome. Signs include slow wound healing, buffalo hump, hirsutism, weight gain, hypertension, acne, moon face, thin arms and legs, and behavioral disturbances. (c); IM; AP; ME; ED; EI

1 Cortisone therapy has a glucocorticoid action, which increases blood glucose levels.

3 Hyperkalemia occurs with Addison's disease; cortisone therapy helps correct fluid and electrolyte imbalances.

4 Hypertension and fluid retention occur.

264. **2** Some cortisol derivatives possess 17-ketosteroid (androgenic) properties, which result in masculinization. (c); IM; AP; ME; ED; EI

1 Masculinization is not part of the disease; it results from the androgens present in cortisol.

3 Saying not to worry denies the client her concerns; masculinization results from the therapy and will not go away.

4 Denies the client's feelings.

265. **1** Development of mood swings and psychosis is possible from overdose of glucocorticoids as a result of fluid and electrolyte alterations. (b); EV; CP; ME; PA; EI

2 This is not a sign of glucocorticoid overdose.

3 This is not a sign of glucocorticoid overdose.

4 This is not a sign of glucocorticoid overdose.

266. **3** Clients with internal radiation for cervical cancer are given low-residue diets and often medications to suppress peristalsis and prevent pressure from BMs. (c); IM; AN; ME; TC; RG

1 The head of the bed can be only slightly elevated to prevent the implant from being dislodged by gravity.

2 A catheter is routinely inserted to prevent bladder distention and possible radiation damage or alteration of implant position.

4 Since the client is the source of radiation, the nurse must limit the time spent with her to avoid excessive exposure.

267. **2** A total abdominal hysterectomy in the premenopausal woman produces artificial onset of menopause. (a); IM; CP; SU; ED; RG

1 Untrue; because the uterus was removed, there will be no uterine endometrial proliferation and no desquamation.

3 Untrue; because the uterus was removed, there will be no uterine endometrial proliferation and no desquamation.

4 Untrue; because the uterus was removed, there will be no uterine endometrial proliferation and no desquamation.

268. **3** Accidental ligation of a ureter is a serious complication of a total abdominal hysterectomy. A decrease in urine output should be reported immediately to the surgeon. (c); EV; CP; SU; TC; RG

1 A nasogastric tube is not routinely inserted.

2 Serosanguineous vaginal drainage is to be expected.

4 An apical rate of 90 falls within normal limits but should be evaluated in relation to the client's previous vital signs.

269. **3** Abdominal distention, caused by retention of flatus, is a frequent postoperative problem. A rectal tube will usually accomplish expulsion of flatus in 20 to 30 minutes. Application of heat, in addition to its vasodilating effect, will relax tensed muscles. (b); IM; AP; SU; PA; RG

1 Although position changes may promote peristalsis, restriction of oral intake will not.

2 Carbonated drinks increase flatulence.

4 Distention usually occurs as a result of flatus in the intestines and would not be alleviated by gastric decompression.

270. **4** Postoperatively a client may wear a girdle to provide abdominal support and/or do exercises to strengthen the abdominal muscles. (a); IM; CP; SU; PA; RG
    1 Constriction may actually impair venous return if not fitted accurately.
    2 Since pressure is being applied to the incision, healing is not directly facilitated.
    3 Abdominal supports do not prevent nausea; may actually induce it if applied too tightly.
271. **2** Fetal death usually occurs in diabetic mothers after 36 weeks of gestation. It results from acidosis and placental dysfunction. The fetus may be delivered by cesarean section or induction as necessary. (c); AN; KN; OB; PA; HP
    1 Exercise and ambulation are needed to promote adequate circulation and prevent thromboembolism.
    3 Fetal growth continues as long as placental functioning is still intact.
    4 This is not a routine procedure; insulin is administered according to need.
272. **1** Usually, as pregnancy progresses, there are alterations in glucose tolerance and in the metabolism and utilization of insulin. The result is an increased need for exogenous insulin. (a); PL; CP; OB; PA; HP
    2 Estrogenic hormones are not administered during pregnancy.
    3 Caloric intake is increased to meet demands of the growing fetus.
    4 Pancreatic enzymes or hormones other than insulin are not affected by pregnancy.
273. **3** The effects of insulin on the fetus are known since the fetal pancreas secretes insulin. However, the effects of oral hypoglycemics are not well known; such agents may be teratogenic. (b); AN; CP; OB; ED; HP
    1 The fetal pancreas does not compensate for the mother's diabetes but hypertrophies because of increased insulin secretion to cover increased circulating glucose.
    2 Hypoglycemics are not insulin; also they may have a teratogenic effect on the fetus.
    4 There is often a need for larger amounts of insulin in the latter part of pregnancy.
274. **4** Feeding difficulties are due to hypoglycemic effects on the fetal CNS. (c); AS; AP; OB; ED; NH
    1 Excessive birthweight is common but does not indicate hypoglycemia.
    2 May be related to hypoxia, not lowered blood sugar.
    3 May be related to prematurity; generally not related to hypoglycemia.
275. **4** The infant of a diabetic mother is a newborn at risk because of the interplay between the maternal disease and the developing fetus. (b); IM; AP; OB; TC; NH
    1 The baby may be prone to hypoglycemia and will need increased glucose.
    2 Infants of diabetic mothers are high risk and are admitted to intensive care nurseries.
    3 Babies are generally hypoglycemic because of oversecretion of insulin by their hypertrophied pancreas.
276. **2** Because of tissue destruction, sodium ions are lost in the interstitial fluid whereas potassium ions are liberated from the injured cells. The result is hyperkalemia. (c); AN; CP; SU; PA; EI
    1 Fluid shifts may cause shock but it is reversible with therapy.
    3 Capillary permeability is increased in burns.
    4 Blood volume decreases, and hypovolemic shock may occur.
277. **4** Because of fluid loss and sodium retention, urinary output is diminished. However, output of less than 30

ml per hour is considered a sign of shock. (c); PL; AP; SU; PA; EI
    1 This amount would cause overload; output is less than 30 ml per hour.
    2 This intake is excessive, as is the output; would not be expected in the newly burned client.
    3 This amount of fluid replacement would be inadequate, and fluid loss excessive, in the newly burned client; very little fluid is left to replace losses during the first few days.
278. **3** Since a great deal of intravascular fluid is lost during the first 48 hours through evaporation and in the exudate and edema, urinary output is not expected to equal the intake but increases from that of the first day. An output of less than 30 ml per hour is an indication of shock. (c); EV; CP; SU; PA; EI
    1 If half the intake is excreted, insufficient fluid is left to replace losses.
    2 This would probably indicate inadequate kidney perfusion, shock, or kidney damage.
    4 This would not allow for replacement of fluid loss due to burns.
279. **3** Vitamin C is essential for wound healing. It provides a component of intercellular ground substance that develops into collagen and is necessary to build supportive tissue. (a); IM; AP; SU; PA; EI
    1 To help in repairing damaged tissue, protein intake should be increased.
    2 Decreasing calories could increase the work of the body; would promote catabolism of body tissue.
    4 To prevent excess fluid retention, which would increase the cardiovascular workload, sodium intake should be regulated.
280. **1** The skin is the first line of defense against infection. When much of it is destroyed, the individual is left vulnerable to infection. (a); PL; CP; SU; PA; EI
    2 Complications such as infection may also occur during the convalescent phase.
    3 Diversional therapy as tolerated may be helpful physically and psychologically.
    4 Removing mirrors can increase anxiety about body image and lead the client to conclude that the situation is even worse than it is.
281. **1** Curling's ulcer (an ulcer of the upper GI tract) is related to the excessive secretion of stress-related hormones. These increase hydrochloric acid production. (a); IM; KN; SU; ED; EI
    2 Not a complication of burns.
    3 Not a complication of burns.
    4 Not a complication of burns.

Comprehensive Test 1: Part 4*

282. **4** The client's rights were violated. Mrs. Coan has the right to a complete and accurate explanation of treatment. (a); AN; AP; OB; PE; HP
    1 When administering treatment, the nurse is responsible for explaining to the client what the treatment is and why it is being done.
    2 The Patient's Bill of Rights states that the client should be informed.
    3 All preparations or procedures should be explained since they are not routine to the client.

---

*A key to the letters following the correct rationale can be found on p. 633.

How to Use Worksheet 1: Errors in Processing Information

Common errors in processing information are listed in the left-hand column of this worksheet. At the top of the worksheet is a row of blank spaces for inserting the number of the question missed. Directly below each number, check any errors you made in answering that question. You may have made more than one type of error in an answer.

Worksheet 1: Errors in processing information

Question number																						
Did not read situation/question carefully																						
Missed important details																						
Confused major and minor points																						
Defined problem incorrectly																						
Could not remember terms/ facts/concepts/principles																						
Defined terms incorrectly																						
Focused on incomplete/incorrect data in assessing situation																						
Interpreted data incorrectly																						
Applied wrong concepts/principles in situation																						
Drew incorrect conclusions																						
Identified wrong goals																						
Identified priorities incorrectly																						
Carried out plan incorrectly/incompletely																						
Was unclear about criteria for evaluating success in achieving goals																						

How to Use Worksheet 2: Knowledge Gaps

Types of common knowledge gaps are listed along the top of this worksheet. Write a brief description of topics you want to review in the spaces provided. For example, if you missed a question on administration of a particular drug, write the drug name and problem (e.g., dosage) in the appropriate space under the column labeled *Pharmacology*.

Worksheet 2: Knowledge gaps

Basic science	Skills/ procedures	Basic human needs	Growth & develop-ment	Normal nutrition	Psycho-social factors	Clinical area/ topic	Stressors/ coping mechanisms	Patho-physiology	Pharma-cology	Therapeutic nutrition	Legal implications	Other

283. **3** To prevent further maternal and fetal complications, clients must be continuously observed for blood loss by the monitoring of external bleeding and the counting and weighing of pads. (b); AS; AP; OB; TC; HP

    1 This would be necessary only if bleeding were continuous and profuse; a cesarean delivery might be necessary.

    2 To minimize further placental separation, the client would be confined to complete bed rest.

    4 Unnecessary; no indication that the client is toxemic or that cerebral irritation is present.

284. **2** A vaginal examination might precipitate severe bleeding, which would be life threatening to the mother and infant and necessitate an immediate cesarean delivery. (b); PL; AP; OB; TC; HP

    1 The vaginal examination might precipitate severe bleeding; there would be no time for induction of labor.

    3 This might lead to further placental separation and severe bleeding before the fetus could be delivered.

    4 Not a priority item after a vaginal examination, which can precipitate severe bleeding; x-ray examination would not reveal placental separation, only fetal size and position.

285. **3** An infant should receive 60 calories and 88.8 ml (3 oz) of fluid per pound daily. (b); PL; AN; OB; ED; NE

    1 Too much; 74 ml (2 to 3 oz) fluid and 60 calories per pound per day required.

    2 Too much; 74 ml (2 to 3 oz) fluid and 60 calories per pound per day required.

    4 Too much; 74 ml (2 to 3 oz) fluid and 60 calories per pound per day required.

286. **4** Development of jaundice before 48 hours after birth may indicate a blood dyscrasia, requiring immediate medical investigation. Jaundice occurring between 48 and 72 hours after birth is a consequence of the normal physiologic breakdown of fetal red cells and immaturity of the liver. (c); EV; AN; OB; ED; NH

    1 Bilirubin studies would be done first to determine whether the amount of bilirubin present warranted phototherapy.

    2 Unless pathologic (occurring in the first 24 hours of life), this is not necessary.

    3 First, the age of the infant must be ascertained to see whether this is physiologic; then, the nurse can do a "heel-stick" to determine the amount of bilirubin.

287. **1** Clients use delusions as a defense and cannot be argued out of them. The nurse's response did not demonstrate acceptance of the client and only added to her anxiety and agitation. (b); EV; AP; PS; PE; MD

    2 There is nothing to indicate that treatment has not been started toward relieving these symptoms.

    3 Mrs. Gold should have a one-to-one relationship with staff before attempting to relate to other clients on the unit.

    4 That would be masking the problem rather than planning more suitable intervention.

288. **3** Electroconvulsive therapy helps relieve severe depression by interrupting established patterns of behavior, thereby limiting possible suicide attempts. (a); EV; AP; PS; PE; MD

    1 This would be used if the client showed little or no response to the antidepressants.

    2 Psychotherapy combined with antidepressants is the treatment of choice; not psychoanalysis.

    4 Psychotherapy is helping the person learn new coping mechanisms and better ways of dealing with problems; the depressed client needs direction to accomplish this.

289. **3** Feelings of hopelessness, helplessness, and isolation dominate the emotional state of the depressed client. The ability to attempt to act out suicide ideation frequently does not occur until psychomotor depression begins to lift. (a); AN; CP; PS; PE; MD

    1 This is not true; they frequently attempt suicide.

    2 This is when the danger is greatest; more energy at this time to follow through on a plan.

    4 A person intent on self-destruction will find a way on any type of unit.

290. **4** Preoccupied clients are usually not aware of events in the environment. The client has not refused to eat but has simply not responded to external stimuli. Taking her by the hand to the dining hall simply puts her where she needs to be. (c); IM; AP; PS; PE; MD

    1 She may be too preoccupied to eat anything; part of intervention is aimed at her nutritional needs.

    2 She probably would not care and will not respond.

    3 This would allow a withdrawal pattern to continue.

291. **1** Spending time with clients communicates to them that the staff members feel they are worthy of their attention and that someone cares. (b); IM; CP; PS; PE; MD

    2 The goal is eventually to have her relate to the other clients not get away from them.

    3 Nothing indicates that she has a delusion regarding food.

    4 It does not give her some special attention, but the goal is to increase her self-esteem and have her believe she is a worthwhile person.

292. **2** The therapeutic level of lithium carbonate is very close to the toxic level. Therefore it is vital that blood levels of the drug be monitored twice a week during the acute phase and bimonthly once the client is on maintenance dosage. (c); EV; AP; PS; PA; MD

    1 Lithium does not affect fluid retention; monitoring daily weights is not necessary.

    3 Psychomotor activity should be normal once the maintenance dosage is achieved; careful monitoring, though, is not a major priority.

    4 Lithium does not affect the leukocyte levels; monitoring the leukocyte count is unnecessary.

293. **4** Lithium decreases sodium reabsorption by the renal tubules. If sodium intake is decreased, sodium depletion can occur. In addition, lithium retention is increased when sodium intake is decreased; a low-sodium intake can lead to lithium toxicity. (c); IM; AP; PS; ED; MD

    1 Clients should never adjust the dosage of prescribed medication without the physician's approval.

    2 This would not have any effect on the lithium therapy.

    3 If the client were well enough to go home for 3 days, participation in controversial discussions would not be contraindicated.

294. **3** Because of its proximity to the heart, the carotid pulse is used to determine whether the ventricles are contracting effectively. The absence of a carotid pulse, in the absence of other vascular problems, indicates ventricular fibrillation or standstill, and immediate cardiopulmonary resuscitation is required to prevent death. (a); AS; AN; ME; PA; CB

    1 If the client has had a cardiac arrest, CPR should be instituted immediately to prevent irreversible brain damage.

    2 If the pulse is absent, there is no BP to be measured.

    4 The presence or absence of the carotid pulse will determine the nature of assistance needed.

295. **3** CPR by one person is less efficient than that performed by two because of the two activities required. The 2:15

ratio is the most efficient way to provide minimally adequate tissue perfusion. (b); IM; KN; ME; PA; CB

1 This ratio would be used when two people were administering CPR.

2 Ineffective; would result in the circulation of unoxygenated blood.

4 Ineffective; blood would not be circulated while four breaths were being administered, and thus hypoxia would result.

296. **2** This provides the best leverage for depressing the sternum. Thus the heart is adequately compressed, and blood is forced into the arteries. Grasping the fingers keeps them off the chest and concentrates the energy expended in the heel of the hand while minimizing the possibility of fracturing ribs. (a); IM; AP; ME; PA; CB

1 Pressure spread over two hands may inadequately compress the heart and fracture the ribs.

3 Application of pressure by the fingers is less effective; inadequate cardiac compression.

4 Both hands must be utilized; pressure on the lower portion of the sternum may fracture the xiphoid process, which can injure vital underlying organs.

297. **1** Hair and oils in the skin may interfere with conduction of electric impulses. Therefore the chest hair immediately around the site may need to be shaved; the area must be scrubbed to remove oils and debris. (c); IM; AP; ME; PA; CB

2 The use of an antimicrobial agent is unnecessary since there will be no break in the skin.

3 Moisture will prevent adherence of the electrodes and thus interfere with impulse conduction.

4 Electrode paste facilitates conduction of electrical impulses and is used regardless of excoriation.

298. **3** When ventricular fibrillation is verified, the first intervention is defibrillation. It is the only measure that will terminate this lethal arrhythmia. (b); EV; AN; ME; PA; CB

1 Digitalis preparations are not used in the treatment of ventricular arrhythmias.

2 If not already in a place, an IV line should be inserted as soon as the client is defibrillated.

4 Elective cardioversion delivers a shock during the R wave; since there is no R wave in ventricular fibrillation, the arrhythmia would continue and death would result.

299. **3** In the absence of oxygen, the body derives its energy anaerobically. This results in a buildup of lactic acid. Sodium bicarbonate, an alkaline drug, will help neutralize the acid, raising the pH back to normal. (a); PL; AP; ME; PA; CB

1 Although potassium is essential for cardiac function, it will not correct acidosis.

2 Calcium gluconate is used primarily in the treatment of hypocalcemia, but its inotropic effect may be utilized in the management of cardiac arrest.

4 Insulin is used in the treatment of diabetes mellitus; it lowers blood sugar by facilitating the transport of glucose across cell membranes.

300. **1** An interference with bile flow into the intestine will lead to increasing inability to tolerate fatty foods. The unemulsified fat remains in the intestine for prolonged periods, and the result is inhibition of stomach emptying with possible gas formation. (a); AS; CP; ME; PA, GI

2 Coffee-ground emesis is usually indicative of gastric bleeding; it is not associated with cholecystitis.

3 Associated with peptic ulcers.

4 Melena is tarry stools associated with upper GI bleeding; diarrhea would be associated with increased intestinal motility, and clay-colored stools associated with obstructive jaundice.

301. **2** Vitamin K is necessary in the formation of prothrombin to prevent bleeding. It is a fat-soluble vitamin and is not absorbed from the GI tract in the absence of bile. (a); AN; KN; SU; TC; GI

1 Bilirubin is the bile pigment formed by the breakdown of erythrocytes.

3 Thromboplastin converts prothrombin to thrombin in the normal coagulation process.

4 Cholecystokinin is the hormone that stimulates pancreatic secretion and contraction of the gallbladder.

302. **2** A nasogastric tube attached to suction removes gastric secretions and prevents vomiting. However, if it becomes clogged, secretions may accumulate, leading to distension, nausea, and vomiting. (b); EV; AN; SU; PA; GI

1 An antiemetic should be administered if nausea persists after the patency of the nasogastric tube is established.

3 To promote drainage of vomitus and prevent aspiration, the client should be initially turned on her side.

4 Deep breathing will not prevent vomiting if the nasogastric tube is not patent.

303. **3** Bleeding disorders are common when bile does not flow through the intestine. Vitamin K, a fat-soluble vitamin requiring bile salts for its absorption, is needed by the liver to synthesize prothrombin. (a); AS; AN; SU; PA; GI

1 Diaphragmatic excursion itself does not put pressure on the suture line; deep breathing does result in pain.

2 Temperature elevation is associated with infection, not with bleeding.

4 Pain is expected because of the location of the incision near the diaphragm.

304. **1** An incision close to the diaphragm (as in surgery of the biliary tract) causes a great deal of pain when the client coughs and deep breathes. These clients tend to take shallow breaths, which leads to inadequate expansion of the lungs, the accumulation of secretions, and infection. (a); AN; AN; SU; PA; GI

2 Cholecystectomy does not require more time than other uncomplicated abdominal surgery.

3 Elevation of serum bilirubin does not affect the immune mechanisms.

4 There is no evidence of an infection present.

305. **3** A full fluid diet ordered by the physician after a cholecystectomy should be verified by the nurse, since there are different schools of thought concerning the use of creamed fluids. Providing a correct diet is the shared responsibility of the physician and the nurse. (b); EV; AP; SU; TC; GI

1 The meal was consistent with the physician's orders; the dietician is not at fault.

2 The nurse is responsible for transcribing the orders and notifying the appropriate departments; unreasonable orders should not be carried out but should be questioned.

4 The client may not be aware of the orders or the significance of such a diet.

306. **4** Although the gallbladder has been removed, the liver will continue to produce and secrete the bile necessary for emulsification of fatty foods. As soon as any inflammation affecting the common bile duct subsides, the bile will flow into the duodenum, but not in concentrated form. (a); IM; AP; SU; ED; GI

1 Since bile is still produced by the liver, a low-fat diet is not continued indefinitely.

2 This is an evasive answer; the surgery was performed to remove an inflamed gallbladder and was successful.

3 This is an evasive answer; the nurse is a resource person and shares the responsibility for client education.

307. **1** Because the client is attached to a machine and movement may alter the tracings, movement is discouraged. (b); AN; CP; OB; PA; IP

    2 Lamaze techniques work well with a monitor.

    3 An external monitor does not necessitate more frequent vaginal examinations.

    4 Placement of the monitor leads does not interfere with the administration of sedatives.

308. **1** Any other action would be invasion of privacy. The marital status has little bearing on the needs of the client at this time. (b); AS; CP; PS; PE; CS

    2 Marital status has no bearing on the course of labor.

    3 This is an invasion of privacy.

    4 No indication at this time that the client requires this referral.

309. **2** Mothers need to explore their infants visually and tactilely to assure themselves that the infant is normal in all respects. (a); AS; CP; OB; ED; IP

    1 Pregnancy and labor have no relationship to "normalcy" of the infant.

    3 Crying is not indicative of congenital defects; a strong cry does not assure "normalcy."

    4 Assumption; closing off communication with the mother at a very opportune moment.

310. **4** The pregnant teenager is more prone to toxemia because of age, poor diet, and often poor prenatal care. (c); AN; AN; OB; PA; PN

    1 False assumption; societal mores vary, and an unwed pregnancy may be totally acceptable.

    2 Unrelated; no proof that teenagers are more diabetogenic than other pregnant women.

    3 May or may not be true.

311. **3** With the head and chest elevated, gravity promotes respiratory excursion; alternating side-lying positions allows for pulmonary drainage and expansion. (b); PL; AP; PE; PA; CB

    1 Would permit the abdominal viscera to impinge on the diaphragm, impeding lung expansion.

    2 Difficult to maintain a 5-week-old infant in this position; also would not promote rest.

    4 Would make it difficult for the lungs to expand, causing difficulty in breathing.

312. **1** Some mottling is expected because of the circulatory disruption and arterial spasm. Further assessment (e.g., palpation of the pedal pulse) is done to rule out total occlusion. (a); EV; AP; PE; PA; CB

    2 Other observations should be made before the physician is notified.

    3 Mottling would occur all over if due to the external temperature; a blanket would interfere with observation.

    4 Elevation of leg would be contraindicated; might support bleeding from the puncture site.

313. **2** A patent airway and adequate pulmonary ventilation are always priorities after surgery. (a); AS; AP; PE; PA; CB

    1 This is important, but adequate ventilation is the priority.

    3 IV lines would be checked once the airway, breathing, and circulation are determined to be functioning well.

    4 Too soon to be a priority; however, it certainly must be assessed later.

314. **1** This provides the best reassurance as long as they know what to expect in the recovery room. (b); IM; AP; PS; PE; CS

    2 If recovery room visit were not possible, this would be the next best action.

    3 This might increase Mrs. Dorn's anxiety; seeing her child would be more therapeutic.

    4 There is an immediate need to reduce anxiety; having coffee will not meet this need.

315. **1** Low gastric acidity predisposes infant to GI infections. (c); AN; CP; PE; ED; GI

    2 There is hydrochloric acid, but not enough to protect the infant.

    3 *E. coli* is the normal intestinal bacterium; not found in the stomach.

    4 The infant is born with passive immunity from maternal antibodies.

316. **4** An increase is the extracellular fluid volume can cause a relatively decrease in the hemoglobin and hematocrit by dilution of the blood. (c); AS; AN; ME; PA; CB

    1 Occurs when pooling of blood in the peripheral vessels causes hypotension; rarely occurs with hypervolemia.

    2 The increased fluid volume in the intravascular compartment (overhydration) will cause the pulse to feel full and bounding.

    3 Headache might accompany overhydration, but rhinitis would not.

317. **1** This defect in bone matrix formation weakens the bones, making them unable to withstand normal stresses. (a); AN; KN; ME; PA; MN

    2 Incorrect; not related to osteoporosis. This occurs during bone healing.

    3 Occurs during normal activity or after minimal injury in bones weakened by disease.

    4 This is death of bone tissue; results from reduced circulation to bone.

318. **2** This regimen limits bone demineralization. It also reduces osteoporitic pain, which promotes increased activity. (c); EV; AN; ME; PA; MN

    1 Would be expected if the client were receiving vitamin C and calcium for capillary fragility.

    3 Not related to osteoporosis or the rationale for therapy.

    4 Would be expected if the client were receiving calcium for hypocalcemia.

319. **4** The client's statement is really saying, "I can manage this myself. I am capable." (c); AS; AN; PS; PE; CS

    1 Nothing in her statement can be interpreted as denial; she has stated, "I know I'm sick."

    2 None of the information given would lead to this conclusion.

    3 Her statement would not be reassuring to the daughter who brought her to the hospital and probably is more reassured having her there.

320. **3** This is normal. It results from the increased pressure of the uterus on venous return. Elevating the legs encourages venous return. (a); IM; AN; OB; ED; HP

    1 Can be harmful; increased circulating blood volume during pregnancy must be maintained.

    2 Contraindicated; salt is necessary to retain fluid for increased circulating blood volume during pregnancy.

    4 Diuretics are not used during pregnancy; may decrease the circulating blood volume.

321. **4** This is recommended to keep weight gain in balance and to control blood pressure. (c); PL; CP; OB; ED; HP

    1 Increasing fats could cause accumulation of unwanted adipose tissue.

    2 Increasing sodium intake is not advised for clients with cardiac problems.

    3 Decreasing protein intake is not advised for clients with cardiac problems.

322. **4** Uteroplacental insufficiency correlates well with a positive OCT (potential fetal distress during delivery). Prompt intervention is indicated. (c); AN; CP; OB; ED; HP
 1 The OCT is unrelated to the mother; it is concerned only with the ability of the fetus to tolerate labor.
 2 An incomplete statement; the occurrence of decelerations and accelerations is also evaluated.
 3 The small dose of oxytocin is too small to test completely the ability of the uterus to contract.

323. **2** The OCT will take 1 to 2 hours, during which time the client is confined to bed. Movement on and off a bedpan should be avoided. (a); IM; AP; OB; ED; HP
 1 Valium could interfere with the results of the OCT since the baby would be sedated.
 3 No food restrictions are indicated.
 4 She may go home 1 hour after the test.

324. **1** This is done to measure baseline variability of the FHR and to observe any alteration in the FHR without oxytocin-induced stress. (c); IM; AP; OB; ED; HP
 2 The semi-Fowler's position with a left-sided tilt is the position of choice.
 3 False; the test involves monitoring the fetal heart during three uterine contractions within a 10-minute period.
 4 There is no indication for this; the test is concerned only with observing the FHR.

325. **3** Touching for pulse and inserting the thermometer increase anxiety and cause elevated vital signs. This sequence is least disturbing. (a); AS; AP; PE; ED; NH
 1 Respirations should be measured first, but temperature should be measured after the pulse rate.
 2 Temperature should be measured last.
 4 Respirations should precede pulse, since the vital signs will change when the baby is touched.

326. **2** Breast milk is digested faster than formula. Breast-fed infants therefore become hungry sooner. (c); PL; CP; OB; ED; NH
 1 An infant may want to nurse hourly if irritable, but this is not a usual feeding pattern.
 3 A breast-fed newborn must be fed more often than this.
 4 All infants must be fed more often than this.

327. **2** Information seeking is the first step in problem solving. (b); IM; AP; PS; PE; CS
 1 The nurse assumes that the husband will solve the problem; violates the confidence between nurse and client.
 3 Shifts the responsibility to the physician.
 4 Presumptuous and expensive; makes the decision for the client.

328. **3** This provides the opportunity for paternal-infant bonding. Handling the infant may reduce some of his anxiety. (c); PL; AP; OB; PE; PP
 1 Does not recognize his anxiety; also he may not be ready to absorb this information.
 2 A simplistic approach to his emotional needs; does not deal with the real situation.
 4 Although helpful, does not meet the need for paternal-infant bonding.

329. **4** Whole milk does not meet the infant's need for vitamin C and iron. Also, it contains high amounts of protein and sodium, which may be harmful. (c); PL; CP; PE; ED; NH
 1 Whole milk contains adequate thiamin; the sodium content is three times that found in human milk.
 2 Whole milk contains adequate carbohydrates; the protein content is three times that found in human milk.

3 Whole milk contains adequate fats; the calcium content is 3½ times that found in human milk.

330. **2** The mismatched blood cells are attacked by antibodies, and the hemoglobin released from the ruptured erythrocytes plugs the kidney tubules; such kidney involvement results in backache. (c); AS; CP; ME; PA; CB
 1 This symptom is not common to transfusion reactions.
 3 This symptom is not common to transfusion reactions.
 4 This symptom is not common to transfusion reactions.

331. **2** The cessation of renal function is usually evidenced by a decrease in output to less than 400 ml/24 hr. (b); AS; AP; ME; PA; CB
 1 Although this symptom is related to the renal system, its presence does not indicate kidney damage.
 3 Although this symptom is related to the renal system, its presence does not indicate kidney damage.
 4 Although this symptom is related to the renal system, its presence does not indicate kidney damage.

332. **1** Perspiration is an involuntary physiologic response. It is mediated by the autonomic nervous system under a variety of circumstances, such as rising ambient temperature, high humidity, stress, and pain. (a); AS, CP; ME; PA; MN
 2 This is a voluntary emotional response.
 3 This is a voluntary action that may limit tension on the abdomen, reducing pain.
 4 This is a reuslt of voluntary contraction of the facial muscles, a common response to pain.

333. **1** The client is assessed and observed. Then the dialysis solutions are instilled, equilibrated, and drained by the nurse. (b); PL; KN; SU; TC; RG
 2 Dialysis may be maintained for longer than 48 hours.
 3 Vital signs may be checked less frequently unless complications occur.
 4 Abdominal discomfort may be relieved by repositioning the client.

334. **3** Peritoneal dialysis uses the peritoneum as a selectively permeable membrane for diffusion of toxins and wastes from the blood into the dialyzing solution. (a); AN; KN; SU; PA; RG
 1 Substitute for kidney function; toxins and wastes pass from the blood into the dialyzing solution by diffusion.
 2 The dialysate does not clean the peritoneal membrane; the semipermeable membrane allows toxins and wastes to pass into the dialysate within the abdominal cavity.
 4 Fluid in the abdominal cavity does not enter the intracellular compartment.

335. **4** Hyperkalemia occurs in renal failure. Because the kidneys are damaged, the body does not excrete K^+. (b); AN; AP; ME; PA; RG
 1 Calcium deficiency would be manifested by tingling of the nose, ears, and fingertips along with muscle spasms and tetany.
 2 Calcium excess would produce renal calculi and pathologic fractures.
 3 Hyponatremia would cause headache, muscle weakness, apathy, and abdominal cramps.

336. **2** Potassium is always low to prevent hyperkalemia. (c); AN; CP; ME; PA; RG
 1 Protein is low, but as high in essential amino acids as possible, forcing synthesis of nonessential amino acids from excess urea nitrogen; this prevents muscle wasting and decreases the production of protein catabolites and azotemia.
 3 Adequate sodium is needed to maintain life; high sodium could cause hypernatremia.

4 Calories are needed to meet metabolic needs and prevent a negative nitrogen balance.

337. **3** If fluid is not draining properly, the client should be positioned from side to side or with the head raised; or manual pressure should be applied to the lower abdomen to facilitate drainage by the use of external pressure and gravity. (c); IM; AP; SU; TC; RG

    1 The client's position may be changed prn; a supine position does not facilitate drainage by the use of gravity.

    2 This deficit is not enough to require notifying the physician.

    4 The physician removes the cannula.

338. **2** When respiratory embarrassment occurs, possibly from pressure of the dialysate on the diaphragm, fluid should be removed and the client's vital signs and status observed. (c); EV; AP; SU; TC; RG

    1 This may be indicated after the solution is drained and the diaphragmatic pressure decreased.

    3 The physician should be notified after immediate action is taken.

    4 Treatment is discontinued only if ordered.

339. **3** All clients who are confined to bed for any considerable period risk losing calcium from bones. This is precipitated in the urine and causes calculi. (b); AN; AP; SU; PA; RG

    1 Although this may occur from inability to assume a normal anatomic position and the emotional impact of using a urinal, it usually does not predispose a client to the development of renal calculi unless fluid intake is low and stasis occurs.

    2 There is no indication that his diet has changed.

    4 The presence of a healing fracture does not increase total calcium metabolism; however, there will be increased deposition of bone at the fracture site.

340. **2** Constriction of circulation decreases venous return and increases pressure within the vessels. Fluid then moves into the interstitial spaces, causing edema. (a); EV; AP; SU; PA; MN

    1 This would indicate infection.

    3 This would indicate infection.

    4 This would indicate infection.

341. **1** Immunosuppressive agents are administered to decrease the immune system's tendency to reject the transplanted organ. (b); IM; AP; ME; ED; RG

    2 Untrue; recreation and exercise are encouraged. Only contact sports should be avoided.

    3 Although fever and edema would occur, hypotension would not; an increased BP would usually be due to fluid retention.

    4 Urine production occurs almost immediately.

342. **3** Inadequate oxygenation increases demands on the heart. This leads to tachycardia as the body tries to compensate. (a); AS; AP; PE; PA; CB

    1 RBC levels are close to normal; suggests anemia caused by iron deficiency rather than by blood loss that could cause cold, clammy skin.

    2 Results from excess carboxyhemoglobin; pallor is more common with anemia.

    4 Not generally an adaptation associated with decreased hemoglobin.

343. **3** The 4-year-old child has developed trust but still needs frequent support from this parents. (a); IM; AP; PE; PE; CB

    1 Appropriate for an infant who is just developing trust in his parents; hospitalization should not interfere with this important aspect of personality development.

    2 The parents may bring a toy; but their presence to provide support and reinforce trust is more important.

4 The parents should participate in their son's care as much as possible, so there will be no interference with the trust relationship and to provide support.

344. **4** Immediate physical safety takes priority. The client must sit down before he falls down. Follow with the supine position. (b); IM; AP; PE; TC; CB

    1 Immediate physical safety takes priority over further assessment.

    2 Although gravity promotes cerebral blood flow in this position, immediate physical safety takes priority; walk at this time is unsafe.

    3 Subjective symptom of dizziness alone does not warrant this; immediate physical safety takes priority.

345. **3** Decreased oxygen-carrying capacity of the blood may lead to hypoxia during exercise, when oxygen demand is greater. (b); AN; CP; PE; PA; CB

    1 Although this may be a cause of the symptom, it is not directly related to anemia.

    2 Although this may be a cause of the symptom, it is not directly related to anemia.

    4 Although this may be a cause of the symptom, it is not directly related to anemia.

346. **3** Liquid iron preparations may stain tooth enamel, so they should be diluted and administered through a straw. (a); IM; AP; PE; PA; CB

    1 To avoid gastric irritation, iron should be given with food.

    2 To improve absorption, iron may be given with orange juice.

    4 Constipation, rather than loose stools, often results.

347. **3** Residual medication on the needle may stain the skin during penetration. (a); IM; AP; PE; PA; CB

    1 Deep penetration is necessary; only the gluteal muscles should be used because of their size and the decreased visibility of staining.

    2 Should be avoided; might cause seepage of drug through the needle track, with subsequent tissue irritation and staining.

    4 Would constrict blood vessels and impair absorption.

348. **4** The 4-year-old can express himself better through play than with words. (b); IM; AP; PE; PE; CB

    1 This may help the nurse understand emotional problems; however, it is not as helpful as play therapy in meeting the child's emotional needs.

    2 Understanding explanations requires abstract thinking; 4-year-olds think in a concrete manner.

    3 A needle is dangerous; even a play syringe would focus the child's attention on one aspect of treatment, without eliciting broader feelings.

349. **1** The added cardiac workload of individuals with anemia receiving transfusions increases the risk of heart failure, leading to pulmonary edema. (b); AN; AN; PE; PA; CB

    2 Untrue; not increased by anemia.

    3 Untrue; not increased by anemia.

    4 Untrue; not increased by anemia.

350. **4** Warm water will often relax the urinary sphincter, enabling a client to void. (b); IM; AP; SU; PA; RG

    1 Since the bladder is already distended, increased fluid intake will only increase pressure and may result in hydronephrosis.

    2 The client has already indicated that he was unable to void.

    3 Pressure over a distended bladder induces pain, which causes muscular contraction of the urinary sphincters.

351. **4** A suprapubic prostatectomy involves an abdominal incision to gain access to the prostate through the bladder. Postoperatively the client has a suprapubic cystot-

omy tube to instill a GU irrigant and drain urine as well as a Foley catheter to limit bleeding, maintain patency, and drain urine. (b); PL; KN; SU; PA; RG

  1 An incision is made into the lower abdomen, a ureteral catheter is not used.

  2 The ureters are not involved in this surgery.

  3 The kidneys are not involved in this surgery.

352. **1** Because of the vascularity of the involved tissue, hemorrhage and shock constitute the immediate postoperative danger after a prostatectomy. (a); AN; CP; SU; PA; RG

  2 Impotence is a relatively rare complication.

  3 Foley is used; leakage of urine may occur for a few days after the Foley is removed due to sphincter trauma.

  4 Bladder spasms may occur but are not potentially life threatening; observing for hemorrhage is a priority.

353. **3** The catheter must be reinserted by the physician to ensure bladder emptying, maintain pressure at the operative site, and prevent hemorrhage. (a); IM; AP; SU; TC; RG

  1 Irrigations require a physician's approval.

  2 Because of the danger of further trauma to the urethra and surgical site, the surgeon should insert the catheter.

  4 In addition to urinary drainage, the balloon of the urethral catheter exerts pressure against the prostate to help control bleeding and should be reinserted.

354. **4** After a suprapubic prostatectomy there is generally leakage of urine around the suprapubic tube, creating an environment in which bacteria can flourish if the dressing is not changed frequently. (b); PL; CP; SU; PA; RG

  1 Uremia is caused by inadequate kidney function; not directly related to bladder infection.

  2 Negative pressure on the bladder may traumatize the delicate tissue; urine should flow by gravity.

  3 Clamping off the tube causes urinary stasis, which increases the risk of infection.

355. **3** Pain after a suprapubic prostatectomy may denote retention of urine as a result of blocked drainage tubes or infection, or it may be a normal response to surgery. The possibility of any complication must first be investigated. (a); EV; AP; SU; TC; RG

  1 Analgesics can be administered after the cause of pain has been investigated; assessment should occur before implementation.

  2 The need for vital signs is dependent upon the analgesic ordered; assessing the cause of pain takes priority.

  4 Encouraging fluids without a patent drainage tube will increase pressure and discomfort; assessment should occur before implementation.

356. **3** Straining applies pressure to the operative site. (c); IM; AN; SU; TC; RG

  1 A retention catheter is routinely in place.

  2 To prevent trauma, negative pressure should not be exerted on the bladder.

  4 A retention catheter is routinely in place.

357. **3** Babies with Down syndrome have decreased muscle tone, which compromises respiratory expansion as well as the adequate drainage of mucus. These factors contribute to increased susceptibility to upper respiratory tract infections. (b); AN; AP; PE; PA; RE

  1 Slowed development is usually apparent shortly after birth.

  2 Cardiac, not circulatory, problems are common in these children.

  4 Impaired hearing is not an expected problem in Down syndrome.

358. **4** A simian crease is a common clinical manifestation. It is readily observable when present. (a); AS; KN; PE; ED; MN

  1 Not a characteristic of children with Down syndrome, but of children with congenital hip dislocation.

  2 Children with Down syndrome usually manifest hypotonicity of skeletal muscles.

  3 Many normal children also have rounded occiputs.

359. **2** Parents' responses to their children may greatly influence decisions regarding future care. Learning about their child and Down syndrome can help lessen guilt feelings. (a); PL; AP; PE; ED; MN

  1 Frequent handling and rocking are essential for all babies.

  3 Important for all babies.

  4 Not particularly necessary for infants with Down syndrome.

360. **2** Babies with Down syndrome have a high incidence of congenital heart disease, especially atrial defects. (b); PL; AP; PE; PA; CB

  1 Deafness is not usually a problem in Down syndrome.

  3 Infants with Down syndrome usually do not have a problem with excessive CSF.

  4 The muscles of infants with Down syndrome are usually hypotonic.

361. **3** When the parents can verbalize the need to change plans they have made for their infant, it usually signifies that they are beginning to face reality. (a); EV; AN; PS; PE; CS

  1 Probably not critically significant to the nurse.

  2 Not usually a problem; is therefore not the most significant factor to the nurse.

  4 Would be after the fact; is not the most significant factor to be considered by the nurse.

362. **2** For a child who is moderately retarded, simple repetitive tasks provide all the challenge needed. (b); IM; AP; PS; PE; CS

  1 Asking too much of a moderately retarded child.

  3 Asking too much of a moderately retarded child.

  4 Moderately retarded children will not be able to follow many instructions given at a single time.

363. **3** When one's efforts toward meeting a goal are blocked or thwarted, frustration results. The child with moderate retardation may be constantly thwarted in trying to meet his needs, especially in an environment where certain achievements beyond his ability are expected. (a); AN; CP; PS; PE; CS

  1 Does not occur frequently.

  2 Does not occur.

  4 An external factor that has little to do with the child's ability to deal with his limitations.

364. **3** This reply encourages the client to discuss fears and anxieties. (a); IM; AP; PS; PE; CS

  1 Does not encourage the client to discuss the situation further; mention of risk may frighten the client.

  2 Opinions or value judgments should not be expressed by the nurse; should deal only with the client's feelings.

  4 Cuts off communication; does not allow the client to express her fears and anxiety.

365. **2** False labor does not produce cervical dilation. Only true labor does. (b); AS; CP; OB; ED; IP

  1 Braxton Hicks contractions may have some regularity.

  3 Urine may appear to leak from the vaginal orifice.

  4 Associated with other situations, such as hemorrhoids, diarrhea, or constipation.

366. **3** The application of back pressure combined with frequent positional changes will help alleviate the discomfort. (a); IM; AP; OB; PA; IP

  1 The supine position places increased pressure on the back; aggravates the pain.

2 Although this may be comfortable for some individuals, rubbing the back and alternating positions are more universally effective.

4 Neuromuscular control exercises are used to teach selective relaxation in childbirth classes; not utilized in labor.

367. **2** Gastric peristalsis often ceases during periods of stress. Abdominal contractions put pressure on the stomach and can cause nausea and vomiting, increasing the risk of aspiration, especially with general anesthesia. (a); IM; CP; OB; TC; IP

1 Gastric activity and digestion cease during periods of tension.

3 Gastric activity and digestion cease during periods of tension.

4 Although food may cause dyspepsia, the primary reason for withholding it is to prevent aspiration.

368. **1** Increased intraabdominal pressure associated with crying, coughing, or straining will cause protrusion of the hernia. (a); AS; AP; OB; ED; NH

2 Does not increase intraabdominal pressure.

3 The lowering of the diaphragm may increase intraabdominal pressure slightly but not enough to cause protrusion of the hernia.

4 Does not increase intraabdominal pressure.

369. **1** Jerky lateral eye movement, particularly toward the involved ear. (b); AS; AN; ME; PA; MN

2 Not usually associated with Ménière's disease.

3 Not usually associated with Ménière's disease.

4 Not usually associated with Ménière's disease.

370. **4** Prepared without salt, this food has the least sodium. (a); PL; AP; ME; ED; MN

1 Have a high sodium content, which promotes fluid retention and increases endolymphatic fluid in the cochlea.

2 Has a high sodium content.

3 Has a high sodium content.

371. **4** Keeping a record of what one eats helps limit unconscious and nervous eating by making the individual aware of food intake. (b); PL; AP; ME; ED; GI

1 Not always practical and is difficult to implement; assessment of dietary habits is the priority.

2 Exercise causes rapid head movements, which may precipitate an attack.

3 Limiting calories to 900 per day requires a physician's order.

372. **1** It has been medically proved that during the first stage of detoxification, nausea, anorexia, and hypertension are experienced. (c); AS; CP; PS; PA; SA

2 Hypertension (not hypotension) and agitation are experienced during this stage.

3 Hypertension, hyperactivity, and tachycardia (not bradycardia) are experienced during this stage.

4 Psychomotor hyperactivity (not lethargy) and hypertension (not hypotension) are experienced during this stage.

373. **1** This would provide some security since the client would know what to expect at different periods during the day. (b); PL; AP; PS; PE; SA

2 Inappropriate; would probably increase anxiety, and there is no one prototype of a client's role.

3 Inappropriate; would be somewhat overwhelming. Many of the regulations would not even apply to Mrs. Bartin.

4 Inappropriate; would increase anxiety and severe little purpose. Necessary limits should be individual, not set by regulation.

374. **1** A well-lit and quiet room helps reduce the fears and illusional experiences of the client during alcoholic withdrawal. (c); PL; AN; PS; PE; SA

2 The nurses' station is usually a busy place; a room nearby is not the ideal location for the alcoholic client experiencing delirium. Noises can be frightening and may stimulate hallucinations or illusions.

3 Bright lights from corridors can cast shadows on the walls and ceiling of a darkened room, increasing stimulation and illusions of frightening objects.

4 Dim lights in the room increase stimulation, producing illusions and hallucinations; strangers may increase the client's fear, restlessness, and confusion.

375. **4** This action would provide the disorganized client with the necessary structure to encourage participation and support of self-image. (b); PL; AP; PS; PE; SA

1 Would increase her anxiety and withdrawal and decrease her level of function.

2 Would increase her anxiety and withdrawal and decrease her level of function.

3 Would increase dependency and add to her self-doubt.

Comprehensive Test 2: Part 1*

1. **4** Gentle pressure is applied against the baby's head as it emerges so it is not delivered too rapidly. The head is never held back, and it should be supported as it emerges so there will be no vaginal lacerations. (b); IM; AP; OB; ED; IP

1 It is impossible to breathe and pant at the same time.

2 Unless she pants and blows breath out, she will push involuntarily.

3 Unless she pants to slow the pushing, she will deliver on the stretcher.

2. **2** Position the baby with head lower than chest and rub the infant's back to stimulate crying so he can oxygenate his lungs. (a); IM; AP; OB; PA; IP

1 This is not the priority at the present moment; the uterus still contains placenta and will not contract.

3 There is no need for haste in cutting the cord; a clear airway is the priority.

4 There is no time, and the mother will not be able to cooperate with a move to the stretcher.

3. **1** Precipitate delivery may be injurious to both mother and infant. The maternal morbidity rate is increased by infection and/or hemorrhage resulting from the trauma of a rapid forceful delivery in a contaminated field. (b); EV; AN; OB; PA; IP

2 This is common to all clients after all types of delivery; due to the change in blood volume.

3 This may be due to the use of oxytocin or to impending toxemia, not to a precipitous delivery.

4 Unless there is some airway obstruction, a precipitous delivery will not have any influence on the baby's respirations.

4. **2** The first hour after delivery is called the fourth stage of labor. During this time the uterus is at the level of the umbilicus, and each day after delivery it descends one finger breadth. (c); AS; CP; OB; PA; IP

1 The uterus descends below the umbilicus, rising above it only if the bladder is full.

---

*A key to the letters following the correct rationale can be found on p.633.

How to Use Worksheet 1: Errors in Processing Information

Common errors in processing information are listed in the left-hand column of this worksheet. At the top of the worksheet is a row of blank spaces for inserting the number of the question missed. Directly below each number, check any errors you made in answering that question. You may have made more than one type of error in an answer.

Worksheet 1: Errors in processing information

Question number																					
Did not read situation/question carefully																					
Missed important details																					
Confused major and minor points																					
Defined problem incorrectly																					
Could not remember terms/facts/concepts/principles																					
Defined terms incorrectly																					
Focused on incomplete/incorrect data in assessing situation																					
Interpreted data incorrectly																					
Applied wrong concepts/principles in situation																					
Drew incorrect conclusions																					
Identified wrong goals																					
Identified priorities incorrectly																					
Carried out plan incorrectly/incompletely																					
Was unclear about criteria for evaluating success in achieving goals																					

How to Use Worksheet 2: Knowledge Gaps

Types of common knowledge gaps are listed along the top of this worksheet. Write a brief description of topics you want to review in the spaces provided. For example, if you missed a question on administration of a particular drug, write the drug name and problem (e.g., dosage) in the appropriate space under the column labeled *Pharmacology.*

Worksheet 2: Knowledge gaps

Basic science	Skills/ procedures	Basic human needs	Growth & develop-ment	Normal nutrition	Psycho-social factors	Clinical area/ topic	Stressors/ coping mechanisms	Patho-physiology	Pharma-cology	Therapeutic nutrition	Legal implications	Other

3 This will happen on the second day postpartum; the uterus descends one finger breadth each day.

4 This will happen on the fourth or fifth day postpartum; the uterus descends one finger breadth per day.

5. **3** The Nurse Practice Act requires nurses to diagnose human responses. (b); AS; KN; OB; TC; NH

1 This is physical assessment, not medical diagnosis, and is within the nurse's role

2 Fortunately not true, since the physician may not be present; the nurse is capable of making physical assessment.

4 Assessment should not differ if done by the nurse.

6. **4** To maintain a patent airway and promote respiration and gaseous exchange, mucus must be removed from the respiratory tract. (b); IM; AN; OB; TC; NH

1 If the airway is obstructed, oxygen will be of no use; therefore suctioning is a priority.

2 This is for aspirating the stomach contents not for airway clearance.

3 Documentation is important but secondary to clearing a passageway for air.

7. **1** Respiratory distress is a frequent response indicative of possible immaturity of the infant's respiratory tract— such as a small lumen, weakness of the respiratory musculature, paucity of functional alveoli, or insufficient calcification of the bony thorax. (b); EV; KN; OB; PA; NH

2 Temperature generally stabilizes after 8 hours, unless the baby is premature.

3 This would not yet be important since the baby's intake is limited in the first 24 hours.

4 Tone (i.e., high, shrill) would be more pertinent than duration.

8. **1** The tonic neck reflex is normal in the newborn and disappears within 3 to 6 months. (b); IM; AN; OB; ED; NH

2 This is a normal newborn response and does not need medical attention.

3 This response disappears between 3 and 4 months.

4 Lack of this reflex may indicate neurologic impairment.

9. **2** Allowing the mother time to inspect the child permits viewing, touching, and holding, promoting bonding. (b); PL; AP; OB; PE; PP

1 The mother should have made this decision before delivery.

3 The client will proceed at her own rate; requiring her to do things is not supportive.

4 This can be done only by allowing the mother ample time to inspect and interact with her baby.

10. **1** The common bile duct enters the duodenum. The pyloric sphincter is located between the end of the stomach and the beginning of the duodenum; therefore, when it is hypertrophied, the tight sphincter prevents any mixing of formula with bile. (b); AS; CP; PE; PA; GI

2 Pyloric stenosis involves hypertrophy and hyperplasia of the muscle of the pyloric sphincter, causing a severe narrowing between the stomach and the duodenal canal.

3 The area obstructed in pyloric stenosis is the pyloric sphincter, between the stomach and duodenum.

4 The bile duct enters the duodenum at a site different from the pyloric sphincter and is uninvolved in pyloric stenosis.

11. **1** The hypertrophied muscle becomes elongated and is palpable as an olive-shaped mass. Because of its normal anatomic location, it is felt in the upper right quadrant of the abdomen. (b); EV; CP; PE; PA; GI

2 Normal transmission of ingested food is interrupted, but normal digestive processes are intact.

3 Food does not reach the lower GI tract.

4 The upper abdomen may be distended since food is unable to leave the stomach and progress through the remainder of the GI tract.

12. **2** Prior to inserting the lavage/gavage tube the nurse measures the anatomic pathway the tube will follow— i.e., from the nose to the earlobe (corresponding to the nasopharynx) to the epigastric area of the abdomen (lower end of stomach). It is then marked and inserted to this point. (b); IM; AN; PE; PA; GI

1 Resistance to the passage of a gastric tube may be felt, and rotation of the tube often changes placement enough to continue insertion to the point marked by measurement.

3 This distance would be much too long.

4 This distance might not place the tube well into the stomach and would increase the risk of aspiration.

13. **2** If the nasogastric tube is accidently passed into the trachea rather than the esophagus, it will occlude the airway, causing cyanosis. (b); EV; AN; PE; PA; RE

1 Choking may occur as the tube passes through the back of the throat.

3 Flushing may result if the infant attempts to fight the passage of the tube.

4 Gagging may occur as the tube passes from the nasal passage through the pharynx.

14. **4** During and after feeding, the position most favoring gravity is employed to promote retention of fluid and prevent vomiting. (c); IM; AP; PE; ED; GI

1 Postoperative positioning with the head elevated helps to assist food passage; the prone position would promote vomiting.

2 Vomiting may continue postoperatively, so limited movement of the child after feedings is suggested.

3 Feeding any child in the supine position greatly increases the risk of aspiration.

15. **3** Offering a new food after giving formula associates this activity with eating and takes advantage of the child's unsatisfied hunger. (b); IM; AP; PE; ED; GI

1 Solid food should be introduced by spoon to acquaint the child to new tastes and textures as well as the use of the spoon.

2 New foods should be initiated one at a time and continued for 4 to 5 days to assess for allergy.

4 Offering food after the regular feeding decreases the chance of success since the infant's hunger is already satisfied.

16. **1** The first solid foods added to the infant's diet should be easily digestible, such as fruits and cereals, and rich sources of iron, such as cereals and egg yolk. (b); IM; AP; PE; ED; GI

2 Egg white is added very late because of the allergic reactions associated with it.

3 Meats are more difficult to digest and so are added later.

4 Sweets have less nutritional value and may make an infant less accepting of other foods later.

17. **1** Excessive thyroid hormones increase the metabolic rate, causing nervousness, weight loss, increased appetite, heat intolerance, and tachycardia. (a); AS; CP; ME; PA; EI

2 Exophthalmos is common in hyperthyroidism; however, the pulse rate is rapid and the client is nervous and hyperactive.

3 Although the appetite is increased, moist skin and rapid pulse rate are associated with hyperthyroidism; a slow pulse rate and dry skin accompany hypothyroidism because of a decreased metabolic rate.

4 Although loss of weight is associated with hyperthyroidism, constipation and listlessness occur with hypothyroidism because of a decreased metabolic rate.

18. **1** The radioactive iodine uptake test involves administering trace amounts of ^{131}I and subsequently evaluating its uptake. In hyperthyroidism, blood levels of both ^{131}I and T_3 (triiodothyronine) are increased. (b); IM; AP; ME; ED; EI

   2 The results with the sequential multichannel autoanalyzer (SMA 12) are not specific to thyroid disease; the protein bound iodine test is not definitive because it is influenced by the intake of exogenous iodine.

   3 X-ray results would not indicate thyroid disease, and elevation of T_4 (thyroxine) might indicate hyperthyroidism; however, this could be a false reading because of the presence of thyroid-binding globulin (TBG) and is inadequate for diagnosis when used alone.

   4 Po_2 is not specific to thyroid disease, and the basal metabolic rate is a measure of energy expenditure, not thyroid function (for which it is inaccurate); results of the BMR would be readily altered by CHF, anemia, caffeine, obesity, and adrenal disease.

19. **3** Promotion of rest to reduce metabolic demands is a challenging but essential task with a client who has hyperthyroidism. (b); PL; CP; ME; TC; EI

   1 Diet can be increased to meet metabolic demands; the client usually has an excellent appetite.

   2 The neatness of linen is not an important aspect of care; the client is usually hyperactive, and it is difficult to promote rest.

   4 Hospital routines should not be considered a nursing problem; routines should always be flexible to meet client needs.

20. **1** Propylthiouracil (Propacil), used in the treatment of hyperthyroidism, blocks the synthesis of thyroid hormones by preventing iodination of tyrosine. (b); IM; CP; ME; PA; EI

   2 Iodine solutions reduce the size and vascularity of the thyroid gland.

   3 Propylthiouracil does not increase the uptake of iodine.

   4 Thyroid-stimulating hormone (TSH), secreted by the anterior pituitary, is not affected by propylthiouracil.

21. **4** Lugol's solution provides iodine, which aids in decreasing the vascularity of the thyroid gland, decreasing the risk of hemorrhage. (b); IM; CP; SU; PA; EI

   1 Calcium is needed to maintain parathyroid function.

   2. Thyroid hormone substitutes will regulate the body's metabolism.

   3 Antithyroid drugs, not iodine, prevent the formation of thyroxine.

22. **1** Medication is regulated to maintain the normal blood levels of thyroxine; therefore ovulation is not affected, and future pregnancy is possible. (c); IM; AN; OB; ED; EI

   2 Pregnancy is not contraindicated after a thyroidectomy.

   3 The client will no longer be hyperthyroid after surgery because the overactive tissue is excised.

   4 Thyroid hormones may have to be increased; however, the alterations in dosage are based on individual needs.

23. **4** Thyroid surgery sometimes results in accidental removal of the parathyroid glands. A resultant hypocalcemia may lead to contraction of the glottis, causing airway obstruction; edema also causes obstruction. (b); IM; AP; SU; TC; EI

   1 Speaking is important in determing the status of the glottis.

2 Although inspection of the dressing is important, the incision cannot normally be visualized without removal of the dressing; the physician usually changes the first dressing 24 to 48 hours after surgery; the airway takes priority.

   3 The client should be maintained in a semi-Fowler's position to maximize respiratory excursion.

24. **3** Thyroid storm refers to a sudden and excessive release of thyroid hormones, which cause pyrexia, tachycardia, and exaggerated symptoms of thyrotoxicosis. Surgery or infection will generally precipitate this life-threatening condition. (b); EV; AN; SU; PA; EI

   1 Temperature would be elevated in thyroid storm because of the sudden excessive release of thyroid hormones, which elevate the basal metabolic rate.

   2 Hypercalcemia is not related to thyroid storm; hypocalcemia may result from accidental removal of the parathyroid glands.

   4 Pulse rate would be rapid in thyroid storm because of the sudden excessive release of thyroid hormones, which elevate the basal metabolic rate.

25. **2** Thyroid trauma, thyroid surgery, or psychologic stress in a client with hyperthyroidism may lead to the release of abnormally high levels of thyroid hormones. This intensifies all symptoms of hyperthyroidism — thyroid storm (increased pulse, elevated temperature, restlessness, vomiting, and often death). (b); AN; CP; SU; PA; EI

   1 Tetany occurs from this inadvertent surgical excision.

   3 Iodine would bind with thyroxine, decreasing the potential storm.

   4 Anesthesia would depress metabolism, not increase it.

26. **4** Introducing May Ann to the nurse who will be primarily working with her on a one-to-one basis is extremely important because the withdrawn client can be assisted back to reality by a caring individual (nurse) who is interested in everything that happens to her. (b); IM; AP; PS; PE; SD

   1 This would be a later action.

   2 Would have no effect, since she is involved with a strong delusional pattern.

   3 How does the nurse know she will not be frightened; false reassurance.

27. **2** A simple statement that the client is not understood provides feedback and points out reality. (b); IM; AN; PS; PE; SD

   1 Neologisms have symbolic meaning only for the client.

   3 This will be of limited help and does not present reality.

   4 There is no one other than herself who can understand the fantasies.

28. **3** May Ann needs someone who has been working with her and whom she trusts to stay with her until she is calmer. She has lost control and needs the protection of another person who will observe her, anticipate her actions, and prevent her from acting out her destructive impulses. (c); PL; AP; PS; TC; SD

   1 It may still be necessary to do this, but staying with her is a better immediate action.

   2 She may not be ready for participation though she does need to be kept in touch with reality.

   4 At this time she cannot be held responsible for her behavior.

29. **1** The nurse demonstrates knowledge of her own perceptions and can accept the client's, even though they are hallucinatory. (b); IM; AP; PS; PE; SD

   2 The client would be unable to accept this; it would only increase her fear.

3 This would increase the client's guilt and fear.

4 Presents reality but negates the client's feelings and asks for unrealistic responses.

30. **2** Once May Ann realizes that the staff members do not recognize her negative behavior (which is a defense against feelings of inferiority) but praise her for real accomplishments, she will no longer need the superior attitude. She will have gained recognition and self-esteem for socially acceptable behavior. (b); PL; AN; PS; PE; SD

   1 Unrealistic, since a goal is to function again in society.

   3 This is expecting too much of her at present.

   4 The withdrawn clients must be protected from her ridicule and sarcasm just as she must be protected.

31. **3** The caffeine in coffee acts as a stimulant to counteract the drowsiness she may experience during the first week of treatment. After the first week, drowsiness may be replaced by a feeling of calmness. (c); IM; AN; PS; PA; SD

   1 Rinsing her mouth would help alleviate the dryness, but increasing her fluid intake would have little effect.

   2 Postural hypotension is a possible side effect, so client teaching is important; but BP should be checked after giving the drug.

   4 Not necessary to give Cogentin unless she starts exhibiting extrapyramidal effects.

32. **1** Tranquilizers reduce anxiety levels and make clients more amenable to looking at new approaches to handling stress. (b); AN; KN; PS; PE; SD

   2 The major tranquilizers are used to treat psychotic symptoms, which may include destructive behavior; however, not the major reason for administration.

   3 They are used to treat severe emotional illness, not neurotic symptoms.

   4 They cannot prevent any secondary complications.

33. **2** Maladaptive behavior that may be accepted in the hospital will not be approved in the community. The nurse's observations can help determine which clients are ready to cope with life's realities and which need further help. The nurse can report the observations to the medical team, and appropriate actions can be taken. (c); EV; CP; PS; PE; SD

   1 A social evening in town would not accomplish this.

   3 A social evening in town would not by itself constitute reality.

   4 There is nothing to indicate that any of these clients needed broadening cultural experiences.

34. **2** Signs of mild to moderate placental separation include uterine discomfort and tenderness because of concealed bleeding. Visible bleeding may be scant, moderate, or heavy. (b); AS; AN; OB; ED; HP

   1 Uterine size may increase because of accumulated blood at the placental site.

   3 There is a great deal of pain because of accumulated blood in the uterine cavity.

   4 Uterine size increases from accumulated blood; vaginal bleeding may be present.

35. **4** The blood cannot escape from behind the placenta. Thus the abdomen becomes boardlike and painful because of the entrapment (b); AN; CP; OB; PA; HP

   1 Symptoms of hemorrhagic shock do not include pain.

   2 This is not an immediate response; may occur later if the client's resistance is lessened.

   3 Blood may be at the site of placental separation but not in the uterine muscle.

36. **1** Clotting defects are common in moderate and severe abruptio placentae because of the loss of fibrinogen from severe internal bleeding. (b); AN; CP; OB; PA; HP

2 Excessive globulin in the blood; unrelated to clotting.

3 Decrease in the number of platelets; bleeding of abruptio is caused by depletion of fibrinogen not platelets.

4 Excessive amount of red blood cells; not related to the depletion of fibrinogen.

37. **4** Parents must be helped to identify their feelings. (a); IM; AP; PS; PE; CS

   1 Answer based on the nurse's religious belief; no indication that the client has the same belief; closes off communication.

   2 Unpredictable; does not encourage the client to explore her feelings.

   3 Many stillborn children are apparently free of any defects.

38. **4** In small children the eustachian tube is shorter, wider, and straighter. Pulling the auricle down and back facilitates passage of fluid to the drum. (b); IM; AP; PE; ED; MN

   1 Pulling the auricle down and back helps straighten the canal for passage of the drops.

   2 Pulling the auricle up and back is used for older children and adults.

   3 Pulling the auricle down and back facilitates passage of the eardrops.

39. **2** The middle ear contains the three ossicles—malleus, incus, and stapes—which, with the tympanic membrane and oval window, form an amplifying system. (b); AN; KN; PE; PA; MN

   1 Normally the eustachian tube, which connects the middle ear and nasopharynx, is closed and flat to prevent organisms from entering the middle ear; however, it allows air into the middle ear and thus equalizes pressure on both sides of the eardrum.

   3 The pressure of sound waves is amplified in the middle ear and transmitted to the cochlea (inner ear), where it is detected by the organ of Corti and transmitted along the acoustic nerve.

   4 The inner ear contains both the organ of hearing (the cochlea) and the organ of balance (the vestibule).

40. **4** Myringotomy relieves pressure and prevents spontaneous rupture of the eardrum by allowing pus and fluid to escape from the middle ear into the external auditory canal, from which the exudate drains. (b); AS; CP; SU; PA; MN

   1 Myringotomy involves drainage of the middle ear through an incision made in the eardrum; the CNS is not involved.

   2 These symptoms might be expected after surgery involving some part of the urinary tract.

   3 The lacrimal glands are the tear-producing glands.

41. **4** Toddlers are ritualistic and do not tolerate change well. Any change in diet should be done matter-of-factly. Because of their characteristic struggle for independence, toddlers should not be forced to eat. (b); AS; KN; PE; TC; GI

   1 This is not always possible in dietary restrictions.

   2 The toddler is still dependent on the parents and therefore responds better to them than to strangers.

   3 The toddler does not have the cognitive capacity to understand reasons for behavior.

42. **1** The toddler is still dependent on the mother, is narcissistic, and still plays alone but is aware of others playing next to him. (a); EV; KN; PE; ED; MN

   2 Competitive play would be seen in school-age children.

   3 Solitary play or onlookers' play is characteristic of the 1-to-2-year-old.

   4 Tumbling-type play is not a commonly accepted term used to refer to how play incorporates other children.

43. **4** Appropriate limit setting and discipline are necessary for children to develop self-control while learning the boundaries of their abilities. (c); AN; KN; PE; ED; MN
    1 Trust and security are tasks that the infant learns.
    2 Roles within society are learned by the schoolage child.
    3 Superego control begins in the preschooler.

44. **2** Third-degree burns are those extending into the subcutaneous tissue. They are not painful, because of nerve destruction. (c); AS; KN; SU; PA; EI
    1 Burns affecting the outer layer of skin are first degree.
    3 Burns extending through the epidermis and involving the corium (the fiberous inner layer of skin just below the epidermis) are second degree.
    4 Burns affecting the underlying fat, muscles, tendons, and bones are fourth degree.

45. **3** By the rule of nines: each arm is 9%, each leg is 18%, and the head is 9%. Therefore the total percentage of burned area on Mr. Jones is 36%. (a); AS; KN; SU; PA; EI
    1 This figure reflects a miscalculation of the rule of nines.
    2 This figure reflects a miscalculation of the rule of nines.
    4 This figure reflects a miscalculation of the rule of nines.

46. **3** In the first 48 hours after a severe burn, fluid moves into the tissues surrounding the injured area. Fluid is also lost in drainage and from evaporation. This results in a decreased blood volume and could lead to shock. (a); PL; AN; SU; PA; EI
    1 The burn wound is generally considered sterile for the first 24 hours; if fluid losses are not replaced immediately, the client may die before infection can set in.
    2 Blood loss is usually minimal; the loss of fluid, colloids, and electrolytes is what causes the hypovolemia.
    4 Although pain relief is an important aspect in the care of clients with burns, the immediate priority is to replace fluid losses to prevent death.

47. **1** The severe pain experienced by the client during debridement of burns places an emotional strain on the relationship. (a); AN; AN; SU; PE; MN
    2 According to Maslow, basic needs of survival and safety take precedence over higher-level needs. Pain becomes all encompassing, and the nurse must help the client cope with it.
    3 This answer is not complete. The frequency with which the nurse must perform tasks is not the problem; rather it is the pain associated with debridement and the nurse's inability to eliminate the pain.
    4 Maintaining sterility is not a problem if the nurse understands surgical asepsis.

48. **2** The mucous membranes of the respiratory tract may be charred after inhalation burns. This is evidenced by the production of sooty sputum. (c); EV; CP; ME; PA; RE
    1 Frothy sputum is usually indicative of pulmonary edema.
    3 This finding may indicate respiratory infection.
    4 This finding may indicate respiratory infection.

49. **3** The shift of plasma proteins into the burned area increases the tissue colloid osmotic pressure (TCOP). This results in fluid diffusion from the intravascular to the interstitial fluid compartment. The result is decreased blood volume and hypovolemic shock. (c); EV; CP; SU; PA; EI
    1 Sodium passes to the burned area and helps cause blister formation.
    2 Decreased glomerular filtration may occur because of hypovolemia; it is not involved in the etiology of hypovolemia.

    4 Extracellular fluid is lost through burned tissue.

50. **3** Cellular catabolism, as in burns, results in the loss of potassium from cells; this raises the K^+ level in the extracellular fluid (normal range, 3.5 to 5.5 mEq/L). Such hyperkalemia may lead to arrhythmias (peaked T wave at 6 mEq) and, as a terminal event, cardiac arrest. (c); AS; CP; SU; PA; EI
    1 Hypokalemia may result on the fourth or fifth postburn day as potassium shifts from the extracellular fluid into the intracellular compartment.
    2 The shift of potassium from the intracellular to the extracellular compartment results in hyperkalemia. In addition, *to excrete* means to eliminate waste matter by a normal discharge; the loss of fluids and electrolytes through a damaged integument is not a normal discharge.
    4 Potassium loss from damaged tissues results in hyperkalemia as the potassium shifts from the intracellular to the extracellular spaces.

51. **2** Showing understanding of and identifying the client's feelings by giving feedback helps in establishing a therapeutic relationship. (b); IM; AN; PS; PE; CS
    1 Negates the person's feelings and cuts off any further communication of feelings.
    3 Too direct; does not allow the client time to reflect and explore feelings.
    4 Encourages dependence; does not allow for exploration of feelings.

52. **4** Emotional support and close surveillance can demonstrate the staff's caring and their attempt to prevent acting out of suicidal ideation. (b); IM; AP; PS; TC; CS
    1 This would be routinely done; by itself not necessarily therapeutic.
    2 This would be punishment for him; he could still find a way to kill himself in his room.
    3 This is not a suicide precaution.

53. **3** The staff's presence provides continued emotional support and helps relieve anxiety. (b); IM; AP; PS; PE; AD
    1 He may not, and if he does it will pass; emphasis on amnesia will increase fear.
    2 They may not make him better; would be false reassurance.
    4 This will be part of explaining the treatments; focus should not be on fear but on having someone with him.

54. **3** The relatively massive electrical energy passing through the cerebral cortex during ECT results in a temporary state of confusion after treatment. (b); EV; AP; PS; PA; AD
    1 Not a usual side effect.
    2 Not a side effect.
    4 Not an expected side effect.

55. **1** Succinylcholine chloride (Anectine) causes paralysis of muscles, including the intercostals and diaphragm, so artificial support of respirations is required to sustain life. (a); AN; KN; PS; PA; AD
    2 This is the purpose of the drug; not a disadvantage.
    3 This is the purpose of the drug; not a disadvantage.
    4 This is the purpose of the drug; not a disadvantage.

56. **2** Succinylcholine chloride temporarily paralyzes the muscles, including those of respiration. Therefore some artificial means of respiration is necessary until the drug is metabolized and excreted. (b), AN; KN; PS; PA; AD
    1 Pentothal decreases the possibility of nausea.
    3 This is necessary to prevent respiratory acidosis.
    4 The most significant therapeutic factor in ECT is the convulsion itself.

57. **2** Depressed clients find it difficult to express anger and hostility because they have internalized these feelings and turned them on themselves. (b); PL; AP; PS; PE; AD
    1 This would develop in time; not really a goal of therapy.
    3 There is nothing to indicate that Mr. Smith has unrealistic goals.
    4 This would be part of the intervention, not a goal.
58. **1** Severely depressed clients are not motivated to take action or to plan ahead. They are unable to direct their energy on the environment. (c); PL; AP; PS; PE; AD
    2 This would be helpful to a severely depressed client, whose attention span is limited.
    3 This would be helpful to a severely depressed client, since it requires little thought and provides gratification and satisfaction.
    4 This would be helpful for a person with depression as well as for the mentally retarded.
59. **3** Before teaching, the nurse must determine the client's areas of concern. Learning increases when anxiety decreases, and it is hoped that knowledge will reduce anxiety. (c); IM; AN; SU; ED; RE
    1 Although this may be part of the information included in preopeartive teaching, the teaching should begin at the client's level.
    2 The client will be dependent on a respirator postoperatively; breathing exercises are not required.
    4 This is not beneficial for all preoperative clients.
60. **2** Poor dental hygiene may predispose a person to oral infections but would be only remotely involved in laryngeal neoplasms. (c); AS; KN; SU; PA; RE
    1 Alcohol is an irritant which may initiate a tissue change that results in a malignant neoplasm.
    3 The irritation of air pollutants may initiate a tissue change that can lead to malignancy.
    4 Tissue alterations caused by repeated microbiologic stress may result in a malignant neoplasm.
61. **3** Secretions are increased because of alterations in structure and function. A patent airway must be maintained. (b); IM; AP; SU; PA; RE
    1 The orthopneic position may cause neck flexion and block the airway.
    2 The outer tube is not removed because the stoma may close.
    4 Whispering can put tension on the suture line; initially nonverbal and written forms of communication should be encouraged.
62. **4** Slow feeding of foods with reduced carbohydrate content helps to prevent rapid peristalsis and subsequent diarrhea. (c); PL; AP; SU; TC; GI
    1 The energy value of food is not related to its effect on intestinal peristalsis; carbohydrates should be reduced to prevent rapid emptying of the stomach and a shift of fluid into the intestinal lumen.
    2 The diarrhea is unrelated to the digestibility of the feedings.
    3 High fluid content shortens the time the feeding will remain in the stomach, leading to increased peristalsis and diarrhea.
63. **2** Food should be avoided until the area is totally healed. This will keep the area from becoming irritated and contaminated and will generally promote healing. (c); IM; AP; SU; ED; GI
    1 Tube feedings are usually required for the first 2 weeks after surgery.
    3 The ability to belch has no bearing on the decision to resume oral feedings.

4 The ability to tolerate oral feedings is not necessarily lost; such feedings are withheld to prevent irritation to the surgical site.
64. **2** The client's concerns will be reduced if he knows the stoma will stay open long enough so another tube can easily be inserted. (b); IM; AN; SU; ED; RE
    1 The client is in no immediate danger and it is not imperative to notify the physician at once.
    3 A permanent opening into the trachea is formed after 2 to 3 weeks and will not close quickly.
    4 A permanent opening into the trachea is formed after 2 or 3 weeks, and a tube need not be promptly reinserted.
65. **3** The procedure should be explained so the client understands that the tracheostomy can serve as an entrance for bacteria and that cleanliness is imperative. (b); PL; AP; SU; ED; RE
    1 Sterile technique is not required; medical aseptic technique is adequate and realistic.
    2 Suctioning must be performed only as needed; a pattern is not necessary.
    4 Laryngectomized clients may no longer swim, since water will flood the lungs.
66. **2** Valium is a tranquilizer and anticonvulsant used to relax smooth muscles during seizures. (a); EV; CP; ME; ED; MN
    1 This in not an effect of Valium.
    3 This is not an effect of Valium.
    4 This is not an effect of Valium.
67. **1** Serum albumin is administered to maintain serum levels and normal oncotic pressures. It does this by pulling fluid from the intestitial spaces into the intravascular compartment, thus decreasing the hematocrit level. (c); EV; CP; ME; PA; GI
    2 Serum albumin will not affect blood ammonia levels; fluid accumulated in the abdominal cavity is best removed via paracentesis.
    3 The administration of albumin results in a shift of fluid from the interstitial to the intravascular compartment; this will probably increase the BP.
    4 Albumin administration does not affect venous stasis or blood urea nitrogen.
68. **1** Albumin acts to elevate the BP to normal levels when it is administered slowly and oral fluid intake is restricted. It causes fluid to move from the interstitial spaces into the circulatory system. (b); IM; AN; ME; TC; GI
    2 Rapid administration could cause circulatory overload; high fluid intake would limit the shift of fluid from the interstitial to the intravascular compartment, interfering with the optimal effects of the drug.
    3 Fluids are restricted to facilitate the optimal effects of the drug, which shifts fluids from the interstitial tissues to the intravascular compartment.
    4 Rapid administration could cause circulatory overload; fluid is restricted, not withheld.
69. **4** Paraldehyde is excreted through the lungs and gives off a specific identifiable odor. (c); EV; AP; ME; PA; MN
    1 Although some of this drug is eliminated through the kidneys, primary excretion is through the lungs.
    2 This drug is eliminated through the lungs and kidneys, not excreted in saliva.
    3 This drug is eliminated through the lungs and kidneys, not through the skin.
70. **2** Neomycin aids in reducing the intestinal flora that act on protein substances, causing the production of ammonia. Ammonia is detoxified in the liver. When the liver is unable to perform this function adequately, blood ammonia levels rise, causing encephalopathy. (c); AN; AP; ME; PA; GI

1 Although immune mechanisms may be limited in alcoholism and cirrhosis, the neomycin is administered to limit ammonia levels.

3 Bacteria in the intestines do not digest urea.

4 This does not occur; neomycin controls protein metabolism, a severe problem in liver disease.

71. **2** When the bladder contains large amounts of urine, it becomes distended and may push upward into the abdominal cavity, where it can be punctured. (a); IM; CP; SU; TC; GU

1 A urine specimen is not necessary; an empty bladder prevents accidental trauma to the bladder during a paracentesis.

3 This is not the rationale for wanting the bladder to be empty.

4 The amount of fluid in the bladder has no relationship to ascites.

72. **4** Elixir of terpin hydrate should be avoided because it contains alcohol and will promote an Antabuse reaction. (a); IM; AN; ME; ED; GI

1 These symptoms do not occur if the client ingests both Antabuse and alcohol.

2 These are not symptoms of an Antabuse reaction.

3 The client will not only be nauseated but also experience violent vomiting.

73. **3** Psychoemotional factors related to chronic illness often affect the individual's compliance with a medical regimen. These feelings must be explored and worked out for acceptance of the treatment plan. (b); IM; AP; PE; PE; EI

1 This may be helpful later, but Jane needs an opportunity now to share her feelings about the disease.

2 Adolescents need control but are capable of handling most of their health care needs.

4 Jane's knowledge and feelings should be explored.

74. **2** Before planning and instituting a teaching plan, the nurse must assess the client's attitudes, experience, knowledge, and understanding of the health problem. (b); IM; AN; PE; ED; EI

1 Before teaching can begin, assessment of the present level of the knowledge is necessary.

3 Before goals can be set, assessment must be carried out.

4 Before teaching begins, assessment and planning must occur.

75. **1** The acquiring of knowledge or understanding aids in developing concepts rather than skills or attitudes and is a basic learning task in the cognitive domain. (b); AN; CP; PE; ED; EI

2 The acquiring of skills and tasks is psychomotor learning.

3 The acquiring of skills and tasks is psychomotor learning.

4 The acquiring of values and attitudes is in the affective domain.

76. **2** As a result of hormones involved in growth and development, clients with juvenile diabetes have different and changing needs regarding nutrition and exogenous insulin. (a); PL; CP; PE; ED; EI

1 Adequate caloric intake is needed by the average-sized adolescent since adolescence is a time of growth.

3 Potatoes bread, and cereal contain necessary fiber and nutrients.

4 Some flexibility is needed to promote adherence to any dietary regimen.

77. **4** An insulin-dependent diabetic client must carry sugar or candy as a ready source of carbohydrate in the event of signs of hypoglycemia. (a); IM; AP; PE; ED; EI

1 This is an unnecessary and time-consuming procedure.

2 This is an unrealistic and unnatural pattern for an adolescent.

3 Jane should be made to feel a part of the family; the diabetic diet will have foods that will be nutritious for the entire family.

78. **2** The protein in milk and cheese may be slowly converted to carbohydrate (gluconeogenesis), providing the body with some glucose during sleep while the NPH is still acting. (b); PL; AP; PE; PA; EI

1 The foods chosen are rich in protein and will be utilized slowly.

3 The purpose of an evening snack is to cover for NPH activity during sleep.

4 Jane's physical size does not indicate a need to gain weight.

79. **3** When a client or family member asks for information, this is a clue identifying readiness for learning. (b); AN; AP; PE; ED; EI

1 Asking this question indicates readiness to learn.

2 Data are not evident to indicate this.

4 The question indicates a desire for more information.

80. **3** Some mothers will respond to mores and pressures by trying to nurse in spite of the fact that they would prefer to give the baby a bottle. The nurse should elicit more information before responding. (b); EV; AP; OB; PE; PP

1 Although true, the mother's statement indicates some reluctance to breast feed and should be further explored.

2 The baby's sucking and emptying the breasts will determine the amount of milk.

4 Untrue; successful breast feeding requires mastery, and many women are unable to do this.

81. **4** Daily washing of the breasts and nipples with water is sufficient for cleanliness; soap may be drying. (b); IM; AP; OB; ED; PP

1 Scrubbing as well as the use of soap may irritate and dry nipples, which may already be tender.

2 Unnecessary to use sterile water; the inside of the baby's mouth is not sterile.

3 Alcohol is drying; may leave a taste that causes the infant to reject the nipple.

82. **3** The pressure and tenderness resulting from accumulated milk can be relieved by manually expressing some of the fluid. (b); IM; AP; OB; ED; PP

1 The nurse is capable of independent action that involves client teaching.

2 Pain medications would be offered only if other measures were unsuccessful; limits transfer of medication to the infant through breast milk.

4 Very unsound advice; the mother needs to drink fluid and keep nursing to ensure the flow of breast milk.

83. **1** Frequently the emotional excitement of going home will diminish lactation and/or the letdown reflex for a brief period. When the mother has knowledge that this may happen and how to cope with it, the problem is apt to be a minor one and easily overcome. (b); IM; AP; OB; ED; PP

2 Lacks an explanation of why it happens as well as concrete instructions for remedying the situation.

3 Many factors (stress) inhibit lactation, and the client should be aware of this; false reassurance.

4 This supply may diminish or stop under stress factors; false reassurance.

84. **3** Most average-sized babies regulate themselves on an approximate 4-hour schedule. However, wide variations do exist. (b); IM; AP; OB; ED; PP

1 Although true, this does not answer the mother's question concerning the time for doing things.

2 It is best to allow the baby to set her own schedule; usually close to hospital routine.

4 Some of the episodes of crying do not indicate that the baby is hungry; the mother will learn the difference.

85. **3** Anovulation occurs in nursing mothers for varying periods. Lactation does affect the degree of infertility, but it is generally not a reliable method of birth control. (a); IM; AP; OB; ED; FS

   1 Untrue; lactation may delay menses but does not reliably suppress ovulation.

   2 Ovulation can occur without menstruation.

   4 Menstrual periods may not occur for several months; this would put undue strain on marital relationships.

86. **3** Ischemia causes tissue injury and the release of chemicals, such as bradykinin, that stimulate sensory nerves and produce pain. (b); AN; CP; ME; PA; CB

   1 Arterial spasm, resulting in tissue hypoxia and pain, is associated with angina pectoris.

   2 Tissue injury and pain occur in the myocardium.

   4 Arteries, not veins, are involved in the etiology of a myocardial infarction.

87. **3** Administration of oxygen increases the transalveolar O_2 gradient, which improves the efficiency of the cardiopulmonary system. This increases the oxygen supply to the heart. (b); AN; CP; ME; PA; CB

   1 This is not a specific or inclusive answer; increased oxygen to the heart cells will improve cardiac output, which may or may not prevent dyspnea.

   2 Pallor is usually associated with myocardial infarction.

   4 Although this may be true, it is not specific to heart cells, which are hypoxic when there has been a myocardial infarction.

88. **1** Until the client's condition has reached some degree of stability after myocardial infarction, routine activities such as changing sheets are avoided so the client's movements will be minimized and the cardiac workload reduced. (b); IM; AP; ME; TC; CB

   2 Changing all the linen causes unnecessary movement, which increases oxygen demands and makes the heart work harder.

   3 Activity is contraindicated because it increases oxygen consumption and cardiac workload.

   4 Any activity is counterproductive to rest; rest must take precedence so the cardiac workload will be reduced.

89. **2** Acute care of the client with a myocardial infarction is aimed at reducing the cardiac workload. Foods that are easily digested help reduce this workload. Sympathetic nervous system involvement causes decreased peristalsis and gastric secretion, so limiting food intake will help prevent gastric distention. (b); AN; CP; ME; PA; CB

   1 Gastric acidity is not reduced by a clear liquid diet.

   3 Weight control is not a concern immediately following coronary occlusion.

   4 Feces are in the intestine generally 4 days after the ingestion of foods. The client's desire to have a bowel movement will be the result of pre-hospitalization meals; the liquid diet will affect future elimination.

90. **2** The body's general inflammatory response to myocardial necrosis causes an elevation of temperature as well as leukocytosis within 24 to 48 hours. (b); EV; CP; ME; PA; CB

   1 This is not an expected finding after tissue damage associated with an infarction

   3 This is not a common complication after myocardial infarction; it is usually associated with phlebitis or multiple fractures.

4 This is not an expected complication after myocardial infarction.

91. **3** Visits by family members can allay anxiety and consequently reduce emotional stress, an important risk factor in cardiovascular disease (a); PL; AP; PS; PE; CS

   1 The client may be disturbed by current news. This would raise the metabolic rate, increasing oxygen demands on the heart.

   2 Family, community, or work problems conveyed by phone may cause anxiety; only vital communications with family should be permitted.

   4 Television programs can cause anxiety or excitement, which would increase the metabolic rate and cardiac output.

92. **3** The presence of a P wave before each QRS complex indicates a sinus rhythm. A heart rate of over 100 beats per minute is referred to as tachycardia. (a); AN; CP; ME; PA; CB

   1 Atrial fibrillation causes irregular rhythm.

   2 Ventricular fibrillation is irregular and shows no PQRST configurations.

   4 Heart block pattern is irregular and slow.

93. **1** Signs of digitalis toxicity include cardiac arrhythmias, anorexia, nausea, vomiting, and visual disturbances. Cardiac arrhythmias result from the inhibition, by digitalis, of myocardial Na^+, K^+, and ATP. Extracardiac effects may be due to CNS or local disturbances. (a); EV; AN; ME; PA; CB

   2 Although nausea and heartblock may occur with lidocaine, these symptoms are rarely seen; drowsiness and CNS disturbances are more common side effects of lidocaine.

   3 Toxic effects of morphine sulfate are slow deep respirations, stupor, and constricted pupils; nausea is a side effect, not a toxic effect.

   4 Nausea is a side effect of meperidine hydrochloride (Demerol); toxic effects include dilated pupils, tremor, confusion, and respiratory depression.

Comprehensive Test 2: Part 2*

94. **2** A low-residue diet limits stool formation. (a); PL; CP; SU; PA; GI

   1 A high-protein diet is indicated postoperatively to promote healing.

   3 Bland diets are usually employed in the management of upper, not lower, GI disturbances.

   4 Although a clear diet is low in residue, it does not meet normal nutritional needs; a poor nutritional status increases the risk of postoperative complications.

95. **3** Sitz baths provide moist heat, which dilates the blood vessels and promotes circulation. It also relieves local inflammation and itching. (b); IM; AP; SU; PA; GI

   1 Medicated suppositories are used preoperatively but not after surgery because of the possibility of causing bleeding.

   2 This would not alleviate pain.

   4 Ice may alleviate pain; but it also causes vasoconstriction, which can impair healing.

96. **1** Moist cotton is not irritating and is the most soothing to the anal mucosa. (b); IM; AP; SU; TC; GI

---

*A key to the letters following the correct rationale can be found on p.633.

How to Use Worksheet 1: Errors in Processing Information

Common errors in processing information are listed in the left-hand column of this worksheet. At the top of the worksheet is a row of blank spaces for inserting the number of the question missed. Directly below each number, check any errors you made in answering that question. You may have made more than one type of error in an answer.

Worksheet 1: Errors in processing information

Question number																					
Did not read situation/question carefully																					
Missed important details																					
Confused major and minor points																					
Defined problem incorrectly																					
Could not remember terms/ facts/concepts/principles																					
Defined terms incorrectly																					
Focused on incomplete/incorrect data in assessing situation																					
Interpreted data incorrectly																					
Applied wrong concepts/principles in situation																					
Drew incorrect conclusions																					
Identified wrong goals																					
Identified priorities incorrectly																					
Carried out plan incorrectly/incompletely																					
Was unclear about criteria for evaluating success in achieving goals																					

How to Use Worksheet 2: Knowledge Gaps

Types of common knowledge gaps are listed along the top of this worksheet. Write a brief description of topics you want to review in the spaces provided. For example, if you missed a question on administration of a particular drug, write the drug name and problem (e.g., dosage) in the appropriate space under the column labeled *Pharmacology*.

Worksheet 2: Knowledge gaps

Basic science	Skills/ procedures	Basic human needs	Growth & develop- ment	Normal nutrition	Psycho- social factors	Clinical area/ topic	Stressors/ coping mechanisms	Patho- physiology	Pharma- cology	Therapeutic nutrition	Legal implications	Other

2 Betadine may cause excessive drying and irritation; the rectum is normally contaminated; external cleansing with Betadine will not appreciably affect the bacteria present.

3 Sterile gauze pads are not needed; the rectal area is considered contaminated.

4 Moist cotton is softer and more effective in removing feces than is dry facial tissue, which is irritating and can cause trauma.

97. **2** The first phase of separation anxiety is protest, which is characterized by loud crying, rejection of all strangers, and inconsolable grief. (a); AS; AP; PE; ED; RE

   1 An 18-month-old is not so easily consoled when separated from parents.

   3 This would be indicative of despair, a more advanced stage of separation anxiety.

   4 Toddlers do not socialize well with peers.

98. **3** The child has progressed to the third phase, detachment, in which he resigns himself to the loss of his mother and superficially appears adjusted to his environment. (c); AN; AP; PE; ED; RE

   1 This is often the mistaken interpretation of such behavior.

   2 Eighteen-month-olds have not outgrown separation anxiety.

   4 Staff members are usually viewed by toddlers as unfamiliar, frightening, and often threatening.

99. **2** Hearing is a sense that is not greatly influenced by emotional response in the young child. (b); AN; CP; PE; PA; MN

   1 Institutionalized children often manifest delays in neuromuscular development.

   3 The emotional trauma of institutionalization will influence the child's cognitive development.

   4 The trauma of institutionalization may also result in speech and other expressive delays.

100. **1** The child experiencing long-term hospitalization is forced to relate to a variety of significant adults instead of to a single figure providing mothering. The lack of continuity creates anxiety. (a); AN; CP; PE; PE; MN

   2 Even with sufficient sensory stimulation, the young child will still suffer from the lack of a mother figure.

   3 Although mother surrogates are helpful, they do not replace the mother figure.

   4 Even with sufficient play objects, the child will still suffer from the lack of a mother figure.

101. **1** The child learns to love others by the love he receives. When her receives love, he feels he is worthy of being loved and can share this feeling with others. (a); AN; CP; PE; PE; MN

   2 These children have difficulties forming attachments to people.

   3 Studies do not address this issue.

   4 Studies do not address this issue.

102. **4** Until trust has been reestablished, the child will be unable to develop an emotional tie to his mother. (b); IM; AP; PE; PE; MN

   1 At this stage of separation anxiety, the child would be too detached to be hostile.

   2 In extreme cases of separation, the child will be withdrawn from his parents.

   3 The child will be despairing and withdrawn.

103. **2** An oral contraceptive program requires taking 1 tablet daily from the fifth day of the cycle and continuing for 20 or 21 days. Interrupting the monthly dosage program may permit release of luteinizing hormone, then ovulation, and then possible pregnancy. (b); IM; AP; OB; PA; FS

   1 Untrue; there is a very high rate of success if the oral contraceptive is taken regularly and correctly.

   3 Too much information being given; also telling the client not to worry may close off communication.

   4 Judgmental; a value statement on the part of the nurse. Contraceptive practice is the client's choice.

104. **3** Knowing that others share the same problems may be comforting. The second part of the nurse's statement is open ended and allows the client to describe her physical and emotional feelings. (a); AN; AP; OB; PA; PN

   1 Telling the client not to worry closes off communication; does not allow exploration of avenues for further discussion.

   2 Too factual; closes off communication. The client needs to explore with the nurse the means for feeling better.

   4 Within the nursing purview; should be handled at this time.

105. **4** Before health teaching is instituted, the nurse should ascertain the client's past experiences; they will influence the teaching plan. (b); AS; AP; OB; ED; PN

   1 This answer does not give the client a chance to discuss her feelings about the examination.

   2 This answer does not give the client a chance to discuss her feelings about the examination; the nurse can only assume that the client's concerns are related to discomfort.

   3 Presupposes a yes or no answer; does not really give the client an opportunity to discuss it further.

106. **3** In calculating the expected date of delivery, subtract 3 months and add 7 days to the date of the last menstrual period. (b); AS; KN; OB; PA; PN

   1 Incorrect; count back 3 months and add 7 days.

   2 Incorrect; count back 3 months and add 7 days.

   4 Incorrect; count back 3 months and add 7 days.

107. **2** Successful dietary teaching usually incorporates, as much as possible, the client's food preferences and dietary patterns. (c); AS; AP; OB; ED; PN

   1 This does not take into consideration the client's likes and dislikes or cultural preferences; would not foster compliance.

   3 Salt is not limited during pregnancy unless a disease process is present or develops; seasoned foods are permissible if the client does not experience discomfort from them.

   4 This presupposes that the client has been eating a normal diet; does not provide for additional caloric or protein requirements of pregnancy.

108. **4** Maintaining the sitting position for prolonged periods may constrict the vessels of the legs, particularly in the popliteal spaces, as well as diminish venous return. Walking contracts the muscles of the legs, which apply gentle pressure to the veins in the legs, and promotes venous return. (b); AN; AP; OB; PA; PN

   1 A better means of improving circulation would be to walk about several times each morning and afternoon; she could also keep her legs elevated while sitting at her desk.

   2 If she is feeling well, there are no contraindications to working until her due date.

   3 Adequate nourishment can be obtained during meal times; she does not require extra nutrition breaks.

109. **4** When the membranes rupture, the potential for infection is increased; and when the contractions are 5 to 8 minutes apart, they are usually of sufficient force to warrant medical supervision. Therefore, for the safety of the mother and fetus, the mother should go to the hospital. (b); PL; AP; OB; PA; PN

1 This is indicative of advanced labor, and the client may have difficulty getting to the hospital at this time.

2 Too early; the client still has a great deal of time and would be better off with her family and moving about at home.

3 These may be early signs of labor or signs of posterior labor.

110. **3** The FHR is usually between 120 and 160 beats per minute. This is to be expected normally, and the mother should be made aware of this fact. (a); IM; AP; OB; ED; PN

1 This is too variable; the normal heart rate for a fetus is 120 to 160 beats per minute.

2 To accommodate to the oxygen needs of the fetus, the heart rate is rapid.

4 Unnecessary information; the mother should be informed only of that which is normal.

111. **2** Lets him know that the nurse understands adjustment will have to be made. It also is open ended enough to let him talk about feelings. (b); IM; AP; PS; PE; CS

1 Has not expressed his feelings enough for the nurse to offer any specific suggestions for help.

3 Not open ended enough to foster expression of feelings about what is bothering him.

4 This may compound his anxiety; also does not let him explore feelings.

112. **1** Since her diabetes appears to be out of control, dietary indiscretions or changes should be ruled out. Information about habits can be elicited only during a client interview. (b); EV; AN; ME; PA; EI

2 This information can be objectively assessed by examination of past and present medical records, which should serve as the primary source for these types of data.

3 This information can be objectively assessed by examination of past and present medical records, which should serve as the primary source for these types of data.

4 This information can be objectively assessed by examination of past and present medical records, which should serve as the primary source for these types of data.

113. **2** Taking a pill may give the client a false sense that the disease is under control, and this can lead to dietary indiscretions. (b); IM; CP; ME; PA; EI

1 A person's ability to follow dietary restrictions is highly individual; the employment setting is not a universal factor in such behaviors.

3 Individuals receiving insulin may also believe that their diabetes is under control and may not adhere to their prescribed diet; having to take any medication every day can be threatening to some people.

4 Diabetes is a chronic disease; and its complications can affect all individuals with the disease, particularly those who do not comply with the prescribed regimen.

114. **4** An understanding of the diet is imperative for compliance. A balance of carbohydrates, proteins, and fats usually apportioned over three main meals and two between-meal snacks needs to be tailored to the client's specific needs, with due regard for activity, diet, and therapy. (b); IM; CP; ME; ED; EI

1 True; however, indigestion is not the basis for the client's problems.

2 Total caloric intake, rather than the distribution of meals, is the major factor in weight gain.

3 Although restriction of calories and sodium is essential, a total dietary regimen must be followed to ensure adequate nutrition and control of the disease.

115. **4** Past experiences have the most meaningful influence on present learning. (b); PL; CP; PS; PE; CS

1 Although this consideration affects learning, its influence is not as great as that of all past experiences.

2 Although this consideration affects learning, its influence is not as great as that of all past experiences.

3 Although this consideration affects learning, its influence is not as great as that of all past experiences.

116. **2** Nonjudgmentally identifying the client's feelings encourages further verbalization about those feelings and the diet. (a); IM; CP; PS; PE; CS

1 The nurse should first acknowledge the client's feelings and then assess the client's level of knowledge before imparting such information.

3 This response is inappropriate; no mention of specific foods.

4 Suggests that adherence the prescribed medical regimen is unnecessary.

117. **2** Fasting prior to the test is indicated for accurate and reliable results. Food will elevate the blood glucose levels through metabolism of the nutrients. (b); IM; AP; ME; ED; EI

1 Medications are withheld because of their influence on blood sugar.

3 Clear fluids contain carbohydrates, which will increase the blood glucose levels.

4 Food should not be ingested; it will raise the serum glucose levels, negating the accuracy of the test.

118. **2** Cough syrup contains a sugar base. This must be taken into account by diabetic clients. (b); IM; AN; ME; ED; EI

1 Additional glucose may increase serum glucose levels without altering sugar and acetone results; once control is achieved, it is unwise to alter dietary intake or medication without supervision.

3 Elixirs have an alcohol base and also contain sweeteners.

4 Although this will loosen secretions, it will not suppress a cough.

119. **4** In diabetes mellitus, progressive thickening of the capillary basement membranes and medial sclerosis of small arteries leading to the eyes gradually occlude the vessel lumina. This significantly reduces retinal perfusion and leads to blindness. (b); AN; AP; ME; PA; EI

1 There is usually an increase in serum glucose with diabetes mellitus; thickening of the capillary basement membranes often occurs, even if the glucose level is maintained within normal limits.

2 There is usually an increase in serum glucose with diabetes mellitus; thickening of capillary basement membranes often occurs, even if the glucose level is maintained within normal limits.

3 Ketones do not usually affect retinal metabolism; retinopathy is due to vascular changes, retinal detachment, and hemorrhage within the eye.

120. **3** Damage to Broca's area, located in the posterior frontal region of the dominant hemisphere, causes problems in the motor aspect of speech. (a); AN; CP; ME; PA; MN

1 This would be associated with receptive aphasia, not expressive aphasia; receptive aphasia is associated with disease of Wernicke's area.

2 This would be associated with receptive aphasia, not expressive aphasia; receptive aphasia is associated with disease of Wernicke's area.

4 Although difficulty writing may be associated with expressive aphasia, understanding speech would be associated with receptive aphasia.

121. **4** Giving adequate time to respond and employing a calm, accepting, deliberate, and interested manner will reduce the client's anxiety and tension as well as increase self-esteem. (a); IM; AP; ME; PE; MN
    1 Sensory pathways are unaffected; she can see, hear, and understand.
    2 Isolation is not therapeutic; the client must be encouraged to remain in contact with others.
    3 The client should continue to speak so she can develop new pathways and gradually improve her speech.
122. **1** Assuming a normal position for voiding reduces tension (physical and psychologic), facilitates the movement of urine into the lower portion of the bladder, and relaxes the external sphincter (increasing pressure and initiating the micturition reflex). (c); IM; AP; ME; PA; MN
    2 Bladder training should be instituted by encouraging voiding every 1 to 2 hours and progressively increasing the time between voiding.
    3 This is an extremely large fluid intake and will result in a large volume of urine, probably increasing the frequency of incontinence.
    4 Voiding should be encouraged at regular and frequent intervals during waking hours, not just in the afternoon.
123. **2** Left-sided paresis creates instability. Using a cane provides a wider base of support and, therefore, greater stability. (a); AN; CP; ME; TC; MN
    1 Activity should not injure but strengthen weakened muscles.
    3 Since inflammation of these joints is not mentioned, this is unnecessary.
    4 The use of a cane will not prevent involuntary movements if they were present.
124. **3** The body is supported partially on the affected limb and partially on the cane as the unaffected limb moves forward. (b); IM; AP; ME; ED; MN
    1 The cane is held on the unaffected side and advanced at the same time as the affected extremity to increase the base of support and provide stability.
    2 Leaning the body will change the center of gravity and cause instability.
    4 Normal ambulation should be approximated; this would produce an awkward gait and instability.
125. **2** Vitamin K stores are almost absent in the newborn because the intestinal flora that produces this vitamin is not present. Vitamin K is an essential precursor of prothrombin, which is part of the clotting mechanism. (b); IM; CP; OB; PA; NH
    1 Increased bilirubin in the blood occurs in newborns because of the rapid breakdown of RBCs and the liver's difficulty in conjugating such large amounts; not influenced by vitamin K.
    3 The normal flora develops as the newborn is exposed to extrauterine living conditions.
    4 The young kidneys operate at a functional level appropriate to the needs of a healthy infant; not influenced by vitamin K.
126. **2** Drug dependence in the newborn is physiologic. As the drug is cleared from the body, symptoms of drug withdrawal become evident. Tremors, irritability, difficulty sleeping, twitching, and convulsions may result. (b); EV; CP; OB; PA; NH
    1 Symptoms of drug withdrawal involve signs of excessive stimulation.
    3 Dehydration is secondary to poor feeding; not a result of withdrawal per se.

    4 Hypertonicity of muscles would be seen.
127. **3** Drug-dependent newborns are poor feeders because of hyperactivity, nausea, vomiting, respiratory distress, excessive mucus, and pyrexia. Small frequent feedings should be given to prevent dehydration. (c); PL; AP; OB; PA; NH
    1 To minimize extraneous stimulation, environmental stimuli should be decreased.
    2 Infants of drug-addicted mothers are prone to hypothermia, not hyperthermia.
    4 Infants need supportive care during the time the drug is leaving their systems; methadone only modifies withdrawal, does not prevent it.
128. **3** The nurse should attempt to support the mother-child relationship. The mother is experiencing a developmental crisis while having to deal with drug addiction and possibly guilt. (a); IM; AP; PS; PE; CS
    1 Melanie needs contact with her new infant to facilitate bonding.
    2 The timing for this is after adjustment to the present situation has begun.
    4 This will make Melanie feel guilty and not facilitate positive action at this point.
129. **4** The immediate postburn period is marked by dramatic alterations in circulation because of large fluid losses through the denuded skin, vasodilation, edema formation, and a direct response on the contractility of the heart muscle. The precipitous drop in cardiac output causes shock. (a); AN; AN; PE; PA; EI
    1 Pneumonia would be a later complication associated with immobility.
    2 Contractures are a later complication associated with scarring and aggravated by improper positioning and splinting.
    3 Fluid dynamics are drastically altered; dehydration is a concern closely following shock in importance.
130. **3** Body weight is used in the calculation of body surface area. It is the main criterion in determining drug dosage and fluid requirements. (b); AN; CP; PE; TC; EI
    1 It is inappropriate to be concerned about growth in the face of an acute situation.
    2 Measurement of the burned surface is determined by parts of the body involved.
    4 Dietary management is a later consideration.
131. **3** High fever and disorientation may be initial indications of dehydration and/or early signs of hypoxia from respiratory complications. (c); AS; AN; PE; PA; EI
    1 Tachycardia is normally associated with the early phases of burn injury; vomiting may be a sign of circulatory collapse or paralytic ileus or may be nonspecific.
    2 High temperatures and increased basal metabolic rate are seen with burns.
    4 Decreased BP is rarely seen unless the client is in severe shock.
132. **2** The minimum urine volume is 10 to 20 ml per hour in children under 2 years and 20 to 40 ml per hour in children over 2 years of age. (b); EV; KN; PE; TC; RG
    1 This is the minimum safe output in children under 2 years.
    3 This volume is higher than minimum.
    4 This volume is higher than minimum.
133. **4** Because their verbal ability is limited, children act out their feelings via play. (a); IM; CP; PE; PE; EI
    1 Acceptance of the hospital situation is not as important as dealing with her own feelings.
    2 Therapeutic play does not necessarily involve other children.
    3 Mary needs to cope with her feelings rather than forget them.

134. **2** By the client's lying on her affected side, the unaffected lung can expand to its fullest potential. Elevation of the head facilitates respirations by reducing the pressure of the abdominal organs on the diaphragm and allowing the diaphragm to descend with gravity. (c); IM; AN; SU; TC; RE

   1 Maximum lung expansion is inhibited when the head is not elevated.

   3 Unclear as to what "left side supported" means. Although it facilitates diaphragmatic movement, it does not assist expansion of the right lung.

   4 Pressure against the right thorax limits right intercostal expansion and gaseous exchange in the right lung; the supine position allows the abdominal viscera to restrict contraction of the diaphragm and does not permit the diaphragm to drop by gravity.

135. **1** The rate and characteristics of respiration should be assessed so the amount of exertion required for breathing can be determined. The nurse should also evaluate signs such as unilateral chest movements that may indicate pneumothorax and tachypnea, which are associated with hypercapnea and acidosis. (b); AS; AN; SU; PA; RE

   2 Excessive blood loss might affect BP, but such bleeding would be indicated first by respiratory changes because the blood would accumulate in the pleural space; pupillary response would be unaffected.

   3 Drainage may accumulate in the pleural space, which is inaccessible for direct assessment.

   4 Although important, it is not a life-threatening symptom.

136. **4** Maintains negative intrathoracic pressure by limiting the amount of air rushing in from the outside. This can result in total pneumothorax and mediastinal shift, severely embarrassing respiration. (b); AN; CP; SU; TC; RE

   1 Major blood vessels are not occluded by a thoracic pressure dressing.

   2 A sterile dressing without pressure would suffice in preventing contamination.

   3 The dressing does not prevent injury to the pleura.

137. **4**

$$\frac{\text{Total amount to be infused} \times \text{Drop factor}}{\text{Total time for infusion (in minutes)}}$$

$$\frac{3000 \times 20}{24 \times 60} = 41.66 \text{ drops/min}$$

   (b); IM; AP; SU; PA; CB

   1 Inaccurate calculation; would not deliver an adequate amount of fluid.

   2 Inaccurate calculation; would not deliver an adequate amount of fluid.

   3 Inaccurate calculation; would not deliver an adequte amount of fluid.

138. **1** Retention of carbon dioxide in the blood lowers the pH, causing respiratory acidosis. Deep breathing maximizes gaseous exchange, ridding the body of excess carbon dioxide. (b); IM; CP; SU; PA; RE

   2 Although regular deep breathing improves the vital capacity, residual volume is unaffected.

   3 Deep breathing improves oxygenation of the blood, but it does not affect volume.

   4 Deep breathing increases the partial pressure of oxygen.

139. **2** Leakage of air into the subcutaneous tissue is evidenced by a crackling sound when the area is gently palpated. This is referred to as crepitus. (c); EV; AN; SU; TC; RE

   1 To minimize the risk of pneumothorax, the dressing is not routinely changed.

   3 The system is kept closed to prevent the pressure of the atmosphere from causing a pneumothorax; drainage levels are marked on the drainage chamber to measure output.

   4 Although hemostats should be readily available for any client with chest tubes in the event of a break in the drainage system, clamping the tube would not be otherwise necessary.

140. **2** Immediately prior to administration, an assessment of vital signs is necessary to determine whether any contraindications to analgesia exist (e.g., hypotension, a respiratory rate of 12 or less). (c); EV; AP; SU; PA; RE

   1 Pain prevents both psychologic and physiologic rest.

   3 Before administration, the nurse must check the physician's orders, the time of the last administration, and the client's vital signs.

   4 Prior to determining the time of the last dose, the nurse should record the client's vital signs; client's status must be evaluated further.

141. **1** Talking in the third person reflects poor ego boundaries and a dissociation from the real self. (a); AN; CP; PS; PE; SD

   2 Reaction formation is the expression of an emotion opposite the one really felt.

   3 Displacement is the attempt to reduce anxiety by transferring the emotions associated with one object or person to another.

   4 Transference is the movement of emotional energy and feelings from one person to another.

142. **2** These clients need sensory stimulation to maintain orientation and should be encouraged to do as much as possible for themselves, depending on their ability. (c); PL; AP; PS; PE; SD

   1 Surroundings should be bright to minimize confusion of stimuli.

   3 Clients are usually not completely out of contact with reality; it is important to differentiate fantasy from reality, but this would not take top priority in care.

   4 Although it is important to make certain that clients receive physical hygiene and comfort, they should be encouraged to help themselves as much as possible.

143. **4** When the client's perceptions are especially frightening, the nurse must let her know that her fears are recognized as real and frightening to her even if the nurse does not share her perceptions. Staying with the client will convey concern as well as reduce her fears. (b); IM; AP; PS; PE; SD

   1 Nontherapeutic; the voices are real to the client.

   2 Nontherapeutic; the client is unable to separate the voices from reality.

   3 The client will be unable to play cards because she cannot concentrate when the voices are speaking to her.

144. **3** This response points out reality while attempting to let the client understand that the nurse sees her as a person of worth. (c); IM; AN; PS; PE; SD

   1 This is a somewhat punitive response; cuts off communication.

   2 Nontherapeutic; the client may indeed see herself as a devil.

   4 Asks the client to explain feelings, an unrealistic goal.

145. **2** Major tranquilizers tend to make the client listless or drowsy and can interfere with the ability to participate in the therapeutic regimen. (b); AN; CP; PS; TC; SD

   1 Major tranquilizers do not really induce sleep; just listlessness.

   3 Major tranquilizers do not appreciably affect diurnal rhythms.

4 Assaultiveness is associated with increased anxiety rather than time.

146. **1** Liver damage is a well-documented toxic side effect of the major tranquilizers. By continuing to administer the drug, the nurse failed to use professional knowledge in the performance of responsibilities as outlined in the Nurse Practice Act. (b); EV; AP; PS; PA; SD

   2 The tranquilizer should be stopped not reduced; liver damage is a well-documented toxic side effect.

   3 False; liver damage, indicated by jaundice, is a well-documented side effect.

   4 False; blood levels must be reduced when signs of liver damage are present.

147. **4** The delusional client can never be argued out of a delusion, since it serves as a defense against reality and is the client's reality. It is best to accept the delusion without discussion. (c); IM; AP; PS; PE; SD

   1 This action can lead to increased feelings of guilt about the delusion since the client will not understand why the nurse is changing the topic.

   2 Encouraging discussion gives credulence to the delusion rather than pointing out reality to the client.

   3 The client would have difficulty getting involved in a repetitive activity, and the activity would not stop the delusion.

148. **1** When an individual expresses interest in physical appearance, it demonstrates a rebuilding of the self-image and the return of feelings of worth and conern for how others see them. (a); EV; CP; PS; PE; SD

   2 The information provided does not demonstrate a need for social reassurance or approval.

   3 The client's response goes further than the nurse's implied suggestion; she is expressing her own needs.

   4 The client's response is well within the normal range; does not indicate the beginning of a hyperactive phase.

149. **1** If the client is to remain at home, she must be aware of when to notify the physician of her symptoms. (b); AS; AN; OB; ED; HP

   2 The actual causes of spontaneous abortion are not known.

   3 This is factual information; will not alleviate anxiety concerning a possible abortion.

   4 Too broad an explanation; unrelated to the worry about abortion.

150. **2** Tension may be the precipitating cause of gastroesophageal reflux early in pregnancy. Displacement of the stomach and delayed emptying of stomach contents because of uterine enlargement may be the cause of heartburn later in pregnancy. (c); IM; AP; OB; ED; PN

   1 This would allow acid to pass into the small intestine.

   3 Gastric motility and acidity are generally decreased in pregnancy.

   4 Increased motility would utilize acid, leaving little or none to be regurgitated.

151. **3** The increase of estrogen during pregnancy causes hyperplasia of the vaginal mucosa, which leads to increased production of mucus by the endocervical glands. The mucus contains exfoliated epithelial cells. (b); IM; AP; OB; ED; PN

   1 Increased metabolism leads to many systemic changes but does not increase vaginal discharge.

   2 Normal functioning of the glands, which lubricate the vagina during intercourse, remains unchanged during pregnancy.

   4 There is no additional supply of sodium chloride to the cells during pregnancy.

152. **1** The antibodies in human milk provide the newborn infant with immunity against all or most of the pathogens that the mother has encountered. (b); IM; CP; OB; ED; PN

   2 Complex carbohydrates are not required by the infant.

   3 Present in commercial formulas.

   4 Present in commercial formulas.

153. **3** Provides the mother an opportunity to express her concerns regarding prophylactic eye medication. (b); IM; AP; OB; PE; NH

   1 Blocks communication; instillation can be delayed for an hour.

   2 Does not respond to the mother's statement.

   4 Does not respond to the mother's statement.

154. **2** Maternal hypotension is a common complication of conduction anesthesia for labor, and nausea is one of the first clues that this has occurred. Elevating the extremities restores blood to the central circulation. (c); EV; AN; OB; TC; IP

   1 If signs and symptoms do not abate after elevation of the legs, the physician should be notified.

   3 If the FHR is being monitored, it is a constant process; if not, the FHR should be monitored every 15 minutes.

   4 This is not a specific observation after caudal anesthesia; it is part of the general nursing care during labor.

155. **1** A neat surgical incision is easier to repair and quicker to heal than an irregular laceration. (a); IM CP; OB; TC; IP

   2 An episiotomy will contribute to rather than limit postpartal discomfort.

   3 Contrariwise; upon healing it will tighten up the perineum.

   4 May or may not influence birth trauma to the fetus; usually reduces trauma to the mother.

156. **3** Respirations are normally abdominal, diaphragmatic, and irregular. The rate is 30 to 50 per minute. (b); AS; CP; OB; PA; NH

   1 The newborn's respirations are abdominal not thoracic.

   2 Retractions are a sign of respiratory distress.

   4 Stertorous breathing may indicate respiratory distress.

157. **3** After the need to survive (air, food, water) the need for comfort and freedom from pain closely follow. Care should be given in order of the client's needs. (b); PL; AN; ME; TC; MN

   1 Joints must be exercised to prevent stiffness, contractures, and muscle atony.

   2 Although bladder training should be included in care, it is not a priority when the client is in pain.

   4 Motivation and learning will not occur unless basic needs, such as freedom from pain, are met.

158. **2** The antiinflammatory action of acetylsalicylic acid (ASA) is effective in reducing the discomfort and pain associated with rheumatoid arthritis. (b); AN; KN; ME; PA; MN

   1 Methocarbamol is a muscle relaxant; it does not reduce the inflammation associated with arthritis.

   3 Cortisone is employed when more conservative treatment fails; its use is avoided because of associated adverse effects (e.g., osteoporosis, gastric ulceration, psychosis, decreased resistance, hirsutism, hyperglycemia, edema, hypertension).

   4 Gold salts are employed if more conservative treatment fails; they must be administered intramuscularly and are highly toxic.

159. **4** Maintenance of joints in extension offsets the deformity often seen in rheumatoid arthritis. It also frequently prevents potentially deforming contractures. (b); PL; AN; ME; PA; MN

1 Clients often assume a fetal position, which results in flexion contractures of all extremities; this should be avoided.

2 Pressure on the popliteal space can impede venous return, increasing the risk of thrombus formation; it can also promote knee flexion contratures.

3 The Fowler's position is not required; respiratory function is unimpaired.

160. **1** Incontinence without a physiologic basis is an act of hostility that the individual uses to deal with anxiety-producing situations. (a); AN; AN; PS; PE; CS

2 Incontinence is rarely the result of conscious effort.

3 Incontinence is not a necessary complication of age and inactivity; can be prevented by a bladder-training program.

4 Incontinence is often seen as a symbol of regression and loss of control.

161. **2** For psychologic equilibrium Mrs. Ryan's environment must be one of novel and changing stimuli, promoting physical activity and effective interaction with others. (b); PL; AP; PS; PE; CS

1 Since the client has been able to regain control of elimination, frequent toileting is unnecessary.

3 To prevent urinary stasis and dehydration, fluid intake should be encouraged.

4 Although stimulation is important, it should be vaired and the client's preferences taken into consideration; radio and television do not promote interaction.

162. **1** Since air-conduction hearing aids utilize the person's own middle ear, they increase hearing acuity in cases of diminished sensitivity of the cochlea. The amplified signal from the hearing aid gives the cochlea greater stimulation and promotes hearing. (b); AN; KN; ME; PA; MN

2 Perforation of the tympanic membrane prevents ossicular conduction, which involves transmission of resonant vibrations from the tympanic membrane to the ossicles to the cochlea; hearing aids will not correct this.

3 Immobilization of the ossicles prevents conduction of resonant vibrations from the tympanic membrane to the cochlea; air-conduction hearing aids will not correct this problem.

4 Destruction of the auditory nerve results in deafness because impulses cannot be transmitted to the brain's auditory center.

163. **4** GI distress causes disturbance in intestinal motility and absorption, acclerating excretion. IV fluids are necessary, since severe dehydration and fluid and electroltye imbalance occur rapidly and can lead to death in infancy because of the infant's large fluid content. (b); IM; AP; PE; PA; GI

1 This test is used to determine blood type when a transfusion is indicated.

2 Intestinal intubation with suction is utilized to remove stomach contents when there is blockage or it is necessary to have the GI tract clear of contents.

3 Isolettes serve to isolate, warm, and if necessary oxygenate small infants and newborns.

164. **2** Loss of fluid as a result of dehydration is most objectively assessed by measuring the child's weight, since total body water accounts for approximately 60% of body weight. (c); EV; CP; PE; PA; GI

1 This is a clinical sign of dehydration but not an accurate way to measure hydration.

3 Decreased urine output is hard to measure in individuals who are not toilet trained.

4 Dry skin may be indicative of conditions other than dehydration.

165. **1** Sodium, potassium, and bicarbonate are the electrolytes most often lost because of diarrhea. They are excreted before they can be absorbed. (b); AS; CP; PE; PA; GI

2 Chloride serves to maintain electrolyte neutrality and accompanies sodium losses or excesses.

3 Calcium serum levels are indicators of parathyroid function and calcium metabolism.

4 Phosphorus levels are determined by calcium metabolism, parathormone, and to a lesser degree intestinal absorption.

166. **3**
$$\frac{\text{Total amount} \times \text{Drop factor}}{\text{Total time (in minutes)}}$$
$$\frac{400 \times 50}{8 \times 60} = \frac{20,000}{480} = 41.6 \text{ or } 42 \text{ gtts}$$

(a); IM; AP; PE; PA; CB

1 Too slow to achieve fluid ordered.

2 Too slow to achieve fluid ordered.

4 Will provide more fluid than ordered.

167. **2** Clear liquids with sugar added provide glucose without bulk. (c); PL; AN; PE; PA; GI

1 Fruit juices may cause fermentation, which can stimulate peristalsis.

3 Ginger ale adds a great deal of unnecessary carbonation.

4 Clear liquids are best tolerated after a gastric upset.

168. **2** Weight is the best indicator of fluid loss if measured each day at the same time, on the same scale, and with the same amount of clothes. (b); EV; AN; PE; PA; GI

1 In cases of severe diarrhea, an IV is usually employed until the diarrhea is controlled; fluids are gradually added as tolerated.

3 Because of the diarrhea, food will not be properly absorbed.

4 This temperature is not unusual in infants.

169. **3** By 12 months of age a child can usually drink from a cup, although fluid may spill and a bottle may be preferred at times. (c); AN; CP; PE; ED; GI

1 The child is just beginning lip control at 5 months and cannot handle a cup.

2 At 7 months a child can handle a bottle but not a cup.

4 Since this skill is present at 12 months, by 18 months most children are quite proficient.

170. **2** In an attempt to ward off anxiety, the client in the manic phase runs headlong into it, becoming totally involved in everything that goes on in the environment. (b); AS; AN; PS; PE; MD

1 Just the opposite is true; psychomotor activity is greatly increased.

3 This would be more indicative of the depressive episode.

4 During this phase there is no insight into behavior.

171. **2** Overactive individuals are stimulated by environmental factors. A responsibility of the nurse is to simplify their surroundings as much as possible. (c); IM; AP; PS; PE; MD

1 During this phase the client needs a decrease in stimuli.

3 During this phase the client needs a decrease in stimuli; two overactive clients together would produce excessive stimuli.

4 The quiet client may become the target of her overactivity.

172. **3** Clients in the manic phase of a bipolar disorder are easily distracted. Rather than placing emphasis on their behavior, staff members should use the easy distractability of these clients to redirect this behavior to more constructive channels. (a); IM; AN; PS; PE; MD

1 Encourages the client to defend the statement rather than what is behind the statement; does not foster communications about feelings.

2 Focuses on the behavior; a punitive response does not foster communications.

4 She would be unable to tell the nurse why she was angry.

173. **2** This approach incorporates the principles of starting where the client is and helping the client verbalize feelings. It also provides for more data collection to carry out the nursing process. (b); IM; AN; PS; PE; MD

1 The cient is obviously not ready to do this.

3 Accepts her right not to be forced back to the group; however, another nursing intervention should be attempted at this time.

4 This would be a second step, after the initial nursing action, to plan future intervention.

174. **4** Because of the severity of side effects and the stress it places on the renal as well as the cardiovascular system, its administration is contraindicated in clients with renal or cardiovascular diseases. (b); AS; AN; PS; TC; MD

1 Not necessary; lithium does not alter neurologic functions.

2 Necessary after the start of lithium administration.

3 Necessary after the start of lithium administration.

175. **1** Metrorrhagia is uterine bleeding at any time other than during the menstrual period. (a); AN; KN; ME; PA; RG

2 Severe menstrual bleeding is menorrhagia.

3 This is menstruation when it occurs in a cyclic pattern after menarche.

4 This is dyspareunia.

176. **2** In a hysterectomy the uterus is removed, but no other female organs. Consequently menstruation ceases but the hypophyseal and ovarian hormone cycles continue. (a); PL; CP; SU; PA; RG

1 An oophorectomy was not performed; ovarian hormones continue to be secreted.

3 Removal of the uterus does not affect the secretion of ovarian hormones.

4 Normally menopause begins gradually; after an oophorectomy it begins immediately. However, an oophorectomy was not performed.

177. **4** Thrombophlebitis, common after pelvic surgery, is inflammation of a vein. The signs include pain, redness, swelling, and heat. It is associated with the formation of a clot (thrombosis). (a); EV; AP; SU; PA; RG

1 Classically thrombophlebitis is usually located in the area of the calf in a deep vein, not over a bony prominence.

2 Itching is not a symptom of phlebitis.

3 Although swelling accompanies thrombophlebitis, it is not a pitting edema.

178. **1** Menstruation is the shedding of the endometrial lining of the uterus. A female who has undergone hysterectomy has had her uterus removed and will no longer menstruate. (b); AN; AN; SU; PA; RG

2 After a hysterectomy there is no endometrial lining to shed.

3 Not a psychosomatic reaction, which would imply the presence of both physical and mental components; there is no uterus.

4 Frank bleeding is not expected postoperatively.

179. **2** Flushing of the head and neck with accompanying diaphoresis is known as hot flashes. It is a symptom of estrogen deprivation. (c); AN; CP; SU; PA; RG

1 Heat intolerance is not a symptom associated with estrogen deprivation.

3 Aging is not accelerated through lack of estrogen.

4 There is no menstruation after this surgery.

180. **2** When the intestine cannot be returned to the body cavity, the hernia is incarcerated. (c); AN; CP; SU; PA; GI

1 This is a strangulated hernia.

3 Erosion of intestinal tissue may be caused by a variety of conditions; usually results in perforation.

4 This is a volvulus.

181. **3** A possible complication of hernias is intestinal obstruction. If an obstruction occurs, there will be no passage of flatus or normal bowel movements. (b); AS; AP; SU; PA; GI

1 The supine position would have no effect on an incarcerated hernia.

2 This is done for all clients; not specific for a client with a hernia. Observation of signs of intestinal obstruction takes priority.

4 This would not assist in the definitive diagnosis of a hernia and its complications.

182. **4** Hernioplasty involves not only the reduction of a hernia but also an attempt to change or strengthen the structure to prevent recurrence. (b); AN; KN; SU; PA; GI

1 Herniorrhaphy is surgical repair of a hernia.

2 Analysis of the word shows that it means an opening cut into the hernia; does not refer to repair of a hernia.

3 There is no such word; hernias are not cut out. They are reduced and/or reinforced to prevent recurrence.

183. **1** After inguinal hernia repair, the scrotum frequently becomes edematous and painful. Drainage is facilitated by elevating the scrotum on a rolled towel or using a scrotal support. (c); IM; AP; SU; PA; GI

2 Obesity is a factor in the development of hernias; high-carbohydrate diets should not be encouraged.

3 Coughing increases intraabdominal pressure and may strain the operative site.

4 An abdominal binder would not support the operative site; the incision is too low.

184. **3** Placing the feet apart creates a wider base of support and brings the center of gravity closer to the ground. This improves stability. (b); IM; CP; SU; TC; GI

1 Bending at the waist should be avoided; strains the lower back muscles.

2 Pressure on the abdomen is prevented by tightening the abdominal and gluteal muscles to form an internal girdle; keeping the body straight does not reduce strain on the abdominal musculature.

4 Relaxing the abdominal muscles with physical activity increases strain on the abdomen.

185. **3** Gamma globulin provides passive immunity in infectious hepatitis. It is given to all individuals who come into direct contact with the client. (b); PL; CP; ME; ED; GI

1 Infectious hepatitis virus is found in the stools of infected individuals before the onset of symptoms and during the first few days of illness.

2 Gamma globulin is available; it is given 2 to 7 days after exposure with a second dose later.

4 Gamma globulin provides passive immunity in infectious hepatitis.

186. **4** Temperature during steaming is never high enough or sustained long enough to kill organisms. (b); IM; CP; ME; ED; GI

1 Because of the extremely high temperature, broiling sufficiently destroys the virus.

2 Not a shellfish; baking would destroy the organisms.

3 Processing destroys the organisms.

187. **4** Relapses are common. They occur after too early ambulation and too much physical activity. (b); PL; CP; ME; ED; GI

How to Use Worksheet 1: Errors in Processing Information

Common errors in processing information are listed in the left-hand column of this worksheet. At the top of the worksheet is a row of blank spaces for inserting the number of the question missed. Directly below each number, check any errors you made in answering that question. You may have made more than one type of error in an answer.

Worksheet 1: Errors in processing information

Question number																				
Did not read situation/question carefully																				
Missed important details																				
Confused major and minor points																				
Defined problem incorrectly																				
Could not remember terms/facts/concepts/principles																				
Defined terms incorrectly																				
Focused on incomplete/incorrect data in assessing situation																				
Interpreted data incorrectly																				
Applied wrong concepts/principles in situation																				
Drew incorrect conclusions																				
Identified wrong goals																				
Identified priorities incorrectly																				
Carried out plan incorrectly/incompletely																				
Was unclear about criteria for evaluating success in achieving goals																				

How to Use Worksheet 2: Knowledge Gaps

Types of common knowledge gaps are listed along the top of this worksheet. Write a brief description of topics you want to review in the spaces provided. For example, if you missed a question on administration of a particular drug, write the drug name and problem (e.g., dosage) in the appropriate space under the column labeled *Pharmacology*.

Worksheet 2: Knowledge gaps

Basic science	Skills/ procedures	Basic human needs	Growth & develop-ment	Normal nutrition	Psycho-social factors	Clinical area/ topic	Stressors/ coping mechanisms	Patho-physiology	Pharma-cology	Therapeutic nutrition	Legal implications	Other

1 Fatigue is a cardinal symptom; if the client is tired at rest, he should not return to work.

2 The majority of clients recover in 3 to 16 weeks with no further problems.

3 Hepatitis is most communicable before the onset of symptoms and during the first few days of fever.

Comprehensive Test 2: Part 3*

188. **3** A normal cardiopulmonary symptom in pregnancy, caused by increased ventricular rate and elevated diaphragm. (b); AS; CP; OB; PA; PN

1 This is pathologic, a sign of impending cardiac decompensation.

2 This is pathologic, a sign of impending cardiac decompensation.

4 This is pathologic, a sign of impending cardiac decompensation.

189. **3** Forceps reduce mother's need to push, conserving energy; regional anesthesia does not compromise cardiovascular function. (b); PL; AN; OB; TC; HP

1 Induced labor is often more stressful and painful than natural labor.

2 Major abdominal surgery is only performed on clients with cardiac problems when absolutely necessary.

4 Forceps reduce mother's need to push, conserving energy; however, general anesthesia would compromise cardiovascular function.

190. **2** This is because of the impedance of venous return by the gravid uterus, which causes hypotension and decreased systemic perfusion. (a); AN; AP; OB; PA; HP

1 This may be partially true, but more significantly, it is the least comfortable position and may cause hypotension.

3 Even if true, this is not significant as a factor of labor.

4 False; it can lead to supine hypotension.

191. **1** The rapid fluid shift causes an increase in cardiac output and blood volume, making the first 48 hours postpartum crucial. (b); PL; AN; OB; PA; HP

2 False; the first 48 hours are crucial because of the rapid fluid shift and need for increased cardiac output.

3 Progressive ambulation starting 48 hours after delivery is recommended.

4 Not recommended, since this will further increase circulating blood volume and necessitate increased cardiac output.

192. **3** This provides for collection of more data. (b); AS; AP; PS; PE; CS

1 This implies that things are not well, and the mother may be to blame.

2 This could make the mother guilty about not meeting her baby's needs.

4 This is a negative comment that closes communication.

193. **4** Suggested activity for a 2- to 3-month-old so that infant can more readily observe environment. (b); IM; AP; PE; ED; MN

1 Suggested activity for a 6- to 9-month-old.

2 Activity for 9- to 12-month-old.

3 Activity for 4- to 6-month-old.

194. **2** Appropriate sequence is fruits, vegetables, meats and table foods. (a); IM; KN; PE; ED; GI

1 Table foods should not be introduced before the infant can chew or bite (6 to 7 months).

3 Vegetables and fruits are introduced before meats because of the generous supply of vitamins and minerals; meats are high in saturated fats.

4 Vegetables or fruits should begin after cereal; avoid table foods until the infant can chew or bite.

195. **2** Streptococcal infections occurring in childhood may result in damage to the heart valves. An autoimmune reaction occurs between antibodies made against the bacteria and the heart valves, particularly the mitral. (b); AS; AN; ME; PA; CB

1 Rubella virus would not affect the valves of the heart.

3 Pleurisy usually follows pulmonary problems unrelated to streptococcal infection; would not result in damage to the heart valve.

4 Cystitis is usually caused by *Escherichia coli,* which would not affect the heart valves.

196. **2** The pulse should be assessed, since a cutdown may interfere with venous flow distal to the site. There is also a danger of phlebitis in the area. (a); IM; AP; SU; TC; CB

1 The client does not usually require additional rest after catheterization.

3 It is not necessary to check the ECG every 30 minutes following the procedure.

4 This would be determined on an individual basis; not routine.

197. **1** Because blood pools in the extremities, there is an increased hazard of peripheral emboli in clients who have received a mitral replacement. (c); EV; AP; SU; TC; CB

2 This is not a danger after mitral replacement.

3 Bleeding is detected by checking the wound dressing and observing for signs of shock (e.g., lowered BP, tachycardia, restlessness).

4 Peripheral pulses alone will not reveal atrial fibrillation; to detect the presence of a pulse deficit, one must compare them with the apical pulses.

198. **3** Temperatures over 102.2° F (38.9° C) lead to increased metabolism and cardiac workload. (a); AN; AN; SU; TC; CB

1 Elevated temperature is not an early sign of developing cerebral edema, although the temperature may rise eventually because of medullary compression.

2 Fever is unrelated to hemorrhage; in hemorrhage with shock, the temperature decreases.

4 These symptoms are caused by an elevated temperature, which is the primary reason for increased metabolism and cardiac workload.

199. **4** Fluid will accumulate in the intrapleural space after thoracic surgery because of trauma and the inflammatory response. During the first 24 hours 500 ml of fluid is not uncommon. Gradually this amount will decrease. (c); AS; AP; SU; PA; CB

1 Excessive amount; may indicate complications.

2 Less than expected; when no air leak is noted and less than 150 ml of fluid is aspirated in 24 hours, the tube may be removed.

3 Excessive amount; may indicate complications.

200. **1** Chills, headache, nausea, and vomiting are all signs of a transfusion reaction. (a); EV; AN; SU; TC; CB

2 The infusion must be stopped before treatment of the symptoms begins.

3 The physician should be notified after the transfusion is stopped.

4 Slowing the infusion will continue the reaction; may lead to kidney damage.

201. **3** Shivering should be prevented. Peripheral vasoconstriction increases the temperature, the circulatory rate, and oxygen consumption. (b); IM; CP; SU; PA; CB

1 Not a response to treatment with hypothermia.

---

*A key to the letters following the correct rationale can be found on p. 633.

2 Not a response to treatment with hypothermia.

4 Not a response to treatment with hypothermia.

202. **3** Different infusion sets deliver different, preset numbers of drops per ml. This number is necessary for calculating the drip rate. (a); IM; AP; SU; PA; CB

   1 This does not determine the drip rate.

   2 This does not determine the drip rate.

   4 This does not determine the drip rate, only the size of the drop.

203. **3** Symptoms are a defense against anxiety resulting from decision making, which triggers old fears; client needs support. (b); IM; AN; PS; PE; PD

   1 Judgmental; she should be encouraged to work through symptoms, not avoid risk.

   2 Judgmental; an increase in anxiety does not necessarily mean the client does not want to attain the goal.

   4 Denies the client's overwhelming anxiety and lacks realistic support.

204. **1** These clients can better work through their underlying conflicts when demands are reduced and the routine is simple. (a); AN; CP; PS; PE; PD

   2 Preventing these clients from carrying out rituals can precipitate panic reactions.

   3 Since anxiety stems from unconscious conflicts, a controlled environment alone is not enough to effect resolution.

   4 The intent of therapy should be to help the client gain control, not to enable others to do the controlling.

205. **4** Sets an unrealistic limit that would increase anxiety by removing a defense the client needs. (c); AN; CP; PS; PE; PD

   1 This is done in therapy as the client's condition improves. Insight is slowly developed to minimzie anxiety.

   2 This would increase self-esteem and self-control, not increase anxiety.

   3 This would reduce not increase anxiety since the client would feel free to express her feelings.

206. **4** It is important to set limits on behavior, but also to involve the client in decision making. (c); IM; AP; PS; PE; PD

   1 This would increase anxiety, since the client uses the ritual as a defense against anxiety.

   2 Nontherapeutic approach; some limits must be set by the client and nurse together.

   3 Nontherapeutic approach; rarely can a client be distracted from a ritual.

207. **3** Platelets are rapidly administered to avoid destruction after hanging IV. (c); IM; AP; PE; TC; CB

   1 Dextrose solution is not appropriate for flushing a blood derivative line because it may clog the tubing.

   2 Platelets should not hang for a long time because of their fragility.

   4 Too long an interval; during infusion of blood derivative, vital signs are more closely monitored.

208. **3** Many vitamins contain folic acid and are contraindicated with methotrexate, a folic acid antagonist. (b); IM; AP; PE; ED; CB

   1 Folic acid interferes with action of methotrexate.

   2 True, but does not answer question and leaves open vitamin use in the near future, which long-term chemotherapy contraindicates.

   4 Inaccurate; vitamin use is contraindicated.

209. **2** The most accurate and age-appropriate response to the child's question. (c); IM; AN; PE; ED; CB

   1 Insensitive to the question and does not provide any explanation.

   3 Inaccurate; not being truthful interferes with the development of trust.

   4 Inaccurate and may instill more fear.

210. **4** Chemotherapy causes severe alteration in mucous membranes; rectal temperatures may easily damage delicate rectal tissue. (a); AN; AN; PE; TC; CB

   1 True, but not the primary reason to avoid rectal temperatures in children with leukemia.

   2 Inaccurate; axillary temperatures are frequently used.

   3 Oral temperatures are accurate, provided the child can hold the thermometer in the mouth correctly and comfortably.

211. **3** Foam is soft, so it will not damage the oral mucosa. (a); PL; AP; PE; TC; CB

   1 Will injure the oral mucosa.

   2 Will irritate the mucosa and has an offensive taste.

   4 May irritate the oral mucosa and should always be diluted.

212. **4** Destroys leukemic cells in the brain because chemotherapeutic agents are poorly absorbed through the blood-brain barrier. (a); AN; CP; PE; PA; CB

   1 Inaccurate; this is not the reason for cranial radiation.

   2 Not the primary reason for the treatment; it is a curative measure.

   3 Inaccurate; ALL is an abnormality of the bone marrow and lymphatic system.

213. **1** Bed rest in the side-lying position keeps the pressure of the fetus off the cervix and enhances uterine perfusion. (b); PL; CP; OB; ED; HP

   2 Used only when cord is prolapsed or client is in shock.

   3 May aid in relieving pressure of fetus on cervix but will not enhance uterine perfusion.

   4 Sitting in bed will increase pressure on cervix; may lead to further dilation.

214. **2** Therapeutic regimen includes bed rest; peace of mind can best be achieved if children are adequately cared for. (c); IM; AP; PS; PE; CS

   1 Explores feelings without including the therapeutic regimen.

   3 Complete bed rest has been prescribed.

   4 This is giving solutions rather than exploring the situation with the client.

215. **2** Prostaglandins in semen may stimulate labor, and penile contact with the cervix may increase myometrial contractibility. (a); PL; AP; OB; TC; HP

   1 Sexual intercourse may cause labor to progress; not desired in week 33 of pregnancy with 2 cm dilation.

   3 Sexual intercourse may cause labor to progress; not desired in week 33 of pregnancy with 2 cm dilation.

   4 Sexual intercourse may cause labor to progress; not desired in week 33 of pregnancy with 2 cm dilation.

216. **2** Hypotension is an expected side effect of ritodrine, a sympathomimetic drug. (c); EV; CP; OB; TC; HP

   1 Reflexes not affected; this is necessary when using magnesium sulfate.

   3 Not given for diuretic action; this is necesary when using magnesium sulfate.

   4 Does not affect client's level of consciousness, merely relaxes uterine musculature.

217. **1** When protein intake is inadequate, the liver is unable to manufacture albumin, the major plasma protein. There is a drop in intravascular colloidal osmotic pressure, with a resulting fluid shift to the interstitial spaces. (c); AN; CP; ME; PA; GI

   2 The renin/aldosterone mechanism is not directly linked to inadequate nutrition.

   3 ADH is secreted when the intravascular osmotic pressure increases, not decreases.

   4 Nitrogen balance is the relationship between intake and output of nitrogen; linked only indirectly to fluid shifts.

218. **1** Total parenteral nutrition should be infused at a slow, constant rate. This will prevent both cellular dehydration from too rapid infusion of hypertonic solutions and hyperglycemia. (b); PL; AP; SU; TC; GI
    2 Monitoring vital signs may indicate a complication such as infection; will not prevent it.
    3 Generally a major vein is selected for administration of total parenteral nutrition; the site is not changed every 24 hours.
    4 Recording intake and output is essential because of the danger of fluid overload; however, will not prevent the complication.

219. **3** A gastrostomy is an opening made directly through the abdominal wall into the stomach. When tube feedings are given via this route, they bypass the upper GI tract and reduce the risk of tracheal aspiration. (b); PL; CP; SU; TC; GI
    1 The amount of feeding is not affected.
    2 Both methods utilize gravity.
    4 Clients can be taught to feed themselves with either method.

220. **4** A rise in the level of formula within the tube indicates a full stomach. (a); EV; AP; SU; PA; GI
    1 Passage of flatus reflects intestinal motility, which does not pose a potential problem.
    2 A rapid inflow is the result of holding the container too high or using a feeding tube with too large a lumen.
    3 Epigastric tenderness is not necessarily caused by a full stomach.

221. **2** Water is administered after the tube feeding to prevent the thicker feeding solution from obstructing the lumen of the tube. (b); IM; AP; SU; ED; GI
    1 Tube feedings are best tolerated at body temperature.
    3 To prevent regurgitation and aspiration, a Fowler's position is recommended.
    4 The feeding tube has been surgically inserted and fixed in place so position does not need to be determined.

222. **1** Since mastication of food is a psychologically satisfying activity, clients are advised to chew their food before putting it in the blender. (c); IM; AP; SU; ED; GI
    2 The texture as well as the taste of food provides a source of satisfaction; not experienced when food enters the stomach directly through a feeding tube.
    3 The texture as well as the taste of food provides a source of satisfaction; not experienced when food enters the stomach directly through a feeding tube.
    4 The texture as well as the taste of food provides a source of satisfaction; chewing gum does not provide this satisfaction.

223. **3** This test allows the physician to perform a biopsy of the gastric mucosa. (c); AS; CP; ME; PA; GI
    1 Done to determine the response of gastric secretion after an intravenous injection of secretin; normally there should be a decrease. This will not confirm the presence of malignant cells.
    2 Will outline structural changes; however, it will not identify the presence of malignant cells.
    4 Not a tissue study; will not confirm the diagnosis of cancer.

224. **3** The nurse was negligent in using a stretcher with worn straps. Such oversight did not reflect the actions of a reasonably prudent nurse. (b); EV; AP; ME; TC; GI
    1 The nurse is responsible for determining the safety of hospital equipment.
    2 The nurse is responsible for own actions and must ascertain the adequate functioning of equipment.

    4 The hospital shares responsibility for safe, functioning equipment.

225. **4** Barium salts used in a GI series and barium enemas coat the inner lining of the GI tract and then absorb x-rays passing through. They thus outline the surface features of the tract on a photographic plate. (a); IM; AP; ME; PA; GI
    1 Barium has no light-emitting properties.
    2 Barium does not fluoresce.
    3 Barium has no properties of a dye.

226. **3** Anxiety or stress causes a hypersecretion of hydrochloric acid. This produces actual physiologic changes in the tissue itself. (a); AN; CP; ME; PA; GI
    1 The changes are the result of psychologic conflicts that cause physiologic changes.
    2 Illness may result from psychologic conflicts but is not a defense mechanism.
    4 Physiologic changes do not cause psychologic changes.

227. **2** Hemorrhage after erosion of blood vessel walls is often the first symptom that leads the client to seek medical assistance. (b); AS; KN; ME; PA; GI
    1 Perforation would occur well after hemorrage, and treatment would have been sought at the time of hemorrhage.
    3 Not a common complication.
    4 Occur because of portal hypertension not peptic ulcers.

228. **2** Applesauce, Cream of Wheat, and milk are bland foods that do not irritate the gastric mucosa. (c); IM; AP; ME; TC; GI
    1 Not considered bland; may be irritating to the mucosal lining.
    3 Not considered bland; may be irritating to the mucosal lining.
    4 Not considered bland; may be irritating to the mucosal lining.

229. **4** Stimulation of the autonomic nervous system is a normal response to cord compression during uterine contraction (a); IM; AP; OB; PA; IP
    1 Requires no intervention at this time.
    2 Requires no intervention at this time.
    3 Done when deceleration occurs.

230. **3** Bradycardia (baseline FHR below 120 beats per minute) indicates fetal distress and requires medical intervention. (a); EV; AP; OB; TC; HP
    1 No indication of maternal distress.
    2 The normal FHR is 120 to 160 beats per minute.
    4 Dangerous; fetus is in distress, and time should not be spent on monitoring.

231. **2** Heat causes vasodilation and an increased blood supply to the area. (a); IM; CP; OB; TC; PP
    1 Sitz baths do not soften the incision site.
    3 Cleansing is done with perineal bottle immediately after voiding and defecating.
    4 Neither relaxation nor tightening of the rectal sphincter will increase healing of an episiotomy.

232. **3** Prevention of infection has priority. (b); PL; AP; OB; ED; PP
    1 Provides comfort but is not the priorty.
    2 Not necessary to stop sitz baths as long as they provide comfort.
    4 Stair climbing may cause some discomfort but is not detrimental to healing.

233. **3** In transfer, the suspected back-injured client should be positioned to keep the vertebral column in perfect alignment (back straight) to prevent further spinal cord damage by vertebral (bone) movements. (a); IM; AP; ME; TC; MN

1 To prevent additional damage to the spinal cord, the vertebral column should be kept in alignment.
2 To prevent additional damage to the spinal cord, the vertebral column should be kept in alignment.
4 To prevent additional damage to the spinal cord, the vertebral column should be kept in alignment.
234. **4** Both legs and generally the lower part of the body are paralyzed in paraplegia. (a); IM; KN; ME; PA; MN
  1 This is quadriplegia.
  2 There is no term to describe this condition; all parts below an injury are affected.
  3 This is hemiplegia.
235. **4** Lack of or reduced movement predisposes the paraplegic or quadriplegic client to urinary tract infection and stone formation. (a); PL; AP; ME; PA; MN
  1 Fluids do not prevent temperature elevation, unless it is elevated because of dehydration.
  2 Administration of fluids does not maintain electrolyte "balance."
  3 All individuals require fluid to prevent dehydration; not why fluids are encouraged for this client.
236. **4** Care should be aimed at encouraging independence. (a); PL; AP; ME; ED; MN
  1 A client with this type of injury will never return to previous function.
  2 Lay persons may be taught to care for clients with a spinal cord injury.
  3 Independence should be encouraged in clients with a chronic disability; they should not rely totally on others for care.
237. **1** The bones respond to the stress of activity (walking, running, etc.) by laying down new bone substance along the lines of stress. Inactivity leads to reduced bone deposition and actual bone decalcification. (b); AN; CP; ME; PA; MN
  2 Calcium intake does not alter bone demineralization in the bedridden client.
  3 Kidney function may be altered as bone decalcification occurs and stones are formed in the kidneys.
  4 Fluid intake has no effect on bone decalcification.
238. **1** Bowel or bladder distention causes autonomic nerve impulses to ascend in the cord to the point of injury. Here the reflex is completed, and autonomic outflow causes piloerection (goosebumps), sweating, and splanchnic vasoconstriction. The last causes hypertension and a pounding headache. (c); AN; AN; ME; PA; MN
  2 Not involved in the sympathetic hyperreflexia mechanism.
  3 Not involved in the sympathetic hyperreflexia mechanism.
  4 Not involved in the sympathetic hyperreflexia mechanism.
239. **2** Oral airways provide direct access to the posterior pharynx for effective suctioning and prevent airway occlusion. (b); IM; AN; PE; TC; MN
  1 A tongue blade will interfere with suctioning and will not necessarily promote breathing.
  3 Cyanosis may indicate an occluded airway; intervention is necessary.
  4 May be unnecessary; opening airway will permit natural oxygenation.
240. **3** Will open airway and not cause injury. (a); IM; AP; PE; TC; MN
  1 Never leave a client having a seizure unattended.
  2 Attempting to open the jaw in this situation wastes precious time and may result in injury.
  4 This may cause airway occlusion by forcing the chin onto the neck. A small flat blanket is more effective.

241. **4** May reduce the risk of gingival hyperplasia, a common side effect of Dilantin. (a); IM; AN; PE; ED; MN
  1 May occur normally during drug excretion; causes no physiologic problems.
  2 Drug is strongly alkaline and should be administered with meals to avoid gastric irritation.
  3 Avoiding overeating and overhydration may result in better seizure control.
242. **2** This behavior is a form of denial that may occur once the seizures are controlled. (b); EV; CP; PE; PA; MN
  1 Drugs are prescribed according to seizure type.
  3 Dosage is not based on activity but on type of seizure.
  4 This is desired and indicates that the drug is effective.
243. **1** Heparin is used because its molecular size is too large to pass the placental barrier. (a); PL; AN; OB; PA; HP
  2 Can pass the placental barrier and cause hemorrhage in the fetus.
  3 Can pass the placental barrier and cause hemorrhage in the fetus.
  4 Can pass the placental barrier and cause hemorrhage in the fetus.
244. **2** Ninety-five seconds is more than twice the normal baseline level of 30 to 35 seconds and may cause prolonged bleeding. (b); EV; AN; OB; TC; HP
  1 It may already to too much, since the PPT is more than twice the normal of 30 to 35 seconds.
  3 An adjustment of dosage, not a change, is required when the PPT is prolonged.
  4 This PPT is not normal but prolonged, since it is twice the normal baseline of 30 to 35 seconds.
245. **3** A full bladder is required for effective visualization in early pregnancy. (b); PL; AP; OB; TC; HP
  1 For this noninvasive procedure nothing is passed through the alimentary tract. Also, fasting is contraindicated during pregnancy.
  2 Noninvasive; in no way can this irritate the uterus and initiate labor.
  4 Unnecessary, since procedure is not done via the colon and will not cause fecal contamination.
246. **4** As the process of effacement occurs in the latter part of pregnancy, placental separation from the uterus occurs, causing bleeding. (b); AN; AP; OB; PA; HP
  1 This occurs in premature separation of a normally implanted placenta.
  2 Not usually the first thing to occur; may occur after the placenta separates.
  3 Generally not associated with placenta previa at its onset; may occur later.
247. **1** Indicates she understands that the well-being of the infant in labor is related to normal fetal heart functioning. (b); EV; AP; OB; PA; HP
  2 Nonstress test does not require any injections; done by external monitoring.
  3 This noninvasive procedure should not affect uterine musculature.
  4 The baby is not affected by the use of external monitoring.
248. **3** An interpersonal relationship based on trust must be established before clients can be helped back to reality. (a); PL; AP; PS; PE; SD
  1 Socialization would come at a later time in her therapy.
  2 There is nothing to indicate an urgency to remove her from her home.
  4 An important part of her treatment and care, but of lesser importance than a trusting relationship.
249. **2** Provides support and security without rejecting the client or placing value judgments on behavior. (b); IM; AP; PS; PE; SD

1 Limits will have to be set in Gail's care, but staying with her and showing acceptance are an immediate nursing action.

3 This would only calm her down; does not try to deal with the problem.

4 This would be ignoring the problem; isolation would imply punishment.

250. **2** This behavior reflects the early fetal position. The individual curls up for both protection and security. (c); AN; CP; PS; PE; SD

1 Does not seem to be in response to an observable stimulus.

3 Behavior does not indicate dissociation or depersonalization.

4 Gail gives no indication of a hallucinatory pattern.

251. **4** When the client who is out of control feels that someone is assuming control, it promotes a feeling of security. As this continues, a sense of trust in this individual is established. (c); IM; AN; PS; PE; SD

1 This would be important in planning care but not in establishing a therapeutic relationship.

2 Less important in the beginning phase of a relationship.

3 She exhibits no self-destructive tendencies at this time.

252. **3** Trust is basic to all other therapy. Without it a therapeutic relationship cannot be established. (b); PL; AN; PS; PE; SD

1 There is nothing to indicate that Gail does not have a sense of identity.

2 Part of treatment is to build on present ego strengths; not a priority goal.

4 Helping her relate to others is a part of her treatment, not a priority goal.

253. **2** This response reassures the client that the staff member is able to help and that the client's feelings are accurate. (b); EV; AP; PS; PE; SD

1 It is a reversible condition that can be treated with benztropine mesylate (Cogentin) or diphenhydramine hydrochloride (Benadryl).

3 It is not a symptom that requires adjusting to; rather one that must be treated.

4 Early treatment to reverse the symptoms is important.

254. **3** Yellow sclerae are a sign of jaundice, indicating liver damage, which can be irreversible if drug therapy is continued. (b); EV; AN; PS; PA; SD

1 Photosensitivity is not a problem as long as the client is cautioned to stay out of the sun.

2 This is Parkinson-type syndrome, which can be reversed with treatment; continuation of medication is permitted.

4 A usually irreversible side effect even when medication is stopped.

255. **2** Close follow-up and continued monitoring of medication, behavior, and emotional state are necessary to enable the client to maintain a positive behavioral change. (a); PL; AP; PS; TC; SD

1 It would depend on what her regular activities were.

3 Would encourage dependence.

4 A self-help group might or might not be effective.

256. **2** Bed rest with leg extended prevents trauma caused by hip flexion and provides time for insertion site to heal. (b); PL; AN; ME; ED; CB

1 Mild sedation and local infiltration are used for adult clients. The client is conscious.

3 With the femoral approach, bed rest is maintained for several hours.

4 The physician will thoroughly review test results and may consult other physicians before answering.

257. **1** When neither rest nor nitroglycerin relieves the pain, there may be acute myocardial infarction. (a); PL; AP; ME; ED; CB

2 Expected; anginal pain can, and often does, radiate.

3 Expected; acute myocardial infarction causes profuse, not mild, diaphoresis, which should be reported.

4 Expected; activity increases cardiac output causing angina.

258. **2** Informed consent means the client must comprehend the surgery, the alternatives, and the consequences. (a); EV; AP; SU; ED; CB

1 This explanation is not within nursing's domain.

3 Nurse's signature documents that client has given informed consent.

4 True, but does not determine client's ability to give informed consent.

259. **4** More than 80% of those who have this surgery have marked relief of their symptoms. (b); IM; CP; SU; ED; CB

1 So far, studies have failed to show that bypass surgery affects life span.

2 The surgery itself does not affect the disease process; clients must also reduce risk factors (obesity, smoking, and poor diet).

3 Depends on client's presurgical condition, not the surgery itself.

260. **3** Clients should be familiar with these people and hear from them what will be experienced. (b); PL; CP; SU; ED; CB

1 Most do not want or need a minutely detailed description.

2 Although discharge plans should be mentioned, they are not the primary focus at this time.

4 The client's whole body will be prepped and shaved.

261. **2** These arrhythmias result from postoperative inflammation around the SA node area. (c); EV; CP; SU; PA; CB

1 This syndrome occurs later, not immediately.

3 This syndrome occurs later in the postoperative period.

4 Hgb and Hct levels usually fall; anemia can be a problem.

262. **2** Since the client is up more at home, edema usually increases. (c); IM; CP; SU; ED; CB

1 Serosanguineous drainage will persist after discharge.

3 These symptoms will persist longer, as it takes 6 to 12 weeks for the sternum to heal.

4 These should not be expected and are, in fact, signs of postpericardotomy syndrome.

263. **2** Abrupt discontinuation of Inderal may cause an acute myocardial infarction. (b); PL; CP; ME; ED; CB

1 Alcohol is contraindicated for clients taking Inderal.

3 The pulse rate can go much lower as long as the client feels well and is not dizzy.

4 Clients should never increase medications without medical direction.

264. **2** The exact reason is unknown, but three factors appear to influence it: child prone to pica, lead in the environment, and a passive mother. (c); AS; CP; PE; PA; MN

1 Child prone to pica is only one of the three etiologic factors.

3 The role of the mother is only one of the three etiologic factors.

4 The environment is only one of the three etiologic factors.

265. **4** Bone marrow is most susceptible to lead toxicity; interference with hemoglobin biosynthesis leads to early signs of anemia. (c); AS; CP; PE; PA; MN

1 Late response indicating CNS involvement.

2 This is a serious late response.

3 Late response indicating kidney shut-down; loss of protein and other substances occurs first.

266. **3** Damaged nerve cells do not regenerate. Once mental retardation has occurred, it is not reversible. (b); AN; CP; PE; PA; MN
   1 Effects of lead in bone marrow are reversible when lead is mobilized for excretion in urine or deposition in bone by chelation therapy.
   2 Damage to kidneys is reversible with treatment.
   4 Skeletal changes are not significant and are reversible as lead leaves the body.

267. **1** The desired outcome is the increased excretion of lead in urine. (c); EV; AP; PE; PA; MN
   2 Expected when lead initially equilibrates to the blood; until lead is excreted in urine, the treatment is not considered a success.
   3 Fecal elimination of lead is not as satisfactory as urinary elimination and is not as successful in ridding the soft tissues of lead.
   4 A desirable effect, but it does not determine success of therapy. Also, amount is difficult to determine.

268. **2** The child should be given an outlet for tension, and needle play is the most appropriate. (c); PL; AP; PE; PE; MN
   1 Part of the preparation, but not the most important; child must be allowed to express feelings.
   3 May ease discomfort, but an outlet for feelings should be provided.
   4 His fear is not directed at unfamiliar adults but at the painful treatments.

269. **2** Applying moist or dry heat relieves muscle pain through vasodilation, increases circulation to the area, and facilitates drug absorption. (b); AN; AP; PE; TC; EI
   1 Movement will most likely be difficult and cause more discomfort.
   3 This will cause more discomfort when the injection site is tender.
   4 This will prolong the discomfort by slowing the rate of absorption of the drug by vasoconstriction.

270. **4** Lead toxicity and Ca EDTA both damage the proximal renal tubules, resulting in the abnormal excretion of protein and other substances. (c); EV; CP; PE; PA; MN
   1 Attributable to the chelating agent only; not likely to occur with the Ca EDTA preparation, which replaces calcium.
   2 Bone marrow damage is caused by lead toxicity only.
   3 Lead encephalopathy causes serious elevation of intracranial pressure.

271. **1** The gross pathology in primary degenerative dementia is brain tissue degeneration with loss of brain neurons. (c); AS; CP; PS; PA; DD
   2 Severe emotional trauma may contribute to but does not necessarily cause primary degenerative dementia.
   3 False; nerve cells do not have the capacity to regenerate. Neural degeneration leads to permanent, not transient, changes.
   4 Poor nutrition may be one of the factors that bring about a general decline of health; however, no direct evidence that avitaminosis causes primary degenerative dementia.

272. **1** The sense of ego integrity comes from satisfaction with life and acceptance of what has been and what is. Despair is due to guilt or remorse over what might have been. (c); AS; AP; PS; PE; DD
   2 Autonomy is developed during the toddler period and corresponds to the child's ability to control the body and environment; doubt can result when made to feel ashamed or embarrassed.

3 During puberty the adolescent attempts to find her/himself and integrate values with those of society; inability to solve conflict results in confusion and hinders mastery of future roles.
   4 During early and middle adulthood the individual is concerned with the ability to produce and to care for that which is produced or created; failure during this stage leads to self-absorption or stagnation.

273. **3** Fears and anxieties about themselves and their possessions are common in aged because of decreased self-concept and altered body image. (c); AN; CP; PS; PE; DD
   1 Aging need not necessarily bring about losing one's ability to cooperate.
   2 The attitude of elderly persons about authority or others in their environment is set; indecision about life situations may be due to insecurity.
   4 The elderly fear the loss they must face in almost every aspect of their lives; this leads to lowering of their self-esteem and faulty reality testing.

274. **3** Impairment of abstract thinking interferes with interpretation and defining of words. Skill in abstract thinking is required to follow directions and select clothes. (c); AN; AN; PS; PE; DD
   1 Primary degenerative dementia does not cause a clouding of consciousness.
   2 Following directions does not require skill in judgement or decision making.
   4 The selection of clothes does not require an intact attention span.

275. **3** Erosion of blood vessels may lead to hemorrhage, a life-threatening situation further complicated by decreased prothrombin production. (c); PL; AP; ME; PA; GI
   1 Increased intraabdominal pressure may cause this; there is no immediate threat to life. Assessment for bleeding takes priority.
   2 Increased intraabdominal pressure may cause this; there is no immediate threat to life. Assessment for bleeding takes priority.
   4 While this may cause gastritis, there is no immediate threat to life; assessment for bleeding takes priority.

276. **4** Enlarged liver impairs venous return, leading to increased portal vein hydrostatic pressure and fluid shift into the abdominal cavity. (b); AN; CP; ME; PA; RE
   1 Ascites is not related to the interstitial fluid compartment.
   2 Increased serum albumin causes hypervolemia, not ascites.
   3 Bile plays an important role in digestion of fats but is not a major factor in fluid balance.

277. **1** The bladder should be empty to avoid injury during insertion of the trocar. (a); IM; AP; SU; TC; GI
   2 Consent may be signed any time before the procedure; it is preferable that the client have time to consider the decision.
   3 The upright position is assumed to allow accumulation of fluid in the lower abdomen by gravity.
   4 Although regular monitoring of girth is important, it is not necessary immediately before this procedure.

278. **1** Fluid may shift from intravascular space to abdomen as fluid is removed, leading to hypovolemia and compensatory tachycardia. (a); EV; AP; SU; PA; GI
   2 A paracentesis should decrease the degree of distention.
   3 Fluid shift can cause hypovolemia with resulting hypotension, not hypertension.
   4 This sign of dehydration may occur, but it is not as vital or immediate as signs of shock.

How to Use Worksheet 1: Errors in Processing Information

Common errors in processing information are listed in the left-hand column of this worksheet. At the top of the worksheet is a row of blank spaces for inserting the number of the question missed. Directly below each number, check any errors you made in answering that question. You may have made more than one type of error in an answer.

Worksheet 1: Errors in processing information

Question number																		
Did not read situation/question carefully																		
Missed important details																		
Confused major and minor points																		
Defined problem incorrectly																		
Could not remember terms/ facts/concepts/principles																		
Defined terms incorrectly																		
Focused on incomplete/incorrect data in assessing situation																		
Interpreted data incorrectly																		
Applied wrong concepts/principles in situation																		
Drew incorrect conclusions																		
Identified wrong goals																		
Identified priorities incorrectly																		
Carried out plan incorrectly/incompletely																		
Was unclear about criteria for evaluating success in achieving goals																		

How to Use Worksheet 2: Knowledge Gaps

Types of common knowledge gaps are listed along the top of this worksheet. Write a brief description of topics you want to review in the spaces provided. For example, if you missed a question on administration of a particular drug, write the drug name and problem (e.g., dosage) in the appropriate space under the column labeled *Pharmacology*.

Worksheet 2: Knowledge gaps

Basic science	Skills/ procedures	Basic human needs	Growth & develop-ment	Normal nutrition	Psycho-social factors	Clinical area/ topic	Stressors/ coping mechanisms	Patho-physiology	Pharma-cology	Therapeutic nutrition	Legal implications	Other

279. **2** Clear cell adenoma of daughters is associated with mothers who took DES or DES-type drugs during pregnancy. (b) AS; KN; OB; PA; PN
    1 DES was prescribed between 1941 and 1971 to reduce the risk of spontaneous abortion in high-risk women.
    3 The client with DES-related problems may exhibit abnormal bleeding or a heavy mucoid vaginal discharge, not lesions on the perineum.
    4 Use of oral contraceptives is not associated with DES exposure.
280. **4** When an Rh-negative mother carries an Rh-positive fetus there is a risk of maternal antibodies against Rh-positive blood; antibodies cross the placenta and destroy the fetal RBCs. (b); IM; AN; OB; PA; PN
    1 Physiologic bilirubinemia is a common occurrence in newborns; it is not associated with the Rh factor.
    2 Testing for Rh factor will not provide information about protein metabolism deficiency.
    3 Determination of the lecithin-sphingomyelin ratio, not the Rh factor, may provide information about the risk of developing RDS.
281. **1** Increasing the client's knowledge of physical and psychologic changes resulting from pregnancy is done during the first teimester. (b); PL; CP; OB; ED; PN
    2 Concerns about role transition to parenthood should be addressed in the third trimester.
    3 Too early; this would be done in the last trimester.
    4 The client should be alerted to danger signs; however, primary teaching is directed toward increasing her knowledge of the normal physiologic changes.

Comprehensive Test 2: Part 4*

282. **2** A rapid delivery does not give the fetal head adequate time for molding, so pressure against the head is increased. (b); AN; CP; OB; PA; NH
    1 This is due to excessive pulling on the head and shoulders during delivery; certainly not incurred in precipitous delivery.
    3 Likely to occur in footling breech delivery.
    4 May occur with pull on the shoulders during delivery; not likely to occur with precipitous delivery.
283. **3** Lacerated tissue does not heal as quickly as a smooth, closely approximated surgical incision. (c); PL; AN; OB; ED; PP
    1 This is a routine postpartum intervention, not specific for clients with perineal lacerations.
    2 The perineum at this time is too sore to be contracted as part of perineal exercise.
    4 High protein would be acceptable, but high roughage would cause large stools and pain on defecation.
284. **3** Tears in the tentorial membrane cause bleeding into the cerebellum, pons, or medulla oblongata. The respiratory regulation centers are located in the medulla and pons. (c); AN; CP; OB; PA; NH
    1 Lethargy would be more indicative of cerebellar injury.
    2 A weak timorous cry would be more indicative of cardiac or respiratory difficulty; a high-pitched shrill cry is usually present with CNS difficulty.
    4 Purpura is unrelated to tentorial or other CNS injuries.

*A key to the letters following the correct rationale can be found on p. 633.

285. **1** The newborn's immature neuromuscular development normally causes dorsiflexion of the big toe and fanning of the remaining toes, a positive Babinski sign. (b); AN; CP; OB; ED; NH
    2 CNS damage from hypoxia can result in a negative Babinski sign, an abnormal finding in an infant.
    3 Hyperreflexia is an abnormal increase in reflexes; a positive Babinski sign is a normal response in the infant.
    4 A positive Babinski sign is a normal response in an infant; its absence may demonstrate neural impairment.
286. **2** Elevation of the head helps decrease intracranial pressure by gravity. (c) IM; AP; OB; TC; NH
    1 Frequent stimulation may cause further irritability to an already traumatized CNS.
    3 This may be disturbing to the infant and impair his ability to rest.
    4 This is done routinely on all neonates; not specific for this injury.
287. **3** Teaching her by example is a nonthreatening approach that allows her to proceed at her own pace. (b); PL; AN; PE; ED; NH
    1 Learning doesn't occur by schedule; must answer questions as they arise.
    2 Mothers need demonstration of appropriate mothering skills, not just discussion.
    4 Satisfying the mother's needs will allow her to develop reserves to give the child; plan should promote security in her role and facilitate more independent caretaking.
288. **3** Sitting down shows the client that the nurse cares enough to spend time. It also opens up channels of communication. (a); IM; AP; PS; PE; CS
    1 The nurse sets dimensions on the mother's feelings; does not promote free expression of feelings.
    2 This statement ignores the mother's need to express feelings; takes a cognitive approach to the problem.
    4 This statement provides false hope; the diagnosis has been made.
289. **2** Braces are used to enable the spastic child to control motions. They also prevent deformities from poor alignment. (a); AN; CP; PE; PA; MN
    1 Since Jimmy is at the age when self-reliance is important (Erikson's stage of industry vs. inferiority) and dependent on his braces for self-care, it is unlikely that he would reject them.
    3 Exercises are used to stretch ligaments and improve muscle strength and tone.
    4 Early ambulation is promoted by maintaining muscle strength and tone.
290. **1** The choice of gait is based on the weight-bearing capabilities of each of the four extremities. (b); AS; CP; PE; PA; MN
    2 The cerebral palsied child uses upper extremity strength for crutch control and lower extremity strength to facilitate some movement.
    3 Under normal circumstances orthostatic circulatory impairment is unlikely in the child with cerebral palsy.
    4 Because of the decreased muscle control in CP, Jimmy will not likely be able to utilize a gait involving complete support of body weight off the floor.
291. **3** The four-point alternate crutch gait is a simple, slow, but stable gait because there are always three points of support on the floor with equal but partial weight bearing on each limb. (b); AN; AN; PE; TC; MN
    1 The four-point gait provides for three points of support.

2 A four-point gait divides weight bearing equally among the limbs.

4 Jimmy has uncoordinated movement in the lower extremities because of the CP.

292. **4** When sensory perceptions are impaired, with resultant lack of effective specific motor responses, an individual will be more vulnerable to skin irritation and trauma. (a); IM; AP; PE; ED; MN

1 Jimmy's lack of sensation makes him more vulnerable to skin irritation from braces; observation of the skin takes priority in sensory loss.

2 Alignment of brace joints to body joints is important to facilitate joint mobility; observation of the skin takes priority in sensory loss.

3 A wide flat shoe will facilitate balance; observation of the skin takes priority in sensory loss.

293. **2** Many behaviors require a background of knowledge, skills, and attitudes (experiential readiness). If this background is not available, then more learning must take place before the individual can function. (c); AN; CP; PE; ED; MN

1 Learning progress varies according to the individual; there are both progressive and regressive periods.

3 Although teaching may facilitate learning, other factors related to readiness for learning and willingness to learn affect whether learning occurs.

4 Jimmy will be able to learn the four-point gait without understanding normal walking.

294. **1** Clients whose thermoreceptive senses are impaired are unable to detect changes or degrees of temperature. They must be taught to test the temperature in any water-related activity to prevent scalding and burning. (a); IM; AP; PE; ED; MN

2 The cerebral palsied child normally has uncontrolled movement of voluntary muscles; makes it unnecesary to reposition on a schedule.

3 Overtightening straps and buckles may lead to circulatory impairment and/or skin breakdown.

4 Dangerous as it alters center of gravity; with practice, Jimmy will be able to place his legs in appropriate positions for walking without looking down.

295. **3** The damage is fixed. It does not become progressively greater. (c); AN; CP; PE; PA; MN

1 Cerebral palsy is a nonprogressive chronic condition.

2 The etiology of CP is related to anoxia in the prenatal, perinatal, or postnatal periods.

4 Although mental retardation may be present in some children with CP, Jimmy cannot be assumed to be mentally retarded.

296. **2** Apple juice and pear nectar have low sodium content and are therefore the better choices for this client. (b); IM; AP; ME; TC; CB

1 The client is permitted juice between meals.

3 Tomato juice has a high sodium content; should be avoided to prevent fluid retention.

4 Low-sodium juices are not contraindicated.

297. **2**

$$\frac{0.2 \text{ mg}}{0.5 \text{ mg}} \times \frac{x}{2 \text{ ml}} \quad 0.2 \text{ mg}: x = 0.5 \text{ mg}: 2 \text{ ml}$$
$$0.5x = 0.4 \quad\quad 0.5x = 0.4$$
$$x = 0.8 \text{ ml} \quad\quad x = 0.8 \text{ ml}$$

(a); IM; AN; ME; PA; CB

1 This would be an overdose.

3 This would be an overdose.

4 This would be an overdose.

298. **2** Elevation of an extremity promotes venous and lymphatic drainage by gravity. (a); PL; AP; ME; PA; CB

1 This is a dependent function of the nurse.

3 This is a dependent function of the nurse.

4 This procedure will have little effect on edema.

299. **2** This combination of foods has the highest sodium content. (b); EV; AP; ME; ED; CB

1 This meal is low in sodium.

3 This meal is low in sodium.

4 This meal is low in sodium.

300. **4** Fluctuation of IV fluid in the manometer with respirations is due to alteration of intrathoracic pressure during inhalation and exhalation. (c); IM; AP; ME; PA; CB

1 The fluid in the manometer must be allowed to rise above the expected reading before the line to the client is opened to premit the fluid in the manometer to drop; when the fluid level stops dropping and fluctuates slightly, it reflects the venous pressure.

2 CVP is a measure of venous, not arterial, pressure.

3 The fluid in the manometer must be allowed to rise above the expected reading before the line to the client is opened to permit the fluid in the manometer to drop; when the fluid level stops dropping and fluctuates slightly, it reflects the venous pressure.

301. **1** Furosemide (Lasix) inhibits sodium reabsorption in the ascending loop of Henle, whereas chlorothiazide (Diuril) inhibits the reabsorption of sodium and chloride. Water and potassium are not reasbsorbed by the distal renal tubules, and dehydration and hypokalemia may result. (b); EV; CP; ME; PA; CB

2 With an increased fluid loss the specific gravity would more likely be lowered.

3 These drugs do not affect protein metabolism.

4 These drugs inhibit the reabsorption of sodium.

302. **1** Digitalis increases the strength of the myocardial contractions (positive inotropic effect) and, by altering the electrophysiologic properties of the heart, slows the heart rate (positive chronotropic effect). (a); AN; AP; ME; PA; CB

2 The PR interval is prolonged.

3 Although this may result from the increased blood supply to the kidneys, it is not the primary reason for administering digitalis.

4 Too general; digitalis increases the strength of the contractions but decreases the heart rate.

303. **3** Preoperative skin preparation includes washing the operative site with an antiseptic agent several times to reduce the number of microorganisms on the skin. (c); PL; AN; SU; TC; EI

1 Although the client should be informed in advance of the care she is to expect, leaning specific exercises would be impeded by high preoperative anxiety level.

2 It is impossible to ascertain how an individual will react to a situation that has not occurred; efforts should be made to establish a therapeutic relationship so that feelings can be ventilated.

4 The client may not require a mastectomy; these arrangements are made postoperatively.

304. **3** Women facing breast surgery often have many feelings relating to their sexuality, change in body image, etc. The nurse plays a vital role in helping the client verbalize feelings and this response keeps channels of communication open. (a); IM; AN; PS; PE; CS

1 The client's concerns are real and such a statement will only block further communication.

2 This can be interpreted as the nurse's reluctance to listen; client may not be able to talk with husband about this.

4 Does not focus on the importance of the client as an individual; each person feels differently.

305. **4** Postoperatively the arm on the operated side is elevated on pillows with the hand higher than the arm to prevent muscle strain and edema. (b); IM; AP; SU; PA; EI
    1 Although the arm is slightly abducted, sand bags are not utilized because complete immobility should be prevented.
    2 This would impair venous return and increase edema.
    3 Total immobilization should be avoided, and adduction may put undue pressure on the operative site.

306. **1** Postmastectomy exercises should be bilateral, using both arms simultaneously to prevent shortening of muscles and contracture of joints. (b); IM; AP; SU; ED; MN
    2 Both arms should be exercised to maintain symmetry of muscle tone and strength.
    3 A sling immobilizes the arm creating joint stiffness and loss of muscle tone.
    4 Exercises of the affected arm are usually started within 24 hours to prevent contractures and muscle atony.

307. **1** Chemotherapeutic agents are not specific for malignant cells. They generally interfere with protein synthesis and cell division in all rapidly dividing cells, including those regenerating traumatized tissue (as in wound healing), bone marrow, and cutaneous and alimentary tract epithelial tissue. (b); AN; CP; SU; PA; EI
    2 The muscles underlying the incision are not primarily involved in vomiting so the integrity of the area is not endangered.
    3 Decreased RBC levels caused by bone marrow depression can be corrected with transfusions.
    4 Chemotherapy would not increase edema.

308. **2** When there is increased pressure within the cranial cavity, the body adapts by increasing the BP and decreasing the pulse. (c); EV; CP; ME; PA; MN
    1 Signs and symptoms reflect the part of brain upon which pressure is exerted, so that changes in behavior, judgment, consciousness and motor function may occur as well as autonomic changes, such as pupil size and reactivity, vital signs, and vomiting.
    3 Signs and symptoms reflect the part of brain upon which pressure is exerted, so that changes in behavior, judgment, consciousness and motor function may occur as well as autonomic changes, such as pupil size and reactivity, vital signs, and vomiting.
    4 Signs and symptoms reflect the part of brain upon which pressure is exerted. Thus changes in behavior, judgment, consciousness, and motor function may occur as well as autonomic changes, such as pupil size and reactivity, vital signs, and vomiting.

309. **4** Rotating tourniquets are used to decrease venous return to the heart and would have no value in the treatment of increased intracranial pressure. (b); AN; AN; ME; TC; MN
    1 Osmotic diuretics such as mannitol may be used to draw fluid from the cerebral tissue into the vascular space to decrease cerebral edema and intracranial pressure.
    2 Elevation of the head helps reduce edema because of gravitational force on the fluid.
    3 Steroids inhibit the inflammatory response, preventing increased edema.

310. **3** If there is no obstruction, pressure on the jugular vein causes increased intracranial pressure. This, in turn, causes an increase in spinal fluid pressure. (b); AS; KN; SU; PA; MN
    1 Chvostek's sign is twitching elicited by tapping the angle of the jaw if hypocalcemia is present.
    2 Romberg's sign is failure to maintain balance when the eyes are closed; indicates cerebellar pathology.

    4 Homan's sign is calf pain elicited by dorsiflexion of the foot if thrombophlebitis is present.

311. **2** The cerebellum is involved in the synergistic control of muscle action. Below the level of consciousness if functions to produce smooth, steady, coordinated, and efficient movements. (b); AS; CP; ME; PA; MN
    1 The brain is not involved in a simple reflex arc.
    3 The cerebrum is responsible for motor function.
    4 The cerebrum is responsible for the level of consciousness.

312. **3** Because of cosmetic concerns, consent must be obtained before a client's head may be shaved. (b); IM; AP; SU; TC; MN
    1 Usually unnecessary; the hair will be shaved to help prevent contamination of surgical site.
    2 The client will not be able to wear a wig until healing occurs; by this time the hair will begin to regrow.
    4 Shaving is usually performed before the client is taken to the surgical suite.

313. **3** Yellow drainage may be CSF and should be reported immediately. (a); EV; AN; SU; TC; MN
    1 Temperature evaluation must be accurate, axillary temperatures are influenced by environmental conditions and are lower than oral or rectal temperatures.
    2 Deep breathing expands the lungs and mobilizes secretions to prevent respiratory complications; secretions may be removed by suctioning to avoid increased intracranial pressure associated with coughing.
    4 Administration of narcotics makes accurate neurologic assessment impossible; narcotics depress the CNS.

314. **2** Near term, most mothers are tired of the pregnant state and anxious for labor to begin. It is helpful to know that this is a common reaction. (c); IM; AP; OB; PE; PN
    1 The client has just told the nurse what is bothering her; this response does not encourage the client to discuss her feelings further.
    3 Narrows the client's verbalization to what the nurse sees as the client's area of concern.
    4 Does not encourage further verbalization, merely closes off communication.

315. **2** Preparation for parenthood classes should help couples develop realistic expectations of the laboring process, including associated discomfort and ways of dealing with it. (b); IM; AP; OB; ED; PN
    1 Untrue and unpredictable; contractions are uncomfortable, but childbirth preparation helps the client cope with discomfort.
    3 Clients are taught what to expect and the proper exercises to expedite labor; focus should not be on pain.
    4 There is no way of predicting whether medication will be needed; however, the client should be assured of its availability.

316. **3** Tension in the woman prevents relaxation and has the greatest influence on how she will progress through labor and on her perception of pain. Tension is related to the expectation of pain, which is based on cultural norms and past experiences. (a); AN; CP; OB; PE; IP
    1 Although the difficulty of labor affects the amount of pain, it does not play a major role in the woman's perception of pain.
    2 Although the woman frequently becomes more uncomfortable and tired near the end of labor, the length of labor does not play a major role in her perception of pain.
    4 Parity does not play a major role in the woman's perception of pain.

317. **2** It is important to listen to the fetal heart rate (FHR) during contractions even though it may be difficult to hear. If the FHR slows during contraction and then resumes the normal rate within 30 seconds after acme, it is not serious. (c); EV; AP; OB; PA; IP

   1 Data are incomplete; during a contraction the FHR may be inaudible or slowed; should be retaken at the end of the contraction to see whether it remains decelerated.

   3 The FHR should not be taken at the height of a contraction; wait until the contraction subsides to obtain the FHR to determine deceleration.

   4 Unless the FHR remains decelerated, there is no sign of hypoxia and oxygen is not necessary.

318. **1** In the advanced stage of labor the presenting part is low in the birth canal and may cause strong sensations of pressure on the rectum. (c); AN; CP; OB; PA; IP

   2 This may occur with persistent posterior pressure; usually not sudden and not a sign of advanced labor.

   3 Transitional or advanced labor begins when the cervix is 8 to 10 cm dilated.

   4 Restlessness and thrashing are generally not present in the early or middle phases of labor; begin during the transitional phase.

319. **3** Immediate action to prevent excessive bleeding is to massage the fundus until it is firm. This stimulates uterine muscle contraction. (a); IM; AP; OB; PA; IP

   1 Not necessary unless bleeding persists after massaging of the uterus.

   2 The immediate action is to promote uterine contraction; obtaining the BP would be indicated if a large amount of bleeding occurred or bleeding persisted.

   4 If the uterus does not contract after massage, the nurse should notify the physician; not just observe the bleeding.

320. **4** Although thrombophlebitis is suspected, prior to a definitive diagnosis the client should be confined to bed so further complications will be avoided. (a); EV; AN; OB; TC; PP

   1 Assessment of the leg may indicate thrombophlebitis; the client should be put to bed.

   2 If a thrombus is present, massage may dislodge it and lead to pulmonary embolism.

   3 May cause extreme vasodilation, which would allow a thrombus to dislodge and circulate freely.

321. **1** The tremendous visual impact of cleft lip on parents may significantly affect the parent-child attachment process and is often considered a reason for early surgical intervention. (c); AN; CP; PE; PE; GI

   2 Feeding can be accomplished by use of special equipment; not an indication for early surgery by itself.

   3 Precautions may be taken to prevent ear and upper respiratory tract infections.

   4 The baby uses the mouth to facilitate breathing; cleft lip does not interfere.

322. **4** An almost universal reaction to birth of an imperfect child is guilt. Encouraging the parents to discuss such feelings, without actually asking whether they feel guilty, allows them an opportunity to express such thoughts. (b); IM; AN; PS; PE; CS

   1 This statement cuts off the parents' expression of feelings.

   2 This statement does not show recognition of the concern the parents are expressing.

   3 This statement lacks sensitivity in dealing with the parents' feelings.

323. **1** Cleft lip and palate demonstrate a familial pattern of inheritance that is significantly increased when a close relative is similarly affected. (b); AS; CP; PE; PA; GI

   2 Mendelian laws of inheritance do not apply to these defects.

   3 The way the young child responds to these defects is dependent on the parental response.

   4 The defects are familial; however, no exact pathogenesis has been found.

324. **1** Because the infant with a cleft lip and palate is unable to form the vacuum needed for sucking, a rubber-tipped syringe or dropper is used. This allows formula to flow along the sides and back of the mouth, minimizing the danger of aspiration. (a); AN; AN; PE; TC; GI

   2 Feeding can be accomplished with the child in an upright position to facilitate swallowing and prevent choking; impaired sucking prevents breast-feeding in most situations.

   3 A soft crosscut nipple may be used with some infants but rapid flow can cause aspiration.

   4 Feeding can be accomplished with special equipment; IV feedings do not supply ample calories.

325. **3** Infants with cleft lip breathe through their mouth, bypassing the natural humidification provided by the nose. As a result, the mucous membranes become dry and cracked and are easily infected. (b); AN; AN; PE; PA; GI

   1 Feeding can be adequate with special epuipment and a slow approach.

   2 Circulation to the area is unimpaired.

   4 The area may be kept clean by washing with water after feeding.

326. **2** After cleft lip repair, infants are always placed supine or slightly on their side to prevent damage to the suture line. (b); IM; AP; PE; TC; GI

   1 Swelling in or near the area traumatized by surgery is a complication that may occur postoperatively.

   3 For maximum healing and minimal scarring, a clean suture line is essential.

   4 Crying may disturb the suture line; the parents should be encouraged to hold the infant to reduce crying.

327. **2** Severe pain accompanied by bleeding at term or close to it is symptomatic of complete premature detachment of the placenta. (b); AS; CP; OB; PA; HP

   1 Bleeding caused by marginal placenta previa should not be painful.

   3 There is no bleeding with vena caval syndrome.

   4 Hydatidiform mole does not usually last until 36 weeks; no severe pain accompanies it.

328. **2** Immediate cesarean section is the treatment of choice for complete placental separation. The risk of fetal death is too high to delay. (a); IM; CP; OB; TC; HP

   1 Too slow; besides, a high forceps delivery is rarely used because the forceps may further complicate the situation by tearing the cervix.

   3 The fetus would probably expire if this course of action were taken.

   4 The fetus would probably expire if this course of action were taken.

329. **3** In an emergency surgical situation when invasive techniques are necessary, it is important to have a consent signed as well as a history of the client's known allergies. (a); IM; AP; OB; TC; HP

   1 An enema is not given to a bleeding client; may stimulate contractions and further bleeding.

   2 An enema is not given to a bleeding client; may stimulate contractions and further bleeding.

   4 Not a priority item in an emergency such as this.

330. **2** Elevating the head of the bed will prevent reflux of gastric contents into the esophagus. (b); IM; AP; ME; PA; GI

1 Eating at bedtime and drinking orange juice would stimulate gastric secretions.

3 Small frequent meals would relieve symptoms of fullness and prevent gastric stimulation.

4 Would delay emptying of the stomach, which would increase gastric secretions and the feeling of fullness.

331. **3** Whole grain cereals and breads are irritating, provide bulk, and should be excluded from a bland diet. (a); IM; KN; ME; ED; GI

1 Eggs are permitted except when fried.

2 Meats are permitted except pork.

4 All cooked vegetables are permitted; raw vegetables should be avoided.

332. **3** Sodium bicarbonate is absorbed and can alter the acid-base balance. Antacids are not readily absorbed, so they do not alter acid-base balance. (c); AN; CP; ME; ED; GI

1 False; these are side effects of nonsystemic antacids.

2 False; nonsystemic antacids are insoluble and not readily absorbed.

4 False; aluminum hydroxide preparations contain sodium and should be used only with caution.

333. **3** Antacids interfere with absorption of drugs such as anticholinergics, barbituates, tetracycline, and digoxin. (b); PL; CP; ME; ED; GI

1 May be taken as frequently as every 1 to 2 hours without adverse effects.

2 Liquid antacids are faster acting and more effective.

4 False; antacids should be given 1 or 2 hours *after* meals and at bedtime.

334. **3** Increased gluconeogenesis may lead to hyperglycemia and glycosuria, which can produce urinary frequency. Protein catabolism will cause muscle weakness. (c); AS; AN; ME; PA; EI

1 These are symptoms of Addison's syndrome; in this case sodium and fluid retention leads to hypervolemia and hypertension.

2 As sodium ions are retained, potassium is excreted; the result is hypokalemia. Edema occurs because of sodium retention.

4 Muscle wasting results from increased protein catabolism; however, hyperglycemia rather than hypoglycemia will result from increased gluconeogenesis.

335. **1** Excess adrenocorticoids cause emotional lability, euphoria, and psychosis. (c); AS; CP; ME; PA; EI

2 Increased secretion of androgens results in hirsutism.

3 Ectomorphism is a term for the tall, thin, genetically determined body type; not related to adaptions to Cushing's syndrome.

4 Capillary fragility results in multiple ecchymotic areas.

336. **2** Steroid therapy is usually instituted preoperatively and continued intraoperatively to prepare for the acute adrenal insufficiency that follows surgery. (b); IM; AP; SU; PA; EI

1 Glucocorticoids must be administered preoperatively to prevent adrenal insufficiency during surgery.

3 The diet must supply ample protein and potassium; however, must be low in calories, carbohydrates, and sodium to promote weight loss and reduce fluid retention.

4 Urine is routinely tested for sugar and acetone, but 24-hour urine is unnecessary.

337. **4** Because of instability of the vascular system and the lability of circulating adrenal hormones after adrenalectomy, hypotension frequently occurs until the hormonal level is controlled by replacement therapy. (c); AS; CP; SU; PA; EI

1 This is a sign of excessive adrenal hormones; after an adrenalectomy, adrenal hormones are not secreted.

2 This is a sign of hyperadrenalism; does not occur after the adrenals are removed.

3 This is an adaptation to excessive adrenal hormones; after an adrenalectomy, adrenal hormones are lowered until replacement therapy is regulated.

338. **3** Administration of adrenocortical hormones causes sodium retention by the kidneys. Dietary intake of salt must therefore be limited. (b); PL; AP; SU; ED; EI

1 Since there is normally an increased secretion of glucocorticoids under stressful situations, dosage must be adjusted accordingly.

2 Insommnia is not an adverse effect of adrenocortical hormones.

4 Since pancreatic function is unimpaired, insulin therapy is not normally indicated.

339. **3** Clients with adrenocortical insufficiency who are receiving steroid therapy usually require increased amounts of medication during periods of stress, since they are unable to produce the excess needed by the body. (c); EV; CP; SU; TC; EI

1 Although sedation may be prescribed, the major concern is the regulation of glucocorticoids in the presence of emotional or physiological stress.

2 Increased stress requires increased glucocorticoids.

4 Although these symptoms may occur and may be minimized by an increase in glucocorticoids, the primary reason for an adjustment in dosage is to assist the body's ability to adapt to stress.

340. **1** Clients with Cushing's syndrome or who are receiving cortical hormones must limit their intake of salt and increase their potassium intake. The kidneys are retaining sodium and excreting potassium. (b); IM; AN; ME; ED; EI

2 Excessive secretion of adrenocortical hormones in Cushing's syndrome not increased or high sodium intake is the problem.

3 Because of steroid therapy, excess sodium may be retained rather than excreted.

4 Although sodium retention causes fluid retention and weight gain, the need for increased potassium must also be considerd.

341. **2** Excess glucocorticoids cause hyperglycemia. Signs of diabetes mellitus may develop. (c); AN; CP; ME; PA; EI

1 Adrenocortical hormones cause sodium retention and subsequent weight gain.

3 Although muscle wasting is associated with excessive corticoid production, this will not cause diabetes mellitus.

4 ACTH affects the adrenal cortex, not the pancreas.

342. **4** The 2-year-old child is extremely fearful of separation as well as intrusive procedures. If parents are present, they should be encouraged to stay and give comfort. (b); IM; AP; PE; PE; RG

1 Two-year-olds are still dependent on their parents; the parent should be encouraged to participate in care.

2 Two-year-olds still depend on their parents for comfort and control.

3 His father may provide comfort to Alex during the procedure as well.

343. **3** If able to handle personal anxiety and give comfort to the child, parents can be a real help to the staff as well as the child. If the parents are extremely anxious, their anxiety can be transmitted, making the child even more anxious. (b); AN; CP; PS; PE; CS

1 It is how the parents cope with the situation, rather than the situation itself, that helps determine how helpful their presence may be.

2 Two-year-olds are cognitively unable to make decisions of this nature.

4 Parents can be helpful to the child and the staff; they often want to participate in the child's care.

344. **3** Infants and small children have small buttocks with a very proximal sciatic nerve. (b); AN; CP; PE; TC; MN

  1 Children of this age fear the procedure no matter what site is chosen.

  2 Children properly restrained can be held still in this position.

  4 Preschoolers tend to associate many treatments, and illness itself, with punishment.

345. **4** It is difficult to apply adequate pressure to this vascular site. Therefore observation for early signs of bleeding is imperative. (b); IM; AP; PE; TC; RG

  1 Fluids should be encouraged as soon as Alex tolerates them.

  2 This simple procedure usually requires minimal or no IV fluid therapy.

  3 Ice packs are not necessary.

346. **3** Superego development reflects the internalized norms of the family and society; the antisocial personality has never achieved this internalization. (b); AN; CP; PS; PE; PD

  1 A person with this behavior has an overdeveloped need to seek pleasure.

  2 The ego is not the problem; the defect is in the superego.

  4 There may be a defect in sexual attitudes but not in sexual development.

347. **1** A sincere, cautious, and consistent attitude limits this individual's ability to manipulate both situations and staff members. (b); PL; AN; PS; PE; PD

  2 An attitude such as this would allow Mr. Jay to rationalize his manipulative behavior to deal with the response he received.

  3 In accepting the person, the nurse should not support negative behavior; a friendly attitude may encourage further problem behavior.

  4 This would only encourage Mr. Jay to continue in his lifestyle rather than learn better ways to relate to his environment.

348. **4** Sets realistic limits on behavior without rejecting the client. (b); IM; AP; PS; PE; PD

  1 This would encourage further manipulation of the staff by Mr. Jay.

  2 This would be rejecting the person rather than the behavior.

  3 The other client is entitled to a special time with the nurse; this is inconsistent limit setting on the part of the nurse.

349. **4** Helps the client focus on feelings rather than just points out that current behavior is unacceptble. (b); IM; AP; PS; PE; PD

  1 Points out the behavior in front of another client.

  2 Gives Mr. Jay an alibi for unacceptable behavior.

  3 The nurse is becoming defensive rather than dealing with the problem directly.

350. **1** Accepts the client while rejecting and setting limits on the behavior the client is using. (b); IM; AP; PS; PE; PD

  2 A confusing message is sent to the client since it is unclear what the nurse did not like.

  3 A rejection of the client instead of the behavior.

  4 Encourages this type of behavior instead of setting limits.

351. **2** Sets limits, points out reality, and places responsibility for behavior on the client. (b); IM; AN; PS; PE; PD

  1 This is a punishing response and endangers the trust relationship.

  3 Clients such as this need limits set; changing the time shows inconsistency.

4 The nurse using this response is showing inconsistency, endangering the trust relationship, and using a threat to gain control.

352. **2** Demonstrates the client's acceptance of the professional role of the nurse as well as the ability to end dependent relationships. (b); EV; AN; PS; PE; PD

  1 Shows an inability to relate to other staff members involved with his care.

  3 This still shows the existence of manipulation on his part.

  4 Shows a childish need to punish the nurse for leaving.

353. **1** This response demonstrates an understanding of the client's feelings and encourages the client to share feelings, which is an immediate need at the moment. (b); IM; AP; PS; PE; SD

  2 This would have the effect of only increasing the fears.

  3 The nurse is entering into the hallucination, thereby reinforcing it.

  4 This response argues with the client, making him defensive and reinforcing the hallucination.

354. **4** You cannot argue a client out of a delusion. Statements made by the nurse show a lack of knowledge and constitute a threat, which is a form of assault. (c); EV; AN; PS; PE; SD

  1 Everyone needs nourishment, but threats accomplish little.

  2 A person cannot be argued out of a delusion.

  3 There is no indication that he needed a reminder to eat.

355. **2** This response recognizes the client's feelings and provides assurance that the staff member will stay with him. (a); IM; AP; PS; PE; SD

  1 Mr. Walter does not know this; if he did, he would not have a delusion.

  3 The client is not ready to accept this; he really believes he is going to be killed.

  4 Locking the client in a room by himself will only increase the fear and delusion.

356. **3** Delusions are protective and can be abandoned only when the individual feels secure and adequate. This response is the only one directed at building the client's security and reducing anxiety. (b); AN; AP; PS; PE; SD

  1 This would be a nursing action to help him develop trust; the goal is to have trust.

  2 This is helpful more in regard to hallucinations than delusions.

  4 He is unable to explain the reason for his feelings.

357. **2** Clients losing control feel frightened and threatened. They need external controls and a reduction in external stimuli. (b); IM; AP; PS; TC; SD

  1 This is helpful for pen-up aggressive behavior but not for agitation associated with delusions.

  3 He may get completely out of control if he is allowed to continue pacing.

  4 He would be unable, at this time, to sit in one place; his agitation is building.

358. **4** Jaundice signifies liver cell damage, a side effect of the phenothiazine drugs, which can be irreversible and life threatening. The nurse should immediately stop the medication if this side effect is noted. (b); EV; CP; PS; TC; SD

  1 A reversible side effect with treatments using benztropine mesylate (Congentin) or diphenhydramine (Benadryl).

  2 A common anticholinergic effect that will pass.

  3 Not a known side effect.

359. **2** This response supports reality and self-awareness while helping the client to look to the future rather than focus on the past. (c); IM; AP; PS; PE; SD

1 May be taken as ridicule of the client; focuses on the past.

3 What made him have this delusion is unimportant at the moment; still focuses on the past.

4 This may or may not be so; the statement dismisses an opportunity for validating how he feels at the present time.

360. **2** The phenothiazine drugs cause photosensitivity. Severe burning can occur on exposure to the sun. (b); PL; CP; PS; ED; SD

  1 No contraindication with aspirin.

  3 No known side effect that would affect night driving.

  4 This would be true if the client were taking an MAO inhibitor.

361. **2** Using Naegele's rule, subtract 3 months and add 7 days to the first day of the last menstrual period, April 11. (b); AN; CP; OB; PA; PN

  1 To have an EDC of January 10, Mrs. Wills' last menstrual period would have begun on April 3.

  3 To have an EDC of February 12, Mrs. Wills' last menstrual period would have begun on May 5.

  4 Even though Mrs. Wills had some spotting on May 8, her last normal menstrual period began April 11.

362. **2** Blood volume increases by approximately 50% during pregnancy. Peak blood volume occurs between 30 and 34 weeks of gestation. (b); AN; CP; OB; PA; PN

  1 The sedimentation rate increases because of a decrease in plasma proteins.

  3 White blood cell values remain stable during the antepartum period.

  4 The hematocrit decreases as a result of hemodilution.

363. **3** AFP in amniotic fluid is elevated in the presence of neural tube defects. (c); AS; CP; OB; PA; PN

  1 Fetal lung maturity cannot be determined until after 35 weeks gestation.

  2 Cardiac disorders cannot be detected.

  4 Fetal diabetes cannot be detected.

364. **3** This response shows empathy and gives the client an opportunity to ventilate her feelings. (b); IM; AP; OB; PE; PN

  1 Closes off any opportunity for discussion.

  2 Important question but may close off communication between the nurse and client.

  4 Ignores the client's feelings; focuses on the husband's desires.

365. **3** Children who have been abused quickly learn that attention-seeking behavior such as crying for comforting provokes more abuse. Therefore they learn to accept the battering silently. (c); AS; AN; PS; PE; CS

  1 Battered children seldom cry.

  2 Battered children rarely cry; tend to seek the approval of strangers.

  4 This may or may not be true.

366. **1** Typically, abusing parents have difficulty showing concern for their child. They are unable to comfort him, such as through touch, and give little indication of realizing how he feels. (b); AS; AN; PS; PE; CS

  2 Rather than guilt, battering parents tend to feel angry at the child for the injury.

  3 Battering parents rarely show concern about the child's care or progress.

  4 This is not particularly a characteristic reaction of abusive parents.

367. **4** In an attempt to block the hospital staff from discovering what happened, abusing parents frequently provide inconsistent accounts. (c); AS; AN; PS; PE; CS

  1 Battering parents tend to be vague about the details of the accident but maintain the child injured himself.

  2 Battering parents tend to show more concern about how the child's condition affects them than about how the child is affected.

  3 This may or may not occur.

368. **4** The first and most important observation should be for respiratory obstruction. If this occurs, treatment must be instituted immediately. (a); EV; CP; SU; TC; EI

  1 Can be due to the anesthesia; however, it is not life threatening and usually passes.

  2 Blood pressure is not significantly affected by this type of surgery; however, surgery itself can have an influence on it. If the BP had significantly dropped, other symptoms would be present.

  3 A later concern; not in the immediate postoperative period.

369. **4** The laryngeal nerve is close to the operative site and can be inadvertently damaged. (b); EV; AN; SU; PA; EI

  1 Loss of the gag reflex occurs with all surgery; the ability to swallow signifies its return.

  2 This might test the seventh cranial (facial) nerve, which would not be affected in thyroid surgery.

  3 Muscles and nerves involved in turning the head are not near the thyroid gland.

370. **3** Soreness is to be expected. A progression to a soft diet will provide nutrients needed for healing and energy and will stimulate the return of bowel activity. Analgesics as ordered will reduce soreness during meals. (c); IM; AN; SU; PA; EI

  1 This is not a nursing function.

  2 Soreness is to be expected; is not an emergency necessitating medical action.

  4 The soreness is not due to drying; a humidifier might help reduce soreness but would not help the client eat the soft diet.

371. **4** This action determines the client's tolerance of turning. Orthostatic hypotension can occur, and the physician should be alerted if the vital signs do not stabilize in 5 to 10 minutes. (b); PL; AP; SU; PA; MN

  1 The neck should be maintained in a neutral position; a roll under the neck causes hyperextension.

  2 The client is maintained in a supine position unless the physician indicates otherwise; a retention catheter is usually inserted.

  3 Sand bags are generally unnecessary; constant pressure is being exerted by skull traction to reduce the fracture.

372. **4** The CircOlectric bed turns clients from a horizontal supine position vertically to a horizontal prone position. It can also remain stationary in a vertical position. The change of position alters the body pressures periodically while the client is confined to the bed. (c); PL; KN; SU; PA; MN

  1 It is possible for one nurse to turn a client in a CircOlectric bed.

  2 Lateral turning is not possible with a CircOlectric bed.

  3 Although in some mattresses a pad can be removed so that a bedpan may be inserted, a receptacle itself would be impractical since the entire bed turns.

373. **2** Asepsis around the site of insertion must be maintained, since it is a break in the first line of defense. (b); IM; AP; SU; TC; MN

  1 Skin care is essential in preventing breakdown; however, it must be administered carefully.

  3 Constant traction must be maintained to reduce the fracture.

  4 The weights must be guided, but not removed during position changes.

How to Use Worksheet 1: Errors in Processing Information

Common errors in processing information are listed in the left-hand column of this worksheet. At the top of the worksheet is a row of blank spaces for inserting the number of the question missed. Directly below each number, check any errors you made in answering that question. You may have made more than one type of error in an answer.

Worksheet 1: Errors in processing information

Question number																					
Did not read situation/question carefully																					
Missed important details																					
Confused major and minor points																					
Defined problem incorrectly																					
Could not remember terms/ facts/concepts/principles																					
Defined terms incorrectly																					
Focused on incomplete/incorrect data in assessing situation																					
Interpreted data incorrectly																					
Applied wrong concepts/principles in situation																					
Drew incorrect conclusions																					
Identified wrong goals																					
Identified priorities incorrectly																					
Carried out plan incorrectly/incompletely																					
Was unclear about criteria for evaluating success in achieving goals																					

How to Use Worksheet 2: Knowledge Gaps

Types of common knowledge gaps are listed along the top of this worksheet. Write a brief description of topics you want to review in the spaces provided. For example, if you missed question on administration of a particular drug, write the drug name and problem (e.g., dosage) in the appropriate space under the column labeled *Pharmacology*.

Worksheet 2: Knowledge gaps

Basic science	Skills/ procedures	Basic human needs	Growth & develop- ment	Normal nutrition	Psycho- social factors	Clinical area/ topic	Stressors/ coping mechanisms	Patho- physiology	Pharma- cology	Therapeutic nutrition	Legal implications	Other

374. **2** The Schwann cells that compose the neurilemma of peripheral nerve fibers (dendrites and axons) are capable of supporting nerve fiber regeneration. (b); AN; KN; SU; PA; MN

    1 The myelin sheath, produced peripherally by the Schwann cells and centrally by the oligodendrocytes, is not involved directly in the regenerative process.

    3 Found in all neurons; not involved in regeneration.

    4 Found in all neurons; not involved in regeneration.

375. **4** The phrenic nerves innervate the diaphragm. Therefore a crushing spinal cord injury above the level of phrenic origin would stop diaphragmatic contractions and result in respiratory paralysis. (b); AN; CP; SU; PA; MN

    1 Cardiac activity would not be affected; the heart is regulated by the autonomic nervous system from fibers originating in the medulla.

    2 Activities regulated by the vagus nerve would be unaffected; the vagi originate in the medulla, which is superior to the cervical region (the phrenic nerves originate from the cervical plexuses).

    3 In a crushing spinal injury both motor and sensory conduction would be affected.

Index

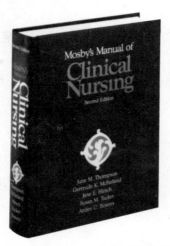